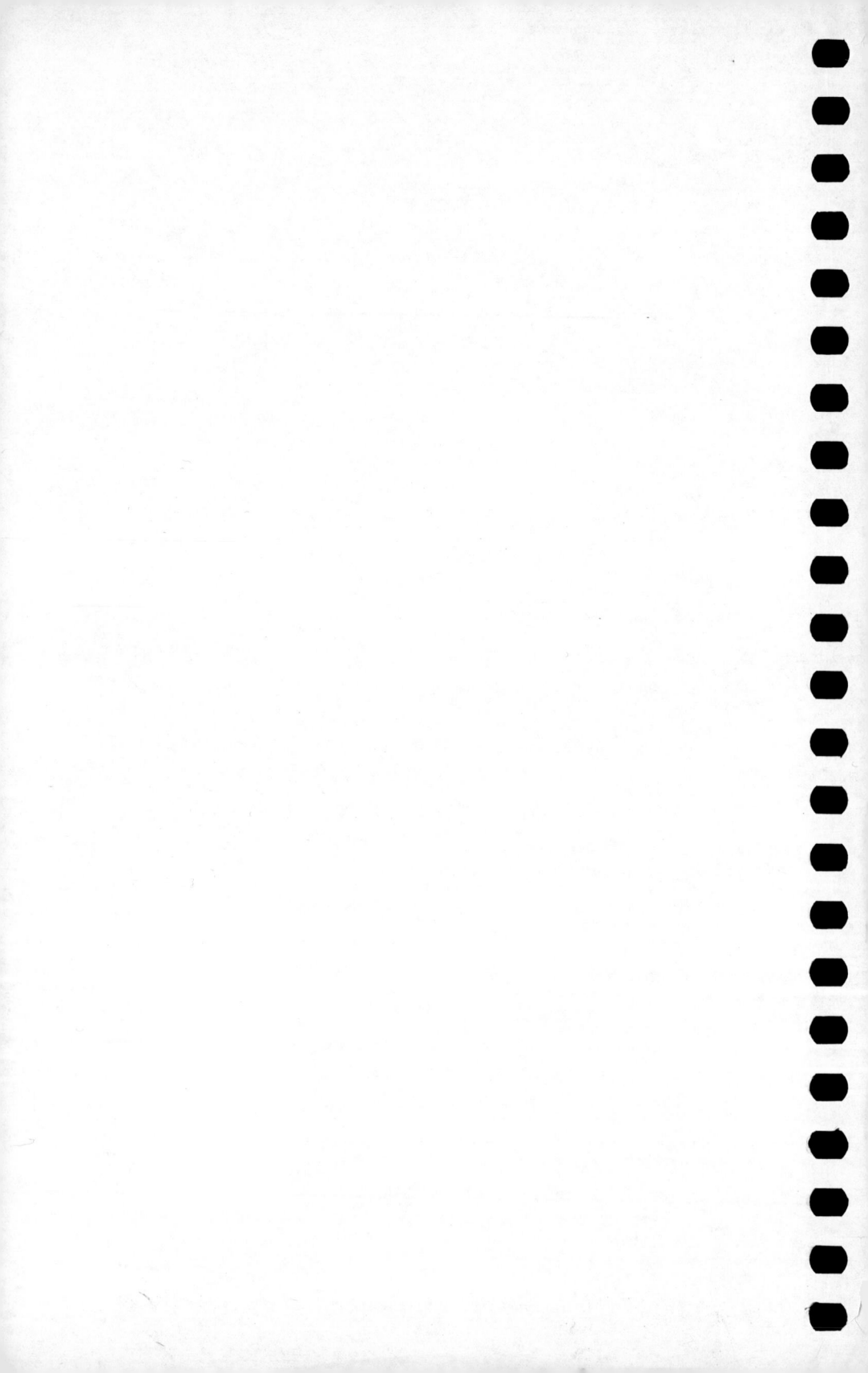

OTHER PMIC TITLES OF INTEREST

CODING AND REIMBURSEMENT TITLES

Collections Made Easy!
CPT & HCPCS Coding Made Easy!
CPT Coding Guides by Medical Specialty
CPT Plus! Coders Choice®
DRG Plus!
E/M Coding Made Easy!
Getting Paid for What You Do
HCPCS Coders Choice®,
Health Insurance Carrier Directory
HIPAA Compliance Manual
ICD-9-CM, Coders Choice®,
ICD-9-CM Coding for Physicians' Offices
ICD-9-CM Coding Made Easy!
ICD-9-CM, Home Health Edition
Medical Fees in the United States
Medicare Compliance Manual
Medicare Rules & Regulations
Physicians Fee Guide
Reimbursement Manual for the Medical Office

PRACTICE MANAGEMENT TITLES

Accounts Receivable Management for the Medical Practice
Achieving Profitability With a Medical Office System
Encyclopedia of Practice and Financial Management
Managed Care Organizations
Managing Medical Office Personnel
Marketing Strategies for Physicians
Medical Marketing Handbook
Medical Office Policy Manual
Medical Practice Forms
Medical Practice Handbook
Medical Staff Privileges
Negotiating Managed Care Contracts
Patient Satisfaction
Performance Standards for the Laboratory
Professional and Practice Development
Promoting Your Medical Practice
Starting in Medical Practice
Working With Insurance and Managed Care Plans

**AVAILABLE FROM YOUR LOCAL MEDICAL
BOOK STORE OR CALL 1-800-MED-SHOP**

OTHER PMIC TITLES OF INTEREST

RISK MANAGEMENT TITLES
Malpractice Depositions
Medical Risk Management
Preparing for Your Deposition
Preventing Emergency Malpractice
Testifying in Court

FINANCIAL MANAGEMENT TITLES
A Physician's Guide to Financial Independence
Business Ventures for Physicians
Financial Valuation of Your Practice
Personal Money Management for Physicians
Personal Pension Plan Strategies for Physicians
Securing Your Assets

DICTIONARIES AND OTHER REFERENCE TITLES
Dictionary of Coding & Billing Terminology
Drugs of Abuse
Health and Medicine on the Internet
Medical Acronyms and Abbreviations
Medical Phrase Index
Medical Word Building
Medico Mnemonica
Medico-Legal Glossary
Spanish/English Handbook for Medical Professionals

MEDICAL REFERENCE AND CLINICAL TITLES
Advance Medical Directives
Clinical Research Opportunities
Gastroenterology: Problems in Primary Care
Manual of IV Therapy
Medical Care of the Adolescent Athlete
Medical Procedures for Referral
Neurology: Problems in Primary Care
Orthopaedics: Problems in Primary Care
Patient Care Emergency Handbook
Patient Care Flowchart Manual
Patient Care Procedures for Your Practice
Physician's Office Laboratory
Pulmonary Medicine: Problems in Primary Care
Questions and Answers on AIDS

**AVAILABLE FROM YOUR LOCAL MEDICAL
BOOK STORE OR CALL 1-800-MED-SHOP**

CPT®·PLUS!

A Comprehensive Guide To Current Procedural Terminology

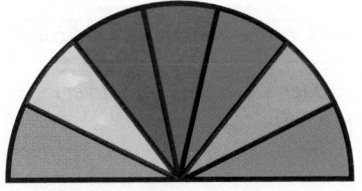

Color Coded

2013

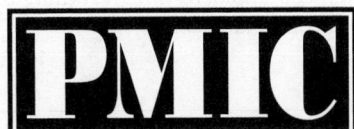

ISBN 978-1-936977-15-4 (Coder's Choice® soft cover)
ISBN 978-1-936977-16-1 (Spiral)
ISBN 978-1-936977-17-8 (e-book)

Practice Management Information Corporation
4727 Wilshire Boulevard
Los Angeles, California 90010
1-800-MED-SHOP
http://pmiconline.com/

Printed in China

INTRODUCTION

CPT® PLUS! 2013 is an enhanced CPT® coding resource which includes all official CPT 2013 codes and complete descriptions plus comprehensive CPT coding instructions, full-color anatomical illustrations, a unique color-coding system to help identify CPT codes subject to special coding rules, and a new and improved alphabetic index.

The CPT coding system includes over 9,000 codes and descriptions for reporting medical services, procedures, supplies and materials. Accurate CPT coding provides an efficient method of communicating medical services and procedures among health care providers, health care facilities, and third party payers and enhances the health care provider's control of the reimbursement process.

The CPT coding system is revised annually by the American Medical Association (AMA). Each year hundreds of additions, changes and deletions are made the CPT coding system. These changes become effective on January 1st. CPT is required by federal law for all health insurance claim forms filed with Medicare, Medicaid, CHAMPUS and Federal Employee Health Plans and is accepted or required by all other third party payers.

CPT® PLUS! 2013 provides valuable instructions, coding tips, and other information to help providers maximize reimbursement while minimizing audit liability. Our objective is to make CPT coding faster, easier and more accurate for medical office, healthcare facility and third party payer coding and billing staff, while setting a new standard for CPT coding references.

James B. Davis, Publisher

DISCLAIMER

This publication is designed to offer basic information regarding coding and reporting of medical services, supplies and procedures using the CPT coding system. The information presented is based on a thorough analysis of the CPT coding system and the experience and interpretations of the editors. Though all of the information has been carefully researched and checked for accuracy and completeness, neither the editors nor the publisher accept any responsibility or liability with regard to errors, omissions, misuse or misinterpretation.

CONTENTS

v

CONTENTS

CPT CODING FUNDAMENTALS

CPT® is an acronym for Current Procedural Terminology. Physicians' Current Procedural Terminology, Fourth Edition, known as CPT-4 or more commonly CPT, is a systematic listing of codes and descriptions which classify medical services and procedures. CPT codes are used by physicians, hospitals, and other health care professionals, to report specific medical, surgical and diagnostic services and procedures for statistical and third party payment purposes.

The CPT coding system is maintained by the American Medical Association (AMA) and a revised edition of the CPT book is published each fall. The new CPT codes become effective on January 1st of the following year. The revisions in each new edition are prepared by the CPT Editorial Panel with the assistance of physicians representing all specialties of medicine.

A thorough understanding of the CPT coding system is essential in order to provide accurate reporting of medical services and procedures, maximize payments from third parties, minimize denials, rejections and reductions from third parties, and to protect the medical practice from audit liability.

KEY POINTS REGARDING THE CPT CODING SYSTEM

- *CPT codes describe medical procedures, services and supplies.*

- *All CPT codes are five digit codes.*

- *CPT codes are mandated by federal law for Medicare, Medicaid, CHAMPUS and Federal Employee Health Plan (FEHP) reporting and are accepted or required by all other third party payers.*

- *CPT codes are self-definitive, eg. with the exception of CPT codes for unlisted procedures and/or the few CPT codes which include the term specify in the description, each CPT code number represents the universal definition of the service or procedure.*

- *CPT codes are revised and updated annually by the AMA and the revisions become effective each January 1st. Hundreds of CPT codes are added, changed or deleted each year. All health care professionals, third party payers, and health care facilities must maintain copies of the current code books.*

- *Accurate CPT coding provides an efficient method of communicating medical, surgical and diagnostic services and procedures among health care professionals, health care facilities, and third party payers.*

- *Accurate CPT coding enhances the health care provider's control of the reimbursement process.*

STRUCTURE OF THE CPT CODING SYSTEM

The CPT coding system includes over 7,900 codes and definitions for medical services, procedures and diagnostic tests. Each procedure or service is identified by a five digit code, followed by the definition.

*The CPT coding system is divided into eight **SECTIONS**. The eight sections of are:*

Evaluation and Management	*99201-99499*
Anesthesiology	*00100-01999, 99100-99140*
Surgery	*10021-69990*
Radiology *(Including Nuclear Med & Dx U/S)*	*70010-79999*
Pathology and Laboratory	*80047-89398*
Medicine *(except Anesthesiology)*	*90281-99199, 99500-99607*
Category II Performance Measurement	*0001F-7025F*
Category III Emerging Technology	*0019T-0318T*

Each section of the CPT book includes subsections with anatomic, procedural, condition, or descriptor subheadings. The Evaluation and Management (E/M) section is presented first because 1) these codes are used by virtually all health care providers and 2) are the most frequently used CPT codes.

HOW TO USE THE CPT CODING SYSTEM

A provider or coder using the CPT coding system first chooses the name and associated code of the procedure or service which most accurately identifies and describes the service(s) performed. The provider or coder then chooses names and codes for additional services or procedures. If necessary, modifiers are chosen and added to the selected service and procedure codes. All services or procedures coded must also be documented in the patient's medical record.

According to CPT, "The listing of a service or procedure and its code number in a specific section of the CPT book does not restrict its use to a specific specialty group. Any procedure or service in any section of the CPT coding system may be used to designate the services rendered by any qualified physician or other qualified health care professional."

The codes and descriptions listed in the CPT coding system are those that are generally consistent with contemporary medical practice and being performed by health care professionals in clinical practice. Inclusion in the CPT coding system does not represent endorsement by the American Medical Association of any particular diagnostic or therapeutic procedure. In addition, inclusion or exclusion

2

of a procedure does not imply any health insurance coverage or reimbursement policy.

CPT FORMAT AND CONVENTIONS

DESCRIPTIONS

The descriptions associated with CPT codes have been developed by the AMA to provide complete descriptions of medical services and procedures.

Many CPT descriptions include the definition of basic procedures followed by supplemental descriptions for variations or modifications of the basic procedure. In the CPT coding book, the basic procedure description ends with a semicolon (;), followed by the additional description.

If a CPT description includes the same basic procedure as the preceding listing, the basic procedure is not listed. Only the supplemental description is listed, preceded by an indentation. For example:

25100   Arthrotomy, wrist joint; with biopsy

25105   with synovectomy

SYMBOLS

● *A filled BLACK CIRCLE preceding a CPT code indicates that the code is new to this revision of the CPT coding system. A symbol key appears on all left-hand pages.*

▲ *A filled BLACK TRIANGLE preceding a CPT code indicates that there is a revision to the description. Wherever possible, the revised text is identified with underlining.*

( ) *CPT codes enclosed within parenthesis have been deleted from the CPT coding system and should no longer be used.*

+ *A bold plus sign preceding a CPT code indicates that the code is an "add-on" code and must be listed in addition to the main CPT code.*

⊘ *This symbol preceding a CPT code indicates that the code is exempt from the use of modifier -51.*

⊙ *This symbol preceding a CPT code indicates that the procedure includes conscious sedation as a part of providing the procedure and that the conscious sedation codes, 99141 or 99142, should not be reported separately.*

Note that a CPT code may be preceded by the add-on, star symbol or modifier-51 exempt symbol, in addition to new or changed code symbols.

3

COLOR CODING

Separate procedure. A procedure or service that is normally performed as an integral component of a total service or procedure. CPT codes identified as separate procedure codes should not be coded in addition to the basic procedure code of which it is considered an integral component.

However, if the procedure or service that is usually designated as a separate procedure is performed independently or is considered to be unrelated or distinct from other procedures or services provided at that time, the separate procedure may be coded by itself. The modifier -59 should be added to the separate procedure code to indicate that the procedure is not considered to be a component of another procedure, but is a distinct, independent procedure.

Unlisted code. Descriptions include the term "unlisted." Use only when a CPT code which specifically describes the service or procedure is unavailable. A report is usually required by third party payers.

Nonspecific code. Descriptions include the term "specify" instructing the coder to include additional information such as the quadrant, the nerve, the muscle, the level of spine, the number of joints, the type of study, the method of dosimetry, the hormone, the receptor, the assay method, the type of kit, the material injected, the type of tests, the number of tests, the doses provided.

CCI comprehensive code. Indicates codes identified as comprehensive codes in the Comprehensive Coding Initiative, revised annually. Per CMS rules, all identifiable component procedures are included in the comprehensive code and should not be billed separately to Medicare.

ITALICIZED AND NON-ITALICIZED TEXT

Italicized text is used throughout this publication to distinguish information authored, contributed or otherwise provided by PMIC.

Non-italicized text *is used to distinguish information reproduced verbatim from* CPT 2013, *published by the American Medical Association.*

SECTION OVERVIEWS

Specific guidelines are presented at the beginning of each of the six sections of the CPT coding system. The guidelines define items that are necessary to interpret and report the procedures and services contained in that section. CPT guidelines also provide explanations regarding terms that apply only to a particular section.

REQUESTS TO UPDATE THE CPT CODING SYSTEM

The American Medical Association (AMA) maintains a CPT Editorial Panel that reviews and approves requests for changes to the CPT coding system. Requests to add, delete or revise specific CPT codes should be addressed to:

CPT Editorial Research & Development
American Medical Association
515 North State Street
Chicago, Illinois 60610

CPT 2013 AVAILABLE IN ELECTRONIC FORMAT

CPT 2013 codes and descriptions with relative value information are available on CD-ROM or as a download. The data files are available in standard ASCII format and may be imported into your billing and health insurance claims software. CPT Plus! 2013 is also available as a PC resident e-book in PDF format. For more information call (800) 633-7467 or visit http://pmiconline.com.

This page intentionally left blank.

CODING & BILLING ISSUES

Most billing, coding and reporting issues involving the CPT® coding system apply generally to all medical specialties and professions. However, there are some specialty specific issues defined in each section of the CPT coding system that apply only to the specific medical specialty represented.

SUPPORTING DOCUMENTATION

Documentation in the patient's medical report must clearly support the procedures, services and supplies coded on the health insurance claim form. Most medical chart reviewers take the position that if something is not documented in the medical record, then the service or procedure was not performed and therefore is not subject to reimbursement.

If a medical practice is selected for an audit by Medicare or other third party payer, the accuracy and completeness of the documentation of the medical records, or lack thereof, will have a significant impact on the outcome of the audit. The current emphasis on "fraud" and "abuse" by Medicare, Medicaid and private third party payer necessitates a review of documentation by all health care professionals.

SPECIAL MEDICARE CONSIDERATIONS

To satisfy Medicare requirements, there must be sufficient documentation in the medical record to verify the services coded and the level of care required. Section 1833(e) of Title XVIII, Social Security Act requires "available information that documents a claim." If there is no documentation to justify the services or level of care, the claim cannot be considered for Medicare benefits.

If there is insufficient documentation to support claims that have already been paid by Medicare, the reimbursement will be considered an overpayment and a refund will be requested by Medicare. Medicare has the authority to review any information, including medical records, when such information pertains to a Medicare claim.

UNLISTED PROCEDURES OR SERVICES

There are services or procedures performed by health care professionals that are not found in the CPT coding system. These services or procedures may be either new procedures which have not yet been assigned a CPT code or simply a variation of a procedure which precludes using the existing CPT code. Each section of the CPT coding system includes codes for reporting these unlisted procedures.

Unlisted procedure codes should not be coded unless the coder has reviewed the CPT coding system carefully to ensure that a more specific code is not available. If a specific CPT code is not located, check for HCPCS codes that may be reportable.

As a rule, a report needs to be enclosed with the health insurance claim form when reporting unlisted procedure codes. Because unlisted procedure codes are subject to manual medical review, payment is usually slower than for normal processing time.

CPT ADDITIONS, CHANGES, AND DELETIONS

Each year hundreds of codes are added, changed or deleted from the CPT coding system. A summary of these changes is found in Appendix B of the CPT code book, which provides a quick reference for coding review. In addition to the summary, these modifications are identified throughout the CPT code book.

ADDITIONS TO THE CPT CODING SYSTEM

New codes are added to the CPT coding system each year. New CPT codes are identified with a small black circle placed to the left of the code number. Examples of new codes found in CPT 2013 include:

- **23473** Revision of total shoulder arthroplasty, including allograft when performed; humeral or glenoid component

- **33361** Transcatheter aortic valve replacement (TAVR/TAVI) with prosthetic valve; percutaneous femoral artery approach

CHANGES TO CPT CODE DEFINITIONS

Each year the definitions of many CPT codes are revised. CPT codes with changed definitions are identified with a small black triangle placed to the left of the code number. Examples of CPT codes with changed definitions in CPT 2012 include:

▲ **15740** Flap; island pedicle requiring identification and dissection of an anatomically named axial vessel

▲ **90660** Influenza virus vaccine, trivalent, live, for intranasal use

The only way to determine exactly what part of the definition has been changed is to compare the current changed definition with the definition from the previous edition of the CPT code book.

DELETIONS FROM THE CPT CODING SYSTEM

Each year some CPT codes are deleted. Deleted CPT codes, and references to replacement codes, if there are any, are enclosed within parentheses. Examples of CPT codes deleted from CPT 2013 include:

(29590   Deleted 2012 [2013 edition].)

(90862   Deleted 2012 [2013 edition]. To report, see 90863 or evaluation and management services codes 99201-99255, 99281-99285, 99304-99337, 99341-99350)

NEW SECTIONS AND SUBSECTIONS

New sections and subsections are frequently added to the CPT coding system to reflect changes in technology or medical practice and to provide additional code sequences for special purposes.

Complex Chronic Care Coordination Services	99487-99489
Transitional Care Management Services	99495-99496
Bronchial Thermoplasty	31660-31661
Stereotactic Radiation Therapy	32701
Multianalyte Assays with Algorithmic Analyses	81500-81599

CATEGORY II PERFORMANCE MEASUREMENT CODES

Category II, Performance Measurement CPT codes, are designed to facilitate outcomes research. This new section was introduced in the 2005 CPT updates. Category II codes include the letter "F" as the fifth digit of the five digit CPT code. These codes are optional, and are not a substitute for Category I codes.

CATEGORY III EMERGING TECHNOLOGY CODES

Emerging technology codes are temporary codes for emerging technology, services and procedures. These codes are designed to permit data collection and assessment of new technologies. All Category III codes include the letter "T" as the fifth digit of the five digit CPT code. The inclusion of a specific service or procedure in this section does not imply or endorse clinical efficacy, safety, or applicability to clinical practice.

STARRED PROCEDURES

Starred procedure designation was removed from CPT 2004.

INSTRUCTIONAL NOTES

Notes found in the CPT coding system give instructions for using codes. When selecting a code, look for instructions in the section guidelines for any additional information necessary to code accurately. Also, instructional notes take the form of parenthetical statements and paragraphs, which may appear at the beginning of subsections, headings and subheadings, or above and below the code itself.

DEFINITION OF NEW AND ESTABLISHED PATIENT

Solely to distinguish between new and established patients, professional services are those face-to-face services rendered by physicians and other qualified health care professionals and coded by a specific CPT code(s). A new patient is one who has not received any professional services from the physician/qualified health care professional or another physician/qualified health care professional of the same specialty who belongs to the same group practice, within the past three years. An established patient is one who has received professional services from the physician/qualified health care professional or another physician/qualified health care professional of the same specialty who belongs to the same group practice, within the past three years.

In the instance where a physician/qualified health care professional is on call for or covering for another physician/qualified health care professional, the patient's encounter will be classified as it would have been by the physician/qualified health care professional who is not available.

No distinction is made between new and established patients in the emergency department. Evaluation and Management services in the emergency department category may be coded for any new or established patient who presents for treatment in the emergency department.

PLACE (LOCATION) OF SERVICE

CPT makes specific distinctions for place (location) of service for evaluation and management codes. Place of service may have considerable impact on reimbursement. This list gives CPT code ranges for some specific places of service:

Office or Other Outpatient Services	*99201-99215*
Hospital Observation Services	*99217-99226*
Hospital Inpatient Services	*99221-99239*
Emergency Department	*99281-99288*
Nursing Facility Services	*99304-99318*
Domiciliary, Rest Home, or Custodial Care Services	*99324-99337*
Domiciliary, Rest Home, or Home Care Plan Oversight Services	*99339-99340*
Home Services	*99341-99350*
Inpatient Neonatal and Pediatric Critical Care	*99468-99476*

PLACE OF SERVICE CODES FOR PROFESSIONAL CLAIMS

Listed below are place of service codes and descriptions. These codes should be used on professional claims to specify the entity where service(s) were rendered. Check with individual payers (e.g., Medicare, Medicaid, other private insurance) for reimbursement policies regarding these codes.

Code	Place Name	Place Description
01	Pharmacy**	A facility or location where drugs and other medically related items and services are sold, dispensed, or otherwise provided directly to patients.
02	Unassigned	N/A
03	School	A facility whose primary purpose is education.
04	Homeless Shelter	A facility or location whose primary purpose is to provide temporary housing to homeless individuals (e.g., emergency shelters, individual or family shelters).
05	Indian Health Service Free-standing Facility	A facility or location, owned and operated by the Indian Health Service, which provides diagnostic, therapeutic (surgical and non-surgical), and rehabilitation services to American Indians and Alaska Natives who do not require hospitalization.
06	Indian Health Service Provider-based Facility	A facility or location, owned and operated by the Indian Health Service, which provides diagnostic, therapeutic (surgical and non-surgical), and rehabilitation services rendered by, or under the supervision of, physicians to American Indians and Alaska Natives admitted as inpatients or outpatients.
07	Tribal 638 Free-Standing Facility	A facility or location owned and operated by a federally recognized American Indian or Alaska Native tribe or tribal organization under a 638 agreement, which provides diagnostic, therapeutic (surgical and non-surgical), and rehabilitation services to tribal members who do not require hospitalization.
08	Tribal 638 Provider-based Facility	A facility or location owned and operated by a federally recognized American Indian or Alaska Native tribe or tribal organization under a 638 agreement, which provides diagnostic, therapeutic (surgical and non-surgical), and rehabilitation services to tribal members admitted as inpatients or outpatients

09	Prison-Correction al Facility	A prison, jail, reformatory, work farm, detention center, or any other similar facility maintained by either Federal, State or local authorities for the purpose of confinement or rehabilitation of adult or juvenile criminal offenders. (effective 7/1/06)
10	Unassigned	N/A
11	Office	Location, other than a hospital, skilled nursing facility (SNF), military treatment facility, community health center, State or local public health clinic, or intermediate care facility (ICF), where the health professional routinely provides health examinations, diagnosis, and treatment of illness or injury on an ambulatory basis.
12	Home	Location, other than a hospital or other facility, where the patient receives care in a private residence.
13	Assisted Living Facility	Congregate residential facility with self-contained living units providing assessment of each resident's needs and on-site support 24 hours a day, 7 days a week, with the capacity to deliver or arrange for services including some health care and other services.
14	Group Home*	A residence, with shared living areas, where clients receive supervision and other services such as social and/or behavioral services, custodial service, and minimal services (e.g., medication administration).
15	Mobile Unit	A facility/unit that moves from place-to-place equipped to provide preventive, screening, diagnostic, and/or treatment services.
16	Temporary lodging	A short-term accomodation such as a hotel, campground, hostel, cruise ship, or resort where the patient receives care, and which is not identified by any other POS code.
17	Walk-in retail health clinic	A walk-in retail health clinic, other than an office, urgent care facility, pharmacy, or independent clinic, which is not described by any other POS code, that is located within a retail operation and provides on an ambulatory basis, preventive and primary care services. (This code is available for use immediately with a final effective date of May 1, 2010)
18-19	Unassigned	N/A

20	Urgent Care Facility	Location, distinct from a hospital emergency room, an office, or a clinic, whose purpose is to diagnose and treat illness or injury for unscheduled, ambulatory patients seeking immediate medical attention.
21	Inpatient Hospital	A facility, other than psychiatric, which primarily provides diagnostic, therapeutic (both surgical and non-surgical), and rehabilitation services by, or under, the supervision of physicians to patients admitted for a variety of medical conditions.
22	Outpatient Hospital	A portion of a hospital which provides diagnostic, therapeutic (both surgical and non-surgical), and rehabilitation services to sick or injured persons who do not require hospitalization or institutionalization.
23	Emergency Room – Hospital	A portion of a hospital where emergency diagnosis and treatment of illness or injury is provided.
24	Ambulatory Surgical Center	A freestanding facility, other than a physician's office, where surgical and diagnostic services are provided on an ambulatory basis.
25	Birthing Center	A facility, other than a hospital's maternity facilities or a physician's office, which provides a setting for labor, delivery, and immediate post-partum care as well as immediate care of new born infants.
26	Military Treatment Facility	A medical facility operated by one or more of the Uniformed Services. Military Treatment Facility (MTF) also refers to certain former U.S. Public Health Service (USPHS) facilities now designated as Uniformed Service Treatment Facilities (USTF).
27-30	Unassigned	N/A
31	Skilled Nursing Facility	A facility which primarily provides inpatient skilled nursing care and related services to patients who require medical, nursing, or rehabilitative services but does not provide the level of care or treatment available in a hospital.
32	Nursing Facility	A facility which primarily provides to residents skilled nursing care and related services for the rehabilitation of injured, disabled, or sick persons, or, on a regular basis, health-related care services above the level of custodial care to other than mentally retarded individuals.

33	Custodial Care Facility	A facility which provides room, board and other personal assistance services, generally on a long-term basis, and which does not include a medical component.
34	Hospice	A facility, other than a patient's home, in which palliative and supportive care for terminally ill patients and their families are provided.
35-40	Unassigned	N/A
41	Ambulance - Land	A land vehicle specifically designed, equipped and staffed for lifesaving and transporting the sick or injured.
42	Ambulance – Air or Water	An air or water vehicle specifically designed, equipped and staffed for lifesaving and transporting the sick or injured.
43-48	Unassigned	N/A
49	Independent Clinic	A location, not part of a hospital and not described by any other Place of Service code, that is organized and operated to provide preventive, diagnostic, therapeutic, rehabilitative, or palliative services to outpatients only. (effective 10/1/03)
50	Federally Qualified Health Center	A facility located in a medically underserved area that provides Medicare beneficiaries preventive primary medical care under the general direction of a physician.
51	Inpatient Psychiatric Facility	A facility that provides inpatient psychiatric services for the diagnosis and treatment of mental illness on a 24-hour basis, by or under the supervision of a physician.
52	Psychiatric Facility-Partial Hospitalization	A facility for the diagnosis and treatment of mental illness that provides a planned therapeutic program for patients who do not require full time hospitalization, but who need broader programs than are possible from outpatient visits to a hospital-based or hospital-affiliated facility.

53	Community Mental Health Center	A facility that provides the following services: outpatient services, including specialized outpatient services for children, the elderly, individuals who are chronically ill, and residents of the CMHC's community mental health area who have been discharged from inpatient treatment at a mental health facility; 24-hour a day emergency care services; day treatment, other partial hospitalization services, or psychosocial rehabilitation services; screening for patients being considered for admission to State mental health facilities to determine the appropriateness of such admission; and consultation and education services.
54	Intermediate Care Facility/Mentally Retarded	A facility which primarily provides health-related care and services above the level of custodial care to mentally retarded individuals but does not provide the level of care or treatment available in a hospital or SNF.
55	Residential Substance Abuse Treatment Facility	A facility which provides treatment for substance (alcohol and drug) abuse to live-in residents who do not require acute medical care. Services include individual and group therapy and counseling, family counseling, laboratory tests, drugs and supplies, psychological testing, and room and board.
56	Psychiatric Residential Treatment Center	A facility or distinct part of a facility for psychiatric care which provides a total 24-hour therapeutically planned and professionally staffed group living and learning environment.
57	Non-residential Substance Abuse Treatment Facility	A location which provides treatment for substance (alcohol and drug) abuse on an ambulatory basis. Services include individual and group therapy and counseling, family counseling, laboratory tests, drugs and supplies, and psychological testing. (effective 10/1/03)
58-59	Unassigned	N/A
60	Mass Immunization Center	A location where providers administer pneumococcal pneumonia and influenza virus vaccinations and submit these services as electronic media claims, paper claims, or using the roster billing method. This generally takes place in a mass immunization setting, such as, a public health center, pharmacy, or mall but may include a physician office setting.

15

61	Comprehensive Inpatient Rehabilitation Facility	A facility that provides comprehensive rehabilitation services under the supervision of a physician to inpatients with physical disabilities. Services include physical therapy, occupational therapy, speech pathology, social or psychological services, and orthotics and prosthetics services.
62	Comprehensive Outpatient Rehabilitation Facility	A facility that provides comprehensive rehabilitation services under the supervision of a physician to outpatients with physical disabilities. Services include physical therapy, occupational therapy, and speech pathology services.
63-64	Unassigned	N/A
65	End-Stage Renal Disease Treatment Facility	A facility other than a hospital, which provides dialysis treatment, maintenance, and/or training to patients or caregivers on an ambulatory or home-care basis.
66-70	Unassigned	N/A
71	Public Health Clinic	A facility maintained by either State or local health departments that provide ambulatory primary medical care under the general direction of a physician. (effective 10/1/03)
72	Rural Health Clinic	A certified facility which is located in a rural medically underserved area that provides ambulatory primary medical care under the general direction of a physician.
73-80	Unassigned	N/A
81	Independent Laboratory	A laboratory certified to perform diagnostic and/or clinical tests independent of an institution or a physician's office.
82-98	Unassigned	N/A
99	Other Place of Service	Other place of service not identified above.

HOSPITAL CARE

Hospital services frequently cause reimbursement problems for health care professionals. The three most common coding errors are:

- *More than one physician submits an initial hospital care code for the same patient.*

- *Follow-up hospital visits are coded incorrectly.*

- *Concurrent care visits by multiple specialists are coded improperly.*

If more than one physician is involved in the process of hospitalizing a patient, for example, surgeon and internist, the physicians must decide which is going to actually admit the patient and report the admission services on the health insurance claim form. If both do, the first health insurance claim form to arrive will be processed and paid, and the second will be rejected.

There are valid reasons for visiting a patient more than once daily while hospitalized, however, many physicians and even some insurance billers do not know that subsequent hospital visit codes are for "daily" services. When a physician visits the patient twice in one day, providing a brief level of service each time, the physician or insurance biller may incorrectly report two hospital visit services for the same day, instead of a higher level code incorporating both visits.

Reporting multiple hospital visits provided on the same day separately on the health insurance claim form usually results in either the entire claim being returned for clarification, or the second visit being denied as an apparent duplication. Unfortunately, insurance billers who are unclear on the proper coding of same day hospital visits may simply accept the rejection without question and write-off the unpaid visit as uncollectible.

The CPT coding system clearly defines subsequent hospital care as "per day", meaning daily services. If the physician visits the patient twice in one day, providing the equivalent of "brief" services each time, report the service using the appropriate evaluation and management code that defines the cumulative level of service provided.

HOSPITAL DISCHARGE

The CPT codes for hospital discharge services are evaluation and management code 99238 and 99239, defined as Hospital Discharge Day Management. Hospital discharge services include final examination of the patient, discussion of the hospital stay, instructions for continuing care, and preparation of discharge records. Many health insurance companies do not recognize and/or do not reimburse this CPT code.

actually provided by the ordering physician. It is also common for the ordering physician to "mark-up" the fee for the purchased service prior to billing. This is referred to as global billing.

Medical equipment companies, particularly those offering electrocardiography, pulmonary diagnostic equipment, and other diagnostic equipment, have used this global billing concept in the past as a method of selling physicians a new "profit center" for their practice. Some even provided technicians, who were not employees of the practice, to perform the diagnostic tests in the physicians office. OBRA 1987 placed severe restrictions on global billing of certain diagnostic tests as of March 1, 1988.

The Medicare regulations apply to diagnostic tests other than clinical laboratory tests including, but not limited to: EKGs, EEGs, cardiac monitoring, X-rays and ultrasound. Global billing is allowed only when the billing physician personally performs or supervises the diagnostic procedure. To qualify under the supervision definition, the person performing the test must be an employee or the physician or group. Ownership interest in an outside supplier does not meet the supervision requirement.

Billing for purchased services under the new requirement is complicated. The provider must provide the supplier's name, address, provider number and net charge on the health insurance claim form. In addition, a HCPCS Level III modifier must be coded to indicate that the service was purchased. Billing for global services usually will also require a HCPCS Level III modifier to indicate that the service was not purchased. This requirement does not apply to the professional component of these services if provided separately.

Providers should discontinue billing for the technical component of diagnostic services that were not provided or supervised by the provider as defined in this regulation for the following reasons:

1. *The provider is no longer making any profit on these procedures;*

2. *Operating costs are higher due to the increased reporting requirements; and*

3. *Risk of audit liability is increased if these services are not coded properly.*

UNBUNDLING

Unbundling is defined as reporting multiple CPT codes when one CPT code is sufficient. For example, it is considered unbundling if incidental surgical procedures are coded separately, or office visits for uncomplicated follow-up care are separately coded. This practice often happens unintentionally. However, most third-party payers currently have software in place to catch unbundling when it occurs. When physicians continually break out or itemize services in this manner, they often find themselves under close scrutiny and even the focus of an audit by the insurance company. It is most important to know the guidelines to prevent unbundling when coding and billing for services and/or procedures.

MODERATE (CONSCIOUS) SEDATION

Moderate (conscious) sedation induces an altered state of consciousness that minimizes pain and discomfort through the use of pain relievers and sedatives. Patients who receive such sedation usually are able to speak and respond to verbal cues throughout the procedure, communicating any discomfort they experience to the provider. A brief period of amnesia may erase any memory of the procedure. Moderate sedation is administered in hospitals, outpatient facilities, for example ambulatory surgery centers, and doctors offices to facilitate procedures such as the following:

- *Breast biopsy*

- *Vasectomy*

- *Minor foot surgery*

- *Minor bone fracture repair*

- *Plastic/reconstructive surgery*

- *Dental prosthetic/reconstructive surgery*

- *Endoscopy*

Procedures That Include Moderate (Conscious) Sedation

Beginning with CPT 2006, surgical and medical procedures that include moderate (conscious)sedation as part of the procedure were identified with a ⊙ symbol to the left of the CPT code. Because these surgical and medical procedures include such sedation, the CPT codes for moderate (conscious) sedation, 99143-99145, should not be reported separately. Following is a list of surgical and medical CPT codes that include moderate (conscious) sedation:

19298	33214	36227	37212	43240	44373
20982	33216	36228	37213	43241	44376
22520	33217	36245	37214	43242	44377
22521	33218	36246	37215	43243	44378
22522	33220	36247	37216	43244	44379
22526	33221	36248	37220	43245	44380
22527	33222	36251	37221	43246	44382
31615	33223	36252	37222	43247	44383
31620	33227	36253	37223	43248	44385
31622	33228	36254	37224	43249	44386
31623	33229	36481	37225	43250	44388
31624	33230	36555	37226	43251	44389
31625	33231	36557	37227	43252	44390
31626	33233	36558	37228	43255	44391
31627	33234	36560	37229	43256	44392
31628	33235	36561	37230	43257	44393
31629	33240	36563	37231	43258	44394
31634	33241	36565	37232	43259	44397
31635	33244	36566	37233	43260	44500
31645	33249	36568	37234	43261	44901
31646	33262	36570	37235	43262	45303
31647	33263	36571	43200	43263	45305
31648	33264	36576	43201	43264	45307
31649	33990	36578	43202	43265	45308
31651	33991	36581	43204	43267	45309
31660	33992	36582	43205	43268	45315
31661	33993	36583	43206	43269	45317
31725	35471	36585	43215	43271	45320
32201	35472	36590	43216	43272	45321
32405	35475	36870	43217	43273	45327
32550	35476	37183	43219	43453	45332
32551	36010	37184	43220	43456	45333
32553	36140	37185	43226	43458	45334
33010	36147	37186	43227	44360	45335
33011	36148	37187	43228	44361	45337
33206	36200	37188	43231	44363	45338
33207	36221	37191	43232	44364	45339
33208	36222	37192	43235	44365	45340
33210	36223	37193	43236	44366	45341
33211	36224	37197	43237	44369	45342
33212	36225	37210	43238	44370	45345
33213	36226	37211	43239	44372	45355

45378	50382	92953	93462	93650
45379	50384	92960	93463	93653
45380	50385	92961	93464	93654
45381	50386	92973	93505	93655
45382	50387	92974	93530	93656
45383	50592	92975	93561	93657
45384	50593	92978	93562	94011
45385	57155	92979	93563	94012
45386	58823	92986	93564	94013
45387	66720	92987	93565	0200T
45391	69300	93312	93566	0201T
45392	77371	93313	93567	0282T
47000	77600	93314	93568	0283T
47011	77605	93315	93571	0284T
47382	77610	93316	93572	0291T
47525	77615	93317	93609	0292T
48511	92920	93318	93613	0293T
49021	92921	93451	93615	0294T
49041	92924	93452	93616	0301T
49061	92925	93453	93618	0302T
49411	92928	93454	93619	0303T
49418	92929	93455	93620	0304T
49440	92933	93456	93621	0307T
49441	92934	93457	93622	0308T
49442	92937	93458	93624	
49446	92938	93459	93640	
50021	92941	93460	93641	
50200	92943	93461	93642	

2013 ADDITIONS, DELETIONS & REVISIONS

Following is a complete list of all additions, deletions and revisions to the CPT 2013 coding system. Indicators to the left of each code define the status of the CPT code as follows:

●   Indicates CPT codes that are new to CPT 2013.

▲   Indicates CPT codes that have been revised in CPT 2013.

( )   Indicates CPT codes that have been deleted from CPT 2013.

Evaluation and Management

▲ 99201   Office or other outpatient visit for the evaluation and management of a new patient, which requires these 3 key components:

- A problem focused history;
- A problem focused examination;
- Straightforward medical decision making.

Counseling and/or coordination of care with other physicians, other qualified health care professionals, or agencies are provided consistent with the nature of the problem(s) and the patient's and/or family's needs.

Usually, the presenting problem(s) are self-limited or minor. Typically, 10 minutes are spent face-to-face with the patient and/or family.

▲ 99202   Office or other outpatient visit for the evaluation and management of a new patient, which requires these 3 key components:

- An expanded problem focused history;
- An expanded problem focused examination;
- Straightforward medical decision making.

Counseling and/or coordination of care with other physicians, other qualified health care professionals, or agencies are provided consistent with the nature of the problem(s) and the patient's and/or family's needs.

Usually, the presenting problem(s) are of low to moderate severity. Typically, 20 minutes are spent face-to-face with the patient and/or family.

▲ 99203   Office or other outpatient visit for the evaluation and management of a new patient, which requires these 3 key components:

- A detailed history;
- A detailed examination;
- Medical decision making of low complexity.

Counseling and/or coordination of care with other physicians, other qualified health care professionals, or agencies are provided consistent with the nature of the problem(s) and the patient's and/or family's needs.

Usually, the presenting problem(s) are of moderate severity. Typically, 30 minutes are spent face-to-face with the patient and/or family.

▲ 99204   Office or other outpatient visit for the evaluation and management of a new patient, which requires these 3 key components:

- A comprehensive history;

- A comprehensive examination;

- Medical decision making of moderate complexity.

Counseling and/or coordination of care with other physicians, other qualified health care professionals, or agencies are provided consistent with the nature of the problem(s) and the patient's and/or family's needs.

Usually, the presenting problem(s) are of moderate to high severity. Typically, 45 minutes are spent face-to-face with the patient and/or family.

▲ 99205   Office or other outpatient visit for the evaluation and management of a new patient, which requires these 3 key components:

- A comprehensive history;

- A comprehensive examination;

- Medical decision making of high complexity.

Counseling and/or coordination of care with other physicians, other qualified health care professionals, or agencies are provided consistent with the nature of the problem(s) and the patient's and/or family's needs.

Usually, the presenting problem(s) are of moderate to high severity. Typically, 60 minutes are spent face-to-face with the patient and/or family.

▲ 99211   Office or other outpatient visit for the evaluation and management of an established patient, that may not require the presence of a physician or other qualified health care professional. Usually, the presenting problem(s) are minimal. Typically, 5 minutes are spent performing or supervising these services.

▲ 99212   Office or other outpatient visit for the evaluation and management of an established patient, which requires at least 2 of these 3 key components:

- A problem focused history;

- A problem focused examination;

- Straightforward medical decision making.

Counseling and/or coordination of care with other physicians, other qualified health care professionals, or agencies are provided consistent with the nature of the problem(s) and the patient's and/or family's needs.

Usually, the presenting problem(s) are self-limited or minor. Typically, 10 minutes are spent face-to- face with the patient and/or family.

▲ 99213   Office or other outpatient visit for the evaluation and management of an established patient, which requires at least 2 of these 3 key components:

- An expanded problem focused history;

- An expanded problem focused examination;

- Medical decision making of low complexity.

Counseling and coordination of care with other physicians, other qualified health care professionals, or agencies are provided consistent with the nature of the problem(s) and the patient's and/or family's needs.

Usually, the presenting problem(s) are of low to moderate severity.
Typically, 15 minutes are spent face-to-face with the patient and/or family.

▲ 99214   Office or other outpatient visit for the evaluation and management of an
established patient, which requires at least 2 of these 3 key components:

■ A detailed history;

■ A detailed examination;

■ Medical decision making of moderate complexity.

Counseling and/or coordination of care with other physicians, other
qualified health care professionals, or agencies are provided consistent with
the nature of the problem(s) and the patient's and/or family's needs.

Usually, the presenting problem(s) are of moderate to high severity.
Typically, 25 minutes are spent face-to-face with the patient and/or family.

▲ 99215   Office or other outpatient visit for the evaluation and management of an
established patient, which requires at least 2 of these 3 key components:

■ A comprehensive history;

■ A comprehensive examination;

■ Medical decision making of high complexity.

Counseling and/or coordination of care with other physicians, other
qualified health care professionals, or agencies are provided consistent with
the nature of the problem(s) and the patient's and/or family's needs.

Usually, the presenting problem(s) are of moderate to high severity.
Typically, 40 minutes are spent face-to-face with the patient and/or family.

▲ 99217   Observation care discharge day management (This code is to be utilized to
report all services provided to a patient on discharge from "observation
status" if the discharge is on other than the initial date of "observation
status." To report services to a patient designated as "observation status" or
"inpatient status" and discharged on the same date, use the codes for
Observation or Inpatient Care Services [including Admission and Discharge
Services, 99234-99236 as appropriate.])

▲ 99218   Initial observation care, per day, for the evaluation and management of a
patient which requires these 3 key components:

■ A detailed or comprehensive history;

■ A detailed or comprehensive examination; and

■ Medical decision making that is straightforward or of low complexity.

Counseling and/or coordination of care with other physicians, other
qualified health care professionals, or agencies are provided consistent with
the nature of the problem(s) and the patient's and/or family's needs.

Usually, the problem(s) requiring admission to "observation status" are of
low severity. Typically, 30 minutes are spent at the bedside and on the
patient's hospital floor or unit.

▲ 99219   Initial observation care, per day, for the evaluation and management of a
patient, which requires these 3 key components:

■ A comprehensive history;

■ A comprehensive examination; and

■ Medical decision making of moderate complexity.

Counseling and/or coordination of care with other physicians, other qualified health care professionals, or agencies are provided consistent with the nature of the problem(s) and the patient's and/or family's needs.

Usually, the problem(s) requiring admission to "observation status" are of moderate severity. Physicians typically spendTypically, 50 minutes are spent at the bedside and on the patient's hospital floor or unit.

▲ 99220   Initial observation care, per day, for the evaluation and management of a patient, which requires these 3 key components:

■ A comprehensive history;

■ A comprehensive examination; and

■ Medical decision making of high complexity.

Counseling and/or coordination of care with other physicians, other qualified health care professionals, or agencies are provided consistent with the nature of the problem(s) and the patient's and/or family's needs.

Usually, the problem(s) requiring admission to "observation status" are of high severity. Typically, 70 minutes are spent at the bedside and on the patient's hospital floor or unit.

▲ 99224   Subsequent observation care, per day, for the evaluation and management of a patient, which requires at least 2 of these 3 key components:

■ Problem focused interval history;

■ Problem focused examination;

■ Medical decision making that is straightforward or of low complexity.

Counseling and/or coordination of care with other physicians, other qualified health care professionals, or agencies are provided consistent with the nature of the problem(s) and the patient's and/or family's needs.

Usually, the patient is stable, recovering, or improving. Typically, 15 minutes are spent at the bedside and on the patient's hospital floor or unit.

▲ 99225   Subsequent observation care, per day, for the evaluation and management of a patient, which requires at least 2 of these 3 key components:

■ An expanded problem focused interval history;

■ An expanded problem focused examination;

■ Medical decision making of moderate complexity.

Counseling and/or coordination of care with other physicians, other qualified health care professionals, or agencies are provided consistent with the nature of the problem(s) and the patient's and/or family's needs.

Usually, the patient is responding inadequately to therapy or has developed a minor complication. Typically, 25 minutes are spent at the bedside and on the patient's hospital floor or unit.

▲ 99226   Subsequent observation care, per day, for the evaluation and management of a patient, which requires at least 2 of these 3 key components:

■ A detailed interval history;

■ A detailed examination;

■ Medical decision making of high complexity.

Counseling and/or coordination of care with other physicians, other qualified health care professionals, or agencies are provided consistent with the nature of the problem(s) and the patient's and/or family's needs.

Usually, the patient is unstable or has developed a significant complication or a significant new problem. Typically, 35 minutes are spent at the bedside and on the patient's hospital floor or unit.

▲ 99221   Initial hospital care, per day, for the evaluation and management of a patient, which requires these 3 key components:

■ A detailed or comprehensive history;

■ A detailed or comprehensive examination; and

■ Medical decision making that is straightforward or of low complexity.

Counseling and/or coordination of care with other physicians, other qualified health care professionals, or agencies are provided consistent with the nature of the problem(s) and the patient's and/or family's needs.

Usually, the problem(s) requiring admission are of low severity. Typically, 30 minutes are spent at the bedside and on the patient's hospital floor or unit.

▲ 99222   Initial hospital care, per day, for the evaluation and management of a patient, which requires these 3 key components:

■ A comprehensive history;

■ A comprehensive examination; and

■ Medical decision making of moderate complexity.

Counseling and/or coordination of care with other physicians, other qualified health care professionals, or agencies are provided consistent with the nature of the problem(s) and the patient's and/or family's needs.

Usually, the problem(s) requiring admission are of moderate severity. Typically, 50 minutes are spent at the bedside and on the patient's hospital floor or unit.

▲ 99223   Initial hospital care, per day, for the evaluation and management of a patient, which requires these 3 key components:

■ A comprehensive history;

■ A comprehensive examination; and

■ Medical decision making of high complexity.

Counseling and/or coordination of care with other physicians, other qualified health care professionals, or agencies are provided consistent with the nature of the problem(s) and the patient's and/or family's needs.

Usually, the problem(s) requiring admission are of high severity. Typically, 70 minutes are spent at the bedside and on the patient's hospital floor or unit.

▲ 99231   Subsequent hospital care, per day, for the evaluation and management of a patient, which requires at least 2 of these 3 key components:

■ A problem focused interval history;

■ A problem focused examination;

■ Medical decision making that is straightforward or of low complexity.

Counseling and/or coordination of care with other physicians, other qualified health care professionals, or agencies are provided consistent with the nature of the problem(s) and the patient's and/or family's needs.

Usually, the patient is stable, recovering or improving. Typically, 15 minutes are spent at the bedside and on the patient's hospital floor or unit.

▲ 99232   Subsequent hospital care, per day, for the evaluation and management of a patient, which requires at least 2 of these 3 key components:

■ An expanded problem focused interval history;

■ An expanded problem focused examination;

■ Medical decision making of moderate complexity.

Counseling and/or coordination of care with other physicians, other qualified health care professionals, or agencies are provided consistent with the nature of the problem(s) and the patient's and/or family's needs.

Usually, the patient is responding inadequately to therapy or has developed a minor complication. Typically, 25 minutes are spent at the bedside and on the patient's hospital floor or unit.

▲ 99233   Subsequent hospital care, per day, for the evaluation and management of a patient, which requires at least 2 of these 3 key components:

■ A detailed interval history;

■ A detailed examination;

■ Medical decision making of high complexity.

Counseling and/or coordination of care with other physicians, other qualified health care professionals, or agencies are provided consistent with the nature of the problem(s) and the patient's and/or family's needs.

Usually, the patient is unstable or has developed a significant complication or a significant new problem. Typically, 35 minutes are spent at the bedside and on the patient's hospital floor or unit.

▲ 99234   Observation or inpatient hospital care, for the evaluation and management of a patient including admission and discharge on the same date, which requires these 3 key components:

■ A detailed or comprehensive history;

■ A detailed or comprehensive examination; and

■ Medical decision making that is straightforward or of low complexity.

Counseling and/or coordination of care with other physicians, other qualified health care professionals, or agencies are provided consistent with the nature of the problem(s) and the patient's and/or family's needs.

Usually the presenting problem(s) requiring admission are of low severity. Typically, 40 minutes are spent at the bedside and on the patient's hospital floor or unit.

▲ 99235   Observation or inpatient hospital care, for the evaluation and management of a patient including admission and discharge on the same date, which requires these 3 key components:

■ A comprehensive history;

■ A comprehensive examination; and

■ Medical decision making of moderate complexity.

28

Counseling and/or coordination of care with other physicians, other qualified health care professionals, or agencies are provided consistent with the nature of the problem(s) and the patient's and/or family's needs.

Usually the presenting problem(s) requiring admission are of moderate severity. Typically, 50 minutes are spent at the bedside and on the patient's hospital floor or unit.

▲ 99236　Observation or inpatient hospital care, for the evaluation and management of a patient including admission and discharge on the same date, which requires these 3 key components:

■ A comprehensive history;

■ A comprehensive examination; and

■ Medical decision making of high complexity.

Counseling and/or coordination of care with other physicians, other qualified health care professionals, or agencies are provided consistent with the nature of the problem(s) and the patient's and/or family's needs.

Usually the presenting problem(s) requiring admission are of high severity. Typically, 55 minutes are spent at the bedside and on the patient's hospital floor or unit.

▲ 99241　Office consultation for a new or established patient, which requires these 3 key components:

■ A problem focused history;

■ A problem focused examination; and

■ Straightforward medical decision making.

Counseling and/or coordination of care with other physicians, other qualified health care professionals, or agencies are provided consistent with the nature of the problem(s) and the patient's and/or family's needs.

Usually, the presenting problem(s) are self limited or minor. Typically, 15 minutes are spent face-to-face with the patient and/or family.

▲ 99242　Office consultation for a new or established patient, which requires these 3 key components:

■ An expanded problem focused history;

■ An expanded problem focused examination; and

■ Straightforward medical decision making.

Counseling and/or coordination of care with other physicians, other qualified health care professionals, or agencies are provided consistent with the nature of the problem(s) and the patient's and/or family's needs.

Usually, the presenting problem(s) are of low severity. Typically, 30 minutes are spent face-to-face with the patient and/or family.

▲ 99243　Office consultation for a new or established patient, which requires these 3 key components:

■ A detailed history;

■ A detailed examination; and

■ Medical decision making of low complexity.

Counseling and/or coordination of care with other physicians, other qualified health care professionals, or agencies are provided consistent with the nature of the problem(s) and the patient's and/or family's needs.

Usually, the presenting problem(s) are of moderate severity. Typically, 40 minutes are spent face-to-face with the patient and/or family.

▲ 99244   Office consultation for a new or established patient, which requires these 3 key components:

■ A comprehensive history;

■ A comprehensive examination; and

■ Medical decision making of moderate complexity.

Counseling and/or coordination of care with other physicians, other qualified health care professionals, or agencies are provided consistent with the nature of the problem(s) and the patient's and/or family's needs.

Usually, the presenting problem(s) are of moderate to high severity. Typically, 60 minutes are spent face-to-face with the patient and/or family.

▲ 99245   Office consultation for a new or established patient, which requires these 3 key components:

■ A comprehensive history;

■ A comprehensive examination; and

■ Medical decision making of high complexity.

Counseling and/or coordination of care with other physicians, other qualified health care professionals, or agencies are provided consistent with the nature of the problem(s) and the patient's and/or family's needs.

Usually, the presenting problem(s) are of moderate to high severity. Typically, 80 minutes are spent face-to-face with the patient and/or family.

▲ 99251   Inpatient consultation for a new or established patient, which requires these 3 key components:

■ A problem focused history;

■ A problem focused examination; and

■ Straightforward medical decision making.

Counseling and/or coordination of care with other physicians, other qualified health care professionals, or agencies are provided consistent with the nature of the problem(s) and the patient's and/or family's needs.

Usually, the presenting problem(s) are self limited or minor. Typically, 20 minutes are spent at the bedside and on the patient's hospital floor or unit.

▲ 99252   Inpatient consultation for a new or established patient, which requires these 3 key components:

■ An expanded problem focused history;

■ An expanded problem focused examination; and

■ Straightforward medical decision making.

Counseling and/or coordination of care with other physicians, other qualified health care professionals, or agencies are provided consistent with the nature of the problem(s) and the patient's and/or family's needs.

Usually, the presenting problem(s) are of low severity. Typically, 40 minutes are spent at the bedside and on the patient's hospital floor or unit.

▲ 99253   Inpatient consultation for a new or established patient, which requires these 3 key components:

■ A detailed history;

■ A detailed examination; and

■ Medical decision making of low complexity.

Counseling and/or coordination of care with other physicians, other qualified health care professionals, or agencies are provided consistent with the nature of the problem(s) and the patient's and/or family's needs.

Usually, the presenting problem(s) are of moderate severity. Typically, 55 minutes are spent at the bedside and on the patient's hospital floor or unit.

▲ 99254   Inpatient consultation for a new or established patient, which requires these 3 key components:

■ A comprehensive history;

■ A comprehensive examination; and

■ Medical decision making of moderate complexity.

Counseling and/or coordination of care with other physicians, other qualified health care professionals, or agencies are provided consistent with the nature of the problem(s) and the patient's and/or family's needs.

Usually, the presenting problem(s) are of moderate to high severity. Typically, 80 minutes are spent at the bedside and on the patient's hospital floor or unit.

▲ 99255   Inpatient consultation for a new or established patient, which requires these 3 key components:

■ A comprehensive history;

■ A comprehensive examination; and

■ Medical decision making of high complexity.

Counseling and/or coordination of care with other physicians, other qualified health care professionals, or agencies are provided consistent with the nature of the problem(s) and the patient's and/or family's needs.

Usually, the presenting problem(s) are of moderate to high severity. Typically, 110 minutes are spent at the bedside and on the patient's hospital floor or unit.

▲ 99281   Emergency department visit for the evaluation and management of a patient, which requires these 3 key components:

■ A problem focused history;

■ A problem focused examination; and

■ Straightforward medical decision making.

Counseling and/or coordination of care with other physicians, other qualified health care professionals, or agencies are provided consistent with the nature of the problem(s) and the patient's and/or family's needs.

Usually, the presenting problem(s) are self limited or minor.

▲ 99282   Emergency department visit for the evaluation and management of a patient, which requires these 3 key components:

■ An expanded problem focused history;

■ An expanded problem focused examination; and

■ Medical decision making of low complexity.

Counseling and/or coordination of care with other physicians, other qualified health care professionals, or agencies are provided consistent with the nature of the problem(s) and the patient's and/or family's needs.

Usually, the presenting problem(s) are of low to moderate severity.

▲ 99283   Emergency department visit for the evaluation and management of a patient, which requires these 3 key components:

■ An expanded problem focused history;

■ An expanded problem focused examination; and

■ Medical decision making of moderate complexity.

Counseling and/or coordination of care with other physicians, other qualified health care professionals, or agencies are provided consistent with the nature of the problem(s) and the patient's and/or family's needs.

Usually, the presenting problem(s) are of moderate severity.

▲ 99284   Emergency department visit for the evaluation and management of a patient, which requires these 3 key components:

■ A detailed history;

■ A detailed examination; and

■ Medical decision making of moderate complexity.

Counseling and/or coordination of care with other physicians, other qualified health care professionals, or agencies are provided consistent with the nature of the problem(s) and the patient's and/or family's needs.

Usually, the presenting problem(s) are of high severity, and require urgent evaluation by the physicians or other health care professionals but do not pose an immediate significant threat to life or physiologic function.

▲ 99285   Emergency department visit for the evaluation and management of a patient, which requires these 3 key components within the constraints imposed by the urgency of the patient's clinical condition and/or mental status:

■ A comprehensive history;

■ A comprehensive examination; and

■ Medical decision making of high complexity.

Counseling and/or coordination of care with other physicians, other qualified health care professionals, or agencies are provided consistent with the nature of the problem(s) and the patient's and/or family's needs.

Usually, the presenting problem(s) are of high severity and pose an immediate significant threat to life or physiologic function.

▲ 99288   Physician or other qualified health care professional direction of emergency medical systems (EMS) emergency care, advanced life support;

▲ 99304 Initial nursing facility care, per day, for the evaluation and management of a patient, which requires these 3 key components:

- A detailed or comprehensive history;

- A detailed or comprehensive examination; and

- Medical decision making that is straightforward or of low complexity.

Counseling and/or coordination of care with other physicians, other qualified health care professionals, or agencies are provided consistent with the nature of the problem(s) and the patient's and/or family's needs.

Usually, the problem(s) requiring admission are of low severity. Typically, 25 minutes are spent at the bedside and on the patient's facility floor or unit.

▲ 99305 Initial nursing facility care, per day, for the evaluation and management of a patient, which requires these 3 key components:

- A comprehensive history;

- A comprehensive examination; and

- Medical decision making of moderate complexity.

Counseling and/or coordination of care with other physicians, other qualified health care professionals, or agencies are provided consistent with the nature of the problem(s) and the patient's and/or family's needs.

Usually, the problem(s) requiring admission are of moderate severity. Typically, 35 minutes are spent at the bedside and on the patient's facility floor or unit.

▲ 99306 Initial nursing facility care, per day, for the evaluation and management of a patient, which requires these 3 key components:

- A comprehensive history;

- A comprehensive examination; and

- Medical decision making of high complexity.

Counseling and/or coordination of care with other physicians, other qualified health care professionals, or agencies are provided consistent with the nature of the problem(s) and the patient's and/or family's needs.

Usually, the problem(s) requiring admission are of high severity. Typically, 45 minutes are spent at the bedside and on the patient's facility floor or unit.

▲ 99307 Subsequent nursing facility care, per day, for the evaluation and management of a patient, which requires at least 2 of these 3 key components

- A problem focused interval history;

- A problem focused examination;

- Straightforward medical decision making.

Counseling and/or coordination of care with other physicians, other qualified health care professionals, or agencies are provided consistent with the nature of the problem(s) and the patient's and/or family's needs.

Usually, the patient is stable, recovering, or improving. Typically, 10 minutes are spent at the bedside and on the patient's facility floor or unit.

▲ 99308 Subsequent nursing facility care, per day, for the evaluation and management of a patient, which requires at least 2 of these 3 key components:

- An expanded problem focused interval history;

- An expanded problem focused examination;

- Medical decision making of low complexity.

Counseling and/or coordination of care with other physicians, other qualified health care professionals, or agencies are provided consistent with the nature of the problem(s) and the patient's and/or family's needs.

Usually, the patient is responding inadequately to therapy or has developed a minor complication. Typically, 15 minutes are spent at the bedside and on the patient's facility floor or unit.

▲ 99309 Subsequent nursing facility care, per day, for the evaluation and management of a patient, which requires at least 2 of these 3 key components:

- A detailed interval history;

- A detailed examination;

- Medical decision making of moderate complexity.

Counseling and/or coordination of care with other physicians, other qualified health care professionals, or agencies are provided consistent with the nature of the problem(s) and the patient's and/or family's needs.

Usually, the patient has developed a significant complication or a significant new problem. Typically, 25 minutes are spent at the bedside and on the patient's facility floor or unit.

▲ 99310 Subsequent nursing facility care, per day, for the evaluation and management of a patient, which requires at least 2 of these 3 key components:

- A comprehensive interval history;

- A comprehensive examination;

- Medical decision making of high complexity.

Counseling and/or coordination of care with other physicians, other qualified health care professionals, or agencies are provided consistent with the nature of the problem(s) and the patient's and/or family's needs.

The patient may be unstable or may have developed a significant new problem requiring immediate physician attention. Typically, 35 minutes are spent at the bedside and on the patient's facility floor or unit.

▲ 99318 Evaluation and management of a patient involving an annual nursing facility assessment, which requires these 3 key components:

- A detailed interval history;

- A comprehensive examination; and

- Medical decision making that is of low to moderate complexity.

Counseling and/or coordination of care with other physicians, other qualified health care professionals, or agencies are provided consistent with the nature of the problem(s) and the patient's and/or family's needs.

Usually, the patient is stable, recovering, or improving. Typically, 30 minutes are spent at the bedside and on the patient's facility floor or unit.

▲ 99324   Domiciliary or rest home visit for the evaluation and management of a new patient, which requires these 3 key components:

■ A problem focused history;

■ A problem focused examination; and

■ Straightforward medical decision making.

Counseling and/or coordination of care with other physicians, other qualified health care professionals, or agencies are provided consistent with the nature of the problem(s) and the patient's and/or family's needs.

Usually, the presenting problem(s) are of low severity. Typically, 20 minutes are spent with the patient and/or family or caregiver

▲ 99325   Domiciliary or rest home visit for the evaluation and management of a new patient, which requires these 3 key components:

■ An expanded problem focused history;

■ An expanded problem focused examination; and

■ Medical decision making of low complexity.

Counseling and/or coordination of care with other physicians, other qualified health care professionals, or agencies are provided consistent with the nature of the problem(s) and the patient's and/or family's needs.

Usually, the presenting problem(s) are of moderate severity. Typically, 30 minutes are spent with the patient and/or family or caregiver

▲ 99326   Domiciliary or rest home visit for the evaluation and management of a new patient, which requires these 3 key components:

■ A detailed history;

■ A detailed examination; and

■ Medical decision making of moderate complexity.

Counseling and/or coordination of care with other physicians, other qualified health care professionals, or agencies are provided consistent with the nature of the problem(s) and the patient's and/or family's needs.

Usually, the presenting problem(s) are of moderate to high severity. Typically, 45 minutes are spent with the patient and/or family or caregiver

▲ 99327   Domiciliary or rest home visit for the evaluation and management of a new patient, which requires these 3 key components:

■ A comprehensive history;

■ A comprehensive examination; and

■ Medical decision making of moderate complexity.

Counseling and/or coordination of care with other physicians, other rsqualified health care professionals, or agencies are provided consistent with the nature of the problem(s) and the patient's and/or family's needs.

Usually, the presenting problem(s) are of high severity. Typically, 60 minutes are spent with the patient and/or family or caregiver

▲ 99328   Domiciliary or rest home visit for the evaluation and management of a new patient, which requires these 3 key components:

- A comprehensive history;

- A comprehensive examination; and

- Medical decision making of high complexity.

Counseling and/or coordination of care with other physicians, other qualified health care professionals, or agencies are provided consistent with the nature of the problem(s) and the patient's and/or family's needs.

Usually, the patient is unstable or has developed a significant new problem requiring immediate physician attention. Pypically, 75 minutes are spent with the patient and/or family or caregiver

▲ 99334   Domiciliary or rest home visit for the evaluation and management of an established patient, which requires at least 2 of these 3 key components:

- A problem focused interval history;

- A problem focused examination;

- Straightforward medical decision making.

Counseling and/or coordination of care with other physicians, other qualified health care professionals, or agencies are provided consistent with the nature of the problem(s) and the patient's and/or family's needs.

Usually, the presenting problem(s) are self-limited or minor. Typically, 15 minutes are spent with the patient and/or family or caregiver

▲ 99335   Domiciliary or rest home visit for the evaluation and management of an established patient, which requires at least 2 of these 3 key components:

- An expanded problem focused interval history;

- An expanded problem focused examination;

- Medical decision making of low complexity.

Counseling and/or coordination of care with other physicians, other qualified health care professionals, or agencies are provided consistent with the nature of the problem(s) and the patient's and/or family's needs.

Usually, the presenting problem(s) are of low to moderate severity. Typically, 25 minutes are spent with the patient and/or family or caregiver

▲ 99336   Domiciliary or rest home visit for the evaluation and management of an established patient, which requires at least 2 of these 3 key components:

- A detailed interval history;

- A detailed examination;

- Medical decision making of moderate complexity.

Counseling and/or coordination of care with other physicians, other qualified health care professionals, or agencies are provided consistent with the nature of the problem(s) and the patient's and/or family's needs.

Usually, the presenting problem(s) are of moderate to high severity. Typically, 40 minutes are spent with the patient and/or family or caregiver

▲ 99337   Domiciliary or rest home visit for the evaluation and management of an established patient, which requires at least 2 of these 3 key components:

■ A comprehensive interval history;

■ A comprehensive examination;

■ Medical decision making of moderate to high complexity.

Counseling and/or coordination of care with other physicians, other qualified health care professionals, or agencies are provided consistent with the nature of the problem(s) and the patient's and/or family's needs.

Usually, the presenting problem(s) are of moderate to high severity. The patient may be unstable or may have developed a significant new problem requiring immediate physician attention. Typically, 60 minutes are spent with the patient and/or family or caregiver

▲ 99341   Home visit for the evaluation and management of a new patient, which requires these 3 key components:

■ A problem focused history;

■ A problem focused examination; and

■ Straightforward medical decision making.

Counseling and/or coordination of care with other physicians, other qualified health care professionals, or agencies are provided consistent with the nature of the problem(s) and the patient's and/or family's needs.

Usually, the presenting problem(s) are of low severity. Typically, 20 minutes are spent face-to-face with the patient and/or family

▲ 99342   Home visit for the evaluation and management of a new patient, which requires these 3 key components:

■ An expanded problem focused history;

■ An expanded problem focused examination; and

■ Medical decision making of low complexity.

Counseling and/or coordination of care with other physicians, other qualified health care professionals, or agencies are provided consistent with the nature of the problem(s) and the patient's and/or family's needs.

Usually, the presenting problem(s) are of moderate severity. Typically, 30 minutes are spent face-to-face with the patient and/or family

▲ 99343   Home visit for the evaluation and management of a new patient, which requires these 3 key components:

■ A detailed history;

■ A detailed examination; and

■ Medical decision making of moderate complexity.

Counseling and/or coordination of care with other physicians, other qualified health care professionals, or agencies are provided consistent with the nature of the problem(s) and the patient's and/or family's needs.

Usually, the presenting problem(s) are of moderate to high severity. Typically, 45 minutes are spent face-to-face with the patient and/or family

▲ 99344   Home visit for the evaluation and management of a new patient, which requires these 3 key components:

■ A comprehensive history;

■ A comprehensive examination; and

■ Medical decision making of moderate complexity.

Counseling and/or coordination of care with other physicians, other qualified health care professionals, or agencies are provided consistent with the nature of the problem(s) and the patient's and/or family's needs.

Usually, the presenting problem(s) are of high severity. Typically, 60 minutes are spent face-to-face with the patient and/or family

▲ 99345   Home visit for the evaluation and management of a new patient, which requires these 3 key components:

■ A comprehensive history;

■ A comprehensive examination; and

■ Medical decision making of high complexity.

Counseling and/or coordination of care with other physicians, other qualified health care professionals, or agencies are provided consistent with the nature of the problem(s) and the patient's and/or family's needs.

Usually, the patient is unstable or has developed a significant new problem requiring immediate physician attention. Typically, 75 minutes are spent face-to-face with the patient and/or family

▲ 99347   Home visit for the evaluation and management of an established patient, which requires at least 2 of these 3 key components:

■ A problem focused interval history;

■ A problem focused examination;

■ Straightforward medical decision making.

Counseling and/or coordination of care with other physicians, other qualified health care professionals, or agencies are provided consistent with the nature of the problem(s) and the patient's and/or family's needs.

Usually, the presenting problem(s) are self limited or minor. Typically, 15 minutes are spent face-to-face with the patient and/or family

▲ 99348   Home visit for the evaluation and management of an established patient, which requires at least 2 of these 3 key components:

■ An expanded problem focused interval history;

■ An expanded problem focused examination;

■ Medical decision making of low complexity.

Counseling and/or coordination of care with other physicians, other qualified health care professionals, or agencies are provided consistent with the nature of the problem(s) and the patient's and/or family's needs.

Usually, the presenting problem(s) are of low to moderate severity. Typically, 25 minutes are spent face-to-face with the patient and/or family

▲ 99349   Home visit for the evaluation and management of an established patient, which requires at least 2 of these 3 key components:

■ A detailed interval history;

■ A detailed examination;

■ Medical decision making of moderate complexity.

Counseling and/or coordination of care with other physicians, other qualified health care professionals, or agencies are provided consistent with the nature of the problem(s) and the patient's and/or family's needs.

Usually, the presenting problem(s) are moderate to high severity. Typically, 40 minutes are spent face-to-face with the patient and/or family

▲ 99350   Home visit for the evaluation and management of an established patient, which requires at least 2 of these 3 key components:

■ A comprehensive interval history;

■ A comprehensive examination;

■ Medical decision making of moderate to high complexity.

Counseling and/or coordination of care with other physicians, other qualified health care professionals, or agencies are provided consistent with the nature of the problem(s) and the patient's and/or family's needs.

Usually, the presenting problem(s) are of moderate to high severity. The patient may be unstable or may have developed a significant new problem requiring immediate physician attention. Typically, 60 minutes are spent face-to-face with the patient and/or family.

▲ 99360   Standby service, requiring prolonged attendance, each 30 minutes (eg, operative standby, standby for frozen section, for cesarean/high risk delivery, for monitoring EEG)

▲ 99374   Supervision of a patient under care of home health agency (patient not present) in home, domiciliary or equivalent environment (eg, Alzheimer's facility) requiring complex and multidisciplinary care modalities involving regular development and/or revision of care plans by that individual, review of subsequent reports of patient status, review of related laboratory and other studies, communication (including telephone calls) for purposes of assessment or care decisions with health care professional(s), family member(s), surrogate decision maker(s) (eg, legal guardian) and/or key caregiver(s) involved in patient's care, integration of new information into the medical treatment plan and/or adjustment of medical therapy, within a calendar month; 15-29 minutes

▲ 99375   30 minutes or more

▲ 99377   Supervision of a hospice patient (patient not present) requiring complex and multidisciplinary care modalities involving regular development and/or revision of care plans by that individual, review of subsequent reports of patient status, review of related laboratory and other studies, communication (including telephone calls) for purposes of assessment or care decisions with health care professional(s), family member(s), surrogate decision maker(s) (eg, legal guardian) and/or key caregiver(s) involved in patient's care, integration of new information into the medical treatment plan and/or adjustment of medical therapy, within a calendar month; 15-29 minutes

▲ 99378   30 minutes or more

▲ 99379   Supervision of a nursing facility patient (patient not present) requiring complex and multidisciplinary care modalities involving regular development and/or revision of care plans by that individual, review of subsequent reports of patient status, review of related laboratory and other studies, communication (including telephone calls) for purposes of assessment or care decisions with health care professional(s), family member(s), surrogate decision maker(s) (eg, legal guardian) and/or key

39

caregiver(s) involved in patient's care, integration of new information into the medical treatment plan and/or adjustment of medical therapy, within a calendar month; 15-29 minutes

▲ 99380   30 minutes or more

▲ 99441   Telephone evaluation and management service by a physician or other qualified health care professional who may report evaluation and management services provided to an established patient, parent, or guardian not originating from a related E/M service provided within the previous 7 days nor leading to an E/M service or procedure within the next 24 hours or soonest available appointment; 5-10 minutes of medical discussion

▲ 99442   11-20 minutes of medical discussion

▲ 99443   21-30 minutes of medical discussion

▲ 99444   Online evaluation and management service provided by a physician or other qualified health care professional who may report an evaluation and management services provided to an established patient, or guardian not originating from a related E/M service provided within the previous 7 days, using the Internet or similar electronic communications network

▲ 99464   Attendance at delivery (when requested by the delivering physician or other qualified health care professional) and initial stabilization of newborn

▲ 99466   Critical care face-to-face services, during an interfacility transport of critically ill or critically injured pediatric patient, 24 months of age or younger; first 30-74 minutes of hands-on care during transport

▲ + 99467   each additional 30 minutes (List separately in addition to code for primary service)

● 99485   Code added

● +99486   Code added

● 99487   Code added

● 99488   Code added

● +99489   Code added

● 99495   Code added

● 99496   Code added

Anesthesia

▲ 01991   Anesthesia for diagnostic or therapeutic nerve blocks and injections (when block or injection is performed by a different physician or other qualified health care professional); other than the prone position

▲ 01992   prone position

Surgery

▲ 15740   Flap; island pedicle requiring identification and dissection of an anatomically named axial vessel

▲ 20665   Removal of tongs or halo applied by another individual

40

▲ ⊙+22522   each additional thoracic or lumbar vertebral body (List separately in addition to code for primary procedure)

● 22586   Code added

● 23473   Code added

● 23474   Code added

● 24370   Code added

● 24371   Code added

▲ 28890   Extracorporeal shock wave, high energy, performed by a physician or other qualified health care professional, requiring anesthesia other than local, including ultrasound guidance, involving the plantar fascia

(29590   Code deleted 2012 [2013 edition])

● ⊙31647   Code added

● ⊙31648   Code added

● ⊙+31649   Code added

● ⊙+31651   Code added

(31656   Code deleted 2012 [2013 edition])

● ⊙31660   Code added

● ⊙31661   Code added

(31715   Code deleted 2012 [2013 edition])

(32420   Code deleted 2012 [2013 edition])

(32421   Code deleted 2012 [2013 edition])

(32422   Code deleted 2012 [2013 edition])

▲ ⊙32551   Tube thoracostomy, includes connection to drainage system (eg, water seal), when performed, open (separate procedure)

● 32554   Code added

● 32555   Code added

● 32556   Code added

● 32557   Code added

● 32701   Code added

▲ +33225   Insertion of pacing electrode, cardiac venous system, for left ventricular pacing, at time of insertion of pacing cardioverter-defibrillator or pacemaker pulse generator (eg, for upgrade to dual chamber system) (List separately in addition to code for primary procedure)

● 33361   Code added

● 33362   Code added

● 33363   Code added

● 33364   Code added

● 33365   Code added

● +33367   Code added

41

- +33368   Code added
- +33369   Code added
- ⊙33990   Code added
- ⊙33991   Code added
- ⊙33992   Code added
- ⊙33993   Code added
- ▲ ⊙36010   Introduction of catheter, superior or inferior vena cava
- ▲ ⊙36140   extremity artery
- ⊙36221   Code added
- ⊙36222   Code added
- ⊙36223   Code added
- ⊙36224   Code added
- ⊙36225   Code added
- ⊙36226   Code added
- ⊙+36227   Code added
- ⊙+36228   Code added
- ▲ 36400   Venipuncture, younger than age 3 years, necessitating the skill of a physician or other qualified health care professional, not to be used for routine venipuncture; femoral or jugular vein
- ▲ 36405   scalp vein
- ▲ 36406   other vein
- ▲ 36410   Venipuncture, age 3 years or older, necessitating the skill of a physician or other qualified health care professional (separate procedure), for diagnostic or therapeutic purposes (not to be used for routine venipuncture)
- ⊙37197   Code added
- (37201   Code deleted 2012 [2013 edition])
- ⊙37211   Code added
- ⊙37212   Code added
- ⊙37213   Code adde
- ⊙37214   Code added
- (37203   Code deleted 2012 [2013 edition])
- (37209   Code deleted 2012 [2013 edition])
- ▲ 38240   Hematopoietic progenitor cell (HPC); allogeneic transplantation per donor
- ▲ 38241   autologous transplantation
- 38243   Code added
- ▲ 38242   Allogenic lymphocyte infusions
- ▲ ⊙43206   Code added
- (43234   Code deleted 2012 [2013 edition])

- ⊙43252   Code added

- 44705   Code added

- 52287   Code added

▲ 59300   Episiotomy or vaginal repair, by other than attending;

▲ 62370   with reprogramming and refill (requiring skill of a physician or other qualified health care professional)

▲ 64561   sacral nerve (transforaminal placement) including image guidance, if performed

▲ 64612   Chemodenervation of muscle(s); muscle(s) innervated by facial nerve, unilateral (eg, for blepharospasm, hemifacial spasm)

▲ 64614   extremity and/or trunk muscle(s) (eg, for dystonia, cerebral palsy, multiple sclerosis)

- 64615   Code added

▲ 65800   Paracentesis of anterior chamber of eye (separate procedure); with removal of aqueous

(65805   Code deleted 2012 [2013 edition])

▲ 67810   Incisional biopsy of eyelid skin including lid margin

Radiology

(71040   Code deleted 2012 [2013 edition])

(71060   Code deleted 2012 [2013 edition])

▲ 72040   Radiologic examination, spine, cervical; 3 views or less

▲ 72050   4 or 5 views

▲ 72052   6 or more views

(75650   Code deleted 2012 [2013 edition])

(75660   Code deleted 2012 [2013 edition])

(75662   Code deleted 2012 [2013 edition])

(75665   Code deleted 2012 [2013 edition])

(75671   Code deleted 2012 [2013 edition])

(75676   Code deleted 2012 [2013 edition])

(75680   Code deleted 2012 [2013 edition])

(75685   Code deleted 2012 [2013 edition])

▲ 75896   Transcatheter therapy, infusion, other than for thrombolysis, radiological supervision and interpretation

▲ 75898   Angiography through existing catheter for follow-up study for transcatheter therapy, embolization or infusion, other than for thrombolysis

(75900   Code deleted 2012 [2013 edition])

(75961   Code deleted 2012 [2013 edition])

▲ 76000   Fluoroscopy (separate procedure), up to 1 hour physician or other qualified health care professional time, other than 71023 or 71034 (eg, cardiac fluoroscopy)

▲ 76001   Fluoroscopy, physician or other qualified health care professional time more than 1 hour, assisting a nonradiologic physician or other qualified health care professional (eg, nephrostolithotomy, ERCP, bronchoscopy, transbronchial biopsy)

▲ 76376   3D rendering with interpretation and reporting of computed tomography, magnetic resonance imaging, ultrasound, or other tomographic modality with image postprocessing under concurrent supervision; not requiring image postprocessing on an independent workstation

▲ 76377   requiring image postprocessing on an independent workstation

▲ 76885   Ultrasound, infant hips, real time with imaging documentation; dynamic (requiring physician or other qualified health care professional manipulation)

▲ 76886   limited, static (not requiring physician or other qualified health care professional manipulation)

▲ +77051   Computer-aided detection (computer algorithm analysis of digital image data for lesion detection) with further review for interpretation, with or without digitization of film radiographic images; diagnostic mammography (List separately in addition to code for primary procedure)

▲ +77052   screening mammography (List separately in addition to code for primary procedure)

▲ 77071   Manual application of stress performed by physician or other qualified health care professional for joint radiography, including contralateral joint if indicated

(78000   Code deleted 2012 [2013 edition])

(78001   Code deleted 2012 [2013 edition])

(78003   Code deleted 2012 [2013 edition])

(78006   Code deleted 2012 [2013 edition])

(78007   Code deleted 2012 [2013 edition])

(78010   Code deleted 2012 [2013 edition])

(78011   Code deleted 2012 [2013 edition])

● 78012   Code added

● 78013   Code added

● 78014   Code added

▲ 78070   Parathyroid planar imaging (including subtraction, when performed)

● 78071   Code added

● 78072   Code added

Pathology and Laboratory

● 81201   Code added

● 81202   Code added

- 81203   Code added
- 81235   Code added
- 81252   Code added
- 81253   Code added
- 81254   Code added
- 81321   Code added
- 81322   Code added
- 81323   Code added
- 81324   Code added
- 81325   Code added
- 81326   Code added
- ▲ 81400   Molecular pathology procedure, Level 1 identification of single germline variant [eg, SNP] by techniques such as restriction enzyme digestion or melt curve analysis)

ABCC8 (ATP-binding cassette, sub-family C [CFTR/MRP], member 8) (eg, familial hyperinsulinism), F1388del variant

ACADM (acyl-CoA dehydrogenase, C-4 to C-12 straight chain, MCAD) (eg, medium chain acyl dehydrogenase deficiency), K304E variant

ACE (angiotensin converting enzyme) (eg, hereditary blood pressure regulation), insertion/deletion variant

AGTR1 (angiotensin II receptor, type 1) (eg, essential hypertension), 1166A>C variant

CCR5 (chemokine C-C motif receptor 5) (eg, HIV resistance), 32-bp deletion mutation/794 825del32 deletion

CLRN1 (clarin 1) (eg, Usher syndrome, type 3), N48K variant

DPYD (dihydropyrimidine dehydrogenase) (eg, 5-fluorouracil/5-FU and capecitabine drug metabolism), IVS14+1G>A variant

F2 (coagulation factor 2) (eg, hereditary hypercoagulability), 1199G>A variant

tF5 (coagulation factor V) (eg, hereditary hypercoagulability), HR2 variant

F7 (coagulation factor VII [serum prothrombin conversion accelerator]) (eg, hereditary hypercoagulability), R353Q variant

F13B (coagulation factor XIII, B polypeptide) (eg, hereditary hypercoagulability), V34L variant

FGB (fibrinogen beta chain) (eg, hereditary ischemic heart disease), -455G>A variant

FGFR3 (fibroblast growth factor receptor 3) (eg, Muenke syndrome), P250R variant

Human Platelet Antigen 1 genotyping (HPA-1), ITGB3 (integrin, beta 3 [platelet glycoprotein IIIa], antigen CD61 [GPIIIa]) (eg, neonatal alloimmune thrombocytopenia [NAIT], post-transfusion purpura), HPA-1a/b (L33P)

45

Human Platelet Antigen 2 genotyping (HPA-2), GP1BA (glycoprotein Ib [platelet], alpha polypeptide [GPIba]) (eg, neonatal alloimmune thrombocytopenia [NAIT], posttransfusion purpura), HPA-2a/b (T145M)

Human Platelet Antigen 3 genotyping (HPA-3), ITGA2B (integrin, alpha 2b [platelet glycoprotein IIb of IIb/IIIa complex], antigen CD41 [GPIIb]) (eg, neonatal alloimmune thrombocytopenia [NAIT], posttransfusion purpura), HPA-3a/b (I843S)

Human Platelet Antigen 4 genotyping (HPA-4), ITGB3 (integrin, beta 3 [platelet glycoprotein IIIa], antigen CD61 [GPIIIa]) (eg, neonatal alloimmune thrombocytopenia [NAIT], post-transfusion purpura), HPA-4a/b (R143Q)

Human Platelet Antigen 5 genotyping (HPA-5), ITGA2 (integrin, alpha 2 [CD49B, alpha 2 subunit of VLA-2 receptor] [GPIa]) (eg, neonatal alloimmune thrombocytopenia [NAIT], post-transfusion purpura), HPA-5a/b (K505E)

Human Platelet Antigen 6 genotyping (HPA-6w), ITGB3 (integrin, beta 3 [platelet glycoprotein IIIa, antigen CD61] [GPIIIa]) (eg, neonatal alloimmune thrombocytopenia [NAIT], post-transfusion purpura), HPA-6a/b (R489Q)

Human Platelet Antigen 9 genotyping (HPA-9w), ITGA2B (integrin, alpha 2b [platelet glycoprotein IIb of IIb/IIIa complex, antigen CD41] [GPIIb]) (eg, neonatal alloimmune thrombocytopenia [NAIT], posttransfusion purpura), HPA-9a/b (V837M)

Human Platelet Antigen 15 genotyping (HPA-15), CD109 (CD109 molecule) (eg, neonatal alloimmune thrombocytopenia [NAIT], post-transfusion purpura), HPA-15a/b (S682Y)

IVD (isovaleryl-CoA dehydrogenase) (eg, isovaleric acidemia), A282V variant

SERPINE1 (serpine peptidase inhibitor clade E, member 1, plasminogen activator inhibitor -1, PAI-1) (eg, thrombophilia), 4G variant

SHOC2 (soc-2 suppressor of clear homolog) (eg, Noonan-like syndrome with loose anagen hair), S2G variant

MN1 (survival of motor neuron 1, telomeric) (eg, spinal muscular atrophy), exon 7 deletion

SRY (sex determining region Y) (eg, 46,XX testicular disorder of sex development, gonadal dysgenesis), gene analysis

TOR1A (torsin family 1, member A [torsin A])(eg, early-onset primary dystonia [DYT1]), 907_909delGAG (904_906delGAG) variant

▲ 81401 Molecular pathology procedure, Level 2 (eg, 2-10 SNPs, 1 methylated variant, or 1 somatic variant [typically using nonsequencing target variant analysis], or detection of a dynamic mutation disorder/triplet repeat)

ABL (c-abl oncogene 1, receptor tyrosine kinase) (eg, acquired imatinib resistance), T315I variant

ACADM (acyl-CoA dehydrogenase, C-4 to C-12 straight chain, MCAD) (eg, medium chain acyl dehydrogenase deficiency), commons variants (eg, K304E, Y42H)

ADRB2 (adrenergic beta-2 receptor surface) (eg, drug metabolism), common variants (eg, G16R, Q27E) APOB (apolipoprotein B) (eg, familial hypercholesterolemia type B), common variants (eg, R3500Q, R3500W)

APOE (apolipoprotein E) (eg, hyperlipoproteinemia type III, cardiovascular disease, Alzheimer disease), common variants (eg, *2, *3, *4)

AR (androgen receptor) (eg, spinal and bulbar muscular atrophy, Kennedy disease, X chromosome inactivation), characterization of alleles (eg, expanded size or methylation status)

ATN1 (atrophin 1) (eg, dentatorubral-pallidoluysian atrophy), evaluation to detect abnormal (eg, expanded) alleles

CBFB/MYH11 (inv(16)) (eg, acute myeloid leukemia), qualitative, and quantitative, if performed

CBS (cystathionine-beta-synthase) (eg, homocystinuria, cystathionine beta-synthase deficiency), common variants (eg, I278T, G307S)

CCND1/IGH (BCL1/IgH, t(11;14)) (eg, mantle cell lymphoma) translocation analysis, major breakpoint, qualitative, and quantitative, if performed

CFH/ARMS2 (complement factor H/age-related maculopathy susceptibility 2) (eg, macular degeneration), common variants (eg, Y402H [CFH], A69S [ARMS2])

CYP3A4 (cytochrome P450, family 3, subfamily A, polypeptide 4) (eg, drug metabolism), common variants (eg, *2, *3, *4, *5, *6)

CYP3A5 (cytochrome P450, family 3, subfamily A, polypeptide 5) (eg, drug metabolism), common variants (eg, *2, *3, *4, *5, *6)

DMPK (dystrophia myotonica-protein kinase) (eg, myotonic dystrophy, type 1), evaluation to detect abnormal (eg, expanded) alleles

E2A/PBX1 (t(1;19)) (eg, acute lymphocytic leukemia), translocation analysis, qualitative, and quantitative, if performed

EML4/ALK (inv(2)) (eg, non-small cell lung cancer), translocation or inversion analysis

ETV6/RUNX1 (t(12;21)) (eg, acute lymphocytic leukemia), translocation analysis, qualitative, and quantitative, if performed

EWSR1/ERG (t(21;22)) (eg, Ewing sarcoma/peripheral neuroectodermal tumor), translocation analysis, qualitative, and quantitative, if performed

EWSR1/FLI1 (t(11;22)) (eg, Ewing sarcoma/peripheral neuroectodermal tumor), translocation analysis, qualitative, and quantitative, if performed

F11 (coagulation factor XI) (eg, coagulation disorder), common variants (eg, E117X [Type II], F283L [Type III], IVS14del14, and IVS14+1G>A [Type I])

FGFR3 (fibroblast growth factor receptor 3) (eg, achondroplasia, hypochondroplasia), common variants (eg, 1138G>A, 1138G>C, 1620C>A, 1620C>G)

FIP1L1/PDGFRA (del[4q12]) (eg, imatinib-sensitive chronic eosinophilic leukemia), qualitative, and quantitative, if performed

FOXO1/PAX3 (t(1;13)) (eg, Ewing sarcoma/peripheral neuroectodermal tumor), translocation analysis, qualitative, and quantitative, if performed

FOXO1/PAX7 (t(2;13)) (eg, Ewing sarcoma/peripheral neuroectodermal tumor), translocation analysis, qualitative, and quantitative, if performed

FXN (frataxin) (eg, Friedreich ataxia), evaluation to detect abnormal (expanded) alleles

GALT (galactose-1-phosphate uridylyltransferase) (eg, galactosemia), common variants (eg, Q188R, S135L, K285N, T138M, L195P, Y209C, IVS2-2A>G, P171S, del5kb, N314D, L218L/N314D)

H19 (imprinted maternally expressed transcript [non-protein coding]) (eg, Beckwith-Wiedemann syndrome), methylation analysis

HBB (hemoglobin, beta) (eg, sickle cell anemia, hemoglobin C, hemoglobin E), common variants (eg, HbS, HbC, HbE)

HTT (huntingtin) (eg, Huntington disease), evaluation to detect abnormal (eg, expanded alleles) expanded

KCNQ1OT1 (KCNQ1 overlapping transcript 1 [non-protein coding]) (eg, Beckwith-Wiedemann syndrome), methylation analysis

MEG3/DLK1 (maternally expressed 3 [non-protein coding]/deltalike 1 homolog [Drosophila]) (eg, intrauterine growth retardation), methylation analysis

MLL/AFF1 (t(4;11)) (eg, acute lymphoblastic leukemia), translocation analysis, qualitative, and quantitative, if performed MLL/MLLT3 (t(9;11)) (eg, acute myeloid leukemia), translocation analysis, qualitative, and quantitative, if performed

MT-RNR1 (mitochondrially encoded 12S RNA) (eg, nonsyndromic hearing loss), common variants (eg, m.1555A>G, m.1494C>T)

MUTYH (mutY homolog [E. coli]) (eg, MYH-associated polyposis), common variants (eg, Y165C, G382D)

MT-ATP6 (mitochondrially encoded ATP synthase 6) (eg, neuropathy with ataxia and retinitis pigmentosa [NARP], Leigh syndrome), common variants (eg, m.8993T>G, m.8993T>C)

MT-ND4, MT-ND6 (mitochondrially encoded NADH dehydrogenase 4, mitochondrially encoded NADH dehydrogenase 6) (eg, Leber hereditary optic neuropathy [LHON]), common variants (eg, m.11778G>A, m.3460G>A, m.14484T>C)

MT-TK (mitochondrially encoded tRNA lysine) (eg, myoclonic epilepsy with ragged-red fibers [MERRF]), common variants (eg, m.8344A>G, m.8356T>C)

MT-TL1 (mitochondrially encoded tRNA leucine 1 [UUA/G]) (eg, diabetes and hearing loss), common variants (eg, m.3243A>G, m.14709 T>C) MT-TL1

MT-ND5 (mitochondrially encoded tRNA leucine 1 [UUA/G], mitochondrially encoded NADH dehydrogenase 5) (eg, mitochondrial encephalopathy with lactic acidosis and stroke-like episodes [MELAS]), common variants (eg, m.3243A>G, m.3271T>C, m.3252A>G, m.13513G>A)

MT-TS1, MT-RNR1 (mitochondrially encoded tRNA serine 1 [UCN], mitochondrially encoded 12S RNA) (eg, nonsyndromic sensorineural deafness [including aminoglycoside-induced nonsyndromic deafness]), common variants (eg, m.7445A>G, m.1555A>G)

NPM1/ALK (t(2;5)) (eg, anaplastic large cell lymphoma), translocation analysis

PAX8/PPARG (t(2;3) (q13;p25)) (eg, follicular thyroid carcinoma), translocation analysis

PRSS1 (protease, serine, 1 [trypsin 1]) (eg, hereditary pancreatitis), common variants (eg, N29I, A16V, R122H)

PYGM (phosphorylase, glycogen, muscle) (eg, glycogen storage disease type V, McArdle disease), common variants (eg, R50X, G205S)

RUNX1/RUNX1T1 (t(8;21)) (eg, acute myeloid leukemia) translocation analysis, qualitative, and quantitative, if performed

SEPT9 (Septin 9) (eg, colon cancer), methylation analysis

SMN1/SMN2 (survival of motor neuron 1, telomeric/survival of motor neuron 2, centromeric) (eg, spinal muscular atrophy), dosage analysis (eg, carrier testing)

TPMT (thiopurine S-methyltransferase) (eg, drug metabolism), common variants (eg, *2, *3)

TYMS (thymidylate synthetase) (eg, 5-fluorouracil/5-FU drug metabolism), tandem repeat variant

VWF (von Willebrand factor) (eg, von Willebrand disease type 2N), common variants (eg, T791M, R816W, R854Q)

▲ 81402   Molecular pathology procedure, Level 3 (eg, >10 SNPs, 2-10 methylated variants, or 2-10 somatic variants [typically using non-sequencing target variant analysis], immunoglobulin and T-cell receptor gene rearrangements, duplication/deletion variants of 1 exon, loss of heterozygosity [LOH], uniparental disomy [UPD])

Chromosome 18q- (eg, D18S55, D18S58, D18S61, D18S64, and D18S69) (eg, colon cancer), allelic imbalance assessment (ie, loss of heterozygosity)

CYP21A2 (cytochrome P450, family 21, subfamily A, polypeptide 2) (eg, congenital adrenal hyperplasia, 21-hydroxylase deficiency), common variants (eg, IVS2-13G, P30L, I172N, exon 6 mutation cluster [I235N, V236E, M238K], V281L, L307FfsX6, Q318X, R356W, P453S, G110VfsX21, 30-kb deletion variant)

ESR1/PGR (receptor 1/progesterone receptor) ratio (eg, breast cancer)

KIT (v-kit Hardy-Zuckerman 4 feline sarcoma viral oncogene homolog) (eg, mastocytosis), common variants (eg, D816V, D816Y, D816F)

MEFV (Mediterranean fever) (eg, familial Mediterranean fever), common variants (eg, E148Q, P369S, F479L, M680I, I692del, M694V, M694I, K695R, V726A, A744S, R761H)

MPL (myeloproliferative leukemia virus oncogene, thrombopoietin receptor, TPOR) (eg, myeloproliferative disorder), common variants (eg, W515A, W515K, W515L, W515R)

TCD@ (T cell antigen receptor, delta) (eg, leukemia and lymphoma), gene rearrangement analysis, evaluation to detect abnormal clonal population

Uniparental disomy (UPD) (eg, Russell-Silver syndrome, Prader-Willi/Angelman syndrome), short tandem repeat (STR) analysis

▲ 81403   Molecular pathology procedure, Level 4 (eg, analysis of single exon by DNA sequence analysis, analysis of >10 amplicons using multiplex PCR in 2 or more independent reactions, mutation scanning or duplication/deletion variants of 2-5 exons)

ABL1 (c-abl oncogene 1, receptor tyrosine kinase) (eg, acquired imatinib tyrosine kinase inhibitor resistance), variants in the kinase domain

ANG (angiogenin, ribonuclease, RNase A family, 5) (eg, amyotrophic lateral sclerosis), full gene sequence

CEBPA (CCAAT/enhancer binding protein [C/EBP], alpha) (eg, acute myeloid leukemia), full gene sequence

CEL (carboxyl ester lipase [bile salt-stimulated lipase]) (eg, maturity-onset diabetes of the young [MODY]), targeted sequence analysis of exon 11 (eg, c.1785delC, c.1686delT)

DAZ/SRY (deleted in azoospermia and sex determining region Y) (eg, male infertility), common deletions (eg, AZFa, AZFb, AZFc, AZFd)

F8 (coagulation factor VIII) (eg, hemophilia A), inversion analysis, intron 1 and intron 22A

FGFR3 (fibroblast growth factor receptor 3) (eg, isolated craniosynostosis), targeted sequence analysis (eg, exon 7) (For targeted sequence analysis of multiple FGFR3 exons, use 81404)

GJB1 (gap junction protein, beta 1) (eg, Charcot-Marie-Tooth X-linked), full gene sequence

HBB (hemoglobin, beta, beta-globin) (eg, beta thalassemia), duplication/deletion analysis

HRAS (v-Ha-ras Harvey rat sarcoma viral oncogene homolog) (eg, Costello syndrome), exon 2 sequence

IDH1 (isocitrate dehydrogenase 1 [NADP+], soluble) (eg, glioma), common exon 4 variants (eg, R132H, R132C)

IDH2 (isocitrate dehydrogenase 2 [NADP+], mitochondrial) (eg, glioma), common exon 4 variants (eg, R140W, R172M)

JAK2 (Janus kinase 2) (eg, myeloproliferative disorder), exon 12 sequence and exon 13 sequence, if performed

Known familial variant not otherwise specified, for gene listed in Tier 1 or Tier 2, DNA sequence analysis, each variant exon (For a known familial variant that is considered a common variant, use specific common variant Tier 1 or Tier 2 code)

KRAS (v-Ki-ras2 Kirsten rat sarcoma viral oncogene) (eg, carcinoma), gene analysis, variant(s) in exon 23 (eg, codon 61)

MPL (myeloproliferative leukemia virus oncogene, thrombopoietin receptor, TPOR) (eg, myeloproliferative disorder), exon 10 sequence

MT-RNR1 (mitochondrially encoded 12S RNA) (eg, nonsyndromic hearing loss), full gene sequence

MT-TS1 (mitochondrially encoded tRNA serine 1) (eg, nonsyndromic hearing loss), full gene sequence

SMN1 (survival of motor neuron 1, telomeric) (eg, spinal muscular atrophy), known familial sequence variant(s)

VHL (von Hippel-Lindau tumor suppressor) (eg, von Hippel-Lindau familial cancer syndrome), deletion/duplication analysis

VWF (von Willebrand factor) (eg, von Willebrand disease types 2A, 2B, 2M), targeted sequence analysis (eg, exon 28)

▲ 81404   Molecular pathology procedure, Level 5 (eg, analysis of 2-5 exons by DNA sequence analysis, mutation scanning or duplication/deletion variants of 6-10 exons, or characterization of a dynamic mutation disorder/triplet repeat by Southern blot analysis)

ACADS (acyl-CoA dehydrogenase, C-2 to C-3 short chain) (eg, short chain acyl-CoA dehydrogenase deficiency), targeted sequence analysis (eg, exons 5 and 6)

AQP2 (aquaporin 2 [collecting duct]) (eg, nephrogenic diabetes insipidus), full gene sequence

ARX (aristaless related homeobox) (eg, X-linked lissencephaly with ambiguous genitalia, X-linked mental retardation), full gene sequence

BTD (biotinidase) (eg, biotinidase deficiencysequence gene full ,)

CAV3 (caveolin 3) (eg, CAV3-related distal myopathy, limb-girdle muscular dystrophy type 1C), full gene sequence

CDKN2A (cyclin-dependent kinase inhibitor 2A) (eg, CDKN2A related cutaneous malignant melanoma, familial atypical molemalignant melanoma syndrome), full gene sequence

CLRN1 (clarin 1) (eg, Usher syndrome, type 3), full gene sequence

CPT2 (carnitine palmitoyltransferase 2) (eg, carnitine palmitoyltransferase II deficiency), full gene sequence

CYP1B1 (cytochrome P450, family 1, subfamily B, polypeptide 1) (eg, primary congenital glaucoma), full gene sequence

DMPK (dystrophia myotonica-protein kinase) (eg, myotonic dystrophy type 1), characterization of abnormal (eg, expanded) alleles

EGR2 (early growth response 2) (eg, Charcot-Marie-Tooth), full gene sequence

FGFR2 (fibroblast growth factor receptor 2) (eg, craniosynostosis, Apert syndrome, Crouzon syndrome), targeted sequence analysis (eg, exons 8, 10)

FGFR3 (fibroblast growth factor receptor 3) (eg, achondroplasia, hypochondroplasia), targeted sequence analysis (eg, exons 8, 11, 12, 13)

FKRP (Fukutin related protein) (eg, congenital muscular dystrophy type 1C [MDC1C], limb-girdle muscular dystrophy [LGMD] type 2I), full gene sequence

FOXG1 (forkhead box G1) (eg, Rett syndrome), full gene sequence

FSHMD1A (facioscapulohumeral muscular dystrophy 1A) (eg, facioscapulohumeral muscular dystrophy), evaluation to detect abnormal (eg, deleted) alleles

FSHMD1A (facioscapulohumeral muscular dystrophy 1A) (eg, facioscapulohumeral muscular dystrophy), characterization of haplotype(s) (ie, chromosome 4A and 4B haplotypes)

FXN (frataxin) (eg, Friedreich ataxia), full gene sequence

HBA1/HBA2 (alpha globin 1 and alpha globin 2) (eg, alpha thalassemia), duplication/deletion analysis

(For common deletion variants of alpha globin 1 and alpha globin 2 genes, use 81257)

HBB (hemoglobin, beta, Beta-Globin) (eg, thalassemia), full gene sequence

51

HNF1B (HNF1 homeobox B) (eg, maturity-onset diabetes of the young [MODY]), duplication/deletion analysis

HRAS (v-Ha-ras Harvey rat sarcoma viral oncogene homolog) (eg, Costello syndrome), full gene sequence

KCNJ10 (potassium inwardly-rectifying channel, subfamily J, member 10) (eg, SeSAME syndrome, EAST syndrome, sensorineural hearing loss), full gene sequence

KIT (C-kit) (v-kit Hardy-Zuckerman 4 feline sarcoma viral oncogene homolog) (eg, GIST, acute myeloid leukemia, melanoma), targeted gene analysis (eg, exons 8, 11, 13, 17, 18)

LITAF (lipopolysaccharide-induced TNF factor) (eg, Charcot-Marie-Tooth), full gene sequence

MEFV (Mediterranean fever) (eg, familial Mediterranean fever), full gene sequence

MEN1 (multiple endocrine neoplasia I) (eg, multiple endocrine neoplasia type 1, Wermer syndrome), duplication/deletion analysis

NRAS (neuroblastoma RAS viral oncogene homolog) (eg, colorectal carcinoma), exon 1 and exon 2 sequences

PDGFRA (platelet-derived growth factor receptor alpha polypeptide) (eg, gastrointestinal stromal tumor), targeted sequence analysis (eg, exons 12, 18)

PDX1 (pancreatic and duodenal homeobox 1) (eg, maturity-onset diabetes of the young [MODY]), full gene sequence

PRNP (prion protein) (eg, genetic prion disease), full gene sequence

PRSS1 (protease, serine, 1 [trypsin 1]) (eg, hereditary pancreatitis), full gene sequence

RAF1 (v-raf-1 murine leukemia viral oncogene homolog 1) (eg, LEOPARD syndrome), targeted sequence analysis (eg, exons 7, 12, 14, 17)

RET (ret proto-oncogene) (eg, multiple endocrine neoplasia, type 2B and familial medullary thyroid carcinoma), common variants (eg, M918T, 2647_2648delinsTT, A883F)

SDHD (succinate dehydrogenase complex, subunit D, integral membrane protein) (eg, hereditary paraganglioma), full gene sequence

SLC25A4 (solute carrier family 25 [mitochondrial carrier; adenine nucleotide translocator], member 4) (eg, progressive external ophthalmoplegia), full gene sequence

TP53 (tumor protein 53) (eg, tumor samples), targeted sequence analysis of 2-5 exons

TTR (transthyretin) (eg, familial transthyretin amyloidosis), full gene sequence

TYR (tyrosinase [oculocutaneous albinism IA]) (eg, oculocutaneous albinism IA), full gene sequence

USH1G (Usher syndrome 1G [autosomal recessive]) (eg, Usher syndrome, type 1), full gene sequence

VHL (von Hippel-Lindau tumor suppressor) (eg, von Hippel-Lindau familial cancer syndrome), full gene sequence

VWF (von Willebrand factor) (eg, von Willebrand disease type 1C), targeted sequence analysis (eg, exons 26, 27, 37)

▲ 81405   Molecular pathology procedure, Level 6 (eg, analysis of 6-10 exons by DNA sequence analysis, mutation scanning or duplication/deletion variants of 11-25 exons)

ABCD1 (ATP-binding cassette, sub-family D [ALD], member 1) (eg, adrenoleukodystrophy), full gene sequence

ACADS (acyl-CoA dehydrogenase, C-2 to C-3 short chain) (eg, short chain acyl-CoA dehydrogenase deficiency), full gene sequence

ACTC1 (actin, alpha, cardiac muscle 1) (eg, familial hypertrophic cardiomyopathy), full gene sequence

APTX (aprataxin) (eg, ataxia with oculomotor apraxia 1), full gene sequence

AR (androgen receptor) (eg, androgen insensitivity syndrome), full gene sequence

CHRNA4 (cholinergic receptor, nicotinic, alpha 4) (eg, nocturnal frontal lobe epilepsy), full gene sequence

CHRNB2 (cholinergic receptor, nicotinic, beta 2 [neuronal]) (eg, nocturnal frontal lobe epilepsy), full gene sequence

CYP21A2 (cytochrome P450, family 21, subfamily A, polypeptide2) (eg, steroid 21-hydroxylase isoform, congenital adrenal hyperplasia), full gene sequence

DFNB59 (deafness, autosomal recessive 59) (eg, autosomal recessive nonsyndromic hearing impairment), full gene sequence

DHCR7 (7-dehydrocholesterol reductase) (eg, Smith-Lemli-Opitz syndrome), full gene sequence

EYA1 (eyes absent homolog 1 [Drosophila]) (eg, branchio-otorenal [BOR] spectrum disorders), duplication/deletion analysis

F9 (coagulation factor IX) (eg, hemophilia B), full gene sequence

FH (fumarate hydratase) (eg, fumarate hydratase deficiency, hereditary leiomyomatosis with renal cell cancer), full gene sequence

FKTN (fukutin) (eg, limb-girdle muscular dystrophy [LGMD] type 2M or 2L), full gene sequence

GFAP (glial fibrillary acidic protein) (eg, Alexander disease), full gene sequence

GLA (galactosidase, alpha) (eg, Fabry disease), full gene equence

HBA1/HBA2 (alpha globin 1 and alpha globin 2) (eg, thalassemia), full gene sequence

HNF1A (HNF1 homeobox A) (eg, maturity-onset diabetes of the young [MODY]), full gene sequence

HNF1B (HNF1 homeobox B) (eg, maturity-onset diabetes of the young [MODY]), full gene sequence

KRAS (v-Ki-ras2 Kirsten rat sarcoma viral oncogene homolog) (eg, Noonan syndrome), full gene sequence

LAMP2 (lysosomal-associated membrane protein 2) (eg, Danon disease), full gene sequence

53

MEN1 (multiple endocrine neoplasia I) (eg, multiple endocrine neoplasia type 1, Wermer syndrome), full gene sequence

MPZ (myelin protein zero) (eg, Charcot-Marie-Tooth), full gene sequence

MYL2 (myosin, light chain 2, regulatory, cardiac, slow) (eg, familial hypertrophic cardiomyopathy), full gene sequence

MYL3 (myosin, light chain 3, alkali, ventricular, skeletal, slow) (eg, familial hypertrophic cardiomyopathy), full gene sequence

MYOT (myotilin) (eg, limb-girdle muscular dystrophy), full gene sequence

NEFL (neurofilament, light polypeptide) (eg, Charcot-Marie-Tooth), full gene sequence

NF2 (neurofibromin 2 [merlin]) (eg, neurofibromatosis, type 2), duplication/deletion analysis

NSD1 (nuclear receptor binding SET domain protein 1) (eg, Sotos syndrome), duplication/deletion analysis

OTC (ornithine carbamoyltransferase) (eg, ornithine transcarbamylase deficiency), full gene sequence

PDHB (pyruvate dehydrogenase [lipoamide] beta) (eg, lactic acidosis), full gene sequence

PSEN1 (presenilin 1) (eg, Alzheimer disease), full gene sequence

RET (ret proto-oncogene) (eg, multiple endocrine neoplasia, type 2A and familial medullary thyroid carcinoma), targeted sequence analysis (eg, exons 10, 11, 13-16)

SDHB (succinate dehydrogenase complex, subunit B, iron sulfur) (eg, hereditary paraganglioma), full gene sequence

SDHC (succinate dehydrogenase complex, subunit C, integral membrane protein, 15kDa) (eg, hereditary paragangliomapheochromocytoma syndrome), full gene sequence

SGCA (sarcoglycan, alpha [50kDa dystrophin-associated glycoprotein]) (eg, limb-girdle muscular dystrophy), full gene sequence

SGCB (sarcoglycan, beta [43kDa dystrophin-associated glycoprotein]) (eg, limb-girdle muscular dystrophy), full gene sequence

SGCD (sarcoglycan, delta [35kDa dystrophin-associated glycoprotein]) (eg, limb-girdle muscular dystrophy), full gene sequence

SGCG (sarcoglycan, gamma [35kDa dystrophin-associated glycoprotein]) (eg, limb-girdle muscular dystrophy), full gene sequence

SHOC2 (soc-2 suppressor of clear homolog) (eg, Noonan-like syndrome with loose anagen hair), full gene sequence

SMN1 (survival of motor neuron 1, telomeric) (eg, spinal muscular atrophy), full gene sequence

SPRED1 (sprouty-related, EVH1 domain containing 1) (eg, Legius syndrome), full gene sequence

TGFBR1 (transforming growth factor, beta receptor 1) (eg, Marfan syndrome), full gene sequence

TGFBR2 (transforming growth factor, beta receptor 2) (eg, Marfan syndrome), full gene sequence

THRB (thyroid hormone receptor, beta) (eg, thyroid hormone resistance, thyroid hormone beta receptor deficiency), full gene sequence or targeted sequence analysis of >5 exons

TNNI3 (troponin I, type 3 [cardiac]) (eg, familial hypertrophic cardiomyopathy), full gene sequence

TP53 (tumor protein 53) (eg, Li-Fraumeni syndrome, tumor samples), full gene sequence or targeted sequence analysis of >5 exons

TPM1 (tropomyosin 1 [alpha]) (eg, familial hypertrophic cardiomyopathy), full gene sequence

TSC1 (tuberous sclerosis 1) (eg, tuberous sclerosis), duplication/ deletion analysis

VWF (von Willebrand factor) (eg, von Willebrand disease type 2N), targeted sequence analysis (eg, exons 18-20, 23-25)

▲ 81406   Molecular pathology procedure, Level 7 (eg, analysis of 11-25 exons by DNA sequence analysis, mutation scanning or duplication/deletion variants of 26-50 exons, cytogenomic array analysis for neoplasia)

ACADVL (acyl-CoA dehydrogenase, very long chain) (eg, very long chain acyl-coenzyme A dehydrogenase deficiency), full gene sequence

ACTN4 (actinin, alpha 4) (eg, focal segmental glomerulosclerosis), full gene sequence

ANO5 (anoctamin 5) (eg, limb-girdle muscular dystrophy), full gene sequence

APP (amyloid beta [A4] precursor protein) (eg, Alzheimer disease), full gene sequence

ATP7B (ATPase, Cu++ transporting, beta polypeptide) (eg, Wilson disease), full gene sequence

BRAF (v-raf murine sarcoma viral oncogene homolog B1) (eg, Noonan syndrome), full gene sequence

CAPN3 (Calpain 3) (eg, limb-girdle muscular dystrophy [LGMD] type 2A, calpainopathy), full gene sequence

CBS (cystathionine-beta-synthase) (eg, homocystinuria, cystathionine beta-synthase deficiency), full gene sequence

CDH1 (cadherin 1, type 1, E-cadherin [epithelial]) (eg, hereditary diffuse gastric cancer), full gene sequence

CDKL5 (cyclin-dependent kinase-like 5) (eg, early infantile epileptic encephalopathy), full gene sequence

Cytogenomic microarray analysis, neoplasia (eg, interrogation of copy number, and loss-of-heterozygosity via single nucleotide polymorphism [SNP]-based comparative genomic hybridization [CGH] microarray analysis)

DLAT (dihydrolipoamide S-acetyltransferase) (eg, pyruvate dehydrogenase E2 deficiency), full gene sequence

DLD (dihydrolipoamide dehydrogenase) (eg, maple syrup urine disease, type III), full gene sequence

EYA1 (eyes absent homolog 1 [Drosophila]) (eg, branchio-otorenal [BOR] spectrum disorders), full gene sequence

F8 (coagulation factor VIII) (eg, hemophilia A), duplication/ deletion analysis

GAA (glucosidase, alpha; acid) (eg, glycogen storage disease type II [Pompe disease]), full gene sequence

GALT (galactose-1-phosphate uridylyltransferase) (eg, galactosemia), full gene sequence

GCDH (glutaryl-CoA dehydrogenase) (eg, glutaricacidemia type 1), full gene sequence

GCK (glucokinase [hexokinase 4]) (eg, maturity-onset diabetes of the young [MODY]), full gene sequence

HADHA (hydroxyacyl-CoA dehydrogenase/3-ketoacyl-CoA thiolase/enoyl-CoA hydratase [trifunctional protein] alpha subunit) (eg, long chain acyl-coenzyme A dehydrogenase deficiency), full gene sequence

HEXA (hexosaminidase A, alpha polypeptide) (eg, Tay-Sachs disease), full gene sequence

HNF4A (hepatocyte nuclear factor 4, alpha) (eg, maturity-onset diabetes of the young [MODY]), full gene sequence

IVD (isovaleryl-CoA dehydrogenase) (eg, isovaleric acidemia), full gene sequence

JAG1 (jagged 1) (eg, Alagille syndrome), duplication/deletion analysis

LDB3 (LIM domain binding 3) (eg, familial dilated cardiomyopathy, myofibrillar myopathy), full gene sequence

LMNA (lamin A/C) (eg, Emery-Dreifuss muscular dystrophy [EDMD1, 2 and 3] limb-girdle muscular dystrophy [LGMD] type 1B, dilated cardiomyopathy [CMD1A], familial partial lipodystrophy [FPLD2]), full gene sequence

MAP2K1 (mitogen-activated protein kinase 1) (eg, cardiofaciocutaneous syndrome), full gene sequence

MAP2K2 (mitogen-activated protein kinase 2) (eg, cardiofaciocutaneous syndrome), full gene sequence

MCCC2 (methylcrotonoyl-CoA carboxylase 2 [beta]) (eg, 3-methylcrotonyl carboxylase deficiency), full gene sequence

MUTYH (mutY homolog [E. coli]) (eg, MYH-associated polyposis), full gene sequence

NF2 (neurofibromin 2 [merlin]) (eg, neurofibromatosis, type 2), full gene sequence

NOTCH3 (notch 3) (eg, cerebral autosomal dominant arteriopathy with subcortical infarcts and leukoencephalopathy [CADASIL]), targeted sequence analysis (eg, exons 1-23)

NSD1 (nuclear receptor binding SET domain protein 1) (eg, Sotos syndrome), full gene sequence

OPA1 (optic atrophy 1) (eg, optic atrophy), duplication/deletion analysis

PAH (phenylalanine hydroxylase) (eg, phenylketonuria), full gene sequence

PALB2 (partner and localizer of BRCA2) (eg, breast and pancreatic cancer), full gene sequence

PAX2 (paired box 2) (eg, renal coloboma syndrome), full gene sequence

PC (pyruvate carboxylase) (eg, pyruvate carboxylase deficiency), full gene sequence

PCCB (propionyl CoA carboxylase, beta polypeptide) (eg, propionic acidemia), full gene sequence

PDHA1 (pyruvate dehydrogenase [lipoamide] alpha 1) (eg, lactic acidosis), full gene sequence

PDHX (pyruvate dehydrogenase complex, component X) (eg, lactic acidosis), full gene sequence

POLG (polymerase [DNA directed], gamma) (eg, Alpers- Huttenlocher syndrome, autosomal dominant progressive external ophthalmoplegia), full gene sequence

POMGNT1 (protein O-linked mannose beta1,2-N acetylglucosaminyltransferase) (eg, muscle-eye-brain disease, Walker-Warburg syndrome), full gene sequence

POMT1 (protein-O-mannosyltransferase 1) (eg, limb-girdle muscular dystrophy [LGMD] type 2K, Walker-Warburg syndrome), full gene sequence

POMT2 (protein-O-mannosyltransferase 2) (eg, limb-girdle muscular dystrophy [LGMD] type 2N, Walker-Warburg syndromesequence gene full)

PRKAG2 (protein kinase, AMP-activated, gamma 2 non-catalytic subunit) (eg, familial hypertrophic cardiomyopathy with Wolff-Parkinson-White syndrome, lethal congenital glycogen storagedisease of heart), full gene sequence

PSEN2 (presenilin 2 [Alzheimer disease 4]) (eg, Alzheimer disease), full gene sequence

PTPN11 (protein tyrosine phosphatase, non-receptor type 11) (eg, Noonan syndrome, LEOPARD syndrome), full gene sequence

PYGM (phosphorylase, glycogen, muscle) (eg, glycogen storage disease type V, McArdle disease), full gene sequence

RAF1 (v-raf-1 murine leukemia viral oncogene homolog 1) (eg, LEOPARD syndrome), full gene sequence

RET (ret proto-oncogene) (eg, Hirschsprung disease), full gene sequence

RYR1 (ryanodine receptor 1, skeletal) (eg, malignant hyperthermia), targeted sequence analysis of exons with functionally-confirmed mutations

SLC9A6 (solute carrier family 9 [sodium/hydrogen exchanger], member 6) (eg, Christianson syndrome), full gene sequence

SLC26A4 (solute carrier family 26, member 4) (eg, Pendred syndrome), full gene sequence

SOS1 (son of sevenless homolog 1) (eg, Noonan syndrome, gingival fibromatosis), full gene sequence

TAZ (tafazzin) (eg, methylglutaconic aciduria type 2, Barth syndrome), full gene sequence

TNNT2 (troponin T, type 2 [cardiac]) (eg, familial hypertrophic cardiomyopathy), full gene sequence

TSC1 (tuberous sclerosis 1) (eg, tuberous sclerosis), full gene sequence

TSC2 (tuberous sclerosis 2) (eg, tuberous sclerosis), duplication/deletion analysis

UBE3A (ubiquitin protein ligase E3A) (eg, Angelman syndrome), full gene sequence

VWF (von Willebrand factor) (von Willebrand disease type 2A), extended targeted sequence analysis (eg, exons 11-16, 24-26, 51, 52)

▲ 81407 Molecular pathology procedure, Level 8 (eg, analysis of 26-50 exons by DNA sequence analysis, mutation scanning or duplication/deletion variants of >50 exons, sequence analysis of multiple genes on one platform)

ABCC8 (ATP-binding cassette, sub-family C [CFTR/MRP], member 8) (eg, familial hyperinsulinism), full gene sequence

CHD7 (chromodomain helicase DNA binding protein 7) (eg, CHARGE syndrome), full gene sequence

F8 (coagulation factor VIII) (eg, hemophilia A), full gene sequence

JAG1 (jagged 1) (eg, Alagille syndrome), full gene sequence

MYBPC3 (myosin binding protein C, cardiac) (eg, familial hypertrophic cardiomyopathy), full gene sequence

MYH6 (myosin, heavy chain 6, cardiac muscle, alpha) (eg, familial dilated cardiomyopathy), full gene sequence

MYH7 (myosin, heavy chain 7, cardiac muscle, beta) (eg, familial hypertrophic cardiomyopathy, Liang distal myopathy), full gene sequence

MYO7A (myosin VIIA) (eg, Usher syndrome, type 1), full gene sequence

NOTCH1 (notch 1) (eg, aortic valve disease), full gene sequence

OPA1 (optic atrophy 1) (eg, optic atrophy), full gene sequence

PCDH15 (protocadherin-related 15) (eg, Usher syndrome, type 1), full gene sequence

SCN1A (sodium channel, voltage-gated, type 1, alpha subunit) (eg, generalized epilepsy with febrile seizures), full gene sequence

SCN5A (sodium channel, voltage-gated, type V, alpha subunit) (eg, familial dilated cardiomyopathy), full gene sequence

TSC2 (tuberous sclerosis 2) (eg, tuberous sclerosis), full gene sequence

USH1C (Usher syndrome 1C [autosomal recessive, severe]) (eg, Usher syndrome, type 1), full gene sequence

▲ 81408 Molecular pathology procedure, Level 9 (eg, analysis of > 50 exons in a single gene by DNA sequence analysis)

ATM (ataxia telangiectasia mutated) (eg, ataxia telangiectasia),full gene sequence

CDH23 (cadherin-related 23) (eg, Usher syndrome, type 1), full gene sequence

COL1A1 (collagen, type I, alpha 1) (eg, osteogenesis imperfecta, type I), full gene sequence

COL1A2 (collagen, type I, alpha 2) (eg, osteogenesis imperfecta, type I), full gene sequence

DYSF (dysferlin, limb girdle muscular dystrophy 2B [autosomal recessive]) (eg, limb-girdle muscular dystrophy), full gene sequence

FBN1 (fibrillin 1) (eg, Marfan syndrome), full gene sequence

NF1 (neurofibromin 1) (eg, neurofibromatosis, type 1), full gene sequence

RYR1 (ryanodine receptor 1, skeletal) (eg, malignant hyperthermia), full gene sequence

USH2A (Usher syndrome 2A [autosomal recessive, mild]) (eg, Usher syndrome, type 2), full gene sequence

VWF (von Willebrand factor) (eg, von Willebrand disease types 1 and 3), full gene sequence;

- 81479   Code added
- 81500   Code added
- 81503   Code added
- 81506   Code added
- 81508   Code added
- 81509   Code added
- 81510   Code added
- 81511   Code added
- 81512   Code added
- 81599   Code added
▲ 82009   Ketone body(s) (eg, acetone, acetoacetic acid, serumbeta-hydroxybutyrate); qualitative
▲ 82010   quantitative
- 82777   Code added
(83890   Code deleted 2012 [2013 edition])
(83891   Code deleted 2012 [2013 edition])
(83892   Code deleted 2012 [2013 edition])
(83893   Code deleted 2012 [2013 edition])
(83894   Code deleted 2012 [2013 edition])
(83896   Code deleted 2012 [2013 edition])
(83897   Code deleted 2012 [2013 edition])
(83898   Code deleted 2012 [2013 edition])
(83900   Code deleted 2012 [2013 edition])
(83901   Code deleted 2012 [2013 edition])
(83902   Code deleted 2012 [2013 edition])
(83903   Code deleted 2012 [2013 edition])
(83904   Code deleted 2012 [2013 edition])
(83905   Code deleted 2012 [2013 edition])
(83906   Code deleted 2012 [2013 edition])

(83907	Code deleted 2012 [2013 edition])
(83908	Code deleted 2012 [2013 edition])
(83909	Code deleted 2012 [2013 edition])
(83912	Code deleted 2012 [2013 edition])
(83913	Code deleted 2012 [2013 edition])
(83914	Code deleted 2012 [2013 edition])
● 86152	Code added
● 86153	Code added
● 86711	Code added
● 86828	Code added
● 86829	Code added
● 86830	Code added
● 86831	Code added
● 86832	Code added
● 86833	Code added
● 86834	Code added
● 86835	Code added
▲ 87498	enterovirus, reverse transcription and amplified probe technique
▲ 87521	hepatitis C, reverse transcription and amplified probe technique
▲ 87522	hepatitis C, reverse transcription and quantification
▲ 87535	HIV-1, reverse transcription and amplified probe technique
▲ 87536	HIV-1, reverse transcription and quantification
▲ 87538	HIV-2, reverse transcription and amplified probe technique
▲ 87539	HIV-2, reverse transcription and quantification
● 87631	Code added
● 87632	Code added
● 87633	Code added
● 87910	Code added
▲ 87901	HIV-1, reverse transcriptase and protease regions
● 87912	Code added
● 88375	Code added
(88384	Code deleted 2012 [2013 edition])
(88385	Code deleted 2012 [2013 edition])
(88386	Code deleted 2012 [2013 edition])

Medicine

● 90653   Code added

▲ 90655   Influenza virus vaccine, trivalent, split virus, preservative free, when administered to children 6-35 months of age, for intramuscular use

▲ 90656   Influenza virus vaccine, trivalent, split virus, preservative free, when administered to individuals 3 years and older, for intramuscular use

▲ 90657   Influenza virus vaccine, trivalent, split virus, when administered to children 6-35 months of age, for intramuscular use

▲ 90658   Influenza virus vaccine, trivalent, split virus, when administered to individuals 3 years of age and older, for intramuscular use

▲ 90660   Influenza virus vaccine, trivalent, live, for intranasal use

● 90672   Code added

(90665   Code deleted 2012 [2013 edition])

(90701   Code deleted 2012 [2013 edition])

(90718   Code deleted 2012 [2013 edition])

● 90739   Code added

▲ 90746   Hepatitis B vaccine, adult dosage (3 dose schedule), for intramuscular use

● 90785   Code added

● 90791   Code added

● 90792   Code added

(90801   Code deleted 2012 [2013 edition])

(90802   Code deleted 2012 [2013 edition])

(90804   Code deleted 2012 [2013 edition])

(90805   Code deleted 2012 [2013 edition])

(90806   Code deleted 2012 [2013 edition])

(90807   Code deleted 2012 [2013 edition])

(90808   Code deleted 2012 [2013 edition])

(90809   Code deleted 2012 [2013 edition])

(90810   Code deleted 2012 [2013 edition])

(90811   Code deleted 2012 [2013 edition])

(90812   Code deleted 2012 [2013 edition])

(90813   Code deleted 2012 [2013 edition])

(90814   Code deleted 2012 [2013 edition])

(90815   Code deleted 2012 [2013 edition])

(90816   Code deleted 2012 [2013 edition])

(90817   Code deleted 2012 [2013 edition])

(90818   Code deleted 2012 [2013 edition])

(90819   Code deleted 2012 [2013 edition])

(90821	Code deleted 2012 [2013 edition])
(90822	Code deleted 2012 [2013 edition])
(90823	Code deleted 2012 [2013 edition])
(90824	Code deleted 2012 [2013 edition])
(90826	Code deleted 2012 [2013 edition])
(90827	Code deleted 2012 [2013 edition])
(90828	Code deleted 2012 [2013 edition])
(90829	Code deleted 2012 [2013 edition])
● 90832	Code added
● +90833	Code added
● 90834	Code added
● +90836	Code added
● 90837	Code added
● +90838	Code added
● 90839	Code added
● +90840	Code added
(90857	Code deleted 2012 [2013 edition])
(90862	Code deleted 2012 [2013 edition])
● +90863	Code added
▲ 90875	Individual psychophysiological therapy incorporating biofeedback training by any modality (face-to-face with the patient), with psychotherapy (eg, insight oriented, behavior modifying or supportive psychotherapy); 30 minutes
▲ 90876	45 minutes
▲ 90889	Preparation of report of patient's psychiatric status, history, treatment, or progress (other than for legal or consultative purposes) for other individuals, agencies, or insurance carriers
▲ 90935	Hemodialysis procedure with single evaluation by a physician or other qualified health care professional
▲ 90945	Dialysis procedure other than hemodialysis (eg, peritoneal dialysis, hemofiltration, or other continuous renal replacement therapies), with single evaluation by a physician or other qualified health care professional
▲ 90947	Dialysis procedure other than hemodialysis (eg, peritoneal dialysis, hemofiltration, or other continuous renal replacement therapies) requiring repeated evaluation by a physician or other qualified health care professional, with or without substantial revision of dialysis prescription
▲ 90951	End-stage renal disease (ESRD) related services monthly, for patients younger than 2 years of age to include monitoring for the adequacy of nutrition, assessment of growth and development, and counseling of parents; with 4 or more face-to-face visits by a physician or other qualified health care professional per month

▲ 90952   with 2-3 face-to-face visits by a physician or other qualified health care professional per month

▲ 90953   with 1 face-to-face visit by a physician or other qualified health care professional per month

▲ 90954   End-stage renal disease (ESRD) related services monthly, for patients 2-11 years of age to include monitoring for the adequacy of nutrition, assessment of growth and development, and counseling of parents; with 4 or more face-to-face visits by a physician or other qualified health care professional per month

▲ 90955   with 2-3 face-to-face visits by a physician or other qualified health care professional per month

▲ 90956   with 1 face-to-face visit by a physician or other qualified health care professional per month

▲ 90957   End-stage renal disease (ESRD) related services monthly, for patients 12-19 years of age to include monitoring for the adequacy of nutrition, assessment of growth and development, and counseling of parents; with 4 or more face-to-face visits by a physician or other qualified health care professional per month

▲ 90958   with 2-3 face-to-face visits by a physician or other qualified health care professional per month

▲ 90959   with 1 face-to-face visit by a physician or other qualified health care professional per month

▲ 90960   End-stage renal disease (ESRD) related services monthly, for patients 20 years of age and older; with 4 or more face-to-face visits by a physician or other qualified health care professional per month

▲ 90961   with 2-3 face-to-face visits by a physician or other qualified health care professional per month

▲ 90962   with 1 face-to-face visit by a physician or other qualified health care professional per month

▲ 91110   Gastrointestinal tract imaging, intraluminal (eg, capsule endoscopy), esophagus through ileum, with interpretation and report

▲ 91111   Gastrointestinal tract imaging, intraluminal (eg, capsule endoscopy), esophagus with interpretation and report

● 91112   Code added

▲ 92286   Anterior segment imaging with interpretation and report; with specular microscopy and endothelial cell analysis

▲ 92287   with fluorescein angiography

▲ 92613   interpretation and report only

▲ 92615   interpretation and report only

▲ 92617   interpretation and report only

(92980   Code deleted 2012 [2013 edition])

(92981   Code deleted 2012 [2013 edition])

(92982   Code deleted 2012 [2013 edition])

(92984	Code deleted 2012 [2013 edition])
(92995	Code deleted 2012 [2013 edition])
(92996	Code deleted 2012 [2013 edition])

- ⊙ 92920 Code added
- ⊙+92921 Code added
- ⊙ 92924 Code added
- ⊙+92925 Code added
- ⊙ 92928 Code added
- ⊙+92929 Code added
- ⊙ 92933 Code added
- ⊙+92934 Code added
- ⊙ 92937 Code added
- ⊙+92938 Code added
- ⊙ 92941 Code added
- ⊙ 92943 Code added
- ⊙+92944 Code added

▲ ⊙+92973 Percutaneous transluminal coronary thrombectomy mechanical (List separately in addition to code for primary procedure)

▲ 93015 Cardiovascular stress test using maximal or submaximal treadmill or bicycle exercise, continuous electrocardiographic monitoring, and/or pharmacological stress; with supervision, with interpretation and report

▲ 93016 supervision only, without interpretation and report

▲ 93224 External electrocardiographic recording up to 48 hours by continuous rhythm recording and storage; includes recording, scanning analysis with report, review and interpretation by a physician or other qualified health care professional

▲ 93227 review and interpretation by a physician or other qualified health care professional

▲ 93228 External mobile cardiovascular telemetry with electrocardiographic recording, concurrent computerized real time data analysis and greater than 24 hours of accessible ECG data storage (retrievable with query) with ECG triggered and patient selected events transmitted to a remote attended surveillance center for up to 30 days; review and interpretation with report by a physician or other qualified health care professional

▲ 93229 technical support for connection and patient instructions for use, attended surveillance, analysis and transmission of daily and emergent data reports as prescribed by a physician or other qualified health care professional

▲ 93268 External patient and, when performed, auto activated electrocardiographic rhythm derived event recording with symptom-related memory loop with remote download capability up to 30 days, 24-hour attended monitoring; includes transmission, review and interpretation by a physician or other qualified health care professional

▲ 93272   review and interpretation by a physician or other qualified health care professional

▲ 93279   Programming device evaluation (in person) with iterative adjustment of the implantable device to test the function of the device and select optimal permanent programmed values with analysis, review and report by a physician or other qualified health care professional; single lead pacemaker system

▲ 93280   dual lead pacemaker system

▲ 93281   multiple lead pacemaker system

▲ 93282   single lead implantable cardioverter-defibrillator system

▲ 93283   dual lead implantable cardioverter-defibrillator system

▲ 93284   multiple lead implantable cardioverter-defibrillator system

▲ 93285   implantable loop recorder system

▲ 93286   Peri-procedural device evaluation (in person) and programming of device system parameters before or after a surgery, procedure, or test with analysis, review and report by a physician or other qualified health care professional; single, dual, or multiple lead pacemaker system

▲ 93287   single, dual, or multiple lead implantable cardioverterdefibrillator system

▲ 93288   Interrogation device evaluation (in person) with analysis, review and report by a physician or other qualified health care professional, includes connection, recording and disconnection per patient encounter; single, dual, or multiple lead pacemaker system

▲ 93289   single, dual, or multiple lead implantable cardioverterdefibrillator system, including analysis of heart rhythm derived data elements

▲ 93290   implantable cardiovascular monitor system, including analysis of 1 or more recorded physiologic cardiovascular data elements from all internal and external sensors

▲ 93291   implantable loop recorder system, including heart rhythm derived data analysis

▲ 93292   wearable defibrillator system

▲ 93293   Transtelephonic rhythm strip pacemaker evaluation(s) single, dual, or multiple lead pacemaker system, includes recording with and without magnet application with analysis, review and report(s) by a physician or other qualified health care professional, up to 90 days

▲ 93294   Interrogation device evaluation(s) (remote), up to 90 days; single, dual, or multiple lead pacemaker system with interim analysis, review(s) and report(s) by a physician or other qualified health care professional

▲ 93295   single, dual, or multiple lead implantable cardioverterdefibrillator system with interim analysis, review(s) and report(s) by a physician or other qualified health care professional

▲ 93297   Interrogation device evaluation(s), (remote) up to 30 days; implantable cardiovascular monitor system, including analysis of 1 or more recorded physiologic cardiovascular data elements from all internal and external sensors, analysis, review(s) and report(s) by a physician or other qualified health care professional

▲ 93298   implantable loop recorder system, including analysis of recorded heart rhythm data, analysis, review(s) and report(s) by a physician or other qualified health care professional

▲ 93351   including performance of continuous electrocardiographic monitoring, with supervision by a physician or other qualified health care professional

(93651   Code deleted 2012 [2013 edition])

(93652   Code deleted 2012 [2013 edition])

● ⊙ 93653   Code added

● ⊙ 93654   Code added

● ⊙+93655   Code added

● ⊙ 93656   Code added

● ⊙+93657   Code added

▲ 93745   Initial set-up and programming by a physician or other qualified health care professional of wearable cardioverter-defibrillator includes initial programming of system, establishing baseline electronic ECG, transmission of data to data repository, patient instruction in wearing system and patient reporting of problems or events

▲ 93750   Interrogation of ventricular assist device (VAD), in person, with physician or other qualified health care professional analysis of device parameters (eg, drivelines, alarms, power surges), review of device function (eg, flow and volume status, septum status, recovery), with programming, if performed, and report

▲ 93790   review with interpretation and report

▲ 93797   Physician or other qualified health care professional services for outpatient cardiac rehabilitation; without continuous ECG monitoring (per session)

▲ 93798   with continuous ECG monitoring (per session)

▲ 94014   Patient-initiated spirometric recording per 30-day period of time; includes reinforced education, transmission of spirometric tracing, data capture, analysis of transmitted data, periodic recalibration and review and interpretation by a physician or other qualified health care professional

▲ 94016   review and interpretation only by a physician or other qualified health care professional

▲ 94452   High altitude simulation test (HAST), with interpretation and report by a physician or other qualified health care professional

▲ 94453   with supplemental oxygen titration

▲ ⊙ 94610   Intrapulmonary surfactant administration by a physician or other qualified health care professional through endotracheal tube

▲ 94774   Pediatric home apnea monitoring event recording including respiratory rate, pattern and heart rate per 30-day period of time; includes monitor attachment, download of data, review, interpretation, and preparation of a report by a physician or other qualified health care professional

▲ 94777   review, interpretation and preparation of report only by a physician or other qualified health care professional

▲ 95004	Percutaneous tests (scratch, puncture, prick) with allergenic extracts, immediate type reaction, including test interpretation and report, specify number of tests
(95010	Code deleted 2012 [2013 edition])
(95015	Code deleted 2012 [2013 edition])
• 95017	Code added
• 95018	Code added
▲ 95024	Intracutaneous (intradermal) tests with allergenic extracts, immediate type reaction, including test interpretation and report , specify number of tests
▲ 95027	Intracutaneous (intradermal) tests, sequential and incremental, with allergenic extracts for airborne allergens, immediate type reaction, including test interpretation and report, specify number of tests
(95075	Code deleted 2012 [2013 edition])
• 95076	Code added
• +95079	Code added
▲ 95120	Professional services for allergen immunotherapy in the office or institution of the prescribing physician or other qualified health care professional, including provision of allergenic extract; single injection
▲ 95125	2 or more injections
▲ 95130	single stinging insect venom
▲ 95131	2 stinging insect venoms
▲ 95132	3 stinging insect venoms
▲ 95133	4 stinging insect venoms
▲ 95134	5 stinging insect venoms
▲ 95808	Polysomnography; any age, sleep staging with 1-3 additional parameters of sleep, attended by a technologist
▲ 95810	age 6 years or older, sleep staging with 4 or more additional parameters of sleep, attended by a technologist
▲ 95811	age 6 years or older, sleep staging with 4 or more additional parameters of sleep, with initiation of continuous positive airway pressure therapy or bilevel ventilation, attended by a technologist
• 95782	Code added
• 95783	Code added
▲ 95830	Insertion by physician or other qualified health care professional of sphenoidal electrodes for electroencephalographic (EEG) recording;
(95900	Code deleted 2012 [2013 edition])
(95903	Code deleted 2012 [2013 edition])
(95904	Code deleted 2012 [2013 edition])
• 95907	Code added
• 95908	Code added

CPT PLUS! 2013

- 95909 Code added
- 95910 Code added
- 95911 Code added
- 95912 Code added
- 95913 Code added
(95920 Code deleted 2012 [2013 edition])
- +95940 Code added
- +95941 Code added
- 95924 Code added
- 95943 Code added
(95934 Code deleted 2012 [2013 edition])
(95936 Code deleted 2012 [2013 edition])
▲ 95954 Pharmacological or physical activation requiring physician or other qualified health care professional attendance during EEG recording of activation phase (eg, thiopental activation test)
▲ 95961 Functional cortical and subcortical mapping by stimulation and/or recording of electrodes on brain surface, or of depth electrodes, to provoke seizures or identify vital brain structures; initial hour of attendance by a physician or other qualified health care professional
▲ +95962 each additional hour of attendance by a physician or other qualified health care professional (List separately in addition to code for primary procedure)
▲ 95991 requiring skill of a physician or other qualified health care professional
▲ 96004 Review and interpretation by physician or other qualified health care professional of comprehensive computerbased motion analysis, dynamic plantar pressure measurements, dynamic surface electromyography during walking or other functional activities, and dynamic fine wire electromyography, with written report
▲ 96020 Neurofunctional testing selection and administration during noninvasive imaging functional brain mapping, with test administered entirely by a physician or other qualified health care professional (ie, psychologist), with review of test results and report
▲ 97530 Therapeutic activities, direct (one-on-one) patient contact (use of dynamic activities to improve functional performance), each 15 minutes
▲ 97532 Development of cognitive skills to improve attention, memory, problem solving (includes compensatory training), direct (one-onone) patient contact, each 15 minutes
▲ 97533 Sensory integrative techniques to enhance sensory processing and promote adaptive responses to environmental demands, direct (one-on-one) patient contact, each 15 minutes
▲ 97535 Self-care/home management training (eg, activities of daily living (ADL) and compensatory training, meal preparation, safety procedures, and instructions in use of assistive technology devices/adaptive equipment) direct one-on-one contact, each 15 minutes

68

▲ 97537   Community/work reintegration training (eg, shopping, transportation, money management, avocational activities and/or work environment/modification analysis, work task analysis, use of assistive technology device/adaptive equipment), direct one-on-one contact, each 15 minutes

▲ 97755   Assistive technology assessment (eg, to restore, augment or compensate for existing function, optimize functional tasks and/or maximize environmental accessibility), direct one-on-one contact, with written report, each 15 minutes

▲ 98969   Online assessment and management service provided by a qualified nonphysician health care professional to an established patient, or guardian, not originating from a related assessment and management service provided within the previous 7 days, using the Internet or similar electronic communications network

▲ 99000   Handling and/or conveyance of specimen for transfer from the office to a laboratory

▲ 99001   Handling and/or conveyance of specimen for transfer from the patient in other than a an office to a laboratory (distance may be indicated)

▲ 99002   Handling, conveyance, and/or any other service in connection with the implementation of an order involving devices (eg, designing, fitting, packaging, handling, delivery or mailing) when devices such as orthotics, protectives, prosthetics are fabricated by an outside laboratory or shop but which items have been designed, and are to be fitted and adjusted by the attending physician or other qualified health care professional

▲ 99070   Supplies and materials (except spectacles), provided by the physician or other qualified health care professional over and above those usually included with the office visit or other services rendered (list drugs, trays, supplies, or materials provided)

▲ 99071   Educational supplies, such as books, tapes, and pamphlets, for the patient's education at cost to physician or other qualified health care professional

▲ 99078   Physician or other qualified health care professional qualified by education, training, licensure/regulation (when applicable) educational services rendered to patients in a group setting (eg, prenatal, obesity, or diabetic instructions)

▲ 99091   Collection and interpretation of physiologic data (eg, ECG, blood pressure, glucose monitoring) digitally stored and/or transmitted by the patient and/or caregiver to the physician or other qualified health care professional, qualified by education, training, licensure/regulation (when applicable) requiring a minimum of 30 minutes of time

▲ 99143   Moderate sedation services (other than those services described by codes 00100-01999) provided by the same physician or other qualified health care professional performing the diagnostic or therapeutic service that the sedation supports, requiring the presence of an independent trained observer to assist in the onitoring of the patient's level of consciousness and physiological status; younger than 5 years of age, first 30 minutes intra-service time

▲ 99144   age 5 years or older, first 30 minutes intra-service time

▲ +99145   each additional 15 minutes intra-service time (List separately in addition to code for primary service)

69

▲ 99148   Moderate sedation services (other than those services described by codes 00100-01999), provided by a physician or other qualified health care professional other than the health care professional performing the diagnostic or therapeutic service that the sedation supports; younger than 5 years of age, first 30 minutes intraservice time

▲ 99149   age 5 years or older, first 30 minutes intra-service time

▲ 99150   each additional 15 minutes intra-service time (List separately in addition to code for primary service)

▲ 99174   Instrumentbased ocular screening (eg, photoscreening, automatedrefraction), bilateral

▲ 99183   Physician or other qualified health care professional attendance and supervision of hyperbaric oxygen therapy, per session

Category II Codes

▲ 1005F   Asthma symptoms evaluated (includes documentation of numeric frequency of symptoms or patient completion of an asthma assessment tool/survey/questionnaire) (NMA –No Measure Associated)

● 1052F   Code added

▲ 2060F   Patient interviewed directly on or before date of diagnosis of major depressive disorder (MDD ADOL)1;

● 3517F   Code added

● 3520F   Code added

● 3750F   Code added

(4009F   Code deleted 2012 [2013 edition])

● 4069F   Code added

● 4142F   Code added

▲ 4240F   Instruction in therapeutic exercise with follow-up provided to patients during episode of back pain lasting longer than 12 weeks (BkP)2;

▲ 5010F   Findings of dilated macular or fundus exam communicated to the physician or other qualified health care professional managing the diabetes care (EC)5;

▲ 5020F   Treatment summary report communicated to physician(s) or other qualified health care professional(s) managing continuing care and to the patient within 1 month of completing treatment (ONC)1;

▲ 5100F   Potential risk for fracture communicated to the referring physician or other qualified health care professional within 24 hours of completion of the imaging study (NUC_MED)1;

● 6150F   Code added

Category III Codes

(0030T   Code deleted 2012 [2013 edition])

(0048T   Code deleted 2012 [2013 edition])

(0050T   Code deleted 2012 [2013 edition])

(0173T	Code deleted 2012 [2013 edition])
▲ 0195T	Arthrodesis, pre-sacral interbody technique, disc space preparation, discectomy, without instrumentation, with image guidance, includes bone graft when performed; L5-S1 interspace
▲ +0196T	L4-L5 interspace (List separately in addition to code for primary procedure)
▲ 0206T	Computerized database analysis of multiple cycles of digitized cardiac electrical data from two or more ECG leads, including transmission to a remote center, application of multiple nonlinear mathematical transformations, with coronary artery obstruction severity assessment
(0242T	Code deleted 2012 [2013 edition])
(0250T	Code deleted 2012 [2013 edition])
(0251T	Code deleted 2012 [2013 edition])
(0252T	Code deleted 2012 [2013 edition])
(0256T	Code deleted 2012 [2013 edition])
(0257T	Code deleted 2012 [2013 edition])
(0258T	Code deleted 2012 [2013 edition])
(0259T	Code deleted 2012 [2013 edition])
(0276T	Code deleted 2012 [2013 edition])
(0277T	Code deleted 2012 [2013 edition])
(0279T	Code deleted 2012 [2013 edition])
(0280T	Code deleted 2012 [2013 edition])
● 0291T	Code added
● 0292T	Code added
● 0293T	Code added
● 0294T	Code added
● 0295T	Code added
● 0296T	Code added
● 0297T	Code added
● 0298T	Code added
● 0299T	Code added
● 0300T	Code added
● 0301T	Code added
● 0302T	Code added
● 0303T	Code added
● 0304T	Code added
● 0305T	Code added
● 0306T	Code added
● 0307T	Code added

- 0308T   Code added
- 0309T   Code added
- 0310T   Code added
- 0311T   Code added
- 0312T   Code added
- 0313T   Code added
- 0314T   Code added
- 0315T   Code added
- 0316T   Code added
- 0317T   Code added
- 0318T   Code added

CPT MODIFIERS

The CPT® coding system includes two-digit modifier codes which are used to report that a service or procedure has been "altered or modified by some specific circumstance" without altering or modifying the basic definition or CPT code.

The proper use of CPT modifiers can speed up claim processing and increase reimbursement, while the improper use of CPT modifiers may result in claim delays or claim denials. In addition, using certain CPT modifiers, for example -22, too frequently may trigger a claims audit.

CPT MODIFIERS

-22 Increased procedural services

When the work required to provide a service is substantially greater than typically required, it may be identified by adding modifier -22 to the usual procedure code. Documentation must support the substantial additional work and the reason for the additional work (ie, increased intensity, time, technical difficulty of procedure, severity of patient's condition, physical and mental effort required). **Note**: This modifier should not be appended to an E/M service.

-23 Unusual anesthesia

Occasionally, a procedure, which usually requires either no anesthesia or local anesthesia, because of unusual circumstances must be done under general anesthesia. This circumstance may be reported by adding the modifier -23 to the procedure code of the basic service.

▲ -24 Unrelated evaluation and management service by the same physician or other qualified health care professional during a postoperative period

The physician or other qualified health care professional may need to indicate that an evaluation and management service was performed during a postoperative period for a reason(s) unrelated to the original procedure. This circumstance may be reported by adding the modifier -24 to the appropriate level of E/M service.

▲ -25 Significant, separately identifiable evaluation and management service by the same physician or other qualified health care professional on the same day of the procedure or other service

---

73

It may be necessary to indicate that on the day a procedure or service identified by a CPT code was performed, the patient's condition required a significant, separately identified E/M service above and beyond the other service provided or beyond the usual preoperative and postoperative care associated with the procedure that was performed. A significant, separately identifiable E/M service is defined or substantiated by documentation that satisfies the relevant criteria for the respective E/M service to be reported (see Evaluation and Management Services Guidelines for instructions on determining level of E/M service). The E/M service may be prompted by the symptom or condition for which the procedure and/or service was provided. As such, different diagnoses are not required for reporting of the E/M service on the same date. This circumstance may be reported by adding modifier -25 to the approprite level of E/M service. **Note**: This modifier is not used to report an E/M service that resulted in a decision to perform surgery. See modifier -57. For significant, separately identifiable non-E/M services, see modifier -59.

▲ -26   Professional component

Certain procedures are a combination of a physician or other qualified health care professional component and a technical component. When the physician or other qualified health care professional component is reported separately, the service may be identified by adding the modifier -26 to the usual procedure number.

-27   Multiple outpatient hospital evaluation and management encounters on the same date

For hospital outpatient reporting purposes, utilization of hospital resources related to separate and distinct E/M encounters performed in multiple outpatient hospital settings on the same date may be reported by adding modifier -27 to each appropriate level outpatient and/or emergency department E/M code(s). This modifier provides a means of reporting circumstances involving evaluation and management services provided by physician(s) in more than one (multiple) outpatient hospital setting(s) (eg, hospital emergency department, clinic). **Note**: This modifier is not to be used for physician reporting of multiple E/M services performed by the same physician on the same date. For physician reporting of all outpatient evaluation and management services provided by the same physician on the same date and performed in multiple outpatient setting(s) (eg, hospital emergency department, clinic), see Evaluation and Management, Emergency Department, or Preventive Medicine Services codes.

-32   Mandated services

Services related to *mandated* consultation and/or related services (eg, third party payer, governmental, legislative or regulatory requirement) may be identified by adding the modifier -32 to the basic procedure.

-33 **Preventive service**

When the primary purpose of the service is the delivery of an evidence based service in accordance with a US Preventive Services Task Force A or B rating in effect and other preventive services identified in preventive services mandates (legislative or regulatory), the service may be identified by adding -33 to the procedure. For separately reported services specifically identified as preventive, the modifier should not be used.

-47 **Anesthesia by surgeon**

Regional or general anesthesia provided by the surgeon may be reported by adding the modifier -47 to the basic service. (This does not include local anesthesia.) **Note**: Modifier -47 would not be used as a modifier for the Anesthesia procedures.

-50 **Bilateral procedure**

Unless otherwise identified in the listings, bilateral procedures that are performed at the same session, should be identified by adding modifier -50 to the appropriate 5 digit code.

This modifier is reported when bilateral procedures requiring a separate incision are performed during the SAME operative session. Proper reporting of this modifier on the CMS1500 health insurance claim form requires the CPT procedure code to be listed two times: first with no modifier, and the second time with modifier -50.

This modifier may not be used if the definition of the basic procedure code includes the term "bilateral."

▲ -51 **Multiple procedures**

When multiple procedures, other than E/M services, Physical Medicine and Rehabilitation services, or provision of supplies (eg, vaccines), are performed at the same session by the same individual, the primary procedure or service may be reported as listed. The additional procedure(s) or service(s) may be identified by appending modifier -51 to the additional procedure or service code(s). **Note**: This modifier should not be appended to designated "add-on" codes.

▲ -52 **Reduced services**

Under certain circumstances a service or procedure is partially reduced or eliminated at the discretion of the physician or other qualified health care professional. Under these circumstances the service provided can be identified by its usual procedure number and the addition of the modifier -52, signifying that the service is reduced. This provides a means of

75

reporting reduced services without disturbing the identification of the basic service. **Note**: For hospital outpatient reporting of a previously scheduled procedure/service that is partially reduced or cancelled as a result of extenuating circumstances or those that threaten the well-being of the patient prior to or after administration of anesthesia, see modifiers -73 and -74 (see modifiers approved for ASC hospital outpatient use).

The intended use of this modifier is to report the reduction of a service without affecting provider profiles maintained by health insurance companies.

Modifier -52 is another frequently misused modifier. Some medical practices mistakenly use modifier -52 to mean "reduced fee" and use it as a discounting method. Not only is this incorrect, the provider may seriously damage their provider profile with health insurance companies. The proper use for modifier -52 is to report that a service was not completed, or some part of a multiple-part service was not performed. A fee reduction may be in order as well; however that is not the primary purpose of the modifier.

▲ -53 Discontinued procedure

Under certain circumstances, the physician or other qualified health care professional may elect to terminate a surgical or diagnostic procedure. Due to extenuating circumstances or those that threaten the well-being of the patient, it may be necessary to indicate that a surgical or diagnostic procedure was started but discontinued. This circumstance may be reported by adding modifier -53 to the code reported by the individual for the discontinued procedure. **Note**: This modifier is not used to report the elective cancellation of a procedure prior to the patient's anesthesia induction and/or surgical preparation in the operating suite. For outpatient hospital/ambulatory surgery center (ASC) reporting of a previously scheduled procedure/service that is partially reduced or cancelled as a result of extenuating circumstances or those that threaten the well-being of the patient prior to or after administration of anesthesia, see modifiers -73 and -74 (see modifiers approved for ASC hospital outpatient use).

▲ -54 Surgical care only

When 1 physician or other qualified health care professional performs a surgical procedure and another provides preoperative and/or postoperative management, surgical services may be identified by adding modifier -54 to the usual procedure number.

▲ -55 Postoperative management only

When 1 physician or other qualified health care professional performed the postoperative management and another performed the surgical procedure, the postoperative component may be identified by adding modifier -55 to the usual procedure number.

▲ -56   **Preoperative management only**

When 1 physician or other qualified health care professional performed the preoperative care and evaluation and another performed the surgical procedure, the preoperative component may be identified by adding modifier -56 to the usual procedure number.

-57   **Decision for surgery**

An evaluation and management service that resulted in the initial decision to perform the surgery may be identified by adding the modifier -57 to the appropriate level of E/M service.

▲ -58   **Staged or related procedure or service by the same physician or other qualified health care professional during the postoperative period**

It may be necessary to indicate that the performance of a procedure or service during the postoperative period was: (a) planned or anticipated (staged); (b) more extensive than the original procedure; or (c) for therapy following a surgical procedure. This circumstance may be reported by adding modifier -58 to the staged or related procedure. **Note**: For treatment of a problem that requires a return to the operating/procedure room (eg, unanticipated clinical condition), see modifier -78.

-59   **Distinct Procedural Service**

Under certain circumstances it may be necessary to indicate that a procedure or service was distinct or independent from other non-E/M services performed on the same day. Modifier -59 is used to identify procedures or services, other than E/M services, that are not normally reported together but are appropriate under the circumstances. Documentation must support a different session, different procedure or surgery, different site or organ system, separate incision or excision, separate lesion, or separate injury (or area of injury in extensive injuries) not ordinarily encountered or performed on the same day by the same individual. However, when another already established modifier is appropriate it should be used rather than modifier -59. Only if no more descriptive modifier is available and the use of modifier -59 bet explains the circumstances should modifier -59 be used. **Note**: Modifier -59 should not be appended to an E/M service. To report a separate and distinct E/M service with a non-E/M service performed on the same date, see modifier -25.

▲ -62   **Two surgeons**

When 2 surgeons work together as primary surgeons performing distinct part(s) of a procedure, each surgeon should report his/her distinct operative work by adding modifier -62 to the procedure code and any associated add-on code(s) for that procedure as long as both surgeons continue to work together as primary surgeons. Each surgeon should report the co-surgery once using the same procedure code. If additional procedure(s) (including add-on procedure(s) are performed during the same surgical session, separate code(s) may also be reported with modifier -62 added. **Note**: If a co-surgeon acts as an assistant in the performance of additional procedure(s), other than those reported with the modifier -62, during the same surgical session, those services may be reported using separate procedure code(s) with modifier -80 or modifier -82 added, as appropriate.

▲ -63   **Procedure performed on infants less than 4 kg**

Procedures performed on neonates and infants up to a present body weight of 4 kg may involve significantly increased complexity and physician or other qualified health care professional work commonly associated with these patients. This circumstance may be reported by adding modifier -63 to the procedure number. **Note**: Unless otherwise designated, this modifier may only be appended to procedures/services listed in the 20005-69990 code series. Modifier -63 should not be appended to any CPT codes listed in the Evaluation and Management Services, Anesthesia, Radiology, Pathology/Laboratory, or Medicine sections.

▲ -66   **Surgical team**

Under some circumstances, highly complex procedures (requiring the concomitant services of several physicians or other qualified health care professionals, often of different specialties, plus other highly skilled specially trained personnel, various types of complex equipment) are carried out under the "surgical team" concept. Such circumstances may be identified by each participating individual with the addition of modifier -66 to the basic procedure number used for reporting services.

-73   **Discontinued out-patient hospital/ambulatory surgery center (ASC) procedure prior to the administration of anesthesia**

Due to extenuating circumstances or those that threaten the well being of the patient, the physician may cancel a surgical or diagnostic procedure subsequent to the patient's surgical preparation (including sedation when provided, and being taken to the room where the procedure is to be performed), but prior to the administration of anesthesia (local, regional block(s) or general). Under these circumstances, the intended service that is prepared for but cancelled can be reported by its usual procedure number and the addition of the modifier -73.

Note: The elective cancellation of a service prior to the administration of anesthesia and/or surgical preparation of the patient should not be reported. For physician reporting of a discontinued procedure, see modifier -53.

-74 **Discontinued out-patient hospital/ambulatory surgery center (ASC) procedure after administration of anesthesia**

Due to extenuating circumstances or those that threaten the well being of the patient, the physician may terminate a surgical or diagnostic procedure after the administration of anesthesia (local, regional block(s), general) or after the procedure was started (incision made, intubation started, scope inserted, etc.). Under these circumstances, the procedure started but terminated can be reported by its usual procedure number and the addition of the modifier -74. **Note**: The elective cancellation of a service prior to the administration of anesthesia and/or surgical preparation of the patient should not be reported. For physician reporting of a discontinued procedure, see modifier -53.

▲ -76 **Repeat procedure or service by same physician or other qualified health care professional**

It may be necessary to indicate that a procedure or service was repeated by the same physician or other qualified health care professional subsequent to the original procedure or service. This circumstance may be reported by adding modifier -76 to the repeated procedure or service. **Note**: This modifier should not be appended to an E/M service.

▲ -77 **Repeat procedure or service by another physician or other qualified health care professional**

It may be necessary to indicate that a basic procedure or service was repeated by another physician or other qualified health care professional subsequent to the original procedure or service. This circumstance may be reported by adding modifier -77 to the repeated procedure or service. **Note**: This modifier should not be appended to an E/M service.

▲ -78 **Unplanned return to the operating/procedure room by the same physician or other qualified health care professional following initial procedure for a related procedure during the postoperative period**

It may be necessary to indicate that another procedure was performed during the postoperative period of the initial procedure (unplanned procedure following initial procedure). When this procedure is related to the first and requires the use of an operating/procedure room, it may be reported by adding modifier -78 to the related procedure. (For repeat procedures, see modifier -76.)

▲ **-79**   **Unrelated procedure or service by the same physician or other qualified health care professional during the postoperative period**

The individual may need to indicate that the performance of a procedure or service during the postoperative period was unrelated to the original procedure. This circumstance may be reported by using modifier -79. (For repeat procedures on the same day, see '-76.')

-80   **Assistant surgeon**

Surgical assistant services may be identified by adding the modifier -80 to the usual procedure number(s).

-81   **Minimum assistant surgeon**

Minimum surgical assistant services are identified by adding the modifier -81 to the usual procedure number.

-82   **Assistant surgeon (when qualified resident surgeon not available)**

The unavailability of a qualified resident surgeon is a prerequisite for use of modifier -82 appended to the usual procedure code number(s).

▲ **-90**   **Reference (outside) laboratory**

When laboratory procedures are performed by a party other than the treating or reporting physician or other qualified health care professional, the procedure may be identified by adding modifier -90 to the usual procedure number.

-91   **Repeat clinical diagnostic laboratory test**

In the course of treatment of the patient, it may be necessary to repeat the same laboratory test on the same day to obtain subsequent (multiple) test results. Under these circumstances, the laboratory test performed can be identified by its usual procedure number and the addition of modifier -91. **Note**: This modifier may not be used when tests are rerun to confirm initial results; due to testing problems with specimens or equipment; or for any other reason when a normal, one-time, reportable result is all that is required. This modifier may not be used when other code(s) describe a series of tests results (eg, glucose tolerance tests, evocative/suppression testing). This modifier may only be used for laboratory test(s) performed more than once on the same day on the same patient.

-92   **Alternative Laboratory Platform Testing**

When laboratory testing is being performed using a kit or transportable instrument that wholly or in part consists of a single use, disposable analytical chamber, the service may be identified by adding modifier 92 to the usual laboratory procedure code (HIV testing 86701-86703, and 87389). The test does not require permanent dedicated space, hence by its design may be hand carried or transported to the vicinity of the patient for immediate testing at that site, although location of the testing is not in itself determinative of the use of this modifier.

-99 **Multiple modifiers**

Under certain circumstances two or more modifiers may be necessary to completely delineate a service. In such situations modifier -99 should be added to the basic procedure, and other applicable modifiers may be listed as part of the description of the service.

ANESTHESIA PHYSICAL STATUS MODIFIERS

The Physical Status modifiers are consistent with the American Society of Anesthesiologists ranking of patient physical status, and distinguishing various levels of complexity of the anesthesia provided. All anesthesia services are reported by use of the anesthesia five-digit procedure code (00100-01999) with the appropriate physical status modifier appended. For example, 00100-P1

Under certain circumstances, when another established modifier(s) is appropriate, it should be used in addition to the physical status modifier. i.e., 00100-P4-53

P1 A normal healthy patient

P2 A patient with mild systemic disease

P3 A patient with severe systemic disease

P4 A patient with severe systemic disaease that is a constant threat to life

P5 A moribund patient who is not expected to survive without the operation

P6 A declared brain-dead patient whose organs are being removed for donor purposes

GENETIC TESTING CODE MODIFIERS

The following modifiers are used with molecular laboratory procedures related to genetic testing. These modifiers should be used with CPT and HCPCS codes to provide diagnostic granularity of service. This allows providers to submit complete and precise genetic testing information without altering test descriptors.

The genetic testing code modifiers are categorized by mutation. The first digit identifies the disease category and the second digit identifies gene type.

Neoplasia (Solid Tumor Excluding Sarcoma and Lymphoma)

0A   BRCA1 (hereditary breast/ovarian cancer)

0B   BRCA2 (hereditary breast cancer)

0C   Neurofibromin (neurofibromatosis, type 1)

0D   Merlin (neurofibromatosis, type 2)

0E   c-RET (multiple endocrine neoplasia, types 2A/B, familial medullary thyroid carcinoma)

0F   VHL (Von Hippel Lindau disease, renal carcinoma)

0G   SDHD (hereditary paraganglioma)

0H   SDHB (hereditary paraganglioma)

0I   ERRB2 - also called Her-2/neu

0J   MLH1 (HNPCC, mismatch repair genes)

0K   MSH2, MSH6, or PMS2 (HNPCC, mismatch repair genes)

0L   APC (hereditary polyposis coli)

0M   Rb (retinoblastoma)

0N   TP53 - also called p53

0O   PTEN (Cowden's syndrome)

0P   KIT, also called CD117 (gastrointestinal stromal tumor)

0Z   Solid tumor gene, not otherwise specified

Neoplasia (Sarcoma)

1A   WT1 or WT2 (Wilm's tumor)

1B   PAX3, PAX7, or FOXO1A (alveolar rhabdomyosarcoma)

1C   FLI1, ERG, ETV1, or EWSR1 (Ewing's sarcoma, desmoplastic round cell)

1D   DDIT3 or FUS (myxoid liposarcoma)

1E   NR4A3, RBF56, or TCF12 (myxoid chondrosarcoma)

1F SSX1, SSX2, or SYT (synovial sarcoma)

1G MYCN (neuroblastoma)

1H COL1A1 or PDGFB (dermatofibrosarcoma protruberans)

1I TFE3 or ASPSCR1 (alveolar soft parts sarcoma)

1J JAZF1 or JJAZ1 (endometrial stromal sarcoma)

1Z Sarcoma gene, not otherwise specified

Neoplasia (Lymphoid/Hemotopoetic)

2A RUNX1 or CBFA2T1 — also called AML1 or ETO, genes associated with t(8;21) AML1 — also ETO (acute myelogenous leukemia)

2B BCR or ABL1, genes associated with t(9;22) (chronic myelogenous or acute leukemia) BCR — also ABL (chronic myeloid, acute lymphoid leukemia)

2C PBX1 or TCF3, genes associated with t(1;19) (acute lymphoblastic leukemia) CGF1

2D CBFB or MYH11, genes associated with inv 16 (acute myelogenous leukemia) CBF beta (leukemia)

2E MLL (acute leukemia)

2F PML or RARA, genes associated with t(15;17) (acute promyelocytic leukemia) PML/RAR alpha (promyelocytic leukemia)

2G ETV6, also called TEL, gene associated with t(12;21) (acute leukemia) TEL (leukemia)

2H BCL2 (B cell lymphoma, follicle center cell origin) bcl-2 (lymphoma)

2I CCND1, also called BCL1, cyclin D1 (Mantle cell lymphoma, myeloma) bcl-1 (lymphoma)

2J MYC (Burkitt lymphoma) c-myc (lymphoma)

2K IgH (lymphoma/leukemia)

2L IGK (lymphoma/leukemia)

2M TRB, T cell receptor beta (lymphoma/leukemia)

2N TRG, T cell receptor gamma (lymphoma/leukemia)

83

2O   SIL or TAL1 (T cell leukemia)

2T   BCL6 (B cell lymphoma)

2Q   API1 or MALT1 (MALT lymphoma)

2R   NPM or ALK, genes associated with t(2;5) (anaplastic large cell lymphoma)

2S   FLT3 (acute myelogenous leukemia)

2Z   Lymphoid/hematopoetic neoplasia, not otherwise specified

Non-Neoplastic Hematology/Coagulation

3A   F5, also called Factor V (Leiden, others) (hypercoagulable state)

3B   FACC (Fanconi anemia)

3C   FACD (Fanconi anemia)

3D   HBB, beta globin (thalassemia, sickle cell anemia, other hemoglobinopathies)

3E   HBA, also called alpha globin (thalassemia)

3F   MTHFR (elevated homocysteine)

3G   F2, commonly called prothrombin (20210, others) (hypercoagulable state) prothrombin (Factor II, 20210A) (hypercoagulable state)

3H   F8, commonly called Factor VIII (hemophilia A/VWF)

3I   F9, commonly called Factor IX (hemophilia B)

3K   F13, commonly called Factor XIII (bleeding or hypercoagulable state) beta globin

3Z   Non-neoplastic hematology/coagulation, not otherwise specified

Histocompatibility/Blood Typing/Identity/Microsatellite

4A   HLA-A*

4B   HLA-B*

4C   HLA-C*

(**4D**   deleted 2011 [2012 edition])

4E HLA-DRB all

4P HLA-DRB1*

4Q HLA-DRB3*

4R HLA-DRB4*

4S HLA-DRB5*

4T HLA-DQA1*

4F HLA-DQB1*

4U HLA-DPA1*

4G HLA-DPB1*

4H Kell

4I Fingerprint for engraftment (post allogeneic progenitor cell transplant)

4J Fingerprint for donor allelotype (allogeneic transplant)

4K Fingerprint for recipient allelotype (allogeneic transplant)

4L Fingerprint for leukocyte chimerism (allogeneic solid organ transplant)

4M Fingerprint for maternal versus fetal origin

4N Microsatellite instability

4O Microsatellite loss (loss of heterozygosity)

4P This code is out of order. See page 51

4Q This code is out of order. See page 51

4R This code is out of order. See page 51

4S This code is out of order. See page 51

4T This code is out of order. See page 51

4U This code is out of order. See page 51

4Z Histocompatibility/typing, not otherwise specified

Neurologic, Non-Neoplastic

5A ASPA, commonly called Aspartoacylase A (Canavan disease)

5B FMR-1 (Fragile X, FRAXA, syndrome)

5C FRDA, commonly called Frataxin (Freidreich's ataxia)

5D HD, commonly called Huntington (Huntington's disease)

5E GABRA5, NIPA1, UBE3A, or ANCR GABRA (Prader Willi-Angelman syndrome)

5F GJB2, commonly called Connexin-26 (hereditary hearing loss) Connexin-32 (GJB2) (hereditary deafness)

5G GJB1, commonly called Connexin-32 (X-linked Charcot-Marie-Tooth disease)

5H SNRPN (Prader Willi-Angelman syndrome)

5I SCA1, commonly called Ataxin-1 (spinocerebellar ataxia, type 1)

5J SCA2, commonly called Ataxin-2 (spinocerebellar ataxia, type 2)

5K MJD, commonly called Ataxin-3 (spinocerebellar ataxia, type 3, Machado-Joseph disease)

5L CACNA1A (spinocerebellar ataxia, type 6)

5M ATXN7 Ataxin-7 (spinocerebellar ataxia, type 7)

5N PMP-22 (Charcot-Marie-Tooth disease, type 1A)

5O MECP2 (Rett syndrome)

5Z Neurologic, non-neoplastic, not otherwise specified

Muscular, Non-Neoplastic

6A DMD, commonly called dystrophin (Duchenne/Becker muscular dystrophy)

6B DMPK (myotonic dystrophy, type 1)

6C ZNF-9 (myotonic dystrophy, type 2)

6D SMN1/SMN2 (autosomal recessive spinal muscular atrophy)

6E   MTTK, commonly called tRNAlys (myotonic epilepsy, MERRF)

6F   MTTL1, commonly called tRNAleu (mitochondrial encephalomyopathy, MELAS)

6Z   Muscular, not otherwise specified

Metabolic, Other

7A   APOE, commonly called apolipoprotein E (cardiovascular disease, Alzheimer's disease)

7B   NPC1 or NPC2, commonly called sphingomyelin phosphodiesterase (Nieman-Pick disease)

7C   GBA, commonly called acid beta glucosidase (Gaucher disease)

7D   HFE (hemochromatosis)

7E   HEXA, commonly called hHexosaminidase A (Tay-Sachs disease)

7F   ACADM (medium chain acyl CoA dehydrogenase deficiency)

7Z   Metabolic, other, not otherwise specified

Metabolic, Transport

8A   CFTR (cystic fibrosis)

8B   PRSS1 (hereditary pancreatitis)

8C   Long QT syndrome, KCN (Jevell and Lange-Nielsen syndromes, types 1, 2, 5, and 6) and SCN (Brugada syndrome, SIDS and type 3)

8Z   Metabolic, transport, not otherwise specified

Metabolic-Pharmacogenetics

9A   TPMT, commonly called thiopurine methyltransferase (patients on antimetabolite therapy)

9B   CYP2 genes, commonly called cytochrome p450 (drug metabolism)

9C   ABCB1, commonly called MDR1 or p-glycoprotein (drug transport)

9D   NAT2 (drug metabolism)

9L   Metabolic-pharmacogenetics, not otherwise specified

Dysmorphology

9M FGFR1 (Pfeiffer and Kallmann syndromes)

9N FGFR2 (Crouzon, Jackson-Weiss, Apert, Saethre-Chotzen syndromes)

9O FGFR3 (achondroplasia, hypochondroplasia, thanatophoric dysplasia, types I and II, Crouzon syndrome with acanthosis nigricans, Muencke syndromes)

9P TWIST (Saethre-Chotzen syndrome)

9Q DGCR, commonly called CATCH-22 (DiGeorge and 22q11 deletion syndromes)

9Z Dysmorphology, not otherwise specified

HCPCS MODIFIERS

HCPCS modifiers, defined and managed by The Centers for Medicare and Medicaid Services (CMS), are two digit modifier codes which may be either alpha (all letters) or alphanumeric (letters plus numbers). Some HCPCS modifiers may be used with CPT codes to modify procedures and services on health insurance claim forms filed for Medicare patients. See the most current edition of HCPCS for a complete list.

This page intentionally left blank.

ANATOMICAL ILLUSTRATIONS

A fundamental knowledge and understanding of basic human anatomy and physiology is a prerequisite for accurate CPT© procedure coding. While a comprehensive treatment of anatomy and physiology is beyond the scope of this text, the large scale, full color anatomical illustrations on the following pages are designed to facilitate the procedure coding process for both beginning and experienced coders.

The illustrations provide an anatomical perspective of procedure coding by providing a side-by-side view of the major systems of the human body and a corresponding list of the most common CPT procedural categories used to report medical, surgical and diagnostic services performed on the illustrated system.

The CPT procedural categories listed on the left facing page of each anatomical illustration are code ranges only and should not be used for coding. These categories are provided as "pointers" to the appropriate section of CPT, where the definitive code may be found.

PLATE 1. SKIN AND SUBCUTANEOUS TISSUE - MALE

SKIN, SUBCUTANEOUS AND ACCESSORY STRUCTURES

Incision and Drainage	10040-10180
Debridement	11000-11047
Paring or Cutting	11055-11057
Biopsy	11100-11101
Removal of Skin Tags	11200-11201
Shaving of Lesions	11300-11313
Excision-Benign Lesions	11400-11471
Excision-Malignant Lesions	11600-11646

Nails	11719-11765

Pilondial Cyst	11770-11772

Repair (Closure)

Repair-Simple	12001-12021
Repair-Intermediate	12031-12057
Repair-Complex	13100-13160
Adjacent Tissue Transfer	14000-14350
Skin Replacement Surgery	15002-15278
Flaps (Skin and/or Deep Tissues)	15570-15777
Pressure Ulcers	15920-15999
Burns, Local Treatment	16000-16036

Destruction

Destruction, Benign or Premalignant Lesions	17000-17250
Destruction, Malignant Lesions	17260-17286
Mohs' Micrographic Surgery	17311-17315
Other Destruction Procedures	17340-17999

Laboratory Services

Skin Tests, Immunology	86485-86580
Skin Tests, Allergy	95004-95199

Visit and Medicine Services

E/M Services	99201-99499
Special Dermatological Procedures	96900-96999

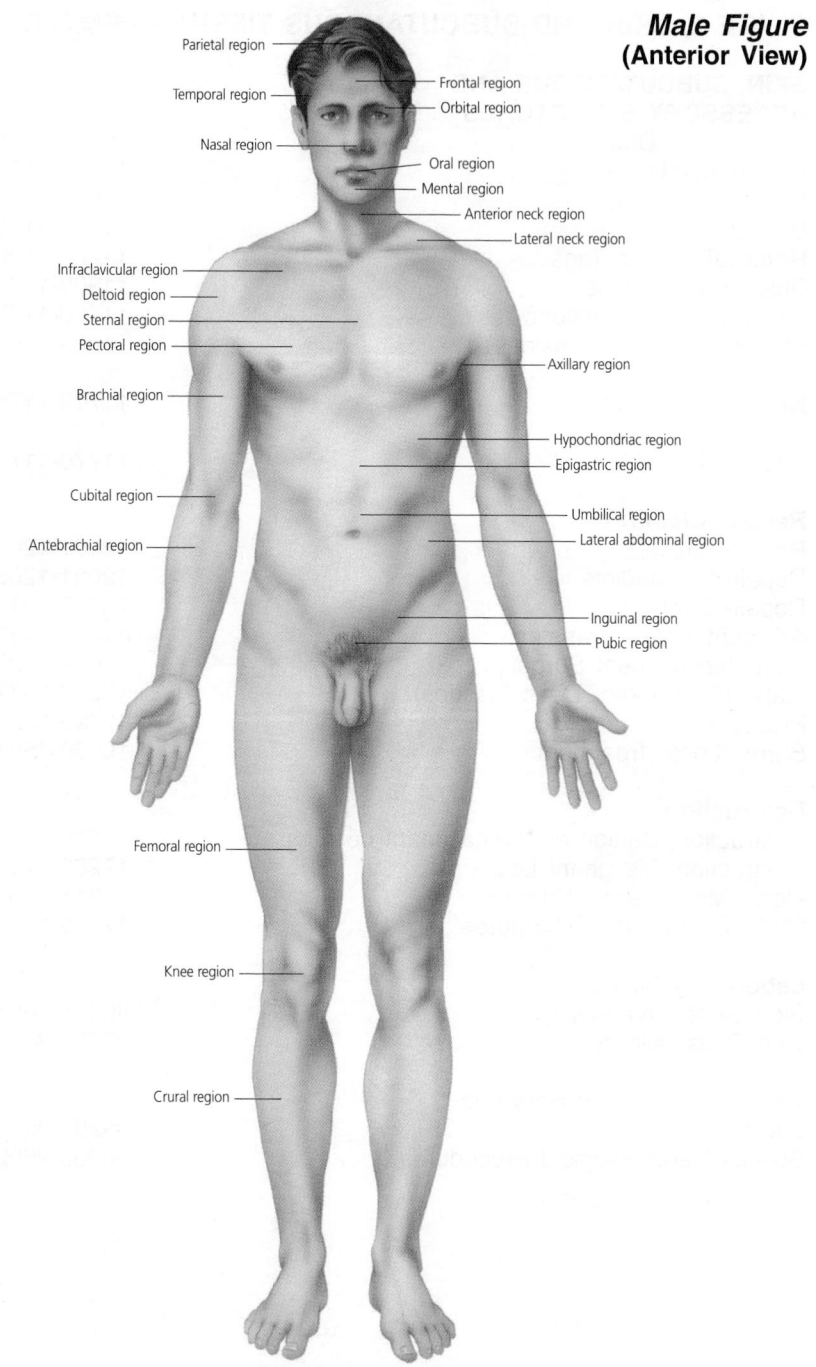

Male Figure
(Anterior View)

Parietal region

Temporal region

Nasal region

Frontal region

Orbital region

Oral region

Mental region

Anterior neck region

Lateral neck region

Infraclavicular region

Deltoid region

Sternal region

Pectoral region

Brachial region

Axillary region

Hypochondriac region

Epigastric region

Cubital region

Umbilical region

Antebrachial region

Lateral abdominal region

Inguinal region

Pubic region

Femoral region

Knee region

Crural region

PLATE 2. SKIN AND SUBCUTANEOUS TISSUE - FEMALE

SKIN, SUBCUTANEOUS AND ACCESSORY STRUCTURES

Incision and Drainage	10040-10180
Debridement	11000-11047
Paring or Cutting	11055-11057
Biopsy	11100-11101
Removal of Skin Tags	11200-11201
Shaving of Lesions	11300-11313
Excision-Benign Lesions	11400-11471
Excision-Malignant Lesions	11600-11646

Nails   11719-11765

Pilondial Cyst   11770-11772

Repair (Closure)

Repair-Simple	12001-12021
Repair-Intermediate	12031-12057
Repair-Complex	13100-13160
Adjacent Tissue Transfer	14000-14350
Skin Replacement Surgery	15002-15278
Flaps (Skin and/or Deep Tissues)	15570-15777
Pressure Ulcers	15920-15999
Burns, Local Treatment	16000-16036

Destruction

Destruction, Benign or Premalignant Lesions	17000-17250
Destruction, Malignant Lesions	17260-17286
Mohs' Micrographic Surgery	17311-17315
Other Destruction Procedures	17340-17999

Laboratory Services

Skin Tests, Immunology	86485-86580
Skin Tests, Allergy	95004-95199

Visit and Medicine Services

E/M Services	99201-99499
Special Dermatological Procedures	96900-96999

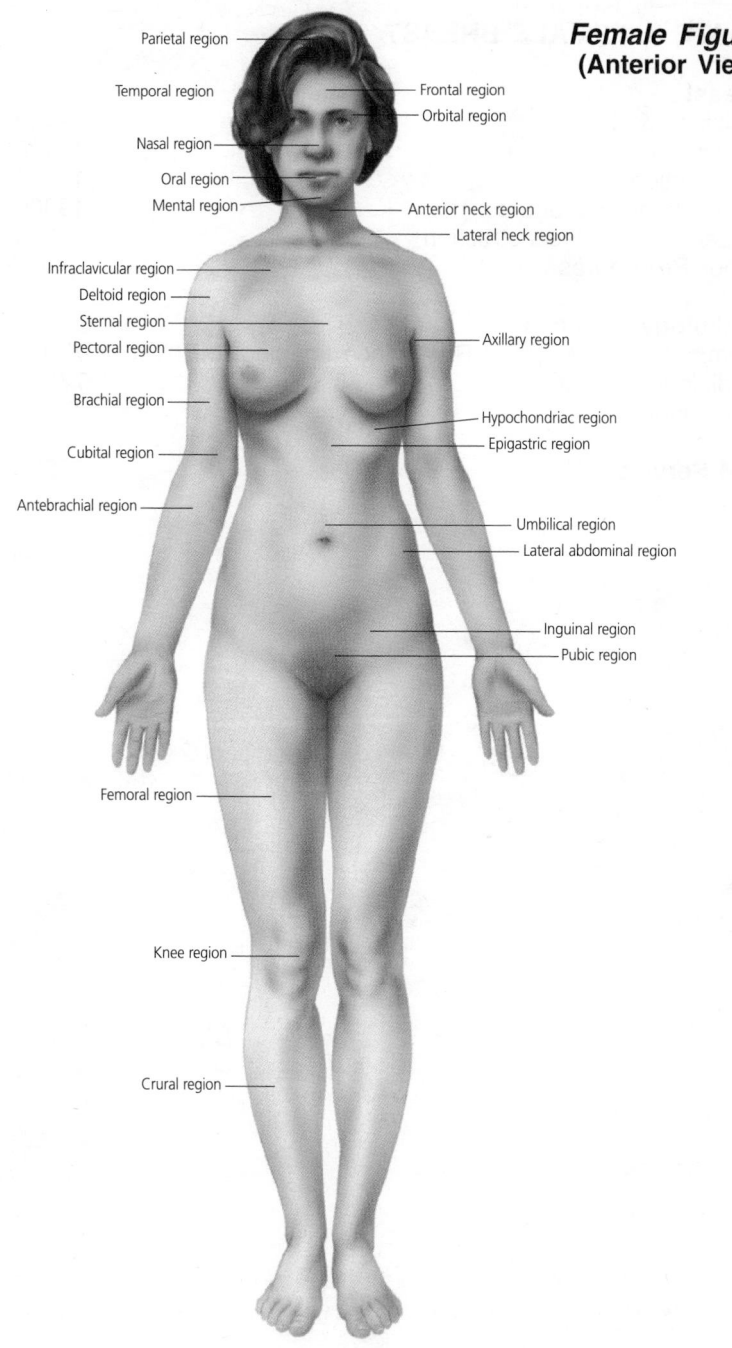

Female Figure
(Anterior View)

Parietal region

Temporal region

Nasal region

Oral region

Mental region

Frontal region

Orbital region

Anterior neck region

Lateral neck region

Infraclavicular region

Deltoid region

Sternal region

Pectoral region

Axillary region

Brachial region

Hypochondriac region

Epigastric region

Cubital region

Antebrachial region

Umbilical region

Lateral abdominal region

Inguinal region

Pubic region

Femoral region

Knee region

Crural region

PLATE 3. FEMALE BREAST

Breast

Incision	19000-19030
Excision	19100-19272
Introduction	19290-19298
Mastectomy Procedures	19300-19307
Repair and/or Reconstruction	19316-19396
Other Procedures	19499

Radiology Services

Mammography/Magnetic Resonance Imaging (MRI)	77051-77059
Radiologic Guidance	77031-77032
Ultrasound	76645

E/M Services 99201-99499

Female Breast

Pectoralis major muscle

Lobule

Lobe

Secondary tubules

Mammary duct

Lactiferous sinus

Lactiferous duct

Nipple

Areola

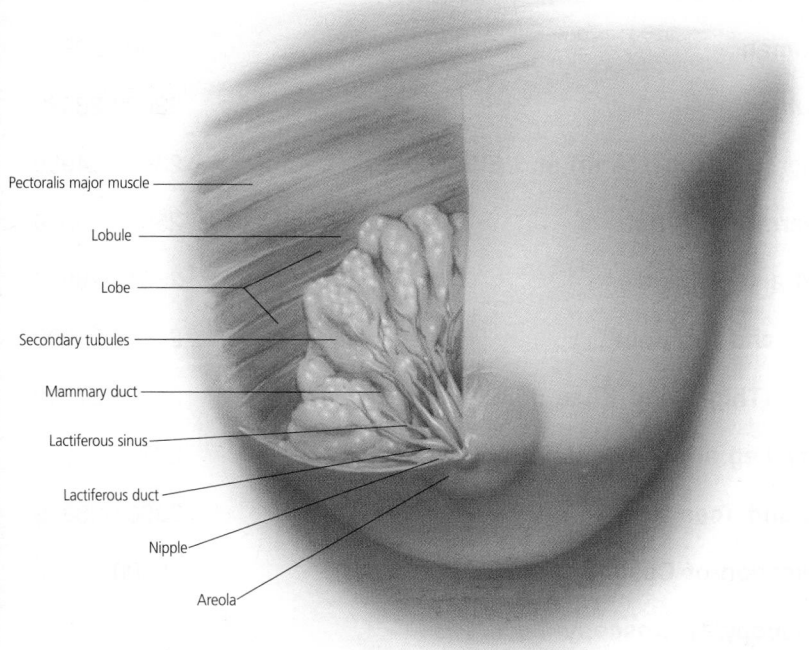

PLATE 4. MUSCULAR SYSTEM AND CONNECTIVE TISSUE - ANTERIOR VIEW

General	20005-20999
Head	21010-21499
Neck (Soft Tissues) and Thorax	21501-21899
Back and Flank	21920-21936
Spine (Vertebral Column)	22010-22899
Abdomen	22900-22999
Shoulder	23000-23929
Humerous (Upper Arm) and Elbow	23930-24999
Forearm and Wrist	25000-25999
Hand and Fingers	26010-26989
Pelvis and Hip Joint	26990-27299
Femur (Thigh) and Knee Joint	27301-27599
Lower Leg and Ankle Joint	27600-27899
Foot and Toes	28001-28899
Application of Casts/Strapping	29000-29799
Endoscopy/Arthroscopy	29800-29999
E/M Services	99201-99499

Muscular System
(Anterior View)

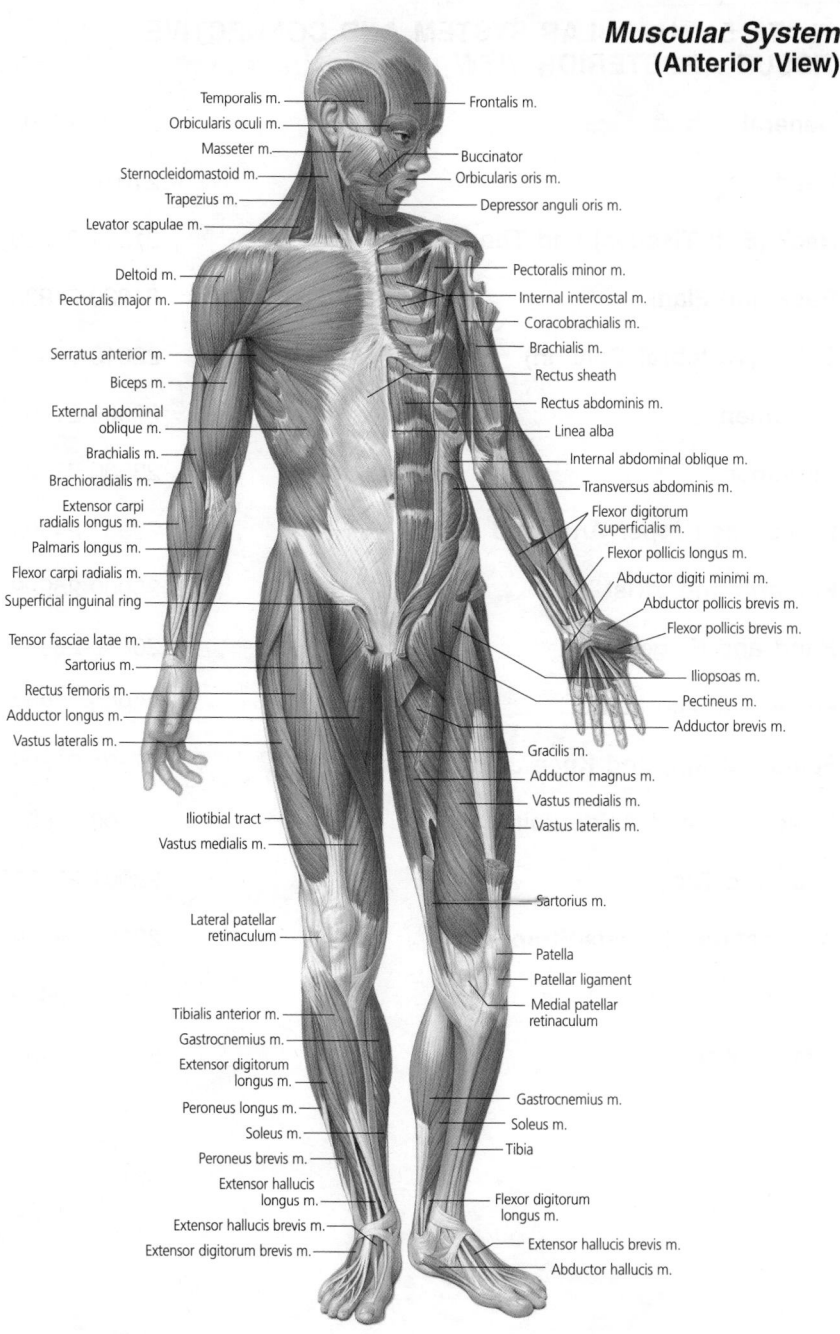

Temporalis m.
Orbicularis oculi m.
Masseter m.
Sternocleidomastoid m.
Trapezius m.
Levator scapulae m.

Frontalis m.
Buccinator
Orbicularis oris m.
Depressor anguli oris m.

Deltoid m.
Pectoralis major m.

Pectoralis minor m.
Internal intercostal m.
Coracobrachialis m.
Brachialis m.

Serratus anterior m.
Biceps m.
External abdominal oblique m.
Brachialis m.
Brachioradialis m.
Extensor carpi radialis longus m.
Palmaris longus m.
Flexor carpi radialis m.
Superficial inguinal ring
Tensor fasciae latae m.
Sartorius m.
Rectus femoris m.
Adductor longus m.
Vastus lateralis m.

Rectus sheath
Rectus abdominis m.
Linea alba
Internal abdominal oblique m.
Transversus abdominis m.
Flexor digitorum superficialis m.
Flexor pollicis longus m.
Abductor digiti minimi m.
Abductor pollicis brevis m.
Flexor pollicis brevis m.
Iliopsoas m.
Pectineus m.
Adductor brevis m.

Gracilis m.
Adductor magnus m.
Vastus medialis m.
Vastus lateralis m.

Iliotibial tract
Vastus medialis m.

Sartorius m.

Lateral patellar retinaculum

Patella
Patellar ligament
Medial patellar retinaculum

Tibialis anterior m.
Gastrocnemius m.
Extensor digitorum longus m.
Peroneus longus m.
Soleus m.
Peroneus brevis m.
Extensor hallucis longus m.
Extensor hallucis brevis m.
Extensor digitorum brevis m.

Gastrocnemius m.
Soleus m.
Tibia
Flexor digitorum longus m.
Extensor hallucis brevis m.
Abductor hallucis m.

99

PLATE 5. MUSCULAR SYSTEM AND CONNECTIVE TISSUE - POSTERIOR VIEW

General	20005-20999
Head	21010-21499
Neck (Soft Tissues) and Thorax	21501-21899
Back and Flank	21920-21936
Spine (Vertebral Column)	22010-22899
Abdomen	22900-22999
Shoulder	23000-23929
Humerous (Upper Arm) and Elbow	23930-24999
Forearm and Wrist	25000-25999
Hand and Fingers	26010-26989
Pelvis and Hip Joint	26990-27299
Femur (Thigh) and Knee Joint	27301-27599
Lower Leg and Ankle Joint	27600-27899
Foot and Toes	28001-28899
Application of Casts/Strapping	29000-29799
Endoscopy/Arthroscopy	29800-29999
E/M Services	99201-99499

Muscular System
(Posterior View)

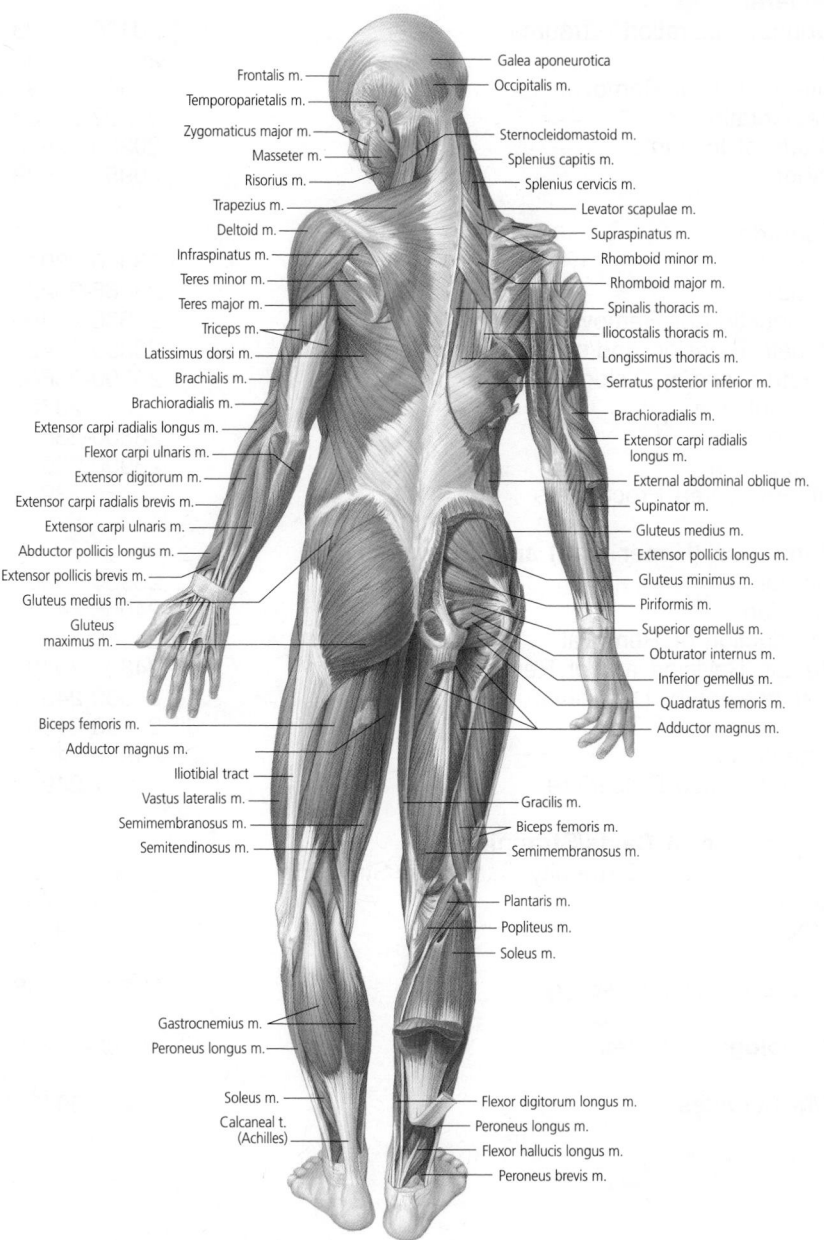

Galea aponeurotica
Occipitalis m.
Frontalis m.
Temporoparietalis m.
Zygomaticus major m.
Masseter m.
Risorius m.
Trapezius m.
Deltoid m.
Infraspinatus m.
Teres minor m.
Teres major m.
Triceps m.
Latissimus dorsi m.
Brachialis m.
Brachioradialis m.
Extensor carpi radialis longus m.
Flexor carpi ulnaris m.
Extensor digitorum m.
Extensor carpi radialis brevis m.
Extensor carpi ulnaris m.
Abductor pollicis longus m.
Extensor pollicis brevis m.
Gluteus medius m.
Gluteus maximus m.
Biceps femoris m.
Adductor magnus m.
Iliotibial tract
Vastus lateralis m.
Semimembranosus m.
Semitendinosus m.
Gastrocnemius m.
Peroneus longus m.
Soleus m.
Calcaneal t. (Achilles)

Sternocleidomastoid m.
Splenius capitis m.
Splenius cervicis m.
Levator scapulae m.
Supraspinatus m.
Rhomboid minor m.
Rhomboid major m.
Spinalis thoracis m.
Iliocostalis thoracis m.
Longissimus thoracis m.
Serratus posterior inferior m.
Brachioradialis m.
Extensor carpi radialis longus m.
External abdominal oblique m.
Supinator m.
Gluteus medius m.
Extensor pollicis longus m.
Gluteus minimus m.
Piriformis m.
Superior gemellus m.
Obturator internus m.
Inferior gemellus m.
Quadratus femoris m.
Adductor magnus m.
Gracilis m.
Biceps femoris m.
Semimembranosus m.
Plantaris m.
Popliteus m.
Soleus m.
Flexor digitorum longus m.
Peroneus longus m.
Flexor hallucis longus m.
Peroneus brevis m.

101

PLATE 6. MUSCULAR SYSTEM - SHOULDER AND ELBOW

General
Wound exploration - Trauma	20100-20103
Excision	20150-20251
Introduction or Removal	20500-20697
Replantation	20802-20838
Grafts of Implants	20900-20938
Other	20950-20999

Shoulder
Incision	23000-23044
Excision	23065-23220
Introduction or Removal	23330-23350
Repair, Revision and/or Reconstruction	23395-23491
Fracture and/or Dislocation	23500-23680
Manipulation	23700
Arthrodesis	23800-23802
Amputation	23900-23921
Other/Unlisted Procedures	23929

Humerous (Upper Arm) and Elbow
Incision	23930-24006
Excision	24065-24155
Introduction or Removal	24160-24220
Repair, Revision and/or Reconstruction	24300-24498
Fracture and/or Dislocation	24500-24685
Arthrodesis	24800-24802
Amputation	24900-24940
Other/Unlisted Procedure	24999

Application of Casts/Strapping
Body and Upper Extremity Casts and Strapping	29000-29280
Removal or Repair	29700-29750
Other	29799

Endoscopy/Arthroscopy
29805-29838

Radiology Services
73000-73225

E/M Services
99201-99499

Shoulder and Elbow
(Anterior View)

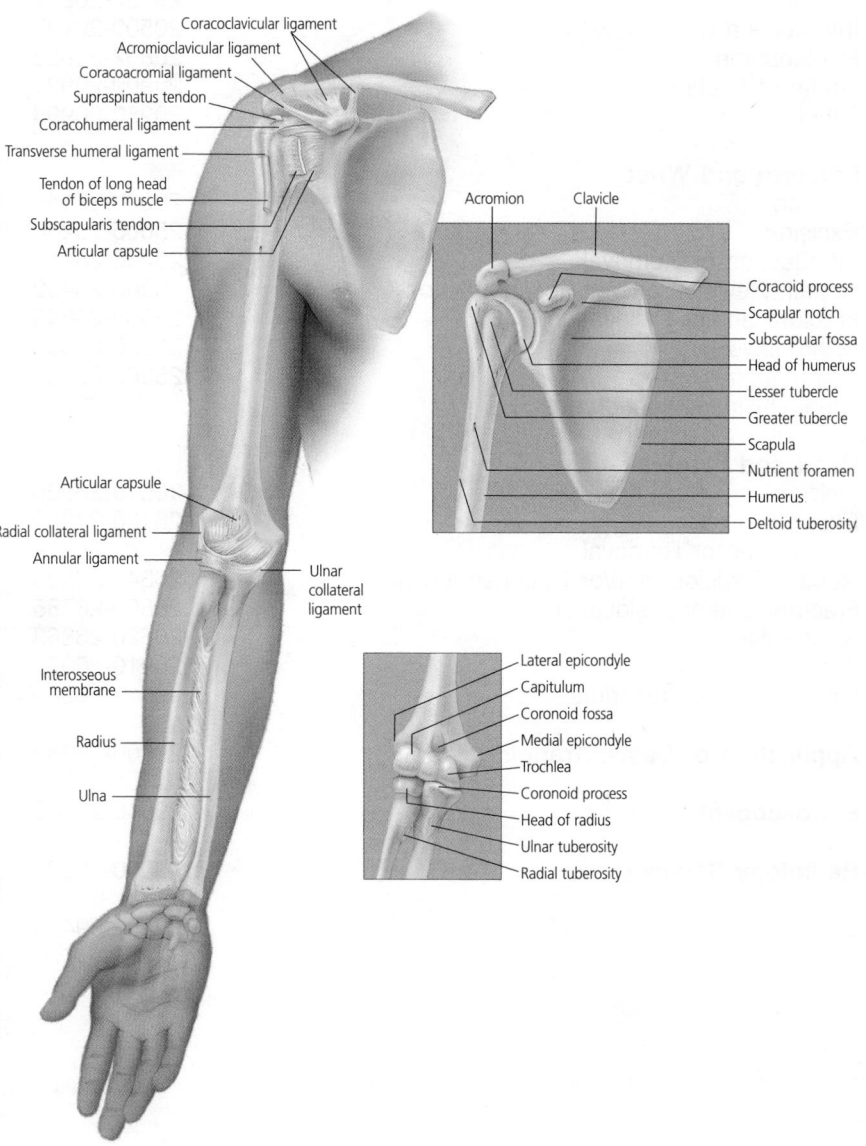

PLATE 7. MUSCULAR SYSTEM - HAND AND WRIST

General

Wound exploration - Trauma	20100-20103
Excision	20150-20251
Introduction or Removal	20500-20697
Replantation	20802-20838
Grafts of Implants	20900-20938
Other	20950-20999

Forearm and Wrist

Incision	25000-25040
Excision	25065-25240
Introduction or Removal	25246-25259
Repair, Revision and/or Reconstruction	25260-25492
Fracture and/or Dislocation	25500-25695
Arthrodesis	25800-25830
Amputation	25900-25931
Other/Unlisted Procedure	25999

Hand and Fingers

Incision	26010-26080
Excision	26100-26262
Introduction or Removal	26320
Repair, Revision, and/or Reconstruction	26340-26596
Fracture and/or Dislocation	26600-26785
Arthrodesis	26820-26863
Amputation	26910-26952
Other/Unlisted Procedure	26989

Application of Casts/Strapping   29000-29280

Endoscopy/Arthroscopy   29840-29848

Radiology Services   73000-73225

E/M Services   99201-99499

Hand and Wrist

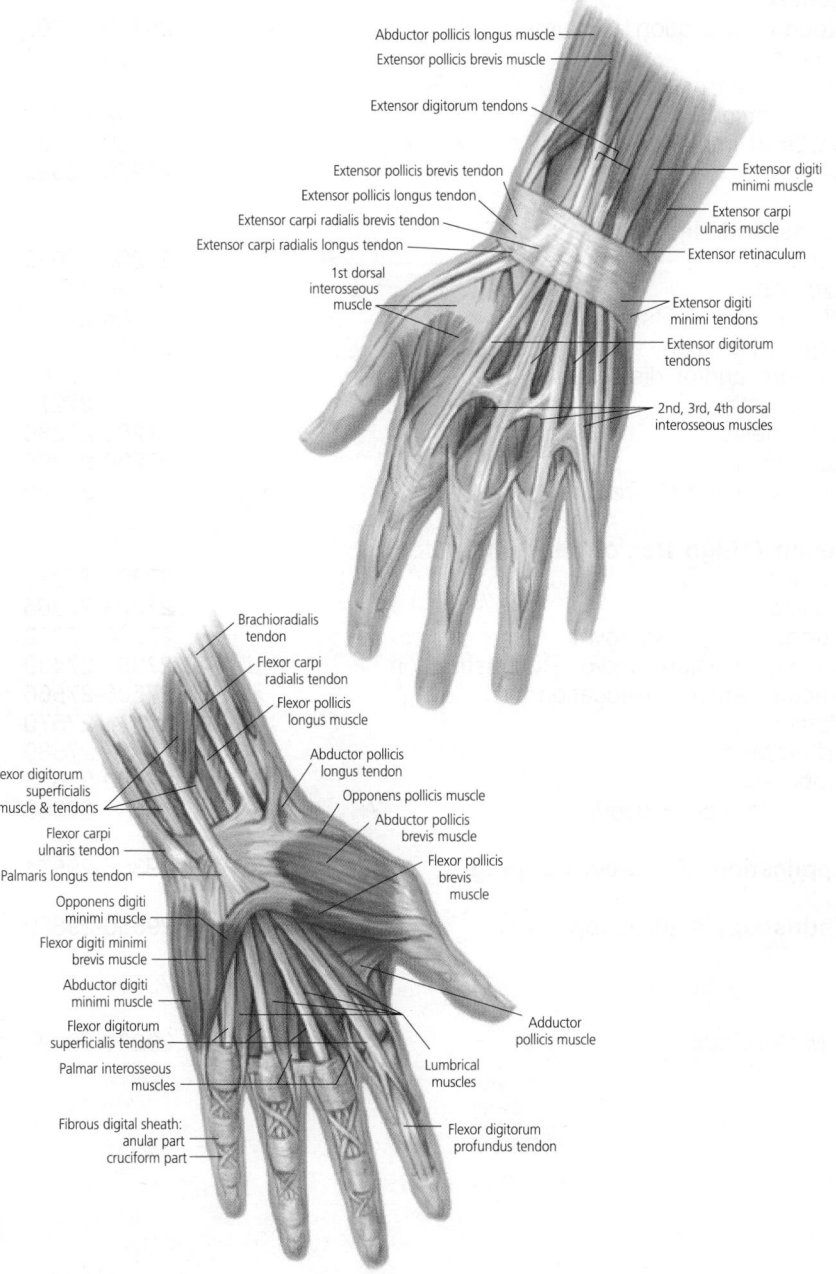

PLATE 8. MUSCULOSKELETAL SYSTEM - HIP AND KNEE

General

Wound exploration - Trauma	20100-20103
Excision	20150-20251
Introduction or Removal	20500-20697
Replantation	20802-20838
Grafts of Implants	20900-20938
Other	20950-20999

Pelvis and Hip Joint

Incision	26990-27036
Excision	27040-27080
Introduction or Removal	27086-27096
Repair, Revision, and/or Reconstruction	27097-27187
Fracture and/or dislocation	27193-27269
Manipulation	27275
Arthrodesis	27280-27286
Amputation	27290-27295
Other/Unlisted Procedure	27299

Femur (Thigh Region) and Knee Joint

Incision	27301-27310
Excision	27323-27365
Introduction or Removal	27370-37372
Repair, Revision, and/or Reconstruction	27380-27499
Fracture and/or Dislocation	27500-27566
Manipulation	27570
Arthrodesis	27580
Amputation	27590-27598
Other/Unlisted Procedure	27599

Application of Casts/Strapping 29305-29584

Endoscopy/Arthroscopy 29850-29889

Radiology Services 73500-73725

E/M Services 99201-99499

Hip and Knee
(Anterior View)

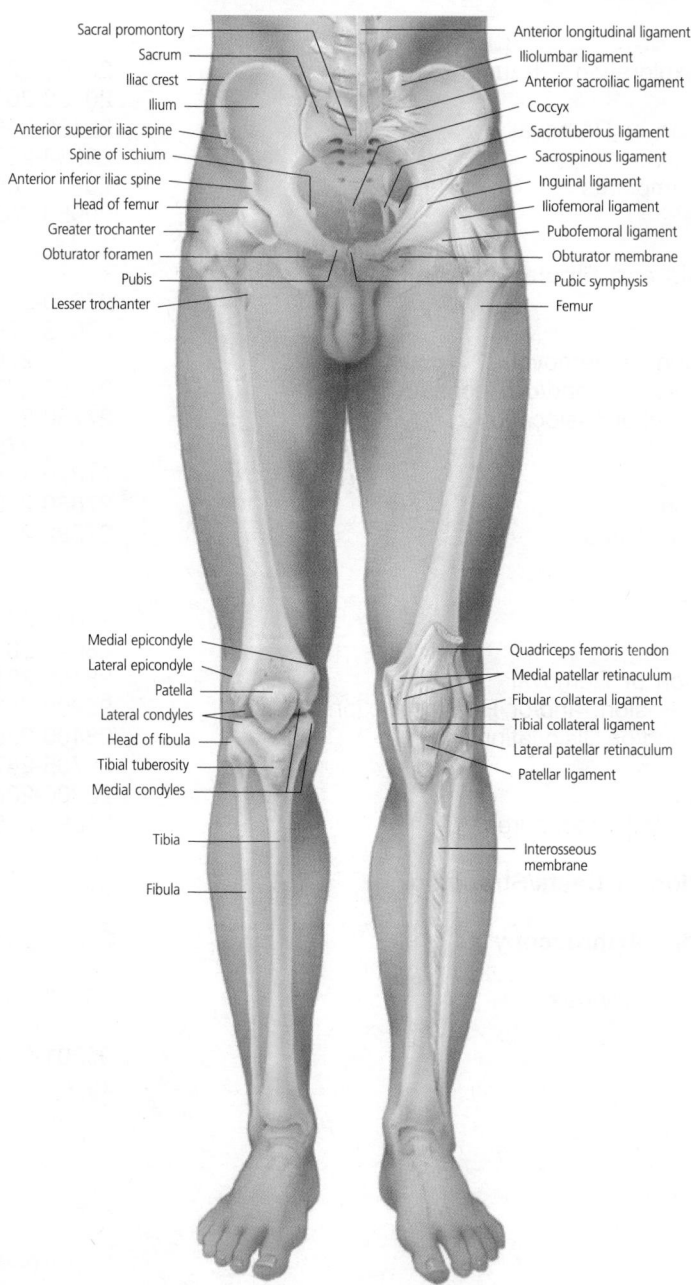

Sacral promontory
Sacrum
Iliac crest
Ilium
Anterior superior iliac spine
Spine of ischium
Anterior inferior iliac spine
Head of femur
Greater trochanter
Obturator foramen
Pubis
Lesser trochanter

Anterior longitudinal ligament
Iliolumbar ligament
Anterior sacroiliac ligament
Coccyx
Sacrotuberous ligament
Sacrospinous ligament
Inguinal ligament
Iliofemoral ligament
Pubofemoral ligament
Obturator membrane
Pubic symphysis
Femur

Medial epicondyle
Lateral epicondyle
Patella
Lateral condyles
Head of fibula
Tibial tuberosity
Medial condyles

Tibia

Fibula

Quadriceps femoris tendon
Medial patellar retinaculum
Fibular collateral ligament
Tibial collateral ligament
Lateral patellar retinaculum
Patellar ligament

Interosseous membrane

107

PLATE 9. MUSCULOSKELETAL SYSTEM - FOOT AND ANKLE

General

Wound exploration - Trauma	20100-20103
Excision	20150-20251
Introduction or Removal	20500-20697
Replantation	20802-20838
Grafts of Implants	20900-20938
Other	20950-20999

Leg (Tibia and Fibula) and Ankle Joint

Incision	27600-27612
Excision	27613-27647
Introduction or Removal	27648
Repair, Revision and/or Reconstruction	27650-27745
Fracture and/or Dislocation	27750-27848
Manipulation	27860
Arthrodesis	27870-27871
Amputation	27880-27889
Other Procedures	27892-27899

Foot and Toes

Incision	28001-28035
Excision	28043-28175
Introduction or Removal	28190-28193
Repair, Revision, and/or Reconstruction	28200-28360
Fracture and/or Dislocation	28400-28675
Arthrodesis	28705-28760
Amputation	28800-28825
Other/Unlisted Procedures	28890-28899

Application of Casts/Strapping	29305-29584
Endoscopy/Arthroscopy	29891-29999
Radiology Services	73500-73725
E/M Services	99201-99499

Foot and Ankle

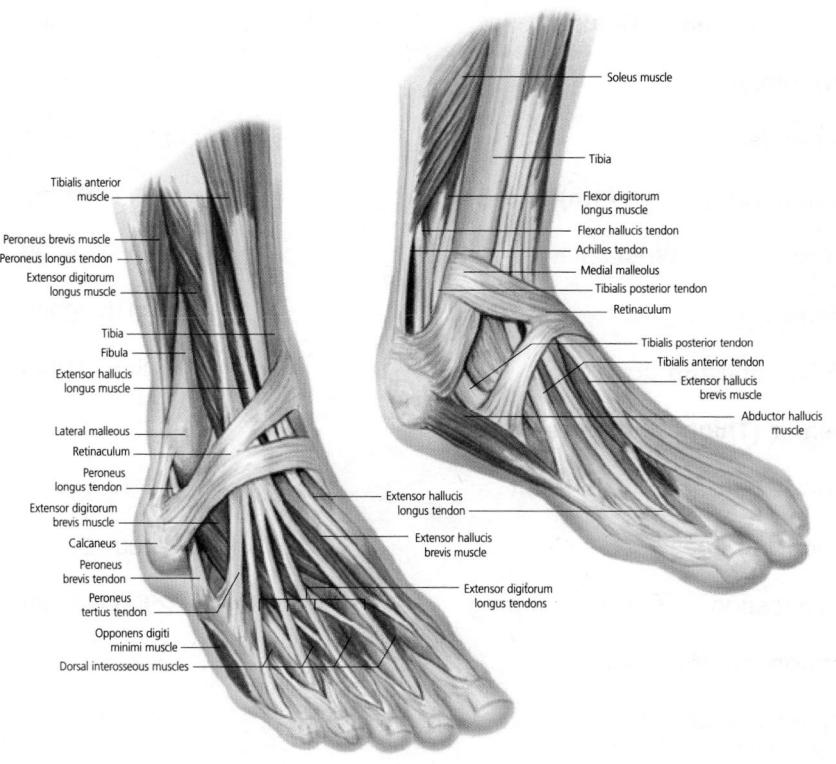

Soleus muscle

Tibia

Flexor digitorum longus muscle

Flexor hallucis tendon

Achilles tendon

Medial malleolus

Tibialis posterior tendon

Retinaculum

Tibialis posterior tendon

Tibialis anterior tendon

Extensor hallucis brevis muscle

Abductor hallucis muscle

Tibialis anterior muscle

Peroneus brevis muscle

Peroneus longus tendon

Extensor digitorum longus muscle

Tibia

Fibula

Extensor hallucis longus muscle

Lateral malleous

Retinaculum

Peroneus longus tendon

Extensor digitorum brevis muscle

Calcaneus

Peroneus brevis tendon

Peroneus tertius tendon

Opponens digiti minimi muscle

Dorsal interosseous muscles

Extensor hallucis longus tendon

Extensor hallucis brevis muscle

Extensor digitorum longus tendons

PLATE 10. SKELETAL SYSTEM - ANTERIOR VIEW

General	20005-20999
Head	21010-21499
Neck (Soft Tissues) and Thorax	21501-21899
Back and Flank	21920-21936
Spine (Vertebral Column)	22010-22899
Abdomen	22900-22999
Shoulder	23000-23929
Humerous (Upper Arm) and Elbow	23930-24999
Forearm and Wrist	25000-25999
Hand and Fingers	26010-26989
Pelvis and Hip Joint	26990-27299
Femur (Thigh) and Knee Joint	27301-27599
Lower Leg and Ankle Joint	27600-27899
Foot and Toes	28001-28899
Application of Casts/Strapping	29000-29799
Endoscopy/Arthroscopy	29800-29999
Radiology Services Bone/Joint Studies	70010-73725 77071-77084
E/M Services	99201-99499

Skeletal System
(Anterior View)

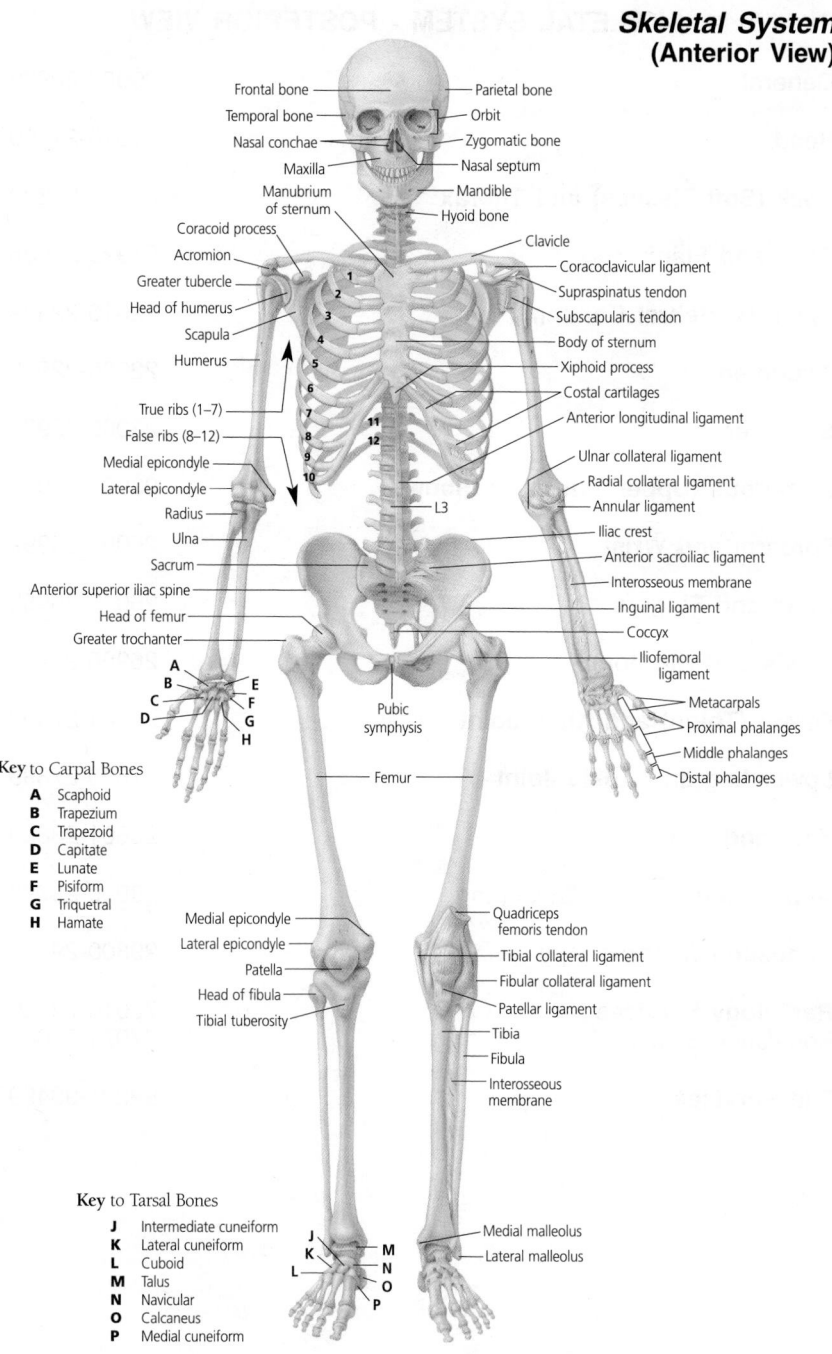

Frontal bone
Temporal bone
Nasal conchae
Maxilla
Manubrium of sternum
Coracoid process
Acromion
Greater tubercle
Head of humerus
Scapula
Humerus
True ribs (1–7)
False ribs (8–12)
Medial epicondyle
Lateral epicondyle
Radius
Ulna
Sacrum
Anterior superior iliac spine
Head of femur
Greater trochanter

Parietal bone
Orbit
Zygomatic bone
Nasal septum
Mandible
Hyoid bone
Clavicle
Coracoclavicular ligament
Supraspinatus tendon
Subscapularis tendon
Body of sternum
Xiphoid process
Costal cartilages
Anterior longitudinal ligament
Ulnar collateral ligament
Radial collateral ligament
Annular ligament
Iliac crest
Anterior sacroiliac ligament
Interosseous membrane
Inguinal ligament
Coccyx
Iliofemoral ligament
Metacarpals
Proximal phalanges
Middle phalanges
Distal phalanges

1 2 3 4 5 6 7 8 9 10 11 12 L3

A B C D E F G H

Pubic symphysis

Femur

Key to Carpal Bones

A	Scaphoid
B	Trapezium
C	Trapezoid
D	Capitate
E	Lunate
F	Pisiform
G	Triquetral
H	Hamate

Medial epicondyle
Lateral epicondyle
Patella
Head of fibula
Tibial tuberosity

Quadriceps femoris tendon
Tibial collateral ligament
Fibular collateral ligament
Patellar ligament
Tibia
Fibula
Interosseous membrane

Key to Tarsal Bones

J	Intermediate cuneiform
K	Lateral cuneiform
L	Cuboid
M	Talus
N	Navicular
O	Calcaneus
P	Medial cuneiform

J K L M N O P

Medial malleolus
Lateral malleolus

111

PLATE 11. SKELETAL SYSTEM - POSTERIOR VIEW

General	20005-20999
Head	21010-21499
Neck (Soft Tissues) and Thorax	21501-21899
Back and Flank	21920-21936
Spine (Vertebral Column)	22010-22899
Abdomen	22900-22999
Shoulder	23000-23929
Humerous (Upper Arm) and Elbow	23930-24999
Forearm and Wrist	25000-25999
Hand and Fingers	26010-26989
Pelvis and Hip Joint	26990-27299
Femur (Thigh) and Knee Joint	27301-27599
Lower Leg and Ankle Joint	27600-27899
Foot and Toes	28001-28899
Application of Casts/Strapping	29000-29799
Endoscopy/Arthroscopy	29800-29999
Radiology Services Bone/Joint Studies	70010-73725 77071-77084
E/M Services	99201-99499

Skeletal System
(Posterior View)

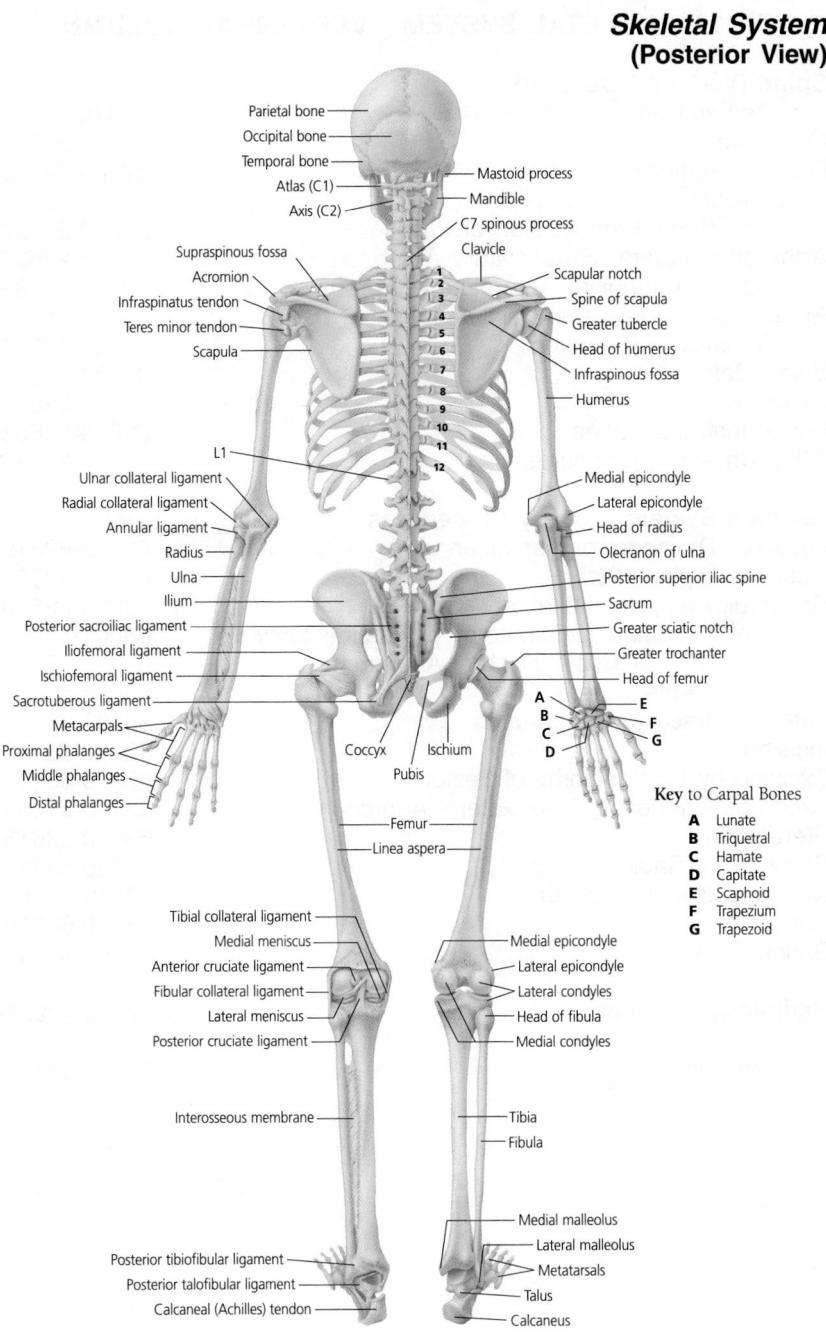

Parietal bone
Occipital bone
Temporal bone
Atlas (C1)
Axis (C2)
Mastoid process
Mandible
C7 spinous process
Clavicle
Supraspinous fossa
Acromion
Infraspinatus tendon
Teres minor tendon
Scapula
Scapular notch
Spine of scapula
Greater tubercle
Head of humerus
Infraspinous fossa
Humerus
L1
Ulnar collateral ligament
Radial collateral ligament
Annular ligament
Radius
Ulna
Ilium
Posterior sacroiliac ligament
Iliofemoral ligament
Ischiofemoral ligament
Sacrotuberous ligament
Metacarpals
Proximal phalanges
Middle phalanges
Distal phalanges
Medial epicondyle
Lateral epicondyle
Head of radius
Olecranon of ulna
Posterior superior iliac spine
Sacrum
Greater sciatic notch
Greater trochanter
Head of femur
Coccyx
Ischium
Pubis
A
B
C
D
E
F
G
Femur
Linea aspera
Tibial collateral ligament
Medial meniscus
Anterior cruciate ligament
Fibular collateral ligament
Lateral meniscus
Posterior cruciate ligament
Medial epicondyle
Lateral epicondyle
Lateral condyles
Head of fibula
Medial condyles
Interosseous membrane
Tibia
Fibula
Medial malleolus
Lateral malleolus
Metatarsals
Talus
Calcaneus
Posterior tibiofibular ligament
Posterior talofibular ligament
Calcaneal (Achilles) tendon

Key to Carpal Bones

A	Lunate
B	Triquetral
C	Hamate
D	Capitate
E	Scaphoid
F	Trapezium
G	Trapezoid

113

PLATE 12. SKELETAL SYSTEM - VERTEBRAL COLUMN

Spine (Vertebral Column)

Incision/Excision	22010-22116
Osteotomy	22206-22226
Fracture and/or Dislocation	22305-22328
Manipulation	22505
Vertebral Body, Embolization or Injection	22520-22527
Arthrodesis-Lateral Extracavitary Approach	22532-22534
Arthrodesis-Anterior or Anterolateral Approach	22548-22585
Arthrodesis-Posterolateral or Lateral Transverse Approach	22590-22634
Spine Deformity	22800-22819
Exploration	22830
Spinal Instrumentation	22840-22865
Other/Unlisted Procedures	22899

Nervous System Surgery Procedures

Injection, Drainage, or Aspiration	62263-62319
Catheter Implantation	62350-62355
Reservoir/Pump Implantation	62360-62370
Posterior Extradural Laminotomy or Laminectomy	63001-63051
Transpedicular or Costovertebral Approach	63055-63066
Anterior or Anterolateral Approach	63075-63091
Lateral Extracavitary Approach	63101-63103
Incision	63170-63200
Excision by Laminectomy of Lesion	63250-63295
Excision, Anterior or Anterolateral Approach	63300-63308
Stereotaxis	63600-63615
Stereotactic Radiosurgery	63620-63621
Neurostimulators (Spinal)	63650-63688
Repair	63700-63710
Shunt, Spinal CSF	63740-63746

Radiology Services 72010-72295

E/M Services 99201-99499

Vertebral Column
(Lateral View)

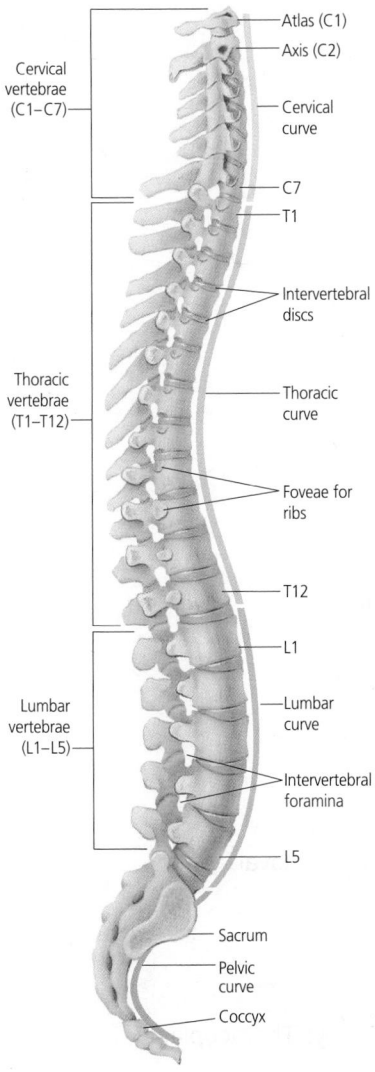

Atlas (C1)

Axis (C2)

Cervical
vertebrae
(C1–C7)

Cervical
curve

C7

T1

Intervertebral
discs

Thoracic
vertebrae
(T1–T12)

Thoracic
curve

Foveae for
ribs

T12

L1

Lumbar
vertebrae
(L1–L5)

Lumbar
curve

Intervertebral
foramina

L5

Sacrum

Pelvic
curve

Coccyx

PLATE 13. RESPIRATORY SYSTEM

Nose
Incision	30000-30020
Excision	30100-30160
Introduction	30200-30220
Removal of Foreign Body	30300-30320
Repair	30400-30630
Destruction	30801-30802
Other	30901-30999

Accessory Sinuses
Incision	31000-31090
Excision	31200-31230
Endoscopy	31231-31297
Other	31299

Larynx
Excision	31300-31420
Introduction	31500-31502
Endoscopy	31505-31579
Repair	31580-31590
Destruction	31595
Other	31599

Trachea and Bronchi
Incision	31600-31614
Endoscopy	31615-31656
Introduction	31715-31730
Excision, Repair	31750-31830
Other	31899

Lungs and Pleura
Incision	32035-32225
Excision/Resection and Removal	32310-32540
Introduction and Removal	32550-32553
Destruction	32560-32562
Thoracoscopy	32601-32674
Repair	32800-32820
Lung Transplantation	32850-32856
Surgical Collapse Therapy; Thoracoplasty	32900-32960
Other	32997-32999

Radiology Services/Chest   71010-71555

E/M Services   99201-99499

Respiratory System

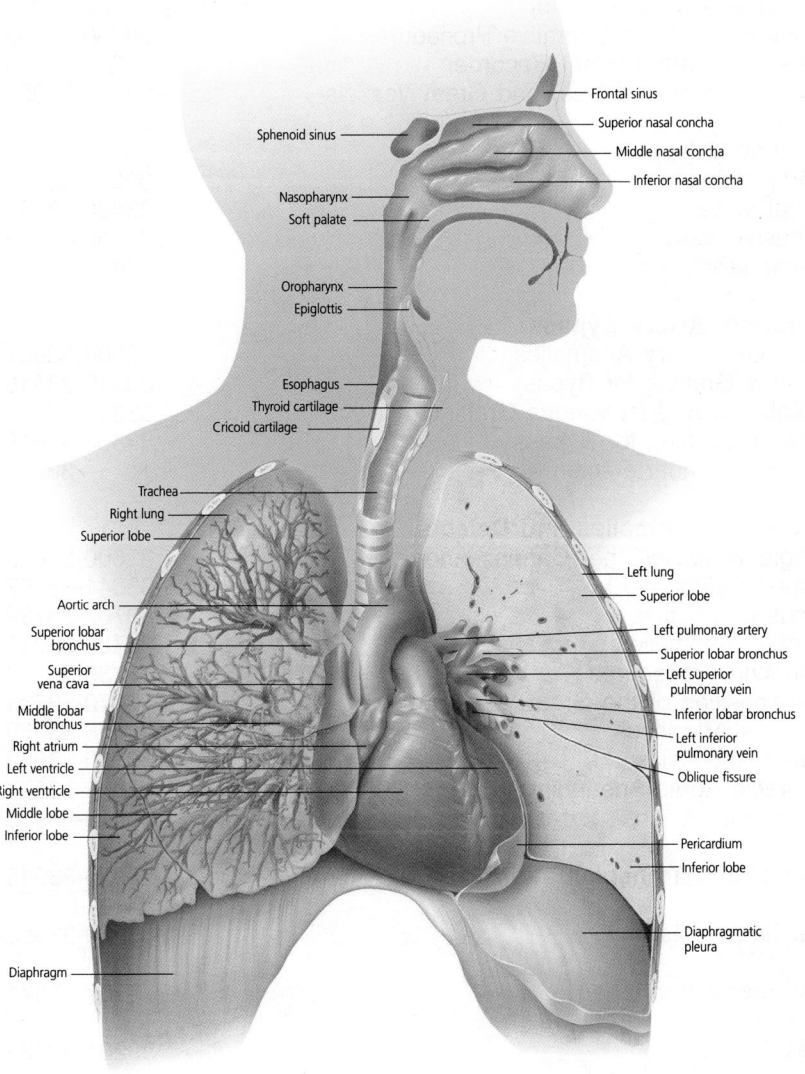

Frontal sinus
Superior nasal concha
Sphenoid sinus
Middle nasal concha
Inferior nasal concha
Nasopharynx
Soft palate
Oropharynx
Epiglottis
Esophagus
Thyroid cartilage
Cricoid cartilage
Trachea
Right lung
Superior lobe
Left lung
Superior lobe
Aortic arch
Left pulmonary artery
Superior lobar bronchus
Superior lobar bronchus
Superior vena cava
Left superior pulmonary vein
Middle lobar bronchus
Inferior lobar bronchus
Right atrium
Left inferior pulmonary vein
Left ventricle
Oblique fissure
Right ventricle
Middle lobe
Inferior lobe
Pericardium
Inferior lobe
Diaphragmatic pleura
Diaphragm

117

PLATE 14. HEART AND PERICARDIUM

General
Pericardium	33010-33050
Cardiac Tumor	33120-33130
Pacemaker or Defibrillator	33202-33249
Electrophysiologic Operative Procedures	33250-33266
Patient Activated Event Recorder	33282-33284
Heart (Including Valves) and Great Vessels	33300-33335

Cardiac Valves
Aortic Valve	33361-33417
Mitral Valve	33420-33430
Tricuspid Valve	33460-33468
Pulmonary Valve	33470-33478

Coronary Artery Bypass
Coronary Artery Anomalies	33500-33507
Venous Grafting for Bypass	33510-33516
Combined Arterial-Venous Grafting	33517-33530
Arterial Grafting for Bypass	33533-33548
Coronary Endarterectomy	33572

Repair of Anomalies and Defects
Single Ventricle/Other Cardiac Anomalies	33600-33622
Septal Defect	33641-33697
Sinus of Valsalva	33702-33722
Venous Anomalies	33724-33732
Shunting Procedures	33735-33768
Transposition of the Great Vessels	33770-33783
Truncus Arteriosus	33786-33788
Aortic Anomalies	33800-33853
Thoracic Aortic Aneurysm	33860-33877
Pulmonary Artery	33910-33926

Heart/Lung Transplantation
33930-33945

Cardiac Assist
33960-33993

Radiology Services/Heart
75557-75574

E/M Services
99201-99499

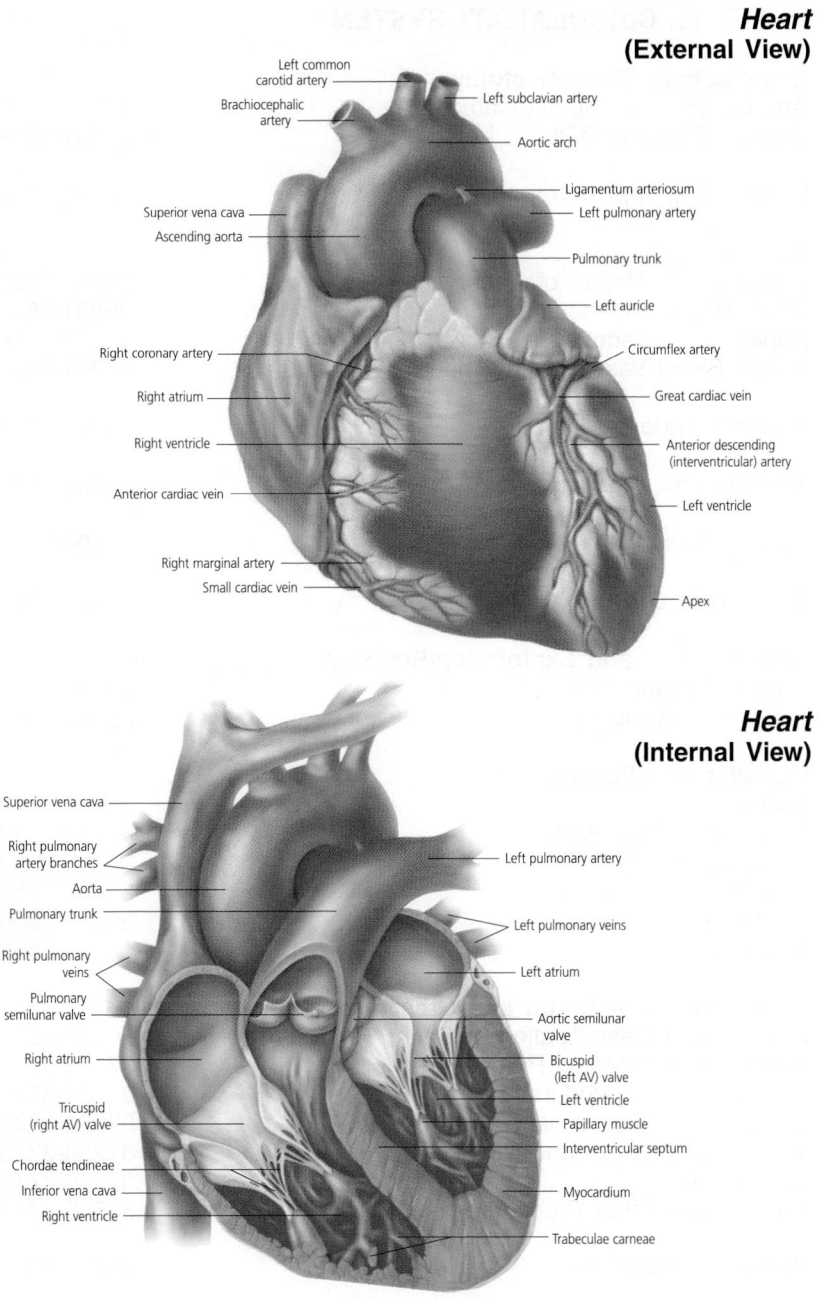

Heart
(External View)

Left common carotid artery
Brachiocephalic artery
Left subclavian artery
Aortic arch
Ligamentum arteriosum
Superior vena cava
Left pulmonary artery
Ascending aorta
Pulmonary trunk
Left auricle
Right coronary artery
Circumflex artery
Right atrium
Great cardiac vein
Right ventricle
Anterior descending (interventricular) artery
Anterior cardiac vein
Left ventricle
Right marginal artery
Small cardiac vein
Apex

Heart
(Internal View)

Superior vena cava
Right pulmonary artery branches
Left pulmonary artery
Aorta
Pulmonary trunk
Left pulmonary veins
Right pulmonary veins
Left atrium
Pulmonary semilunar valve
Aortic semilunar valve
Right atrium
Bicuspid (left AV) valve
Left ventricle
Tricuspid (right AV) valve
Papillary muscle
Interventricular septum
Chordae tendineae
Inferior vena cava
Myocardium
Right ventricle
Trabeculae carneae

119

PLATE 15. CIRCULATORY SYSTEM

Embolectomy/Thrombectomy
Arterial, With or Without Catheter	34001-34203
Venous, Direct or With Catheter	34401-34490

Venous Reconstruction 34501-34530

Repair
Endovascular Repair of Aneurysm	34800-34900
Direct Repair of Aneurysm	35001-35152
Repair Arteriovenous Fistula	35180-35190
Repair Blood Vessel Other Than for Fistula	35201-35286

Thromboendarterectomy 35301-35390

Transluminal Angioplasty 35450-35476

Bypass Graft 35500-35671

Composite Grafts 35681-35683

Transposition and Exploration/Revision
Arterial Transposition	35691-35697
Exploration/Revision	35700-35907

Vascular Injection Procedures
Intravenous	36000-36015
Intra-Arterial/Intra-Aortic	36100-36299
Venous	36400-36522
Central Venous Access	36555-36598
Arterial	36600-36660
Intraosseous	36680

Cannulization or Shunt and Other Procedures
Intervascular Cannulization or Shunt	36800-36870
Portal Decompression Procedures	37140-37183
Transcatheter Procedures	37184-37216
Endovascular Revascularization	37220-37235
Intravascular Ultrasound Services	37250-37251
Endoscopy	37500-37501
Ligation and Other Procedures	37565-37799

Radiology Services 75600-75989

E/M Services 99201-99499

Vascular System

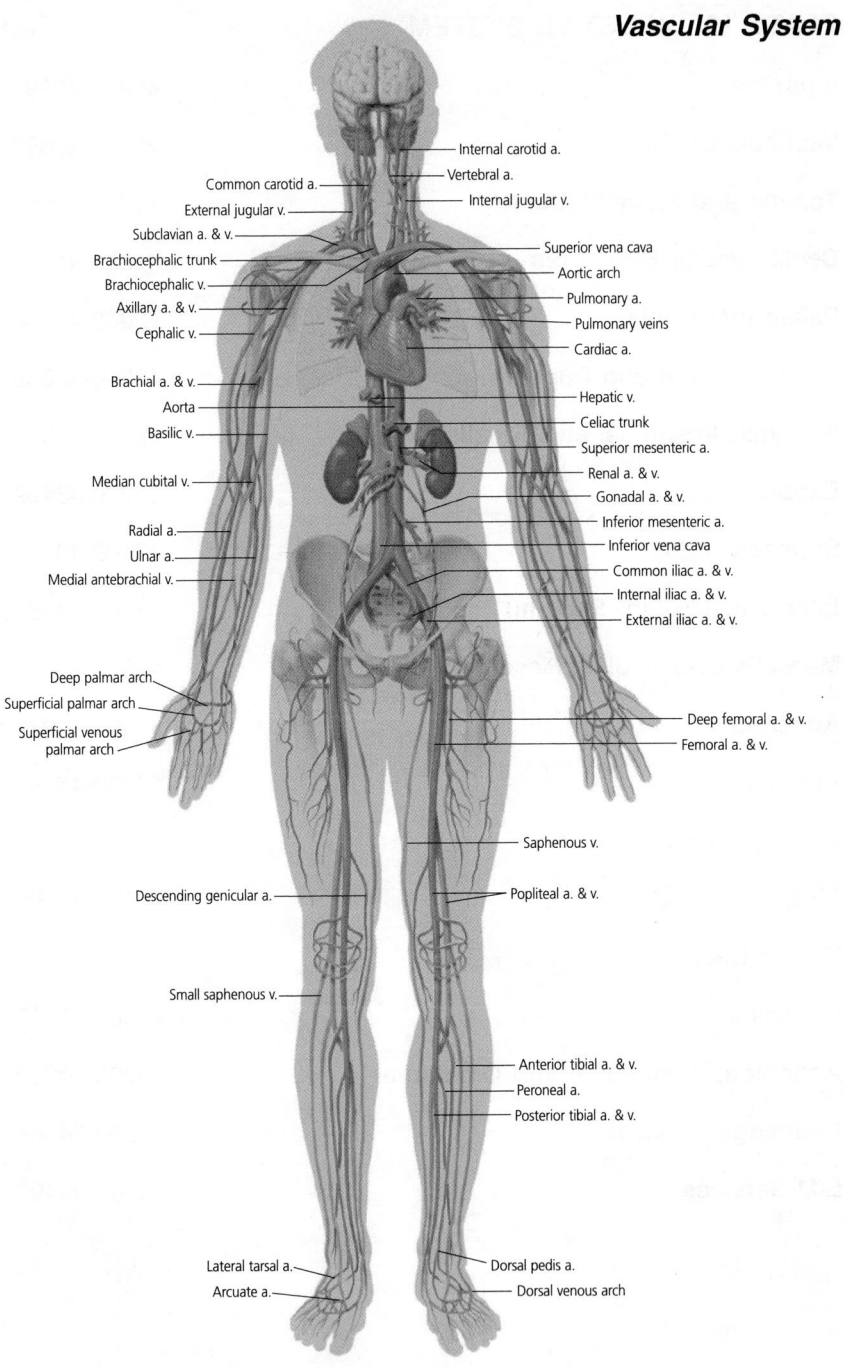

Internal carotid a.
Vertebral a.
Common carotid a.
Internal jugular v.
External jugular v.
Subclavian a. & v.
Superior vena cava
Brachiocephalic trunk
Aortic arch
Brachiocephalic v.
Pulmonary a.
Axillary a. & v.
Pulmonary veins
Cephalic v.
Cardiac a.
Brachial a. & v.
Hepatic v.
Aorta
Celiac trunk
Basilic v.
Superior mesenteric a.
Median cubital v.
Renal a. & v.
Gonadal a. & v.
Radial a.
Inferior mesenteric a.
Ulnar a.
Inferior vena cava
Medial antebrachial v.
Common iliac a. & v.
Internal iliac a. & v.
External iliac a. & v.
Deep palmar arch
Superficial palmar arch
Superficial venous palmar arch
Deep femoral a. & v.
Femoral a. & v.
Saphenous v.
Descending genicular a.
Popliteal a. & v.
Small saphenous v.
Anterior tibial a. & v.
Peroneal a.
Posterior tibial a. & v.
Lateral tarsal a.
Dorsal pedis a.
Arcuate a.
Dorsal venous arch

PLATE 16. DIGESTIVE SYSTEM

Lips	40490-40799
Vestibule of Mouth	40800-40899
Tongue and Floor of Mouth	41000-41599
Dentoalveolar Structures	41800-41899
Palate and Uvula	42000-42299
Salivary Gland and Ducts	42300-42699
Pharynx, Adenoids, and Tonsils	42700-42999
Esophagus	43020-43499
Stomach	43500-43999
Intestines (Except Rectum)	44005-44799
Meckel's Diverticulum/Mesentery	44800-44899
Appendix	44900-44979
Rectum	45000-45999
Anus	46020-46999
Liver	47000-47399
Biliary Tract	47400-47999
Pancreas	48000-48999
Abdomen, Peritoneum and Omentum	49000-49999
Radiology Services	74000-74363
E/M Services	99201-99499

Digestive System

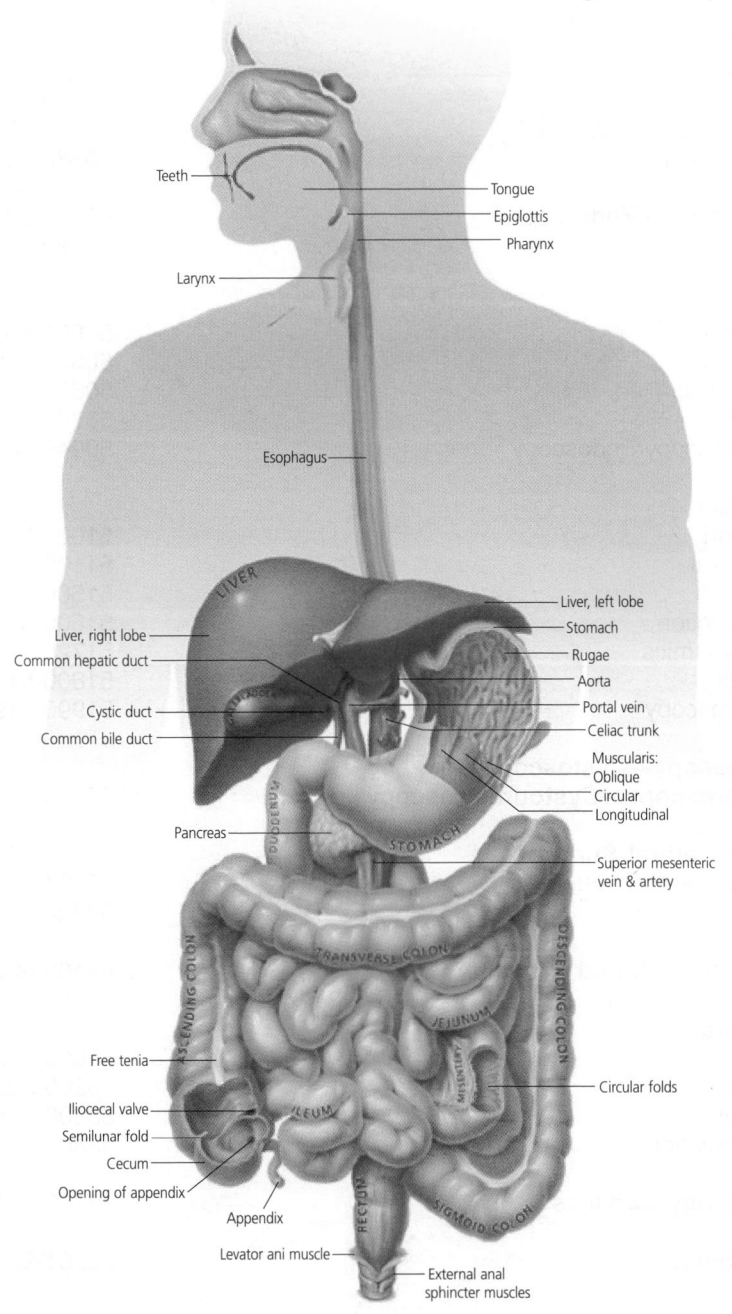

PLATE 17. GENITOURINARY SYSTEM

Kidney

Incision	50010-50135
Excision	50200-50290
Renal Transplantation	50300-50380
Introduction	50382-50398
Repair	50400-50540
Laparoscopy/Endoscopy	50541-50580
Other	50590-50593

Ureter

Incision	50600-50630
Excision	50650-50660
Introduction	50684-50690
Repair	50700-50940
Laparoscopy/Endoscopy	50945-50980

Bladder

Incision	51020-51080
Removal	51100-51102
Excision	51500-51597
Introduction	51600-51720
Urodynamics	51725-51798
Repair	51800-51980
Laparoscopy	51990-51999

**Endoscopy—Cystoscopy—
Urethroscopy—Cystourethroscopy**   52000-52010

Transurethral Surgery

Urethra and Bladder	52204-52318
Ureter and Pelvis	52320-52355

Vesical Neck and Prostate   52400-52700

Urethra

Incision	53000-53085
Excision	53200-53275
Repair	53400-53520
Manipulation	53600-53665

Radiology Services   74400-74485

E/M Services   99201-99499

Urinary System

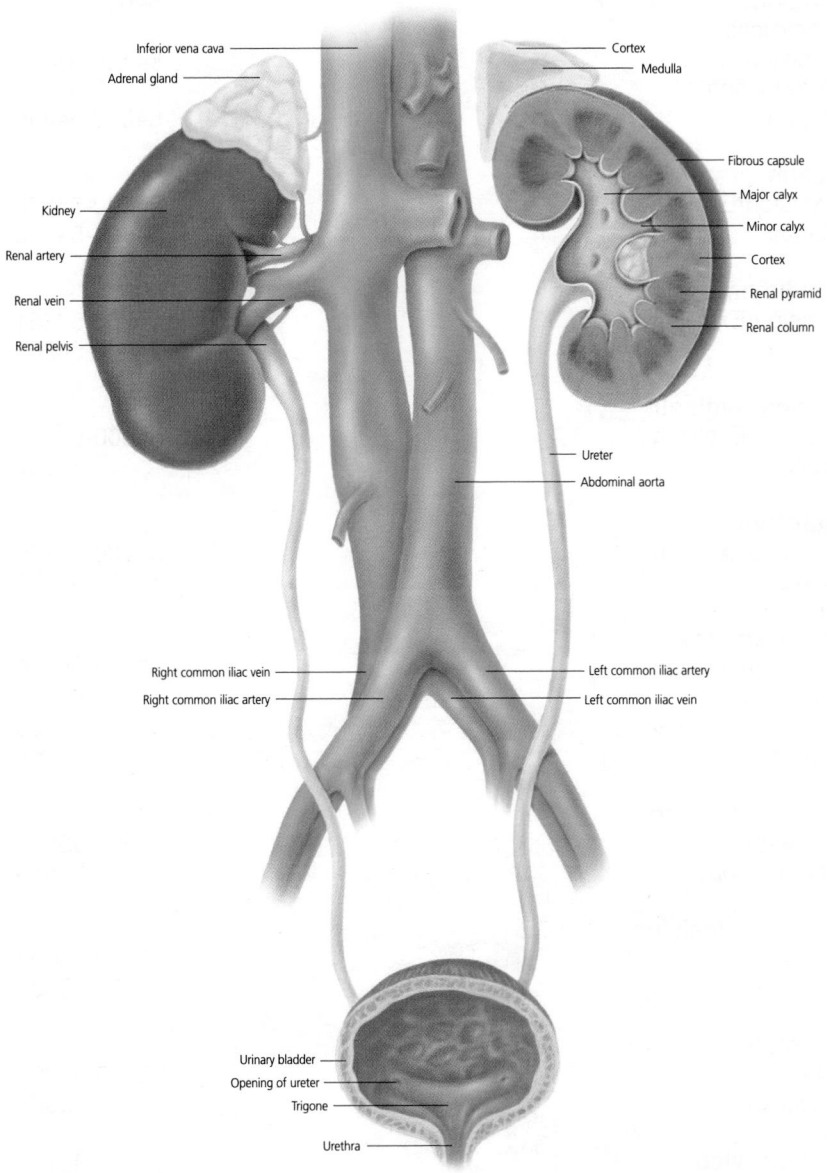

PLATE 18. MALE REPRODUCTIVE SYSTEM

Penis
Incision   54000-54015
Destruction   54050-54065
Excision   54100-54164
Introduction   54200-54250
Repair   54300-54440

Testis
Excision/Exploration   54500-54560
Repair   54600-54680

Epididymis
Incision/Excision   54700-54861
Repair   54900-54901

Tunica Vaginalis
Incision/Excision   55000-55041
Repair   55060

Scrotum
Incision/Excision   55100-55150
Repair   55175-55180

Vas Deferens
Incision/Excision   55200-55250
Introduction   55300
Repair   55400
Suture   55450

Spermatic Cord
Excision   55500-55540
Laparoscopy   55550-55559

Seminal Vesicles
Incision   55600-55605
Excision   55650-55680

Prostate
Incision   55700-55725
Excision   55801-55865

E/M Services   99201-99499

Male Reproductive System

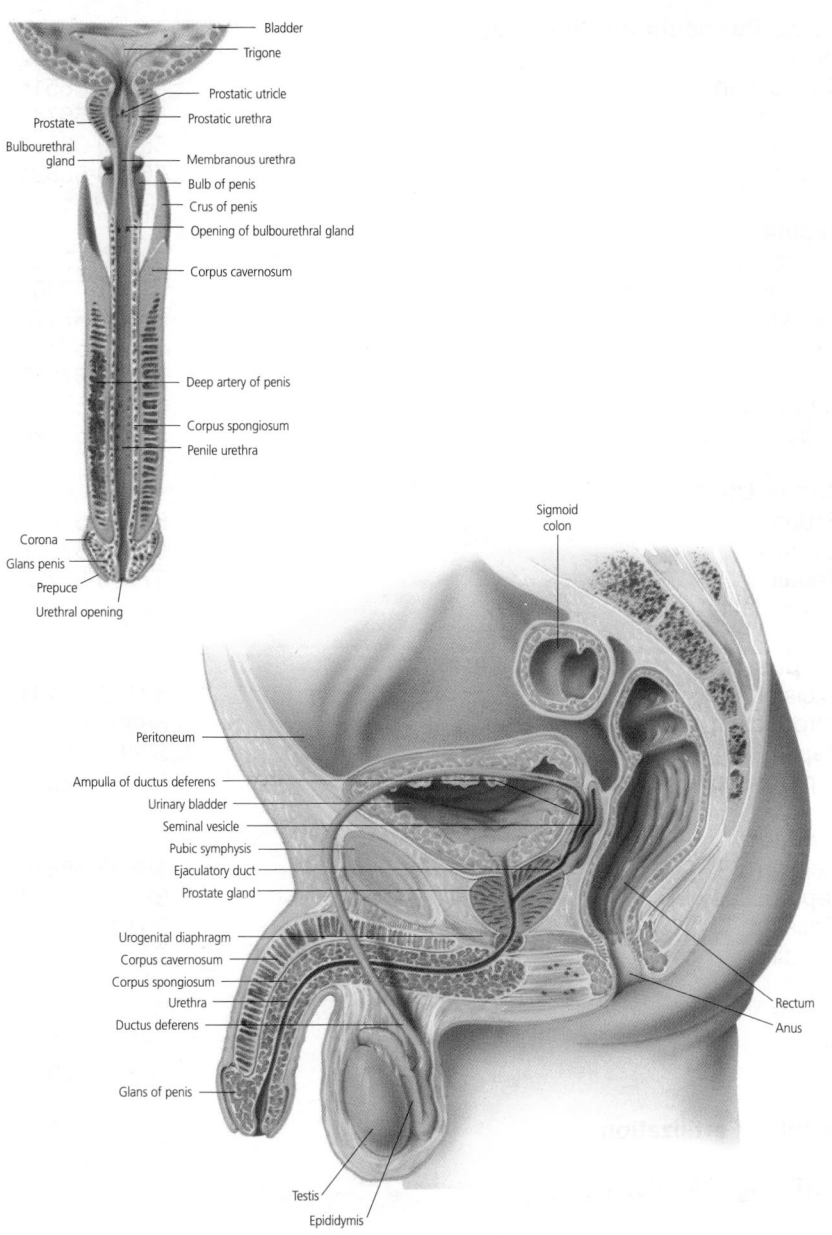

PLATE 19. FEMALE REPRODUCTIVE SYSTEM

Vulva, Perineum and Introitus

Incision	56405-56442
Destruction	56501-56515
Excision	56605-56740
Repair	56800-56810
Endoscopy	56820-56821

Vagina

Incision	57000-57023
Destruction	57061-57065
Excision	57100-57135
Introduction	57150-57180
Repair	57200-57335
Manipulation	57400-57415
Endoscopy/Laparoscopy	57420-57426

Cervix Uteri

Endoscopy	57452-57461
Excision	57500-57558
Repair	57700-57720
Manipulation	57800

Corpus Uteri

Excision	58100-58294
Introduction	58300-58356
Repair	58400-58540
Laparoscopy/Hysteroscopy	58541-58579

Oviduct

Incision	58600-58615
Laparoscopy	58660-58679
Excision	58700-58720
Repair	58740-58770

Ovary

Incision	58800-58825
Excision	58900-58960

In Vitro Fertilization   58970-58999

Radiology Services   74710-74775

E/M Services   99201-99499

Female Reproductive System

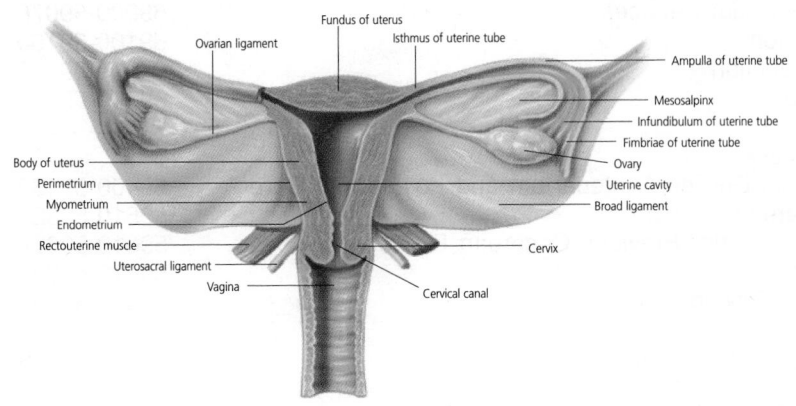

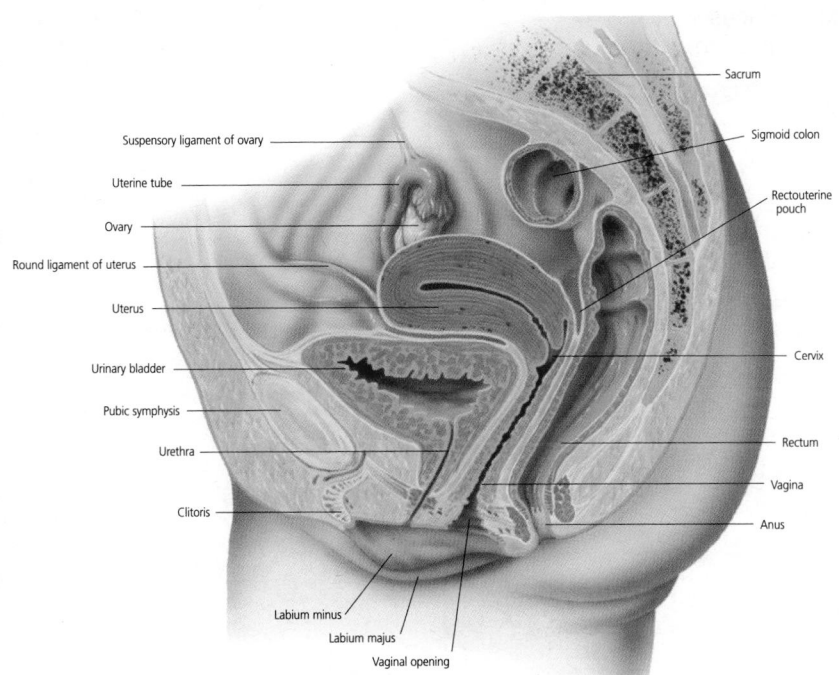

PLATE 20. PREGNANCY, CHILDBIRTH AND THE PUERPERIUM

Antepartum Services
Antepartum Services	59000-59076
Excision	59100-59160
Introduction	59200
Repair	59300-59350

Delivery
Vaginal Delivery, Antepartum and Postpartum Care	59400-59430
Cesarean Delivery	59510-59525
Delivery after Previous Cesarean Delivery	59610-59622
Abortion	59812-59857
Other Procedures	59866-59899

Radiology Services
74710-74775

E/M Services
E/M Services	99201-99499
Newborn Care	99460-99465

Female Reproductive System: Pregnancy
(Lateral View)

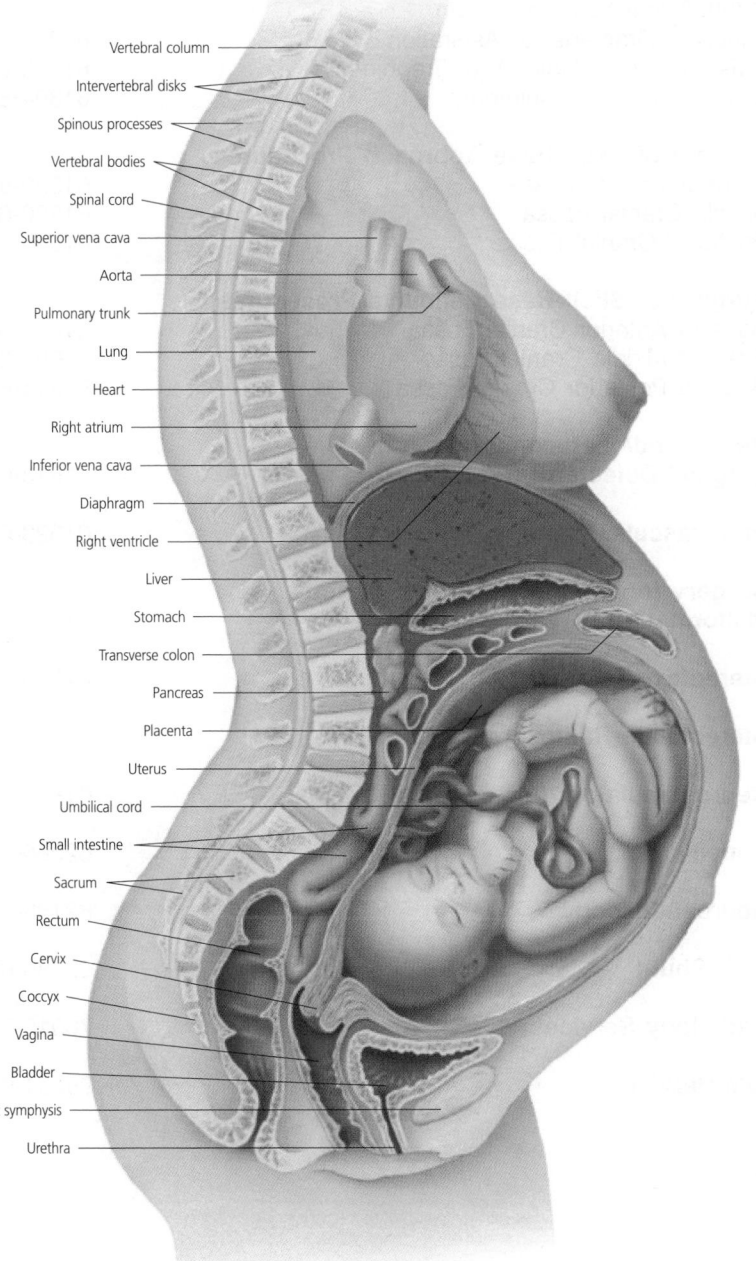

Vertebral column
Intervertebral disks
Spinous processes
Vertebral bodies
Spinal cord
Superior vena cava
Aorta
Pulmonary trunk
Lung
Heart
Right atrium
Inferior vena cava
Diaphragm
Right ventricle
Liver
Stomach
Transverse colon
Pancreas
Placenta
Uterus
Umbilical cord
Small intestine
Sacrum
Rectum
Cervix
Coccyx
Vagina
Bladder
Pubic symphysis
Urethra

PLATE 21. NERVOUS SYSTEM - BRAIN

Skull, Meninges, and Brain

Injection, Drainage, or Aspiration	61000-61070
Twist Drill, Burr Hole(s), or Trephine	61105-61253
Craniectomy or Craniotomy	61304-61576

Surgery of Skull Base Approach Procedures

Anterior Cranial Fossa	61580-61586
Middle Cranial Fossa	61590-61592
Posterior Cranial Fossa	61595-61598

Surgery of Skull Base Definitive Procedures

Base of Anterior Cranial Fossa	61600-61601
Base of Middle Cranial Fossa	61605-61613
Base of Posterior Cranial Fossa	61615-61616

Repair and/or Reconstruction of Surgical Defects of Skull Base	61618-61619
Endovascular Therapy	61623-61642
Surgery for Aneurysm, Arterio-Venous Malformation or Vascular Disease	61680-61711
Stereotaxis	61720-61791
Stereotactic Radiosurgery (Cranial)	61796-61800
Neurostimulators (Intra-Cranial)	61850-61888
Repair	62000-62148
Neuroendoscopy	62160-62165
CSF Shunt	62180-62258
Radiology Services	70010-70559
E/M Services	99201-99499

Brain
(Base View)

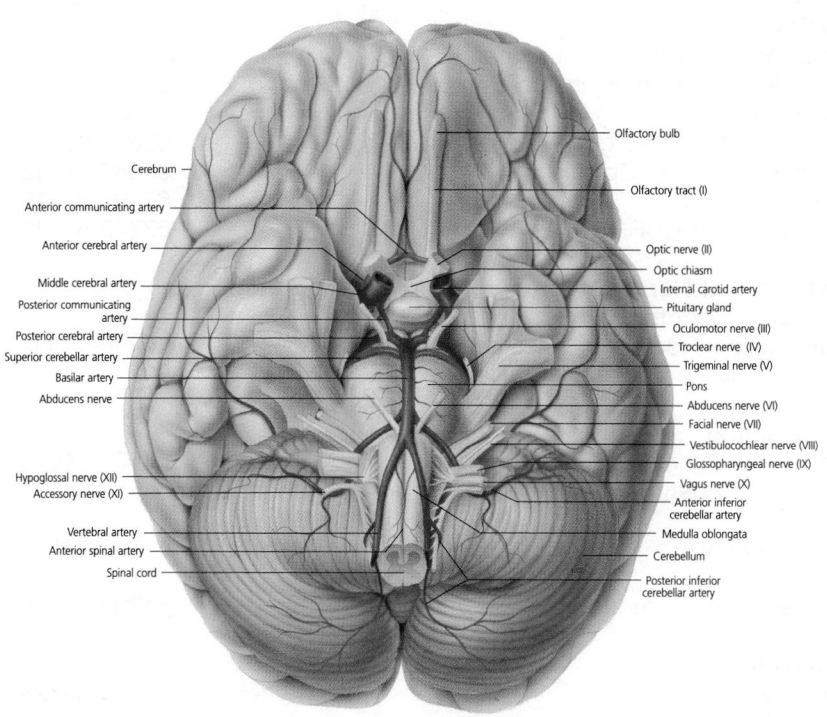

Olfactory bulb

Cerebrum

Anterior communicating artery

Anterior cerebral artery

Middle cerebral artery

Posterior communicating artery

Posterior cerebral artery

Superior cerebellar artery

Basilar artery

Abducens nerve

Hypoglossal nerve (XII)

Accessory nerve (XI)

Vertebral artery

Anterior spinal artery

Spinal cord

Olfactory tract (I)

Optic nerve (II)

Optic chiasm

Internal carotid artery

Pituitary gland

Oculomotor nerve (III)

Troclear nerve (IV)

Trigeminal nerve (V)

Pons

Abducens nerve (VI)

Facial nerve (VII)

Vestibulocochlear nerve (VIII)

Glossopharyngeal nerve (IX)

Vagus nerve (X)

Anterior inferior cerebellar artery

Medulla oblongata

Cerebellum

Posterior inferior cerebellar artery

133

PLATE 22. NERVOUS SYSTEM

Spine and Spinal Cord
Injection, Drainage or Aspiration	62263-62319
Catheter, Reservoir, Pump Implantation	62350-62370
Posterior Extradural Laminotomy or Laminectomy	63001-63051
Transpedicular or Costovertebral Approach	63055-63066
Anterior or Anterolateral Approach	63075-63091
Lateral Extracavitary Approach	63101-63103
Incision	63170-63200
Excision by Laminectomy of Lesion	63250-63295
Excision, Anterior or Anterolateral Approach Intraspinal Lesion	63300-63308
Stereotaxis	63600-63615
Sterotactic Radiosurgery (Spinal)	63620-63621
Neurostimulators (Spinal)	63650-63688
Repair	63700-63710
Shunt, Spinal CSF	63740-63746

Extracranial Nerves, Peripheral Nerves and Autonomic Nervous System
Introduction/Injection of Anesthetic Agent	64400-64530
Neurostimulators (Peripheral Nerve)	64550-64595

Destruction
Neurolytic Agent — Somatic Nerves	64600-64640
Neurolytic Agent — Sympathetic Nerves	64650-64681

Neuroplasty
64702-64727

Transection or Avulsion
64732-64772

Excision
Somatic Nerves	64774-64795
Sympathetic Nerves	64802-64823

Neurorrhaphy
Without Nerve Graft	64831-64876
With Nerve Graft	64885-64911

E/M Services
99201-99499

Nervous System

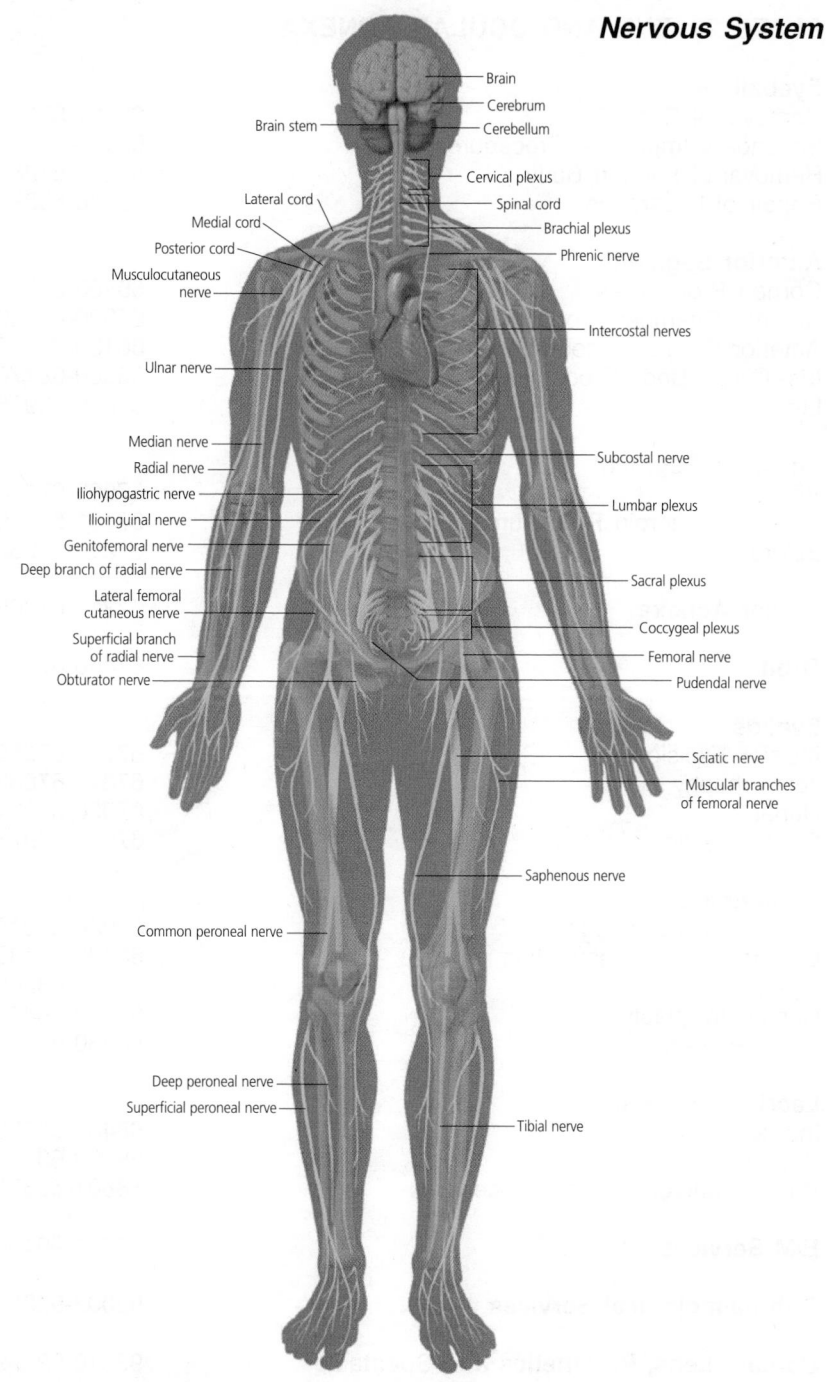

- Brain
- Cerebrum
- Cerebellum
- Brain stem
- Cervical plexus
- Lateral cord
- Spinal cord
- Medial cord
- Brachial plexus
- Posterior cord
- Phrenic nerve
- Musculocutaneous nerve
- Intercostal nerves
- Ulnar nerve
- Median nerve
- Subcostal nerve
- Radial nerve
- Iliohypogastric nerve
- Lumbar plexus
- Ilioinguinal nerve
- Genitofemoral nerve
- Deep branch of radial nerve
- Sacral plexus
- Lateral femoral cutaneous nerve
- Coccygeal plexus
- Superficial branch of radial nerve
- Femoral nerve
- Obturator nerve
- Pudendal nerve
- Sciatic nerve
- Muscular branches of femoral nerve
- Saphenous nerve
- Common peroneal nerve
- Deep peroneal nerve
- Superficial peroneal nerve
- Tibial nerve

135

PLATE 23. EYE AND OCULAR ADNEXA

Eyeball
Removal of Eye 65091-65114
Secondary Implant(s) Procedures 65125-65175
Removal of Foreign Body 65205-65265
Repair of Laceration 65270-65290

Anterior Segment
Cornea Procedures 65400-65782
Anterior Chamber Procedures 65800-66030
Anterior Sclera Procedures 66130-66250
Iris, Ciliary Body Procedures 66500-66770
Lens Procedures 66820-66986

Posterior Segment
Vitreous 67005-67043
Retina or Choroid Procedures 67101-67229
Sclera 67250-67255

Ocular Adnexa 67311-67399

Orbit 67400-67599

Eyelids
Incision/Excision 67700-67850
Tarsorrhaphy 67875-67882
Repair 67900-67924
Reconstruction 67930-67975

Conjunctiva
Incision and Drainage 68020-68040
Excision and/or Destruction 68100-68135
Injection 68200
Conjunctivoplasty 68320-68340
Other Procedures 68360-68399

Lacrimal System
Incision/Excision 68400-68550
Repair 68700-68770
Probing and/or Related Procedures 68801-68850

E/M Services 99201-99499

Ophthalmological Services 92002-92287

Contact Lens, Prosthetics and Spectacles .. 92310-92499

Right Eye
(Horizontal Section)

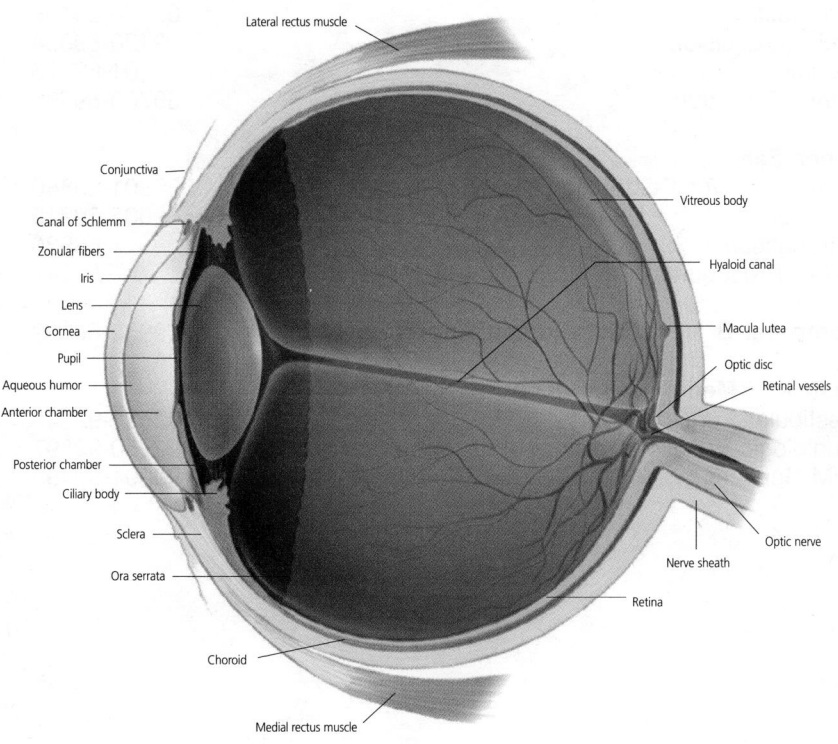

Lateral rectus muscle

Conjunctiva

Canal of Schlemm

Zonular fibers

Iris

Lens

Cornea

Pupil

Aqueous humor

Anterior chamber

Posterior chamber

Ciliary body

Sclera

Ora serrata

Choroid

Medial rectus muscle

Vitreous body

Hyaloid canal

Macula lutea

Optic disc

Retinal vessels

Optic nerve

Nerve sheath

Retina

PLATE 24. AUDITORY SYSTEM

External Ear

Incision	69000-69090
Excision	69100-69155
Removal of Foreign Body	69200-69222
Repair	69300-69320
Other Procedures	69399

Middle Ear

Introduction	69400-69405
Incision/Excision	69420-69554
Repair	69601-69676
Other Procedures	69700-69799

Inner Ear

Incision and/or Destruction	69801-69840
Excision	69905-69915
Introduction	69930
Other Procedures	69949

Temporal Bone, Middle Fossa Approach	69950-69979

Visit and Medicine Services

Vestibular Function Tests	92531-92548
Audiologic Function Tests	92550-92597
E/M Services	99201-99499

The Ear

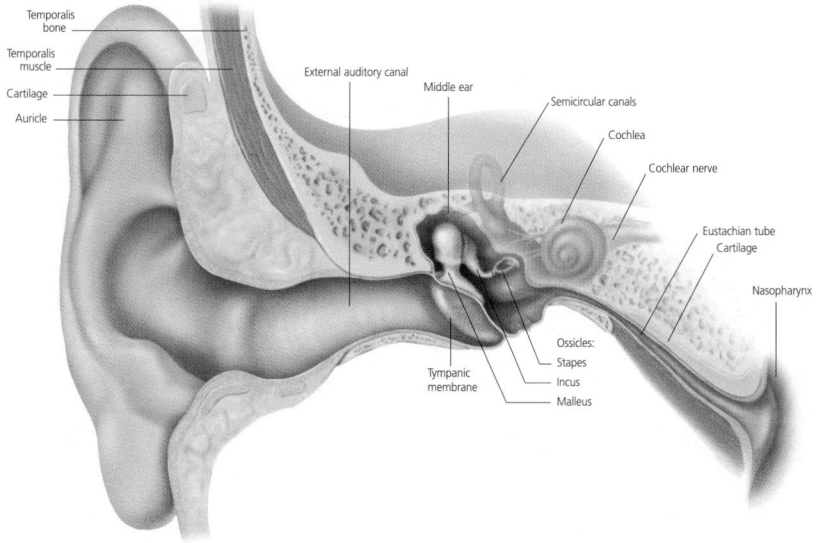

Temporalis bone
Temporalis muscle
Cartilage
Auricle
External auditory canal
Middle ear
Semicircular canals
Cochlea
Cochlear nerve
Eustachian tube
Cartilage
Nasopharynx
Ossicles:
Stapes
Incus
Malleus
Tympanic membrane

This page intentionally left blank.

EVALUATION & MANAGEMENT GUIDELINES

EVALUATION AND MANAGEMENT (E/M) SERVICES OVERVIEW

The first section of the CPT coding system is the evaluation and management (E/M) section, which includes procedure codes for visits and special care services. Within each subsection, the CPT codes are arranged first by patient category, then by the level of service.

The evaluation and management section of the CPT coding system includes codes for reporting visits, consultations, prolonged service, case management services, preventive medicine services, newborn care, and special services. The section is divided into categories such as office visits, hospital visits and consultations. Most of the categories are further divided into two or more subcategories.

The subcategories for evaluation and management services are further classified into levels of service that are identified by specific codes. The level of service classification is important because the physician work required to provide the service varies by the type of service, the place of service, and the patient's clinical status.

The basic format of the evaluation and management service codes and definitions is the same for most categories.

- *A unique five-digit CPT code number is listed*

- *The place and/or type of service is specified, for example "office consultation"*

- *The content of the service is defined, eg. "comprehensive history and comprehensive examination"*

- *The nature of the presenting problem(s) usually associated with a given level is described.*

- *The time typically required to provide the service is specified.*

EVALUATION AND MANAGEMENT SERVICES SUBSECTIONS

The Evaluation and Management section of the CPT book is divided into the following subsections:

Office or Other Outpatient Services	
New Patient	99201-99205
Established Patient	99211-99215
Hospital Observation Services	
Observation Discharge Services	99217
Initial Observation Care	99218-99220
Susbequent Observation Care	99224-99226
Hosptial Inpatient Services	
Initial Hospital Care	99221-99223
Subsequent Hosptial Care	99231-99233
Observation or Inpatient Care (including admission and discharge)	99234-99236
Hosptial Discharge Services	99238-99239
Consultations	
Office or Other Outpatient Consultations	99241-99245
Inpatient Consultation	99251-99255
Emergency Department Services	99281-99288
Critical Care Services, Adult	99291-99292
Nursing Facility Services	
Initial Nursing Facility Care	99304-99306
Subsequent Nursing Facility Care	99307-99310
Nursing Facility Discharge Services	99315-99316
Other Nursing Facility Services	99318
Domiciliary, Rest Home, or Custodial Care Services	
New Patient	99324-99328
Established Patient	99334-99337
Domiciliary, Rest Home, or Home Care Plan Oversight	99339-99340
Home Services	
New Patient	99341-99345
Established Patient	99347-99350
Prolonged Services	
With Direct Patient Contact	99354-99357
Without Direct Patient Contact	99358-99359
Standby Services	99360
Case Management Services	
Anticoagulent Management	99363-99364
Medical Team Conferences	99366-99368
Care Plan Oversight Services	99374-99380
Preventive Medicine Services	
New Patient	99381-99387
Established Patient	99391-99397

Individual Counseling	99401-99404
Behavior Change Intervention	99406-99409
Group Counseling	99411-99412
Other	99420-99429
Non Face-to-Face Physician Services	
Telephone Services	99441-99443
Online Medical Evaluation	99444
Special Evaluation and Management Services	99450-99456
Newborn Care	99460-99463
Delivery/Birthing Room Attendance	99464-99465
Inpatient Neonatal Intensive Care Services and Pediatric and Neonatal Critical Care Services	
Pediatric Critical Care Patient Transport	99466-99467, 99485-99486
Inpatient Neonatal and Pediatric Critical Care	99468-99476
Initial and Continuing Intensive Care Services	99477-99480
Complex Chronic Care Coordination Services	99487-99489
Transitional Care Management Services	99495-99496
Other Evaluation and Management Services	99499

All of these subsections have extensive notes that should be reviewed carefully prior to selecting codes for services located within the section.

CLASSIFICATION OF EVALUATION AND MANAGEMENT SERVICES

The E/M section is divided into broad categories such as office visits, hospital visits, and consultations. Most of the categories are further divided into two or more subcategories of E/M services. For example, there are two subcategories of office visits (new patient and established patient) and there are two subcategories of hospital visits (initial and subsequent). The subcategories of E/M services are further classified into levels of E/M services that are identified by specific codes. This classification is important because the nature of work varies by type of service, place of service, and the patient's status.

The basic format of the levels of evaluation and management services is the same for most categories. First, a unique code number is listed. Second, the place and/or type of service is specified, eg, office consultation. Third, the content of the service is defined, eg, comprehensive history and comprehensive examination. Fourth, the nature of the presenting problem(s) usually associated with a given level is described. Fifth, the time typically required to provide the service is specified.

DEFINITIONS OF COMMONLY USED TERMS

Certain key words and phrases are used throughout the Evaluation and Management section. The following definitions are intended to reduce the potential for differing interpretations and to increase the consistency of reporting by physicians in differing specialties. E/M services may also be reported by other qualified health care professionals who are authorized to perform such services within the scope of their practice.

NEW AND ESTABLISHED PATIENTS

Solely for the purposes of distinguishing between new and established patients, professional services are those face-to-face services rendered by physicians and other qualified health care professionals who may report evaluation and management services reported by a specific CPT code(s). A new patient is one who has not received any professional services from the physician/qualified health care professional or another physician/qualified health care professional of the exact same specialty and subspecialty who belongs to the same group practice, within the past three years.

An established patient is one who has received professional services from the physician/qualified health care professional or another physician/qualified health care professional of the exact same specialty and subspecialty who belongs to the same group practice, within the past three years. See Decision Tree.

In the instance where a physician/qualified health care professional is on call for or covering for another physician/qualified health care professional, the patient's encounter will be classified as it would have been by the physician/qualified health care professional who is not available. When advanced practice nurses and physician assistants are working with physicians, they are considered as working in the exact same specialty and exact same subspecialties as the physician

No distinction is made between new and established patients in the emergency department. Evaluation and Management services in the emergency department category may be coded for any new or established patient who presents for treatment in the emergency department.

The decision tree on the next page is provided to aid in determining whether to report the E/M service provided as a new or as an established patient encounter.

CHIEF COMPLAINT

A chief complaint is a concise statement describing the symptom, problem, condition, diagnosis or other factor that is the reason for the encounter, usually stated in the patient's words.

Decision Tree for New vs Established Patients

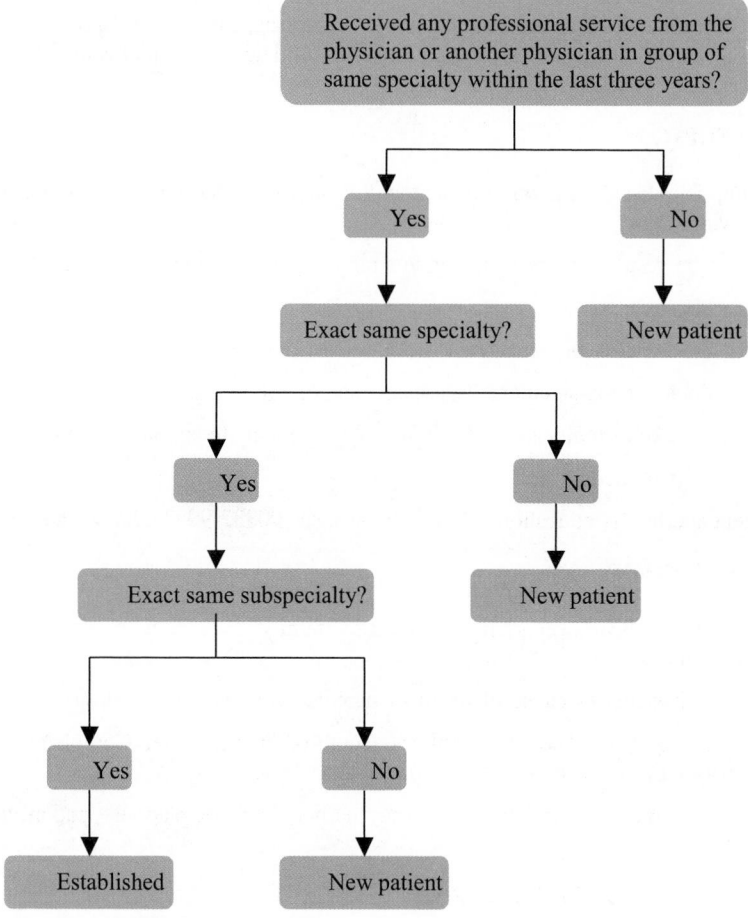

CONCURRENT CARE AND TRANSFER OF CARE

Concurrent care is the provision of similar services (eg, hospital visits) to the same patient by more than one physician or other qualified health care professional on the same day. When concurrent care is provided, no special reporting is required. Transfer of care is the process whereby a physician or other qualified health care professional who is providing management for some or all of a patient's problems relinquishes this responsibility to another physician or other qualified health care professional who explicitly agrees to accept this responsibility and who, from the initial encounter, is not providing consultative services. The physician or other qualified health care professional transferring care is then no longer providing care for these problems though he or she may continue providing care for other conditions when appropriate. Consultation codes should not be reported by the physician or other qualified health care professional who has agreed to accept transfer of care before an initial evaluation but are appropriate to report if the decision to accept transfer of care cannot be made until after the initial consultation evaluation, regardless of site of service.

COUNSELING

Counseling is a discussion with a patient and/or family concerning one or more of the following areas:

- Diagnostic results, impressions, and/or recommended diagnostic studies;
- Prognosis;
- Risks and benefits of management (treatment) options;
- Instructions for management (treatment) and/or follow-up;
- Importance of compliance with chosen management (treatment) options;
- Risk factor reduction; and
- Patient and family education. (Psychotherapy, see 90832-90834,90836-90840)

FAMILY HISTORY

A review of medical events in the patient's family that includes significant information about:

- The health status or cause of death of parents, siblings, and children;
- Specific diseases related to problems identified in the Chief Complaint or History of the Present Illness, and/or System Review;
- Discases of family members which may be hereditary or place the patient at risk.

HISTORY OF PRESENT ILLNESS

A chronological description of the development of the patient's present illness from the first sign and/or symptom to the present. This includes a description of location, quality, severity, timing, context, modifying factors and associated signs and symptoms significantly related to the presenting problem(s).

LEVELS OF EVALUATION AND MANAGEMENT SERVICES

Within each category or subcategory of evaluation and management service, there are three to five levels of evaluation and management services available for reporting purposes. Levels of evaluation and management services are **not** interchangeable among the different categories or subcategories of service. For example, the first level of evaluation and management services in the subcategory of office visit, new patient, does not have the same definition as the first level of evaluation and management services in the subcategory of office visit, established patient.

The levels of E/M services encompass the wide variations in skill, effort, time, responsibility, and medical knowledge required for the prevention or diagnosis and treatment of illness or injury and the promotion of optimal health. Each level of E/M services may be used by all physicians or other qualified health care professionals.

The descriptors for the levels of evaluation and management services recognize seven components, six of which are used in defining the levels of evaluation and management services. These components are:

- History;
- Examination;
- Medical decision making;
- Counseling;
- Coordination of care;
- Nature of presenting problem; and
- Ttime.

The first three of these components (history, examination, and medical decision making) are considered the **key** components in selecting a level of evaluation and management services. (See "Determine the Extent of History Obtained")

The next three components (counseling, coordination of care, and the nature of the presenting problem) are considered **contributory** factors in the majority of encounters. Although the first two of these contributory factors are important evaluation and management services, it is not required that these services be provided at every patient encounter.

Coordination of care with other physicians, other health care professionals, or agencies without a patient encounter on that day is coded using the case management codes.

The final component, time, is discussed in detail later in the chapter.

Any specifically identifiable procedure (ie, identified with a specific cpt code) performed on or subsequent to the date of initial or subsequent evaluation and management services should be reported separately.

The actual performance and/or interpretation of diagnostic tests/studies ordered during a patient encounter are not included in the levels of evaluation and management services. Physician performance of diagnostic tests/studies for which specific CPT codes are available may be reported separately, in addition to the appropriate evaluation and management code. The physician's interpretation of the results of diagnostic tests/studies (ie, professional component) with preparation of a separate distinctly identifiable signed written report may also be reported separately, using the appropriate CPT code with the modifier 26 appended.

The physician or other qualified health care professional may need to indicate that on the day a procedure or service identified by a CPT code was performed, the patient's condition required a significant separately identifiable E/M service above and beyond other services provided or beyond the usual preservice and postservice care associated with the procedure that was performed. The E/M service may be caused or prompted by the symptoms or condition for which the procedure and/or service was provided. This circumstance may be reported by adding modifier 25 to the appropriate level of E/M service. As such, different diagnoses are not required for reporting of the procedure and the E/M services on the same date.

NATURE OF PRESENTING PROBLEM

A presenting problem is a disease, condition, illness, injury, symptom, sign, finding, complaint, or other reason for encounter, with or without a diagnosis being established at the time of the encounter. The evaluation and management codes recognize five types of presenting problems that are defined as follows:

Minimal: a problem that may not require the presence of the physician or other qualified health care professional, but service is provided under the physician's or other qualified health care professional's supervision.

Self-limited or minor: a problem that runs a definite and prescribed course, is transient in nature, and is not likely to permanently alter health status OR has a good prognosis with management/compliance.

Low severity: a problem where the risk of morbidity without treatment is low; there is little to no risk of mortality without treatment; full recovery without functional impairment is expected.

Moderate severity: a problem where the risk of morbidity without treatment is moderate; there is moderate risk of mortality without treatment; uncertain prognosis OR increased probability of prolonged functional impairment.

High severity: a problem where the risk of morbidity without treatment is high to extreme; there is a moderate to high risk of mortality without treatment OR high probability of severe, prolonged functional impairment.

PAST HISTORY

A review of the patient's past experiences with illnesses, injuries, and treatments that includes significant information about:

- prior major illnesses and injuries;
- prior operations;

- prior hospitalizations;
- current medications;
- allergies (eg, drug, food);
- age appropriate immunization status;
- age appropriate feeding/dietary status.

SOCIAL HISTORY

An age appropriate review of past and current activities that includes significant information about:

- marital status and/or living arrangements;
- current employment;
- occupational history;
- use of drugs, alcohol, and tobacco;
- level of education;
- sexual history;
- other relevant social factors

SYSTEM REVIEW (REVIEW OF SYSTEMS)

An inventory of body systems obtained through a series of questions seeking to identify signs and/or symptoms that the patient may be experiencing or has experienced. For the purposes of the CPT codebook, the following elements of a system review have been identified:

- Constitutional symptoms (fever, weight loss, etc.)
- Eyes
- Ears, nose, mouth, throat
- Cardiovascular
- Respiratory
- Gastrointestinal
- Genitourinary
- Musculoskeletal
- Integumentary (skin and/or breast)
- Neurological
- Psychiatric
- Endocrine
- Hematologic/lymphatic

- Allergic/immunologic

The review of systems helps define the problem, clarify the differential diagnosis, identify needed testing, or serves as baseline data on other systems that might be affected by any possible management options.

TIME

The inclusion of time in the definitions of levels of E/M services has been implicit in prior editions of the CPT codebook. The inclusion of time as an explicit factor beginning in CPT 1992 is done to assist in selecting the most appropriate level of E/M services. It should be recognized that the specific times expressed in the visit ode descriptors are averages and, therefore, represent a range of times that may be higher or lower depending on actual clinical circumstances.

Time is **not** a descriptive component for the emergency department levels of E/M services because emergency department services are typically provided on a variable intensity basis, often involving multiple encounters with several patients over an extended period of time.Therefore, it is often difficult to provide accurate estimates of the time spent face-to-face with the patient.

Studies to establish levels of E/M services employed surveys of practicing physicians to obtain data on the amount of time and work associated with typical E/M services. Since "work" is not easily quantifiable, the codes must rely on other objective, verifiable measures that correlate with physicians' estimates of their "work." It has been demonstrated that estimations of **intraservice** time (as explained on the next page), both within and across specialties, is a variable that is predictive of the "work" of E/M services. This same research has shown there is a strong relationship between intraservice time and total time for E/M services. Intraservice time, rather than total time, was chosen for inclusion with the codes because of its relative ease of measurement and because of its direct correlation with measurements of the total amount of time and work associated with typical E/M services.

Intraservice times are defined as **face-to-face** time for office and other outpatient visits and as **unit/floor** time for hospital and other inpatient visits. This distinction is necessary because most of the work of typical office visits takes place during the face-to-face time with the patient, while most of the work of typical hospital visits takes place during the time spent on the patient's floor or unit. When prolonged time occurs in either the office or the inpatient areas, the appropriate add-on code should be reported.

Face-to-face time (office and other outpatient visits and office consultations): for coding purposes, face-to-face time for these services is defined as only that time spent face-to-face with the patient and/or family. This includes the time performing such tasks as obtaining a history, performing an examination, and counseling the patient.

Time is also spent doing work before or after the face-to-face time with the patient, performing such tasks as reviewing records and tests, arranging for further services, and communicating further with other professionals and the patient through written reports and telephone contact.

This **non-face-to-face** time for office services—also called pre- and post-encounter time—is not included in the time component described in the evaluation and management codes. However, the pre- and post-non-face-to-face work associated with an encounter was included in calculating the total work of typical services in physician surveys. Thus, the face-to-face time associated with the services described by any evaluation and management code is a valid proxy for the total work done before, during, and after the visit.

Unit/floor time (hospital observation services, inpatient hospital care, initial inpatient hospital consultations, nursing facility): for reporting purposes, intraservice time for these services is defined as unit/floor time, which includes the time present on the patient's hospital unit and at the bedside rendering services for that patient. This includes the time to establish and/or review the patient's chart, examine the patient, write notes, and communicate with other professionals and the patient's family.

In the hospital, pre- and post-time includes time spent off the patient's floor performing such tasks as reviewing pathology and radiology findings in another part of the hospital.

This pre- and post-visit time is not included in the time component described in these codes. However, the pre- and post-work performed during the time spent off the floor or unit was included in calculating the total work of typical services in physician surveys.

Thus, the unit/floor time associated with the services described by any code is a valid proxy for the total work done before, during, and after the visit.

UNLISTED SERVICE

An evaluation and management service may be provided that is not listed in this section of CPT. When reporting such a service, the appropriate "Unlisted" code may be used to indicate the service, identifying it by "Special Report", as discussed in the following paragraph. The "Unlisted Services" and accompanying codes for the evaluation and management section are as follows:

99429   Unlisted preventive medicine service
99499   Unlisted evaluation and management service

SPECIAL REPORT

An unlisted service or one that is unusual, variable, or new may require a special report demonstrating the medical appropriateness of the service. Pertinent information should include an adequate definition or description of the nature, extent, and need for the procedure; and the time, effort, and equipment necessary to provide the service. Additional items which may be included are complexity of symptoms, final diagnosis, pertinent physical findings, diagnostic and therapeutic procedures, concurrent problems, and follow-up care.

CLINICAL EXAMPLES

Clinical examples of the codes for E/M services are provided to assist in understanding the meaning of the descriptors and selecting the correct code. The clinical examples are listed in Appendix C of the AMA's book. Each example was developed by the specialties shown.

The same problem, when seen by different specialties, may involve different amounts of work. Therefore, the appropriate level of encounter should be reported using the descriptors rather than the examples.

HOW TO SELECT A LEVEL OF E/M SERVICE

IDENTIFY THE CATEGORY AND SUBCATEGORY OF SERVICE

The categories and subcategories of codes available for reporting evaluation and management services are shown in Table 1 below and continued on the next page.

Table 1: Categories and subcategories of service

Category/subcategory	Code Numbers
Office or other outpatient services	
New patient	99201-99205
Established patient	99211-99215
Hospital observation services	
Observation care discharge services	99217
Initial observation care services	99218-99220
Subsequent observation care	99224-99226
Hospital inpatient services	
Initial hospital care	99221-99223
Subsequent hospital care	99231-99233
Observation or inpatient care (including admission and discharge)	99234-99236
Hospital discharge services	99238-99239
Consultations	
Office or other outpatient consultations	99241-99245
Inpatient consultations	99251-99255
Emergency department services	99281-99288
Critical care services	
Adult (over 24 months of age)	99291-99292
Nursing facility services	
Initial nursing facility care	99304-99306
Subsequent nursing facility care	99307-99310
Nursing facility discharge services	99315-99316
Other nursing facility services	99318

Domiciliary, rest home or custodial care services
    New patient   99324-99328
    Established patient   99334-99337

Domiciliary, rest home or custodial care services	
New patient	99324-99328
Established patient	99334-99337
Domiciliary, rest home or home care plan oversight services	99339-99340
Home services	
New patient	99341-99345
Established patient	99347-99350
Prolonged services	
With direct patient contact	99354-99357
Without direct patient contact	99358-99359
Standby services	99360
Case management services	
Anticoagulant management	99363-99364
Medical team conferences	99366-99368
Care plan oversight services	99374-99380
Preventive medicine services	
New patient	99381-99387
Established patient	99391-99397
Individual counseling	99401-99404
Behavioral change	99406-99409
Group counseling	99411-99412
Other	99420-99429
Non-face-to-face physician services	
Telephone services	99441-99443
Online medical evaluation	99444
Special E/M Services	99450-99456
Newborn care	99460-99463
Delivery/birthing room attendance	99464-99465
Inpatient neonatal intensive care and pediatric and neonatal critical care services	
Pediatric critical care patient transport	99466-99467, 99485-99486
Inpatient neonatal and pediatric critical care	99468-99476
Initial and continuing intensive care services	99477-99480
Complex chronic care coordination services	99487-99489
Transitional care management services	99495-99496
Other E/M services	99499

REVIEW THE REPORTING INSTRUCTIONS FOR THE SELECTED CATEGORY OR SUBCATEGORY

Most of the categories and many of the subcategories of service have special guidelines or instructions unique to that category or subcategory. Where these are indicated, eg, "Inpatient Hospital Care," special instructions will be presented preceding the levels of evaluation and management services.

REVIEW THE LEVEL OF E/M SERVICE DESCRIPTORS AND EXAMPLES IN THE SELECTED CATEGORY OR SUBCATEGORY

The descriptors for the levels of evaluation and management services recognize seven components, six of which are used in defining the levels of evaluation and management services. These components are:

- history;

- examination;

- medical decision making;

- counseling;

- coordination of care;

- nature of presenting problem; and

- time.

The first three of these components (ie, history, examination, and medical decision making) should be considered the **key** components in selecting the level of evaluation and management services. An exception to this rule is in the case of visits which consist predominantly of counseling or coordination of care.

The nature of the presenting problem and time are provided in some levels to assist the physician in determining the appropriate level of E/M service.

DETERMINE THE EXTENT OF HISTORY OBTAINED

The extent of the history is dependent upon clinical judgment and on the nature of presenting problems(s). The levels of evaluation and management services recognize four types of history that are defined as follows:

Problem focused: chief complaint; brief history of present illness or problem.

Expanded problem focused: chief complaint; brief history of present illness; problem pertinent system review.

Detailed: chief complaint; extended history of present illness; problem pertinent system review extended to include a review of a limited number of additional systems; **pertinent** past, family, and/or social history **directly related to the patient's problems**.

Comprehensive: chief complaint; extended history of present illness; review of systems which is directly related to the problem(s) identified in the history of the present illness plus a review of all additional body systems; **complete** past, family, and social history.

The comprehensive history obtained as part of the preventive medicine evaluation and management service is not problem-oriented and does not involve a chief complaint or present illness. It does, however, include a comprehensive system review and comprehensive or interval past, family, and social history as well as a comprehensive assessment/history of pertinent risk factors.

DETERMINE THE EXTENT OF EXAMINATION PERFORMED

The extent of the examination performed is dependent on clinical judgment and on the nature of the presenting problem(s). The levels of evaluation and management services recognize four types of examination that are defined as follows:

Problem focused: a limited examination of the affected body area or organ system.

Expanded problem focused: a limited examination of the affected body area or organ system and other symptomatic or related organ system(s).

Detailed: an extended examination of the affected body area(s) and other symptomatic or related organ system(s).

Comprehensive: a general multi-system examination or a complete examination of a single organ system. **Note:** the comprehensive examination performed as part of the preventive medicine evaluation and management service is multisystem, but its extent is based on age and risk factors identified.

For the purposes of these CPT definitions, the following body areas are recognized:

- Head, including the face
- Neck
- Chest, including breasts and axilla
- Abdomen
- Genitalia, groin, buttocks
- Back
- Each extremity

For the purposes of these CPT definitions, the following organ systems are recognized:

- Eyes
- Ears, nose, mouth, and throat
- Cardiovascular
- Respiratory
- Gastrointestinal
- Genitourinary
- Musculoskeletal
- Skin
- Neurologic

155

- Psychiatric

- Hematologic/lymphatic/immunologic

DETERMINE COMPLEXITY OF MEDICAL DECISION MAKING

Medical decision making refers to the complexity of establishing a diagnosis and/or selecting a management option as measured by:

- the number of possible diagnoses and/or the number of management options that must be considered;

- the amount and/or complexity of medical records, diagnostic tests, and/or other information that must be obtained, reviewed, and analyzed; and

- the risk of significant complications, morbidity, and/or mortality, as well as comorbidities, associated with the patient's presenting problems(s), the diagnostic procedure(s) and/or the possible management options.

Four types of medical decision making are recognized: straightforward; low complexity; moderate complexity; and high complexity. To qualify for a given type of decision making, two of the three elements in Table 2 below must be met or exceeded.

Table 2: Complexity of Medical Decision Making

Number of diagnoses or management options	Amount and/or complexity of data to be reviewed	Risk of complications and/or morbidity or mortality	Type of decision making
Minimal	Minimal or none	Minimal	**Straightforward**
Limited	Limited	Low	**Low complexity**
Multiple	Moderate	Moderate	**Moderate complexity**
Extensive	Extensive	High	**High complexity**

Comorbidities/underlying diseases, in and of themselves, are not considered in selecting a level of evaluation and management services unless their presence significantly increases the complexity of the medical decision making.

SELECT THE APPROPRIATE LEVEL OF EVALUATION AND MANAGEMENT SERVICES BASED ON THE FOLLOWING

1. For the following categories/subcategories, **all of the key components**, (ie, history, examination, and medical decision making), must meet or exceed the stated requirements to qualify for a particular level of evaluation and management service: office, new patient; hospital observation services; initial hospital care; office consultations; initial inpatient consultations; emergency

department services; initial nursing facility care; domiciliary care, new patient; and home, new patient.

2. For the following categories/subcategories, **two of the three key components** (ie, history, examination, and medical decision making) must meet or exceed the stated requirements to qualify for a particular level of evaluation and management services: office, established patient; subsequent hospital care; subsequent nursing facility care; domiciliary care, established patient; and home, established patient.

3. When counseling and/or coordination of care dominates (more than 50%) the encounter with the patient and/or family (face-to-face time in the office or other outpatient setting or floor/unit time in the hospital or nursing facility), then **time** shall be considered the key or controlling factor to qualify for a particular level of E/M services. This includes time spent with parties who have assumed responsibility for the care of the patient or decision making whether or not they are family members (eg, foster parents, person acting in locum parentis, legal guardian). The extent of counseling and/or coordination of care must be documented in the medical record.

OTHER DEFINITIONS OF NATURE OF THE PRESENTING PROBLEM

In addition to the above five specific definitions found in the CPT coding system, there are other definitions found in the E.M Service codes used to report Subsequent Hospital Care and Follow-Up Inpatient Consultations. See Table 3 for these additional definitions.

DIAGNOSTIC TESTS OR STUDIES

The performance of diagnostic tests or studies for which specific CPT codes are available is not included in the levels of evaluation and management services. Any diagnostic tests or studies performed by the physician for which specific CPT codes are available should be coded separately, in addition to the appropriate evaluation and management service code.

Table 3: Other Definitions of Nature of Presenting Problems

Evaluation and Management Codes	Nature of Presenting Problem(s) Defined	Equivalent To
99231	Stable, recovering or improving	Self-limited or minor
99232	Inadequate response or minor complication	Low to moderate severity
99233	Significant complication or new problem	Moderate to high severity

EVALUATION AND MANAGEMENT SERVICES MODIFIERS

Evaluation and management services may be modified under certain circumstances. When applicable, the modifying circumstance should be identified by reporting the appropriate modifier code in addition to the basic service. Modifiers which may be used with evaluation and management service codes are:

-24 Unrelated evaluation and management service by the same physician during a postoperative period

-25 Significant, separately identifiable evaluation and management service by the same physician on the same day of the procedure or other service

-32 Mandated services

-52 Reduced services

-57 Decision for surgery

HOW TO CHOOSE EVALUATION AND MANAGEMENT CODE(S)

Choosing the correct evaluation and management service code to report is a nine step process. The most important steps, in terms of both reimbursement and audit liability, are verifying compliance and documentation.

1. Identify the Category of Service

Where was the patient seen and what category of services were provided?

- ☐ *Office or Other Outpatient Services*
- ☐ *Hospital Observation Services*
- ☐ *Hospital Inpatient Services*
- ☐ *Consultations*
- ☐ *Emergency Department Services*
- ☐ *Pediatric Patient Transport*
- ☐ *Critical Care Services*
- ☐ *Neonatal Intensive Care*
- ☐ *Nursing Facility Services*
- ☐ *Domiciliary, Rest Home or Custodial Care Services*
- ☐ *Home Services*
- ☐ *Prolonged Services*
- ☐ *Standby Services*
- ☐ *Case Management Services*

- ☐ *Care Plan Oversight Services*
- ☐ *Preventive Medicine Services*
- ☐ *Special or Other E/M Services*

2.   Identify the Subcategory of Service

Is the patient a new patient or established patient?
Is the service initial care, subsequent care or follow-up?

- ☐ *New Patient*
- ☐ *Established Patient*
- ☐ *Initial Care*
- ☐ *Subsequent Care*
- ☐ *Follow-up*

3.   Determine the Extent of History Obtained

What level of history was taken on this patient?

- ☐ *Problem Focused*
- ☐ *Expanded Problem Focused*
- ☐ *Detailed*
- ☐ *Comprehensive*

4.   Determine the Extent of Examination Performed

What level of physician examination was performed?

- ☐ *Problem Focused*
- ☐ *Expanded Problem Focused*
- ☐ *Detailed*
- ☐ *Comprehensive*

5.   Determine the Complexity of Medical Decision Making

What level of medical decision making was required?
- ☐ *Straightforward*
- ☐ *Low Complexity*
- ☐ *Moderate Complexity*
- ☐ *High Complexity*

6. **Record the Approximate Amount of Time**

How much time was spent either face-to-face with the patient for office visits and consults, or unit or floor time for hospital care, hospital consults, and nursing facilities?

If counseling and/or coordination of care exceeds 50 percent of the total face-to-face physician/patient encounter, then TIME is considered to be the key or controlling factor which qualifies the choice of a particular level of evaluation and management service. The extent of counseling and/or coordination of care must be documented in the medical record.

7. **Verify Compliance with Reporting Requirements**

All Three Key Components Required

To report services for new patients, initial care, office or confirmatory consultations, emergency department services, and comprehensive nursing facility assessments, all three key components must meet or exceed the stated requirements.

- ☐ *History component met or exceeded*
- ☐ *Examination component met or exceeded*
- ☐ *Medical decision making component met or exceeded*

Two of Three Key Components Required

To report services to established patients, subsequent or follow-up care, two of the three key components must meet or exceed the stated requirements.

- ☐ *History component met or exceeded; and/or*
- ☐ *Examination component met or exceeded; and/or*
- ☐ *Medical decision making component met or exceeded*

8. **Verify Documentation**

Make sure that the medical record includes proper documentation of the history, examination, medical decision making, the nature of the problem(s), the approximate amount of time, and when appropriate, the extent of counseling and/or coordination of care.

9. **Assign the Code**

The following is an example of the code selection process.

EXAMPLE OF THE CODE SELECTION PROCESS

1. Category of Service	*Office*
2. Subcategory	*New patient*
3. History	*Problem focused*
4. Examination	*Problem focused*
5. Medical Decision Making	*Straightforward*
6. Intra-service Time	*10 minutes*
7. Key Components	*Met or exceeded*
8. Documentation	*Met or exceeded*
9. Assign the Code	**99201**

EVALUATION AND MANAGEMENT SERVICES DOCUMENTATION GUIDELINES

Documentation in the medical record of all services provided is critical for reimbursement and audit liability. If the provider reported a service or procedure on the health insurance claim form but did not document it, or document it completely, in the patient's medical records, from the point of view of Medicare or private health insurance company auditors, the service was not performed, can't be reported, and therefore will not be paid for.

Millions of dollars are reclaimed from physicians and other medical professionals annually by Medicare and other third party payers because the medical record documentation does not support the services and procedures reported. Providers can protect their medical practices from audit liability by following the most current documentation guidelines published by CMS.

The following documentation guidelines for evaluation and management services were developed jointly by the American Medical Association (AMA) and CMS. The stated goal of CMS in publishing these guidelines is to provide physicians and health insurance claims reviewers with advice about preparing or reviewing documentation for evaluation and management services.

In developing and testing the validity of these guidelines, special emphasis was placed on assuring that they:

- *are consistent with the clinical descriptors and definitions contained in CPT,*

- *would be widely accepted by clinicians and minimize any changes in record-keeping practices; and*

- *would be interpreted and applied uniformly by users across the country.*

WHAT IS DOCUMENTATION AND WHY IS IT IMPORTANT?

Medical record documentation is required to record pertinent facts, findings, and observations about an individual's health history including past and present illnesses, examinations, tests, treatments, and outcomes. The medical record chronologically documents the care of the patient and is an important element contributing to high quality care. The medical record facilitates:

- *the ability of the physician and other medical professionals to evaluate and plan the patient's immediate treatment, and to monitor his/her health care over time;*

- *communication and continuity of care among physicians and other medical professionals involved in the patient's care;*

- *accurate and timely claims review and payment;*

- *appropriate utilization review and quality of care evaluations; and*

- *collection of data that may be useful for research and education.*

An appropriately documented medical record can reduce many of the hassles associated with claims processing and may serve as a legal document to verify the care provided, if necessary.

WHAT DO THIRD PARTY PAYERS WANT AND WHY?

Because payers have a contractual obligation to enrollees, they may require reasonable documentation that services are consistent with the insurance coverage provided. They may request information to validate:

- *the site of service;*

- *the medical necessity and appropriateness of the diagnostic and/or therapeutic services provided; and/or*

- *that services provided have been accurately reported.*

GENERAL PRINCIPLES OF MEDICAL RECORD DOCUMENTATION

The principles of documentation listed below are applicable to all types of medical and surgical services in all settings. For evaluation and management (E/M) services, the nature and amount of physician work and documentation varies by type of service, place of service and the patient's status. The general principles listed below may be modified to account for these variable circumstances in providing evaluation and management services.

1. *The medical record should be complete and legible.*

2. *The documentation of each patient encounter should include:*

    • *the reason for the encounter as well as relevant history, physical examination findings and prior diagnostic test results;*

    • *an assessment, clinical impression or diagnosis;*

    • *a plan for care; and*

    • *the date and legible identity of the observer.*

3. *If not documented, the rationale for ordering diagnostic and other ancillary services should be easily inferred.*

4. *Past and present diagnoses should be accessible to the treating and/or consulting physician.*

5. *Appropriate health risk factors should be identified.*

6. *The patient's progress, response to and changes in treatment, and revision of diagnosis should be documented.*

7. *CPT and ICD-9-CM codes reported on the health insurance claim form or patient billing statement should be supported by the documentation in the medical record.*

DOCUMENTATION OF EVALUATION AND MANAGEMENT SERVICES

This section provides definitions and documentation guidelines for the three key components of evaluation and management services and for visits which consist predominately of counseling or coordination of care. The three key components—history, examination, and medical decision making—appear in the descriptors for office and other outpatient services, hospital observation services, hospital inpatient services, consultations, emergency department services, nursing facility services, domiciliary care services, and home services. Note that Documentation Guidelines are identified by the symbol •DG.

The E/M descriptors recognize seven components which are used in defining the levels of service. These components are:

• *History*

• *Examination*

• *Medical decision making*

• *Counseling*

• *Coordination of care*

• *Nature of presenting problem*

• *Time*

163

The first three (i.e., history, examination and medical decision making) are the key components in selecting the level of evaluation and management services. However, with visits that consist predominantly of counseling or coordination of care, <u>time</u> is the key or controlling factor to qualify for a particular level of evaluation and management service.

Because the level of evaluation and management service is dependent on two or three key components, performance and documentation of one component (e.g., examination) at the highest level does not necessarily mean that the encounter in its entirety qualifies for the highest level of evaluation and management service.

These documentation guidelines for evaluation and management services reflect the needs of the typical adult population. For certain groups of patients, the recorded information may vary slightly from that described here.

Specifically, the medical records of infants, children, adolescents and pregnant women may have additional or modified information recorded in each history and examination area.

As an example, newborn records may include under history of the present illness, the details of the mother's pregnancy and the infant's status at birth; social history focused on family structure; family history focused on congenital anomalies and hereditary disorders in the family. In addition, the content of a pediatric examination will vary with the age and development of the child. Although not specifically defined in these documentation guidelines, these patient group variations on history and examination are appropriate.

DOCUMENTATION OF HISTORY

The levels of evaluation and management services are based on four types of history (Problem Focused, Expanded Problem Focused, Detailed, and Comprehensive). Each type of history includes some or all of the following elements:

- *Chief complaint*
- *History of present illness*
- *Review of systems*
- *Past, family and/or social history*

The extent of history of present illness, review of systems and past, family and/or social history that is obtained and documented is dependent upon clinical judgement and the nature of the presenting problem(s).

Present History	Review of Systems	Past, Family or Social History	Type of History
Brief	N/A	N/A	Problem Focused
Brief	Problem Pertinent	N/A	Expanded Problem Focused
Extended	Extended	Pertinent	Detailed
Extended	Complete	Complete	Comprehensive

The above chart shows the progression of the elements required for each type of history. To qualify for a given type of history all three elements in the table must be met. (A chief complaint is indicated at all levels.)

●*DG:* The chief complaint, review of systems and past, family and/or social history may be listed as separate elements of history, or they may be included in the description of the history of the present illness.

●*DG:* A review of systems and/or a past, family and/or social history obtained during an earlier encounter does not need to be re-recorded if there is evidence that the physician reviewed and updated the previous information. This may occur when a physician updates his or her own record or in an institutional setting or group practice where many physicians use a common record. The review and update may be documented by:

 • describing any new review of systems and/or past, family and/or social history information or noting there has been no change in the information; and

 • noting the date and location of the earlier review of systems and/or past, family and/or social history.

●*DG:* The review of systems and/or past, family and/or social history may be recorded by ancillary staff or on a form completed by the patient. To document that the physician reviewed the information, there must be a notation supplementing or confirming the information recorded by others.

●*DG:* If the physician is unable to obtain a history from the patient or other source, the record should describe the patient's condition or other circumstance which precludes obtaining a history.

Definitions and specific documentation guidelines for each of the elements of history are listed below.

CHIEF COMPLAINT

The chief complaint is "a concise statement describing the symptom, problem, condition, diagnosis, or other factor that is the reason for the encounter, usually stated in the patient's words."

●*DG:* *The medical record should clearly reflect the chief complaint.*

HISTORY OF PRESENT ILLNESS

The history of present illness is "a chronological description of the development of the patient's present illness from the first sign and/or symptom to the present." It includes the following elements:

● *Location*

● *Quality*

● *Severity*

● *Duration*

● *Timing*

● *Context*

● *Modifying factors*

● *Associated signs and symptoms*

Brief *and* ***extended*** *history of present illnesses are distinguished by the amount of detail needed to accurately characterize the clinical problem(s). A* ***brief*** *history of present illness consists of one to three elements of the history of present illness.*

●*DG:* *The medical record should describe at least one to three elements of the present illness (history of present illness).*

An ***extended*** *history of present illness consists of at least four elements of the history of present illness or the status of at least three chronic or inactive conditions.*

●*DG:* *Medical record should describe at least four elements of the present illness (history of present illness), or the status of at least three chronic or inactive conditions.*

REVIEW OF SYSTEMS

A review of systems is "an inventory of body systems obtained through a series of questions seeking to identify signs and/or symptoms which the patient may be experiencing or has experienced." For purposes of review of systems, the following systems are recognized:

● *Constitutional symptoms (e.g., fever, weight loss)*

- *Eyes*
- *Ears, Nose, Mouth, Throat*
- *Neck*
- *Cardiovascular*
- *Respiratory*
- *Gastrointestinal*
- *Genitourinary*
- *Musculoskeletal*
- *Integumentary (skin and/or breast)*
- *Neurological*
- *Psychiatric*
- *Endocrine*
- *Hematologic/Lymphatic*
- *Allergic/Immunologic*

A **problem pertinent** review of systems inquires about the system directly related to the problem(s) identified in the history of present illness.

●*DG:*   The patient's positive responses and pertinent negatives for the system related to the problem should be documented.

An **extended** review of systems inquires about the system directly related to the problem(s) identified in the history of present illness and a limited number of additional systems.

●*DG:*   The patient's positive responses and pertinent negatives for two to nine systems should be documented.

A **complete** review of systems inquires about the system(s) directly related to the problem(s) identified in the history of present illness plus all additional body systems.

●*DG:*   At least ten organ systems must be reviewed. Those systems with positive or pertinent negative responses must be individually documented. For the remaining systems, a notation indicating all other systems are negative is permissible. In the absence of such a notation, at least ten systems must be individually documented.

PAST, FAMILY AND/OR SOCIAL HISTORY

The past, family and/or social history consists of a review of the following areas:

- *Past history: the patient's past experiences with illnesses, operations, injuries and treatments.*

- *Family history: a review of medical events in the patient's family, including diseases which may be hereditary or place the patient at risk.*

- *Social history: an age appropriate review of past and current activities.*

For certain categories of evaluation and management services that include only an interval history, it is not necessary to record information about the past, family and/or social history. Those categories are subsequent hospital care, follow-up inpatient consultations and subsequent nursing facility care.

*A **pertinent** past, family and/or social history is a review of the history area(s) directly related to the problem(s) identified in the history of present illness.*

●DG: At least one specific item from any of the three history areas must be documented for a pertinent past, family and/or social history

*A **complete** past, family and/or social history is of a review of two or all three of the past, family and/or social history areas, depending on the category of the evaluation and management service. A review of all three history areas is required for services that by their nature include a comprehensive assessment or reassessment of the patient. A review of two of the three history areas is sufficient for other services.*

●DG: At least one specific item from two of the three history areas must be documented for a complete past, family and/or social history for the following categories of evaluation and management services: office or other outpatient services, established patient; emergency department; domiciliary care, established patient; and home care, established patient.

●DG: At least one specific item from each of the three history areas must be documented for a complete past, family and/or social history for the following categories of evaluation and management services: office or other outpatient services, new patient; hospital observation services; hospital inpatient services, initial care; consultations; comprehensive nursing facility assessments; domiciliary care, new patient; and home care, new patient.

DOCUMENTATION OF EXAMINATION

The levels of E/M services are based on four types of examination:

- *Problem Focused — "a limited examination of the affected body area or organ system."*

- *Expanded Problem Focused — "a limited examination of the affected body area or organ system and any other symptomatic or related body organ system(s)."*

- *Detailed — "an extended examination of the affected body area(s) and other symptomatic or related organ system(s)."*

- *Comprehensive — "a general multi-system examination, or complete examination of a single organ system."*

These types of examinations have been defined for general multi-system and the following single organ systems:

- *Cardiovascular*

- *Ears, Nose, Mouth and Throat*

- *Eyes*

- *Genitourinary (Female)*

- *Genitourinary (Male)*

- *Hematologic/Lymphatic/Immunologic*

- *Musculoskeletal*

- *Neurological*

- *Psychiatric*

- *Respiratory*

- *Skin*

A general multi-system examination or a single organ system examination may be performed by any physician regardless of specialty. The type (general multi-system or single organ system) and content of examination are selected by the examining physician and are based upon clinical judgement, the patient's history, and the nature of the presenting problem(s).

The content and documentation requirements for each type and level of examination are summarized below and described in detail in tables beginning on page 116. In the tables, organ systems and body areas recognized by CPT for purposes of describing examinations are shown in the left column. The content, or individual elements, of the examination pertaining to that body area or organ system are identified by bullets (●) in the right column.

Parenthetical examples, (e.g., ...), have been used for clarification and to provide guidance regarding documentation. Documentation for each element must satisfy any numeric requirements (such as "Measurement of any three of the following seven...") included in the description of the element. Elements with multiple components but with no specific numeric requirement (such as "Examination of liver and spleen") require documentation of at least one component. It is possible for a given examination to be expanded beyond what is defined here. When that occurs, findings related to the additional systems and/or areas should be documented.

●*DG:* *Specific abnormal and relevant negative findings of the examination of the affected or symptomatic body area(s) or organ system(s) should be documented. A notation of "abnormal" without elaboration is insufficient.*

●*DG:* *Abnormal or unexpected findings of the examination of any asymptomatic body area(s) or organ system(s) should be described.*

●*DG:* *A brief statement or notation indicating "negative" or "normal" is sufficient to document normal findings related to unaffected area(s) or asymptomatic organ system(s).*

GENERAL MULTI-SYSTEM EXAMINATIONS

To qualify for a given level of multi-system examination, the following content and documentation requirements should be met:

● *Problem Focused Examination — should include performance and documentation of one to five elements identified by a bullet (●) in one or more organ system(s) or body area(s).*

● *Expanded Problem Focused Examination — should include performance and documentation of at least six elements identified by a bullet (●) in one or more organ system(s) or body area(s).*

● *Detailed Examination — should include at least six organ systems or body areas. For each system/area selected, performance and documentation of at least two elements identified by a bullet (●) is expected. Alternatively, a detailed examination may include performance and documentation of at least twelve elements identified by a bullet (●) in two or more organ systems or body areas.*

● *Comprehensive Examination — should include at least nine organ systems or body areas. For each system/area selected, all elements of the examination identified by a bullet (●) should be performed, unless specific directions limit the content of the examination. For each area/system, documentation of at least two elements identified by a bullet is expected.*

SINGLE ORGAN SYSTEM EXAMINATIONS

Variations among single organ system examinations in the organ systems and body areas identified in the left columns and in the elements of the examinations described in the right columns reflect differing emphases among specialties. To qualify for a given level of single organ system examination, the following content and documentation requirements should be met:

- *Problem Focused Examination — should include performance and documentation of one to five elements identified by a bullet (●), whether in a box with a shaded or unshaded border.*

- *Expanded Problem Focused Examination — should include performance and documentation of at least six elements identified by a bullet (●), whether in a box with a shaded or unshaded border.*

- *Detailed Examination — examinations other than the eye and psychiatric examinations should include performance and documentation of at least twelve elements identified by a bullet (●), whether in box with a shaded or unshaded border.*

  Eye and psychiatric examinations should include the performance and documentation of at least nine elements identified by a bullet (●), whether in a box with a shaded or unshaded border.

- *Comprehensive Examination — should include performance of all elements identified by a bullet (●), whether in a shaded or unshaded box. Documentation of every element in each box with a shaded border and at least one element in each box with an unshaded border is expected.*

Documentation of every element in each box with a shaded border and at least one element in each box with an unshaded border is expected.

GENERAL MULTI-SYSTEM EXAMINATION

SYSTEM/BODY AREA	ELEMENTS OF EXAMINATION
Constitutional	• *Measurement of any three of the following seven vital signs: 1) sitting or standing blood pressure, 2) supine blood pressure, 3) pulse rate and regularity, 4) respiration, 5) temperature, 6) height, 7) weight (May be measured and recorded by ancillary staff)* • *General appearance of patient (e.g., development, nutrition, body habitus, deformities, attention to grooming)*
Eyes	• *Inspection of conjunctivae and lids* • *Examination of pupils and irises (e.g., reaction to light and accommodation, size and symmetry)* • *Ophthalmoscopic examination of optic discs (e.g., size, C/D ratio, appearance) and posterior segments (e.g., vessel changes, exudates, hemorrhages)*
Ears, Nose, Mouth, Throat	• *External inspection of ears and nose (e.g., overall and appearance, scars, lesions, masses)* • *Otoscopic examination of external auditory canals and tympanic membranes* • *Assessment of hearing (e.g., whispered voice, finger rub, tuning fork)* • *Inspection of nasal mucosa, septum and turbinates* • *Inspection of lips, teeth and gums* • *Examination of oropharynx: oral mucosa, salivary glands, hard and soft palates, tongue, tonsils and posterior pharynx*
Neck	• *Examination of neck (e.g., masses, overall appearance, symmetry, tracheal position, crepitus)* • *Examination of thyroid (e.g., enlargement, tenderness, mass)*

Respiratory	• *Assessment of respiratory effort (e.g., intercostal retractions, use of accessory muscles, diaphragmatic movement)* • *Percussion of chest (e.g., dullness, flatness, hyperresonance)* • *Palpation of chest (e.g., tactile fremitus)* • *Auscultation of lungs (e.g., breath sounds, adventitious sounds, rubs)*
Cardiovascular	• *Palpation of heart (e.g., location, size, thrills)* • *Auscultation of heart with notation of abnormal sounds and murmurs* *Examination of:* • *Carotid arteries (e.g., pulse amplitude, bruits)* • *Abdominal aorta (e.g., size, dbruits)* • *Femoral arteries (e.g., pulse amplitude, bruits)* • *Pedal pulses (e.g., pulse amplitude)* • *Extremities for edema and/or varicosities*
Chest (Breasts)	• *Inspection of breasts (e.g., symmetry, nipple discharge)* • *Palpation of breasts and axillae (e.g., masses or lumps, tenderness)*
Gastrointestinal (Abdomen)	• *Examination of abdomen with notation of presence of masses or tenderness* • *Examination of liver and spleen* • *Examination for presence or absence of hernia* • *Examination (when indicated) of anus, perineum and rectum, including sphincter tone, presence of hemorrhoids, rectal masses* • *Obtain stool sample for occult blood test when indicated*
Genitourinary Male	• *Examination of the scrotal contents (e.g., hydrocele, spermatocele, tenderness of cord, testicular mass)* *continued* • *Examination of the penis*

173

- *Digital rectal examination of prostate gland (e.g., size, symmetry, nodularity, tenderness)*

Genitourinary Female

- *Pelvic examination (with or without specimen collection for smears and cultures), including:*

- *Examination of external genitalia (e.g., general appearance, hair distribution, lesions) and vagina (e.g., general appearance, estrogen effect, discharge, lesions, pelvic support, cystocele, rectocele)*

- *Examination of urethra (e.g., masses, tenderness, scarring)*

- *Examination of bladder (e.g., fullness, masses, tenderness)*

- *Cervix (e.g., general appearance, lesions, discharge)*

- *Uterus (e.g., size, contour, position, mobility, tenderness, consistency, descent or support)*

- *Adnexa/parametria (e.g., masses, tenderness, organomegaly, nodularity)*

Lymphatic

Palpation of lymph nodes in two or more areas:

- *Neck*
- *Axillae*
- *Groin*
- *Other*

Musculoskeletal

- *Examination of gait and station*

- *Inspection and/or palpation of digits and nails (eg clubbing, cyanosis, inflammatory conditions, petechiae, ischemia, infections, nodes)*

- *Examination of joints, bones and muscles of one or more of the following six areas: 1) head and neck; 2) spine, ribs and pelvis; 3) right upper extremity; 4) left upper extremity; 5) right lower extremity; and 6) left lower extremity. The examination of a given area includes:*

- *Inspection and/or palpation with notation of presence of any misalignment, asymmetry,* crepitation, defects, tenderness, masses, effusions

- Assessment of range of motion with notation of any pain, crepitation or contracture

- Assessment of stability with notation of any dislocation (luxation), subluxation or laxity

- Assessment of muscle strength and tone (e.g., flaccid, cog wheel, spastic) with notation of any atrophy or abnormal movements

Skin

- Inspection of skin and subcutaneous tissue (e.g., rashes, lesions, ulcers)

- Palpation of skin and subcutaneous tissue (e.g., induration, subcutaneous nodules, tightening)

Neurologic

- Test cranial nerves with notation of any deficits

- Examination of deep tendon reflexes with notation of pathological reflexes (e.g., Babinski)

- Examination of sensation (e.g., by touch, pin, vibration, proprioception)

Psychiatric

- Description of patient's judgment and insight

Brief assessment of mental status including:

- Orientation to time, place and person

- Recent and remote memory

- Mood and affect (e.g., depression, anxiety, agitation)

CONTENT AND DOCUMENTATION REQUIREMENTS

Level of Exam	Perform and Document:
Problem Focused	One to five elements identified by a bullet.
Expanded Problem Focused	At least six elements identified by a bullet.
Detailed	At least two elements identified by a bullet from each of six areas/systems OR at least twelve elements identified by a bullet in two or more areas/systems.
Comprehensive	Perform all elements identified by a bullet in at least nine organ systems or body areas and document at least two elements identified by a bullet from each of nine areas/systems.

CARDIOVASCULAR EXAMINATION

SYSTEM/BODY AREA	ELEMENTS OF EXAMINATION
Constitutional	• *Measurement of any three of the following seven vital signs: 1) sitting or standing blood pressure, 2) supine blood pressure, 3) pulse rate and regularity, 4) respiration, 5) temperature, 6) height, 7) weight (May be measured and recorded by ancillary staff)* • *General appearance of patient (e.g., development, nutrition, body habitus, deformities, attention to grooming)*
Head and Face	
Eyes	• *Inspection of conjunctivae and lids (e.g., xanthelasma)*
Ears, Nose, Mouth and Throat	• *Inspection of teeth, gums and palate* • *Inspection of oral mucosa with notation of presence of pallor or cyanosis*
Neck	• *Examination of jugular veins (e.g., distension; a, v or cannon a waves)* • *Examination of thyroid (e.g., enlargement, tenderness, mass)*
Respiratory	• *Assessment of respiratory effort (e.g., intercostal retractions, use of accessory muscles, diaphragmatic movement)* • *Auscultation of lungs (e.g., breath sounds, adventitious sounds, rubs)*
Cardiovascular	• *Palpation of heart (e.g., location, size and forcefulness of the point of maximal impact; thrills; lifts; palpable S3 or S4)* • *Auscultation of heart including sounds, abnormal sounds and murmurs*

continued

Cardiovascular (continued)	• *Measurement of blood pressure in two or more extremities when indicated (e.g., aortic dissection, coarctation)*
	Examination of:
	• *Carotid arteries (e.g., waveform, pulse amplitude, bruits, apical-carotid delay)*
	• *Abdominal aorta (e.g., size, bruits)*
	• *Femoral arteries (e.g., pulse amplitude, bruits)*
	• *Pedal pulses (e.g., pulse amplitude)*
	• *Extremities for peripheral edema and/or varicosities*

Chest (Breasts)

Gastrointestinal (Abdomen)	• *Examination of abdomen with notation of presence (Abdomen) of masses or tenderness*
	• *Examination of liver and spleen*
	• *Obtain stool sample for occult blood from patients who are being considered for thrombolytic or anticoagulant therapy*

Genitourinary

Lymphatic

Musculoskeletal	• *Examination of the back with notation of kyphosis or scoliosis*
	• *Examination of gait with notation of ability to undergo exercise testing and/or participation in exercise programs*
	• *Assessment of muscle strength and tone (e.g., flaccid, cog wheel, spastic) with notation of any atrophy and abnormal movements*

| *Extremities* | • Inspection and palpation of digits and nails (e.g., clubbing, cyanosis, inflammation, petechiae, ischemia, infections, Osler's nodes) |

| *Skin* | • Inspection and/or palpation of skin and subcutaneous tissue (e.g., stasis dermatitis, ulcers, scars, xanthomas) |

| *Neurological/Psychiatric* | Brief assessment of mental status including: |

• Orientation to time, place and person

• Mood and affect (e.g., depression, anxiety, agitation)

CONTENT AND DOCUMENTATION REQUIREMENTS

Level of Exam	*Perform and Document:*
Problem Focused	One to five elements identified by a bullet.
Expanded Problem Focused	At least six elements identified by a bullet.
Detailed	At least twelve elements identified by a bullet.
Comprehensive	Perform all elements identified by a bullet; document every element in each box with a shaded border and at least one element in each box with an unshaded border.

EAR, NOSE AND THROAT EXAMINATION

SYSTEM/BODY AREA	ELEMENTS OF EXAMINATION
Constitutional	• *Measurement of any three of the following seven vital signs: 1) sitting or standing blood pressure, 2) supine blood pressure, 3) pulse rate and regularity, 4) respiration, 5) temperature, 6) height, 7) weight (May be measured and recorded by ancillary staff)* • *General appearance of patient (e.g., development, nutrition, body habitus, deformities, attention to grooming)* • *Assessment of ability to communicate (e.g., use of sign language or other communication aids) and quality of voice*
Head and Face	• *Inspection of head and face (e.g., overall appearance, scars, lesions and masses)* • *Palpation and/or percussion of face with notation of presence or absence of sinus tenderness* • *Examination of salivary glands* • *Assessment of facial strength*
Eyes	• *Test ocular motility including primary gaze alignment*
Ears, Nose, Mouth and Throat	• *Otoscopic examination of external auditory canals and tympanic membranes including pneumo-otoscopy with notation of mobility of membranes* • *Assessment of hearing with tuning forks and clinical speech reception thresholds (e.g., whispered voice, finger rub)* • *External inspection of ears and nose (e.g., overall appearance, scars, lesions and masses)* • *Inspection of nasal mucosa, septum and turbinates* • *Inspection of lips, teeth and gums*

continued

ENMT (continued)	• *Examination of oropharynx: oral mucosa, hard and soft palates, tongue, tonsils and posterior pharynx (e.g., asymmetry, lesions, hydration of mucosal surfaces)*
	• *Inspection of pharyngeal walls and pyriform sinuses (e.g., pooling of saliva, asymmetry, lesions)*
	• *Examination by mirror of larynx including the condition of the epiglottis, false vocal cords, true vocal cords and mobility of larynx (Use of mirror not required in children)*
	• *Examination by mirror of nasopharynx including appearance of the mucosa, adenoids, posterior choanae and eustachian tubes (Use of mirror not required in children)*
Neck	• *Examination of neck (e.g., masses, overall appearance, symmetry, tracheal position, crepitus)*
	• *Examination of thyroid (e.g., enlargement, tenderness, mass)*
Respiratory	• *Inspection of chest including symmetry, expansion and/or assessment of respiratory effort (e.g., intercostal retractions, use of accessory muscles, diaphragmatic movement)*
	• *Auscultation of lungs (e.g., breath sounds, adventitious sounds, rubs)*
Cardiovascular	• *Auscultation of heart with notation of abnormal sounds and murmurs*
	• *Examination of peripheral vascular system by observation (e.g., swelling, varicosities) and palpation (e.g., pulses, temperature, edema, tenderness)*
Chest (Breasts)	
Gastrointestinal (Abdomen)	
Genitourinary	

181

| **Lymphatic** | ● *Palpation of lymph nodes in neck, axillae, groin and/or other location* |

Musculoskeletal

Extremities

Skin

Neurological/Psychiatric	● *Test cranial nerves with notation of any deficits*
	Brief assessment of mental status including:
	● *Orientation to time, place and person*
	● *Mood and affect (e.g., depression, anxiety, agitation)*

CONTENT AND DOCUMENTATION REQUIREMENTS

Level of Exam	*Perform and Document:*
Problem Focused	*One to five elements identified by a bullet.*
Expanded Problem Focused	*At least six elements identified by a bullet.*
Detailed	*At least twelve elements identified by a bullet.*
Comprehensive	*Perform all elements identified by a bullet; document every element in each box with a shaded border and at least one element in each box with an unshaded border.*

182

EYE EXAMINATION

SYSTEM/BODY AREA	ELEMENTS OF EXAMINATION
Constitutional	
Head and Face	

Eyes	
	• *Test visual acuity (Does not include determination of refractive error)*
	• *Gross visual field testing by confrontation*
	• *Test ocular motility including primary gaze alignment*
	• *Inspection of bulbar and palpebral conjunctivae*
	• *Examination of ocular adnexae including lids (e.g., ptosis or lagophthalmos), lacrimal glands, lacrimal drainage, orbits and preauricular lymph nodes*
	• *Examination of pupils and irises including shape, direct and consensual reaction (afferent pupil), size (e.g., anisocoria) and morphology*
	• *Slit lamp examination of the corneas including epithelium, stroma, endothelium, and tear film*
	• *Slit lamp examination of the anterior chambers including depth, cells, and flare*
	• *Slit lamp examination of the lenses including clarity, anterior and posterior capsule, cortex, and nucleus*
	• *Measurement of intraocular pressures (except in children and patients with trauma or infectious disease)*
	• *Ophthalmoscopic examination through dilated pupils (unless contraindicated) of*
	• *Optic discs including size, C/D ratio, appearance (e.g., atrophy, cupping, tumor elevation) and nerve fiber layer*
	• *Posterior segments including retina and vessels (e.g., exudates and hemorrhages)*

Ears, Nose, Mouth and Throat

Neck

Respiratory

Cardiovascular

Chest (Breasts)

Gastrointestinal (Abdomen)

Genitourinary

Lymphatic

Musculoskeletal

Extremities

Skin

Neurological/Psychiatric	Brief assessment of mental status including:
	• Orientation to time, place and person
	• Mood and affect (e.g., depression, anxiety, agitation)

CONTENT AND DOCUMENTATION REQUIREMENTS

Level of Exam	*Perform and Document:*
Problem Focused	*One to five elements identified by a bullet.*
Expanded Problem Focused	*At least six elements identified by a bullet.*
Detailed	*At least nine elements identified by a bullet.*
Comprehensive	*Perform all elements identified by a bullet; document every element in each box with a shaded border and at least one element in each box with an unshaded border.*

GENITOURINARY EXAMINATION

SYSTEM/BODY AREA	ELEMENTS OF EXAMINATION
Constitutional	• Measurement of any three of the following seven vital signs: 1) sitting or standing blood pressure, 2) supine blood pressure, 3) pulse rate and regularity, 4) respiration, 5) temperature, 6) height, 7) weight (May be measured and recorded by ancillary staff) • General appearance of patient (e.g., development, nutrition, body habitus, deformities, attention to grooming)
Head and Face	
Eyes	
Ears, Nose, Mouth and Throat	
Neck	• Examination of neck (e.g., masses, overall appearance, symmetry, tracheal position, crepitus) • Examination of thyroid (e.g., enlargement, tenderness, mass)
Respiratory	• Assessment of respiratory effort (e.g., intercostal retractions, use of accessory muscles, diaphragmatic movement) • Auscultation of lungs (e.g., breath sounds, adventitious sounds, rubs)
Cardiovascular	• Auscultation of heart with notation of abnormal sounds and murmurs • Examination of peripheral vascular system by observation (e.g., swelling, varicosities) and palpation (e.g., pulses, temperature, edema, tenderness)
Chest (Breasts)	[See genitourinary (female)]

Gastrointestinal (Abdomen)	• *Examination of abdomen with notation of presence of masses or tenderness*
	• *Examination for presence or absence of hernia*
	• *Examination of liver and spleen*
	• *Obtain stool sample for occult blood test when indicated*
Genitourinary (male)	• *Inspection of anus and perineum*
	Examination (with or without specimen collection for smears and cultures) of genitalia including:
	• *Scrotum (e.g., lesions, cysts, rashes)*
	• *Epididymides (e.g., size, symmetry, masses)*
	• *Testes (e.g., size, symmetry, masses)*
	• *Urethral meatus (e.g., size, location, lesions, discharge)*
	• *Penis (e.g., lesions, presence or absence of foreskin, foreskin retractability, plaque, masses, scarring, deformities)*
	Digital rectal examination including:
	• *Prostate gland (e.g., size, symmetry, nodularity, tenderness)*
	• *Seminal vesicles (e.g., symmetry, tenderness, masses, enlargement)*
	• *Sphincter tone, presence of hemorrhoids, rectal masses*
Genitourinary (female)	*Includes at least seven of the following eleven elements identified by bullets:*
	• *Inspection and palpation of breasts (e.g., masses or lumps, tenderness, symmetry, nipple discharge)*
	• *Digital rectal examination including sphincter tone, presence of hemorrhoids, rectal masses*
	Pelvic examination (with or without specimen collection for smears and cultures) including:
	• *External genitalia (e.g., general appearance, hair distribution, lesions)*

Genitourinary (continued)	• *Urethral meatus (e.g., size, location, lesions, prolapse)*
	• *Urethra (e.g., masses, tenderness, scarring)*
	• *Bladder (e.g., fullness, masses, tenderness)*
	• *Vagina (e.g., general appearance, estrogen effect, discharge, lesions, pelvic support, cystocele, rectocele)*
	• *Cervix (e.g., general appearance, lesions, discharge)*
	• *Uterus (e.g., size, contour, position, mobility, tenderness, consistency, descent or support)*
	• *Adnexa/parametria (e.g., masses, tenderness, organomegaly, nodularity)*
	• *Anus and perineum*
Lymphatic	• *Palpation of lymph nodes in neck, axillae, groin and/or other location*
Musculoskeletal	
Extremities	
Skin	• *Inspection and/or palpation of skin and subcutaneous tissue (e.g., rashes, lesions, ulcers)*
Neurological/Psychiatric	*Brief assessment of mental status including:*
	• *Orientation (e.g., time, place and person) and*
	• *Mood and affect (e.g., depression, anxiety, agitation)*

CONTENT AND DOCUMENTATION REQUIREMENTS

Level of Exam	Perform and Document:
Problem Focused	One to five elements identified by a bullet.
Expanded Problem Focused	At least six elements identified by a bullet.
Detailed	At least twelve elements identified by a bullet.
Comprehensive	Perform all elements identified by a bullet; document every element in each box with a shaded border and at least one element in each box with an unshaded border.

HEMATOLOGIC, LYMPHATIC, AND/OR IMMUNOLOGIC EXAMINATION

SYSTEM/BODY AREA	ELEMENTS OF EXAMINATION
Constitutional	• Measurement of any three of the following seven vital signs: 1) sitting or standing blood pressure, 2) supine blood pressure, 3) pulse rate and regularity, 4) respiration, 5) temperature, 6) height, 7) weight (May be measured and recorded by ancillary staff) • General appearance of patient (e.g., development, nutrition, body habitus, deformities, attention to grooming)
Head and Face	• Palpation and/or percussion of face with notation of presence or absence of sinus tenderness
Eyes	• Inspection of conjunctivae and lids
Ears, Nose, Mouth and Throat	• Otoscopic examination of external auditory canals and tympanic membranes • Inspection of nasal mucosa, septum and turbinates • Inspection of teeth and gums • Examination of oropharynx (e.g., oral mucosa, hard and soft palates, tongue, tonsils, posterior pharynx)
Neck	• Examination of neck (e.g., masses, overall appearance, symmetry, tracheal position, crepitus) • Examination of thyroid (e.g., enlargement, tenderness, mass)
Respiratory	• Assessment of respiratory effort (e.g., intercostal retractions, use of accessory muscles, diaphragmatic movement) • Auscultation of lungs (e.g., breath sounds, adventitious sounds, rubs)

Cardiovascular	• *Auscultation of heart with notation of abnormal sounds and murmurs* • *Examination of peripheral vascular system by observation (e.g., swelling, varicosities) and palpation (e.g., pulses, temperature, edema, tenderness)*
Chest (Breasts)	
Gastrointestinal (Abdomen)	• *Examination of abdomen with notation of presence of masses or tenderness* • *Examination of liver and spleen*
Genitourinary	
Lymphatic	• *Palpation of lymph nodes in neck, axillae, groin, and/or other location*
Musculoskeletal	
Extremities	• *Inspection and palpation of digits and nails (e.g., clubbing, cyanosis, inflammation, petechiae, ischemia, infections, nodes)*
Skin	• *Inspection and/or palpation of skin and subcutaneous tissue (e.g., rashes, lesions, ulcers, ecchymoses, bruises)*
Neurological/Psychiatric	*Brief assessment of mental status including:* • *Orientation to time, place and person* • *Mood and affect (e.g., depression, anxiety, agitation)*

CONTENT AND DOCUMENTATION REQUIREMENTS

Level of Exam	Perform and Document:
Problem Focused	One to five elements identified by a bullet.
Expanded Problem Focused	At least six elements identified by a bullet.
Detailed	At least twelve elements identified by a bullet.
Comprehensive	Perform all elements identified by a bullet; document every element in each box with a shaded border and at least one element in each box with an unshaded border.

MUSCULOSKELETAL EXAMINATION

SYSTEM/BODY AREA	ELEMENTS OF EXAMINATION
Constitutional	• Measurement of any three of the following seven vital signs: 1) sitting or standing blood pressure, 2) supine blood pressure, 3) pulse rate and regularity, 4) respiration, 5) temperature, 6) height, 7) weight (May be measured and recorded by ancillary staff) • General appearance of patient (e.g., development, nutrition, body habitus, deformities, attention to grooming)
Head and Face	
Eyes	
Ears, Nose, Mouth and Throat	
Neck	
Respiratory	
Cardiovascular	• Examination of peripheral vascular system by observation (e.g., swelling, varicosities) and palpation (e.g., pulses, temperature, edema, tenderness)
Chest (Breasts)	
Gastrointestinal (Abdomen)	
Genitourinary	
Lymphatic	• Palpation of lymph nodes in neck, axillae, groin and/or other location

Musculoskeletal	• *Examination of gait and station*
	• *Examination of joint(s), bone(s) and muscle(s)/ tendon(s) of four of the following six areas: 1) head and neck; 2) spine, ribs and pelvis; 3) right upper extremity; 4) left upper extremity; 5) right lower extremity; and 6) left lower extremity. The examination of a given area includes:*
	• *Inspection, percussion and/or palpation with notation of any misalignment, asymmetry, crepitation, defects, tenderness, masses or effusions*
	• *Assessment of range of motion with notation of any pain (e.g., straight leg raising), crepitation or contracture*
	• *Assessment of stability with notation of any dislocation (luxation), subluxation or laxity*
	• *Assessment of muscle strength and tone (e.g., flaccid, cog wheel, spastic) with notation of any atrophy or abnormal movements*

NOTE: For the comprehensive level of examination, all four of the elements identified by a bullet must be performed and documented for each of four anatomic areas. For the three lower levels of examination, each element is counted separately for each body area. For example, assessing range of motion in two extremities constitutes two elements.

Extremities	*[See musculoskeletal and skin]*

Skin	• *Inspection and/or palpation of skin and subcutaneous tissue (e.g., scars, rashes, lesions, cafe-au-lait spots, ulcers) in four of the following six areas: 1) head and neck; 2) trunk; 3) right upper extremity; 4) left upper extremity; 5) right lower extremity; and 6) left lower extremity.*

NOTE: For the comprehensive level, all four areas must be examined and documented. For the three lower levels, each body area is counted separately. For example, inspection and/or palpation of the skin and subcutaneous tissue of two extremities constitutes two elements.

Neurological/Psychiatric	• *Test coordination (e.g., finger/nose, heel/knee/shin, rapid alternating movements in the upper and lower extremities, evaluation of fine motor coordination in young children)*
	• *Examination of deep tendon reflexes and/or nerve stretch test with notation of pathological reflexes (e.g., Babinski)*
	• *Examination of sensation (e.g., by touch, pin, vibration, proprioception)*
	Brief assessment of mental status including
	• *Orientation to time, place and person*
	• *Mood and affect (e.g., depression, anxiety, agitation)*

CONTENT AND DOCUMENTATION REQUIREMENTS

Level of Exam	*Perform and Document:*
Problem Focused	*One to five elements identified by a bullet.*
Expanded Problem Focused	*At least six elements identified by a bullet.*
Detailed	*At least twelve elements identified by a bullet.*
Comprehensive	*Perform all elements identified by a bullet; document every element in each box with a shaded border and at least one element in each box with an unshaded border.*

NEUROLOGICAL EXAMINATION

SYSTEM/BODY AREA	*ELEMENTS OF EXAMINATION*
Constitutional	• *Measurement of any three of the following seven vital signs: 1) sitting or standing blood pressure, 2) supine blood pressure, 3) pulse rate and regularity, 4) respiration, 5) temperature, 6) height, 7) weight (May be measured and recorded by ancillary staff)* • *General appearance of patient (e.g., development, nutrition, body habitus, deformities, attention to grooming)*
Head and Face	
Eyes	• *Ophthalmoscopic examination of optic discs (e.g., size, C/D ratio, appearance) and posterior segments (e.g., vessel changes, exudates, hemorrhages)*
Ears, Nose, Mouth and Throat	
Neck	
Respiratory	
Cardiovascular	• *Examination of carotid arteries (e.g., pulse amplitude, bruits)* • *Auscultation of heart with notation of abnormal sounds and murmurs* • *Examination of peripheral vascular system by observation (e.g., swelling, varicosities) and palpation (e.g., pulses, temperature, edema, tenderness)*
Chest (Breasts)	
Gastrointestinal (Abdomen)	
Genitourinary	
Lymphatic	

195

Musculoskeletal	• *Examination of gait and station*
	Assessment of motor function including:
	• *Muscle strength in upper and lower extremities*
	• *Muscle tone in upper and lower extremities (e.g., flaccid, cog wheel, spastic) with notation of any atrophy or abnormal movements (e.g., fasciculation, tardive dyskinesia)*
Extremities	*[See musculoskeletal]*
Skin	
Neurological/Psychiatric	*Evaluation of higher integrative functions including:*
	• *Orientation to time, place and person*
	• *Recent and remote memory*
	• *Attention span and concentration*
	• *Language (e.g., naming objects, repeating phrases, spontaneous speech)*
	• *Fund of knowledge (e.g., awareness of current events, past history, vocabulary)*
	Test the following cranial nerves:
	• *2nd cranial nerve (e.g., visual acuity, visual fields, fundi)*
	• *3rd, 4th and 6th cranial nerves (e.g., pupils, eye movements)*
	• *5th cranial nerve (e.g., facial sensation, corneal reflexes)*
	• *7th cranial nerve (e.g., facial symmetry, strength)*
	• *8th cranial nerve (e.g., hearing with tuning fork, whispered voice and/or finger rub)*
	• *9th cranial nerve (e.g., spontaneous or reflex palate movement)*

continued

Neurological/Psychiatric *(continued)*	• *11th cranial nerve (e.g., shoulder shrug strength)* • *12th cranial nerve (e.g., tongue protrusion)* • *Examination of sensation (e.g., by touch, pin, vibration, proprioception)* • *Examination of deep tendon reflexes in upper and lower extremities with notation of pathological reflexes (e.g., Babinski)* • *Test coordination (e.g., finger/nose, heel/knee/shin, rapid alternating movements in the upper and lower extremities, evaluation of fine motor coordination in young children)*

CONTENT AND DOCUMENTATION REQUIREMENTS

Level of Exam	Perform and Document:
Problem Focused	One to five elements identified by a bullet.
Expanded Problem Focused	At least six elements identified by a bullet.
Detailed	At least twelve elements identified by a bullet.
Comprehensive	Perform all elements identified by a bullet; document every element in each box with a shaded border and at least one element in each box with an unshaded border.

PSYCHIATRIC EXAMINATION

SYSTEM/BODY AREA	ELEMENTS OF EXAMINATION
Constitutional	• *Measurement of any three of the following seven vital signs: 1) sitting or standing blood pressure, 2) supine blood pressure, 3) pulse rate and regularity, 4) respiration, 5) temperature, 6) height, 7) weight (May be measured and recorded by ancillary staff)* • *General appearance of patient (e.g., development, nutrition, body habitus, deformities, attention to grooming)*
Head and Face	
Eyes	
Ears, Nose, Mouth and Throat	
Neck	
Respiratory	
Cardiovascular	
Chest (Breasts)	
Gastrointestinal (Abdomen)	
Genitourinary	
Lymphatic	
Musculoskeletal	• *Assessment of muscle strength and tone (e.g., flaccid, cog wheel, spastic) with notation of any atrophy and abnormal movements* • *Examination of gait and station*
Extremities	
Skin	

Neurological

Psychiatric

- *Description of speech including: rate; volume; articulation; coherence; and spontaneity with notation of abnormalities (e.g., perseveration, paucity of language)*

- *Description of thought processes including: rate of thoughts; content of thoughts (e.g., logical vs. illogical, tangential); abstract reasoning; and computation*

- *Description of associations (e.g., loose, tangential, circumstantial, intact)*

- *Description of abnormal or psychotic thoughts including: hallucinations; delusions; preoccupation with violence; homicidal or suicidal ideation; and obsessions*

- *Description of the patient's judgment (e.g., concerning everyday activities and social situations) and insight (e.g., concerning psychiatric condition)*

Complete mental status examination including:

- *Orientation to time, place and person*

- *Recent and remote memory*

- *Attention span and concentration*

- *Language (e.g., naming objects, repeating phrases)*

- *Fund of knowledge (e.g., awareness of current events, past history, vocabulary)*

- *Mood and affect (e.g., depression, anxiety, agitation, hypomania, lability)*

CONTENT AND DOCUMENTATION REQUIREMENTS

Level of Exam	Perform and Document:
Problem Focused	One to five elements identified by a bullet.
Expanded Problem Focused	At least six elements identified by a bullet.
Detailed	At least nine elements identified by a bullet.
Comprehensive	Perform all elements identified by a bullet; document every element in each box with a shaded border and at least one element in each box with an unshaded border.

RESPIRATORY EXAMINATION

SYSTEM/BODY AREA	*ELEMENTS OF EXAMINATION*
Constitutional	• *Measurement of any three of the following seven vital signs: 1) sitting or standing blood pressure, 2) supine blood pressure, 3) pulse rate and regularity, 4) respiration, 5) temperature, 6) height, 7) weight (May be measured and recorded by ancillary staff)* • *General appearance of patient (e.g., development, nutrition, body habitus, deformities, attention to grooming)*
Head and Face	
Eyes	
Ears, Nose, Mouth and Throat	• *Inspection of nasal mucosa, septum and turbinates* • *Inspection of teeth and gums* • *Examination of oropharynx (e.g., oral mucosa, hard and soft palates, tongue, tonsils and posterior pharynx)*
Neck	• *Examination of neck (e.g., masses, overall appearance, symmetry, tracheal position, crepitus)* • *Examination of thyroid (e.g., enlargement, tenderness, mass)* • *Examination of jugular veins (e.g., distension; a, v or cannon a waves)*
Respiratory	• *Inspection of chest with notation of symmetry and expansion* • *Assessment of respiratory effort (e.g., intercostal retractions, use of accessory muscles, diaphragmatic movement)* • *Percussion of chest (e.g., dullness, flatness, hyperresonance)*

continued

Respiratory (continued)	• *Palpation of chest (e.g., tactile fremitus)*
	• *Auscultation of lungs (e.g., breath sounds, adventitious sounds, rubs)*
Cardiovascular	• *Auscultation of heart including sounds, abnormal sounds and murmurs*
	• *Examination of peripheral vascular system by observation (e.g., swelling, varicosities) and palpation (e.g., pulses, temperature, edema, tenderness)*
Chest (Breasts)	
Gastrointestinal (Abdomen)	• *Examination of abdomen with notation of presence of masses or tenderness*
	• *Examination of liver and spleen*
Genitourinary	
Lymphatic	• *Palpation of lymph nodes in neck, axillae, groin and/or other location*
Musculoskeletal	• *Assessment of muscle strength and tone (e.g., flaccid, cog wheel, spastic) with notation of any atrophy and abnormal movements*
	• *Examination of gait and station*
Extremities	• *Inspection and palpation of digits and nails (e.g., clubbing, cyanosis, inflammation, petechiae, ischemia, infections, nodes)*
Skin	• *Inspection and/or palpation of skin and subcutaneous tissue (e.g., rashes, lesions, ulcers)*
Neurological/Psychiatric	*Brief assessment of mental status including:*
	• *Orientation to time, place and person*
	• *Mood and affect (e.g., depression, anxiety, agitation)*

CONTENT AND DOCUMENTATION REQUIREMENTS

Level of Exam	Perform and Document:
Problem Focused	One to five elements identified by a bullet.
Expanded Problem Focused	At least six elements identified by a bullet.
Detailed	At least twelve elements identified by a bullet.
Comprehensive	Perform all elements identified by a bullet; document every element in each box with a shaded border and at least one element in each box with an unshaded border.

SKIN EXAMINATION

SYSTEM/BODY AREA	ELEMENTS OF EXAMINATION
Constitutional	• *Measurement of any three of the following seven vital signs: 1) sitting or standing blood pressure, 2) supine blood pressure, 3) pulse rate and regularity, 4) respiration, 5) temperature, 6) height, 7) weight (May be measured and recorded by ancillary staff)*
	• *General appearance of patient (e.g., development, nutrition, body habitus, deformities, attention to grooming)*
Head and Face	
Eyes	• *Inspection of conjunctivae and lids*
Ears, Nose, Mouth and Throat	• *Inspection of lips, teeth and gums*
	• *Examination of oropharynx (e.g., oral mucosa, hard and soft palates, tongue, tonsils, posterior pharynx)*
Neck	• *Examination of thyroid (e.g., enlargement, tenderness, mass)*
Respiratory	
Cardiovascular	• *Examination of peripheral vascular system by observation (e.g., swelling, varicosities) and palpation (e.g., pulses, temperature, edema, tenderness)*
Chest (Breasts)	
Gastrointestinal (Abdomen)	• *Examination of liver and spleen*
	• *Examination of anus for condyloma and other lesions*
Genitourinary	

Lymphatic
- *Palpation of lymph nodes in neck, axillae, groin and/or other location*

Musculoskeletal

Extremities
- *Inspection and palpation of digits and nails (e.g., clubbing, cyanosis, inflammation, petechiae, ischemia, infections, nodes)*

Skin
- *Palpation of scalp and inspection of hair of scalp, eyebrows, face, chest, pubic area (when indicated) and extremities*

  Inspection and/or palpation of skin and subcutaneous tissue (e.g., rashes, lesions, ulcers, susceptibility to and presence of photo damage) in eight of the following ten areas:

- *Head, including the face and*
- *Neck*
- *Chest, including breasts and axillae*
- *Abdomen*
- *Genitalia, groin, buttocks*
- *Back*
- *Right upper extremity*
- *Left upper extremity*
- *Right lower extremity*
- *Left lower extremity*

NOTE: For the comprehensive level, the examination of at least eight anatomic areas must be performed and documented. For the three lower levels of examination, each body area is counted separately. For example, inspection and/or palpation of the skin and subcutaneous tissue of the right upper extremity and the left upper extremity constitutes two elements.

- *Inspection of eccrine and apocrine glands of skin and subcutaneous tissue with identification and location of any hyperhidrosis, chromhidroses or bromhidrosis*

Neurological/Psychiatric

Brief assessment of mental status including:

- *Orientation to time, place and person*
- *Mood and affect (e.g., depression, anxiety, agitation)*

CONTENT AND DOCUMENTATION REQUIREMENTS

Level of Exam	*Perform and Document:*
Problem Focused	*One to five elements identified by a bullet.*
Expanded Problem Focused	*At least six elements identified by a bullet.*
Detailed	*At least twelve elements identified by a bullet.*
Comprehensive	*Perform all elements identified by a bullet; document every element in each box with a shaded border and at least one element in each box with an unshaded border.*

DOCUMENTATION OF THE COMPLEXITY OF MEDICAL DECISION MAKING

The levels of evaluation and management services recognize four types of medical decision making (straight-forward, low complexity, moderate complexity and high complexity). Medical decision making refers to the complexity of establishing a diagnosis and/or selecting a management option as measured by:

- the number of possible diagnoses and/or the number of management options that must be considered;

- the amount and/or complexity of medical records, diagnostic tests, and/or other information that must be obtained, reviewed and analyzed; and

- the risk of significant complications, morbidity and/or mortality, as well as comorbidities, associated with the patient's presenting problem(s), the diagnostic procedure(s) and/or the possible management options.

The following chart illustrates the progression of the elements required for each level of medical decision making. To qualify for a given type of decision making, two of the three elements in the table must be either met or exceeded.

NUMBER OF DIAGNOSES OR MANAGEMENT OPTIONS

The number of possible diagnoses and/or the number of management options that must be considered is based on the number and types of problems addressed during the encounter, the complexity of establishing a diagnosis and the management decisions that are made by the physician.

Generally, decision making with respect to a diagnosed problem is easier than that for an identified but undiagnosed problem. The number and type of diagnostic tests employed may be an indicator of the number of possible diagnoses. Problems which are improving or resolving are less complex than those which are worsening or failing to change as expected. The need to seek advice from others is another indicator of complexity of diagnostic or management problems.

- **●DG:** *For each encounter, an assessment, clinical impression, or diagnosis should be documented. It may be explicitly stated or implied in documented decisions regarding management plans and/or further evaluation.*

  - *For a presenting problem with an established diagnosis, the record should reflect whether the problem is: a) improved, well controlled, resolving or resolved; or, b) inadequately controlled, worsening, or failing to change as expected.*

  - *For a presenting problem without an established diagnosis, the assessment or clinical impression may be stated in the form of differential diagnoses or as a "possible", "probable", or "rule out" (R/O) diagnosis.*

207

Number of Diagnoses	Amount of Data to Review	Risk of Complication	Type of Decision Making
Minimal	Minimal or None	Minimal	**Straightforward**
Limited	Limited	Low	**Low Complexity**
Multiple	Moderate	Moderate	**Moderate Complexity**
Extensive	Extensive	High	**High Complexity**

Each of the elements of medical decision making is described below

●*DG:* The initiation of, or changes in, treatment should be documented. Treatment includes a wide range of management options including patient instructions, nursing instructions, therapies, and medications.

●*DG:* If referrals are made, consultations requested or advice sought, the record should indicate to whom or where the referral or consultation is made or from whom the advice is requested.

AMOUNT AND/OR COMPLEXITY OF DATA TO BE REVIEWED

The amount and complexity of data to be reviewed is based on the types of diagnostic testing ordered or reviewed. A decision to obtain and review old medical records and/or obtain history from sources other than the patient increases the amount and complexity of data to be reviewed.

Discussion of contradictory or unexpected test results with the physician who performed or interpreted the test is an indication of the complexity of data being reviewed. On occasion the physician who ordered a test may personally review the image, tracing or specimen to supplement information from the physician who prepared the test report or interpretation; this is another indication of the complexity of data being reviewed.

●*DG:* If a diagnostic service (test or procedure) is ordered, planned, scheduled, or performed at the time of the evaluation and management encounter, the type of service, e.g., lab or x-ray, should be documented.

●*DG:* The review of lab, radiology and/or other diagnostic tests should be documented. A simple notation such as "WBC elevated" or "chest x-ray unremarkable" is acceptable. Alternatively, the review may be documented by initialing and dating the report containing the test results.

●*DG:* A decision to obtain old records or decision to obtain additional history from the family, caretaker or other source to supplement that obtained from the patient should be documented.

●*DG:* *Relevant findings from the review of old records, and/or the receipt of additional history from the family, caretaker or other source to supplement that obtained from the patient should be documented. If there is no relevant information beyond that already obtained, that fact should be documented. A notation of "Old records reviewed" or "additional history obtained from family" without elaboration is insufficient.*

●*DG:* *The results of discussion of laboratory, radiology or other diagnostic tests with the physician who performed or interpreted the study should be documented.*

●*DG:* *The direct visualization and independent interpretation of an image, tracing or specimen previously or subsequently interpreted by another physician should be documented.*

RISK OF SIGNIFICANT COMPLICATIONS, MORBIDITY AND/OR MORTALITY

The risk of significant complications, morbidity, and/or mortality is based on the risks associated with the presenting problem(s), the diagnostic procedure(s), and the possible management options.

●*DG:* *Comorbidities/underlying diseases or other factors that increase the complexity of medical decision making by increasing the risk of complications, morbidity, and/or mortality should be documented.*

●*DG:* *If a surgical or invasive diagnostic procedure is ordered, planned or scheduled at the time of the evaluation and management encounter, the type of procedure, e.g., laparoscopy, should be documented.*

●*DG:* *If a surgical or invasive diagnostic procedure is performed at the time of the evaluation and management encounter, the specific procedure should be documented.*

●*DG:* *The referral for or decision to perform a surgical or invasive diagnostic procedure on an urgent basis should be documented or implied.*

The Table of Risk on the following page may be used to help determine whether the risk of significant complications, morbidity, and/or mortality is minimal, low, moderate, or high. Because the determination of risk is complex and not readily quantifiable, the table includes common clinical examples rather than absolute measures of risk. The assessment of risk of the presenting problem(s) is based on the risk related to the disease process anticipated between the present encounter and the next one. The assessment of risk of selecting diagnostic procedures and management options is based on the risk during and immediately following any procedures or treatment. The highest level of risk in any one category (presenting problem(s), diagnostic procedure(s), or management options) determines the overall risk.

DOCUMENTATION OF AN ENCOUNTER DOMINATED BY COUNSELING OR COORDINATION OF CARE

In the case where counseling and/or coordination of care dominates (more than 50%) of the physician/patient and/or family encounter (face-to-face time in the office or other or outpatient setting, floor/unit time in the hospital or nursing facility), time is considered the key or controlling factor to qualify for a particular level of evaluation and management services.

●*DG:* *If the physician elects to report the level of service based on counseling and/or coordination of care, the total length of time of the encounter (face-to-face or floor time, as appropriate) should be documented and the record should describe the counseling and/or activities to coordinate care.*

TABLE OF RISK

LEVEL OF RISK	PRESENTING PROBLEM(S)	DIAGNOSTIC PROCEDURES	MANAGEMENT OPTIONS
Minimal	● *One self-limited or minor problem, (eg, cold, insect bite, tinea corporis)*	● *Laboratory tests requiring venipuncture* ● *Chest x-rays* ● *EKG/EEG* ● *Urinalysis* ● *Ultrasound, (eg, echocardiography)* ● *KOH prep*	● *Rest* ● *Gargles* ● *Elastic bandages* ● *Superficial dressings*
Low	● *Two or more self-limited or minor problems* ● *One stable chronic illness, (eg, well controlled hypertension, non-insulin dependent diabetes, cataract, BPH)* ● *Acute uncomplicated illness or injury, (eg, cystitis, allergic rhinitis, simple sprain)*	● *Physiologic tests not under stress, (eg, pulmonary function tests)* ● *Non-cardiovascular imaging studies with contrast,(eg, barium enema)* ● *Superficial needle biopsies* ● *Clinical laboratory tests requiring arterial puncture* ● *Skin biopsies*	● *Over-the-counter drugs* ● *Minor surgery with no identified risk factors* ● *Physical therapy* ● *Occupational therapy* ● *IV fluids without additives*

continued

TABLE OF RISK *(continued)*

LEVEL OF RISK	PRESENTING PROBLEM(S)	DIAGNOSTIC PROCEDURES	MANAGEMENT OPTIONS
Moderate	• One or more chronic illnesses with mild exacerbation, progression, or side effects of treatment • Two or more stable chronic illnesses • Undiagnosed new problem with uncertain prognosis, (eg, lump in breast) • Acute illness with systemic symptoms, (eg, pyelonephritis, pneumonitis, colitis) • Acute complicated injury, (eg, head injury with brief loss of consciousness)	• Physiologic tests under stress, (eg, cardiac stress test, fetal contraction stress test) • Diagnostic endoscopies with no identified risk factors • Deep needle or incisional biopsy • Cardiovascular imaging studies with contrast and no identified risk factors, (eg, arteriogram, cardiac catheterization) • Obtain fluid from body cavity, (eg, lumbar puncture, thoracentesis, culdocentesis)	• Minor surgery with identified risk factors • Elective major surgery (open, percutaneous or endoscopic) with no identified risk factors • Prescription drug management • Therapeutic nuclear medicine • IV fluids with additives • Closed treatment of fracture or dislocation without manipulation
High	• One or more chronic illnesses with severe exacerbation, progression, or side effects of treatment • Acute or chronic illnesses or injuries that pose a threat to life or bodily function, (eg, multiple trauma, acute MI, pulmonary embolus, severe respiratory distress, progressive severe rheumatoid arthritis, psychiatric illness with potential threat to self or others, peritonitis, acute renal failure) • An abrupt change in neurologic status, (eg, seizure, TIA, weakness, sensory loss)	• Cardiovascular imaging studies with contrast with identified risk factors • Cardiac electrophysiological tests • Diagnostic endoscopies with identified risk factors • Discography	• Elective major surgery (open, percutaneous or endoscopic) with identified risk factors • Emergency major surgery (open, percutaneous or endoscopic) • Parenteral controlled substances • Drug therapy requiring intensive monitoring for toxicity • Decision not to resuscitate or to de-escalate care because of poor prognosis

EVALUATION AND MANAGEMENT CODING VISUAL MATRIX

Many people are visually oriented, which means they perceive and learn better when presented with pictures, graphics, shapes and colors. The following Evaluation and Management Coding Visual Matrix is designed to assist visually oriented readers to quickly grasp the sections and choices available.

The Evaluation and Management Coding Visual Matrix reinforces that each Evaluation and Management code is selected from a choice of 1) history, 2) medical decision making and 3) presenting problem components. Some Evaluation and Management codes include a time unit; measured as either face-to-face time or bedside/floor or unit time.

Color Key   **Significance**

Components required

History & exam choices

Medical decision making choices

Presenting problem (severity) choices

Office/Other Outpatient Services (New Patients)

Components required: 3 of 3	99201	99202	99203	99204	99205
History & Exam					
Problem focused	●				
Expanded problem focused		●			
Detailed			●		
Comprehensive				●	●
Medical Decision Making					
Straightforward	●	●			
Low			●		
Moderate				●	
High					●
Presenting Problem (Severity)					
Self-limited or minor	●				
Low to moderate		●			
Moderate			●		
Moderate to high				●	●
Typical Time: Face-to-Face	10	20	30	45	60

Office/Other Outpatient Services (Established Patients)

Components required: 3 of 3	99211	99212	99213	99214	99215
History & Exam					
Problem focused		●			
Expanded problem focused			●		
Detailed				●	
Comprehensive					●
Medical Decision Making					
Straightforward		●			
Low			●		
Moderate				●	
High					●
Presenting Problem (Severity)					
Self-limited or minor	●				
Low to moderate		●			
Moderate			●		
Moderate to high				●	●
Typical Time: Face-to-Face	5	10	15	35	40

Initial Observation Care (New/Established Patients)

Components required: 3 of 3	99218	99219	99220
History & Exam			
Detailed or comprehensive	●		
Comprehensive		●	●
Straightforward or low	●		
Moderate		●	
High			●
Presenting Problem (Severity)			
Low	●		
Moderate		●	
High			●
Typical Time: Bedside/Floor/Unit	30	50	70

Subsequent Observation Care (New/Established Patients)

Components required: 2 of 3	99224	99225	99226
History & Exam			
Problem focused	●		
Expanded problem focused		●	
Detailed			●
Medical Decision Making			
Straightforward or low	●		
Moderate		●	
High			●
Presenting Problem (Severity)			
Stable/recovering/improving	●		
Responding inadequately/minor complication		●	
Unstable/significant complication/new problem			●
Typical Time: Bedside/Floor/Unit	15	25	35

Initial Hospital Care (New/Established Patients)

Components required: 3 of 3	99221	99222	99223
History & Exam			
Detailed or comprehensive	●		
Comprehensive		●	●
Straightforward or low	●		
Moderate		●	
High			●
Presenting Problem (Severity)			
Low	●		
Moderate		●	
High			●
Typical Time: Bedside/Floor/Unit	30	50	70

Subsequent Hospital Care (New/Established Patients)

Components required: 2 of 3	99231	99232	99233
History & Exam			
Problem focused	●		
Expanded problem focused		●	
Detailed			●
Medical Decision Making			
Straightforward or low	●		
Moderate		●	
High			●
Presenting Problem (Severity)			
Stable/recovering/improving	●		
Responding inadequately/minor complication		●	
Unstable/significant complication/new problem			●
Typical Time: Bedside/Floor/Unit	15	25	35

Observation/Inpatient Care Services (New/Established Patients) (Including Admission And Discharge Services)

Components required: 3 of 3	99234	99235	99236
History & Exam			
Detailed or comprehensive	●		
Comprehensive		●	●
Straightforward or low	●		
Moderate		●	
High			●
Presenting Problem (Severity)			
Low	●		
Moderate		●	
High			●
Typical Time:	--	--	--

Office/Other Outpatient Consultations (New/Established Patients)

Components required: 3 of 3	99241	99242	99243	99244	99245
History & Exam					
Problem focused	●				
Expanded problem focused		●			
Detailed			●		
Comprehensive				●	●
Medical Decision Making					
Straightforward	●	●			
Low			●		
Moderate				●	
High					●
Presenting Problem (Severity)					
Self-limited or minor	●				
Low		●			
Moderate			●		
Moderate to high				●	●
Typical Time: Face-to-Face	15	30	40	60	80

Inpatient Consultations (New/Established Patients)

Components required: 3 of 3	99251	99252	99253	99254	99255
History & Exam					
Problem focused	●				
Expanded problem focused		●			
Detailed			●		
Comprehensive				●	●
Medical Decision Making					
Straightforward	●	●			
Low			●		
Moderate				●	
High					●
Presenting Problem (Severity)					
Self-limited or minor	●				
Low		●			
Moderate			●		
Moderate to high				●	●
Typical Time: Bedside/Floor/Unit	20	40	55	80	110

Emergency Department Services (New/Established Patients)

Components required: 3 of 3	99281	99282	99283	99284	99285
History & Exam					
Problem focused	●				
Expanded problem focused		●	●		
Detailed				●	
Comprehensive					●
Medical Decision Making					
Straightforward	●				
Low		●			
Moderate			●	●	
High					●
Presenting Problem (Severity)					
Self-limited or minor	●				
Low to moderate		●			
Moderate			●		
High				●	
High severity/immediate significant threat to life or physiological function					●
Typical Time:	--	--	--	--	--

Initial Nursing Facility Care (New/Established Patients)

Components required: 3 of 3	99304	99305	99306
History & Exam			
Detailed or comprehensive	●		
Comprehensive		●	●
Medical Decision Making			
Straightforward or low	●		
Moderate		●	
High			●
Presenting Problem (Severity)			
Low	●		
Moderate		●	
High			●
Typical Time: Bedside/Floor/Unit	25	35	45

Subsequent Nursing Facility Services

Components required: 2 of 3	99307	99308	99309	99310
History & Exam				
Problem focused	●			
Expanded problem focused		●		
Detailed			●	
Comprehensive				●
Medical Decision Making				
Straightforward	●			
Low		●		
Moderate			●	
High				●
Presenting Problem (Severity)				
Stable/recovering/improving	●			
Responding inadequately to therapy/minor complication		●		
Significant complication/significant new problem			●	
Unstable/significant new problem requiring immediate physician attention				●
Typical Time: Bedside/Floor/Unit	10	15	25	35

Domiciliary, Rest Home, Or Custodial Care Services

Components required: 3 of 3	99324	99325	99326	99327	99328
History & Exam					
Problem focused	●				
Expanded problem focused		●			
Detailed			●		
Comprehensive				●	●
Medical Decision Making					
Straightforward	●				
Low		●			
Moderate			●	●	
High					●
Presenting Problem (Severity)					
Low	●				
Moderate		●			
Moderate to high			●		
High				●	
Unstable/significant new problem requiring immediate attention					●
Typical Time: Face-to-Face	20	30	45	60	75

Domiciliary, Rest Home, or Custodial Care Services

Components required: 2 of 3	99334	99335	99336	99337
History & Exam				
Problem focused	●			
Expanded problem focused		●		
Detailed			●	
Comprehensive				●
Medical Decision Making				
Straightforward	●			
Low		●		
Moderate			●	
Moderate to high				●
Presenting Problem (Severity)				
Self-limited or minor	●			
Low to moderate		●		
Moderate to high			●	
Moderate to high/unstable/significant new problem				●
Typical Time: Face-to-Face	15	25	40	60

Home Services (New Patients)

Components required: 3 of 3	99341	99342	99343	99344	99345
History & Exam					
Problem focused	●				
Expanded problem focused		●			
Detailed			●		
Comprehensive				●	●
Medical Decision Making					
Straightforward	●				
Low		●			
Moderate			●	●	
High					●
Presenting Problem (Severity)					
Low	●				
Moderate		●			
Moderate to high			●		
High				●	
Unstable/significant new problem					●
Typical Time: Face-to-Face	20	30	45	60	75

Home Services (Established Patient)

Components required: 2 of 3	99347	99348	99349	99350
History & Exam				
Problem focused	●			
Expanded problem focused		●		
Detailed			●	
Comprehensive				●
Medical Decision Making				
Straightforward	●			
Low		●		
Moderate			●	
Moderate to high				●
Presenting Problem (Severity)				
Self-limited or minor	●			
Low to moderate		●		
Moderate to high			●	
Moderate to high/unstable/significant new problem				●
Typical Time: Face-to-Face	15	25	40	60

EVALUATION AND MANAGEMENT

OFFICE OR OTHER OUTPATIENT SERVICES

The key coding issues are the extent of history obtained, the extent of examination performed, and the complexity of medical decision making. Additional reporting issues include counseling and/or coordination of care, the nature of presenting problem(s), and the duration of face-to-face time spent with the patient and/or family.

CODING RULES

1. *A patient is considered an outpatient until admitted as an inpatient to a health care facility.*

2. *If outpatient evaluation and management services are provided in conjunction with, or result in, an inpatient admission, the service is reported using CPT codes for initial hospital care.*

3. *CPT codes in this section may also be used to report the services provided by a physician to a patient in an observation area of a hospital.*

4. *Laboratory tests, radiology services, and diagnostic or therapeutic procedures performed in conjunction with evaluation and management services are reported in addition to the basic evaluation and management service.*

5. *Supplies and materials provided by the physician over and above those usually included with the evaluation and management or other services rendered may be listed separately. List all drugs, trays, supplies and materials provided.*

The following codes are used to report evaluation and management services provided in the office or in an outpatient or other ambulatory facility. A patient is considered an outpatient until inpatient admission to a health care facility occurs.

To report services provided to a patient who is admitted to a hospital or nursing facility in the course of an encounter in the office or other ambulatory facility, see the notes for initial hospital inpatient care, or initial nursing facility care.

For services provided in the emergency department, see 99281-99285.

For observation care, see 99217-99226.

221

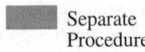 Separate Procedure   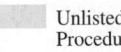 Unlisted Procedure   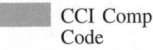 CCI Comp. Code   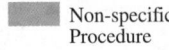 Non-specific Procedure

For observation or inpatient care services (including admission and discharge services), see 99234-99236.

NEW PATIENT

▲ **99201**　Office or other outpatient visit for the evaluation and management of a new patient, which requires these three key components:

- a problem focused history;
- a problem focused examination; and
- straightforward medical decision making.

Counseling and/or coordination of care with other physicians, other qualified health care professionals, or agencies are provided consistent with the nature of the problem(s) and the patient's and/or family's needs.

Usually, the presenting problems are self limited or minor. Typically 10 minutes are spent face-to-face with the patient and/or family.

▲ **99202**　Office or other outpatient visit for the evaluation and management of a new patient, which requires these three key components:

- an expanded problem focused history;
- an expanded problem focused examination; and
- straightforward medical decision making.

Counseling and/or coordination of care with other physicians, other qualified health care professionals, or agencies are provided consistent with the nature of the problem(s) and the patient's and/or family's needs.

Usually, the presenting problem(s) are of low to moderate severity. Typically 20 minutes are spent face-to-face with the patient and/or family.

▲ **99203**　Office or other outpatient visit for the evaluation and management of a new patient, which requires these three key components:

- a detailed history;
- a detailed examination; and
- medical decision making of low complexity.

Counseling and/or coordination of care with other physicians, other qualified health care professionals, or agencies are

● New
　Code

▲ Revised
　Code

＋ Add-On
　Code

⊘ Modifier -51
　Exempt

⊙ Moderate
　Sedation

provided consistent with the nature of the problem(s) and the patient's and/or family's needs.

Usually, the presenting problem(s) are of moderate severity. Typically 30 minutes are spent face-to-face with the patient and/or family.

▲ 99204　Office or other outpatient visit for the evaluation and management of a new patient, which requires these three key components:

- a comprehensive history;

- a comprehensive examination; and

- medical decision making of moderate complexity.

Counseling and/or coordination of care with other physicians, other qualified health care professionals, or agencies are provided consistent with the nature of the problem(s) and the patient's and/or family's needs.

Usually, the presenting problem(s) are of moderate to high severity. Typically 45 minutes are spent face-to-face with the patient and/or family.

▲ 99205　Office or other outpatient visit for the evaluation and management of a new patient, which requires these three key components:

- a comprehensive history;

- a comprehensive examination; and

- medical decision making of high complexity.

Counseling and/or coordination of care with other physicians, other qualified health care professionals, or agencies are provided consistent with the nature of the problem(s) and the patient's and/or family's needs.

Usually, the presenting problem(s) are of moderate to high severity. Typically 60 minutes are spent face-to-face with the patient and/or family.

ESTABLISHED PATIENT

▲ 99211　Office or other outpatient visit for the evaluation and management of an established patient, that may not require the presence of a physician or other qualified health care professional. Usually, the presenting problem(s) are minimal. Typically, 5 minutes are spent performing or supervising these services.

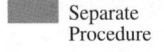 Separate Procedure
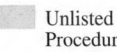 Unlisted Procedure
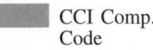 CCI Comp. Code
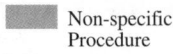 Non-specific Procedure

223

▲ **99212**   Office or other outpatient visit for the evaluation and management of an established patient, which requires at least two of these three key components:

- a problem focused history;

- a problem focused examination;

- straightforward medical decision making.

Counseling and/or coordination of care with other physicians, other qualified health care professionals, or agencies are provided consistent with the nature of the problem(s) and the patient's and/or family's needs.

Usually, the presenting problem(s) are self limited or minor. Typically 10 minutes are spent face-to-face with the patient and/or family.

▲ **99213**   Office or other outpatient visit for the evaluation and management of an established patient, which requires at least two of these three key components:

- an expanded problem focused history;

- an expanded problem focused examination;

- medical decision making of low complexity.

Counseling and coordination of care with other physicians, other qualified health care professionals, or agencies are provided consistent with the nature of the problem(s) and the patient's and/or family's needs.

Usually, the presenting problem(s) are of low to moderate severity. Typically 15 minutes are spent face-to-face with the patient and/or family.

▲ **99214**   Office or other outpatient visit for the evaluation and management of an established patient, which requires at least two of these three key components:

- a detailed history;

- a detailed examination;

- medical decision making of moderate complexity.

Counseling and/or coordination of care with other physicians, other qualified health care professionals, or agencies are provided consistent with the nature of the problem(s) and the patient's and/or family's needs.

● New Code   ▲ Revised Code   + Add-On Code   ⊘ Modifier -51 Exempt   ⊙ Moderate Sedation

Usually, the presenting problem(s) are of moderate to high severity. Typically 25 minutes are spent face-to-face with the patient and/or family.

▲ 99215   Office or other outpatient visit for the evaluation and management of an established patient, which requires at least two of these three key components:

● a comprehensive history;

● a comprehensive examination;

● medical decision making of high complexity.

Counseling and/or coordination of care with other physicians, other qualified health care professionals, or agencies are provided consistent with the nature of the problem(s) and the patient's and/or family's needs.

Usually, the presenting problem(s) are of moderate to high severity. Typically 40 minutes are spent face-to-face with the patient and/or family.

HOSPITAL OBSERVATION SERVICES

Occasionally a physician will watch or "observe" a patient in an area of an inpatient hospital designated as an "observation" area. This area is frequently located in or near the emergency room, and the observation typically after any acute care is rendered.

The purpose of the observation is to determine if the patient's condition requires inpatient hospitalization. Patients considered under observation status may be discharged from the observation area or admitted to the hospital as an inpatient.

All observation care services are "per day" and should be coded only once per date of service. CPT code 99217 is used to report all services provided on discharge from "observation status" if the discharge is on other than the initial date of "observation status."

The following codes are used to report evaluation and management services provided to patients designated/admitted as "observation status" in a hospital. It is not necessary that the patient be located in an observation area designated by the hospital.

If such an area does exist in a hospital (as a separate unit in the hospital, in the emergency department, etc.), these codes are to be utilized if the patient is placed in such an area.

For definitions of key components and commonly used terms, please see Evaluation and Management Services Guidelines.

| ▆ Separate Procedure | ▒ Unlisted Procedure | ▆ CCI Comp. Code | ▆ Non-specific Procedure | **225** |

OBSERVATION CARE DISCHARGE SERVICES

Observation care discharge of a patient from "observation status" includes final examination of the patient, discussion of the hospital stay, instructions for continuing care, and preparation of dishcarge records. For observation or inpatient hospital care including the admission and discharge of the patient on the same date, see codes 99234-99236 as appropriate.

▲ 99217   Observation care discharge day management (This code is to be utilized to report all services provided to a patient on discharge from "observation status" if the discharge is on other than the initial date of "observation status." To report services to a patient designated as "observation status" or "inpatient status" and discharged on the same date, use codes for Observation or Inpatient Care Services [including Admission and Discharge Services, 99234-99236 as appropriate]).

INITIAL OBSERVATION CARE

NEW OR ESTABLISHED PATIENT

The following codes are used to report the encounter(s) by the supervising physician or other qualified health care professional with the patient when designated as "observation status." This refers to the initiation of observation status, supervision of the care plan for observation, and performance of periodic reassessments. For observation encounters by other physicians, see office or other outpatient consultation codes (99241-99245) or subsequent observation care codes (99224-99226) as appropriate.

To report services provided to a patient who is admitted to the hospital after receiving hospital observation care services on the same date, see the notes for initial hospital inpatient care (later in this section). For observation care services on other than the initial or discharge date, see subsequent observation services codes (99224-99226). For a patient admitted to the hospital on a date subsequent to the date of observation status, the hospital admission would be reported with the appropriate initial hospital care code (99221-99223). For a patient admitted and discharged from observation or inpatient status on the same date, the services should be reported with codes 99234-99236 as appropriate. Do not report observation discharge (99217) in conjunction with a hospital admission (99221-99223).

When "observation status" is initiated in the course of an encounter in another site of service (eg, hospital emergency department, office, nursing facility) all evaluation and management services provided by the supervising physician or other qualified health care professional in conjunction with initiating "observation status" are considered part of the initial observation care when performed on the same date. The observation care level of service reported by the supervising physician or other qualified health care professional should include the services

● New Code   ▲ Revised Code   + Add-On Code   ⊘ Modifier -51 Exempt   ⊙ Moderate Sedation

related to initiating "observation status" provided in the other sites of service as well as in the observation setting.

Evaluation and management services including new or established patient office or other outpatient services (99201-99215), emergency department services (99281-99285), nursing facility services (99304-99318), domiciliary, rest home or custodial care services (99324-99337), home services (99341-99350), and preventive medicine services (99381-99429) on the same date related to the admission to "observation status" should **not** be reported separately.

These codes may not be utilized for post-operative recovery if the procedure is considered part of the surgical "package." These codes apply to all evaluation and management services that are provided on the same date of initiating "observation status."

▲ **99218** Initial observation care, per day, for the evaluation and management of a patient which requires these 3 key components:

- A detailed or comprehensive history;

- A detailed or comprehensive examination; and

- Medical decision making that is straightforward or of low complexity.

Counseling and/or coordination of care with other physicians, other qualified health care professionals, or agencies are provided consistent with the nature of the problem(s) and the patient's and/or family's needs.

Usually, the problem(s) requiring admission to "observation status" are of low severity. Typically 30 minutes are spent at the bedside and on the patient's hospital floor or unit.

▲ **99219** Initial observation care, per day, for the evaluation and management of a patient, which requires these 3 key components:

- A comprehensive history;

- A comprehensive examination; and

- Medical decision making of moderate complexity.

Counseling and/or coordination of care with other physicians, other qualified health care professionals, or agencies are provided consistent with the nature of the problem(s) and the patient's and/or family's needs.

Usually, the problem(s) requiring admission to "observation status" are of moderate severity. Typically 50 minutes are spent at the bedside and on the patient's hospital floor or unit.

227

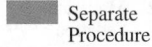 Separate Procedure   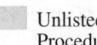 Unlisted Procedure   ▨ CCI Comp. Code   ▨ Non-specific Procedure

99220   Initial observation care, per day, for the evaluation and management of a patient, which requires these 3 key components:

- A comprehensive history;

- A comprehensive examination; and

- Medical decision making of high complexity.

Counseling and/or coordination of care with other physicians, other qualified health care professionals, or agencies are provided consistent with the nature of the problem(s) and the patient's and/or family's needs.

Usually, the problem(s) requiring admission to "observation status" are of high severity. Typically 70 minutes are spent at the bedside and on the patient's hospital floor or unit.

SUBSEQUENT OBSERVATION CARE

All levels of subsequent observation care include reviewing the medical record and reviewing the results of diagnostic studies and changes in the patient's status (ie., changes in history, physical condition, and response to management) since the last assessment.

▲ **99224**   Subsequent observation care, per day, for the evaluation and management of a patient, which requires at least 2 of these 3 key components:

- problem focused interval history;

- problem focused examination;

- medical decision making that is straightforward or of low complexity.

Counseling and/or coordination of care with other physicians, other qualified health care professionals, or agencies are provided consistent with the nature of the problem(s) and the patient's and/or family's needs.

Usually, the patient is stable, recovering, or improving. Typically 15 minutes are spent at the bedside and on the patient's hospital floor or unit.

▲ **99225**   Subsequent observation care, per day, for the evaluation and management of a patient, which requires at least 2 of these 3 key components:

- an expanded problem focused interval history;

- an expanded problem focused examination;

228   ● New   ▲ Revised   + Add-On   ⊘ Modifier -51   ⊙ Moderate
Code   Code   Code   Exempt   Sedation

- medical decision making of moderate complexity

Counseling and/or coordination of care with other physicians, other qualified health care professionals, or agencies are provided consistent with the nature of the problem(s) and the patient's and/or family's needs.

Usually, the patient is responding inadequately to therapy or has developed a minor complication. Typically 25 are spent minutes at the bedside and on the patient's hospital floor or unit.

▲ **99226** Subsequent observation care, per day, for the evaluation and management of a patient, which requires at least 2 of these 3 key components:

- a detailed interval history;
- a detailed examination
- medical decision making of high complexity.

Counseling and/or coordination of care with other physicians, other qualified health care professionals, or agencies are provided consistent with the nature of the problem(s) and the patient's and/or family's needs.

Usually, the patient is unstable or has developed a significant complication or a significant new problem. Typically 35 minutes are spent at the bedside and on the patient's hospital floor or unit.

HOSPITAL INPATIENT SERVICES

Hospital inpatient services refer to hospital visits during the course of an inpatient hospital stay. The services may be provided by the patient's primary physician and/or other physicians in the event of multiple illnesses or injuries. Evaluation and management codes 99221-99239 are used to report services provided in the hospital. The key coding issues are the extent of history obtained, the extent of examination performed, and the complexity of medical decision making. Additional reporting issues include counseling and/or coordination of care, the nature of presenting problem(s), and the time spent at the bedside and on the patient's facility floor or unit.

CODING RULES

1. *CPT codes defined as Initial Hospital Care are used to report the first hospital inpatient encounter with the patient by the admitting physician.*

2. *The admitting physician should report all service related to the admission provided in all other locations.*

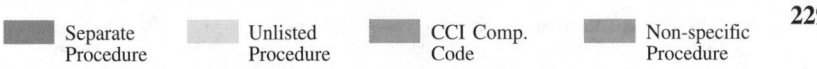

	Separate Procedure		Unlisted Procedure		CCI Comp. Code		Non-specific Procedure

229

3. *For observation care or inpatient hospital care services provided to patients who are admitted and discharged on the same date, report with CPT codes 99234-99236 from the Observation or Inpatient Care services subsections.*

The following codes are used to report evaluation and management services provided to hospital inpatients. Hospital inpatient services include those services provided to patients in a "partial hospital" setting. These codes are to be used to report these partial hospitalization services. See also psychiatry notes in the full text of the CPT code set.

For definitions of key components and commonly used terms, please see Evaluation and Management Services Guidelines. For Hospital Observation Services, see 99218-99220, 99224-99226. For a patient admitted and discharged from observation or inpatient status on the same date, the services should be reported with codes 99234-99236 as appropriate.

INITIAL HOSPITAL CARE

NEW OR ESTABLISHED PATIENT

The following codes are used to report the first hospital inpatient encounter with the patient by the admitting physician.

For initial inpatient encounters by physicians other than the admitting physician, see initial inpatient consultation codes (99251-99255) or subsequent hospital care codes (99231-99233) as .appropriate.

For admission services for the neonate (28 days of age or younger) requiring intensive observation, frequent interventions, and other intensive care services, see 99477.

When the patient is admitted to the hospital as an inpatient in the course of an encounter in another site of service (eg, hospital emergency department, observation status in a hospital, office, nursing facility), all evaluation and mangement services provided by that physician in conjunction with that admission are considered part of the initial hospital care when performed on the same date as the admission. The inpatient care level of service reported by the admitting physician should include the services related to the admission he/she provided in the other sites of service as well as in the inpatient setting.

Evaluation and management services including new or established patient office or other outpatient services (99201-99215), emergency department services (99281-99285), nursing facility services (99304-99318), domiciliary, rest home, or custodial care services (99324-99337), home services (99341-99350), and preventive medicine services (99381-99397) on the same date related to the admission to "observation status" should **not** be reported separately. For a patient admitted and discharged from observation or inpatient status on the same date, the services should be reported with codes 99234-99236 as appropriate.

● New   ▲ Revised   + Add-On   ⊘ Modifier -51   ⊙ Moderate
          Code   Code   Code   Exempt   Sedation

▲ **99221**   Initial hospital care, per day, for the evaluation and management of a patient which requires these three key components:

- a detailed or comprehensive history;

- a detailed or comprehensive examination; and

- medical decision making that is straightforward or of low complexity.

Counseling and/or coordination of care with other physicians, other qualified health care professionals, or agencies are provided consistent with the nature of the problem(s) and the patient's and/or family's needs.

Usually, the problem(s) requiring admission are of low severity. Typically 30 minutes are spent at the bedside and on the patient's hospital floor or unit.

▲ **99222**   Initial hospital care, per day, for the evaluation and management of a patient, which requires these three key components:

- a comprehensive history;

- a comprehensive examination; and

- medical decision making of moderate complexity.

Counseling and/or coordination of care with other physicians, other qualified health care professionals, or agencies are provided consistent with the nature of the problem(s) and the patient's and/or family's needs.

Usually, the problem(s) requiring admission are of moderate severity. Typically 50 minutes are spent at the bedside and on the patient's hospital floor or unit.

▲ **99223**   Initial hospital care, per day, for the evaluation and management of a patient, which requires these three key components:

- a comprehensive history;

- a comprehensive examination; and

- medical decision making of high complexity.

Counseling and/or coordination of care with other physicians, other qualified health care professionals, or agencies are provided consistent with the nature of the problem(s) and the patient's and/or family's needs.

Usually, the problem(s) requiring admission are of high severity. Typically 70 minutes are spent at the bedside and on the patient's hospital floor or unit.

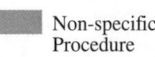

	Separate Procedure		Unlisted Procedure		CCI Comp. Code		Non-specific Procedure

231

99224 This code is out of order. See page 228

99225 This code is out of order. See page 228

99226 This code is out of order. See page 229

SUBSEQUENT HOSPITAL CARE

All levels of subsequent hospital care include reviewing the medical record and reviewing the results of diagnostic studies and changes in the patient's status (i.e., changes in history, physical condition and response to management) since the last assessment.

▲ **99231** Subsequent hospital care, per day, for the evaluation and management of a patient, which requires at least two of these three key components:

- a problem focused interval history;

- a problem focused examination;

- medical decision making that is straightforward or of low complexity.

Counseling and/or coordination of care with other physicians, other qualified health care professionals, or agencies are provided consistent with the nature of the problem(s) and the patient's and/or family's needs.

Usually, the patient is stable, recovering or improving. Typically 15 minutes are spent at the bedside and on the patient's hospital floor or unit.

▲ **99232** Subsequent hospital care, per day, for the evaluation and management of a patient, which requires at least two of these three key components:

- an expanded problem focused interval history;

- an expanded problem focused examination;

- medical decision making of moderate complexity.

Counseling and/or coordination of care with other physicians, other qualified health care professionals, or agencies are provided consistent with the nature of the problem(s) and the patient's and/or family's needs.

Usually, the patient is responding inadequately to therapy or has developed a minor complication. Typically 25 minutes are spent at the bedside and on the patient's hospital floor or unit.

● New Code	▲ Revised Code	+ Add-On Code	⊘ Modifier -51 Exempt	⊙ Moderate Sedation

▲ **99233** Subsequent hospital care, per day, for the evaluation and management of a patient, which requires at least two of these three key components:

- a detailed interval history;
- a detailed examination;
- medical decision making of high complexity.

Counseling and/or coordination of care with other physicians, other qualified health care professionals, or agencies are provided consistent with the nature of the problem(s) and the patient's and/or family's needs.

Usually, the patient is unstable or has developed a significant complication or a significant new problem. Typically 35 minutes are spent at the bedside and on the patient's hospital floor or unit.

OBSERVATION OR INPATIENT CARE SERVICES (INCLUDING ADMISSION AND DISCHARGE SERVICES)

The following codes are used to report observation or inpatient hospital care services provided to patients admitted and discharged on the same date of sevice. When a patient is admitted to the hospital from observation status on the same date, only the initial hospital care code should be reported. The initial hospital care code reported by the admitting physician or other qualified health care professional should include the services related to the observation status services he/she provided on the same date of inpatient admission.

When "observation status" is initiated in the course of an encounter in another site of service (eg, hospital emergency department, office, nursing facility), all evaluation and management services provided by the supervising physician or other qualified health care professional in conjunction with initiating "observation status" are considered part of the initial observation care when performed on the same date. The observation care level of service should include the services related to initiating "observation status" provided in the other sites of services as well as in the observation setting when provided by the same individual.

For patients admitted to observation or inpatient care and discharged on a different date, see codes 99218-99220, 99224-99226, 99217, or 99221-99223, 99238, and 99239.

▲ **99234** Observation or inpatient hospital care, for the evaluation and management of a patient including admission and discharge on the same date which requires these three key components:

- a detailed or comprehensive history;
- a detailed or comprehensive examination; and

233

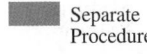 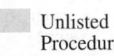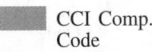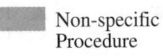

- medical decision making that is straightforward or of low complexity.

Counseling and/or coordination of care with other physicians, other qualified health care professionals, or agencies are provided consistent with the nature of the problem(s) and the patient's and/or family's needs.

Usually the presenting problem(s) requiring admission are of low severity. Typically 40 minutes are spent at the bedside and on the patient's hospital floor or unit.

▲ 99235　Observation or inpatient hospital care, for the evaluation and management of a patient including admission and discharge on the same date which requires these three key components:

- a comprehensive history;

- a comprehensive examination; and

- medical decision making of moderate complexity.

Counseling and/or coordination of care with other physicians, other qualified health care professionals, or agencies are provided consistent with the nature of the problem(s) and the patient's and/or family's needs.

Usually the presenting problem(s) requiring admission are of moderate severity. Typically, 50 minutes are spent at the bedside and on the patient's hospital floor or unit.

▲ 99236　Observation or inpatient hospital care, for the evaluation and management of a patient including admission and discharge on the same date which requires these three key components:

- a comprehensive history;

- a comprehensive examination; and

- medical decision making of high complexity.

Counseling and/or coordination of care with other physicians, other qualified health care professionals, or agencies are provided consistent with the nature of the problem(s) and the patient's and/or family's needs.

Usually the presenting problem(s) requiring admission are of high severity. Typically, 55 minutes are spent at the bedside and on the patient's floor or unit.

HOSPITAL DISCHARGE SERVICES

The hospital discharge day management codes are to be used to report the total duration of time spent by a physician for final hospital discharge of a patient. The codes include, as appropriate, final examination of the patient, discussion of the hospital stay, even if the time spent by the physician on that date is not continuous, instructions for continuing care to all relevant caregivers, and preparation of discharge records, prescriptions and referral forms. For a patient admitted and discharged from observation or inpatient status on the same date, the services should be reported with codes 99234-99236 as appropriate.

99238   Hospital discharge day management; 30 minutes or less

99239   more than 30 minutes

(These codes are to be utilized to report all services provided to a patient on the date of discharge, if other than the initial date of inpatient status. To report services to a patient who is admitted as an inpatient and discharged on the same date, see codes 99234-99236 for observation or inpatient hospital care including the admission and discharge of the patient on the same date. To report concurrent care services provided by a physician[s] other than the ordering physician or another qualified health care professional, use subsequent hospital care codes [99231-99233] on the day of discharge.)

(For Observation Care Discharge, use 99217)

(For observation or inpatient hospital care including the admission and discharge of the patient on the same date, see 99234-99236)

(For Nursing Facility Care Discharge, 99315, 99316)

(For discharge services provided to newborns admitted and discharged on the same date, use 99463)

CONSULTATIONS

A consultation is a type of evaluation and management service provided at the request of another physician or appropriate source to either recommend care for a specific condition or problem or to determine whether to accept responsibility for ongoing management of the patient's entire care or for the care of a specific condition or problem.

A physician consultant may initiate diagnostic and/or therapeutic services at the same or subsequent visit.

A "consultation" initiated by a patient and/or family, and not requested by a physician or other appropriate source (eg, physician assistant, nurse practitioner, doctor of chiropractic, physical therapist, occupational therapist, speech-language pathologist, psychologist, social worker, lawyer, or insurance company) is not

235

| Separate Procedure | Unlisted Procedure | CCI Comp. Code | Non-specific Procedure |

reported using the consultation codes, but may be reported using the office visit, home service, or domiciliary/rest home care codes as appropriate.

The written or verbal request for consult may be made by a physician or other appropriate source and documented in the patient's medical record by either the consulting or requesting physician or appropriate source. The consultant's opinion and any services that were ordered or performed must also be documented in the patient's medical record and sommunicated by written report to the requesting physician or other appropriate source.

If a consultation is mandated (eg, by a third-party payer) modifier 32 should also be reported.

Any specifically identifiable procedure (ie, identified with a specific CPT code) performed on or subsequent to the date of the initial consultation should be reported separately.

If subsequent to the completion of a consultation the consultant assumes responsibility for management of a portion or all of the patient's condition(s), the appropriate Evaluation and Management services code for the site of service should be reported. In the hospital or nursing facility setting, the consulting consultant should use the appropriate inpatient consultation code for the initial encounter and then subsequent hospital or nursing facility care codes. In the office setting, the consultant should use the appropriate office or other outpatient consultation codes and then the established patient office or other outpatient services codes.

To report services provided to a patient who is admitted to a hospital or nursing facility in the course of an encounter in the office or other ambulatory facility, see the notes for Initial Hospital Inpatient Care or Initial Nursing Facility Care. For definitions of key components and commonly used terms, please see Evaluation and Management Services Guidelines.

CODING GUIDELINES

A consultation is the process of taking a history, performing a physical examination, and ordering and interpreting appropriate diagnostic tests for the purpose of rendering an expert opinion about a patient's illness and/or injury. E/M service codes 99241-99275 are used to report office, inpatient, and confirmatory consultation services provided to new or established patients. The key coding issues are the location of the service, the extent of history obtained, the extent of examination performed, and the complexity of medical decision making. Additional reporting issues include counseling and/or coordination of care, the nature of presenting problem(s), and the time, depending on location, spent either face to face with the patient and/or family or at the bedside and on the patient's facility floor or unit.

● New Code   ▲ Revised Code   + Add-On Code   ⊘ Modifier -51 Exempt   ⊙ Moderate Sedation

Coding Rules

1. The request for a consultation from the attending physician or other appropriate source and the need for a consultation must be documented in the patient's medical record.

2. The consultant's opinion and any services that were ordered or performed must be documented in the patient's medical record and communicated to the requesting physician or source.

3. Consultations that are initiated by request from the patient and/or family may be reported using codes for confirmatory consultations or office services as appropriate.

4. If a confirmatory consultation is required by a third party, such as a Peer Review Organization (PRO), modifier -32 should be added to the basic service.

5. Any specifically identifiable procedure performed on or subsequent to the date of the initial consultation is reported separately.

6. If the consultant subsequently assumes responsibility for management of all or a portion of the patient's condition(s), then either hospital services or office services are used as appropriate.

Consultation service codes may not be billed to Medicare for services rendered on or after January 1, 2010. Physicians must use visit/outpatient or inpatient hospital evaluation and management codes to bill Medicare for consultation services. Telehealth consultation may be reported using the appropriate HCPCS G-codes.

Medicare Cross-Walk from Consultation Codes to Outpatient/Hospital Codes

CMS published a cross-walk from consultation codes to outpatient/hospital codes for the purpose of establishing budget neutrality. According to CMS the cross-walks are not billing guidance and physicians should bill the E/M code appropriate for the service provided.

For office based consultations, the selection of E/M visit codes is based on whether the patient is a new or established patient. For hospital consultations, the selection of appropriate E/M codes is based on the location of the consultation in either an acute care hospital or nursing home and the level of history, exam, and medical decision making.

| | Separate Procedure | | Unlisted Procedure | | CCI Comp. Code | | Non-specific Procedure | **237** |

Office Consultation Codes			Inpatient Consultation Codes		
Source	Destination	Mapping*	Source	Destination	Mapping*
99241	99201	50%	99251	99221	70%
	99211	50%		99304	30%
99242	99202	50%	99252	99221	35%
	99212	50%		99222	35%
99243	99203	50%		99304	15%
	99213	50%		99305	15%
99244	99204	50%	99253	99222	70%
	99214	50%		99305	30%
99245	99205	50%	99254	99222	35%
	99215	50%		99223	35%
				99305	15%
				99306	15%
			99255	99223	70%
				99306	30%

*Refers to the CMS estimated frequency of conversion from the consultation code to the visit code.

OFFICE OR OTHER OUTPATIENT CONSULTATIONS

NEW OR ESTABLISHED PATIENT

The following codes are used to report consultations provided in the office or in an outpatient or other ambulatory facility, including hospital observation services, home services, domiciliary, rest home or emergency department (see the preceding consultation definition above). Follow-up visits in the consultant's office or other outpatient facility that are initiated by the consultant or patient are reported using the appropriate codes for established patients, office visits (99211-99215), domiciliary, rest home (99334-99337), or home (99347-99350). If an additional request for an opinion or advice regarding the same or a new problem is received from another physician or other appropriate source and documented in the medical record, the office consultation codes may be used again. Services that constitute transfer of care (ie, are provided for the managment of the patient's entire care or for the care of a specific condition or problem) are reported with the appropriate new or established patient codes for office or other outpatient visits, domiciliary, rest home services, or home services.

● New Code   ▲ Revised Code   + Add-On Code   ⊘ Modifier -51 Exempt   ⊙ Moderate Sedation

▲ **99241** Office consultation for a new or established patient, which requires these three key components:

- a problem focused history;

- a problem focused examination; and

- straightforward medical decision making.

Counseling and/or coordination of care with other physicians, other qualified health care professionals, or agencies are provided consistent with the nature of the problem(s) and the patient's and/or family's needs.

Usually, the presenting problem(s) are self limited or minor. Typically 15 minutes are spent face-to-face with the patient and/or family.

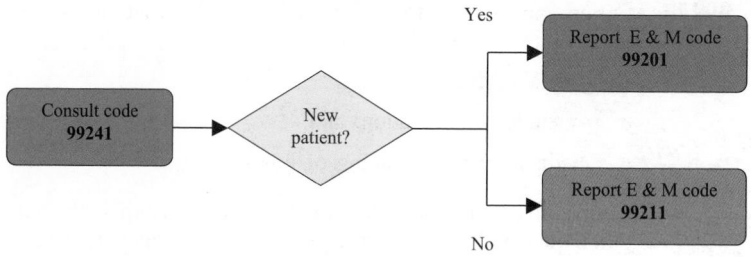

Medicare Cross-Walk:

Report 99201 instead of 99241 for new patients.
Report 99211 instead of 99241 for established patients.

▲ **99242** Office consultation for a new or established patient, which requires these three key components:

- an expanded problem focused history;

- an expanded problem focused examination; and

- straightforward medical decision making.

Counseling and/or coordination of care with other physicians, other qualified health care professionals, or agencies are provided consistent with the nature of the problem(s) and the patient's and/or family's needs.

Usually, the presenting problem(s) are of low severity. Typically 30 minutes are spent face-to-face with the patient and/or family.

239

	Separate Procedure		Unlisted Procedure		CCI Comp. Code		Non-specific Procedure

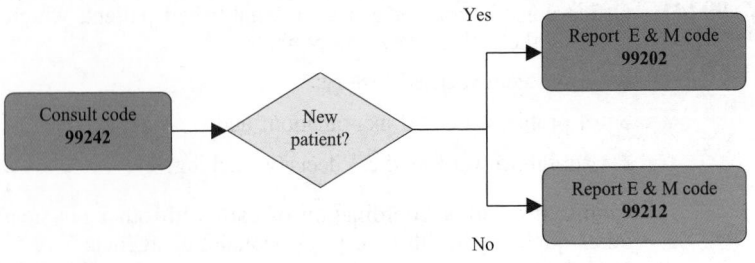

Medicare Cross-Walk:

Report 99202 instead of 99242 for new patients.
Report 99212 instead of 99242 for established patients.

▲ **99243**   Office consultation for a new or established patient, which
requires these three key components:

- a detailed history;

- a detailed examination; and

- medical decision making of low complexity.

Counseling and/or coordination of care with other physicians,
other qualified health care professionals, or agencies are
provided consistent with the nature of the problem(s) and the
patient's and/or family's needs.

Usually, the presenting problem(s) are of moderate severity.
Typically 40 minutes are spent face-to-face with the patient
and/or family.

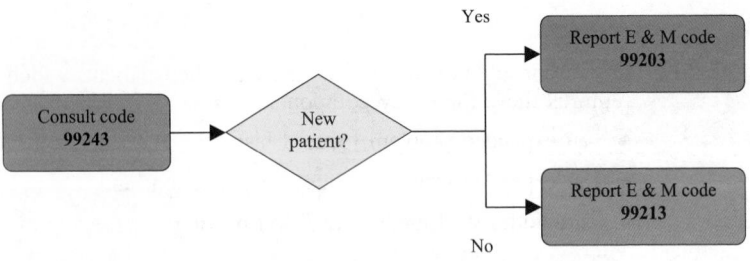

Medicare Cross-Walk:

Report 99203 instead of 99243 for new patients.
Report 99213 instead of 99243 for established patients

● New Code   ▲ Revised Code   + Add-On Code   ⊘ Modifier -51 Exempt   ⊙ Moderate Sedation

▲ **99244** Office consultation for a new or established patient, which requires these three key components:

- a comprehensive history;

- a comprehensive examination; and

- medical decision making of moderate complexity.

Counseling and/or coordination of care with other physicians, other qualified health care professionals, or agencies are provided consistent with the nature of the problem(s) and the patient's and/or family's needs.

Usually, the presenting problem(s) are of moderate to high severity. Typically 60 minutes are spent face-to-face with the patient and/or family.

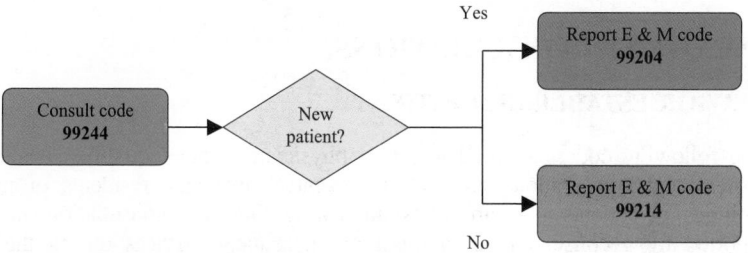

Medicare Cross-Walk:

Report 99204 instead of 99244 for new patients.
Report 99214 instead of 99244 for established patients.

▲ **99245** Office consultation for a new or established patient, which requires these three key components:

- a comprehensive history;

- a comprehensive examination; and

- medical decision making of high complexity.

Counseling and/or coordination of care with other physicians, other qualified health care professionals, or agencies are provided consistent with the nature of the problem(s) and the patient's and/or family's needs.

Usually, the presenting problem(s) are of moderate to high severity. Typically 80 minutes are spent face-to-face with the patient and/or family.

241

	Separate Procedure		Unlisted Procedure		CCI Comp. Code		Non-specific Procedure

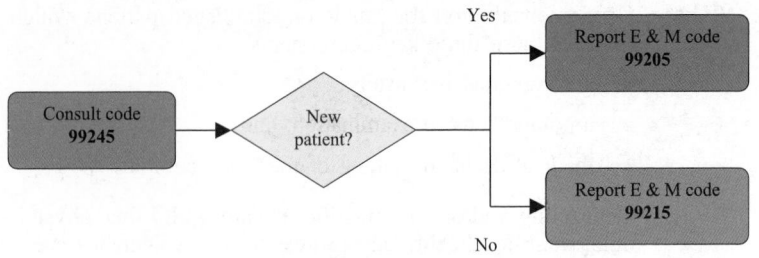

Medicare Cross-Walk:

Report 99205 instead of 99245 for new patients.
Report 99215 instead of 99245 for established patients.

INPATIENT CONSULTATIONS

NEW OR ESTABLISHED PATIENT

The following codes are used to report physician or other qualified health care professional consultations provided to hospital inpatients, residents of nursing facilities, or patients in a partial hospital setting. Only one consultation should be reported by a consultant per admission. Subsequent services during the same admission are reported using Subsequent Hospital Care codes (99231-99233) or Subsequent Nursing Facility Care codes (99307-99310), including services to complete the initial consultation, monitor progress, revise recommendations, or address a new problem. Use subsequent hospital care codes (99231-99233) or subsequent nursing facility care codes (99307-99310) to report transfer of care services.

When an inpatient consultation is performed on a date that a patient is admitted to a hospital or nursing facility, all E/M services provided by the consultant related to the admission are reported with the inpatient consultation service code (99251-99255). If a patient is admitted after an oupatient consultation (office, emergency department, etc.), and the patient is not seen on the unit on the date of admission, only report the outpatient consultation code (99241-99245). If the patient is seen by the consultant on the unit on the date of admission, report all E/M services provided by the consultant related to the admission with either the inpatient consultation code (99251-99255) or with the initial inpatient admission service code (99221-99223). Do not report both an outpatient consultation (99241-99245) and inpatient consultation (99251-99255) for services related to the same inpatient stay. When transfer of care services are provided on a date subsequent to the outpatient consultation, use the subsequent hospital care codes (99231-99233) or subsequent nursing facility care codes (99307-99310).

● New Code	▲ Revised Code	+ Add-On Code	⊘ Modifier -51 Exempt	⊙ Moderate Sedation

▲ **99251** Inpatient consultation for a new or established patient, which requires these three key components:

- a problem focused history;

- a problem focused examination; and

- straightforward medical decision making.

Counseling and/or coordination of care with other physicians, other qualified health care professionals, or agencies are provided consistent with the nature of the problem(s) and the patient's and/or family's needs.

Usually, the presenting problem(s) are self limited or minor. Typically 20 minutes are spent at the bedside and on the patient's hospital floor or unit.

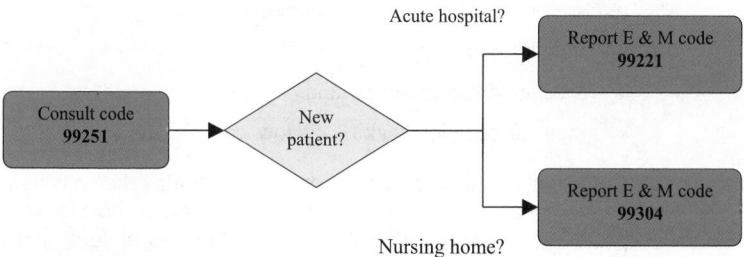

Medicare Cross-Walk:

Report 99221 instead of 99251 for acute hospital consultations.
Report 99304 instead of 99251 for nursing home consultations.

▲ **99252** Inpatient consultation for a new or established patient, which requires these three key components:

- an expanded problem focused history;

- an expanded problem focused examination; and

- straightforward medical decision making.

Counseling and/or coordination of care with other physicians, other qualified health care professionals, or agencies are provided consistent with the nature of the problem(s) and the patient's and/or family's needs.

Usually, the presenting problem(s) are of low severity. Typically 40 minutes are spent at the bedside and on the patient's hospital floor or unit.

Separate Procedure	Unlisted Procedure	CCI Comp. Code	Non-specific Procedure

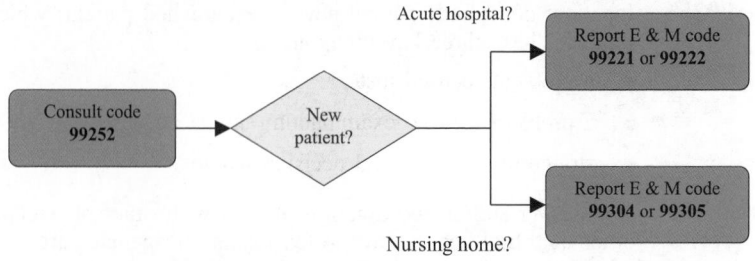

Medicare Cross-Walk:

Report 99221 or 99222 instead of 99252 for acute hospital consultations.
Report 99304 or 99305 instead of 99252 for nursing home consultations.

▲ **99253** Inpatient consultation for a new or established patient, which requires these three key components:

- a detailed history;

- a detailed examination; and

- medical decision making of low complexity.

Counseling and/or coordination of care with other physicians, other qualified health care professionals, or agencies are provided consistent with the nature of the problem(s) and the patient's and/or family's needs.

Usually, the presenting problem(s) are of moderate severity. Typically 55 minutes are spent at the bedside and on the patient's hospital floor or unit.

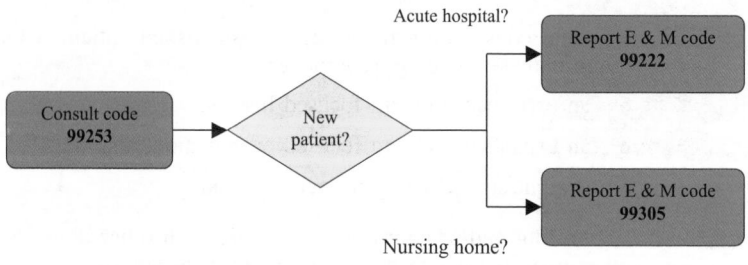

Medicare Cross-Walk:

Report 99222 instead of 99253 for acute hospital consultations.
Report 99305 instead of 99253 for nursing home consultations

● New Code	▲ Revised Code	✚ Add-On Code	⊘ Modifier -51 Exempt	⊙ Moderate Sedation

▲ **99254**   Inpatient consultation for a new or established patient, which requires three key components:

- a comprehensive history;

- a comprehensive examination; and

- medical decision making of moderate complexity.

Counseling and/or coordination of care with other physicians, other qualified health care professionals, or agencies are provided consistent with the nature of the problem(s) and the patient's and/or family's needs.

Usually, the presenting problem(s) are of moderate to high severity. Typically 80 minutes are spent at the bedside and on the patient's hospital floor or unit.

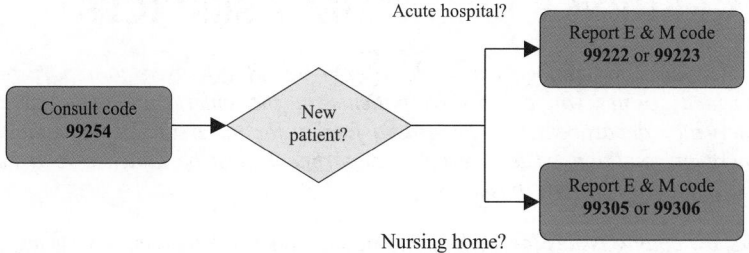

Medicare Cross-Walk:

Report 99222 or 99223 instead of 99254 for acute hospital consultations.
Report 99305 or 99306 instead of 99254 for nursing home consultations.

▲ **99255**   Inpatient consultation for a new or established patient, which requires these three key components:

- a comprehensive history;

- a comprehensive examination; and

- medical decision making of high complexity.

Counseling and/or coordination of care with other physicians, other qualified health care professionals, or agencies are provided consistent with the nature of the problem(s) and the patient's and/or family's needs.

Usually, the presenting problem(s) are of moderate to high severity. Typically 110 minutes are spent at the bedside and on the patient's hospital floor or unit.

| | Separate Procedure | | Unlisted Procedure | | CCI Comp. Code | | Non-specific Procedure |

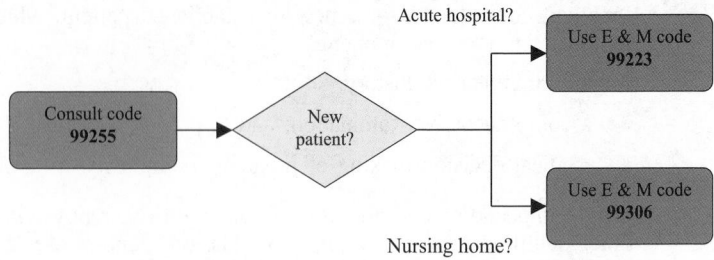

Medicare Cross-Walk:

Report 99223 instead of 99255 for acute hospital consultations.
Report 99306 instead of 99255 for nursing home consultations.

EMERGENCY DEPARTMENT SERVICES

Evaluation and management codes 99281-99288 are used to report services provided to new or established patients in the emergency department. The emergency department is defined as a facility for the treatment of patients with emergent conditions. The emergency department must be attached to a hospital and operate on a 24/7 basis.

The key coding issues for evaluation and management emergency services are the extent of history obtained, the extent of examination performed, and the complexity of medical decision making. Additional reporting issues include counseling and/or coordination of care, and the nature of presenting problem(s).

Time is not a descriptive component for evaluation and management services provided in the emergency department. These services are typically provided on a variable intensity basis, often involving multiple encounters with several patients over an extended period of time. Therefore, it is difficult for physicians to provide accurate estimates of the time spent face-to-face with the patient in the emergency department.

CODING RULES

1. *No distinction is made between new and established patients in the emergency department.*

2. *If the emergency department is used for observation or inpatient care services, report using codes from the Observation Care services subsection of the CPT coding system.*

3. *For critical care services provided in the emergency department, use the appropriate codes from the Critical Care subsection of the CPT coding system.*

● New Code ▲ Revised Code + Add-On Code ⊘ Modifier -51 Exempt ⊙ Moderate Sedation

EMERGENCY DEPARTMENT SERVICES

NEW OR ESTABLISHED PATIENT

The following codes are used to report evaluation and management services provided in the emergency department. No distinction is made between new and established patients in the emergency department.

An emergency department is defined as an organized hospital-based facility for the provision of unscheduled episodic services to patients who present for immediate medical attention. The facility must be available 24 hours a day.

For critical care services provided in the emergency department, see Critical Care notes and 99291, 99292.

For E/M services provided to a patient in an observation area of a hospital, see 99217-99220.

For observation or inpatient care services (including admission and discharge services), see 99234-99236.

▲ **99281** Emergency department visit for the evaluation and management of a patient, which requires these three key components:

- a problem focused history;
- a problem focused examination; and
- straightforward medical decision making.

Counseling and/or coordination of care with other physicians, other qualified health care professionals, or agencies are provided consistent with the nature of the problem(s) and the patient's and/or family's needs.

Usually, the presenting problem(s) are self limited or minor.

▲ **99282** Emergency department visit for the evaluation and management of a patient, which requires these three key components:

- an expanded problem focused history;
- an expanded problem focused examination; and
- medical decision making of low complexity.

Counseling and/or coordination of care with other physicians, other qualified health care professionals, or agencies are provided consistent with the nature of the problem(s) and the patient's and/or family's needs.

Usually, the presenting problem(s) are of low to moderate severity.

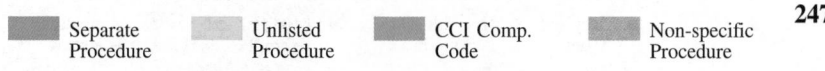

247

| | Separate Procedure | | Unlisted Procedure | | CCI Comp. Code | | Non-specific Procedure |

▲ **99283** Emergency department visit for the evaluation and management of a patient, which requires these three key components:

- an expanded problem focused history;
- an expanded problem focused examination; and
- medical decision making of moderate complexity.

Counseling and/or coordination of care with other physicians, other qualified health care professionals, or agencies are provided consistent with the nature of the problem(s) and the patient's and/or family's needs.

Usually, the presenting problem(s) are of moderate severity.

▲ **99284** Emergency department visit for the evaluation and management of a patient, which requires these three key components:

- a detailed history;
- a detailed examination; and
- medical decision making of moderate complexity.

Counseling and/or coordination of care with other physicians, other qualified health care professionals, or agencies are provided consistent with the nature of the problem(s) and the patient's and/or family's needs.

Usually, the presenting problem(s) are of high severity, and require urgent evaluation by the physician or other qualified health care professional but do not pose an immediate significant threat to life or physiologic function.

▲ **99285** Emergency department visit for the evaluation and management of a patient, which requires these three key components within the constraints imposed by the urgency of the patient's clinical condition and/or mental status:

- a comprehensive history;
- a comprehensive examination; and
- medical decision making of high complexity.

Counseling and/or coordination of care with other physicians, other qualified health care professionals, or agencies are provided consistent with the nature of the problem(s) and the patient's and/or family's needs.

Usually, the presenting problem(s) are of high severity and pose an immediate significant threat to life or physiologic function.

● New Code ▲ Revised Code + Add-On Code ⊘ Modifier -51 Exempt ⊙ Moderate Sedation

OTHER EMERGENCY SERVICES

In directed emergency care, advanced life support, the physician or other qualified health care professional is located in a hospital emergency or critical care department, and is in two-way voice communication with ambulance or rescue personnel outside the hospital. Direction of the performance of necessary medical procedures includes but is not limited to: telemetry of cardiac rhythm; cardiac and/or pulmonary resuscitation; endotracheal or esophageal obturator airway intubation; administration of intravenous fluids and/or administration of intramuscular, intratracheal or subcutaneous drugs; and/or electrical conversion of arrhythmia.

▲ **99288**   Physician or other qualified health care professional direction of emergency medical systems (EMS) emergency care, advanced life support

(99289   deleted 2009 edition, see 99466)

(99290   deleted 2009 edition, see 99467)

CRITICAL CARE SERVICES

Critical care is the direct delivery by a physician(s) or other qualified health care professional of medical care for a critically ill or critically injured patient. A critical illness or injury acutely impairs one or more vital organ systems such that there is a high probability of imminent or life threatening deterioration in the patient's condition. Critical care involves high complexity decision making to assess, manipulate, and support vital system function(s) to treat single or multiple vital organ system failure and/or to prevent further life threatening deterioration of the patient's condition. Examples of vital organ system failure include, but are not limited to: central nervous system failure, circulatory failure, shock, renal, hepatic, metabolic, and/or respiratory failure. Although critical care typically requires interpretation of multiple physiologic parameters and/or application of advanced technology(s), critical care may be provided in life threatening situations when these elements are not present. Critical care may be provided on multiple days, even if no changes are made in the treatment rendered to the patient, provided that the patient's condition continues to require the level of attention described above.

Providing medical care to a critically ill, injured, or post-operative patient qualifies as a critical care service only if both the illness or injury and the treatment being provided meet the above requirements. Critical care is usually, but not always, given in a critical care area, such as the coronary care unit, intensive care unit, pediatric intensive care unit, respiratory care unit, or the emergency care facility.

Inpatient critical care services provided to infants 29 days through 71 months of age are reported with pediatric critical care codes 99471-99476. The pediatric critical care codes are reported as long as the infant/young child qualifies for

249

| Separate Procedure | Unlisted Procedure | CCI Comp. Code | Non-specific Procedure |

critical care services during the hospital stay through 71 months of age. Inpatient critical care services provided to neonates (28 days of age or younger) are reported with the neonatal critical care codes 99468 and 99469. The neonatal critical care codes are reported as long as the neonate qualifies for critical care services during the hospital stay through the 28th postnatal day. The reporting of the pediatric and neonatal critical care services is not based on time or the type of unit (eg, pediatric or neonatal critical care unit) and it is not dependent upon the type of physician or other qualified health care professional delivering the care. To report critical care services provided in the outpatient setting (eg, emergency department or office), for neonates and pediatric patients up through 71 months of age, see the critical care codes 99291, 99292. If the same individual provides critical care services for a neonatal or pediatric patient in both the outpatient and inpatient settings on the same day, report only the appropriate neonatal or pediatric critical care code 99468-99472 for all critical care services provided on that day. Also report 99291-99292 for neonatal or pediatric critical care services provided by the individual providing critical care at one facility but transferring the patient to another facility. Critical care services provided by a second individual of a different specialty not reporting a per day neonatal or pediatric critical care code can be reported with codes 99291-99292. For additional instructions reporting these services, see the Neonatal and Pediatric Critical Care section and codes 99468-99476.

Services for a patient who is not critically ill but happens to be in a critical care unit are reported using other appropriate E/M codes. Critical care and other E/M services may be provided to the same patient on the same date by the same physician.

Critical care and other E/M services may be provided to the same patient on the same date by the same individual.

For reporting by professionals, the following services are included in critical care when performed during the critical period by the physician(s) providing critical care: the interpretation of cardiac output measurements (93561, 93562), chest X-rays (71010, 71015, 71020), pulse oximetry (94760, 94761, 94762), blood gases, and information data stored in computers (eg., ECGs, blood pressures, hematologic data [99090]); gastric intubation (43752, 43753); temporary transcutaneous pacing (92953); ventilatory management (94002-94004, 94660, 94662); and vascular access procedures (36000, 36410, 36415, 36591, 36600). Any services performed that are not included in this listing should be reported separately. Facilities may report the above services separately.

Codes 99291, 99292 should be reported for the attendance during the transport of critically ill or critically injured patients older than 24 months of age to or from a facility or hospital. For transport services of critically ill or critically injured pediatric patients 24 months of age or younger, see 99466, 99467.

Codes 99291, 99292 are used to report the total duration of time spent in provision of critical care services to a critically ill or critically injured patient, even if the time

| • New Code | ▲ Revised Code | + Add-On Code | ⊘ Modifier -51 Exempt | ⊙ Moderate Sedation |

spent providing care on that date is not continuous. For any given period of time spent providing critical care services, the individual must devote his or her full attention to the patient and, therefore, cannot provide services to any other patient during the same period of time.

Time spent with the individual patient should be recorded in the patient's record. The time that can be reported as critical care is the time spent engaged in work directly related to the individual patient's care whether that time was spent at the immediate bedside or elsewhere on the floor or unit. For example, time spent on the unit or at the nursing station on the floor reviewing test results or imaging studies, discussing the critically ill patient's care with other medical staff or documenting critical care services in the medical record would be reported as critical care, even though it does not occur at the bedside. Also, when the patient is unable to lacks capacity to participate in discussions, time spent on the floor or unit with family members or surrogate decision makers obtaining a medical history, reviewing the patient's condition or prognosis, or discussing treatment or limitation(s) of treatment may be reported as critical care, provided that the conversation bears directly on the management of the patient.

Time spent in activities that occur outside of the unit or off the floor (eg, telephone calls whether taken at home, in the office or elsewhere in the hospital) may not be reported as critical care since the individual is not immediately available to the patient. Time spent in activities that do not directly contribute to the treatment of the patient may not be reported as critical care, even if they are performed in the critical care unit (eg, participation in administration meetings or telephone calls to discuss other patients). Time spent performing separately reportable procedures or services should not be included in the time reported as critical care time. No individual may report remote real-time interactive video-conferenced critical care services (0188T, 0189T) for the period in which any other physician or qualified health care professional reports codes 99291, 99292.

Code 99291 is used to report the first 30-74 minutes of critical care on a given date. It should be used only once per date even if the time spent by the individual is not continuous on that date. Critical care of less than 30 minutes total duration on a given date should be reported with the appropriate E/M code.

Code 99292 is used to report additional block(s) of time, of up to 30 minutes each beyond the first 74 minutes. (See table)

| | Separate Procedure | | Unlisted Procedure | | CCI Comp. Code | | Non-specific Procedure | **251** |

CORRECT CODING CHART FOR CRITICAL CARE SERVICES

DURATION OF CRITICAL CARE	CODE(S) TO REPORT
less than 30 minutes	appropriate E/M codes
30- 74 minutes	99291 once
75-104 minutes	99291 once and 99292 once
105-134 minutes	99291 once and 99292 twice
135-164 minutes	99291 once and 99292 three times
165-194 minutes	99291 once and 99292 four times
195 minutes or longer	99291 and 99292 as appropriate (see illustrated reporting examples above)

CODING RULES

1. *The critical care CPT codes are used to report the total duration of time spent by a physician providing constant attention to a critically ill patient.*

2. *Critical care code 99291 is used to report the first 30-74 minutes of critical care on a given day. It should be reported only once per day even if the time spent is not continuous on that day.*

3. *Critical care 99292 is used to report each additional 30 minutes beyond the first 74 minutes.*

4. *Other procedures which are not considered included in the critical care services, for example, suturing of lacerations, setting of fractures, reduction of joint dislocations, lumbar puncture, peritoneal lavage and bladder tap, are reported separately.*

CRITICAL CARE SERVICES

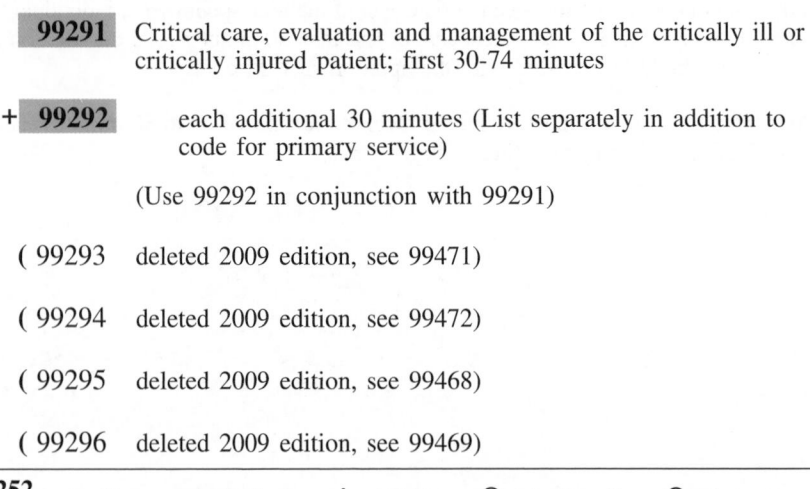

99291   Critical care, evaluation and management of the critically ill or critically injured patient; first 30-74 minutes

+ 99292   each additional 30 minutes (List separately in addition to code for primary service)

(Use 99292 in conjunction with 99291)

(99293   deleted 2009 edition, see 99471)

(99294   deleted 2009 edition, see 99472)

(99295   deleted 2009 edition, see 99468)

(99296   deleted 2009 edition, see 99469)

● New Code   ▲ Revised Code   + Add-On Code   ⊘ Modifier -51 Exempt   ⊙ Moderate Sedation

(99298   deleted 2009 edition, see 99478)

(99299   deleted 2009 edition, see 99479)

(99300   deleted 2009 edition, see 99480)

NURSING FACILITY SERVICES

The following codes are used to report evaluation and management services to patients in nursing facilities (formerly called skilled nursing facilities [SNFs], intermediate care facilities [ICFs], or long-term care facilities [LTCFs]).

These codes should also be used to report evaluation and management services provided to a patient in a psychiatric residential treatment center (a facility or a distinct part of a facility for psychiatric care, which provides a 24-hour therapeutically planned and professionally staffed group living and learning environment). If procedures such as medical psychotherapy are provided in addition to evaluation and management services, these should be reported in addition to the E/M services provided.

Nursing facilities that provide convalescent, rehabilitative, or long-term care are required to conduct comprehensive accurate, standardized, and reproducible assessments of each resident's functional capacity using a Resident Assessment Instrument (RAI). All RAIs include the Minimum Data Set (MDS), Resident Assessment Protocols (RAPs), and utilization guidelines. The MDS is the primary screening and assessment tool; the RAPs trigger the identification of potential problems and provide guidelines for follow-up assessments.

Physicians have a central role in assuring that all residents receive thorough assessments and that medical plans of care are instituted or revised to enhance or maintain the resident's physical and psychosocial functioning. This role includes providing input in the development of the MDS and a multi-disciplinary plan of care, as required by regulations pertaining to the care of nursing facility residents.

Two major subcategories of nursing facility services are recognized: Initial Nursing Facility Care, and Subsequent Nursing Facility Care. Both subcategories apply to new or established patients.

For definitions of key components and commonly used terms, please see Evaluation and Management Services Guidelines.

(For care plan oversight services provided to nursing facility residents, see 99379-99380)

Separate Procedure   Unlisted Procedure   CCI Comp. Code   Non-specific Procedure   **253**

CODING RULES

1. *If a patient is admitted to the nursing facility after receiving services in the physician's office or hospital emergency department, all evaluation and management services are considered inclusive in the initial nursing facility care.*

2. *With the exception of hospital discharge services, evaluation and management service on the same date provided in locations other than the nursing facility that are related to the admission should not be coded separately.*

3. *When reporting these CPT codes to Medicare include the HCPCS Level II modifier -SP or -MP, or HCPCS Level III modifier if specified by the local Medicare carrier.*

INITIAL NURSING FACILITY CARE

NEW OR ESTABLISHED PATIENT

When the patient is admitted to the nursing facility in the course of an encounter in another site of service (eg, hospital emergency department, office), all evaluation and management services provided by that physician in conjunction with that admission are considered part of the initial nursing facility care when performed on the same date as the admission or readmission. The nursing facility care level of service reported by the admitting physician should include the services related to the admission he/she provided in the other sites of service as well as in the nursing facility setting.

Hospital discharge or observation discharge services performed on the same date of nursing facility admission or readmission may be reported separately. For a patient discharged from inpatient status on the same date of nursing facility admission or readmission, the hospital discharge services should be reported with codes 99238, 99239 as appropriate. For a patient discharged from observation status on the same date of nursing facility admission or readmission, the observation care discharge services should be reported with code 99217. For a patient admitted and discharged from observation or inpatient status on the same date, see codes 99234-99236.

(For nursing facility care discharge, see 99315, 99316)

▲ 99304 Initial nursing facility care, per day, for the evaluation and management of a patient which requires these three key components:

- a detailed or comprehensive history;
- a detailed or comprehensive examination;

| ● New Code | ▲ Revised Code | + Add-On Code | ⊘ Modifier -51 Exempt | ⊙ Moderate Sedation |

- and medical decision making that is straightforward or of low complexity.

Counseling and/or coordination of care with other physicians, other qualified health care professionals, or agencies are provided consistent with the nature of the problem(s) and the patient's and/or family's needs.

Usually, the problem(s) requiring admission are of low severity. Typically 25 minutes are spent at the bedside and on the patient's facility floor or unit.

▲ 99305   Initial nursing facility care, per day, for the evaluation and management of a patient which requires these three key components:

- a comprehensive history;

- a comprehensive examination;

- and medical decision making of moderate complexity.

Counseling and/or coordination of care with other physicians, other qualified health care professionals, or agencies are provided consistent with the nature of the problem(s) and the patient's and/or family's needs.

Usually, the problem(s) requiring admission are of moderate severity. Typically 35 minutes are spent at the bedside and on the patient's facility floor or unit.

▲ 99306   Initial nursing facility care, per day, for the evaluation and management of a patient, which requires these three key components:

- a comprehensive history;

- a comprehensive examination;

- and medical decision making of high complexity.

Counseling and/or coordination of care with other physicians, other qualified health care professionals, or agencies are provided consistent with the nature of the problem(s) and the patient's and/or family's needs.

Usually, the problem(s) requiring admission are of high severity. Typically 45 minutes are spent at the bedside and on the patient's facility floor or unit.

SUBSEQUENT NURSING FACILITY CARE

All levels of subsequent nursing facility care include reviewing the medical record and reviewing the results of diagnostic studies and changes in the patient's status

	Separate Procedure		Unlisted Procedure		CCI Comp. Code		Non-specific Procedure

(ie, changes in history, physical condition, and response to management) since the last assessment by the physician or other qualified health care professional.

▲ **99307** Subsequent nursing facility care, per day, for the evaluation and management of a patient, which requires at least two of these three key components:

- a problem focused interval history;
- a problem focused examination;
- straightforward medical decision making.

Counseling and/or coordination of care with other physicians, other qualified health care professionals, or agencies are provided consistent with the nature of the problem(s) and the patient's and/or family's needs.

Usually, the patient is stable, recovering, or improving. Typically 10 minutes are spent at the bedside and on the patient's facility floor or unit.

▲ **99308** Subsequent nursing facility care, per day, for the evaluation and management of a patient, which requires at least two of these three key components:

- an expanded problem focused interval history;
- an expanded problem focused examination;
- medical decision making of low complexity.

Counseling and/or coordination of care with other physicians, other qualified health care professionals, or agencies are provided consistent with the nature of the problem(s) and the patient's and/or family's needs.

Usually, the patient is responding inadequately to therapy or has developed a minor complication. Typically 15 minutes are spent at the bedside and on the patient's facility floor or unit.

▲ **99309** Subsequent nursing facility care, per day, for the evaluation and management of a patient, which requires at least two of these three key components:

- a detailed interval history;
- a detailed examination;
- medical decision making of moderate complexity.

Counseling and/or coordination of care with other physicians, other qualified health care professionals, or agencies are provided consistent with the nature of the problem(s) and the patient's and/or family's needs.

● New Code   ▲ Revised Code   + Add-On Code   ⊘ Modifier -51 Exempt   ⊙ Moderate Sedation

Usually, the patient has developed a significant complication or a significant new problem. Typically 25 minutes are spent at the bedside and on the patient's facility floor or unit.

▲ **99310** Subsequent nursing facility care, per day, for the evaluation and management of a patient, which requires at least two of these three key components:

- a comprehensive interval history;
- a comprehensive examination;
- medical decision making of high complexity.

Counseling and/or coordination of care with other physicians, other qualified health care professionals, or agencies are provided consistent with the nature of the problem(s) and the patient's and/or family's needs.

The patient may be unstable or may have developed a significant new problem requiring immediate physician attention. Typically 35 minutes are spent at the bedside and on the patient's facility floor or unit.

NURSING FACILITY DISCHARGE SERVICES

The nursing facility discharge day management codes are to be used to report the total duration of time spent by a physician or other qualified health care professional for the final nursing facility discharge of a patient. The codes include, as appropriate, final examination of the patient, discussion of the nursing facility stay, even if the time spent on that date is not continuous. Instructions are given for continuing care to all relevant caregivers, and preparation of discharge records, prescriptions and referral forms.

99315 Nursing facility discharge day management; 30 minutes or less

99316 more than 30 minutes

OTHER NURSING FACILITY SERVICES

▲ **99318** Evaluation and management of a patient involving an annual nursing facility assessment, which requires these three key components:

- a detailed interval history;
- a comprehensive examination;
- and medical decision making that is of low to moderate complexity.

	Separate Procedure		Unlisted Procedure		CCI Comp. Code		Non-specific Procedure

Counseling and/or coordination of care with other physicians, other qualified health care professionals, or agencies are provided consistent with the nature of the problem(s) and the patient's and/or family's needs.

Usually, the patient is stable, recovering, or improving. Typically 30 minutes are spent at the bedside and on the patient's facility floor or unitr.

(Do not report 99318 on the same date of service as nursing facility services codes 99304-99316)

DOMICILIARY, REST HOME (eg, BOARDING HOME), OR CUSTODIAL CARE SERVICES

E/M service codes 99324-99340 are used to report services provided to a new or established patient in domiciliary, rest home or custodial care facility. The key coding issues are the extent of history obtained, the extent of examination performed, and the complexity of medical decision making. Additional reporting issues include counseling and/or coordination of care, and the nature of presenting problems.

When reporting these CPT codes to Medicare include HCPCS modifier -SP or -MP to indicate single or multiple patients seen during the visit. Consult the local Medicare intermediary before using these modifiers.

The following codes are used to report evaluation and management services in a facility which provides room, board and other personal assistance services, generally on a long-term basis. The also are used to report evaluation and management services in an assisted living facility. The facility's services do not include a medical component.

For definitions of key components and commonly used terms, please see Evaluation and Management Services Guidelines.

(For care plan oversight services provided to a patient in a domiciliary facility under the care of a home health agency, see 99374, 99375, and for hospice agency, see 99377, 99378. For care plan oversight provided to a patient under hospice or home health agency care, see 99339, 99340)

NEW PATIENT

▲ **99324** Domiciliary or rest home visit for the evaluation and management of a new patient, which requires these three key components:

- a problem focused history;

---

258 ● New Code   ▲ Revised Code   ＋ Add-On Code   ⊘ Modifier -51 Exempt   ⊙ Moderate Sedation

- a problem focused examination; and

- straightforward medical decision making.

Counseling and/or coordination of care with other physicians, other qualified health care professionals, or agencies are provided consistent with the nature of the problem(s) and the patient's and/or family's needs.

Usually, the presenting problem(s) are of low severity. Typically 20 minutes are spent with the patient and/or family or caregiver.

▲ **99325** Domiciliary or rest home visit for the evaluation and management of a new patient, which requires these three key components:

- an expanded problem focused history;

- an expanded problem focused examination; and

- medical decision making of low complexity.

Counseling and/or coordination of care with other physicians, other qualified health care professionals, or agencies are provided consistent with the nature of the problem(s) and the patient's and/or family's needs.

Usually, the presenting problem(s) are of moderate severity. Typically 30 minutes are spent with the patient and/or family or caregiver.

▲ **99326** Domiciliary or rest home visit for the evaluation and management of a new patient, which requires these three key components:

- a detailed history;

- a detailed examination; and

- medical decision making of moderate complexity.

Counseling and/or coordination of care with other physicians, other qualified health care professionals, or agencies are provided consistent with the nature of the problem(s) and the patient's and/or family's needs.

Usually, the presenting problem(s) are of moderate to high severity. Typically 45 minutes are spent with the patient and/or family or caregiver.

▲ **99327** Domiciliary or rest home visit for the evaluation and management of a new patient, which requires these three key components:

- a comprehensive history;

	Separate Procedure		Unlisted Procedure		CCI Comp. Code		Non-specific Procedure

- a comprehensive examination; and

- medical decision making of moderate complexity.

Counseling and/or coordination of care with other physicians, other qualified health care professionals, or agencies are provided consistent with the nature of the problem(s) and the patient's and/or family's needs.

Usually, the presenting problem(s) are of high severity. Typically 60 minutes are spent with the patient and/or family or caregiver.

▲ **99328** Domiciliary or rest home visit for the evaluation and management of a new patient, which requires these three key components:

- a comprehensive history;

- a comprehensive examination; and

- medical decision making of high complexity.

Counseling and/or coordination of care with other physicians, other qualified health care professionals, or agencies are provided consistent with the nature of the problem(s) and the patient's and/or family's needs.

Usually, the patient is unstable or has developed a significant new problem requiring immediate physician attention. Typically 75 minutes are spent with the patient and/or family or caregiver.

ESTABLISHED PATIENT

▲ **99334** Domiciliary or rest home visit for the evaluation and management of an established patient, which requires at least two of these three key components:

- a problem focused interval history;

- a problem focused examination;

- straightforward medical decision making.

Counseling and/or coordination of care with other physicians, other qualified health care professionals, or agencies are provided consistent with the nature of the problem(s) and the patient's and/or family's needs.

Usually, the presenting problem(s) are self-limited or minor. Typically 15 minutes are spent with the patient and/or family or caregiver.

● New Code	▲ Revised Code	+ Add-On Code	⊘ Modifier -51 Exempt	⊙ Moderate Sedation

▲ **99335** Domiciliary or rest home visit for the evaluation and management of an established patient, which requires at least two of these three key components:

- an expanded problem focused interval history;
- an expanded problem focused examination;
- medical decision making of low complexity.

Counseling and/or coordination of care with other physicians, other qualified health care professionals, or agencies are provided consistent with the nature of the problem(s) and the patient's and/or family's needs.

Usually, the presenting problem(s) are of low to moderate severity. Typically 25 minutes are spent with the patient and/or family or caregiver.

▲ **99336** Domiciliary or rest home visit for the evaluation and management of an established patient, which requires at least two of these three key components:

- a detailed interval history;
- a detailed examination;
- medical decision making of moderate complexity.

Counseling and/or coordination of care with other physicians, other qualified health care professionals, or agencies are provided consistent with the nature of the problem(s) and the patient's and/or family's needs.

Usually, the presenting problem(s) are of moderate to high severity. Typically 40 minutes are spent with the patient and/or family or caregiver.

▲ **99337** Domiciliary or rest home visit for the evaluation and management of an established patient, which requires at least two of these three key components:

- a comprehensive interval history;
- a comprehensive examination;
- and medical decision making of moderate to high complexity.

Counseling and/or coordination of care with other physicians, other qualified health care professionals, or agencies are provided consistent with the nature of the problem(s) and the patient's and/or family's needs.

Usually, the presenting problem(s) are of moderate to high severity. The patient may be unstable or may have developed a

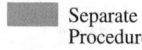 Separate Procedure

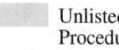 Unlisted Procedure

CCI Comp. Code

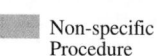 Non-specific Procedure

261

significant new problem requiring immediate physician attention. Typically 60 minutes are spent with the patient and/or family or caregiver.

DOMICILIARY, REST HOME (eg, ASSISTED LIVING FACILITY), OR HOME CARE PLAN OVERSIGHT SERVICES

(For instructions on the use of 99339, 99340, see introductory notes for 99374-99380)

(For care plan oversight services for patients under the care of a home health agency, hospice, or nursing facility, see 99374-99380)

(Do not report 99339, 99340 for time reported with 98966-98969, 99441-99444)

99339 Individual physician supervision of a patient (patient not present) in home, domiciliary or rest home (eg, assisted living facility) requiring complex and multidisciplinary care modalities involving regular physician development and/or revision of care plans, review of subsequent reports of patient status, review of related laboratory and other studies, communication (including telephone calls) for purposes of assessment or care decisions with health care professional(s), family member(s), surrogate decision maker(s) (eg, legal guardian) and/or key caregiver(s) involved in patient's care, integration of new information into the medical treatment plan and/or adjustment of medical therapy, within a calendar month; 15-29 minutes

99340   30 minutes or more

(Do not report 99339, 99340 for patients under the care of a home health agency, enrolled in a hospice program, or for nursing facility residents)

(Do not report 99339, 99340 during the same month with 99487-99489)

(Do not report 99339, 99340 when performed during the service time of codes 99495 or 99496)

HOME SERVICES

The following codes are used to report evaluation and management services provided in a private residence.

● New Code ▲ Revised Code + Add-On Code ⊘ Modifier -51 Exempt ⊙ Moderate Sedation

For definitions of key components and commonly used terms, please see Evaluation and Management Services Guidelines.

> (For care plan oversight services provided to a patient in the home under the care of a home health agency, see 99374-99375, and for hospice agency, see 99377, 99378. For care plan oversight provided to a patient under hospice or home health agency care, see 99339, 99340))

NEW PATIENT

▲ **99341**   Home visit for the evaluation and management of a new patient, which requires these three key components:

- a problem focused history;

- a problem focused examination; and

- straightforward medical decision making.

Counseling and/or coordination of care with other physicians, other qualified health care professionals, or agencies are provided consistent with the nature of the problem(s) and the patient's and/or family's needs.

Usually, the presenting problem(s) are of low severity. Typically 20 minutes are spent face-to-face with the patient and/or family.

▲ **99342**   Home visit for the evaluation and management of a new patient, which requires these three key components:

- an expanded problem focused history;

- an expanded problem focused examination; and

- medical decision making of low complexity.

Counseling and/or coordination of care with other physicians, other qualified health care professionals, or agencies are provided consistent with the nature of the problem(s) and the patient's and/or family's needs.

Usually, the presenting problem(s) are of moderate severity. Typically 30 minutes are spent face-to-face with the patient and/or family.

▲ **99343**   Home visit for the evaluation and management of a new patient, which requires these three key components:

- a detailed history;

- a detailed examination; and

- medical decision making of moderate complexity.

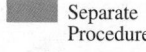 Separate Procedure   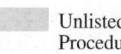 Unlisted Procedure   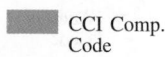 CCI Comp. Code   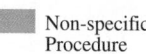 Non-specific Procedure

263

Counseling and/or coordination of care with other physicians, other qualified health care professionals, or agencies are provided consistent with the nature of the problem(s) and the patient's and/or family's needs.

Usually, the presenting problem(s) are of moderate to high severity. Typically 45 minutes ar spent face-to-face with the patient and/or family.

▲ 99344   Home visit for the evaluation and management of a new patient, which requires these three components:

- a comprehensive history;
- a comprehensive examination; and
- medical decision making of moderate complexity.

Counseling and/or coordination of care with other physicians, other qualified health care professionals, or agencies are provided consistent with the nature of the problem(s) and the patient's and/or family's needs.

Usually, the presenting problem(s) are of high severity. Typically 60 minutes are spent face-to-face with the patient and/or family.

▲ 99345   Home visit for the evaluation and management of a new patient, which requires these three key components:

- a comprehensive history;
- a comprehensive examination; and
- medical decision making of high complexity.

Counseling and/or coordination of care with other physicians, other qualified health care professionals, or agencies are provided consistent with the nature of the problem(s) and the patient's and/or family's needs.

Usually, the patient is unstable or has developed a significant new problem requiring immediate physician attention. Typically 75 minutes are spent face-to-face with the patient and/or family.

ESTABLISHED PATIENT

▲ 99347   Home visit for the evaluation and management of an established patient, which requires at least two of these three key components:

- a problem focused interval history;
- a problem focused examination;

- straightforward medical decision making.

Counseling and/or coordination of care with other physicians, other qualified health care professionals, or agencies are provided consistent with the nature of the problem(s) and the patient's and/or family's needs.

Usually, the presenting problem(s) are self-limited or minor. Typically 15 minutes are spent face-to-face with the patient and/or family.

▲ **99348** Home visit for the evaluation and management of an established patient, which requires at least two of these three key components:

- an expanded problem focused interval history;

- an expanded problem focused examination;

- medical decision making of low complexity.

Counseling and/or coordination of care with other physicians, other qualified health care professionals, or agencies are provided consistent with the nature of the problem(s) and the patient's and/or family's needs.

Usually, the presenting problem(s) are of low to moderate severity. Typically 25 minutes are spent face-to-face with the patient and/or family.

▲ **99349** Home visit for the evaluation and management of an established patient, which requires at least two of these three key components:

- a detailed interval history;

- a detailed examination;

- medical decision making of moderate complexity.

Counseling and/or coordination of care with other physicians, other qualified health care professionals, or agencies are provided consistent with the nature of the problem(s) and the patient's and/or family's needs.

Usually, the presenting problem(s) are moderate to high severity. Typically 40 minutes are spent face-to-face with the patient and/or family.

▲ **99350** Home visit for the evaluation and management of an established patient, which requires at least two of these three key components:

- a comprehensive interval history;

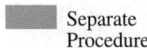
Separate
Procedure

Unlisted
Procedure

CCI Comp.
Code

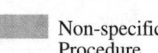
Non-specific
Procedure

265

- a comprehensive examination;

- medical decision making of moderate to high complexity.

Counseling and/or coordination of care with other physicians, other qualified health care professionals, or agencies are provided consistent with the nature of the problem(s) and the patient's and/or family's needs.

Usually, the presenting problem(s) are of moderate to high severity. The patient may be unstable or may have developed a significant new problem requiring immediate physician attention. Typically 60 minutes are spent face-to-face with the patient and/or family.

PROLONGED SERVICES

PROLONGED SERVICE WITH DIRECT PATIENT CONTACT

Codes 99354-99357 are used when a physician or other qualified health care professional provides prolonged service involving direct patient contact that is provided beyond the usual service in either the inpatient or outpatient setting. Direct patient contact is face-to-face and includes additional non-face-to-face services on the patient's floor or unit in the hospital or nursing facility during the same session. This service is reported in addition to the designated evaluation and management services at any level and any other services provided at the same session as evaluation and management services. Appropriate codes should be selected for supplies provided or procedures performed in the care of the patient during this period.

Codes 99354-99355 are used to report the total duration of face-to-face time spent by a physician or other qualified health care professional on a given date providing prolonged service in the office or other outpatient setting, even if the time spent by the physician or other qualified health care professional on that date is not continuous. Codes 99356-99357 are used to report the total duration of time spent by a physician or other qualified health care professional at the bedside and on the patient's floor or unit, in the hospital or nursing facility on a given date providing prolonged service to a patient, even if the time spent by the physician or other qualified health care professional on that date is not continuous.

Code 99354 or 99356 is used to report the first hour of prolonged service on a given date, depending on the place of service.

Either code should be used only once per date, even if the time spent by the physician or other qualified health care professional is not continuous on that date. Prolonged service of less than 30 minutes total duration on a given date is not separately reported because the work involved is included in the total work of the evaluation and management codes.

● New Code ▲ Revised Code + Add-On Code ⊘ Modifier -51 Exempt ⊙ Moderate Sedation

Code 99355 or 99357 is used to report each additional 30 minutes beyond the first hour, depending on the place of service. Either code may also be used to report the final 15-30 minutes of prolonged service on a given date. Prolonged service of less than 15 minutes beyond the first hour or less than 15 minutes beyond the final 30 minutes is not reported separately.

The use of the time based add-on codes requires that the primary evaluation and management service have a typical or specified time published in the CPT codebook.

The following examples illustrate the correct reporting of prolonged physician or other qualified health care professional service with direct patient contact in the office setting:

TOTAL DURATION OF PROLONGED SERVICE	CODE(S) TO REPORT
less than 30 minutes	not reported separately
30- 74 minutes	99354 once
75-104 minutes	99354 once and 99355 once
105 or more	99354 once and 99355 twice or more for each additional 30 minutes

+ **99354** Prolonged service in the office or other outpatient setting requiring direct patient contact beyond the usual service; first hour (List separately in addition to code for office or other outpatient Evaluation and Management service)

(Use 99354 in conjunction with 99201-99215, 99241-99245, 99324-99337, 99341-99350)

+ **99355** each additional 30 minutes (List separately in addition to code for prolonged physician service)

(Use 99355 in conjunction with 99354)

+ **99356** Prolonged service in the inpatient or observation setting, requiring unit/floor time beyond the usual service; first hour (List separately in addition to code for inpatient Evaluation and Management service)

(Use 99356 in conjunction with codes 99218-99220, 99221-99223, 99224-99226, 99231-99233, 99234-99236, 99251-99255, 99304-99310)

+ **99357** each additional 30 minutes (List separately in addition to code for prolonged physician service)

(Use 99357 in conjunction with 99356)

	Separate Procedure		Unlisted Procedure		CCI Comp. Code		Non-specific Procedure

PROLONGED SERVICE WITHOUT DIRECT PATIENT CONTACT

Codes 99358 and 99359 are used when a prolonged service is provided that is neither face-to-face time in the office or outpatient setting, nor additional unit/floor time in the hospital or nursing facility setting during the same session of an evaluation and management service and is beyond the usual physician or other qualified health care professional service time.

This service is to be reported in relation to other physician or other qualified health care professional services, including evaluation and management services at any level. This prolonged service may be reported on a different date than the primary service to which it is related. For example, extensive record review may relate to a previous evaluation and management service performed earlier and commences upon receipt of past records. However, it must relate to a service or patient where (face-to-face) patient care has occurred or will occur and relate to ongoing patient management. A typical time for the primary service need not be established within CPT code set.

Codes 99358 and 99359 are used to report the total duration of non-face-to-face time spent by a physician or other qualified health care professional on a given date providing prolonged service, even if the time spent by the physician or other qualified health care professional on that date is not continuous. Code 99358 is used to report the first hour of prolonged service on a given date regardless of the place of service. It should be used only once per date.

Prolonged service of less than 30 minutes total duration on a given date is not separately reported.

Code 99359 is used to report each additional 30 minutes beyond the first hour regardless of the place of service. It may also be used to report the final 15 to 30 minutes of prolonged service on a given date.

Prolonged service of less than 15 minutes beyond the first hour or less than 15 minutes beyond the final 30 minutes is not reported separately.

Do not report 99358-99359 for time spent in care plan oversight services (99339, 99340, 99374-99380), anticoagulant management (99363, 99364), medical team conferences (99366-99368), on-line medical evaluatinos (99444), or other non face-to-face services that have more specific codes and no upper time limit in the CPT code set. Codes 99358, 99359 may be reported when related to other non face-to-face service codes that have a published maximum time (eg, telephone services).

99358   Prolonged evaluation and management service before and/or after direct patient care; first hour

● New Code   ▲ Revised Code   + Add-On Code   ⊘ Modifier -51 Exempt   ⊙ Moderate Sedation

+ 99359 each additional 30 minutes (List separately in addition to code for prolonged physician service)

(Use 99359 in conjunction with 99358)

(Do not report 99358, 99359 during the same month with 99487-99489)

(Do note report 99358, 99359 when performed during the service time of codes 99495 or 99496)

STANDBY SERVICES

Code 99360 is used to report physician or other qualified health care professional standby services that are requested by another individual and that involve prolonged attendance without direct (face-to-face) patient contact. Care or services may not be provided to other patients during this period. This code is not used to report time spent proctoring another individual. It is also not used if the period of standby ends with the performance of a procedure subject to a surgical package by the individual who was on standby.

Code 99360 is used to report the total duration of time spent on a given date on standby. Standby service of less than 30 minutes total duration on a given date is not reported separately.

Second and subsequent periods of standby beyond the first 30 minutes may be reported only if a full 30 minutes of standby was provided for each unit of service reported.

▲ 99360 Standby service, requiring prolonged attendance, each 30 minutes (eg, operative standby, standby for frozen section, for cesarean/high risk delivery, for monitoring EEG)

(For hospital mandated on call services, see 99026, 99027)

(99360 may be reported in addition to 99460, 99465 as appropriate)

(Do not report 99360 in conjunction with 99464)

CASE MANAGEMENT SERVICES

Case management is a process in which a physician or another qualified health care professional is responsible for direct care of a patient and, additionally, for coordinating, managing access to, initiating, and/or supervising other health care services needed by the patient. .

	Separate Procedure		Unlisted Procedure		CCI Comp. Code		Non-specific Procedure

269

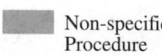

ANTICOAGULANT MANAGEMENT

Anticoagulant services are intended to describe the outpatient management of warfarin therapy, including ordering, review and interpretation of International Normalized Ratio (INR) testing, communication with patient, and dosage adjustments as appropriate.

When reporting these services, the work of anticoagulant management may not be used as a basis for reporting an evaluation and management (E/M) service or care plan oversight time during the reporting period. Do not report these services with 98966-98969, 99441-99444 when telephone or on-line services address anticoagulation with warfarin management. If a significant separately identifiable E/M service is performed, report the appropriate E/M service code using modifier 25.

These services are outpatient services only. When anticoagulation therapy is initiated or continued in the inpatient or observation setting, a new period begins after discharge and is reported with 99364. Do not report 99363-99364 with 99217-99239, 99291-99292, 99304-99318, 99471-99480 or other codes for physician review, interpretation, and patient management of home INR testing for a patient with mechanical heart valves.

Any period less than 60 continuous outpatient days is not reported. If less than the specified minimum number of services per period are performed, do not report the anticoagulation management services (99363-99364).

99363   Anticoagulant management for an outpatient taking warfarin, physician review and interpretation of International Normalized Ratio (INR) testing, patient instructions, dosage adjustment (as needed), and ordering of additional tests; initial 90 days of therapy (must include a minimum of 8 INR measurements)

99364   each subsequent 90 days of therapy (must include a minimum of 3 INR measurements)

(Do not report 99363, 99364 during the same month with 99487-99489)

(Do not report 99363, 99364 when performed during the service time of codes 99495 or 99496)

MEDICAL TEAM CONFERENCES

Medical team conferences include face-to-face participation by a minimum of three qualified health care professionals from different specialties or disciplines (each of whom provide direct care to the patient), with or without the presence of the patient, family member(s), community agencies, surrogate decision maker(s) (eg., legal guardian), and/or caregiver(s). The participants are actively involved in the

● New Code   ▲ Revised Code   + Add-On Code   ⊘ Modifier -51 Exempt   ⊙ Moderate Sedation

development, revision, coordination, and implementation of health care services needed by the patient. Reporting participants shall have performed face-to-face evaluations or treatments of the patient, independent of any team conference, within the previous 60 days.

Physicians or other qualified health care professionals who may report evaluation and management services should report their time spent in a team conference with the patient and/or family present using evaluation and management (E/M) codes (and time as the key controlling factor for code selection when counseling and/or coordination of care dominates the service). These introductory guidelines do not apply to services reported using E/M codes (see E/M services guidelines). However, the individual must be directly involved with the patient, providing face-to-face services outside of the conference visit with other physicians, other qualified health care professionals, or agencies.

Reporting participants shall document their participation in the team conference as well as their contributed information and subsequent treatment recommendations.

No more than one individual from the same specialty may report 99366-99368 at the same encounter.

Individuals should not report 99366-99368 when their participation in the medical team conference is part of a facility or organizational service contractually provided by the organizational or facility.

The team conference starts at the beginning of the review of an individual patient and ends at the conclusion of the review. Time related to record keeping and report generation is not reported. The reporting participant shall be present for all time reported. The time reported is not limited to the time that the participant is communicating to the other team members or patient and/or family. Time reported for medical team conferences may not be used in the determination of time for other services such as care plan oversight (99374-99380), home, domiciliary, or rest home care plan oversight (99339-99340), prolonged services (99354-99359), psychotherapy, or any E/M service. For team conferences where the patient is present for any part of the duration of the conference, nonphysician qualified health care professionals (eg, speech-language pathologists, physical therapists, occupational therapist, social workers, dieticians) report the team conference face-to-face code 99366.

MEDICAL TEAM CONFERENCE, DIRECT (FACE-TO-FACE) CONTACT WITH PATIENT AND/OR FAMILY

99366   Medical team conference with interdisciplinary team of health care professionals, face-to-face with patient and/or family, 30 minutes or more, participation by nonphysician qualified health care professional

(Team conference services of less than 30 minutes duration are not reported separately)

	Separate Procedure		Unlisted Procedure		CCI Comp. Code		Non-specific Procedure	**271**

(For team conference services by a physician with patient and/or family present, see Evaluation and Management services)

(Do not report 99366 during the same month with 99487-99489)

(Do not report 99366 when performed during the service time of codes 99495 or 99496)

MEDICAL TEAM CONFERENCE, WITHOUT DIRECT (FACE-TO-FACE) CONTACT WITH PATIENT AND/OR FAMILY

99367   Medical team conference with interdisciplinary team of health care professionals, patient and/or family not present, 30 minutes or more; participation by physician

99368   participation by nonphysician qualified health care professional

(Team conference services of less than 30 minutes duration are not reported separately)

(Do not report 99367, 99368 during the same month with 99487-99489)

(Do not report 99367, 99368 when performed during the service time of codes 99495 or 99496)

CARE PLAN OVERSIGHT SERVICES

Care plan oversight services are reported separately from codes for office/outpatient, hospital, home, nursing facility or domiciliary or non face-to-face services. The complexity and approximate time of the care plan oversight services provided within a 30-day period determine code selection. Only one individual may report services for a given period of time, to reflect the sole or predominant supervisory role with a particular patient. These codes should not be reported for supervision of patients in nursing facilities or under the care of home health agencies unless they require recurrent supervision of therapy.

The work involved in providing very low intensity or infrequent supervision services is included in the pre- and post-encounter work for home, office/outpatient and nursing facility or domiciliary visit codes.

CODING RULES

1.   *Evaluation and management services are not inclusive of care plan oversight services. Care plan oversight is coded separately.*

● New Code   ▲ Revised Code   + Add-On Code   ⊘ Modifier -51 Exempt   ⊙ Moderate Sedation

2. *Care plan oversight services may be coded only by a single physician for each patient during a specific period of time.*

    (For care plan oversight services of patients in the home, domiciliary, or rest home [eg, assisted living facility] see 99339, 99340, and for hospice agency, see 99377, 99378))

    (Do not report 99374-99380 for time reported with 98966-98969, 99441-99444)

    (Do not report 99374-99378 during the same month with 99487-99489)

    (Do not report 99374-99380 when performed during the service time of codes 99495 or 99496)

▲ **99374**   Supervision of a patient under care of home health agency (patient not present) in home, domiciliary or equivalent environment (eg, Alzheimer's facility) requiring complex and multidisciplinary care modalities involving regular development and/or revision of care plans by that individual, review of subsequent reports of patient status, review of related laboratory and other studies, communication (including telephone calls) for purposes of assessment or care decisions with health care professional(s), family member(s), surrogate decision maker(s) (eg., legal guardian) and/or key caregiver(s) involved in patient's care, integration of new information into the medical treatment plan and/or adjustment of medical therapy, within a calendar month; 15-29 minutes

▲ **99375**   30 minutes or more

▲ **99377**   Supervision of a hospice patient (patient not present) requiring complex and multidisciplinary care modalities involving regular development and/or revision of care plans by that individual, review of subsequent reports of patient status, review of related laboratory and other studies, communication (including telephone calls) for purposes of assessment or care decisions with health care professional(s), family member(s), surrogate decision maker(s) (eg, legal guardian) and/or key caregiver(s) involved in patient's care, integration of new information into the medical treatment plan and/or adjustment of medical therapy, within a calendar month; 15-29 minutes

▲ **99378**   30 minutes or more

▲ **99379**   Supervision of a nursing facility patient (patient not present) requiring complex and multidisciplinary care modalities involving regular development and/or revision of care plans by that individual, review of subsequent reports of patient status,

| | Separate Procedure | | Unlisted Procedure | | CCI Comp. Code | | Non-specific Procedure | **273** |

review of related laboratory and other studies, communication (including telephone calls) for purposes of assessment or care decisions with health care professional(s), family member(s), surrogate decision maker(s) (eg, legal guardian) and/or key caregiver(s) involved in patient's care, integration of new information into the medical treatment plan and/or adjustment of medical therapy, within a calendar month; 15-29 minutes

▲ **99380**   30 minutes or more

PREVENTIVE MEDICINE SERVICES

The following codes are used to report the preventive medicine evaluation and management of infants, children, adolescents, and adults.

The extent and focus of the services will largely depend on the age of the patient.

If an abnormality is encountered or a pre-existing problem is addressed in the process of performing this preventive medicine evaluation and management service, and if the problem or abnormality is significant enough to require additional work to perform the key components of a problem-oriented E/M service, then the appropriate Office/Outpatient code 99201-99215 should also be reported. Modifier 25 should be added to the Office/Outpatient code to indicate that a significant, separately identifiable evaluation and management service was provided on the same day as the preventive medicine service. The appropriate preventive medicine service is additionally reported.

An insignificant or trivial problem/abnormality that is encountered in the process of performing the preventive medicine evaluation and management service and which does not require additional work and the performance of the key components of a problem-oriented E/M service should not be reported.

The "comprehensive" nature of the Preventive Medicine Services codes 99381-99397 reflects an age and gender appropriate history/exam and is NOT synonymous with the "comprehensive" examination required in Evaluation and Management codes 99201-99350.

Codes 99381-99397 include counseling/anticipatory guidance/risk factor reduction interventions which are provided at the time of the initial or periodic comprehensive preventive medicine examination. (Refer to codes 99401-99412 for reporting those counseling/anticipatory guidance/risk factor reduction internventions that are provided at an encounter separate from the preventive medicine examination.)

Vaccine/toxoid products, immunization administrations, ancillary studies involving laboratory, radiology, other procedures, or screening tests (eg, vision, hearing, developmental) identified with a specific CPT code are reported separately. For

● New Code   ▲ Revised Code   + Add-On Code   ⊘ Modifier -51 Exempt   ⊙ Moderate Sedation

immunization administration and vaccine risk/benefit counseling, see 90460, 90461, 90470-90474. For vaccine/toxoid products, see 90476-90749.

CODING RULES

1. *The selection of Preventive Medicine codes is mostly dependent upon the age of the patient.*

2. *Preventive medicine codes are coded only in the absence of illness. If illness, injury is discovered during provision of a preventive medicine service, office/outpatient evaluation and management codes are coded.*

3. *Immunizations and diagnostic studies involving laboratory or radiology, or other procedures are not included in the preventive medicine service and should be coded separately.*

NEW PATIENT

99381 Initial comprehensive preventive medicine evaluation and management of an individual including an age and gender appropriate history, examination, counseling/anticipatory guidance/risk factor reduction interventions, and the ordering of laboratory/diagnostic procedures, new patient; infant (age under 1 year)

99382 early childhood (age 1 through 4 years)

99383 late childhood (age 5 through 11 years)

99384 adolescent (age 12 through 17 years)

99385 18-39 years

99386 40-64 years

99387 65 years and over

ESTABLISHED PATIENT

99391 Periodic comprehensive preventive medicine reevaluation and management of an individual including an age and gender appropriate history, examination, counseling/anticipatory guidance/risk factor reduction interventions, and the ordering of laboratory/diagnostic procedures, established patient; infant (age under 1 year)

99392 early childhood (age 1 through 4 years)

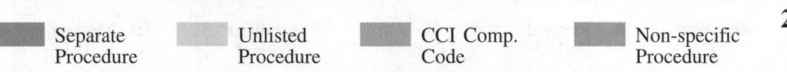

| Separate Procedure | Unlisted Procedure | CCI Comp. Code | Non-specific Procedure |

99393   late childhood (age 5 through 11 years)

99394   adolescent (age 12 through 17 years)

99395   18-39 years

99396   40-64 years

99397   65 years and over

COUNSELING RISK FACTOR REDUCTION AND BEHAVIOR CHANGE INTERVENTION

NEW OR ESTABLISHED PATIENT

These codes are used to report services provided face-to-face by a physician or other qualified health care professional for the purpose of promoting health and preventing illness or injury. They are distinct from evaluation and management (E/M) services that may be reported separately when performed. Risk factor reduction services are used for persons without a specific illness for which the counseling might otherwise be used as part of treatment.

Preventive medicine counseling and risk factor reduction interventions will vary with age and should address such issues as family problems, diet and exercise, substance use, sexual practices, injury prevention, dental health, and diagnostic and laboratory test results available at the time of the encounter.

Behavior change interventions are for persons who have a behavior that is often considered an illness itself, such as tobacco use and addiction, substance abuse/misuse, or obesity. Behavior change services may be reported when performed as part of the treatment of condition(s) related to or potentially exacerbated by the behavior or when performed to change the harmful behavior that has not yet resulted in illness. Any E/M services reported on the same day must be distinct, and time spent providing these services may not be used as a basis for the E/M code selection. Behavior change services involve specific validated interventions of assessing readiness for change and barriers to change, advising a change in behavior, assisting by providing specific suggested actions and motivational counseling, and arranging for services and follow-up.

For counseling groups of patients with symptoms or established illness, use 99078.

Health and Behavior Assessment/Intervention services (96150-96155) should not be reported on the same day as codes 99401-99412).

● New Code   ▲ Revised Code   + Add-On Code   ⊘ Modifier -51 Exempt   ⊙ Moderate Sedation

Preventive Medicine, Individual Counseling

99401 Preventive medicine counseling and/or risk factor reduction intervention(s) provided to an individual (separate procedure); approximately 15 minutes

99402 approximately 30 minutes

99403 approximately 45 minutes

99404 approximately 60 minutes

Behavior Change Interventions, Individual

99406 Smoking and tobacco use cessation counseling visit; intermediate, greater than 3 minutes up to 10 minutes

99407 intensive, greater than 10 minutes

(Do not report 99407 in conjunction with 99406)

99408 Alcohol and/or substance (other than tobacco) abuse structured screening (eg, AUDIT, DAST), and brief intervention (SBI) services; 15 to 30 minutes

(Do not report services of less than 15 minutes with 99408)

99409 greater than 30 minutes

(Do not report 99409 in conjunction with 99408)

(Do not report 99408, 99409 in conjunction with 99420)

(Use 99408, 99409 only for initial screening and brief intervention)

Preventive Medicine, Group Counseling

99411 Preventive medicine counseling and/or risk factor reduction intervention(s) provided to individuals in a group setting (separate procedure); approximately 30 minutes

99412 approximately 60 minutes

OTHER PREVENTIVE MEDICINE SERVICES

99420 Administration and interpretation of health risk assessment instrument (eg, health hazard appraisal)

277

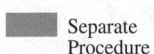 Separate Procedure 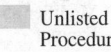 Unlisted Procedure 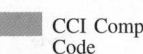 CCI Comp. Code 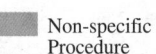 Non-specific Procedure

99429	Unlisted preventive medicine service
(99431	deleted 2009 edition, see 99460)
(99432	deleted 2009 edition, see 99461)
(99433	deleted 2009 edition, see 99462)
(99435	deleted 2009 edition, see 99463)
(99436	deleted 2009 edition, see 99464)
(99440	deleted 2009 edition, see 99465)

NON-FACE-TO-FACE PHYSICIAN SERVICES

TELEPHONE SERVICES

Telephone services are non-face-to-face evaluation and management (E/M) services provided to a patient using the telephone by a physician or other qualified health care professiona, who may report E/M sevices. These codes are used to report episodes of patient care initiated by an established patient or guardian of an established patient. If the telephone service ends with a decision to see the patient within 24 hours or next available urgent visit appointment, the code is not reported; rather the encounter is considered part of the preservice work of the subsequent E/M service, procedure and visit. Likewise, if the telephone call refers to an E/M service performed and reported by that individual within the previous seven days (either requested or unsolicited patient follow-up) or within the postoperative period of the previously completed procedure, then the service(s) are considered part of that previous E/M service or procedure. (Do not report 99441-99443 if reporting 99441-99444 performed in the previous seven days.)

> (For telephone services provided by a qualified nonphysician health care professional who may not report evaluation and management services [eg, speech-language pathologists, physical therapists, occupational therapists, social workers, dieticians], see 98966-98968)

▲ **99441** Telephone evaluation and management service by a physician or other qualified health care professional who may report evaluation and management services provided to an established patient, parent, or guardian not originating from a related E/M service provided within the previous 7 days nor leading to an E/M service or procedure within the next 24 hours or soonest available appointment; 5-10 minutes of medical discussion

▲ **99442** 11-20 minutes of medical discussion

278

● New Code	▲ Revised Code	+ Add-On Code	⊘ Modifier -51 Exempt	⊙ Moderate Sedation

▲ **99443**   21-30 minutes of medical discussion

> (Do not report 99441-99443 when using 99339-99340, 99374-99380 for the same call[s])

> (Do not report 99441-99443 for anticoagulation management when reporting 99363-99364)

> (Do not report 99441-99443 during the same month with 99487-99489)

> (Do not report 99441-99443 when performed during the service time of codes 99495 or 99496)

ON-LINE MEDICAL EVALUATION

An on-line electronic medical evaluation is a non-face-to-face evaluation and management (E/M) service by a physician to a patient using Internet resources in response to a patient's on-line inquiry. Reportable services involve the physician's personal timely response to the patient's inquiry and must involve permanent storage (electronic or hard coy) of the encounter. This service is reported only once for the same episode of care during a seven-day period, although multiple physicians could report their exchange with the same patient. If the on-line medical evaluation refers to an E/M service previously performed and reported by the physician within the previous seven days (either physician requested or un solicited patient follow-up) or within the postoperative period of the previously completed procedure, then the service(s) are considered covered by the previous E/M service or procedure. A reportable service encompasses the sum of communication (eg, related telephone calls, prescription provision, laboratory orders) pertaining to the on-line patient encounter.

> (For an on-line medical evaluation provided by a qualified nonphysician health care professional, use 98969)

▲ **99444** Online evaluation and management service provided by a physician or other qualified health care professional who may report evaluation and management services provided to an established patient or guardian, not originating from a related E/M service provided within the previous 7 days, using the Internet or similar electronic communications network

> (Do not report 99444 when using 99339-99340, 99374-99380 for the same communication[s])

> (Do not report 99444 for anticoagulation management when reporting 99363, 99364)

> (Do not report 99444 during the same month with 99487-99489)

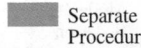 Separate Procedure   Unlisted Procedure   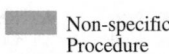 CCI Comp. Code   Non-specific Procedure

(Do not report 99444 when performed during the service time of codes 99495 or 99496)

SPECIAL EVALUATION AND MANAGEMENT SERVICES

The following codes are used to report evaluations performed to establish baseline information prior to life or disability insurance certificates being issued. This service is performed in the office or other setting, and applies to both new and established patients When using these codes, no active management of the problem(s) is undertaken during the encounter..

If other evaluation and management services and/or procedures are performed on the same date, the appropriate E/M or procedure code(s) should be reported in addition to these codes.

BASIC LIFE AND/OR DISABILITY EVALUATION SERVICES

99450 Basic life and/or disability examination that includes:

- measurement of height, weight and blood pressure;

- completion of a medical history following a life insurance pro forma;

- collection of blood sample and/or urinalysis complying with "chain of custody" protocols; and

- completion of necessary documentation/certificates.

WORK RELATED OR MEDICAL DISABILITY EVALUATION SERVICES

99455 Work related or medical disability examination by the treating physician that includes:

- completion of a medical history commensurate with the patient's condition;

- performance of an examination commensurate with the patient's condition;

- formulation of a diagnosis, assessment of capabilities and stability, and calculation of impairment;

- development of future medical treatment plan; and

- completion of necessary documentation/certificates and report.

● New Code ▲ Revised Code + Add-On Code ⊘ Modifier -51 Exempt ⊙ Moderate Sedation

99456   Work related or medical disability examination by other than the treating physician that includes:

- completion of a medical history commensurate with the patient's condition;

- performance of an examination commensurate with the patient's condition;

- formulation of a diagnosis, assessment of capabilities and stability, and calculation of impairment;

- development of future medical treatment plan; and

- completion of necessary documentation/certificates and report.

(Do not report 99455, 99456 in conjunction with 99080 for the completion of Workman's Compensation forms)

NEWBORN CARE SERVICES

The following codes are used to report the services provided to newborns (birth through the first 28 days) in several different settings. Use of the normal newborn codes is limited to the initial care of the newborn in the first days after birth prior to home discharge.

Evaluation and Management (E/M) services for the newborn include maternal and/or fetal and newborn history, newborn physical examination(s), ordering of diagnostic tests and treatments, meetings with the family, and documentation in the medical record.

When delivery room attendance services (99464) or delivery room resuscitation services (99465) are required, report these in addition to normal newborn services E/M codes.

For E/M services provided to newborns who are other than normal, see codes for hospital inpatient services (99221-99233) and neonatal intensive and critical care services (99466-99469, 99477-99480). When normal newborn services are provided by the same individual on the same date that the newborn later becomes ill and receives additional intensive or critical care services, report the appropriate E/M code with modifier 25 for these services in addition to the normal newborn code..

Procedures (eg, 54150, newborn circumcision) are not included with the normal newborn codes, and when performed, should be reported in addition to the newborn services.

When newborns are seen in follow-up after the date of discharge in the office or outpatient setting, see 99201-99215, 99381, 99391 as appropriate.

	Separate Procedure		Unlisted Procedure		CCI Comp. Code		Non-specific Procedure

99460   Initial hospital or birthing center care, per day, for evaluation and management of normal newborn infant

99461   Initial care, per day, for evaluation and management of normal newborn infant seen in other than hospital or birthing center

99462   Subsequent hospital care, per day, for evaluation and management of normal newborn

99463   Initial hospital or birthing center care, per day, for evaluation and management of normal newborn infant admitted and discharged on the same date

(For newborn hosptial discharge services provided on a date subsequent to the admission date, see 99238, 99239)

DELIVERY/BIRTHING ROOM ATTENDANCE AND RESUSCITATION SERVICES

▲ **99464**   Attendance at delivery (when requested by the delivering physician or other qualified health care professional) and initial stabilization of newborn

(99464 may be reported in conjunction with 99460, 99468, 99477)

(Do not report 99464 in conjunction with 99465)

99465   Delivery/birthing room resuscitation, provision of positive pressure ventilation and/or chest compressions in the presence of acute inadequate ventilation and/or cardiac output

(99465 may be reported in conjunction with 99460, 99468, 99477)

(Do not report 99465 in conjunction with 99464)

(Procedures that are performed as a necessary part of the resuscitation [eg, intubation, vascular lines] are reported separately in addition to 99465. In order to report these procedures, they must be performed as a necessary component of the resuscitation and not as a convenience before admission to the neonatal intensive care unit)

● New Code   ▲ Revised Code   + Add-On Code   ⊘ Modifier -51 Exempt   ⊙ Moderate Sedation

INPATIENT NEONATAL INTENSIVE CARE SERVICES AND PEDIATRIC AND NEONATAL CRITICAL CARE SERVICES

PEDIATRIC CRITICAL CARE PATIENT TRANSPORT

Codes 99466, 99467 are used to report the physical attendance and direct face-to-face care by a physician during the interfacility transport of a critically ill or critically injured pediatric patient 24 months of age or younger. Codes 99485, 99486 are used to report the control physician's non-face-to-face supervision of interfacility transport of a critically ill or critically injured pediatric patient 24 months of age or younger. These codes are not reported together for the same patient by the same physician. For the purpose of reporting 99466 and 99467, face-to-face care begins when the physician assumes primary responsibility of the pediatric patient at the referring facility, and ends when the receiving facility accepts responsibility for the pediatric patient's care. Only the time the physician spends in direct face-to-face contact with the patient during the transport should be reported. Pediatric patient transport services involving less than 30 minutes of face-to-face physician care should not be reported using 99466, 99467. Procedure(s) or services(s) performed by other members of the transporting team may not be reported by the supervising physician.

Codes 99485, 99486 are used to report control physician's non-face-to-face supervision of interfacility pediatric critical care transport, which includes all two-way communication between the control physician and the specialized transport team prior to transport, at the referring facility and during transport of the patient back to the receiving facility. The "control" physician is the physician directing transport services. These codes do not include pretransport communication between the control physician and the referring facility before or following patient transport. These codes are only reported for patients 24 month of age or younger who are critically ill or critically injured. The control physician provides treatment advice to a specialized transport team who are present and delivering the hand-on patient care. The control physician does not report any services provided by the specialized transport team. The control physician's non-face-to-face time begins with the first contact by the control physician with the specialized transport team and ends when the patient's care is handed over to the receiving facility team. Refer to 99466 and 99467 for face-to-face transport care of the critically ill/injured patient. Time spent with the individual patient's transport team and reviewing data submissions should be recorded. Code 99485 is used to report the first 16-45 minutes of direction on a given date and should only be used once even if time spent by the physician is discontinuous. Do not report services of 15 minutes or less or any time when another physician is reporting 99466, 99467. Do not report 99485 or 99486 in conjunction with 99466, 99467 when performed by the same physician.

For the definition of the critically injured pediatric patient, see the Neonatal and Pediatric Critical Care Services section.

283

Separate Procedure	Unlisted Procedure	CCI Comp. Code	Non-specific Procedure

The non-face-to-face direction of emergency care to a patient's transporting staff by a physician located in a hospital or other facility by two-way communication is not considered direct face-to-face care and should not be reported with 99466, 99467. Physician-directed non-face-to-face emergency care through outside voice communication to transporting staff personnel is reported with 99288 or 99485, 99486 based upon the age and clinical condition of the patient.

Emergency department services (99281-99285), initial hospital care (99221-99223), critical care (99291, 99292), initial date neonatal intensive (99477) or critical care (99468) are only reported after the patient has been admitted to the emergency department, the inpatient floor, or the critical care unit of the receiving facility. If inpatient critical care services are reported in the referring facility prior to transfer to the receiving hospital, use the critical care codes (99291, 99292).

Services provided by the specialized transport team during non-face-to-face transport supervision are not reported by the control physician.

Code 99485 is used to report the first 30 minutes of non-face-to-face supervision of an interfacility transport of a critically ill or critically injured pediatric patient and should be reported only once per date of service. Code 99486 is used to report each additional 30 minutes beyond the initial 30 minutes. Non-face-to-face interfacility transport of 15 minutes or less is not reported..

(For total body cooling of neonates, see 0260T, 0261T)

▲ **99466**   Critical care face-to-face services, during an interfacility transport of critically ill or critically injured pediatric patient, 24 months of age or less; first 30-74 minutes of hands-on care during transport

▲**+99467**   each additional 30 minutes (list separately in addition to code for primary service)

(Use 99467 in conjunction with 99466)

(Critical care of less than 30 minutes total duration should be reported with the appropriate E/M code)

● **99485**   Supervision by a control physician of interfacility transport care of the critically ill or critically injured pediatric patient, 24 month of age or younger, includes two-way communication with transport team before transport, at the referring facility and during the transport, including data interpretation and report, first 30 minutes.

●**+99486**   each additional 30 minutes (List separately in addition to code for primary procedure)

(Use 99486 in conjunction with 99485)

● New Code   ▲ Revised Code   + Add-On Code   ⊘ Modifier -51 Exempt   ⊙ Moderate Sedation

(For physician direction of emergency medical systems supervision for a pediatric patient older than 24 months of age, or at any age if not critically ill or injured, use 99288)

(Do not report 99485, 99486 with any other services reported by the control physician for the same period)

(Do not report 99485, 99486 in conjunction with 99466, 99467 when performed by the same physician)

INPATIENT NEONATAL AND PEDIATRIC CRITICAL CARE

The same definitions for critical care services apply to the adult, child and neonate.

Codes 99468, 99469 are used to report services of directing the inpatient care of a critically ill neonate or infant 28 days of age or younger. They represent care starting with the date of admission (99468) to a critical care unite and subsequent day(s) (99469) that the neonate remains critical. These codes may be reported only by a single individual and only once per day, per patient, per hospital stay in a given facility. If readmitted to the neonatal critical care unit during the same day, report the subsequent day(s) code 99469 for the first day of readmission to critical care, and 99469 for each day of critical care following readmission.

The initial day neonatal critical care code (99468) can be used in addition to 99464 or 99465 as appropriate, when the physician or other qualified health care professional is present for the delivery (99464), or resuscitation (99465) is required. Other procedures performed as a necessary part of the resuscitation (eg., endotracheal intubation [31500]) are also reported separately when performed as part of the pre-admission delivery room care. In order to report these procedures separately, they must be performed as a necessary component of the resuscitation and not simply as a convenience before admission to the neonatal intensive care unit.

Codes 99471-99476 are used to report direction of the inpatient care of a critically ill infant or young child from 29 days of postnatal age through less than 6 years of age. They represent care starting with the date of admission (99471, 99475) and subsequent day(s) (99472, 99476) the infant or child remains critical. These codes may be reported only by a single individual, and only once per day, per patient in a given setting. Service for the critically ill or critically injured child 6 years of age or older would be reported with the time based critical care codes (99291, 99292). Report 99471, 99475 only once per hospital stay in a given facility. If readmitted to the pediatric critical care unit during the same stay, report 99472 or 99476 for the first day of readmission to critical care and 99472 for each day of critical care following readmission.

The pediatric and neonatal critical care codes include those procedures listed for the critical care codes (99291, 99292). In addition, the following procedures are also included (and are not separately reported by professionals, but may be

| | Separate Procedure | | Unlisted Procedure | | CCI Comp. Code | | Non-specific Procedure | **285** |

reported by facilities) in the pediatric and neonatal critical care service codes (99468-99472, 99475, 99476), and the intensive care services codes (99477-99480):

Any services performed that are not included in these listings may be reported separately. Facilities may report the included services separately.

Invasive or non-invasive electronic monitoring of vital signs

Vascular access procedures

> Peripheral vessel catheterization (36000)
> Other arterial catheters (36140, 36620)
> Umbilical venous catheters (36510)
> Central vessel catheterization (36555)
> Vascular access procedures (36400, 36405, 36406)
> Vascular punctures (36420, 36600)
> Umbilical arterial catheters (36660)

Airway and ventilation management

> Endotracheal intubation (31500)
> Ventilatory management (94002-94004)
> Bedside pulmonary function testing (94375)
> Surfactant administration (94610)
> Continuous positive airway pressure (CPAP) (94660)

Monitoring or interpretation of blood gases or oxygen saturation (94760-94762)

Car Seat Evaluation (94780-94781)

Transfusion of blood components (36430, 36440)

Oral or nasogastric tube placement (43752)

Suprapubic bladder aspiration (51100)

Bladder catheterization (51701, 51702)

Lumbar puncture (62270)

Any services performed which are not listed above may be reported separately.

When a neonate or infant is not critically ill but requires intensive observation, frequent interventions, and other intensive care services, the Continuing Intensive Care Services codes (99477-99480) should be used to report these services.

To report critical care services provided in the outpatient setting (eg., emergency department or office) for neonates and pediatric patients of any age, see the Critical

● New Code ▲ Revised Code + Add-On Code ⊘ Modifier -51 Exempt ⊙ Moderate Sedation

Care codes 99291, 99292. If the same individual provides critical care services for a neonatal or pediatric patient less than 6 years of age in both the outpatient and inpatient settings on the same day, report only the appropriate Neonatal or Pediatric Critical Care codes 99468-99476 for all critical care services provided on that day. Critical care services provided by a second individual of a different specialty not reporting a per-day neonatal or pediatric critical care code can be reported with 99291, 99292.

When critical care services are provided to neonates or pediatric patients less than 6 years of age at two separate institutions by an individual from a different group on the same date of service, the individual from the referring institution should report their critical care services with the critical care codes (99291, 99292) and the receiving institution should report the appropriate initial day of care code 99468, 99471, 99475 for the same date of service.

Critical care services to a pediatric patient six years of age or older are reported with the critical care codes 99291, 99292.

When the critically ill neonate or pediatric patient improves and is transferred to a lower level of care to another individual in another group within the same facility, the transferring individual does not report a per day critical care service. subsequent hospital care (99231-99233) or time-based critical care services (99291-99292) is reported, as appropriate based upon the condition of the neonate or child. The receiving individual reports subsequent intensive care (99478- 99480) or subsequent hospital care (99231-99233) services, as appropriate based upon the condition of the neonate or child.

When the neonate or infant becomes critically ill on a day when initial or subsequent intensive care services (99477-99480), hospital services (99221-99233), or normal newborn services (99460, 99461, 99462) have been performed by one individual and is transferred to a critical care level of care provided by a different individual in a different group, the transferring individual reports either the time-based critical care services performed (99291, 99292) for the time spent providing critical care to the patient, the intensive care service (99477-99480), hospital care services (99221-99233), or normal newborn service ((99460, 99461, 99462) performed, but only one service. The receiving individual reports initial or subsequent inpatient neonatal or pediatric critical care (99468-99476), as appropriate based upon the patient's age and whether this is the first or subsequent admission to the critical care unit for the hospital stay.

When a newborn becomes critically ill on the same day they have already received normal newborn care (99460, 99461, 99462), and the same individual or group assumes critical care, report initial critical care service (99468) with modifier 25 in addition to the normal newborn code.

When a neonate, infant, or child requires initial critical care services on the same day the patient already has received hospital care or intensive care services by the

	Separate Procedure		Unlisted Procedure		CCI Comp. Code		Non-specific Procedure

same individual or group, only the initial critical care service code (99468, 99471, 99475) is reported.

Time-based critical care services (99291, 99292) are not reportable by the same individual or different individual within the same group when neonatal or pediatric critical care services (9468-99476) are reported for the same patient on the same day.

No individual may report remote real-time videoconferenced critical care (0188T, 0189T) when neonatal or pediatric intensive or critical care services (99468-99476) are reported.

99468 Initial inpatient neonatal critical care, per day, for the evaluation and management of a critically ill neonate, 28 days of age or less

99469 Subsequent inpatient neonatal critical care, per day, for the evaluation and management of a critically ill neonate, 28 days of age or less

99471 Initial inpatient pediatric critical care, per day, for the evaluation and management of a critically ill infant or young child, 29 days through 24 months of age

99472 Subsequent inpatient pediatric critical care, per day, for the evaluation and management of a critically ill infant or young child, 29 days through 24 months of age

99475 Initial inpatient pediatric critical care, per day, for the evaluation and management of a critically ill infant or young child, 2 through 5 years of age

99476 Subsequent inpatient pediatric critical care, per day, for the evaluation and management of a critically ill infant or young child, 2 through 5 years of age

INITIAL AND CONTINUING INTENSIVE CARE SERVICES

Code 99477 represents the initial day of inpatient care for the child who is not critically ill but requires intensive observation, frequent interventions, and other intensive care services. Codes 99478-99480 are used to report the subsequent day services of directing the continuing intensive care of the low birth weight (LBW 1500-2500 grams) present body weight infant, very low birth weight (VLBW less than 1500 grams) present body weight infant, or normal (2501-5000 grams) present body weight newborn who does not meet the definition of critically ill but continues to require intensive observation, frequent interventions, and other intensive care services. These services are for infants and neonates who are not critically ill but continue to require intensive cardiac and respiratory monitoring, continuous and/or frequent vital sign monitoring, heat maintenance, enteral and/or parenteral nutritional adjustments, laboratory and oxygen monitoring, and constant observation by the health care team under direct supervision of the physician or other qualified health care professional. Codes 99477-99480 may be reported by a single individual and only once per day, per patient in a given facility. If readmitted to the intensive care unit during the same hospital stay, report 99478-99480 for the first day of intensive care and for each successive day that the child requires intensive care services.

These codes include the same procedures that are outlined in the Neonatal and Pediatric Critical Care Services section and these services should not be separately reported.

The initial day neonatal intensive care code (99477) can be used in addition to 99464 or 99465 as appropriate, when the physician or other qualified health care professional is present for the delivery (99464) or resuscitation (99465) is required. In this situation, report 99477 with modifier 25. Other procedures performed as a necessary part of the resuscitation (eg, endotracheal intubation [31500]) are also reported separately when performed as part of the pre-admission delivery room care. In order to report these procedures separately, they must be performed asa necessary component of the resuscitation and not simply as a convenience before admission to the neonatal intensive care unit.

The same procedures are included as bundled services with the neonatal intensive care codes as those listed for the neonatal (99468, 99469) and pediatric (99471-99476) critical care codes.

When the neonate or infant improves after the initial day and no longer requires intensive care services and is transferred to a lower level of care, the transferring individual does not report a per day intensive care service. Subsequent hospital care (99231-99233) or subsequent normal newborn care (99460, 99462) is reported as appropriate based upon the condition of the neonate or infant. If the transfer to a lower level of care occurs on the same day as initial intensive care services were provided by the transferring individual, 99477 may be reported.

When the neonate or infant is transferred after the initial day within the same facility to the care of another individual in a different group, both individuals report subsequent hospital care (99231-99233) services. The receiving individual reports subsequent hospital care (99231-99233) or subsequent normal newborn care (99462).

When the neonate or infant becomes critically ill on a day when initial or subsequent intensive care services (99477-99480) have been reported by one individual and is transferred to a critical care level of care provided by a different individual from a different group, the transferring individual reports either the time-based critical care services performed (99291-99292) for the time spent

289

	Separate Procedure		Unlisted Procedure		CCI Comp. Code		Non-specific Procedure

providing critical care to the patient, or the initial or subsequent intensive care (99477-99480) services, but not both. The receiving individual reports initial or subsequent inpatient neonatal or pediatric critical care (99468-99476) based upon the patient's age and whether this is the first or subsequent admission to critical care for the same hospital stay.

When the neonate or infant becomes critically ill on a day when initial or subsequent intensive care services (99477-99480) have been performed by the same individual or group, report only initial or subsequent inpatient neonatal or pediatric critical care (99468-99476) based upon the patient's age and whether this is the first or subsequent admission to critical care for the same hospital stay.

For the subsequent care of the sick neonate younger than 28 days of age, but more than 5000 grams who does not require intensive or critical care services, use 99231-99233.

99477 Initial hospital care, per day, for the evaluation and management of the neonate, 28 days of age or less, who requires intensive observation, frequent interventions, and other intensive care services

(For the initiation of inpatient care of the normal newborn, report 99460)

(For the initiation of care of the critically ill neonate, use 99468)

(For initiation of inpatient hospital care of the ill neonate not requiring intensive observation, frequent interventions, and other intensive care services, see 99221-99223)

99478 Subsequent intensive care, per day, for the evaluation and management of the recovering very low birth weight infant (present body weight less than 1500 grams)

99479 Subsequent intensive care, per day, for the evaluation and management of the recovering low birth weight infant (present body weight of 1500-2500 grams)

99480 Subsequent intensive care, per day, for the evaluation and management of the recovering infant (present body weight of 2501-5000 grams)

99485 This code is out of order. See page 284

99486 This code is out of order. See page 284

● New Code   ▲ Revised Code   ✚ Add-On Code   ⊘ Modifier -51 Exempt   ⊙ Moderate Sedation

COMPLEX CHRONIC CARE COORDINATION SERVICES

Complex chronic care coordination services are patient-centered management and support services provided by physicians, other qualified health care professionals, and clinical staff to an individual who resides at home or in a domiciliary, rest home, or assisted living facility. These services typically involve clinical staff implementing a care plan directed by the physician or other qualified health care professional. These services address the coordination of care by multiple disciplines and community service agencies. The reporting individual provides or oversees the management and/or coordination of services, as needed, for all medical conditions, psychosocial needs, and activities of daily living.

Patients who require complex chronic care coordination services may be identified by algorithms that utilize reported conditions and services (eg, predictive modeling risk score or repeat admissions or emergency department use) or by clinician judgment. Typical patients have 1 or more chronic continuous or episodic health conditions expected to last at least 12 months, or until the death of the patient, that place the patient at significant risk of death, acute exacerbation/decompensation, or functional decline. Because of the complex nature of their diseases and morbidities, these patients commonly require the coordination of a number of specialties and services. Patients may have medical and psychiatric behavioral co-morbidities (eg, dementia and chronic obstructive pulmonary disease or substance abuse and diabetes) that complicate their care. Social support weaknesses or access to care difficulties may cause a need for these services. Medical, functional, and/or psychosocial problems that require medical decision making of moderate or high complexity and extensive clinical staff support are expected. Medical decision making as defined in the Evaluation and Management (E/M) guidelines is not only applied to the face-to-face services but it determined by the nature of the problems addresses by the reporting individual during the month. A plan of care should be documented and shared with the patient and/or caregiver.

Codes 99487-99489 are reported only once per calendar month and include all non-face-to-face complex chronic care coordination services and none or 1 face-to-face office or other outpatient, home, or domiciliary visit. Codes 99487-99489 may only be reported by the single physician or other qualified health care professional who assumes the care coordination role with a particular patient for the calendar month.

Code selection is as follows:

Code 99487 is reported when, during the calendar month, there is no face-to-face visit with the physician or other qualified health care professional and at least 31 minutes of clinical staff time is spent in care coordination activities. Code 99488 is reported when, during the calendar month, there is a face-to-face visit with the physician or other qualified health care professional and at least 31 minutes of clinical staff time is spent in care coordination activities.

291

	Separate Procedure		Unlisted Procedure		CCI Comp. Code		Non-specific Procedure

The face-to-face and non-face-to-face time spent by the clinical staff in communicating with the patient and/or family, caregivers, other professionals and agencies; revising, documenting and implementing the care plan; or teaching self-management is used in determining the complex chronic care coordination clinical staff time for the month. Note: Do not count any clinical staff time on the date of the first visit or on a day when the physician or qualified health care professional reports an E/M service (office or other outpatient services 99211-99215; domiciliary, rest home services 99334-99337; home services 99347-99350).

Care coordination activities performed by clinical staff may include:

- communication (with patient, family members, guardian or caretaker, surrogate decision makers, and/or other professionals) regarding aspects of care;

- communication with home health agencies and other community services utilized by the patient;

- collection of health outcomes data and registry documentation;

- patient and/or family/caretaker education to support self-management, independent living, and activities of daily living;

- assessment and support for treatment regimen adherence and medication management;

- identification of available community and health resources;

- facilitating access to care and services needed by the patient and/or family;

- development and maintenance of a comprehensive care plan.

If a face-to-face visit was provided during the month by the physician or other qualified health care professional, report 99488. Additional E/M services beyond the first visit may be reported separately by the same physician or other qualified health care professional during the same calendar month. Complex care coordination services include care plan oversight services (99339, 99340, 99374-99378), prolonged services without direct patient contact (99358, 99359), anticoagulant management (99363, 99364), medical team conferences (99366-99368), education and training (98960-98962, 99071, 99078), telephone services (98966-98968, 99441-99443), on-line medical evaluation (98969, 99444), preparation of special reports (99080), analysis of data (99090, 99091), transitional care management services (99495, 99496), medication therapy management services (99605-99607), and if performed, these services may not be reported separately during the month for which 99487-99489 are reported. All other services may be reported. Do not report 99487-99489 if reporting ESRD services (90951-90970) during the same month. If the complex chronic care coordination services are performed within the postoperative period of a reported surgery, the same individual may not report 99487-99489.

● New Code   ▲ Revised Code   + Add-On Code   ⊘ Modifier -51 Exempt   ⊙ Moderate Sedation

Complex chronic care coordination can be reported in any calendar month during which the clinical staff time requirements are met. If care coordination resumes after a discharge during a new month, start a new period or report transitional care management services (99495, 99496) as appropriate. If discharge occurs in the same month, continue the reporting period or report transitional care management services. Do not report 99487-99489 for any post-discharge complex chronic care coordination services for any days within 30 days of discharge, if reporting 99495, 99496.

Total Duration of Staff Care Coordination Services	Codes
Less than 30 minutes	Not reported separately
31 to 74 minutes (31 minutes to 1 hr. 14 min.)	99487 or 99488 x 1
75 to 104 minutes (1 hr. 15 min. to 1 hr. 44 min.)	99487 or 99488 x 1 AND 99489 x 1
105 minutes or more (1 hr. 45 min. or more)	99487 or 99488 x 1 AND 99489 x 2 or more for each additional 30 minutes

- **99487** Complex chronic care coordination services; first hour of clinical staff time directed by a physician or other qualified health care professional with no face-to-face visit, per calendar month

- **99488** first hour of clinical staff time directed by a physician or other qualified health care professional with one face-to-face visit, per calendar month

- **+99489** each additional 30 minutes of clinical staff time directed by a physician or other qualified health care professional, per calendar month (List separately in addition to code for primary procedure)

(Report 99489 in conjunction with 99487, 99488)

(Do not report 99487-99489 during the same month with 90951-90970, 98960-98962, 98966-98969, 99071, 99078, 99080, 99090, 99091, 99339, 99340, 99358, 99359, 99363, 99364, 99366-99368, 99374-99378, 99441-99444, 99495, 99496, 99605-99607)

TRANSITIONAL CARE MANAGEMENT SERVICES

Codes 99495 and 99496 are used to report transitional care management services (TCM). These services are for an established patient whose medical and/or physchosocial problems require moderate or high complexity medical decision making during transitions in care from an inpatient hospital setting (including acute

Separate Procedure   Unlisted Procedure   CCI Comp. Code   Non-specific Procedure

hospital, rehabilitation hospital, long-tem acute care hospital), partial hospital, observation status in a hospital, or skilled nursing facility/nursing facility, to the patient's community setting (home, domiciliary, rest home or assisted living). TCM commences upon the date of discharge and continues for the next 29 days.

TCM is comprised of one face-to-face visit within the specified time frames, in combination with non-face-to-face services that may be performed by the physician or other qualified health care professional and/or licensed clinical staff under his/her direction.

Non-face-to-face services provided by clinical staff, under the direction of the physician or other qualified health care professional, may include:

- communication (with patient, family members, guardian or caretaker, surrogate decision makers, and/or other professionals) regarding aspects of care;

- communication with home health agencies and other community services utilized by the patient;

- patient and/or family/caretaker education to support self-management, independent living, and activities of daily living;

- assessment and support for treatment regimen adherence and medication management;

- identification of available community and health resources;

- facilitating access to care and services needed by the patient and/or family.

Non-face-to-face services provided by the physician or other qualified health care professional may include:

- obtaining and reviewing the discharge information (eg, discharge summary, as available, or continuity of care documents);

- reviewing need for or follow-up on pending diagnostic tests and treatments;

- interaction with other qualified health care professionals who will assume or reassume care of the patient's system-specific problems;

- education of patient, family, guardian, and/or caregiver;

- establishment or reestablishment of referrals and arranging for needed community resources;

- assistance in scheduling any required follow-up with community providers and services.

TCM requires a face-to-face visit, initial patient contact, and medication reconciliation within specified time frames. The first face-to-face visit is part of the TCM service and not reported separately. Additional E/M services after the first face-to-face visit may be reported separately. TCM requires an interactive contact with the patient or caregiver, as appropriate, within two business days of discharge.

294 ● New Code ▲ Revised Code + Add-On Code ⊘ Modifier -51 Exempt ⊙ Moderate Sedation

CPT codes and descriptions only ©2012 American Medical Association. All rights reserved.

The contact may be direct (face-to-face), by telephone, or by electronic means. Medication reconciliation and management must occur no later than the date of the face-to-face visit.

These services address any needed coordination of care performed by multiple disciplines and community service agencies. The reporting individual provides or oversees the management and/or coordination of services, as needed, for all medical conditions, psychosocial needs, and activities of daily living support by providing first contact and continuous access.

Medical decision making and the date of the first face-to-face visit are used to select and report the appropriate TCM code. For 99496, the face-to-face visit must occur within 7 calendar days of the date of discharge, and medical decision making must be of high complexity. For 99495, the face-to-face visit must occur within 14 calendar days of the date of discharge, and medical decision making must be of at least moderate complexity.

Type of Medical Decision Making	Face-to-face visit within 7 days	Face-to-face visit within 8 to 14 days
Moderate complexity	99495	99495
High complexity	99496	99495

Medical decision making is defined by the E/M Services Guidelines. The medical decision making over the service period reported is used to define the medical decision making of TCM. Documentation includes the timing of the initial post-discharge communication with the patient or caregivers, date of the face-to-face visit, and the complexity of the medical decision making.

Only one individual may report these services and only once per patient within 30 days of discharge. Another TCM may not be reported by the same individual or group for any subsequent discharge(s) within the 30 days. The same individual may report hospital or observation discharge services and TCM. The same individual should not report TCM services provided in the postoperative period.

A physician or other qualified health care professional who reports codes 99495, 99496 may not report care plan oversight services (99339, 99340, 99374-99380), prolonged services without direct patient contact (99358, 99359), anticoagulant management (99363, 99364), medical team conferences (99366-99368), education and training (98960-98962, 99071, 99078), telephone services (98966-98968, 99441-99443), end stage renal disease services (90951-90970), online medical evaluation services 98969, 99444), preparation of special reports (99080), analysis of data (99090, 99091), complex chronic care coordination services (99487-99489), or medication therapy management services (99605-99607) during the time period covered by the transitional care management services codes.

Separate Procedure | Unlisted Procedure | CCI Comp. Code | Non-specific Procedure

● **99495**   Transitional care management services with the following required elements:

  ● Communication (direct contact, telephone, electronic) with the patient and/or caregiver within 2 business days of discharge

  ● Medical decision making of at least moderate complexity during the service period

  ● Face-to-face visit withing 14 calendar days of discharge

● **99496**   Transitional care management services with the following required elements:

  ● Communication (direct contact, telephone, electronic) with the patient and/or caregiver within 2 business days of discharge

  ● Medical decision making of high complexity during the service period

  ● Face-to-face visit within 7 calendar days of discharge

(Do note report 90951-90970, 98960-98962, 98966-98969, 99071, 99078, 99080, 99090, 99091, 99339, 99340, 99358, 99359, 99363, 99364, 99366-99368, 99374-99380, 99441-99444, 99487-99489, 99605-99607 when performed during the service time of codes 99495 or 99496)

OTHER EVALUATION AND MANAGEMENT SERVICES

99499   Unlisted evaluation and management service

● New Code   ▲ Revised Code   + Add-On Code   ⊘ Modifier -51 Exempt   ⊙ Moderate Sedation

ANESTHESIA

ANESTHESIA OVERVIEW

The second section of the CPT coding system is the anesthesia section, which includes service codes for the delivery of anesthesia. Within each subsection, the CPT codes are arranged by anatomical site.

The Anesthesiologist provides pain relief and maintenance, or restoration, of a stable condition during and immediately following an operation, an obstetric or diagnostic procedure. The Anesthesiologist assesses the risk of the patient undergoing surgery and optimizes the patient's condition prior to, during, and after surgery.

Reporting of anesthesia services is dependent on the third party payer involved. Anesthesia services covered by Medicare are coded using codes from the ANESTHESIA section of the CPT coding system. For most other third party payers, anesthesia services are coded using codes from the SURGERY section of the CPT coding system to describe the major surgical procedure.

Anesthesia services may be coded by anesthesiologists or anesthetists working under the supervision of the anesthesiologist. Anesthesia services include pre- and post-op visits, anesthesia delivery, giving fluids and/or blood needed during a procedure, and monitoring. Anesthesia delivery includes general, regional, supplementing local anesthesia, and other supportive services.

To report moderate (conscious) sedation provided by a physician also performing the service for which conscious sedation is being provided, see codes 99143-99145.

For the procedures listed in Appendix G, when a second physician other than the health care professional performing the diagnostic or therapeutic services provides moderate (conscious) sedation in the facility setting (eg, hospital, outpatient hospital/ambulatory surgery center, skilled nursing facility), the second physician reports the associated moderate sedation procedure/service 99148-99150; when these services are performed by the second physician in the nonfacility setting (eg, physician office, freestanding imaging center), codes 99148-99150 would not be reported. Moderate sedation does not include minimal sedation (anxiolysis), deep sedation, or monitored anesthesia care (00100-01999).

KEY POINTS ABOUT ANESTHESIA CODING

1. *Time recording for anesthesia services starts with patient preparation for anesthesia induction and ends when the anesthesiologist or anesthetist has*

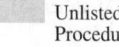

	Separate Procedure		Unlisted Procedure		CCI Comp. Code		Non-specific Procedure

completed his/her services and transfers responsibility for postoperative supervision.

2. Consultations and/or other evaluation and management services which are not included in the administration or supervising the administration of anesthesia, regardless of location provided, are reporting using CPT codes from the evaluation and management section of the CPT book.

3. Any supplies and/or materials provided by the anesthesiologist or anesthetist which are not considered to be included in the standard service may be coded separately.

4. Multiple procedures provided on the same date of service should be coded separately.

5. Any service which may be considered rare, unusual, variable or not defined should be supported with a special report which clearly defines the need for the unusual service. These services are generally coded with an unlisted CPT code or by adding modifier -22 to the CPT code which defines the procedure.

ANESTHESIA SERVICE MODIFIERS

A physical status modifier must be added to all CPT codes when reporting anesthesia services. The physical status modifier defines the physical condition of the patient and ranges from a normal health patient to a declared brain-dead patient whose organs are being harvested for a transplant.

PHYSICAL STATUS MODIFIERS

-P1 A normal healthy patient.

-P2 A patient with a mild systemic disease.

-P3 A patient with severe systemic disease.

-P4 A patient with severe systemic disease that is a constant threat to life.

-P5 A moribund patient who is not expected to survive without the operation.

-P6 A declared brain-dead patient whose organs are being removed for donor purposes.

● New Code　　▲ Revised Code　　+ Add-On Code　　⊘ Modifier -51 Exempt　　⊙ Moderate Sedation

OTHER ANESTHESIA SERVICE MODIFIERS

Under certain circumstances, medical services and procedures may need to be further modified. Other CPT coding system modifiers commonly used with ANESTHESIA services include:

-22   Unusual services

-23   Anesthesia

-32   Mandated services

-51   Multiple procedures

QUALIFYING CIRCUMSTANCES FOR ANESTHESIA

In the case of difficult and/or extraordinary circumstances such as extreme youth or age, extraordinary condition of the patient, and/or unusual risk factors it may be appropriate to report one or more of the following qualifying circumstances in addition to the anesthesia services.

+ 99100   Anesthesia for patient of extreme age, younger than one year and older 70 (List separately in addition to code for primary anesthesia procedure)

(For procedure performed on infants younger than 1 year of age at time of surgery, see 00326, 00561, 00834, 00836)

+ 99116   Anesthesia complicated by utilization of total body hypothermia (List separately in addition to code for primary anesthesia procedure)

+ 99135   Anesthesia complicated by utilization of controlled hypotension (List separately in addition to code for primary anesthesia procedure)

+ 99140   Anesthesia complicated by emergency conditions (specify) (List separately in addition to code for primary anesthesia procedure)

(An emergency is defined as existing when delay in treatment of the patient would lead to a significant increase in the threat to life or body part.)

	Separate Procedure		Unlisted Procedure		CCI Comp. Code		Non-specific Procedure

This page intentionally left blank.

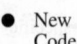

● New Code	▲ Revised Code	✛ Add-On Code	⊘ Modifier -51 Exempt	⊙ Moderate Sedation

ANESTHESIA CODES

HEAD

00100 Anesthesia for procedures on salivary glands, including biopsy

00102 Anesthesia for procedures on plastic repair of cleft lip

00103 Anesthesia for reconstructive procedures of eyelid (eg, blepharoplasty, ptosis surgery)

00104 Anesthesia for electroconvulsive therapy

00120 Anesthesia for procedures on external, middle, and inner ear including biopsy; not otherwise specified

00124   otoscopy

00126   tympanotomy

00140 Anesthesia for procedures on eye; not otherwise specified

00142   lens surgery

00144   corneal transplant

00145   vitreoretinal surgery

00147   iridectomy

00148   ophthalmoscopy

00160 Anesthesia for procedures on nose and accessory sinuses; not otherwise specified

00162   radical surgery

00164   biopsy, soft tissue

00170 Anesthesia for intraoral procedures, including biopsy; not otherwise specified

00172   repair of cleft palate

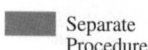 Separate Procedure

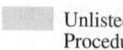 Unlisted Procedure

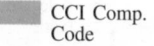 CCI Comp. Code

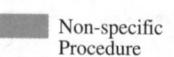 Non-specific Procedure

00174	excision of retropharyngeal tumor
00176	radical surgery
00190	Anesthesia for procedures on facial bones or skull; not otherwise specified
00192	radical surgery (including prognathism)
00210	Anesthesia for intracranial procedures; not otherwise specified
00211	craniotomy or craniectomy for evacuation of hematoma
00212	subdural taps
00214	burr holes, including ventriculography
00215	cranioplasty or elevation of depressed skull fracture, extradural (simple or compound)
00216	vascular procedures
00218	procedures in sitting position
00220	cerebrospinal fluid shunting procedures
00222	electrocoagulation of intracranial nerve

NECK

00300	Anesthesia for all procedures on the integumentary system, muscles and nerves of head, neck, and posterior trunk, not otherwise specified
00320	Anesthesia for all procedures on esophagus, thyroid, larynx, trachea and lymphatic system of neck; not otherwise specified, age 1 year or older
00322	needle biopsy of thyroid
	(For procedures on cervical spine and cord, see 00600, 00604, 00670)
00326	Anesthesia for all procedures on the larynx and trachea in children less than 1 year of age

● New Code ▲ Revised Code + Add-On Code ⊘ Modifier -51 Exempt ⊙ Moderate Sedation

(Do not report 00326 in conjunction with code 99100)

00350 Anesthesia for procedures on major vessels of neck; not otherwise specified

00352 simple ligation

(For arteriography, use 01916)

THORAX (CHEST WALL AND SHOULDER GIRDLE)

00400 Anesthesia for procedures on the integumentary system on the extremities, anterior trunk and perineum; not otherwise specified

00402 reconstructive procedures on breast (eg, reduction or augmentation mammoplasty, muscle flaps)

00404 radical or modified radical procedures on breast

00406 radical or modified radical procedures on breast with internal mammary node dissection

00410 electrical conversion of arrhythmias

00450 Anesthesia for procedures on clavicle and scapula; not otherwise specified

00452 radical surgery

00454 biopsy of clavicle

00470 Anesthesia for partial rib resection; not otherwise specified

00472 thoracoplasty (any type)

00474 radical procedures (eg, pectus excavatum)

INTRATHORACIC

00500 Anesthesia for all procedures on esophagus

00520 Anesthesia for closed chest procedures; (including bronchoscopy) not otherwise specified

---

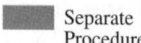 Separate Procedure   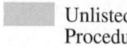 Unlisted Procedure   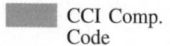 CCI Comp. Code   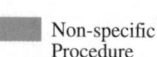 Non-specific Procedure

00522   needle biopsy of pleura

00524   pneumocentesis

00528   mediastinoscopy and diagnostic thoracoscopy not utilizing 1 lung ventilation

(For tracheobronchial reconstruction, use 00539)

00529   mediastinoscopy and diagnostic thoracoscopy utilizing 1 lung ventilation

00530 Anesthesia for permanent transvenous pacemaker insertion

00532 Anesthesia for access to central venous circulation

00534 Anesthesia for transvenous insertion or replacement of pacing cardioverter/defibrillator

(For transthoracic approach, use 00560)

00537 Anesthesia for cardiac electrophysiologic procedures including radiofrequency ablation

00539 Anesthesia for tracheobronchial reconstruction

00540 Anesthesia for thoracotomy procedures involving lungs, pleura, diaphragm, and mediastinum (including surgical thoracoscopy); not otherwise specified

00541   utilizing 1 lung ventilation

(For thoracic spine and cord anesthesia procedures via an anterior transthoracic approach, see 00625-00626)

00542   decortication

00546   pulmonary resection with thoracoplasty

00548   intrathoracic procedures on the trachea and bronchi

00550 Anesthesia for sternal debridement

00560 Anesthesia for procedures on heart, pericardial sac, and great vessels of chest; without pump oxygenator

00561   with pump oxygenator, younger than one year of age

   ● New Code   ▲ Revised Code   + Add-On Code   ⊘ Modifier -51 Exempt   ⊙ Moderate Sedation

(Do not report 00561 in conjunction with 99100, 99116, and 99135)

00562 with pump oxygenator, age 1 year or older, for all non-coronary bypass procedures (eg. valve procedures) or for re-operation for coronary bypass more than 1 month after original operation)

00563 with pump oxygenator with hypothermic circulatory arrest

00566 Anesthesia for direct coronary artery bypass grafting; without pump oxygenator

00567 with pump oxygenator

00580 Anesthesia for heart transplant or heart/lung transplant

SPINE AND SPINAL CORD

00600 Anesthesia for procedures on cervical spine and cord; not otherwise specified

(For percutaneous image-guided spine and spinal cord anesthesia procedures, see 01935, 01936)

00604 procedures with patient in the sitting position

00620 Anesthesia for procedures on thoracic spine and cord; not otherwise specified

00622 thoracolumbar sympathectomy

00625 Anesthesia for procedures on the thoracic spine and cord, via an anterior transthoracic approach; not utilizing 1 lung ventilation

00626 utilizing 1 lung ventilation

(For anesthesia for thoractomy procedures other than spinal, see 00540-00541)

00630 Anesthesia for procedures in lumbar region; not otherwise specified

00632 lumbar sympathectomy

00634 chemonucleolysis

Separate Procedure Unlisted Procedure CCI Comp. Code Non-specific Procedure **305**

00635   diagnostic or therapeutic lumbar puncture

00640   Anesthesia for manipulation of the spine or for closed procedures on the cervical, thoracic or lumbar spine

00670   Anesthesia for extensive spine and spinal cord procedures (eg, spinal instrumentation or vascular procedures)

UPPER ABDOMEN

00700   Anesthesia for procedures on upper anterior abdominal wall; not otherwise specified

00702   percutaneous liver biopsy

00730   Anesthesia for procedures on upper posterior abdominal wall

00740   Anesthesia for upper gastrointestinal endoscopic procedures, endoscope introduced proximal to duodenum

00750   Anesthesia for hernia repairs in upper abdomen; not otherwise specified

00752   lumbar and ventral (incisional) hernias and/or wound dehiscence

00754   omphalocele

00756   transabdominal repair of diaphragmatic hernia

00770   Anesthesia for all procedures on major abdominal blood vessels

00790   Anesthesia for intraperitoneal procedures in upper abdomen including laparoscopy; not otherwise specified

00792   partial hepatectomy or management of liver hemorrhage (excluding liver biopsy)

00794   pancreatectomy, partial or total (eg, Whipple procedure)

00796   liver transplant (recipient)

     (For harvesting of liver, use 01990)

00797   gastric restrictive procedure for morbid obesity

   ● New Code   ▲ Revised Code   + Add-On Code   ⊘ Modifier -51 Exempt   ⊙ Moderate Sedation

LOWER ABDOMEN

00800 Anesthesia for procedures on lower anterior abdominal wall; not otherwise specified

00802 panniculectomy

00810 Anesthesia for lower intestinal endoscopic procedures, endoscope introduced distal to duodenum

00820 Anesthesia for procedures on lower posterior abdominal wall

00830 Anesthesia for hernia repairs in lower abdomen; not otherwise specified

00832 ventral and incisional hernias

(For hernia repairs in the infant 1 year of age or younger, see 00834, 00836)

00834 Anesthesia for hernia repairs in the lower abdomen not otherwise specified, under 1 year of age

(Do not report 00834 in conjunction with code 99100)

00836 Anesthesia for hernia repairs in the lower abdomen not otherwise specified, infants less than 37 weeks gestational age at birth and less than 50 weeks gestational age at time of surgery

(Do not report 00836 in conjunction with code 99100)

00840 Anesthesia for intraperitoneal procedures in lower abdomen including laparoscopy; not otherwise specified

00842 amniocentesis

00844 abdominoperineal resection

00846 radical hysterectomy

00848 pelvic exenteration

00851 tubal ligation/transection

00860 Anesthesia for extraperitoneal procedures in lower abdomen, including urinary tract; not otherwise specified

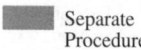 Separate Procedure   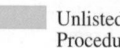 Unlisted Procedure   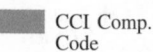 CCI Comp. Code   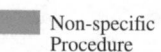 Non-specific Procedure

307

| 00862 | renal procedures, including upper 1/3 of ureter, or donor nephrectomy |

| 00864 | total cystectomy |

| 00865 | radical prostatectomy (suprapubic, retropubic) |

| 00866 | adrenalectomy |

| 00868 | renal transplant (recipient) |

(For donor nephrectomy, use 00862)

(For harvesting kidney from brain-dead patient, use 01990)

| 00870 | cystolithotomy |

| 00872 | Anesthesia for lithotripsy, extracorporeal shock wave; with water bath |

| 00873 | without water bath |

| 00880 | Anesthesia for procedures on major lower abdominal vessels; not otherwise specified |

| 00882 | inferior vena cava ligation |

PERINEUM

(For perineal procedures on the integumentary system, muscles and nerves, see 00300, 00400)

| 00902 | Anesthesia for; anorectal procedure |

| 00904 | radical perineal procedure |

| 00906 | vulvectomy |

| 00908 | perineal prostatectomy |

| 00910 | Anesthesia for transurethral procedures (including urethrocystoscopy); not otherwise specified |

| 00912 | transurethral resection of bladder tumor(s) |

| 00914 | transurethral resection of prostate |

● New Code   ▲ Revised Code   + Add-On Code   ⊘ Modifier -51 Exempt   ⊙ Moderate Sedation

00916   post-transurethral resection bleeding

00918   with fragmentation, manipulation and/or removal of ureteral calculus

00920   Anesthesia for procedures on male genitalia (including open urethral procedures); not otherwise specified

00921   vasectomy, unilateral or bilateral

00922   seminal vesicles

00924   undescended testis, unilateral or bilateral

00926   radical orchiectomy, inguinal

00928   radical orchiectomy, abdominal

00930   orchiopexy, unilateral or bilateral

00932   complete amputation of penis

00934   radical amputation of penis with bilateral inguinal lymphadenectomy

00936   radical amputation of penis with bilateral inguinal and iliac lymphadenectomy

00938   insertion of penile prosthesis (perineal approach)

00940   Anesthesia for vaginal procedures (including biopsy of labia, vagina, cervix or endometrium); not otherwise specified

00942   colpotomy, vaginectomy, colporrhaphy and open urethral procedures

00944   vaginal hysterectomy

00948   cervical cerclage

00950   culdoscopy

00952   hysteroscopy and/or hysterosalpingography

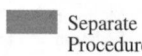 Separate Procedure   Unlisted Procedure   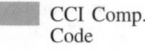 CCI Comp. Code   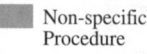 Non-specific Procedure

309

PELVIS (EXCEPT HIP)

01112 Anesthesia for bone marrow aspiration and/or biopsy, anterior or posterior iliac crest

01120 Anesthesia for procedures on bony pelvis

01130 Anesthesia for body cast application or revision

01140 Anesthesia for interpelviabdominal (hindquarter) amputation

01150 Anesthesia for radical procedures for tumor of pelvis, except hindquarter amputation

01160 Anesthesia for closed procedures involving symphysis pubis or sacroiliac joint

01170 Anesthesia for open procedures involving symphysis pubis or sacroiliac joint

01173 Anesthesia for open repair of fracture disruption of pelvis or column fracture involving acetabulum

01180 Anesthesia for obturator neurectomy; extrapelvic

01190 intrapelvic

UPPER LEG (EXCEPT KNEE)

01200 Anesthesia for all closed procedures involving hip joint

01202 Anesthesia for arthroscopic procedures of hip joint

01210 Anesthesia for open procedures involving hip joint; not otherwise specified

01212 hip disarticulation

01214 total hip arthroplasty

01215 revision of total hip arthroplasty

01220 Anesthesia for all closed procedures involving upper 2/3 of femur

---

● New Code   ▲ Revised Code   + Add-On Code   ⃠ Modifier -51 Exempt   ⊙ Moderate Sedation

01230 Anesthesia for open procedures involving upper 2/3 of femur; not otherwise specified

01232 amputation

01234 radical resection

01250 Anesthesia for all procedures on nerves, muscles, tendons, fascia, and bursae of upper leg

01260 Anesthesia for all procedures involving veins of upper leg, including exploration

01270 Anesthesia for procedures involving arteries of upper leg, including bypass graft; not otherwise specified

01272 femoral artery ligation

01274 femoral artery embolectomy

KNEE AND POPLITEAL AREA

01320 Anesthesia for all procedures on nerves, muscles, tendons, fascia, and bursae of knee and/or popliteal area

01340 Anesthesia for all closed procedures on lower 1/3 of femur

01360 Anesthesia for all open procedures on lower 1/3 of femur

01380 Anesthesia for all closed procedures on knee joint

01382 Anesthesia for diagnostic arthroscopic procedures of knee joint

01390 Anesthesia for all closed procedures on upper ends of tibia, fibula, and/or patella

01392 Anesthesia for all open procedures on upper ends of tibia, fibula, and/or patella

01400 Anesthesia for open or surgical arthroscopic procedures on knee joint; not otherwise specified

01402 total knee arthroplasty

01404 disarticulation at knee

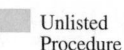 Separate Procedure   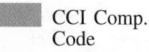 Unlisted Procedure   CCI Comp. Code   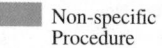 Non-specific Procedure

01420 Anesthesia for all cast applications, removal, or repair involving knee joint

01430 Anesthesia for procedures on veins of knee and popliteal area; not otherwise specified

01432 arteriovenous fistula

01440 Anesthesia for procedures on arteries of knee and popliteal area; not otherwise specified

01442 popliteal thromboendarterectomy, with or without patch graft

01444 popliteal excision and graft or repair for occlusion or aneurysm

LOWER LEG (BELOW KNEE, INCLUDES ANKLE AND FOOT)

01462 Anesthesia for all closed procedures on lower leg, ankle, and foot

01464 Anesthesia for arthroscopic procedures of ankle and/or foot

01470 Anesthesia for procedures on nerves, muscles, tendons, and fascia of lower leg, ankle, and foot; not otherwise specified

01472 repair of ruptured Achilles tendon, with or without graft

01474 gastrocnemius recession (eg, Strayer procedure)

01480 Anesthesia for open procedures on bones of lower leg, ankle, and foot; not otherwise specified

01482 radical resection (including below knee amputation)

01484 osteotomy or osteoplasty of tibia and/or fibula

01486 total ankle replacement

01490 Anesthesia for lower leg cast application, removal, or repair

01500 Anesthesia for procedures on arteries of lower leg, including bypass graft; not otherwise specified

312   ● New Code   ▲ Revised Code   + Add-On Code   ⊘ Modifier -51 Exempt   ⊙ Moderate Sedation

01502   embolectomy, direct or with catheter

01520   Anesthesia for procedures on veins of lower leg; not otherwise specified

01522   venous thrombectomy, direct or with catheter

SHOULDER AND AXILLA

Includes humeral head and neck, sternoclavicular joint, acromioclavicular joint, and shoulder joint

01610   Anesthesia for all procedures on nerves, muscles, tendons, fascia, and bursae of shoulder and axilla

01620   Anesthesia for all closed procedures on humeral head and neck, sternoclavicular joint, acromioclavicular joint, and shoulder joint

01622   Anesthesia for diagnostic arthroscopic procedures of shoulder joint

01630   Anesthesia for open or surgical arthroscopic procedures on humeral head and neck, sternoclavicular joint, acromioclavicular joint, and shoulder joint; not otherwise specified

(01632   Deleted 2009 [2010 edition]; see 01630, 01638)

01634   shoulder disarticulation

01636   interthoracoscapular (forequarter) amputation

01638   total shoulder replacement

01650   Anesthesia for procedures on arteries of shoulder and axilla; not otherwise specified

01652   axillary-brachial aneurysm

01654   bypass graft

01656   axillary-femoral bypass graft

01670   Anesthesia for all procedures on veins of shoulder and axilla

---

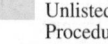 Separate Procedure   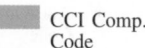 Unlisted Procedure   CCI Comp. Code   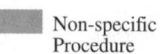 Non-specific Procedure   **313**

01680 Anesthesia for shoulder cast application, removal or repair; not otherwise specified

01682   shoulder spica

UPPER ARM AND ELBOW

01710 Anesthesia for procedures on nerves, muscles, tendons, fascia, and bursae of upper arm and elbow; not otherwise specified

01712   tenotomy, elbow to shoulder, open

01714   tenoplasty, elbow to shoulder

01716   tenodesis, rupture of long tendon of biceps

01730 Anesthesia for all closed procedures on humerus and elbow

01732 Anesthesia for diagnostic arthroscopic procedures of elbow joint

01740 Anesthesia for open or surgical arthroscopic procedures of the elbow; not otherwise specified

01742   osteotomy of humerus

01744   repair of nonunion or malunion of humerus

01756   radical procedures

01758   excision of cyst or tumor of humerus

01760   total elbow replacement

01770 Anesthesia for procedures on arteries of upper arm and elbow; not otherwise specified

01772   embolectomy

01780 Anesthesia for procedures on veins of upper arm and elbow; not otherwise specified

01782   phleborrhaphy

● New Code ▲ Revised Code + Add-On Code ⊘ Modifier -51 Exempt ⊙ Moderate Sedation

FOREARM, WRIST, AND HAND

01810 Anesthesia for all procedures on nerves, muscles, tendons, fascia, and bursae of forearm, wrist, and hand

01820 Anesthesia for all closed procedures on radius, ulna, wrist, or hand bones

01829 Anesthesia for diagnostic arthroscopic procedures on the wrist

01830 Anesthesia for open or surgical arthroscopic/endoscopic procedures on distal radius, distal ulna, wrist, or hand joints; not otherwise specified

01832 total wrist replacement

01840 Anesthesia for procedures on arteries of forearm, wrist, and hand; not otherwise specified

01842 embolectomy

01844 Anesthesia for vascular shunt, or shunt revision, any type (eg, dialysis)

01850 Anesthesia for procedures on veins of forearm, wrist, and hand; not otherwise specified

01852 phleborrhaphy

01860 Anesthesia for forearm, wrist, or hand cast application, removal, or repair

RADIOLOGICAL PROCEDURES

01916 Anesthesia for diagnostic arteriography/venography

(Do not report 01916 in conjunction with therapeutic codes 01924-01926, 01930-01933)

01920 Anesthesia for cardiac catheterization including coronary angiography and ventriculography (not to include Swan-Ganz catheter)

01922 Anesthesia for non-invasive imaging or radiation therapy

---

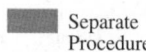 Separate Procedure   Unlisted Procedure   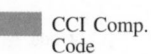 CCI Comp. Code   Non-specific Procedure

315

01924 Anesthesia for therapeutic interventional radiologic procedures involving the arterial system; not otherwise specified

01925 carotid or coronary

01926 intracranial, intracardiac, or aortic

01930 Anesthesia for therapeutic interventional radiologic procedures involving the venous/lymphatic system (not to include access to the central circulation); not otherwise specified

01931 intrahepatic or portal circulation (eg, transvenous intrahepatic portosystemic shunt(s) (TIPS))

01932 intrathoracic or jugular

01933 intracranial

01935 Anesthesia for percutaneous image guided procedures on the spine and spinal cord; diagnostic

01936 therapeutic

BURN EXCISIONS OR DEBRIDEMENT

01951 Anesthesia for second and third degree burn excision or debridement with or without skin grafting, any site, for total body surface area (TBSA) treated during anesthesia and surgery; less than four percent total body surface area

01952 between four and nine percent of total body surface area

+ **01953** each additional nine percent total body surface area or part thereof (List separately in addition to code for primary procedure)

(Use 01953 in conjunction with code 01952)

OBSTETRIC

01958 Anesthesia for external cephalic version procedure

01960 Anesthesia for vaginal delivery only

01961 Anesthesia for cesarean delivery only

● New Code   ▲ Revised Code   + Add-On Code   ⊘ Modifier -51 Exempt   ⊙ Moderate Sedation

01962 Anesthesia for urgent hysterectomy following delivery

01963 Anesthesia for cesarean hysterectomy without any labor analgesia/anesthesia care

01965 Anesthesia for incomplete or missed abortion procedures

01966 Anesthesia for induced abortion procedures

01967 Neuraxial labor analgesia/anesthesia for planned vaginal delivery (this includes any repeat subarachnoid needle placement and drug injection and/or any necessary replacement of an epidural catheter during labor)

+ **01968** Anesthesia for cesarean delivery following neuraxial labor analgesia/anesthesia (List separately in addition to code for primary procedure performed)

(Use 01968 in conjunction with code 01967)

+ **01969** Anesthesia for cesarean hysterectomy following neuraxial labor analgesia/anesthesia (List separately in addition to code for primary procedure performed)

(Use 01969 in conjunction with code 01967)

OTHER PROCEDURES

01990 Physiological support for harvesting of organ(s) from brain-dead patient

▲ **01991** Anesthesia for diagnostic or therapeutic nerve blocks and injections (when block or injection is performed by a different physician or other qualified health care professional); other than the prone position

▲ **01992** prone position

(Do not report code 01991 or 01992 in conjunction with 99141)

(When regional intravenous administration of local anesthetic agent or other medication in the upper or lower extremity is used as the anesthetic for a surgical procedure, report the appropriate anesthesia code. To report a Bier block for pain management, use 64999.)

317

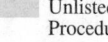 Separate Procedure   Unlisted Procedure   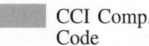 CCI Comp. Code   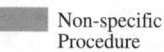 Non-specific Procedure

(For intra-arterial or intravenous therapy for pain management, see 96373, 96374.)

01996 Daily hospital management of epidural or subarachnoid continuous drug administration

(Report code 01996 for daily hospital management of continuous epidural or subarachnoid drug administration performed after insertion of an epidural or subarachnoid catheter placed primarily for anesthesia administration during an operative session, but retained for post-operative pain management)

01999 Unlisted anesthesia procedure(s)

● New Code	▲ Revised Code	✚ Add-On Code	⊘ Modifier -51 Exempt	☉ Moderate Sedation

SURGERY

SURGERY SECTION OVERVIEW

The third section of the CPT coding system is the surgery section, and it includes surgical procedure codes for all body areas. Within each subsection, the CPT codes are arranged by anatomical site.

It is essential to understand the organization of the CPT surgery section in order to locate the correct procedure code. Understanding other or alternative terms which may apply to a procedure, injury, illness or condition may also make the location of the appropriate procedure easier and faster.

All procedures listed in the surgery section of the CPT book include local, metacarpal/digital block or topical anesthesia if used, the surgical procedure, and normal uncomplicated follow-up care. For diagnostic surgical procedures, follow-up care includes only the care related to recovery from the diagnostic procedure. For therapeutic surgical procedures, follow-up care includes only the care which would usually be included in the surgical service. Any complications resulting in additional services are not considered to be included and should be coded separately.

KEY POINTS ABOUT SURGERY SERVICES

- *Evaluation and management services provided by surgeons in the office, home or hospital, plus consultations and other medical services are coded using evaluation and management service codes.*

- *Any supplies and/or materials provided by the surgeon which are not considered to be included in the standard service may be coded separately.*

GLOBAL SURGICAL PACKAGE

Third-party payers differ in their definition of a surgical or global surgical package concept. Medicare defines the global surgical package as follows:

- *The surgeon's initial evaluation or consultation will be paid separately.*

- *There is a one day preoperative period covered under the global surgical package.*

- *Included in the package are all intraoperative services that are considered to be usual and necessary. Separate billing of these services would be considered unbundling.*

- *Any treatment of complications by the surgeon not requiring a return to the operating room is included in the package.*

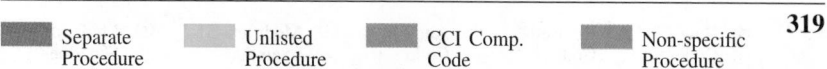

| Separate Procedure | Unlisted Procedure | CCI Comp. Code | Non-specific Procedure |

319

- *The surgical package contains a standard 90-day postoperative period which includes all visits to the physician during that time unless the visit is for a totally different reason than that for the surgery.*

- *In cases of organ transplant, immunosuppressive therapy is not included in the global package.*

- *Minor surgical procedures are those with a 0 or 10-day postoperative period, and are excluded from the surgical package definition.*

SPECIAL REPORT

Surgical procedures which are rarely provided, unusual or vary significantly from the standard definition may require a special report. When preparing reports to accompany health insurance claim forms the provider should include a description of the nature, extent, and need for the procedure, and the time, effort, and equipment necessary to provides the service. Try to keep these reports as brief and simple as possible. Additional items which may be needed are:

- *complexity of symptoms*

- *final diagnosis*

- *pertinent physical findings*

- *diagnostic and therapeutic procedures*

- *concurrent problems*

- *follow-up care*

MULTIPLE SURGICAL PROCEDURES

It is common for several surgical procedures to be performed at the same operative session. When multiple procedures are performed on the same day or at the same session, the "major" procedure or service is listed first followed by secondary, additional, or "lessor" procedures or services. CPT modifier -51 is added to all procedures following the first one.

Reporting multiple procedures incorrectly may have a serious impact on reimbursement from health insurance payers. An inexperienced health insurance biller may simply list the procedures on the health insurance claim form in the order dictated or described in the operative report.

There are two critical decisions related to reporting multiple surgical procedures correctly; namely: 1) The order in which the procedures are listed on the health insurance claim form, and 2) whether or not to list the additional procedures with full or reduced fees.

● New Code   ▲ Revised Code   + Add-On Code   ⊘ Modifier -51 Exempt   ⊙ Moderate Sedation

ORDER OF LISTING MULTIPLE PROCEDURES

The first procedure to be listed when reporting services under the multiple procedure rule is the procedure with the highest fee. Additional procedures should be listed in descending order by fee. Modifier -51 should be added to each additional procedure.

All third party payers will reduce the allowance for the additional procedures, typically by 50 percent for the second procedure, and 50 to 75 percent for the third and subsequent procedures. Listing the procedures in descending order by fee minimizes the possibility of an incorrect reduction.

21. DIAGNOSIS OR NATURE OF ILLNESS OR INJURY. (RELATE ITEMS 1,2,3 OR 4 TO ITEM 24E BY LINE)		
1. 952 . 10	3.	
2.	4.	

24 A DATE(S) OF SERVICE	B Place of Service	C Type of Service	D PROCEDURES, SERVICES, OR SUPPLIES CPT/HCPCS MODIFIER	E DIAGNOSIS CODE
06 15 13	21		63046	
06 15 13	21		62223 51	

BILLING FULL VERSUS REDUCED FEES

The full fee should be listed for each procedure coded on the health insurance claim form as part of multiple surgical procedures. Third party payers will automatically reduce the allowances for the additional procedures by a specific formula. Listing all multiple procedures with full fees in descending fee order (the procedure with the highest fee first, the procedure with the next highest fee second, et cetera) will result in the maximum total allowable reimbursement for the provider or the insured.

After the maximum benefit has been paid by the health insurance company, the balance remaining, less any patient co-insurance or deductible requirements, should be written off. Note that billing practices vary in different areas of the country. Providers should continue to use the method that is customary or required by third party payers in the provider's practice location.

321

Separate Procedure   Unlisted Procedure   CCI Comp. Code   Non-specific Procedure

SEPARATE PROCEDURE

Some surgical procedures are considered to be an integral part of a more extensive surgical procedure. In this circumstance, the integral procedure is not coded. When the integral procedure is performed independently and is unrelated to other services, it should be listed as a "separate procedure."

SURGERY SUBSECTIONS

The SURGERY section of the CPT coding system is divided into 19 subsections:

General	10021-10022
Integumentary System	10040-19499
Musculoskeletal System	20005-29999
Respiratory System	30000-32999
Cardiovascular System	33010-37799
Hemic and Lymphatic Systems	38100-38999
Mediastinum and Diaphragm	39000-39599
Digestive System	40490-49999
Urinary System	50010-53899
Male Genital System	54000-55899
Reproductive System Procedures	55920
Intersex Surgery	55970-55980
Female Genital Surgery	56405-58999
Maternity Care and Delivery	59000-59899
Endocrine System	60000-60699
Nervous System	61000-64999
Eye and Ocular Adnexa	65091-68899
Auditory System	69000-69979
Operating Microscope	69990

Each sub-section of the SURGERY section of the CPT coding system is divided into organs then into procedures involving anatomic sites. Each anatomic site is further separated into surgical processes such as incision, excision, repair, removal, amputation, etc.

SURGERY SECTION MODIFIERS

Due to various circumstances, surgical procedures may be considered to be modified in comparison to the full or complete procedure. Modified procedures are identified by reporting a two-digit modifier to the CPT procedure code(s). The following CPT modifiers may be coded with surgical procedures:

-22 Unusual Procedural Services

-26 Professional Component

-32 Mandated Services

322 ● New Code ▲ Revised Code ✛ Add-On Code ⊘ Modifier -51 Exempt ⊙ Moderate Sedation

-47 Anesthesia by Surgeon

-50 Bilateral Procedure

-51 Multiple Procedures

-52 Reduced Services

-54 Surgical Care Only

-55 Postoperative Management Only

-56 Preoperative Management Only

-57 Decision for Surgery

-58 Staged or Related Procedure or Service by the Same Physician During the Postoperative Period

-62 Two Surgeons

-66 Surgical Team

-76 Repeat Procedure by Same Physician

-77 Repeat Procedure by Another Physician

-78 Return to the Operating Room for a Related Procedure During the Postoperative Period

-79 Unrelated Procedure or Service by the Same Physician During the Postoperative Period

-80 Assistant Surgeon

-81 Minimum Assistant Surgeon

-82 Assistant Surgeon (when qualified resident surgeon not available)

-90 Reference (Outside) Laboratory

-99 Multiple modifiers

| Separate Procedure | Unlisted Procedure | CCI Comp. Code | Non-specific Procedure |

ADD-ON CODES

Many surgical procedures are performed secondary to primary surgical procedures. These procedures are classified as "additional" or "supplemental" procedures and are designated as "add-on" codes in the CPT coding system. "Add-on" CPT codes are identified in the CPT code book by a black plus sign "+" placed to the left of the code number.

Many of the CPT "Add-on" codes are further identified by phrases included within the descriptions of the definition of the CPT code or include the phrase "(List separately in addition to primary procedure)" following the definition. Examples of CPT codes identified as "add-on" codes include:

+ **11008** Removal of prosthetic material or mesh, abdominal wall for infection (eg, for chronic or recurrent mesh infection or necrotizing soft tissue infection) (list separately in addition to code for primary procedure)

+ **19295** Image guided placement, metallic localization clip, percutaneous, during breast biopsy/aspiration (List separately in addition to code for primary procedure)

STARRED PROCEDURES

CPT used to define minor surgical procedures by placing a star (*) after the procedure code number. This designation was removed in CPT 2004.

MEDICAL AND SURGICAL SUPPLIES

HCPCS Level II codes for medical and surgical supplies, A4000-A4999, may be used to report supplies and materials provided to Medicare patients if the supplies and materials are not considered to be included with or part of the basic service(s) or procedure(s).

● New Code   ▲ Revised Code   + Add-On Code   ⊘ Modifier -51 Exempt   ⊙ Moderate Sedation

SURGERY CODES

GENERAL

10021 Fine needle aspiration; without imaging guidance

10022 with imaging guidance

(For placement of percutaneous localization clip during breast biopsy, use 19295)

(For radiological supervision and interpretation, see 76942, 77002, 77012, 77021)

(For percutaneous needle biopsy other than fine needle aspiration, see 20206 for muscle, 32400 for pleura, 32405 for lung or mediastinum, 42400 for salivary gland, 47000 for liver, 48102 for pancreas, 49180 for abdominal or retroperitoneal mass, 50200 for kidney, 54500 for testis, 54800 for epididymis, 60100 for thyroid, 62267 for nucleus pulposus, intervertebral disc, or paravertebral tissue, 62269 for spinal cord)

(For evaluation of fine needle aspirate, see 88172, 88173)

Separate Procedure · Unlisted Procedure · CCI Comp. Code · Non-specific Procedure

This page intentionally left blank.

INTEGUMENTARY SYSTEM

SKIN, SUBCUTANEOUS AND ACCESSORY STRUCTURES

INCISION AND DRAINAGE

(For excision, see 11400, et seq)

10040 Acne surgery (eg, marsupialization, opening or removal of multiple milia, comedones, cysts, pustules)

10060 Incision and drainage of abscess (eg, carbuncle, suppurative hidradenitis, cutaneous or subcutaneous abscess, cyst, furuncle, or paronychia); simple or single

10061 complicated or multiple

10080 Incision and drainage of pilonidal cyst; simple

10081 complicated

(For excision of pilonidal cyst, see 11770-11772)

10120 Incision and removal of foreign body, subcutaneous tissues; simple

10121 complicated

(To report wound exploration due to penetrating trauma without laparotomy or thoracotomy, see 20100-20103, as appropriate)

(To report debridement associated with open fracture(s) and/or dislocation(s), use 11010-11012, as appropriate)

10140 Incision and drainage of hematoma, seroma or fluid collection

(If imaging guidance is performed, see 76942, 77012, 77021)

10160 Puncture aspiration of abscess, hematoma, bulla, or cyst

(If imaging guidance is performed, see 76942, 77012, 77021)

10180 Incision and drainage, complex, postoperative wound infection

(For secondary closure of surgical wound, see 12020, 12021, 13160)

INTEG
10000

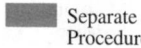 Separate Procedure   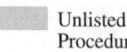 Unlisted Procedure   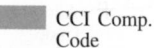 CCI Comp. Code   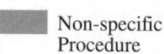 Non-specific Procedure

327

DEBRIDEMENT

Wound debridements (11042-11047) are reported by depth of tissue that is removed and by surface area of the wound. These services may be reported for injuries, infections, wounds and chronic ulcers. When performing debridement of a single wound, report depth using the deepest level of tissue removed. In multiple wounds, sum the surface area of those wounds that are at the same depth, but do not combine sums from different depths. For example: When bone is debrided from a 4 sq cm heel ulcer and from a 10 sq cm ischial ulcer, report the work with a single code, 11044. When subcutaneous tissue is debrided from a 16 sq cm dehisced abdominal wound and a 10 sq cm thigh wound, report the work with 11042 for the first 20 sq cm and 11045 for the second 6 sq cm. If all four wounds were debrided on the same day, use modifier 59 with 11042 or 11044 as appropriate.

(For dermabrasions, see 15780-15783)

(For nail debridement, see 11720-11721)

(For burn(s), see 16000-16035)

(For pressure ulcers, see 15920-15999)

11000   Debridement of extensive eczematous or infected skin; up to 10% of body surface

(For abdominal wall or genitalia debridement for necrotizing soft tissue infection, see 11004-11006)

+ **11001**   each additional 10% of the body surface, or part thereof (List separately in addition to code for primary procedure)

(Use 11001 in conjunction with code 11000)

11004   Debridement of skin, subcutaneous tissue, muscle and fascia for necrotizing soft tissue infection; external genitalia and perineum

11005   abdominal wall, with or without fascial closure

11006   external genitalia, perineum and abdominal wall, with or without fascial closure

(If orchiectomy is performed, use 54520)

(If testicular transplantation is performed, use 54680)

+ **11008**   Removal of prosthetic material or mesh, abdominal wall for infection (eg, for chronic or recurrent mesh infection or necrotizing soft tissue infection) (list separately in addition to code for primary procedure)

(Use 11008 in conjunction with 10180, 11004-11006)

(Do not report 11008 in conjunction with 11000-11001, 11010-11044)

(Report skin grafts or flaps separately when performed for closure at the same session as 11004-11008)

(When insertion of mesh is used for closure, use 49568)

11010 Debridement including removal of foreign material at the site of an open fracture and/or an open dislocation (eg, excisional debridement); skin and subcutaneous tissues

11011 skin, subcutaneous tissue, muscle fascia, and muscle

11012 skin, subcutaneous tissue, muscle fascia, muscle, and bone

(11040 deleted 2010 [2011 edition])

(11041 deleted 2010 [2011 edition])

(For debridement of skin, ie, epidermis and/or dermis only, see 97597, 97598)

(For active wound care management, see 97597, 97598)

(For debridement of burn wounds, see 16020-16030)

11042 Debridement, subcutaneous tissue (includes epidermis and dermis, if performed); first 20 sq cm or less

(For debridement of skin [ie., epidermis and/or dermis only], see 97597, 97598)

+ **11045** each additional 20 sq cm or part thereof (list separately in addition to code for primary procedure)

(Use 11045 in conjunction with 11042)

11043 Debridement, muscle and/or fascia (includes epidermis, dermis, and subcutaneous tissue, if performed); first 20 sq cm or less

+ **11046** each additional 20 sq cm, or part thereof (list separately in addition to code for primary procedure)

(Use 11046 in conjunction with 11043)

329

	Separate Procedure		Unlisted Procedure		CCI Comp. Code		Non-specific Procedure

11044   Debridement, bone (includes epidermis, dermis, subcutaneous tissue, muscle and/or fascia, if performed); first 20 sq cm or less

11045   This code is out of order. See page 329

11046   This code is out of order. See page 329

+ **11047**   each additional 20 sq cm, or part thereof (list separately in addition to code for primray procedure

(Do not report 11042-11047 in conjunction with 97597-97602 for the same wound)

(Use 11047 in conjunction with 11044)

PARING OR CUTTING

(To report destruction, see 17000-17004)

11055   Paring or cutting of benign hyperkeratotic lesion (eg, corn or callus); single lesion

11056   two to four lesions

11057   more than four lesions

BIOPSY

During certain surgical procedures in the integumentary system, such as excision, destruction, or shave removals, the removed tissue is often submitted for pathologic examination. The obtaining of tissue for pathology during the course of these procedures is a routine component of such procedures. This obtaining of tissue is not considered a separate biopsy procedure and is not separately reported. The use of a biopsy procedure code (eg., 11100, 11101) indicates that the procedure to obtain tissue for pathologic examination was performed independently, or was unrelated or distinct from other procedures/services provided at that time. Such biopsies are not considered components of other procedures when performed on different lesions or different sites on the same date, and are to be reported separately.

(For biopsy of conjunctiva, use 68100; eyelid, use 67810)

11100   Biopsy of skin, subcutaneous tissue and/or mucous membrane (including simple closure), unless otherwise listed; single lesion

● New Code   ▲ Revised Code   + Add-On Code   ⊘ Modifier -51 Exempt   ⊙ Moderate Sedation

+ 11101   each separate/additional lesion (List separately in addition to code for primary procedure)

(Use 11101 in conjunction with code 11100)

REMOVAL OF SKIN TAGS

11200   Removal of skin tags, multiple fibrocutaneous tags, any area; up to and including 15 lesions

+ 11201   each additional 10 lesions, or part thereof (List separately in addition to code for primary procedure)

(Use 11201 in conjunction with code 11200)

SHAVING OF EPIDERMAL OR DERMAL LESIONS

Many of the procedure codes listed in the integumentary system subsection of the CPT manual are designated in centimeters or square centimeters. Many physicians document sizes using inches or millimeters. Make sure to verify, and convert if necessary, measurements before assigning a code.

To be able to code lesion removal appropriately, the site, size in centimeters, method of removal and morphology must be documented in the medical record. Always code morphology from the pathology report.

Excision of lesion codes are determined by the diameter of the actual lesion, not the specimen sent to pathology. However, the size of the specimen can be used when the size of the lesion cannot be located in the operative report or elsewhere in the medical record.

When more than one dimension of a lesion is provided in the documentation, select the code based on the largest size. For example, if the dimensions indicated are 3 cm x 2 cm x 1.5 cm, the lesion should be coded as 3 cm. Excision of benign and malignant lesions includes anesthesia and simple repair of the defect site.

Shaving is the sharp removal by transverse incision or horizontal slicing to remove epidermal and dermal lesions without a full-thickness dermal excision. This includes local anesthesia, chemical or electrcauterization ofthe wound. The wound does not require suture closure.

11300   Shaving of epidermal or dermal lesion, single lesion, trunk, arms or legs; lesion diameter 0.5 cm or less

11301   lesion diameter 0.6 to 1.0 cm

11302   lesion diameter 1.1 to 2.0 cm

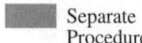 Separate Procedure   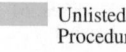 Unlisted Procedure   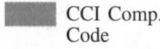 CCI Comp. Code   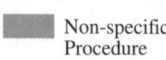 Non-specific Procedure

331

11303	lesion diameter over 2.0 cm
11305	Shaving of epidermal or dermal lesion, single lesion, scalp, neck, hands, feet, genitalia; lesion diameter 0.5 cm or less
11306	lesion diameter 0.6 to 1.0 cm
11307	lesion diameter 1.1 to 2.0 cm
11308	lesion diameter over 2.0 cm
11310	Shaving of epidermal or dermal lesion, single lesion, face, ears, eyelids, nose, lips, mucous membrane; lesion diameter 0.5 cm or less
11311	lesion diameter 0.6 to 1.0 cm
11312	lesion diameter 1.1 to 2.0 cm
11313	lesion diameter over 2.0 cm

EXCISION OF BENIGN LESIONS

Excision (including simple closure) of benign lesions of skin (eg., neoplasm, cicatricial, fibrous, inflammatory, congenital, cystic lesions) includes local anesthesia. See appropriate size and area below. For shave removal, see 11300 et seq., and for electrosurgical and other methods, see 17000 et seq..

Excision is defined as full-thickness (through the dermis) removal of a lesion, inlcuding margins, and includes simple (non-layered) closure when performed. Report separately each benign lesion excised. Code selection is determined by measuring the greatest clinical diameter of the apparent lesion plus that margin required for complete excision (lesion diameter plus the most narrow margins required equals the excised diameter). The margins refer to the most narrow margin required to adequately excise the lesion, based on the individual judgment. The measurement of lesion plus margin is made prior to excision. The excised diameter is the same whether the surgical defect is repaired in a linear fashion, or reconstructed (eg, with a skin graft).

The closure of defects created by incision, excision, or trauma may require intermediate or complex closure. Repair by intermediate or complex closure should be reported separately. For excision of benign lesions requiring more than simple closure, i.e., requiring intermediate or complex closure, report 11400-11446 in addition to appropriate intermediate (12031-12057) or complex closure (13100-13153) codes. For reconstructive closure, see 15002-15261, 15570-15770. For excision performed in conjunction with adjacent tissue transfer, report only the

● New Code   ▲ Revised Code   + Add-On Code   ⊘ Modifier -51 Exempt   ⊙ Moderate Sedation

adjacent tissue transfer code (14000-14302). Excision of lesion (11400-11446) is not separately reportable with adjacent tissue transfer.

11400 Excision, benign lesion including margins, except skin tag (unless listed elsewhere), trunk, arms or legs; excised diameter 0.5 cm or less

11401 excised diameter 0.6 to 1.0 cm

11402 excised diameter 1.1 to 2.0 cm

11403 excised diameter 2.1 to 3.0 cm

11404 excised diameter 3.1 to 4.0 cm

11406 excised diameter over 4.0 cm

(For unusual or complicated excision, add modifier -22)

11420 Excision, benign lesion including margins, except skin tag (unless listed elsewhere), scalp, neck, hands, feet, genitalia; excised diameter 0.5 cm or less

11421 excised diameter 0.6 to 1.0 cm

11422 excised diameter 1.1 to 2.0 cm

11423 excised diameter 2.1 to 3.0 cm

11424 excised diameter 3.1 to 4.0 cm

11426 excised diameter over 4.0 cm

(For unusual or complicated excision, add modifier -22)

11440 Excision, other benign lesion including margins (unless listed elsewhere), face, ears, eyelids, nose, lips, mucous membrane; excised diameter 0.5 cm or less

11441 excised diameter 0.6 to 1.0 cm

11442 excised diameter 1.1 to 2.0 cm

11443 excised diameter 2.1 to 3.0 cm

11444 excised diameter 3.1 to 4.0 cm

	Separate Procedure		Unlisted Procedure		CCI Comp. Code		Non-specific Procedure

333

11446   excised diameter over 4.0 cm

(For unusual or complicated excision, add modifier -22)

(For eyelids involving more than skin, see also 67800 et seq.)

11450 Excision of skin and subcutaneous tissue for hidradenitis, axillary; with simple or intermediate repair

11451   with complex repair

11462 Excision of skin and subcutaneous tissue for hidradenitis, inguinal; with simple or intermediate repair

11463   with complex repair

11470 Excision of skin and subcutaneous tissue for hidradenitis, perianal, perineal, or umbilical; with simple or intermediate repair

11471   with complex repair

(When skin graft or flap is used for closure, use appropriate procedure code in addition)

(For bilateral procedure, add modifier -50)

EXCISION OF MALIGNANT LESIONS

Excision (including simple closure) of malignant lesions of skin (eg., basal cell carcinoma, squamous cell carcinoma, melanoma) includes local anesthesia. (See appropriate size and body area below.) For destruction of malignant lesions of skin, see destruction codes 17260-17286.

The closure of defects created by incision, excision, or trauma may require intermediate or complex closure. Repair by intermediate or complex closure should be reported separately. For excision of malignant lesions requiring more than simple closure, i.e., requiring intermediate or complex closure, report 11600-11646 in addition to appropriate intermediate (12031-12057) or complex closure (13100-13153) codes. For reconstructive closure, see 15002-15261, 15570-15770. For excision performed in conjunction with adjacent tissue transfer, report only the adjacent tissue transfer code (14000-14302). Excision of lesion (11600-11646) is not separately reportable with adjacent tissue transfer.

To report a subsequent operative session, see codes 11600-11646, as appropriate. Append modifier 58 if the re-excision procedure is performed during the postoperative period of the primary excision procedure.

| 11600 | Excision, malignant lesion including margins, trunk, arms, or legs; excised diameter 0.5 cm or less |

| 11601 | excised diameter 0.6 to 1.0 cm |

| 11602 | excised diameter 1.1 to 2.0 cm |

| 11603 | excised diameter 2.1 to 3.0 cm |

| 11604 | excised diameter 3.1 to 4.0 cm |

| 11606 | excised diameter over 4.0 cm |

| 11620 | Excision, malignant lesion including margins, scalp, neck, hands, feet, genitalia; excised diameter 0.5 cm or less |

| 11621 | excised diameter 0.6 to 1.0 cm |

| 11622 | excised diameter 1.1 to 2.0 cm |

| 11623 | excised diameter 2.1 to 3.0 cm |

| 11624 | excised diameter 3.1 to 4.0 cm |

| 11626 | excised diameter over 4.0 cm |

| 11640 | Excision, malignant lesion including margins, face, ears, eyelids, nose, lips; excised diameter 0.5 cm or less |

| 11641 | excised diameter 0.6 to 1.0 cm |

| 11642 | excised diameter 1.1 to 2.0 cm |

| 11643 | excised diameter 2.1 to 3.0 cm |

| 11644 | excised diameter 3.1 to 4.0 cm |

| 11646 | excised diameter over 4.0 cm |

(For eyelids involving more than skin, see also 67800 et seq)

NAILS

(For drainage of paronychia or onychia, see 10060, 10061)

| 11719 | Trimming of nondystrophic nails, any number |

Separate Procedure / Unlisted Procedure / CCI Comp. Code / Non-specific Procedure

335

11720	Debridement of nail(s) by any method(s); 1 to 5
11721	6 or more
11730	Avulsion of nail plate, partial or complete, simple; single
+ 11732	each additional nail plate (List separately in addition to code for primary procedure)

(Use 11732 in conjunction with code 11730)

11740	Evacuation of subungual hematoma
11750	Excision of nail and nail matrix, partial or complete, (eg, ingrown or deformed nail) for permanent removal;
11752	with amputation of tuft of distal phalanx

(For skin graft, if used, use 15050)

11755	Biopsy of nail unit (eg, plate, bed, matrix, hyponychium, proximal and lateral nail folds) (separate procedure)
11760	Repair of nail bed
11762	Reconstruction of nail bed with graft
11765	Wedge excision of skin of nail fold (eg, for ingrown toenail)

PILONIDAL CYST

11770	Excision of pilonidal cyst or sinus; simple
11771	extensive
11772	complicated

(For incision of pilonidal cyst, see 10080, 10081)

INTRODUCTION

11900	Injection, intralesional; up to and including seven lesions
11901	more than seven lesions

(11900, 11901 are not to be used for preoperative local anesthetic injection)

336

● New Code	▲ Revised Code	+ Add-On Code	⊘ Modifier -51 Exempt	⊙ Moderate Sedation

(For veins, see 36470, 36471)

(For intralesional chemotherapy administration, see 96405, 96406)

11920 Tattooing, intradermal introduction of insoluble opaque pigments to correct color defects of skin, including micropigmentation; 6.0 sq cm or less

11921 6.1 to 20.0 sq cm

+ 11922 each additional 20.0 sq cm or part thereof (List separately in addition to code for primary procedure)

(Use 11922 in conjunction with code 11921)

11950 Subcutaneous injection of filling material (eg, collagen); 1 cc or less

11951 1.1 to 5.0 cc

11952 5.1 to 10.0 cc

11954 over 10.0 cc

11960 Insertion of tissue expander(s) for other than breast, including subsequent expansion

(For breast reconstruction with tissue expander(s), use 19357)

11970 Replacement of tissue expander with permanent prosthesis

11971 Removal of tissue expander(s) without insertion of prosthesis

(11975 deleted 2011 [2012 edition]. Te report insertion of non-biodegradable drug delivery implant for contraception, use 11981)

11976 Removal, implantable contraceptive capsules

(11977 deleted 2011 [2012 edition]. To report removal of implantable contraceptive capsules with subsequent insertion of non-biodegradable drug delivery implant, use 11976 and 11981)

11980 Subcutaneous hormone pellet implantation (implantation of estradiol and/or testosterone pellets beneath the skin)

	Separate Procedure		Unlisted Procedure		CCI Comp. Code		Non-specific Procedure

| 11981 | Insertion, non-biodegradable drug delivery implant |

| 11982 | Removal, non-biodegradable drug delivery implant |

| 11983 | Removal with reinsertion, non-biodegradable drug delivery implant |

REPAIR (CLOSURE)

To be able to code wound repair appropriately, the site, length of wound in centimeters and type of repair must be documented in the medical record. Review the definitions of simple, intermediate and complex repair in the current CPT coding system.

Use the codes in this section to designate wound closure utilizing sutures, staples, or tissue adhesives (eg., 2-cyanoacrylate), either singly or in combination with each other, or in combination with adhesive strips. Wound closure utilizing adhesive strips as the sole repair material should be coded using the appropriate E/M code.

Definitions

Simple repair is used when the wound is superficial, eg., involving primarily epidermis or dermis, or subcutaneous tissues without significant involvement of deeper structures, and requires simple one layer closure. This includes local anesthesia and chemical or electrocauterization of wounds not closed.

Intermediate repair includes the repair of wounds that, in addition to the above, require layered closure of one or more of the deeper layers of subcutaneous tissue and superficial (non-muscle) fascia, in addition to the skin (epidermal and dermal) closure. Single-layer closure of heavily contaminated wounds that have required extensive cleaning or removal of particulate matter also constitutes intermediate repair.

Complex repair includes the repair of wounds requiring more than layered closure, viz., scar revision, debridement (eg., traumatic lacerations or avulsions), extensive undermining, stents or retention sutures. Necessary preparation includes creation of a limited defect for repairs or the debridement of complicated lacerations or avulsions. Complex repair does not include excision of benign (11400-11446) or malignant (11600-11646) lesions, excisional preparation of a wound bed (15002-15005) or debridement of an open fracture or open dislocation.

Instuctions for listing services at time of wound repair:

1. The repaired wound(s) should be measured and recorded in centimeters, whether curved, angular or stellate.

2. When multiple wounds are repaired, add together the lengths of those in the same classification (see above) and from all anatomic sites that are grouped

● New Code   ▲ Revised Code   + Add-On Code   ⊘ Modifier -51 Exempt   ⊙ Moderate Sedation

together into the same code descriptor. For example, add together the lengths of intermediate repairs to the trunk and extremities Do not add lengths of repairs from different groupings of anatomic sites (eg, face and extremities). Also, do not add together lengths of different classifications (eg, intermediate and complex repairs).

When more than one classification of wounds is repaired, list the more complicated as the primary procedure and the less complicated as the secondary procedure, using modifier 59.

3. Decontamination and/or debridement: Debridement is considered a separate procedure only when gross contamination requires prolonged cleansing, when appreciable amounts of devitalized or contaminated tissue are removed, or when debridement is carried out separately without immediate primary closure.

> (For extensive debridement of soft tissue and/or bone, not associated with open fracture(s) and/or dislocation(s) resulting from penetrating and/or blunt trauma, see 11042-11047.)

> (For extensive debridement of subcutaneous tissue, muscle fascia, muscle, and/or bone associated with open fracture(s) and/or dislocation(s), see 11010-11012.)

4. Involvement of nerves, blood vessels and tendons: Report under appropriate system (Nervous, Cardiovascular, Musculoskeletal) for repair of these structures. The repair of these associated wounds is included in the primary procedure unless it qualifies as a complex repair, in which case modifier 59 applies.

Simple ligation of vessels in an open wound is considered as part of any wound closure.

Simple "exploration" of nerves, blood vessels, or tendons exposed in an open wound is also considered part of the essential treatment of the wound and is not a separate procedure unless appreciable dissection is required. If the wound requires enlargement, extension of dissection (to determine penetration), debridement, removal of foreign body(s), ligation or coagulation of minor subcutaneous and/or muscular blood vessel(s) of the subcutaneous tissue, muscle fascia, and/or muscle, not requiring thoracotomy or laparotomy, use codes 20100-20103, as appropriate.

REPAIR — SIMPLE

Sum of lengths of repairs for each group of anatomic sites.

12001   Simple repair of superficial wounds of scalp, neck, axillae, external genitalia, trunk and/or extremities (including hands and feet); 2.5 cm or less

12002   2.6 cm to 7.5 cm

12004   7.6 cm to 12.5 cm

	Separate Procedure		Unlisted Procedure		CCI Comp. Code		Non-specific Procedure	**339**

12005	12.6 cm to 20.0 cm
12006	20.1 cm to 30.0 cm
12007	over 30.0 cm
12011	Simple repair of superficial wounds of face, ears, eyelids, nose, lips and/or mucous membranes; 2.5 cm or less
12013	2.6 cm to 5.0 cm
12014	5.1 cm to 7.5 cm
12015	7.6 cm to 12.5 cm
12016	12.6 cm to 20.0 cm
12017	20.1 cm to 30.0 cm
12018	over 30.0 cm
12020	Treatment of superficial wound dehiscence; simple closure
12021	with packing

(For extensive or complicated secondary wound closure, use 13160)

REPAIR — INTERMEDIATE

Sum of lengths of repairs for each group of anatomic sites.

12031	Repair, intermediate of wounds of scalp, axillae, trunk and/or extremities (excluding hands and feet); 2.5 cm or less
12032	2.6 cm to 7.5 cm
12034	7.6 cm to 12.5 cm
12035	12.6 cm to 20.0 cm
12036	20.1 cm to 30.0 cm
12037	over 30.0 cm

● New Code   ▲ Revised Code   + Add-On Code   ⊘ Modifier -51 Exempt   ⊙ Moderate Sedation

12041 Repair, intermediate wounds of neck, hands, feet and/or external genitalia; 2.5 cm or less

12042 2.6 cm to 7.5 cm

12044 7.6 cm to 12.5 cm

12045 12.6 cm to 20.0 cm

12046 20.1 cm to 30.0 cm

12047 over 30.0 cm

12051 Repair, intermediate wounds of face, ears, eyelids, nose, lips and/or mucous membranes; 2.5 cm or less

12052 2.6 cm to 5.0 cm

12053 5.1 cm to 7.5 cm

12054 7.6 cm to 12.5 cm

12055 12.6 cm to 20.0 cm

12056 20.1 cm to 30.0 cm

12057 over 30.0 cm

REPAIR — COMPLEX

Reconstructive procedures, complicated wound closure. Sum of lengths of repairs for each group of anatomic sites.

(For full thickness repair of lip or eyelid, see respective anatomical subsections)

13100 Repair, complex, trunk; 1.1 cm to 2.5 cm

(For 1.0 cm or less, see simple or intermediate repairs)

13101 2.6 cm to 7.5 cm

+ **13102** each additional 5 cm or less (List separately in addition to code for primary procedure)

(Use 13102 in conjunction with code 13101)

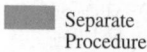 Separate Procedure

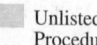 Unlisted Procedure

CCI Comp. Code

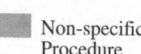 Non-specific Procedure

341

13120   Repair, complex, scalp, arms, and/or legs; 1.1 cm to 2.5 cm

(For 1.0 cm or less, see simple or intermediate repairs)

13121   2.6 cm to 7.5 cm

+ **13122**   each additional 5 cm or less (List separately in addition to code for primary procedure)

(Use 13122 in conjunction with 13121)

13131   Repair, complex, forehead, cheeks, chin, mouth, neck, axillae, genitalia, hands and/or feet; 1.1 cm to 2.5 cm

(For 1.0 cm or less, see simple or intermediate repairs)

13132   2.6 cm to 7.5 cm

+ **13133**   each additional 5 cm or less (List separately in addition to code for primary procedure)

(Use 13133 in conjunction with 13132)

13150   Repair, complex, eyelids, nose, ears and/or lips; 1.0 cm or less

(See also 40650-40654, 67961-67975)

13151   1.1 cm to 2.5 cm

13152   2.6 cm to 7.5 cm

+ **13153**   each additional 5 cm or less (List separately in addition to code for primary procedure)

(Use 13153 in conjunction with code 13152)

13160   Secondary closure of surgical wound or dehiscence, extensive or complicated

(For packing or simple secondary wound closure, see 12020, 12021)

ADJACENT TISSUE TRANSFER OR REARRANGEMENT

For full-thickness repair of lip or eyelid, see respective anatomical subsections.

Codes 14000-14302 are used for excision (including lesion) and/or repair by adjacent tissue transfer or rearrangement (eg., Z-plasty, W-plasty, V-Y plasty, rotation flap, random island flap, advancement flap). When applied in repairing

342   ● New Code   ▲ Revised Code   + Add-On Code   ⊘ Modifier -51 Exempt   ⊙ Moderate Sedation

lacerations, the procedures listed must be performed by the surgeon to accomplish the repair. They do not apply to direct closure or rearrangement of traumatic wounds incidentally resulting in these configurations. Undermining alone of adjacent tissues to achieve closure, without additional incisions, does not constitute adjacent tissue transfer. See complex repair codes 13100-13160. The excision of a benign lesion (11400-11446) or a malignant lesion (11600-11646) is not separately reportable with codes 14000-14302.

Skin graft necessary to close secondary defect is considered an additional procedure. For purposes of code selection, the term "defect" includes the primary and secondary defects. The primary defect resulting from the excision and the secondary defect resulting from flap design to perform the reconstruction are measured together to determine the code.

14000 Adjacent tissue transfer or rearrangement, trunk; defect 10 sq cm or less

14001 defect 10.1 sq cm to 30.0 sq cm

14020 Adjacent tissue transfer or rearrangement, scalp, arms and/or legs; defect 10 sq cm or less

14021 defect 10.1 sq cm to 30.0 sq cm

14040 Adjacent tissue transfer or rearrangement, forehead, cheeks, chin, mouth, neck, axillae, genitalia, hands and/or feet; defect 10 sq cm or less

14041 defect 10.1 sq cm to 30.0 sq cm

14060 Adjacent tissue transfer or rearrangement, eyelids, nose, ears and/or lips; defect 10 sq cm or less

14061 defect 10.1 sq cm to 30.0 sq cm

(For eyelid, full thickness, see 67961 et seq)

(14300 Deleted 2009 [2010 edition]; use 14301, 14302)

14301 Adjacent tissue transfer or rearrangement, any area; defect 30.1 sq cm to 60.0 sq cm

+ **14302** each additional 30.0 sq cm, or part thereof (List separately in addition to code for primary procedure)

(Use 14302 in conjunction with 14301)

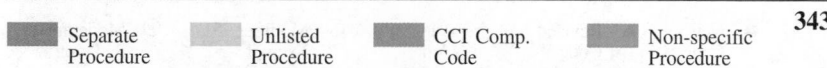

Separate Procedure	Unlisted Procedure	CCI Comp. Code	Non-specific Procedure

343

14350   Filleted finger or toe flap, including preparation of recipient site

SKIN REPLACEMENT SURGERY

Skin replacement surgery consists of surgical preparation and topical placement of an autograft (including tissue cultured autograft) or skin substitute graft (ie, homograft, allograft, xenograft). The graft is anchored using the individual's choice of fixation. When services are performed in the office, routine dressing supplies are not reported separately.

The following definition should be applied to those codes that reference "100 sq cm or 1% of body area of infants and children" when determining the involvement of body size: The measurement of 100 sq cm is applicable to adults and children 10 years of age and older; and percentages of body surface area apply to infants and children younger than 10 years of age. The measurements apply to the size of the recipient area.

Procedures involving wrist and/or ankle are reported with codes that include arm or leg in the descriptor.

When a primary procedure requires a skin substitute or skin autograft for definitive skin closure (eg, orbitectomy, radical mastectomy, or deep tumor removal) use 15100-15278 in conjunction with primary procedure.

For biological implant for soft tissue reinforcement, use 15777 in conjunction with primary procedure.

The supply of skin substitute graft(s) should be reported separately in conjunction with 15271-15278.

Definitions

Surgical preparation codes 15002-15005 for skin replacement surgery describe the initial services related to preparing a clean and viable wound surface for placement of an autograft, flap, skin substitute graft or for negatie pressure wound therapy. In come cases, closure may be possible using adjacent tissue transfer (14000-14061) or complex repair (13100-13153). In add cases, appreciable nonviable tissue is removed to treat a burn, traumatic wound or a necrotizing infection. The clean wound bed may also be created by incisional release of a scar contracture resulting in a surface defect from separation of tissues. The intent is to heal the wound by primary intention, or by the use of negative pressure wound therapy. Patient conditions may require the closure or application of graft, flap, or skin substitute to be delayed, but in all cases the intent is to include these treatments or negative pressure wound therapy to heal the wound. Do not report 15002-15005 for removal of nonviable tissue/debris in a chronic wound (eg, venous or diabetic) when the wound is left to heal by secondary intention. See active wound management codes (97597, 97598) and debridement codes (11042-11047) for this service. For necrotizing soft tissue infections in specific anatomic locations, see 11004-11008.

Select the appropriate code from 15002-15005 based upon location and size of the resultant defect. For multiple wounds, sum the surface area of all wounds from all anatomic sites that are grouped together into the same code descriptor. For example, sum the surface area of all wounds on the trunk and arms. Do not sum wounds from different groupings of anatomic sites (eg, face and arms). Use 15002 or 15004, as appropriate, for excisions and incisional releases resulting in wounds up to and including 100 sq cm of surface area. Use 15003 or 15005 for each additional 100 sq cm or part thereof.

Autografts/tissue cultured autografts include the harvest and or application of an autologous skin graft. Repair of donor site requiring skin graft or local flaps is reported separately. Removal of current graft and/or simple cleansing of the wound is included, when performed. Do not report 97602. Debridement is considered a separate procedure only when gross contamination requires prolonged cleansing, when appreciable amounts of devialized or contaminated tissue ar removed, or when debridement is carried out separately without immediate primary closure.

Selecte the appropriate code from 15040-15261 based upon type of autograft and location and size of the defect. The measurements apply to the size of the recipient area. For multiple wounds, sum teh surface area of all wounds from all anatomic sites that are grouped together into the same code descriptor.

Skin substitute grafts include non-autologous human skin (dermal or epidermal, cellular and acellular) grafts (eg, homograft, allograft), non human skin substitute grafts (ie, xenograft), and biological products that form a sheet scaffolding for skin growth. These codes are not to be reported for application of non-graft wound dressings (eg, gel, ointment, foam, liquid) or injected skin substitutes. Removal of current graft and/or simple cleansing of the wound is included, when performed. Do not report 97602. Debridement is considered a separate procedure only when gross contamination requires prolonged cleansing, when appreciable amounts of devitalized or contaminated tissue are removed, or when debridement is carried out separately without immediate primary closure.

Select the appropriate code from 15271-15278 based upon location and size of the defect. For multiple wounds, sum the surface area of all wounds from all anatomic sites that are grouped together into the same code descriptor.

Surgical Preparation

15002   Surgical preparation or creation of recipient site by excision of open wounds, burn eschar, or scar (including subcutaneous tissues), or incisional release of scar contracture, trunk, arms, legs; first 100 sq cm or 1% of body area of infants and children

(For linear scar revision, see 13100-13153)

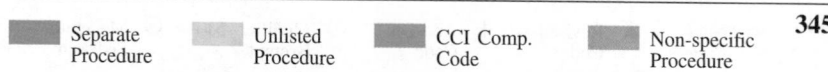

Separate Procedure	Unlisted Procedure	CCI Comp. Code

Non-specific Procedure

345

+ 15003 each additional 100 sq cm, or part thereof, or each additional 1% of body area of infants and children (List separately in addition to code for primary procedure)

(Use 15003 in conjunction with 15002)

15004 Surgical preparation or creation of recipient site by excision of open wounds, burn eschar, or scar (including subcutaneous tissues), or incisional release of scar contracture, face, scalp, eyelids, mouth, neck, ears, orbits, genitalia, hands, feet and/or multiple digits; 1500405 first 100 sq cm or 1% of body area of infants and children

+ 15005 each additional 100 sq cm or part thereof, or each additional 1% of body area of infants and children (List separately in addition to code for primary procedure)

(Use 15005 in conjunction with 15004)

Autografts/Tissue Cultured Autograft

15040 Harvest of skin for tissue cultured skin autograft, 100 sq cm or less

15050 Pinch graft, single or multiple, to cover small ulcer, tip of digit, or other minimal open area (except on face), up to defect size 2 cm diameter

15100 Split-thickness autograft, trunk, arms, legs; first 100 sq cm or less, or one percent of body area of infants and children (except 15050)

+ 15101 each additional 100 sq cm, or each additional one percent of body area of infants and children, or part thereof (List separately in addition to code for primary procedure)

(Use 15101 in conjunction with code 15100)

15110 Epidermal autograft, trunk, arms, legs; first 100 sq cm or less, or one percent of body area of infants and children

+ 15111 each additional 100 sq cm, or each additional one percent of body area of infants and children, or part thereof (List separately in addition to code for primary procedure)

(Use 15111 in conjunction with 15110)

● New Code ▲ Revised Code + Add-On Code ⊘ Modifier -51 Exempt ⊙ Moderate Sedation

15115 Epidermal autograft, face, scalp, eyelids, mouth, neck, ears, orbits, genitalia, hands, feet, and/or multiple digits; first 100 sq cm or less, or one percent of body area of infants and children

+ **15116** each additional 100 sq cm, or each additional one percent of body area of infants and children, or part thereof (List separately in addition to code for primary procedure)

(Use 15116 in conjunction with 15115)

15120 Split-thickness autograft, face, scalp, eyelids, mouth, neck, ears, orbits, genitalia, hands, feet, and/or multiple digits; first 100 sq cm or less, or one percent of body area of infants and children (except 15050)

+ **15121** each additional 100 sq cm, or each additional one percent of body area of infants and children, or part thereof (List separately in addition to code for primary procedure)

(Use 15121 in conjunction with code 15120)

(For eyelids, see also 67961-67975)

15130 Dermal autograft, trunk, arms, legs; first 100 sq cm or less, or one percent of body area of infants and children

+ **15131** each additional 100 sq cm, or each additional one percent of body area of infants and children, or part thereof (List separately in addition to code for primary procedure)

(Use 15131 in conjunction with 15130)

15135 Dermal autograft, face, scalp, eyelids, mouth, neck, ears, orbits, genitalia, hands, feet, and/or multiple digits; first 100 sq cm or less, or one percent of body area of infants and children

+ **15136** each additional 100 sq cm, or each additional one percent of body area of infants and children, or part thereof (List separately in addition to code for primary procedure)

(Use 15136 in conjunction with 15135)

15150 Tissue cultured skin autograft, trunk, arms, legs; first 25 sq cm or less

+ **15151** additional 1 sq cm to 75 sq cm (List separately in addition to code for primary procedure)

(Do not report 15151 more than once per session)

347

 Separate Procedure   Unlisted Procedure   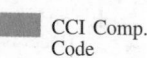 CCI Comp. Code   Non-specific Procedure

(Use 15151 in conjunction with 15150)

+ 15152   each additional 100 sq cm, or each additional 1% of body area of infants and children, or part thereof (List separately in addition to code for primary procedure)

(Use 15152 in conjunction with 15151)

15155   Tissue cultured skin autograft, face, scalp, eyelids, mouth, neck, ears, orbits, genitalia, hands, feet, and/or multiple digits; first 25 sq cm or less

+ 15156   additional 1 sq cm to 75 sq cm (List separately in addition to code for primary procedure)

(Do not report 15156 more than once per session)

(Use 15156 in conjunction with 15155)

+ 15157   each additional 100 sq cm, or each additional 1% of body area of infants and children, or part thereof (List separately in addition to code for primary procedure)

(Use 15157 in conjunction with 15156)

(15170   deleted 2011 [2012 edition]. To report, see 15271-15278)

(15171   deleted 2011 [2012 edition]. To report, see 15271-15278)

(15175   deleted 2011 [2012 edition]. To report, see 15271-15278)

(15176   deleted 2011 [2012 edition]. To report, see 15271-15278)

15200   Full thickness graft, free, including direct closure of donor site, trunk; 20 sq cm or less

+ 15201   each additional 20 sq cm or part thereof (List separately in addition to code for primary procedure)

(Use 15201 in conjunction with 15200)

15220   Full thickness graft, free, including direct closure of donor site, scalp, arms, and/or legs; 20 sq cm or less

+ 15221   each additional 20 sq cm or part thereof (List separately in addition to code for primary procedure)

(Use 15221 in conjunction with 15220)

15240 Full thickness graft, free, including direct closure of donor site, forehead, cheeks, chin, mouth, neck, axillae, genitalia, hands, and/or feet; 20 sq cm or less

(For finger tip graft, use 15050)

(For repair of syndactyly, fingers, see 26560-26562)

+ 15241 each additional 20 sq cm or part thereof (List separately in addition to code for primary procedure)

(Use 15241 in conjunction with code 15240)

15260 Full thickness graft, free, including direct closure of donor site, nose, ears, eyelids, and/or lips; 20 sq cm or less

+ 15261 each additional 20 sq cm or part thereof (List separately in addition to code for primary procedure)

(Use 15261 in conjunction with code 15260)

(For eyelids, see also 67961-67975)

(Repair of donor site requiring skin graft or local flaps is considered a separate procedure)

Skin Substitute Grafts

The supply of skin substitute graft(s) should be reported separately in conjunction with 15271-15278. For biologic implant for soft tissue reinforcement, use 15777 in conjunction with code for primary procedure.

15271 Application of skin substitute graft to trunk, arms, legs, total wound surface area up to 100 sq cm; first 25 sq cm or less wound surface area

+ 15272 each additional 25 sq cm wound surface area, or part thereof (List separately in addition to code for primary procedure)

(Use 15272 in conjunction with 15271)

(For total wound surface area greater than or equal to 100 sq cm, see 15273, 15274)

(Do not report 15271, 15272 in conjunction with 15273, 15274)

15273 Application of skin substitute graft to trunk, arms, legs, total wound surface area greater than or equal to 100 sq cm; first 100 sq cm wound surface area, or 1% of body area of infants and children

349

| | Separate Procedure | | Unlisted Procedure | | CCI Comp. Code | | Non-specific Procedure |

+ 15274   each additional 100 sq cm wound surface area, or part thereof, or each additional 1% of body area of infants and children, or part thereof (List separately in addition to code for primary procedure)

(Use 15274 in conjunction with 15273)

(For total wound surface area up to 100 sq cm, see 15271, 15272)

15275   Application of skin substitute graft to face, scalp, eyelids, mouth, neck, ears, orbits, genitalia, hands, feet, and/or multiple digits, total wound surface area up to 100 sq cm; first 25 sq cm or less wound surface area

+ 15276   each additional 25 sq cm wound surface area, or part thereof (List separately in addition to code for primary procedure)

(Use 15276 in conjunction with 15275)

(For total wound surface area greater than or equal to 100 sq cm, see 15277, 15278)

(Do not report 15275, 15276 in conjunction with 15277, 15278)

15277   Application of skin substitute graft to face, scalp, eyelids, mouth, neck, ears, orbits, genitalia, hands, feet, and/or multiple digits, total wound surface area greater than or equal to 100 sq cm; first 100 sq cm wound surface area, or 1% of body area of infants and children

+ 15278   each additional 100 sq cm wound surface area, or part thereof, or each additional 1% of body area of infants and children, or part thereof (List separately in addition to code for primary procedure)

(Use 15278 in conjunction with 15277)

(For total wound surface area up to 100 sq cm, see 15275, 15276)

(Do not report 15271-15278 in conjunction with 97602)

(15300   deleted 2011 [2012 edition]. To report, see 15271-15274)

(15301   deleted 2011 [2012 edition]. To report, see 15271-15274)

(15320   deleted 2011 [2012 edition]. To report, see 15275-15278)

(15321   deleted 2011 [2012 edition]. To report, see 15275-15278)

(15330   deleted 2011 [2012 edition]. To report, see 15271-15274)

(15331   deleted 2011 [2012 edition]. To report, see 15271-15274)

(15335   deleted 2011 [2012 edition]. To report, see 15275-15278)

(15336   deleted 2011 [2012 edition]. To report, see 15275-15278)

(15340   deleted 2011 [2012 edition]. To report, see 15271-15278)

(15341   deleted 2011 [2012 edition]. To report, see 15271-15278)

(15360   deleted 2011 [2012 edition]. To report, see 15271-15274)

(15361   deleted 2011 [2012 edition]. To report, see 15271-15274)

(15365   deleted 2011 [2012 edition]. To report, see 15275-15278)

(15366   deleted 2011 [2012 edition]. To report, see 15275-15278)

(15400   deleted 2011 [2012 edition]. To report, see 15271-15274)

(15401   deleted 2011 [2012 edition]. To report, see 15271-15274)

(15420   deleted 2011 [2012 edition]. To report, see 15275-15278)

(15421   deleted 2011 [2012 edition]. To report, see 15275-15278)

(15430   deleted 2011 [2012 edition]. To report, see 15271-15278)

(15431   deleted 2011 [2012 edition]. To report, see 15271-15278)

FLAPS (SKIN AND/OR DEEP TISSUES)

Codes 15732-15738 are described by donor site of the muscle, myocutaneous, or fasciocutaneous flap.

Codes 15570-15738 do not include extensive immobilization (eg., large plaster casts and other immobilizing devices are considered additional separate procedures).

A repair of a donor site requiring a skin graft or local flaps is considered an additional separate procedure.

351

| Separate Procedure | Unlisted Procedure | CCI Comp. Code | Non-specific Procedure |

(For microvascular flaps, see 15756-15758)

(For flaps without inclusion of a vascular pedicle, see 15570-15576)

(For adjacent tissue transfer flaps, see 14000-14302)

15570 Formation of direct or tubed pedicle, with or without transfer; trunk

15572 scalp, arms, or legs

15574 forehead, cheeks, chin, mouth, neck, axillae, genitalia, hands or feet

15576 eyelids, nose, ears, lips, or intraoral

15600 Delay of flap or sectioning of flap (division and inset); at trunk

15610 at scalp, arms, or legs

15620 at forehead, cheeks, chin, neck, axillae, genitalia, hands, or feet

15630 at eyelids, nose, ears, or lips

15650 Transfer, intermediate, of any pedicle flap (eg, abdomen to wrist, Walking tube), any location

(For eyelids, nose, ears, or lips, see also anatomical area)

(For revision, defatting or rearranging of transferred pedicle flap or skin graft, see 13100-14302)

15731 Forehead flap with preservation of vascular pedicle (eg, axial pattern flap, paramedian forehead flap)

(For muscle, myocutaneous, or fasciocutaneous flap of the head or neck, see 15732)

15732 Muscle, myocutaneous, or fasciocutaneous flap; head and neck (eg, temporalis, masseter muscle, sternocleidomastoid, levator scapulae)

(For forehead flap with preservation of vascular pedicle, use 15731)

15734 trunk

15736   upper extremity

15738   lower extremity

OTHER FLAPS AND GRAFTS

Code 15740 describes a cutaneous flap, transposed into a nearby but not immediately adjacent defect, with a pedicle that incorporates an anatomically named axial vessel into its design. The flap is typically transferred through a tunnel underneath the skin and sutured into its new position. The donor site is closed directly.

Neurovascular pedicle procedures are reported with 15750. This code includes not only skin but also a functional motor or sensory nerve(s). The flap serves to reinnervate a damaged portion of the body dependent on touch or movement (eg, thumb).

Repair of donor site requiring skin graft or local flaps should be reported as an additional procedure.

For random island flaps, V-Y subcutaneous flaps, advancement flaps, and other flaps from adjacent areas without clearly defined anatomically named axial vessels, see 14000-14302.

▲ **15740**   Flap; island pedicle requiring identification and dissection of an anatomically named axial vessel

15750   neurovascular pedicle

15756   Free muscle or myocutaneous flap with microvascular anastomosis

          (Do not report code 69990 in addition to code 15756)

15757   Free skin flap with microvascular anastomosis

          (Do not report code 69990 in addition to code 15757)

15758   Free fascial flap with microvascular anastomosis

          (Do not report code 69990 in addition to code 15758)

15760   Graft; composite (eg, full thickness of external ear or nasal ala), including primary closure, donor area

15770   derma-fat-fascia

15775   Punch graft for hair transplant; 1 to 15 punch grafts

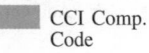

	Separate Procedure		Unlisted Procedure		CCI Comp. Code		Non-specific Procedure

353

15776   more than 15 punch grafts

            (For strip transplant, use 15220)

+ 15777   Implantation of biologic implant (eg, acellular dermal matrix)
          for soft tissue reinforcement (eg, breast, trunk) (List separately
          in addition to code for primary procedure)

          (For bilateral breast procedure, report 15777 with modifier 50)

          (For implantation of mesh or other prosthesis for open
          incisional or ventral hernia repair, use 49568 in conjunction
          with 49560-49566)

          (For insertion of mesh or other prosthesis for closure of a
          necrotizing soft tissue infectino wound, use 49568 in
          conjunction with 11004-11006)

          (For topical application of skin substitute graft to a wound
          surface, see 15271-15278)

          (For repair of anorectal fistula with plug (eg, porcine small
          intestine submucosa [SIS]), use 46707)

          (For insertion of mesh or other prosthesis for repair of pelvic
          floor defect, use 57267)

          (The supply of biologic implant should be reported separately
          in conjunction with 15777)

OTHER PROCEDURES

15780   Dermabrasion; total face (eg, for acne scarring, fine wrinkling,
         rhytids, general keratosis)

15781   segmental, face

15782   regional, other than face

15783   superficial, any site, (eg, tattoo removal)

15786   Abrasion; single lesion (eg, keratosis, scar)

+ 15787   each additional 4 lesions or less (List separately in addition
            to code for primary procedure)

            (Use 15787 in conjunction with code 15786)

15788   Chemical peel, facial; epidermal

● New   ▲ Revised   + Add-On   ⊘ Modifier -51   ⊙ Moderate
        Code   Code   Code   Exempt   Sedation

15789   dermal

15792   Chemical peel, nonfacial; epidermal

15793   dermal

15819   Cervicoplasty

15820   Blepharoplasty, lower eyelid;

15821   with extensive herniated fat pad

15822   Blepharoplasty, upper eyelid;

15823   with excessive skin weighting down lid

    (For bilateral blepharoplasty, add modifier -50)

15824   Rhytidectomy; forehead

    (For repair of brow ptosis, use 67900)

15825   neck with platysmal tightening (platysmal flap, P-flap)

15826   glabellar frown lines

15828   cheek, chin, and neck

15829   superficial musculoaponeurotic system (SMAS) flap

    (For bilateral rhytidectomy, add modifier -50)

15830   Excision, excessive skin and subcutaneous tissue (includes lipectomy); abdomen, infraumbilical panniculectomy

    (Do not report 15830 in conjunction wtih 12031, 12032, 12034, 12035, 12036, 12037, 13100, 13101, 13102, 14000-14001, 14302)

15832   thigh

15833   leg

15834   hip

15835   buttock

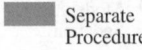 Separate Procedure   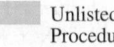 Unlisted Procedure   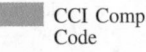 CCI Comp. Code   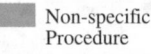 Non-specific Procedure

15836   arm

15837   forearm or hand

15838   submental fat pad

15839   other area

(For bilateral procedure, add modifier -50)

15840   Graft for facial nerve paralysis; free fascia graft (including obtaining fascia)

(For bilateral procedure, add modifier -50)

15841   free muscle graft (including obtaining graft)

15842   free muscle flap by microsurgical technique

(Do not report code 69990 in addition to code 15842)

15845   regional muscle transfer

(For intravenous fluorescein examination of blood flow in graft or flap, use 15860)

(For nerve transfers, decompression, or repair, see 64831-64876, 64905, 64907, 69720, 69725, 69740, 69745, 69955)

+ 15847   Excision, excessive skin and subcutaneous tissue (includes lipectomy), abdomen (eg, abdominoplasty) (includes umbilical transposition and fascial plication) (List separately in addition to code for primary procedure)

(Use 15847 in conjunction with 15830)

(For abdominal wall hernia repair, see 49491-49587)

(To report other abdominoplasty, use 17999)

15850   Removal of sutures under anesthesia (other than local), same surgeon

15851   Removal of sutures under anesthesia (other than local), other surgeon

15852   Dressing change (for other than burns) under anesthesia (other than local)

● New Code   ▲ Revised Code   + Add-On Code   ⊘ Modifier -51 Exempt   ⊙ Moderate Sedation

15860 Intravenous injection of agent (eg, fluorescein) to test vascular flow in flap or graft

15876 Suction assisted lipectomy; head and neck

15877   trunk

15878   upper extremity

15879   lower extremity

PRESSURE ULCERS (DECUBITUS ULCERS)

15920 Excision, coccygeal pressure ulcer, with coccygectomy; with primary suture

15922   with flap closure

15931 Excision, sacral pressure ulcer, with primary suture;

15933   with ostectomy

15934 Excision, sacral pressure ulcer, with skin flap closure;

15935   with ostectomy

15936 Excision, sacral pressure ulcer, in preparation for muscle or myocutaneous flap or skin graft closure;

15937   with ostectomy

(For repair of defect using muscle or myocutaneous flap, use code(s) 15734 and/or 15738 in addition to 15936, 15937. For repair of defect using split skin graft, use codes 15100 and/or 15101 in addition to 15936, 15937)

15940 Excision, ischial pressure ulcer, with primary suture;

15941   with ostectomy (ischiectomy)

15944 Excision, ischial pressure ulcer, with skin flap closure;

15945   with ostectomy

15946 Excision, ischial pressure ulcer, with ostectomy, in preparation for muscle or myocutaneous flap or skin graft closure

357

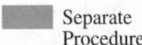 Separate Procedure
 Unlisted Procedure
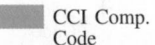 CCI Comp. Code
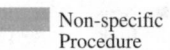 Non-specific Procedure

(For repair of defect using muscle or myocutaneous flap, use code(s) 15734 and/or 15738 in addition to 15946. For repair of defect using split skin graft, use codes 15100 and/or 15101 in addition to 15946)

15950 Excision, trochanteric pressure ulcer, with primary suture;

15951 with ostectomy

15952 Excision, trochanteric pressure ulcer, with skin flap closure;

15953 with ostectomy

15956 Excision, trochanteric pressure ulcer, in preparation for muscle or myocutaneous flap or skin graft closure;

15958 with ostectomy

(For repair of defect using muscle or myocutaneous flap, use code(s) 15734 and/or 15738 in addition to 15956, 15958. For repair of defect using split skin graft, use codes 15100 and/or 15101 in addition to 15956, 15958)

15999 Unlisted procedure, excision pressure ulcer

(For free skin graft to close ulcer or donor site, see 15002 et seq)

BURNS, LOCAL TREATMENT

Procedures 16000-16036 refer to local treatment of burned surface only. Codes 16020-16030 include the application of materials (eg, dressings) not described in 15100-15278.

List percentage of body surface involved and depth of burn.

For necessary related medical services (eg., hospital visits, detention) in management of burned patients, see appropriate services in E/M and Medicine sections.

For the application of skin grafts or skin substitutes, see 15100-15650.

16000 Initial treatment, first degree burn, when no more than local treatment is required

16020 Dressings and/or debridement of partial-thickness burns, initial or subsequent; small (less than 5% total body surface area)

16025   medium (eg, whole face or whole extremity, or 5% to 10% total body surface area)

16030   large (eg, more than 1 extremity, or greater than 10% total body surface area)

16035   Escharotomy; initial incision

+ 16036   each additional incision (List separately in addition to code for primary procedure)

        (Use 16036 in conjunction with code 16035)

        (For debridement, curettement of burn wound, see 16020-16030)

DESTRUCTION

        (For destruction of lesion(s) in specific anatomic sites, see 40820, 46900-46917, 46924, 54050-54057, 54065, 56501, 56515, 57061, 57065, 67850, 68135)

        (For laser treatment for inflammatory skin disease, see 96920-96922)

        (For paring or cutting of benign hyperkeratotic lesions (eg, corns or calluses), see 11055-11057)

        (For sharp removal or electrosurgical destruction of skin tags and fibrocutaneous tags, see 11200, 11201)

        (For cryotherapy of acne, use 17340)

        (For initiation or follow-up care of topical chemotherapy (eg, 5-FU or similar agents), see appropriate office visits)

        (For shaving of epidermal or dermal lesions, see 11300-11313)

DESTRUCTION, BENIGN OR PREMALIGNANT LESIONS

17000   Destruction (eg, laser surgery, electrosurgery, cryosurgery, chemosurgery, surgical curettement), premalignant lesions (eg, actinic keratoses); first lesion

+ 17003   second through 14 lesions, each (List separately in addition to code for first lesion)

        (Use 17003 in conjunction with 17000)

        (For destruction of common or plantar warts, see 17110-17111)

359

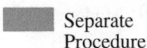 Separate Procedure   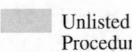 Unlisted Procedure   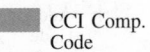 CCI Comp. Code   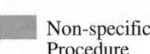 Non-specific Procedure

⊘ **17004** Destruction (eg, laser surgery, electrosurgery, cryosurgery, chemosurgery, surgical curettement), premalignant lesions (eg, actinic keratoses), 15 or more lesions

(Do not report 17004 in conjunction with codes 17000-17003)

17106 Destruction of cutaneous vascular proliferative lesions (eg, laser technique); less than 10 sq cm

17107 10.0 to 50.0 sq cm

17108 over 50.0 sq cm

17110 Destruction (eg, laser surgery, electrosurgery, cryosurgery, chemosurgery, surgical curettement), of benign lesions other than skin tags or cutaneous vascular proliferative lesions; up to 14 lesions

17111 15 or more lesions

17250 Chemical cauterization of granulation tissue (proud flesh, sinus or fistula)

(17250 is not to be used with removal or excision codes for the same lesion)

DESTRUCTION, MALIGNANT LESIONS, ANY METHOD

17260 Destruction, malignant lesion (eg, laser surgery, electrosurgery, cryosurgery, chemosurgery, surgical curettement), trunk, arms or legs; lesion diameter 0.5 cm or less

17261 lesion diameter 0.6 to 1.0 cm

17262 lesion diameter 1.1 to 2.0 cm

17263 lesion diameter 2.1 to 3.0 cm

17264 lesion diameter 3.1 to 4.0 cm

17266 lesion diameter over 4.0 cm

17270 Destruction, malignant lesion (eg, laser surgery, electrosurgery, cryosurgery, chemosurgery, surgical curettement), scalp, neck, hands, feet, genitalia; lesion diameter 0.5 cm or less

17271 lesion diameter 0.6 to 1.0 cm

● New Code ▲ Revised Code + Add-On Code ⊘ Modifier -51 Exempt ⊙ Moderate Sedation

17272	lesion diameter 1.1 to 2.0 cm
17273	lesion diameter 2.1 to 3.0 cm
17274	lesion diameter 3.1 to 4.0 cm
17276	lesion diameter over 4.0 cm
17280	Destruction, malignant lesion, (eg, laser surgery, electrosurgery, cryosurgery, chemosurgery, surgical curettement), face, ears, eyelids, nose, lips, mucous membrane; lesion diameter 0.5 cm or less
17281	lesion diameter 0.6 to 1.0 cm
17282	lesion diameter 1.1 to 2.0 cm
17283	lesion diameter 2.1 to 3.0 cm
17284	lesion diameter 3.1 to 4.0 cm
17286	lesion diameter over 4.0 cm

MOHS MICROGRAPHIC SURGERY

Mohs micrographic surgery involves removing a skin cancer one layer at a time and examining these layers under a microscope immediately after they are removed. This procedure allows for a close examination of each layer of skin to detect cancer cells. It also allows a minimal amount of tissue to be removed while ensuring complete removal of all the cancer cells. A local anesthetic is injected into the skin before the surgery. The physician begins to remove the skin cancer and a small amount of healthy tissue, one layer of skin at a time. Each tissue layer is prepared and examined under the microscope for cancer cells. Surgery is complete when no more cancer cells are detected.

- *If repair is performed, report separate repair, flap, or graft codes.*

- *If a biopsy of a suspected skin cancer is performed on the same day as Mohs surgery, report diagnostic skin biopsy (11100, 11101) and frozen section pathology (88331) with modifier -59 to distinguish from the subsequent definitive surgical procedure of Mohs surgery.*

If repair is performed, use separate repair, flap, or graft codes. If a biopsy of a suspected skin cancer is performed on the same day as Mohs surgery because there was no prior pathology confirmation of a diagnosis, then report diagnostic skin biopsy (11100, 11101) and frozen section pathology (88331) with modifier 59 to distinguish from the subsequent definitive surgical procedure of Mohs surgery.

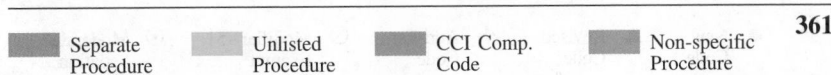

361

| ■ Separate Procedure | ■ Unlisted Procedure | ■ CCI Comp. Code | ■ Non-specific Procedure |

(If additional special pathology procedures, stains or immunostains are required, use 88311-88314, 88342)

(Do not report 88314 in conjunction with 17311-17315 for routine frozen section stain (eg., hematoxylin and eosin, toluidine blue) performed during Mohs surgery. When a nonroutine histochemical stain on frozen tissue is utilized, report 88314 with modifier -59)

(Do not report 88302-88309 on the same specimen as part of the Mohs surgery)

17311 Mohs micrographic technique, including removal of all gross tumor, surgical excision of tissue specimens, mapping, color coding of specimens, microscopic examination of specimens by the surgeon, and histopathologic preparation including routine stain(s) (eg, hematoxylin and eosin, toluidine blue), head, neck, hands, feet, genitalia, or any location with surgery directly involving muscle, cartilage, bone, tendon, major nerves, or vessels; first stage, up to 5 tissue blocks

+ 17312 each additional stage after the first stage, up to 5 tissue blocks (List separately in addition to code for primary procedure)

(Use 17312 in conjunction with 17311)

17313 Mohs micrographic technique, including removal of all gross tumor, surgical excision of tissue specimens, mapping, color coding of specimens, microscopic examination of specimens by the surgeon, and histopathologic preparation including routine stain(s) (eg, hematoxylin and eosin, toluidine blue), of the trunk, arms, or legs; first stage, up to 5 tissue blocks

+ 17314 each additional stage after the first stage, up to 5 tissue blocks (List separately in addition to code for primary procedure)

(Use 17314 in conjunction with 17313)

+ 17315 Mohs micrographic technique, including removal of all gross tumor, surgical excision of tissue specimens, mapping, color coding of specimens, microscopic examination of specimens by the surgeon, and histopathologic preparation including routine stain(s) (eg, hematoxylin and eosin, toluidine blue), each additional block after the first 5 tissue blocks, any stage (List separately in addition to code for primary procedure)

(Use 17315 in conjunction with 17311-17314)

362   ● New Code   ▲ Revised Code   **+** Add-On Code   ⊘ Modifier -51 Exempt   ⊙ Moderate Sedation

OTHER PROCEDURES

17340 Cryotherapy (CO_2 slush, liquid N_2) for acne

17360 Chemical exfoliation for acne (eg, acne paste, acid)

17380 Electrolysis epilation, each 1/2 hour

(For actinotherapy, use 96900)

17999 Unlisted procedure, skin, mucous membrane and subcutaneous tissue

BREAST

Fine needle aspiration biopsies, core biopsies, open incisional or excisional biopsies, and related procedures performed to procure tissue from a lesion for which an established diagnosis exists are not to be reported separately at the time of a lesion excision unless performed on a different lesion or on the contralateral breast. However, if a diagnosis is not established, and the decision to perform the excision or mastectomy is dependent on the results of the biopsy, then the biopsy is separately reported. Modifier -58 may be used appropriately to indicate that the biopsy and the excision or mastectomy are staged or planned procedures.

Because excision of lesions occurs in the course of performing a mastectomy, breast excisions are not separately reported from a mastectomy unless performed to establish the malignant diagnosis before proceeding to the mastectomy. Specifically CPT codes 19110-19126 (breast excision) are in general included in all mastectomy CPT codes 19140-19240 of the same side. However, if the excision is performed to obtain tissue to determine pathologic diagnosis of malignancy prior to proceeding to a mastectomy, the excision is separately reportable with the mastectomy. Modifier -58 should be utilized in this situation.

Use of other integumentary codes for incision and closure are included in the codes describing various breast excision or mastectomy codes. Because of the frequent need to excise lymph node or muscle tissue in conjunction with mastectomies, these procedures have been included in the CPT coding for mastectomy. It would be inappropriate to separately report ipsilateral lymph node excision in conjunction with the appropriate mastectomy codes. However, sentinel lymph node biopsy is separately reported when performed prior to a localized excision of breast or a mastectomy with or without lymphadenectomy.

Open biopsy or excision of sentinel lymph node(s) should be reported as follows: axillary (CPT codes 38500 or 38525), deep cervical (CPT code 38510), internal mammary (CPT code 38530). (CPT code 38740(axillary lymphadenectomy; superficial) should not be reported for a sentinel lymph node biopsy.

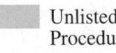 Separate Procedure

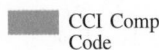 Unlisted Procedure

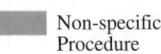 CCI Comp. Code

Non-specific Procedure

363

Sentinel lymph node biopsy of superficial axillary lymph node(s) is correctly reported as CPT code 38500 (biopsy or excision of lymph node(s), superficial) which includes the removal of one or more discretely identified superficial lymph nodes. By contrast a superficial axillary lymphadenectomy (CPT code 38740) requires removal of all superficial axillary adipose tissue with all lymph nodes in this adipose tissue.)

In the circumstance where a breast lesion is identified and it is determined to be medically necessary to biopsy or excise the contralateral lymph nodes, use of the biopsy or lymph node dissection codes (using the appropriate anatomic modifier, -LT or -RT for left or right) would be acceptable. Additionally, breast reconstruction codes that include the insertion of a prosthetic implant are not to be reported with CPT codes that describe the insertion of a breast prosthesis only.

The CPT coding for breast procedures generally refers to unilateral procedures; when performed bilaterally, modifier -50 would be appropriate. This is identified parenthetically, where appropriate, in the CPT narrative.

INCISION

19000   Puncture aspiration of cyst of breast;

+ **19001**   each additional cyst (List separately in addition to code for primary procedure)

(Use 19001 in conjunction with code 19000)

(If imaging guidance is performed, see 76942, 77021, 77031, 77032)

19020   Mastotomy with exploration or drainage of abscess, deep

19030   Injection procedure only for mammary ductogram or galactogram

(For radiological supervision and interpretation, see 77053, 77054)

EXCISION

Breast biopsies are reported using codes 19100-19103. The open excision of breast lesions (eg., lesions of the breast ducts, cysts, benign or malignant tumors), without specific attention to adequate surgical margins, with or without the preoperative placement of radiological markers, is reported using codes 19110-19126. Partial mastectomy procedures (eg., lumpectomy, tylectomy, quadrantectomy, or segmentectomy) describe open excisions of breast tissue with specific attention to adequate surgical margins.

364

● New Code	▲ Revised Code	+ Add-On Code	⊘ Modifier -51 Exempt	⊙ Moderate Sedation

Partial mastectomy procedures are reported using codes 19301 or 19302 as appropriate. Documentation for partial mastectomy procedures includes attention to the removal of adequate surgical margins surrounding the breast mass or lesion.

Total mastectomy procedures include simple mastectomy, complete mastectomy, subcutaneous mastectomy, modified radical mastectomy, radical mastectomy, and more extended procedures (eg., Urban type operation). Total mastectomy procedures are reported using codes 19303-19307 as appropriate.

Excisions or resections of chest wall tumors including ribs, with or without reconstruction, with or without mediastinal lymphadenectomy, are reported using codes 19260, 19271 or 19272. Codes 19260-19272 are not restricted to breast tumors and are used to report resections of chest wall tumors originating from any chest wall component. (For excision of lung or pleura, see 32310 et seq.)

> (To report bilateral procedures, report modifier -50 with the procedure code)

19100 Biopsy of breast; percutaneous, needle core, not using imaging guidance (separate procedure)

> (For fine needle aspiration, use 10021)

> (For image guided breast biopsy, see 19102, 19103, 10022)

19101 open, incisional

19102 percutaneous, needle core, using imaging guidance

> (For placement of percutaneous localization clip, use 19295)

19103 percutaneous, automated vacuum assisted or rotating biopsy device, using imaging guidance

> (For imaging guidance performed in conjunction with 19102, 19103, see 76942, 77012, 77021, 77031, 77032)

> (For placement of percutaneous localization clip, use 19295)

19105 Ablation, cryosurgical, of fibroadenoma, including ultrasound guidance, each fibroadenoma

> (Do not report 19105 in conjunction with 76940, 76942)

> (For adjacent lesions treated with one cryoprobe insertion, report once)

19110 Nipple exploration, with or without excision of a solitary lactiferous duct or a papilloma lactiferous duct

---

| | Separate Procedure | | Unlisted Procedure | | CCI Comp. Code | | Non-specific Procedure | **365** |

19112   Excision of lactiferous duct fistula

19120   Excision of cyst, fibroadenoma, or other benign or malignant tumor, aberrant breast tissue, duct lesion, nipple or areolar lesion (except 19300), open, male or female, 1 or more lesions

19125   Excision of breast lesion identified by preoperative placement of radiological marker, open; single lesion

+ 19126   each additional lesion separately identified by a preoperative radiological marker (List separately in addition to code for primary procedure)

     (Use 19126 in conjunction with code 19125)

19260   Excision of chest wall tumor including ribs

19271   Excision of chest wall tumor involving ribs, with plastic reconstruction; without mediastinal lymphadenectomy

19272   with mediastinal lymphadenectomy

     (Do not report 19260, 19271, 19272 in conjunction with 32100, 32503, 32504, 32551, 32554, 32555)

INTRODUCTION

19290   Preoperative placement of needle localization wire, breast;

+ 19291   each additional lesion (List separately in addition to code for primary procedure)

     (Use 19291 in conjunction with code 19290)

     (For radiological supervision and interpretation, see 76942, 77031, 77032)

+ 19295   Image guided placement, metallic localization clip, percutaneous, during breast biopsy/aspiration (List separately in addition to code for primary procedure)

     (Use 19295 in conjunction with 10022, 19102, 19103)

19296   Placement of radiotherapy afterloading expandable catheter (single or multichannel) into the breast for interstitial radioelement application following partial mastectomy, includes imaging guidance; on date separate from partial mastectomy

   ● New Code   ▲ Revised Code   + Add-On Code   ⊘ Modifier -51 Exempt   ⊙ Moderate Sedation

+ **19297** concurrent with partial mastectomy (List separately in addition to code for primary procedure)

(Use 19297 in conjunction with 19160 or 19162)

⊙ **19298** Placement of radiotherapy afterloading brachytherapy catheters (multiple tube and button type) into the breast for interstitial radioelement application following (at the time of or subsequent to) partial mastectomy, includes imaging guidance

MASTECTOMY PROCEDURES

19300 Mastectomy for gynecomastia

19301 Mastectomy, partial (eg, lumpectomy, tylectomy, quadrantectomy, segmentectomy);

19302 with axillary lymphadenectomy

(For placement of radiotherapy afterloading balloon/brachytherapy catheters, see 19296-19298)

19303 Mastectomy, simple, complete

(For immediate or delayed insertion of implant, see 19340, 19342)

(For gynecomastia, use 19300)

19304 Mastectomy, subcutaneous

(For immediate or delayed insertion of implant, see 19340, 19342)

19305 Mastectomy, radical, including pectoral muscles, axillary lymph nodes

(For immediate or delayed insertion of implant, see 19340, 19342)

19306 Mastectomy, radical, including pectoral muscles, axillary and internal mammary lymph nodes (Urban type operation)

(For immediate or delayed insertion of implant, see 19340, 19342)

19307 Mastectomy, modified radical, including axillary lymph nodes, with or without pectoralis minor muscle, but excluding pectoralis major muscle

---

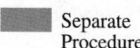 Separate Procedure   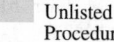 Unlisted Procedure   CCI Comp. Code   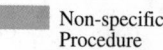 Non-specific Procedure

367

(For immediate or delayed insertion of implant, see 19340, 19342)

REPAIR AND/OR RECONSTRUCTION

(To report bilateral procedures, report modifier -50 with the procedure code)

(For biologic implant for soft tissue reinforcement, use 15777 in conjunction with primary procedure)

19316 Mastopexy

19318 Reduction mammaplasty

19324 Mammaplasty, augmentation; without prosthetic implant

19325 with prosthetic implant

(For flap or graft, use also appropriate number)

19328 Removal of intact mammary implant

19330 Removal of mammary implant material

19340 Immediate insertion of breast prosthesis following mastopexy, mastectomy or in reconstruction

19342 Delayed insertion of breast prosthesis following mastopexy, mastectomy or in reconstruction

(For supply of implant, use 99070)

(For preparation of custom breast implant, use 19396)

19350 Nipple/areola reconstruction

19355 Correction of inverted nipples

19357 Breast reconstruction, immediate or delayed, with tissue expander, including subsequent expansion

19361 Breast reconstruction with latissimus dorsi flap, without prosthetic implant

(For insertion of prosthesis, use also 19340)

19364 Breast reconstruction with free flap

● New Code ▲ Revised Code + Add-On Code ⊘ Modifier -51 Exempt ⊙ Moderate Sedation

(Do not report code 69990 in addition to code 19364)

(19364 includes harvesting of the flap, microvascular transfer, closure of the donor site, and inset shaping the flap into a breast)

19366 Breast reconstruction with other technique

(For operating microscope, use 69990)

(For insertion of prosthesis, use also 19340 or 19342)

19367 Breast reconstruction with transverse rectus abdominis myocutaneous flap (TRAM), single pedicle, including closure of donor site;

19368 with microvascular anastomosis (supercharging)

(Do not report code 69990 in addition to code 19368)

19369 Breast reconstruction with transverse rectus abdominis myocutaneous flap (TRAM), double pedicle, including closure of donor site

19370 Open periprosthetic capsulotomy, breast

19371 Periprosthetic capsulectomy, breast

19380 Revision of reconstructed breast

19396 Preparation of moulage for custom breast implant

OTHER PROCEDURES

19499 Unlisted procedure, breast

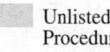 Separate Procedure

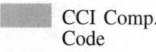 Unlisted Procedure

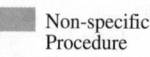 CCI Comp. Code

Non-specific Procedure

This page intentionally left blank.

● New
Code

▲ Revised
Code

+ Add-On
Code

⊘ Modifier -51
Exempt

⊙ Moderate
Sedation

MUSCULOSKELETAL SYSTEM

Musculoskeletal procedure codes include the application and removal of the initial cast or traction device. Use codes in range 29000 to 29999 to report subsequent cast or traction-device applications. Review the instructional notes under the "Application of Casts and Strapping" to identify other uses for these codes.

The procedures and services listed in this section of the CPT coding system include the application and removal of the first cast or traction device only. Subsequent replacement of the cast and/or traction device may be coded using the cast and strapping procedure CPT codes appearing at the end of the section.

MISCELLANEOUS CODING RULES

Most bone, cartilage and fascia graft procedures include obtaining of the graft by the operating surgeon. When a surgical associate obtains the graft for the operating surgeon, the additional service should be coded and coded separately using CPT codes from the 20900-20926 range. In addition, a surgical modifier for assistant surgeon or co-surgeon should be included when reporting the associates services.

CPT codes 20100-20103 relate to treatment of wounds resulting from penetrating trauma (e.g., gunshot, stab wound). Use these codes for wound explorations only if the procedure does not require a thoracotomy or laparotomy and/or repairs to major structure(s) or major blood vessels.

The term "complicated" appears in some narratives in the musculoskeletal subsection. This term implies that an infection occurred, treatment was delayed, or the surgery took longer than usual to perform. Send supporting documentation when the codes containing this descriptor are assigned.

An intermediate repair associated with a musculoskeletal surgery is an integral portion of the surgery and should not be coded separately.

Code the injection codes according to the location of the joint injected or aspirated. Example: small joint = fingers, toes; intermediate joint = wrist, elbow; and major joint = shoulder, hip, or knee.

When removing a foreign body or performing soft tissue biopsy, determine the site and whether or not the foreign body/biopsy is superficial or deep.

FRACTURES

Remember to differentiate between the type of fracture and the type of treatment when coding fractures. Review the meanings of open and closed treatment of fractures. Dislocations must also be coded with emphasis on whether the treatment is open or closed.

MUSC-SKEL 20000

371

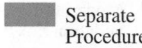 Separate Procedure   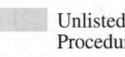 Unlisted Procedure   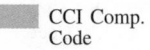 CCI Comp. Code   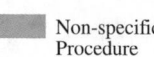 Non-specific Procedure

When coding the re-reduction of a fracture and/or dislocation performed by the primary physician, add modifier -76 to the procedure code. If the re-reduction were performed by another physician, then modifier -77 would be added to the procedure code.

DEFINITIONS

In orthopedic medicine, fractures are classified as closed or open (compound) and simple or multi-fragmentary (formerly comminuted).

Closed treatment

Closed fractures are those in which the skin is intact, i.e. not surgically open. A closed reduction re-aligns a bone by manipulation without surgery. Sometimes it is not possible for the physician to get the bones in the right position with a closed reduction. If this happens, traction can be put on the bones to gently pull them into position. Traction is usually used for a short period of time and before other forms of treatment are used.

Open treatment

Open (compound) fractures involve wounds that communicate with the fracture and may expose bone to contamination. Open injuries carry an elevated risk of infection; they require antibiotic treatment and usually urgent surgical treatment (debridement). This involves removal of all dirt, contamination, and dead tissue. An open reduction and internal fixation of the bone requires an orthopedic surgeon. The surgery requires cutting open the skin of the area over the fracture so bone fragments can be put back into place and the bone fixated or held in place. The bone fragments are held in place with special screws or by attaching metal plates to the bone. Pins that go through the bone or rods that go inside the length of the bone are used to keep the bone in place.

Percutaneous skeletal fixation

Percutaneous skeletal fixation defines fracture treatment which is neither open or closed. Prior to fixation a closed reduction may be performed if necessary for alignment of the broken bones. Pins or screws are then put through the skin and bone above and below the fracture, usually under x-ray guidance. The pins or screws are connected to metal bars on the outside of the skin to form a frame around the fracture. This frame keeps the bone pieces in place.

Simple fractures

Simple fractures are fractures that occur along one line, splitting the bone into two pieces, while multi-fragmentary fractures involve the bone splitting into multiple pieces. A simple, closed fracture is much easier to treat and has a much better prognosis than an open, contaminated fracture. Other considerations in fracture care are displacement (fracture gap) and angulation. If angulation or displacement

● New Code ▲ Revised Code + Add-On Code ⊘ Modifier -51 Exempt ⊙ Moderate Sedation

is large, reduction (manipulation) of the bone may be required and, in adults, frequently requires surgical care. These injuries may take longer to heal than injuries without displacement or angulation

Additional coding rules

- *Codes for obtaining autogenous bone grafts, cartilage, tendon, fascia lata grafts or other tissues through separate incisions are to be used only when the graft is not already listed as part of the basic procedure.*

- *Re-reduction of a fracture and/or dislocation performed in the primary physician may be identified by the addition of modifier -76 to the usual procedure.*

- *Codes for external fixation are to be used only when external fixation is not already listed as part of the basic procedure.*

GENERAL

INCISION

(20000   deleted 2010 [2011 edition])

(For incision and drainage procedures, cutaneous/subcutaneous, see 10060, 10061)

20005   Incision and drainage of soft tissue abscess, subfascial, (ie, involves the soft tissue below the deep fascia)

WOUND EXPLORATION—TRAUMA (EG, PENETRATING GUNSHOT, STAB WOUND)

20100-20103 relate to wound(s) resulting from penetrating trauma. These codes describe surgical exploration and enlargement of the wound, extension of dissection (to determine penetration), debridement, removal of foreign body(s), ligation or coagulation of minor subcutaneous and/or muscular blood vessel(s), of the subcutaneous tissue, muscle fascia, and/or muscle, not requiring thoracotomy or laparotomy. If a repair is done to major structure(s) or major blood vessel(s) requiring thoracotomy or laparotomy, then those specific code(s) would supersede the use of codes 20100-20103. To report simple, intermediate, or complex repair of wound(s) that do not require enlargement of the wound, extension of dissection, etc., as stated above, use specific Repair code(s) in the Integumentary System section.

20100   Exploration of penetrating wound (separate procedure); neck

20101   chest

20102   abdomen/flank/back

| Separate Procedure | Unlisted Procedure | CCI Comp. Code | Non-specific Procedure |

20103   extremity

EXCISION

20150 Excision of epiphyseal bar, with or without autogenous soft tissue graft obtained through same fascial incision

(For aspiration of bone marrow, use 38220)

20200 Biopsy, muscle; superficial

20205   deep

20206 Biopsy, muscle, percutaneous needle

(If imaging guidance is performed, see 76942, 77012, 77021)

(For fine needle aspiration, use 10021 or 10022)

(For evaluation of fine needle aspirate, see 88172-88173)

(For excision of muscle tumor, deep, see specific anatomic section)

20220 Biopsy, bone, trocar, or needle; superficial (eg, ilium, sternum, spinous process, ribs)

20225   deep (eg, vertebral body, femur)

(For bone marrow biopsy, use 38221)

(For radiologic supervision and interpretation, see 77002, 77012, 77021)

20240 Biopsy, bone, open; superficial (eg, ilium, sternum, spinous process, ribs, trochanter of femur)

20245   deep (eg, humerus, ischium, femur)

20250 Biopsy, vertebral body, open; thoracic

20251   lumbar or cervical

(For sequestrectomy, osteomyelitis or drainage of bone abscess, see anatomical area)

● New Code   ▲ Revised Code   + Add-On Code   ⊘ Modifier -51 Exempt   ⊙ Moderate Sedation

INTRODUCTION OR REMOVAL

(For injection procedure for arthrography, see anatomical area)

20500 Injection of sinus tract; therapeutic (separate procedure)

20501 diagnostic (sinogram)

(For radiological supervision and interpretation, use 76080)

(For contrast injection[s] and radiological assessment of gastrostomy, duodenostomy, jejunostomy, gastrojejunostomy, or cecostomy [or other colonic] tube including fluoroscopic imaging guidance, use 49465)

20520 Removal of foreign body in muscle or tendon sheath; simple

20525 deep or complicated

20526 Injection, therapeutic (eg, local anesthetic, corticosteroid), carpal tunnel

20527 Injection, enzyme (eg, collagenase), palmar fascial cord (ie, Dupuytren's contracture)

(For manipulation of palmar fascial cord (ie, Dupuytren's cord) post enzyme injection (eg, collagenase), use 26341)

20550 Injection(s); single tendon sheath, or ligament, aponeurosis (eg, plantar "fascia")

(For injection of Morton's neuroma, see 64455, 64632)

20551 single tendon origin/insertion

(Do not report 20550, 20551 in conjunction with 0232T)

(For injection(s) of platelet rich plasma, use 0232T)

20552 Injection(s); single or multiple trigger point(s), 1 or 2 muscle(s)

20553 single or multiple trigger point(s), 3 or more muscle(s)

(If imaging guidance is performed, see 76942, 77002, 77021)

20555 Placement of needles or catheters into muscle and/or soft tissue for subsequent interstitial radioelement application (at the time of or subsequent to the procedure)

375

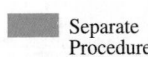

| Separate Procedure | Unlisted Procedure | CCI Comp. Code | Non-specific Procedure |

(For placement of devices into the breast for interstitial radioelement application, see 19296-19298)

(For placement of needles, catheters, or devices into muscle or soft tissue of the head and neck, for interstitial radioelement application, use 41019)

(For placement of needles or catheters for interstitial radioelement application into prostate, use 55875)

(For placement of needles or catheters into the pelvic organs or genitalia [except prostate] for interstitial radioelement application, use 55920)

(For interstitial radioelement application, see 77776-77778, 77785-77787)

(For imaging guidance, see 76942, 77002, 77012, 77021)

20600 Arthrocentesis, aspiration and/or injection; small joint or bursa (eg, fingers, toes)

20605 intermediate joint or bursa (eg, temporomandibular, acromioclavicular, wrist, elbow or ankle, olecranon bursa)

20610 major joint or bursa (eg, shoulder, hip, knee joint, subacromial bursa)

(If imaging guidance is performed, see 76942, 77002, 77012, 77021)

20612 Aspiration and/or injection of ganglion cyst(s) any location

(To report multiple ganglion cyst aspirations/injections, use 20612 and append modifier -59)

20615 Aspiration and injection for treatment of bone cyst

20650 Insertion of wire or pin with application of skeletal traction, including removal (separate procedure)

20660 Application of cranial tongs, caliper, or stereotactic frame, including removal (separate procedure)

20661 Application of halo, including removal; cranial

20662 pelvic

20663 femoral

20664 Application of halo, including removal, cranial, 6 or more pins placed, for thin skull osteology (eg, pediatric patients, hydrocephalus, osteogenesis imperfecta)

▲ **20665** Removal of tongs or halo applied by another individual

20670 Removal of implant; superficial, (eg, buried wire, pin or rod) (separate procedure)

20680 deep (eg, buried wire, pin, screw, metal band, nail,rod or plate)

20690 Application of a uniplane (pins or wires in 1 plane), unilateral, external fixation system

20692 Application of a multiplane (pins or wires in more than 1 plane), unilateral, external fixation system (eg, Ilizarov, Monticelli type)

20693 Adjustment or revision of external fixation system requiring anesthesia (eg, new pin[s] or wire[s] and/or new ring[s] or bar[s])

20694 Removal, under anesthesia, of external fixation system

20696 Application of multiplane (pins or wires in more than 1 plane), unilateral, external fixation with stereotactic computer-assisted adjustment (eg, spatial frame), including imaging; initial and subsequent alignment(s), assessment(s), and computation(s) of adjustment schedule(s)

(Do not report 20696 in conjunction with 20692, 20697)

⊘ **20697** exchange (ie, removal and replacement) of strut, each)

(Do not report 20697 in conjunction with 20692, 20696)

REPLANTATION

20802 Replantation, arm (includes surgical neck of humerus through elbow joint), complete amputation

(To report replantation of incomplete arm amputation, see specific code(s) for repair of bone(s), ligament(s), tendon(s), nerve(s), or blood vessel(s) with modifier -52)

20805 Replantation, forearm (includes radius and ulna to radial carpal joint), complete amputation

---

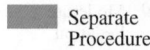 Separate Procedure   Unlisted Procedure   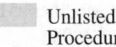 CCI Comp. Code   Non-specific Procedure   **377**

(To report replantation of incomplete forearm amputation, see specific code(s) for repair of bone(s), ligament(s), tendon(s), nerve(s), or blood vessel(s) with modifier -52)

20808 Replantation, hand (includes hand through metacarpophalangeal joints), complete amputation

(To report replantation of incomplete hand amputation, see specific code(s) for repair of bone(s), ligament(s), tendon(s), nerve(s), or blood vessel(s) with modifier -52)

20816 Replantation, digit, excluding thumb (includes metacarpophalangeal joint to insertion of flexor sublimis tendon), complete amputation

(To report replantation of incomplete digit amputation excluding thumb, see specific code(s) for repair of bone(s), ligament(s), tendon(s), nerve(s), or blood vessel(s) with modifier -52)

20822 Replantation, digit, excluding thumb (includes distal tip to sublimis tendon insertion), complete amputation

(To report replantation of incomplete digit amputation excluding thumb, see specific code(s) for repair of bone(s), ligament(s), tendon(s), nerve(s), or blood vessel(s) with modifier -52)

20824 Replantation, thumb (includes carpometacarpal joint to MP joint), complete amputation

(To report replantation of incomplete thumb amputation, see specific code(s) for repair of bone(s), ligament(s), tendon(s), nerve(s), or blood vessel(s) with modifier -52)

20827 Replantation, thumb (includes distal tip to MP joint), complete amputation

(To report replantation of incomplete thumb amputation, see specific code(s) for repair of bone(s), ligament(s), tendon(s), nerve(s), or blood vessel(s) with modifier -52)

(To report replantation of complete leg amputation see specific code(s) for repair of bone(s), ligament(s), tendon(s), nerve(s), or blood vessel(s) with modifier -52)

(To report replantation of incomplete leg amputation, see specific code(s) for repair of bone(s), ligament(s), tendon(s), nerve(s), or blood vessel(s) with modifier -52)

20838 Replantation, foot, complete amputation

● New Code   ▲ Revised Code   ✛ Add-On Code   ⊘ Modifier -51 Exempt   ⊙ Moderate Sedation

(To report replantation of incomplete foot amputation, see specific code(s) for repair of bone(s), ligament(s), tendon(s), nerve(s), or blood vessel(s) with modifier -52)

GRAFTS (OR IMPLANTS)

Codes for obtaining autogenous bone, cartilage, tendon, fascia lata grafts, or other tissues through separate skin/fascial incisions should be reported separately unless the code descriptor references the harvesting of the graft or implant (eg., includes obtaining graft).

Do not append modifier 62 to bone graft codes 20900-20938.

(For spinal surgery bone graft(s) see codes 20930-20938)

20900 Bone graft, any donor area; minor or small (eg, dowel or button)

20902 major or large

20910 Cartilage graft; costochondral

20912 nasal septum

(For ear cartilage, use 21235)

20920 Fascia lata graft; by stripper

20922 by incision and area exposure, complex or sheet

20924 Tendon graft, from a distance (eg, palmaris, toe extensor, plantaris)

20926 Tissue grafts, other (eg, paratenon, fat, dermis)

(For injection(s) of platelet rich plasma, use 0232T)

+ **20930** Allograft, morselized, or placement of osteopromotive material, for spine surgery only (List separately in addition to code for primary procedure)

(Use 20930 in conjunction with 22319, 22532, 22533, 22548-22558, 22590-22612, 22630, 22633, 22634, 22800-22812)

+ **20931** Allograft, structural, for spine surgery only (List separately in addition to code for primary procedure)

	Separate Procedure		Unlisted Procedure		CCI Comp. Code		Non-specific Procedure

(Use 20931 in conjunction with 22319, 22532-22533,
22548-22558, 22590-22612, 22630, 22633, 22634,
22800-22812)

+ 20936 Autograft for spine surgery only (includes harvesting the graft);
local (eg, ribs, spinous process, or laminar fragments) obtained
from same incision (List separately in addition to code for
primary procedure)

(Use 20936 in conjunction with 22319, 22532, 22533,
22548-22558, 22590-22612, 22630, 22633, 22634,
22800-22812)

+ 20937 morselized (through separate skin or fascial incision) (List
separately in addition to code for primary procedure)

(Use 20937 in conjunction with 22319, 22532, 22533,
22548-22558, 22590-22612, 22630, 22633, 22634,
22800-22812)

+ 20938 structural, bicortical or tricortical (through separate skin or
fascial incision) (List separately in addition to code for
primary procedure)

(Use 20938 in conjunction with 22319, 22532-22533,
22548-22558, 22590-22612, 22630, 22633, 22634,
22800-22812)

(For needle aspiration of bone marrow for the purpose of bone
grafting, use 38220. Do not report 38220-38230 for bone
marrow aspiration for platelet rich stem cell injection. For bone
marrow aspiration for platelet rich stem cell injection, use
0232T.)

OTHER PROCEDURES

20950 Monitoring of interstitial fluid pressure (includes insertion of
device,eg, wick catheter technique, needle manometer technique)
in detection of muscle compartment syndrome

20955 Bone graft with microvascular anastomosis; fibula

20956 iliac crest

20957 metatarsal

20962 other than fibula, iliac crest, or metatarsal

(Do not report code 69990 in addition to codes 20955-20962)

● New Code   ▲ Revised Code   + Add-On Code   ⊘ Modifier -51 Exempt   ⊙ Moderate Sedation

20969   Free osteocutaneous flap with microvascular anastomosis; other than iliac crest, metatarsal, or great toe

20970   iliac crest

20972   metatarsal

20973   great toe with web space

(Do not report code 69990 in addition to codes 20969-20973)

(For great toe, wrap-around procedure, use 26551)

⊘ **20974**   Electrical stimulation to aid bone healing; noninvasive (nonoperative)

⊘ **20975**   invasive (operative)

20979   Low intensity ultrasound stimulation to aid bone healing, noninvasive (nonoperative)

⊙ **20982**   Ablation, bone tumor(s) (eg, osteoid osteoma, metastasis) radiofrequency, percutaneous, including computed tomographic guidance

(Do not report 20982 in conjunction with 77013)

+ **20985**   Computer-assisted surgical navigational procedure for musculoskeletal procedures - image-less (List separately in addition to code for primary procedure)

(Do not report 20985 in conjunction with 61781-61783)

(20986   deleted 2009 edition)

(20987   deleted 2009 edition)

(For computer-assisted navigational procedures with image guidance based on pre-operative and intraoperatively obtained images, see 0054T, 0055T)

20999   Unlisted procedure, musculoskeletal system, general

HEAD

Skull, facial bones, and temporomandibular joint.

INCISION

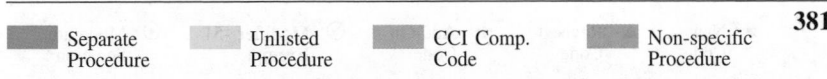

Separate Procedure	Unlisted Procedure	CCI Comp. Code	Non-specific Procedure

381

(For incision and drainage of superficial abscess and hematoma, see 10060, 10061)

(For incision and drainage of soft tissue abscess, use 20005)

(For removal of embedded foreign body from dentoalveolar structure, see 41805, 41806)

21010 Arthrotomy, temporomandibular joint

(To report bilateral procedures, report 21010 with modifier -50)

EXCISION

21011 Excision, tumor, soft tissue of face or scalp, subcutaneous; less than 2 cm

21012 2 cm or greater

21013 Excision, tumor, soft tissue of face and scalp, subfascial (eg, subgaleal, intramuscular); less than 2 cm

21014 2 cm or greater

21015 Radical resection of tumor (eg, malignant neoplasm), soft tissue of face or scalp; less than 2 cm

(To report excision of skull tumor for osteomyelitis, use 61501)

21016 2 cm or greater

21025 Excision of bone (eg, for osteomyelitis or bone abscess); mandible

21026 facial bone(s)

21029 Removal by contouring of benign tumor of facial bone (eg, fibrous dysplasia)

21030 Excision of benign tumor or cyst of maxilla or zygoma by enucleation and curettage

21031 Excision of torus mandibularis

21032 Excision of maxillary torus palatinus

21034 Excision of malignant tumor of maxilla or zygoma

---

382   ● New   ▲ Revised   ＋ Add-On   ⊘ Modifier -51   ⊙ Moderate
              Code   Code   Code   Exempt   Sedation

21040 Excision of benign tumor or cyst of mandible, by enucleation and/or curettage

(For enucleation and/or curettage of benign cysts or tumors of mandible not requiring osteotomy, use 21040)

(For excision of benign tumor or cyst of mandible requiring osteotomy, see 21046-21047)

21044 Excision of malignant tumor of mandible;

21045 radical resection

(For bone graft, use 21215)

21046 Excision of benign tumor or cyst of mandible; requiring intra-oral osteotomy (eg, locally aggressive or destructive lesion(s))

21047 requiring extra-oral osteotomy and partial mandibulectomy (eg, locally aggressive or destructive lesion(s))

21048 Excision of benign tumor or cyst of maxilla; requiring intra-oral osteotomy (eg, locally aggressive or destructive lesion(s))

21049 requiring extra-oral osteotomy and partial maxillectomy (eg, locally aggressive or destructive lesion(s))

21050 Condylectomy, temporomandibular joint (separate procedure)

(For bilateral procedures, report 21050 with modifier -50)

21060 Meniscectomy, partial or complete, temporomandibular joint (separate procedure)

(For bilateral procedures, report 21060 with modifier -50)

21070 Coronoidectomy (separate procedure)

(For bilateral procedures, report 21070 with modifier -50)

MANIPULATION

21073 Manipulation of temporomandibular joint(s) (TMJ), therapeutic, requiring an anesthesia service (ie, general or monitored anesthesia care)

383

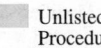 Separate Procedure   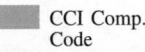 Unlisted Procedure   CCI Comp. Code   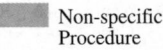 Non-specific Procedure

(For TMJ manipulation without an anesthesia service [ie, general or monitored anesthesia care], see 97140, 98925-98929, 98943)

(For closed treatment of temporomandibular dislocation, see 21480, 21485)

HEAD PROSTHESIS

Codes 21076-21089 describe professional services for the rehabilitation of patients with oral, facial, or other anatomical deficiencies by means of prostheses, such as an artificial eye, ear, or nose or intraoral obturator to close a cleft. Codes 21076-21089 should only be used when the physician or other qualified health care professional actually designs and prepares the prosthesis (ie., not prepared by an outside laboratory).

(For application or removal of caliper or tongs, see 20660, 20665)

21076	Impression and custom preparation; surgical obturator prosthesis
21077	orbital prosthesis
21079	interim obturator prosthesis
21080	definitive obturator prosthesis
21081	mandibular resection prosthesis
21082	palatal augmentation prosthesis
21083	palatal lift prosthesis
21084	speech aid prosthesis
21085	oral surgical splint
21086	auricular prosthesis
21087	nasal prosthesis
21088	facial prosthesis

Other Procedures

| 21089 | Unlisted maxillofacial prosthetic procedure |

● New Code　▲ Revised Code　+ Add-On Code　⊘ Modifier -51 Exempt　⊙ Moderate Sedation

INTRODUCTION OR REMOVAL

21100 Application of halo type appliance for maxillofacial fixation, includes removal (separate procedure)

21110 Application of interdental fixation device for conditions other than fracture or dislocation, includes removal

(For removal of interdental fixation by another individual, see 20670-20680)

21116 Injection procedure for temporomandibular joint arthrography

(For radiological supervision and interpretation, use 70332. Do not report 77002 in addition to 70332)

REPAIR, REVISION AND/OR RECONSTRUCTION

(For cranioplasty, see 21179, 21180 and 62116, 62120, 62140-62147)

21120 Genioplasty; augmentation (autograft, allograft, prosthetic material)

21121 sliding osteotomy, single piece

21122 sliding osteotomies, 2 or more osteotomies (eg, wedge excision or bone wedge reversal for asymmetrical chin)

21123 sliding, augmentation with interpositional bone grafts (includes obtaining autografts)

21125 Augmentation, mandibular body or angle; prosthetic material

21127 with bone graft, onlay or interpositional (includes obtaining autograft)

21137 Reduction forehead; contouring only

21138 contouring and application of prosthetic material or bone graft (includes obtaining autograft)

21139 contouring and setback of anterior frontal sinus wall

21141 Reconstruction midface, LeFort I; single piece, segment movement in any direction (eg, for Long Face Syndrome), without bone graft

---

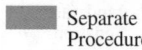 Separate Procedure

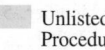 Unlisted Procedure

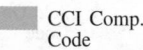 CCI Comp. Code

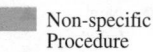 Non-specific Procedure

385

21142   2 pieces, segment movement in any direction, without bone graft

21143   3 or more pieces, segment movement in any direction, without bone graft

21145   single piece, segment movement in any direction, requiring bone grafts (includes obtaining autografts)

21146   2 pieces, segment movement in any direction, requiring bone grafts (includes obtaining autografts) (eg, ungrafted unilateral alveolar cleft)

21147   3 or more pieces, segment movement in any direction, requiring bone grafts (includes obtaining autografts) (eg, ungrafted bilateral alveolar cleft or multiple osteotomies)

21150   Reconstruction midface, LeFort II; anterior intrusion (eg, Treacher-Collins Syndrome)

21151   any direction, requiring bone grafts (includes obtaining autografts)

21154   Reconstruction midface, LeFort III (extracranial), any type, requiring bone grafts (includes obtaining autografts); without LeFort I

21155   with LeFort I

21159   Reconstruction midface, LeFort III (extra and intracranial) with forehead advancement (eg, mono bloc), requiring bone grafts (includes obtaining autografts); without LeFort I

21160   with LeFort I

21172   Reconstruction superior-lateral orbital rim and lower forehead, advancement or alteration, with or without grafts (includes obtaining autografts)

        (For frontal or parietal craniotomy performed for craniosynostosis, use 61556)

21175   Reconstruction, bifrontal, superior-lateral orbital rims and lower forehead, advancement or alteration (eg, plagiocephaly, trigonocephaly, brachycephaly), with or without grafts (includes obtaining autografts)

---

386   ● New Code   ▲ Revised Code   + Add-On Code   ⊘ Modifier -51 Exempt   ⊙ Moderate Sedation

(For bifrontal craniotomy performed for craniosynostosis, use 61557)

21179 Reconstruction, entire or majority of forehead and/or supraorbital rims; with grafts (allograft or prosthetic material)

21180 with autograft (includes obtaining grafts)

(For extensive craniectomy for multiple suture craniosynostosis, use only 61558 or 61559)

21181 Reconstruction by contouring of benign tumor of cranial bones (eg, fibrous dysplasia), extracranial

21182 Reconstruction of orbital walls, rims, forehead, nasoethmoid complex following intra- and extracranial excision of benign tumor of cranial bone (eg, fibrous dysplasia), with multiple autografts (includes obtaining grafts); total area of bone grafting less than 40 sq cm

21183 total area of bone grafting greater than 40 sq cm but less than 80 sq cm

21184 total area of bone grafting greater than 80 sq cm

(For excision of benign tumor of cranial bones, see 61563, 61564)

21188 Reconstruction midface, osteotomies (other than LeFort type) and bone grafts (includes obtaining autografts)

21193 Reconstruction of mandibular rami, horizontal, vertical, C, or L osteotomy; without bone graft

21194 with bone graft (includes obtaining graft)

21195 Reconstruction of mandibular rami and/or body, sagittal split; without internal rigid fixation

21196 with internal rigid fixation

21198 Osteotomy, mandible, segmental;

21199 with genioglossus advancement

(To report total osteotomy of the maxilla, see 21141-21160)

21206 Osteotomy, maxilla, segmental (eg, Wassmund or Schuchard)

				387
Separate Procedure	Unlisted Procedure	CCI Comp. Code	Non-specific Procedure	

21208 Osteoplasty, facial bones; augmentation (autograft, allograft, or prosthetic implant)

21209 reduction

21210 Graft, bone; nasal, maxillary or malar areas (includes obtaining graft)

(For cleft palate repair, see 42200-42225)

21215 mandible (includes obtaining graft)

21230 Graft; rib cartilage, autogenous, to face, chin, nose or ear (includes obtaining graft)

21235 ear cartilage, autogenous, to nose or ear (includes obtaining graft)

(To report graft augmentation of facial bones, use 21208)

21240 Arthroplasty, temporomandibular joint, with or without autograft (includes obtaining graft)

21242 Arthroplasty, temporomandibular joint, with allograft

21243 Arthroplasty, temporomandibular joint, with prosthetic joint replacement

21244 Reconstruction of mandible, extraoral, with transosteal bone plate (eg, mandibular staple bone plate)

21245 Reconstruction of mandible or maxilla, subperiosteal implant; partial

21246 complete

21247 Reconstruction of mandibular condyle with bone and cartilage autografts (includes obtaining grafts) (eg, for hemifacial microsomia)

21248 Reconstruction of mandible or maxilla, endosteal implant (eg, blade, cylinder); partial

21249 complete

(To report midface reconstruction, see 21141-21160)

● New Code   ▲ Revised Code   + Add-On Code   ⊘ Modifier -51 Exempt   ⊙ Moderate Sedation

21255 Reconstruction of zygomatic arch and glenoid fossa with bone and cartilage (includes obtaining autografts)

21256 Reconstruction of orbit with osteotomies (extracranial) and with bone grafts (includes obtaining autografts) (eg, micro-ophthalmia)

21260 Periorbital osteotomies for orbital hypertelorism, with bone grafts; extracranial approach

21261 combined intra- and extracranial approach

21263 with forehead advancement

21267 Orbital repositioning, periorbital osteotomies, unilateral, with bone grafts; extracranial approach

21268 combined intra- and extracranial approach

21270 Malar augmentation, prosthetic material

(For malar augmentation with bone graft, use 21210)

21275 Secondary revision of orbitocraniofacial reconstruction

21280 Medial canthopexy (separate procedure)

(For medial canthoplasty, use 67950)

21282 Lateral canthopexy

21295 Reduction of masseter muscle and bone (eg, for treatment of benign masseteric hypertrophy); extraoral approach

21296 intraoral approach

OTHER PROCEDURES

21299 Unlisted craniofacial and maxillofacial procedure

FRACTURE AND/OR DISLOCATION

(For operative repair of skull fracture, see 62000-62010)

(To report closed treatment of skull fracture, use the appropriate Evaluation and Management code)

21310 Closed treatment of nasal bone fracture without manipulation

	Separate Procedure		Unlisted Procedure		CCI Comp. Code		Non-specific Procedure

389

21315 Closed treatment of nasal bone fracture; without stabilization

21320 with stabilization

21325 Open treatment of nasal fracture; uncomplicated

21330 complicated, with internal and/or external skeletal fixation

21335 with concomitant open treatment of fractured septum

21336 Open treatment of nasal septal fracture, with or without stabilization

21337 Closed treatment of nasal septal fracture, with or without stabilization

21338 Open treatment of nasoethmoid fracture; without external fixation

21339 with external fixation

21340 Percutaneous treatment of nasoethmoid complex fracture, with splint, wire or headcap fixation, including repair of canthal ligaments and/or the nasolacrimal apparatus

21343 Open treatment of depressed frontal sinus fracture

21344 Open treatment of complicated (eg, comminuted or involving posterior wall) frontal sinus fracture, via coronal or multiple approaches

21345 Closed treatment of nasomaxillary complex fracture (LeFort II type), with interdental wire fixation or fixation of denture or splint

21346 Open treatment of nasomaxillary complex fracture (LeFort II type); with wiring and/or local fixation

21347 requiring multiple open approaches

21348 with bone grafting (includes obtaining graft)

21355 Percutaneous treatment of fracture of malar area, including zygomatic arch and malar tripod, with manipulation

---

● New Code   ▲ Revised Code   ✛ Add-On Code   ⊘ Modifier -51 Exempt   ⊙ Moderate Sedation

21356 Open treatment of depressed zygomatic arch fracture (eg, Gillies approach)

21360 Open treatment of depressed malar fracture, including zygomatic arch and malar tripod

21365 Open treatment of complicated (eg, comminuted or involving cranial nerve foramina) fracture(s) of malar area, including zygomatic arch and malar tripod; with internal fixation and multiple surgical approaches

21366 with bone grafting (includes obtaining graft)

21385 Open treatment of orbital floor blowout fracture; transantral approach (Caldwell-Luc type operation)

21386 periorbital approach

21387 combined approach

21390 periorbital approach, with alloplastic or other implant

21395 periorbital approach with bone graft (includes obtaining graft)

21400 Closed treatment of fracture of orbit, except blowout; without manipulation

21401 with manipulation

21406 Open treatment of fracture of orbit, except blowout; without implant

21407 with implant

21408 with bone grafting (includes obtaining graft)

21421 Closed treatment of palatal or maxillary fracture (LeFort I type), with interdental wire fixation or fixation of denture or splint

21422 Open treatment of palatal or maxillary fracture (LeFort I type);

21423 complicated (comminuted or involving cranial nerve foramina), multiple approaches

---

391

 Separate Procedure   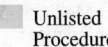 Unlisted Procedure   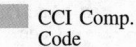 CCI Comp. Code   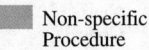 Non-specific Procedure

21431   Closed treatment of craniofacial separation (LeFort III type) using interdental wire fixation of denture or splint

21432   Open treatment of craniofacial separation (LeFort III type); with wiring and/or internal fixation

21433   complicated (eg, comminuted or involving cranial nerve foramina), multiple surgical approaches

21435   complicated, utilizing internal and/or external fixation techniques (eg, head cap, halo device, and/or intermaxillary fixation)

(For removal of internal or external fixation device, use 20670)

21436   complicated, multiple surgical approaches, internal fixation, with bone grafting (includes obtaining graft)

21440   Closed treatment of mandibular or maxillary alveolar ridge fracture (separate procedure)

21445   Open treatment of mandibular or maxillary alveolar ridge fracture (separate procedure)

21450   Closed treatment of mandibular fracture; without manipulation

21451   with manipulation

21452   Percutaneous treatment of mandibular fracture, with external fixation

21453   Closed treatment of mandibular fracture with interdental fixation

21454   Open treatment of mandibular fracture with external fixation

21461   Open treatment of mandibular fracture; without interdental fixation

21462   with interdental fixation

21465   Open treatment of mandibular condylar fracture

21470   Open treatment of complicated mandibular fracture by multiple surgical approaches including internal fixation, interdental fixation, and/or wiring of dentures or splints

---

392

   ● New   ▲ Revised   + Add-On   ⊘ Modifier -51   ⊙ Moderate
      Code   Code   Code   Exempt   Sedation

21480 Closed treatment of temporomandibular dislocation; initial or subsequent

21485 complicated (eg, recurrent requiring intermaxillary fixation or splinting), initial or subsequent

21490 Open treatment of temporomandibular dislocation

(For interdental wire fixation, use 21497)

21495 Open treatment of hyoid fracture

(For laryngoplasty with open reduction of fracture, use 31584)

(To report treatment of closed fracture of larynx, use the applicable Evaluation and Management codes)

21497 Interdental wiring, for condition other than fracture

OTHER PROCEDURES

21499 Unlisted musculoskeletal procedure, head

(For unlisted craniofacial or maxillofacial procedure, use 21299)

NECK (SOFT TISSUES) AND THORAX

(For cervical spine and back, see 21920 et seq)

(For injection of fracture site or trigger point, use 20550)

INCISION

(For incision and drainage of abscess or hematoma, superficial, see 10060, 10140)

21501 Incision and drainage, deep abscess or hematoma, soft tissues of neck or thorax;

(For posterior spine subfascial incision and drainage, see 22010-22015)

21502 with partial rib ostectomy

21510 Incision, deep, with opening of bone cortex (eg, for osteomyelitis or bone abscess), thorax

EXCISION

(For bone biopsy, see 20220-20251)

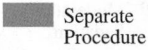 Separate Procedure

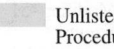 Unlisted Procedure

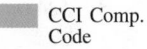 CCI Comp. Code

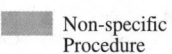 Non-specific Procedure

21550 Biopsy, soft tissue of neck or thorax

(For needle biopsy of soft tissue, use 20206)

21552 This code is out of order. See page 394

21554 This code is out of order. See page 394

21555 Excision, tumor, soft tissue of neck or anterior thorax, subcutaneous; less than 3 cm

21552 3 cm or greater

21556 Excision, tumor, soft tissue of neck or anterior thorax, subfascial (eg, intramuscular); less than 5 cm

21554 5 cm or greater

21557 Radical resection of tumor (eg, malignant neoplasm), soft tissue of neck or anterior thorax; less than 5 cm

21558 5 cm or greater

21600 Excision of rib, partial

(For radical resection of chest wall and rib cage for tumor, use 19260)

(For radical debridement of chest wall and rib cage for injury, see 11044, 11047)

21610 Costotransversectomy (separate procedure)

21615 Excision first and/or cervical rib;

21616 with sympathectomy

21620 Ostectomy of sternum, partial

21627 Sternal debridement

(For debridement and closure, use 21750)

21630 Radical resection of sternum;

21632 with mediastinal lymphadenectomy

● New Code   ▲ Revised Code   + Add-On Code   ⊘ Modifier -51 Exempt   ⊙ Moderate Sedation

REPAIR, REVISION, AND/OR RECONSTRUCTION

(For superficial wound, see Integumentary System section under Repair, Simple)

21685 Hyoid myotomy and suspension

21700 Division of scalenus anticus; without resection of cervical rib

21705   with resection of cervical rib

21720 Division of sternocleidomastoid for torticollis, open operation; without cast application

(For transection of spinal accessory and cervical nerves, see 63191, 64722)

21725   with cast application

21740 Reconstructive repair of pectus excavatum or carinatum; open

21742   minimally invasive approach (Nuss procedure), without thoracoscopy

21743   minimally invasive approach (Nuss procedure), with thoracoscopy

21750 Closure of median sternotomy separation with or without debridement (separate procedure)

FRACTURE AND/OR DISLOCATION

21800 Closed treatment of rib fracture, uncomplicated, each

21805 Open treatment of rib fracture without fixation, each

21810 Treatment of rib fracture requiring external fixation (flail chest)

21820 Closed treatment of sternum fracture

21825 Open treatment of sternum fracture with or without skeletal fixation

(For sternoclavicular dislocation, see 23520-23532)

OTHER PROCEDURES

21899 Unlisted procedure, neck or thorax

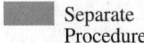 Separate Procedure   Unlisted Procedure   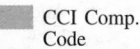 CCI Comp. Code   Non-specific Procedure

395

BACK AND FLANK

EXCISION

21920 Biopsy, soft tissue of back or flank; superficial

21925 deep

(For needle biopsy of soft tissue, use 20206)

21930 Excision, tumor, soft tissue of back or flank, subcutaneous; less than 3 cm

21931 3 cm or greater

21932 Excision, tumor, soft tissue of back or flank, subfascial (eg, intramuscular); less than 5 cm

21933 5 cm or greater

21935 Radical resection of tumor (eg, malignant neoplasm), soft tissue of back or flank; less than 5 cm

21936 5 cm or greater

SPINE (VERTEBRAL COLUMN)

To report bone grafts performed after arthrodesis, see 20930-20938. Do not append modifier 62 to bone graft codes 20900-20938.

For example, posterior arthrodesis of L5-S1 for degenerative disc disease utilizing morselized autogenous iliac bone graft harvested through a separate fascial incision. Report as 22612 and 20937.

Within the spine section, instrumentation is reported separately and in addition to arthrodesis. To report instrumentation procedures performed with definitive vertebral procedure(s), see 22840-22855. Instrumentation procedure codes 22840-22848 and 22851 are reported in addition to the definitive procedure(s). Modifier 62 may not be appended to the definitive or add-on spinal instrumentation procedure code(s) 22840-22848 and 22850-22852.

For example, posterior arthrodesis of L4-S1 utilizing morselized autogenous iliac bone graft harvested through separate fascial incision, and pedicle screw fixation. Report as 22612, 22614, 22842 and 20937.

When arthrodesis is performed in addition to another procedure, the arthrodesis should be reported in addition to the original procedure with modifier 51 (multiple

● New Code   ▲ Revised Code   + Add-On Code   ⊘ Modifier -51 Exempt   ⊙ Moderate Sedation

procedures). Examples are after osteotomy, fracture care, vertebral corpectomy, and laminectomy. Bone grafts and instrumentation are never performed without arthrodesis.

For example, treatment of a burst fracture of L2 by corpectomy followed by arthrodesis of L1-L3, utilizing anterior instrumentation L1-L3 and structural allograft. Report as 63090, 22558-51, 22585, 22845, and 20931.

When two surgeons work together as primary surgeons performing distinct part(s) of a single reportable procedure, each surgeon should report his/her distince operative work by appending modifier 62 to the single definitive procedure code. If additional procedure(s) (including add-on procedure[s]) are performed during the same surgical session, separate code(s) may be reported by each co-surgeon, with modifier 62 appended (see Appendix A).

> (Do not append modifier -62 to bone graft code 20931)
>
> (For injection procedure for myelography, use 62284)
>
> (For injection procedure for discography, see 62290, 62291)
>
> (For injection procedure, chemonucleolysis, single or multiple leveles, use 62292)
>
> (For injection procedure for facet joints, see 64490-64495, 64633--22-64636)
>
> (For needle or trocar biopsy, see 20220-20225)

INCISION

22010 Incision and drainage, open, of deep abscess (subfascial), posterior spine; cervical, thoracic, or cervicothoracic

22015   lumbar, sacral, or lumbosacral

> (Do not report 22015 in conjunction with 22010)
>
> (Do not report 22015 in conjunction with instrumentation removal, 10180, 22850, 22852)
>
> (For incision and drainage of abscess or hematoma, superficial, see 10060, 10140)

EXCISION

For the following codes, when two surgeons work together as primary surgeons performing distinct part(s) of partial vertebral body excision, each surgeon should report his/her distinct operative work by appending modifier 62 to the procedure code. In this situation, modifier 62 may be appended to the procedure code(s) 22100-22102, 22110-22114 and, as appropriate, to the associated additional

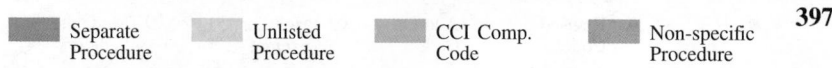

	Separate Procedure		Unlisted Procedure		CCI Comp. Code		Non-specific Procedure

vertebral segment add-on code(s) 22103, 22116 as long as both surgeons continue to work together as primary surgeons.

(For bone biopsy, see 20220-20251)

(To report soft tissue biopsy of back or flank, see 21920-21925)

(For needle biopsy of soft tissue, use 20206)

(To report excision of soft tissue tumor of back or flank, use 21930)

22100 Partial excision of posterior vertebral component (eg, spinous process, lamina or facet) for intrinsic bony lesion, single vertebral segment; cervical

22101 thoracic

22102 lumbar

(For insertion of posterior spinous process distraction devices, see 0171T, 0172T)

+ 22103 each additional segment (List separately in addition to code for primary procedure)

(Use 22103 in conjunction with codes 22100, 22101, 22102)

22110 Partial excision of vertebral body, for intrinsic bony lesion, without decompression of spinal cord or nerve root(s), single vertebral segment; cervical

22112 thoracic

22114 lumbar

+ 22116 each additional vertebral segment (List separately in addition to code for primary procedure)

(Use 22116 in conjunction with codes 22110, 22112, 22114)

(For complete or near complete resection of vertebral body, see vertebral corpectomy, 63081-63091)

(For spinal reconstruction with bone graft (autograft, allograft) and/or methacrylate of cervical vertebral body, use 63081 and 22554 and 20931 or 20938)

(For spinal reconstruction with bone graft (autograft, allograft) and/or methacrylate of thoracic vertebral body, use 63085 or 63087 and 22556 and 20931 or 20938)

● New Code ▲ Revised Code + Add-On Code ⊘ Modifier -51 Exempt ⊙ Moderate Sedation

(For spinal reconstruction with bone graft (autograft, allograft) and/or methacrylate of lumbar vertebral body, use 63087 or 63090 and 22558 and 20931 or 20938)

(For spinal reconstruction following vertebral body resection, use 63082 or 63086 or 63088 or 63091, and 22585)

(For harvest of bone autograft for vertebral reconstruction, see 20931 or 20938)

(For cervical spinal reconstruction with prosthetic replacement of resected vertebral bodies, see codes 63081 and 22554 and 20931 or 20938 and 22851)

(For thoracic spinal reconstruction with prosthetic replacement of resected vertebral bodies, see codes 63085 or 63087 and 22556 and 20931 or 20938 and 22851)

(For lumbar spinal reconstruction with prosthetic replacement of resected vertebral bodies, see codes 63087 or 63090 and 22558, and 20931 or 20938 and 22851)

(For osteotomy of spine, see 22210-22226)

OSTEOTOMY

To report arthrodesis, see codes 22590-22632. (Report in addition to code[s] for the definitive procedure with modifier -51.)

To report instrumentation procedures, see 22840-22855. (Report in addition to code[s] for the definitive procedure[s].) Do not append modifier -62 to spinal instrumentation codes 22840-22848 and 22850-22852.

To report bone graft procedures, see 20930-20938. (Report in addition to code[s] for the definitive procedure[s].) Do not append modifier -62 to bone graft codes 20900-20938.

For the following codes, when two surgeons work together as primary surgeons performing distinct part(s) of an anterior spine osteotomy, each surgeon should report his/her distinct operative work by appending modifier 62 to the procedure code. In this situation, modifier 62 may be appended to the procedure code(s) 22210-22214, 22220-22224 and, as appropriate, to associated additional segment add-on code(s) 22216, 22226 as long as both surgeons continue to work together as primary surgeons.

Spinal osteotomy procedures are reported when a portion(s) of the vertebral segment(s) is cut and removed in preparation for re-aligning the spine as part of a spinal deformity correction. For excision of an intrinsic lesion of the vertebra without deformity correction, see 22100-22116. For decompression of the spinal cord and/or nerve roots, see 63001-63308.

▉ Separate Procedure	▉ Unlisted Procedure	▉ CCI Comp. Code	▉ Non-specific Procedure

22206 Osteotomy of spine, posterior or posterolateral approach, 3 columns, 1 vertebral segment (eg, pedicle/vertebral body subtraction); thoracic

(Do not report 22206 in conjunction with 22207)

22207 lumbar

(Do not report 22207 in conjunction with 22206)

+ 22208 each additional vertebral segment (List separately in addition to code for primary procedure)

(Use 22208 in conjunction with 22206, 22207)

(Do not report 22206, 22207, 22208 in conjunction with 22210-22226, 22830, 63001-63048, 63055-63066, 63075-63091, 63101-63103, when performed at the same level)

22210 Osteotomy of spine, posterior or posterolateral approach, 1 vertebral segment; cervical

22212 thoracic

22214 lumbar

+ 22216 each additional vertebral segment (List separately in addition to primary procedure)

(Use 22216 in conjunction with codes 22210, 22212, 22214)

22220 Osteotomy of spine, including diskectomy, anterior approach, single vertebral segment; cervical

22222 thoracic

22224 lumbar

+ 22226 each additional vertebral segment (List separately in addition to code for primary procedure)

(Use 22226 in conjunction with codes 22220, 22222, 22224)

(For vertebral corpectomy, see 63081-63091)

FRACTURE AND/OR DISLOCATION

To report arthrodesis, see codes 22590-22632. (Report in addition to code[s] for the definitive procedure with modifier -51.)

---

400 ● New Code ▲ Revised Code ✛ Add-On Code ⊘ Modifier -51 Exempt ⊙ Moderate Sedation

To report instrumentation procedures, see 22840-22855. (Report in addition to code[s} for the definitive procedure[s].) Do not append modifier -62 to spinal instrumentation codes 22840-22848 and 22850-22852.

To report bone graft procedures, see 20930-20938. (Report in addition to code[s] for the definitive procedure[s].) Do not append modifier -62 to bone graft codes 20900-20938.

For the following codes, when two surgeons work together as primary surgeons performing distinct part(s) of open fracture and/or dislocation procedure(s), each surgeon should report his/her distinct operative work by appending modifier 62 to the procedure code. In this situation, modifier 62 may be appended to the procedure code(s) 22318-22327 and, as appropriate, the associated additional fracture vertebrae or dislocated segment add-on code 22328 as long as both surgeons continue to work together as primary surgeons.

22305　Closed treatment of vertebral process fracture(s)

22310　Closed treatment of vertebral body fracture(s), without manipulation, requiring and including casting or bracing

22315　Closed treatment of vertebral fracture(s) and/or dislocation(s) requiring casting or bracing, with and including casting and/or bracing, by manipulation or traction

(For spinal subluxation, use 97140)

22318　Open treatment and/or reduction of odontoid fracture(s) and or dislocation(s) (including os odontoideum), anterior approach, including placement of internal fixation; without grafting

22319　　with grafting

22325　Open treatment and/or reduction of vertebral fracture(s) and/or dislocation(s), posterior approach, 1 fractured vertebrae or dislocated segment; lumbar

22326　　cervical

22327　　thoracic

+ **22328**　　each additional fractured vertebrae or dislocated segment (List separately in addition to code for primary procedure)

(Use 22328 in conjunction with codes 22325, 22326, 22327)

| | Separate Procedure | | Unlisted Procedure | | CCI Comp. Code | | Non-specific Procedure | **401** |

(For treatment of vertebral fracture by the anterior approach, see corpectomy 63081-63091, and appropriate arthrodesis, bone graft and instrument codes)

(For decompression of spine following fracture, see 63001-63091; for arthrodesis of spine following fracture, see 22548-22632)

MANIPULATION

(For spinal manipulation without anesthesia, use 97140)

22505 Manipulation of spine requiring anesthesia, any region

VERTEBRAL BODY, EMBOLIZATION OR INJECTION

⊙ **22520** Percutaneous vertebroplasty (bone biopsy included when performed), 1 vertebral body, unilateral or bilateral injection; thoracic

⊙ **22521** lumbar

▲⊙+**22522** each additional thoracic or lumbar vertebral body (List separately in addition to code for primary procedure)

(Do not report 22520-22522 in conjunction with 20225, 22310-22315, 22325, 22327 when performed at the same level as 22520-22522)

(Use 22522 in conjunction with codes 22520, 22521 as appropriate)

(For radiological supervision and interpretation, see 72291, 72292)

22523 Percutaneous vertebral augmentation, including cavity creation (fracture reduction and bone biopsy included when performed) using mechanical device, 1 vertebral body, unilateral or bilateral cannulation (eg, kyphoplasty); thoracic

22524 lumbar

+ **22525** each additional thoracic or lumbar vertebral body (List separately in addition to code for primary procedure)

(Do not report 22523-22525 in conjunction with 20225, 22310-22315, 22325, 22327 when performed at the same level as 22523-22525)

(Use 22525 in conjunction with 22523, 22524)

● New Code   ▲ Revised Code   + Add-On Code   ⊘ Modifier -51 Exempt   ⊙ Moderate Sedation

(For radiological supervision and interpretation, see 72291, 72292)

⊙ **22526** Percutaneous intradiscal electrothermal annuloplasty, unilateral or bilateral including fluoroscopic guidance; single level

⊙+**22527** 1 or more additional levels (List separately in addition to code for primary procedure)

(Use 22527 in conjunction with 22526)

(Do not report codes 22526, 22527 in conjunction with 77002, 77003)

(For percutaneous intradiscal annuloplasty using method other than electrothermal, use 22899)

ARTHRODESIS

Arthrodesis may be performed in the absence of other procedures and therefore when it is combined with another definitive procedure (eg., osteotomy, fracture care, vertebral corpectomy, or laminectomy), modifier 51 is appropriate. However, arthrodesis codes 22585, 22614, and 22632 are considered add-on procedure codes and should not be used with modifier 51.

To report instrumentation procedures, see 22840-22855. (Codes 22840-22848, 22851 are reported in conjunction with code[s] for the definitive procedure[s]. When instrumentation reinsertion or removal is reported in conjunction with other definitive procedures including arthrodesis, decompression, and exploration of fusion, append modifier -51 to 22849, 22850, 22852, and 22855.) To report exploration of fusion, use 22830. (When exploration is reported in conjunction with other definitive procedures, including arthrodesis and decompression, append modifier -51 to 22830.) Do not append modifier -62 to spinal instrumentation codes 22840-22848 and 22850-22852.

To report bone graft procedures, see 20930-20938. (Report in addition to code[s] for the definitive procedure[s].) Do not append modifier -62 to bone graft codes 20900-20938.

Lateral Extracavitary Approach Technique

22532 Arthrodesis, lateral extracavitary technique, including minimal diskectomy to prepare interspace (other than for decompression); thoracic

22533 lumbar

+ **22534** thoracic or lumbar, each additional vertebral segment (List separately in addition to code for primary procedure)

	Separate Procedure		Unlisted Procedure		CCI Comp. Code		Non-specific Procedure

(Use 22534 in conjunction with 22532 and 22533)

Anterior or Anterolateral Approach Technique

Procedure codes 22554-22558 are for SINGLE interspace; for additional interspaces, use 22585. A vertebral interspace is the non-bony compartment between two adjacent vertebral bodies, which contains the intervertebral disc, and includes the nucleus pulposus, annulus fibrosus, and two cartilagenous endplates.

For the following codes, when two surgeons work together as primary surgeons performing distinct part(s) of an anterior interbody arthrodesis, each surgeon should report his/her distinct operative work by appending modifier 62 to the procedure code. In this situation, modifier 62 may be appended to the procedure code(s) 22548-22558 and, as appropriate, to the associated additional interspace add-on code 22585 as long as both surgeons continue to work together as primary surgeons.

22548 Arthrodesis, anterior transoral or extraoral technique, clivus-C1-C2 (atlas-axis), with or without excision of odontoid process

(For intervertebral disc excision by laminotomy or laminectomy, see 63020-63042)

22551 Arthrodesis, anterior interbody, including disc space preparation, discectomy, osteophytectomy and decompression of spinal cord and/or nerve roots, cervical below C2;

+ 22552 each additional interspace (list separately in addition to code for separate procedure)

(Use 22552 in conjunction with 22551)

22554 Arthrodesis, anterior interbody technique, including minimal diskectomy to prepare interspace (other than for decompression); cervical below C2

(Do not report 22554 in conjunction with 63075, even if performed by a separate individual. To report anterior cervical discectomy and interbody fusion at the same level during the same session, use 22551)

22556 thoracic

22558 lumbar

(For arthrodesis using pre-sacral interbody technique, see 22586, 0195T)

● New Code ▲ Revised Code + Add-On Code ⊘ Modifier -51 Exempt ⊙ Moderate Sedation

+ 22585   each additional interspace (List separately in addition to code for primary procedure)

(Use 22585 in conjunction with codes 22554, 22556, 22558)

(Do not report 22585 in conjunction with 63075 even if performed by a separate individual. To report anterior cervical discectomy and interbody fusion at the same level during the same session, use 22552)

● **22586**   Arthrodesis, pre-sacral interbody technique, including disc space preparation, discectomy, with posterior instrumentation, wiht image guidance, includes bone graft when performed, L5-S1 interspace

(Do not report 22586 in conjunction with 20930-20938, 22840, 22848, 72275, 77002, 77003, 77011, 77012)

Posterior, Posterolateral or Lateral Transverse Process Technique

To report instrumentation procedures, see 22840-22855. (Report in addition to code[s] for the definitive procedure[s].) Do not append modifier -62 to spinal instrumentation codes 22840-22848 and 22850-22852.

To report bone graft procedures, see 20930-20938. (Report in addition to code[s] for the definitive procedure[s].) Do not append modifier -62 to bone graft codes 20900-20938.

22590   Arthrodesis, posterior technique, craniocervical (occiput-C2)

22595   Arthrodesis, posterior technique, atlas-axis (C1-C2)

22600   Arthrodesis, posterior or posterolateral technique, single level; cervical below C2 segment

22610   thoracic (with lateral transverse technique, when performed)

22612   lumbar (with lateral transverse technique, when performed)

(Do not report 22612 in conjunction with 22630 for the same interspace and segment, use 22633)

+ 22614   each additional vertebral segment (List separately in addition to code for primary procedure)

(Use 22614 in conjunction with 22600, 22610, 22612, 22630 or 22633 when performed at a different level. When performing a posterior or posterolateral technique for fusion/arthrodesis at an additional level, use 22614. When performing a posterior interbody fusion arthrodesis at an additional level, use 22632.

405

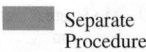 Separate Procedure   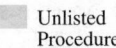 Unlisted Procedure   CCI Comp. Code   Non-specific Procedure

When performing a combined posterior or posterolateral technique with posterior interbody arthrodesis at an additional level, use 22634)

(For facet joint fusion, see 0219T-0222T)

(For placement of a posterior intrafacet implant, see 0219T-0222T)

22630 Arthrodesis, posterior interbody technique, including laminectomy and/or diskectomy to prepare interspace (other than for decompression), single interspace; lumbar

(Do not report 22630 in conjunction with 22612 for the same interspace and segment, use 22633)

+ 22632 each additional interspace (List separately in addition to code for primary procedure)

(Use 22632 in conjunction with 22612, 22630, or 22633 when performed at a different level. When peforming a posterior interbody fusion arthrodesis at an additional level, use 22632. When performing a posterior or posterolateral technique for fusion/arthrodesis at an additional level, use 22614. When performing a combined posterior or posterolateral technique with posterior interbody arthrodesis at an additional level, use 22634)

22633 Arthrodesis, combined posterior or posterolateral technique with posterior interbody technique including laminectomy and/or discectomy sufficient to prepare interspace (other than for decompression), single interspace and segment; lumbar

(Do not report with 22612 or 22630 at the same level)

+ 22634 each additional interspace and segment (List separately in addition to code for primary procedure)

(Use 22634 in conjunction with 22633)

Spine Deformity (eg, Scoliosis, Kyphosis)

To report instrumentation procedures, see 22840-22855. (Report in addition to code[s] for the definitive procedure[s].) Do not append modifier -62 to spinal instrumentation codes 22840-22848 and 22850-22852.

To report bone graft procedures, see 20930-20938. (Report in addition to code[s] for the definitive procedure[s].) Do not append modifier -62 to bone graft codes 20900-20938.

● New Code   ▲ Revised Code   + Add-On Code   ⊘ Modifier -51 Exempt   ⊙ Moderate Sedation

For the following codes, when two surgeons work together as primary surgeons performing distinct part(s) of an arthrodesis for spinal deformity, each surgeon should report his/her distinct operative work by appending modifier 62 to the procedure code. In this situation, modifier 62 may be appended to procedure code(s) 22800-22819 as long as both surgeons continue to work together as primary surgeons.

22800   Arthrodesis, posterior, for spinal deformity, with or without cast; up to 6 vertebral segments

22802   7 to 12 vertebral segments

22804   13 or more vertebral segments

22808   Arthrodesis, anterior, for spinal deformity, with or without cast; 2 to 3 vertebral segments

22810   4 to 7 vertebral segments

22812   8 or more vertebral segments

22818   Kyphectomy, circumferential exposure of spine and resection of vertebral segment(s) (including body and posterior elements); single or 2 segments

22819   3 or more segments

(To report arthrodesis, see 22800-22804 and add modifier -51)

EXPLORATION

To report instrumentation procedures, see 22840-22855. (Codes 22840-22848 and 22851 are reported in conjunction with code[s] for the definitive procedure[s]. When instrumentation reinsertion or removal is reported in conjunction with other definitive procedures including arthrodesis, decompression, and exploration of fusion, append modifier -51 to 22849, 22850, 22852 and 22855.)

Code 22849 shoould not be reported with 22850, 22852, and 22855 at the same spinal levels. To report exploration of fusion, see 22830. (When exploration is reported in conjunction with other definitive procedures, including arthrodesis and decompression, append modifier -51 to 22830.)

(To report bone graft procedures, see 20930-20938)

22830   Exploration of spinal fusion

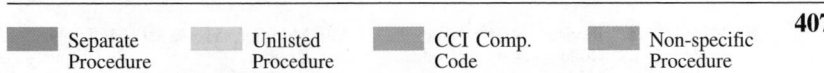

| | Separate Procedure | | Unlisted Procedure | | CCI Comp. Code | | Non-specific Procedure |

SPINAL INSTRUMENTATION

Insertion of spinal instrumentation is reported separately and in addition to arthrodesis. Instrumentation procedure codes 22840-22848 and 22851 are reported in addition to the definitive procedure(s). Do not append modifier -62 to spinal instrumentation codes 22840-22848 and 22850-22852.

To report bone graft procedures, see 20930-20938. (Report in addition to code[s] for definitive procedure[s].) Do not append modifier -62 to bone graft codes 20900-20938.

Codes 22849, 22850, 22852, and 22855 are subject to modifier 51 if reported with other definitive procedure(s), including arthrodesis, decompression, and exploration of fusion. Code 22849 should not be reported in conjincyion with 22850, 22852, and 22855 at the same spinal levels. Only the appropriate insertion code (22840-22848) should be reported when previously placed spinal instrumentation is being removed or revised during the same session where new instrumentation is inserted at levels including all or part of the previously instrumented segments. Do not report the reinsertion (22849) or removal (22850, 22852, 22855) procedures in addition to the insertion of the new instrumentation (22840-22848).

+ 22840 Posterior non-segmental instrumentation (eg, Harrington rod technique, pedicle fixation across 1 interspace, atlantoaxial transarticular screw fixation, sublaminar wiring at C1, facet screw fixation) (List separately in addition to code for primary procedure)

(Use 22840 in conjunction with 22100-22102, 22110-22114, 22206, 22207, 22210-22214, 22220-22224, 22305-22327, 22532, 22533, 22548-22558, 22590-22612, 22630, 22633, 22634, 22800-22812, 63001-63030, 63040-63042, 63045-63047, 63050-63056, 63064, 63075, 63077, 63081, 63085, 63087, 63090, 63101, 63102, 63170-63290, 63300-63307)

(For insertion of posterior spinous process distraction devices, see 0171T, 0172T)

+ 22841 Internal spinal fixation by wiring of spinous processes (List separately in addition to code for primary procedure)

(Use 22841 in conjunction with 22100-22102, 22110-22114, 22206, 22207, 22210-22214, 22220-22224, 22305-22327, 22532, 22533, 22548-22558, 22590-22612, 22630, 22633, 22634, 22800-22812, 63001-63030, 63040-63042, 63045-63047, 63050-63056, 63064, 63075, 63077, 63081, 63085, 63087, 63090, 63101, 63102, 63170-63290, 63300-63307)

+ 22842 Posterior segmental instrumentation (eg, pedicle fixation, dual rods with multiple hooks and sublaminar wires); 3 to 6 vertebral segments (List separately in addition to code for primary procedure)

(Use 22842 in conjunction with 22100-22102, 22110-22114, 22206, 22207, 22210-22214, 22220-22224, 22305-22327, 22532, 22533, 22548-22558, 22590-22612, 22630, 22633, 22634, 22800-22812, 63001-63030, 63040-63042, 63045-63047, 63050-63056, 63064, 63075, 63077, 63081, 63085, 63087, 63090, 63101, 63102, 63170-63290, 63300-63307)

+ 22843 7 to 12 vertebral segments (List separately in addition to code for primary procedure)

(Use 22843 in conjunction with 22100-22102, 22110-22114, 22206, 22207, 22210-22214, 22220-22224, 22305-22327, 22532, 22533, 22548-22558, 22590-22612, 22630, 22633, 22634, 22800-22812, 63001-63030, 63040-63042, 63045-63047, 63050-63056, 63064, 63075, 63077, 63081, 63085, 63087, 63090, 63101, 63102, 63170-63290, 63300-63307)

+ 22844 13 or more vertebral segments (List separately in addition to code for primary procedure)

(Use 22844 in conjunction with 22100-22102, 22110-22114, 22206, 22207, 22210-22214, 22220-22224, 22305-22327, 22532, 22533, 22548-22558, 22590-22612, 22630, 22633, 22634, 22800-22812, 63001-63030, 63040-63042, 63045-63047, 63050-63056, 63064, 63075, 63077, 63081, 63085, 63087, 63090, 63101, 63102, 63170-63290, 63300-633077)

+ 22845 Anterior instrumentation; 2 to 3 vertebral segments (List separately in addition to code for primary procedure)

(Use 22845 in conjunction with 22100-22102, 22110-22114, 22206, 22207, 22210-22214, 22220-22224, 22305-22327, 22532, 22533, 22548-22558, 22590-22612, 22630, 22633, 22634, 22800-22812, 63001-63030, 63040-63042, 63045-63047, 63050-63056, 63064, 63075, 63077, 63081, 63085, 63087, 63090, 63101, 63102, 63170-63290, 63300-63307)

+ 22846 4 to 7 vertebral segments (List separately in addition to code for primary procedure)

(Use 22846 in conjunction with 22100-22102, 22110-22114, 22206, 22207, 22210-22214, 22220-22224, 22305-22327, 22532, 22533, 22548-22558, 22590-22612, 22630, 22633, 22634, 22800-22812, 63001-63030, 63040-63042, 63045-63047,

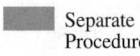 Separate Procedure   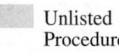 Unlisted Procedure   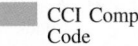 CCI Comp. Code   Non-specific Procedure

63050-63056, 63064, 63075, 63077, 63081, 63085, 63087, 63090, 63101, 63102, 63170-63290, 63300-63307)

+ 22847   8 or more vertebral segments (List separately in addition to code for primary procedure)

(Use 22847 in conjunction with 22100-22102, 22110-22114, 22206, 22207, 22210-22214, 22220-22224, 22305-22327, 22532, 22533, 22548-22558, 22590-22612, 22630, 22633, 22634, 22800-22812, 63001-63030, 63040-63042, 63045-63047, 63050-63056, 63064, 63075, 63077, 63081, 63085, 63087, 63090, 63101, 63102, 63170-63290, 63300-63307)

+ 22848   Pelvic fixation (attachment of caudal end of instrumentation to pelvic bony structures) other than sacrum (List separately in addition to code for primary procedure)

(Use 22848 in conjunction with 22100-22102, 22110-22114, 22206, 22207, 22210-22214, 22220-22224, 22305-22327, 22532, 22533, 22548-22558, 22590-22612, 22630, 22633, 22634, 22800-22812, 63001-63030, 63040-63042, 63045-63047, 63050-63056, 63064, 63075, 63077, 63081, 63085, 63087, 63090, 63101, 63102, 63170-63290, 63300-63307)

22849   Reinsertion of spinal fixation device

22850   Removal of posterior nonsegmental instrumentation (eg, Harrington rod)

+ 22851   Application of intervertebral biomechanical device(s) (eg, synthetic cage(s), methylmethacrylate) to vertebral defect or interspace (List separately in addition to code for primary procedure)

(Use 22851 in conjunction with 22100-22102, 22110-22114, 22206, 22207, 22210-22214, 22220-22224, 22305-22327, 22532, 22533, 22548-22558, 22590-22612, 22630, 22633, 22634, 22800-22812, 63001-63030, 63040-63042, 63045-63047, 63050-63056, 63064, 63075, 63077, 63081, 63085, 63087, 63090, 63101, 63102, 63170-63290, 63300-63307)

(For application of an intervertebral bone device/graft, see 20930-20938)

(For insertion of posterior spinous process distraction devices, see 0171T, 0172T)

22852   Removal of posterior segmental instrumentation

22855   Removal of anterior instrumentation

410

● New Code	▲ Revised Code	+ Add-On Code	⊘ Modifier -51 Exempt	⊙ Moderate Sedation

22856 Total disc arthroplasty (artificial disc), anterior approach, including discectomy with end plate preparation (includes osteophytectomy for nerve root or spinal cord decompression and microdissection), single interspace, cervical

(Do not report 22856 in conjunction with 22554, 22845, 22851, 63075 when performed at the same level)

(Do not report 22856 in conjunction with 69990)

(For additional interspace cervical total disc arthroplasty, use 0092T)

22857 Total disc arthroplasty (artificial disc), anterior approach, including discectomy to prepare interspace (other than for decompression), single interspace, lumbar

(Do not report 22857 in conjunction with 22558, 22845, 22851, 49010 when performed at the same level)

(For additional interspace, use Category III code 0163T)

22861 Revision including replacement of total disc arthroplasty (artificial disc), anterior approach, single interspace; cervical

(Do not report 22861 in conjunction with 22845, 22851, 22864, 63075 when performed at the same level)

(Do not report 22861 in conjunction with 69990)

(For additional interspace revision of cervical total disc arthroplasty, use 0098T)

22862 lumbar

(Do not report 22862 in conjunction with 22558, 22845, 22851, 22865, 49010 when performed at the same level)

(For additional interspace, use Category III code 0165T)

22864 Removal of total disc arthroplasty (artificial disc), anterior approach single interspace; cervical

(Do not report 22864 in conjunction with 22861, 69990)

(For additional interspace removal of cervical total disc arthroplasty, use 0095T)

22865 lumbar

(Do not report 22865 in conjunction with 49010)

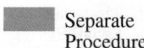 Separate
Procedure

Unlisted
Procedure

CCI Comp.
Code

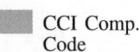 Non-specific
Procedure

411

(For additional interspace, use Category III code 0164T)

(22856-22865 include fluoroscopy when performed)

(For decompression, see 63001-63048)

OTHER PROCEDURES

22899 Unlisted procedure, spine

ABDOMEN

EXCISION

22900 Excision, tumor, soft tissue of abdominal wall, subfascial (eg, intramuscular); less than 5 cm

22901 5 cm or greater

22902 Excision, tumor, soft tissue of abdominal wall, subcutaneous; less than 3 cm

22903 3 cm or greater

22904 Radical resection of tumor (eg, malignant neoplasm), soft tissue of abdominal wall; less than 5 cm

22905 5 cm or greater

OTHER PROCEDURES

22999 Unlisted procedure, abdomen, musculoskeletal system

SHOULDER

INCISION

23000 Removal of subdeltoid calcareous deposits, open

(For arthroscopic removal of bursal deposits, use 29999)

23020 Capsular contracture release (eg, Sever type procedure)

(For incision and drainage procedures, superficial, see 10040-10160)

23030 Incision and drainage, shoulder area; deep abscess or hematoma

---

● New Code   ▲ Revised Code   + Add-On Code   ⊘ Modifier -51 Exempt   ⊙ Moderate Sedation

23031   infected bursa

23035   Incision, bone cortex (eg, osteomyelitis or bone abscess), shoulder area

23040   Arthrotomy, glenohumeral joint, including exploration, drainage, or removal of foreign body

23044   Arthrotomy, acromioclavicular, sternoclavicular joint, including exploration, drainage, or removal of foreign body

EXCISION

23065   Biopsy, soft tissue of shoulder area; superficial

23066   deep

          (For needle biopsy of soft tissue, use 20206)

23071   This code is out of order. See page 413

23073   This code is out of order. See page 413

23075   Excision, tumor, soft tissue of shoulder area, subcutaneous; less than 3 cm

23071   3 cm or greater

23076   Excision, tumor, soft tissue of shoulder area, subfascial (eg, intramuscular); less than 5 cm

23073   5 cm or greater

23077   Radical resection of tumor (eg, malignant neoplasm), soft tissue of shoulder area; less than 5 cm

23078   5 cm or greater

23100   Arthrotomy, glenohumeral joint, including biopsy

23101   Arthrotomy, acromioclavicular joint or sternoclavicular joint, including biopsy and/or excision of torn cartilage

23105   Arthrotomy; glenohumeral joint, with synovectomy, with or without biopsy

---

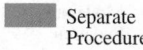 Separate Procedure   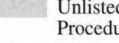 Unlisted Procedure   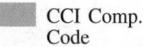 CCI Comp. Code   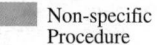 Non-specific Procedure   **413**

23106   sternoclavicular joint, with synovectomy, with or without biopsy

23107   Arthrotomy, glenohumeral joint, with joint exploration, with or without removal of loose or foreign body

23120   Claviculectomy; partial

(For arthroscopic procedure, use 29824)

23125   total

23130   Acromioplasty or acromionectomy, partial, with or without coracoacromial ligament release

23140   Excision or curettage of bone cyst or benign tumor of clavicle or scapula;

23145   with autograft (includes obtaining graft)

23146   with allograft

23150   Excision or curettage of bone cyst or benign tumor of proximal humerus;

23155   with autograft (includes obtaining graft)

23156   with allograft

23170   Sequestrectomy (eg, for osteomyelitis or bone abscess), clavicle

23172   Sequestrectomy (eg, for osteomyelitis or bone abscess), scapula

23174   Sequestrectomy (eg, for osteomyelitis or bone abscess), humeral head to surgical neck

23180   Partial excision (craterization, saucerization, or diaphysectomy) bone (eg, osteomyelitis), clavicle

23182   Partial excision (craterization, saucerization, or diaphysectomy) bone (eg, osteomyelitis), scapula

23184   Partial excision (craterization, saucerization, or diaphysectomy) bone (eg, osteomyelitis), proximal humerus

23190   Ostectomy of scapula, partial (eg, superior medial angle)

● New Code   ▲ Revised Code   + Add-On Code   ⊘ Modifier -51 Exempt   ⊙ Moderate Sedation

SURGERY

23195 Resection, humeral head

(For replacement with implant, use 23470)

23200 Radical resection of tumor; clavicle

23210 scapula

23220 Radical resection of tumor, proximal humerus

(23221 Deleted 2009 [2010 edition])

(23222 Deleted 2009 [2010 edition])

INTRODUCTION OR REMOVAL

(For arthrocentesis or needling of bursa, use 20610)

(For K-wire or pin insertion or removal, see 20650, 20670, 20680)

23330 Removal of foreign body, shoulder; subcutaneous

23331 deep (eg, Neer hemiarthroplasty removal)

23332 complicated (eg, total shoulder)

(Do not report 23331, 23332 in conjunction with 23473, 23474 if a prosthesis [ie, humeral and/or glenoid component(s)] is being removed adn replaced in the same shoulder)

23350 Injection procedure for shoulder arthrography or enhanced CT/MRI shoulder arthrography

(For radiographic arthrography, radiological supervision and interpretation, use 73040. Fluoroscopy [77002] is inclusive of radiographic arthrography)

(When fluoroscopic guided injection is performed for enhanced CT arthrography, use 23350, 77002 and 73201 or 73202)

(When fluoroscopic guided injection is performed for enhanced MR arthrography, use codes 23350, 77002, and 73222 or 73223)

(For enhanced CT or enhanced MRI arthrography, use 77002 and either 73201, 73202, 73222 or 73223)

(To report biopsy of the shoulder and joint, see 29805-29826)

415

Separate Procedure | Unlisted Procedure | CCI Comp. Code | Non-specific Procedure

CPT codes and descriptions only ©2012 American Medical Association. All rights reserved.

REPAIR, REVISION AND/OR RECONSTRUCTION

23395   Muscle transfer, any type, shoulder or upper arm; single

23397   multiple

23400   Scapulopexy (eg, Sprengels deformity or for paralysis)

23405   Tenotomy, shoulder area; single tendon

23406   multiple tendons through same incision

23410   Repair of ruptured musculotendinous cuff (eg, rotator cuff) open; acute

23412   chronic

(For arthroscopic procedure, use 29827)

23415   Coracoacromial ligament release, with or without acromioplasty

(For arthroscopic procedure, use 29826)

23420   Reconstruction of complete shoulder (rotator) cuff avulsion, chronic (includes acromioplasty)

23430   Tenodesis of long tendon of biceps

(For arthroscopic biceps tenodesis, use 29828)

23440   Resection or transplantation of long tendon of biceps

23450   Capsulorrhaphy, anterior; Putti-Platt procedure or Magnuson type operation

(To report arthroscopic thermal capsulorrhaphy, use 29999)

23455   with labral repair (eg, Bankart procedure)

(For arthroscopic procedure, use 29806)

23460   Capsulorrhaphy, anterior, any type; with bone block

23462   with coracoid process transfer

(To report open thermal capsulorrhaphy, use 23929)

---

416   ● New Code   ▲ Revised Code   + Add-On Code   ⊘ Modifier -51 Exempt   ⊙ Moderate Sedation

23465 Capsulorrhaphy, glenohumeral joint, posterior, with or without bone block

(For sternoclavicular and acromioclavicular reconstruction, see 23530, 23550)

23466 Capsulorrhaphy, glenohumeral joint, any type multi-directional instability

23470 Arthroplasty, glenohumeral joint; hemiarthroplasty

23472 total shoulder (glenoid and proximal humeral replacement (eg, total shoulder))

(For removal of total shoulder implants, see 23331, 23332)

(For osteotomy, proximal humerus, use 24400)

● **23473** Revision of total shoulder arthroplasty, including allograft when performed; humeral **or** glenoid component

● **23474** humeral **and** glenoid component

(Do not report 23473, 23474 in conjunction with 23331, 23332 if a prosthesis [ie, humeral and/or glenoid component(s)] is being removed and replaced in the same shoulder)

23480 Osteotomy, clavicle, with or without internal fixation;

23485 with bone graft for nonunion or malunion (includes obtaining graft and/or necessary fixation)

23490 Prophylactic treatment (nailing, pinning, plating or wiring) with or without methylmethacrylate; clavicle

23491 proximal humerus

FRACTURE AND/OR DISLOCATION

23500 Closed treatment of clavicular fracture; without manipulation

23505 with manipulation

23515 Open treatment of clavicular fracture, includes internal fixation, when performed

23520 Closed treatment of sternoclavicular dislocation; without manipulation

	Separate Procedure		Unlisted Procedure		CCI Comp. Code		Non-specific Procedure

23525   with manipulation

23530   Open treatment of sternoclavicular dislocation, acute or chronic;

23532   with fascial graft (includes obtaining graft)

23540   Closed treatment of acromioclavicular dislocation; without manipulation

23545   with manipulation

23550   Open treatment of acromioclavicular dislocation, acute or chronic;

23552   with fascial graft (includes obtaining graft)

23570   Closed treatment of scapular fracture; without manipulation

23575   with manipulation, with or without skeletal traction (with or without shoulder joint involvement)

23585   Open treatment of scapular fracture (body, glenoid or acromion) includes internal fixation when performed

23600   Closed treatment of proximal humeral (surgical or anatomical neck) fracture; without manipulation

23605   with manipulation, with or without skeletal traction

23615   Open treatment of proximal humeral (surgical or anatomical neck) fracture, includes internal fixation, when performed includes repair of tuberosity(-ies) when performed;

23616   with proximal humeral prosthetic replacement

23620   Closed treatment of greater humeral tuberosity fracture; without manipulation

23625   with manipulation

23630   Open treatment of greater humeral tuberosity fracture, includes internal fixation, when performed

23650   Closed treatment of shoulder dislocation, with manipulation; without anesthesia

---

418   ● New Code   ▲ Revised Code   + Add-On Code   ⊘ Modifier -51 Exempt   ⊙ Moderate Sedation

23655   requiring anesthesia

23660   Open treatment of acute shoulder dislocation

(Repairs for recurrent dislocations, see 23450-23466)

23665   Closed treatment of shoulder dislocation, with fracture of greater humeral tuberosity, with manipulation

23670   Open treatment of shoulder dislocation, with fracture of greater humeral tuberosity, includes internal fixation, when performed

23675   Closed treatment of shoulder dislocation, with surgical or anatomical neck fracture, with manipulation

23680   Open treatment of shoulder dislocation, with surgical or anatomical neck fracture, includes internal fixation, when performed

MANIPULATION

23700   Manipulation under anesthesia, shoulder joint, including application of fixation apparatus (dislocation excluded)

ARTHRODESIS

23800   Arthrodesis, glenohumeral joint;

23802   with autogenous graft (includes obtaining graft)

AMPUTATION

23900   Interthoracoscapular amputation (forequarter)

23920   Disarticulation of shoulder;

23921   secondary closure or scar revision

OTHER PROCEDURES

23929   Unlisted procedure, shoulder

| | Separate Procedure | | Unlisted Procedure | | CCI Comp. Code | | Non-specific Procedure |

HUMERUS (UPPER ARM) AND ELBOW

The elbow area includes the head and neck of the radius and olecranon process.

INCISION

(For incision and drainage procedures, superficial, see 10040-10160)

23930 Incision and drainage, upper arm or elbow area; deep abscess or hematoma

23931 bursa

23935 Incision, deep, with opening of bone cortex (eg, for osteomyelitis or bone abscess), humerus or elbow

24000 Arthrotomy, elbow, including exploration, drainage, or removal of foreign body

24006 Arthrotomy of the elbow, with capsular excision for capsular release (separate procedure)

EXCISION

24065 Biopsy, soft tissue of upper arm or elbow area; superficial

24066 deep (subfascial or intramuscular)

(For needle biopsy of soft tissue, use 20206)

24071 This code is out of order. See page 420

24073 This code is out of order. See page 420

24075 Excision, tumor, soft tissue of upper arm or elbow area, subcutaneous; less than 3 cm

24071 3 cm or greater

24076 Excision, tumor, soft tissue of upper arm or elbow area, subfascial (eg, intramuscular); less than 5 cm

24073 5 cm or greater

24077 Radical resection of tumor (eg, malignant neoplasm), soft tissue of upper arm or elbow area; less than 5 cm

● New Code   ▲ Revised Code   + Add-On Code   ⊘ Modifier -51 Exempt   ⊙ Moderate Sedation

24079   5 cm or greater

24100   Arthrotomy, elbow; with synovial biopsy only

24101   with joint exploration, with or without biopsy, with or without removal of loose or foreign body

24102   with synovectomy

24105   Excision, olecranon bursa

24110   Excision or curettage of bone cyst or benign tumor, humerus;

24115   with autograft (includes obtaining graft)

24116   with allograft

24120   Excision or curettage of bone cyst or benign tumor of head or neck of radius or olecranon process;

24125   with autograft (includes obtaining graft)

24126   with allograft

24130   Excision, radial head

         (For replacement with implant, use 24366)

24134   Sequestrectomy (eg, for osteomyelitis or bone abscess), shaft or distal humerus

24136   Sequestrectomy (eg, for osteomyelitis or bone abscess), radial head or neck

24138   Sequestrectomy (eg, for osteomyelitis or bone abscess), olecranon process

24140   Partial excision (craterization, saucerization, or diaphysectomy) bone (eg, osteomyelitis), humerus

24145   Partial excision (craterization, saucerization, or diaphysectomy) bone (eg, osteomyelitis), radial head or neck

24147   Partial excision (craterization, saucerization, or diaphysectomy) bone (eg, osteomyelitis), olecranon process

---

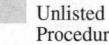 Separate Procedure   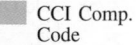 Unlisted Procedure   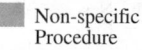 CCI Comp. Code   Non-specific Procedure

24149 Radical resection of capsule, soft tissue, and heterotopic bone, elbow, with contracture release (separate procedure)

(For capsular and soft tissue release only, use 24006)

24150 Radical resection of tumor, shaft or distal humerus

(24151 Deleted 2009 [2010 edition])

24152 Radical resection of tumor, radial head or neck

(24153 Deleted 2009 [2010 edition])

24155 Resection of elbow joint (arthrectomy)

INTRODUCTION OR REMOVAL

(For K-wire or pin insertion or removal, see 20650, 20670, 20680)

(For arthrocentesis or needling of bursa or joint, use 20605)

24160 Implant removal; elbow joint

(Do not report 24160 in conjunction with 24370 or 24371 if a prosthesis [ie, humeral and/or ulnar component(s)] is being removed and replaced in the same elbow)

24164 radial head

24200 Removal of foreign body, upper arm or elbow area; subcutaneous

24201 deep (subfascial or intramuscular)

24220 Injection procedure for elbow arthrography

(For radiological supervision and interpretation, use 73085. Do not report 77002 in addition to 73085)

(For injection of tennis elbow, use 20550)

REPAIR, REVISION, AND/OR RECONSTRUCTION

24300 Manipulation, elbow, under anesthesia

(For application of external fixation, see 20690 or 20692)

● New Code   ▲ Revised Code   + Add-On Code   ⊘ Modifier -51 Exempt   ⊙ Moderate Sedation

24301 Muscle or tendon transfer, any type, upper arm or elbow, single (excluding 24320-24331)

24305 Tendon lengthening, upper arm or elbow, each tendon

24310 Tenotomy, open, elbow to shoulder, each tendon

24320 Tenoplasty, with muscle transfer, with or without free graft, elbow to shoulder, single (Seddon-Brookes type procedure)

24330 Flexor-plasty, elbow (eg, Steindler type advancement);

24331   with extensor advancement

24332 Tenolysis, triceps

24340 Tenodesis of biceps tendon at elbow (separate procedure)

24341 Repair, tendon or muscle, upper arm or elbow, each tendon or muscle, primary or secondary (excludes rotator cuff)

24342 Reinsertion of ruptured biceps or triceps tendon, distal, with or without tendon graft

24343 Repair lateral collateral ligament, elbow, with local tissue

24344 Reconstruction lateral collateral ligament, elbow, with tendon graft (includes harvesting of graft)

24345 Repair medial collateral ligament, elbow, with local tissue

24346 Reconstruction medial collateral ligament, elbow, with tendon graft (includes harvesting of graft)

24357 Tenotomy, elbow, lateral or medial (eg, epicondylitis, tennis elbow, golfer's elbow); percutaneous

24358   debridement, soft tissue and/or bone, open

24359   debridement, soft tissue and/or bone, open with tendon repair or reattachment

(Do not report 24357-24359 in conjunction with 29837, 29838)

24360 Arthroplasty, elbow; with membrane (eg, fascial)

Separate Procedure | Unlisted Procedure | CCI Comp. Code | Non-specific Procedure

24361	with distal humeral prosthetic replacement
24362	with implant and fascia lata ligament reconstruction
24363	with distal humerus and proximal ulnar prosthetic replacement (eg, total elbow)

(For revision of total elbow implant, see 24370, 24371)

24365	Arthroplasty, radial head;
24366	with implant

● **24370** Revision of total elbow arthroplasty, including allograft when performed; humeral **or** ulnar component

● **24371** humeral **and** ulnar component

(Do not report 24370, 24371 in conjunction with 24160 if a prosthesis [ie, humeral and/or ulnar component(s)] is being removed and replaced in the same elbow)

24400	Osteotomy, humerus, with or without internal fixation
24410	Multiple osteotomies with realignment on intramedullary rod, humeral shaft (Sofield type procedure)
24420	Osteoplasty, humerus (eg, shortening or lengthening) (excluding 64876)
24430	Repair of nonunion or malunion, humerus; without graft (eg, compression technique)
24435	with iliac or other autograft (includes obtaining graft)

(For proximal radius and/or ulna, see 25400-25420)

24470	Hemiepiphyseal arrest (eg, cubitus varus or valgus, distal humerus)
24495	Decompression fasciotomy, forearm, with brachial artery exploration
24498	Prophylactic treatment (nailing, pinning, plating or wiring), with or without methylmethacrylate, humeral shaft

---

● New Code   ▲ Revised Code   + Add-On Code   ⊘ Modifier -51 Exempt   ⊙ Moderate Sedation

FRACTURE AND/OR DISLOCATION

24500 Closed treatment of humeral shaft fracture; without manipulation

24505 with manipulation, with or without skeletal traction

24515 Open treatment of humeral shaft fracture with plate/screws, with or without cerclage

24516 Treatment of humeral shaft fracture, with insertion of intramedullary implant, with or without cerclage and/or locking screws

24530 Closed treatment of supracondylar or transcondylar humeral fracture, with or without intercondylar extension; without manipulation

24535 with manipulation, with or without skin or skeletal traction

24538 Percutaneous skeletal fixation of supracondylar or transcondylar humeral fracture, with or without intercondylar extension

24545 Open treatment of humeral supracondylar or transcondylar fracture, includes internal fixation, when performed; without intercondylar extension

24546 with intercondylar extension

24560 Closed treatment of humeral epicondylar fracture, medial or lateral; without manipulation

24565 with manipulation

24566 Percutaneous skeletal fixation of humeral epicondylar fracture, medial or lateral, with manipulation

24575 Open treatment of humeral epicondylar fracture, medial or lateral, includes internal fixation, when performed

24576 Closed treatment of humeral condylar fracture, medial or lateral; without manipulation

24577 with manipulation

24579 Open treatment of humeral condylar fracture, medial or lateral, includes internal fixation, when performed

	Separate Procedure		Unlisted Procedure		CCI Comp. Code		Non-specific Procedure

425

(To report closed treatment of fractures without manipulation, see 24530, 24560, 24576, 24650, 24670)

(To report closed treatment of fractures with manipulation, see 24535, 24565, 24577, 24675)

24582 Percutaneous skeletal fixation of humeral condylar fracture, medial or lateral, with manipulation

24586 Open treatment of periarticular fracture and/or dislocation of the elbow (fracture distal humerus and proximal ulna and/or proximal radius);

24587 with implant arthroplasty

(See also 24361)

24600 Treatment of closed elbow dislocation; without anesthesia

24605 requiring anesthesia

24615 Open treatment of acute or chronic elbow dislocation

24620 Closed treatment of Monteggia type of fracture dislocation at elbow (fracture proximal end of ulna with dislocation of radial head), with manipulation

24635 Open treatment of Monteggia type of fracture dislocation at elbow (fracture proximal end of ulna with dislocation of radial head), includes internal fixation, when performed

24640 Closed treatment of radial head subluxation in child, nursemaid elbow, with manipulation

24650 Closed treatment of radial head or neck fracture; without manipulation

24655 with manipulation

24665 Open treatment of radial head or neck fracture, includes internal fixation or radial head excision, when performed;

24666 with radial head prosthetic replacement

24670 Closed treatment of ulnar fracture, proximal end (eg, olecranon or coronoid process[es]); without manipulation

● New Code   ▲ Revised Code   + Add-On Code   ⊘ Modifier -51 Exempt   ⊙ Moderate Sedation

24675   with manipulation

24685   Open treatment of ulnar fracture proximal end (eg, olecranon or coronoid process[es]), includes internal fixation, when performed

(Do not report 24685 in conjunction with 24100-24102)

ARTHRODESIS

24800   Arthrodesis, elbow joint; local

24802   with autogenous graft (includes obtaining graft)

AMPUTATION

24900   Amputation, arm through humerus; with primary closure

24920   open, circular (guillotine)

24925   secondary closure or scar revision

24930   re-amputation

24931   with implant

24935   Stump elongation, upper extremity

24940   Cineplasty, upper extremity, complete procedure

OTHER PROCEDURES

24999   Unlisted procedure, humerus or elbow

FOREARM AND WRIST

INCISION

25000   Incision, extensor tendon sheath, wrist (eg, deQuervains disease)

(For decompression median nerve or for carpal tunnel syndrome, use 64721)

25001   Incision, flexor tendon sheath, wrist (eg, flexor carpi radialis)

427

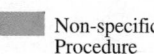

| ▮ Separate Procedure | ▮ Unlisted Procedure | ▮ CCI Comp. Code | ▮ Non-specific Procedure |

25020 Decompression fasciotomy, forearm and/or wrist, flexor OR extensor compartment; without debridement of nonviable muscle and/or nerve

25023 with debridement of nonviable muscle and/or nerve

(For decompression fasciotomy with brachial artery exploration, use 24495)

(For incision and drainage procedures, superficial, see 10040-10160)

(For debridement, see also 11000-11044)

25024 Decompression fasciotomy, forearm and/or wrist, flexor AND extensor compartment; without debridement of nonviable muscle and/or nerve

25025 with debridement of nonviable muscle and/or nerve

25028 Incision and drainage, forearm and/or wrist; deep abscess or hematoma

25031 bursa

25035 Incision, deep, bone cortex, forearm and/or wrist (eg, osteomyelitis or bone abscess)

25040 Arthrotomy, radiocarpal or midcarpal joint, with exploration, drainage, or removal of foreign body

EXCISION

25065 Biopsy, soft tissue of forearm and/or wrist; superficial

25066 deep (subfascial or intramuscular)

(For needle biopsy of soft tissue, use 20206)

25071 This code is out of order. See page 428

25073 This code is out of order. See page 429

25075 Excision, tumor, soft tissue of forearm and/or wrist area, subcutaneous; less than 3 cm

25071 3 cm or greater

25076 Excision, tumor, soft tissue of forearm and/or wrist area, subfascial (eg, intramuscular); less than 3 cm

25073 3 cm or greater

25077 Radical resection of tumor (eg, malignant neoplasm), soft tissue of forearm and/or wrist area; less than 3 cm

25078 3 cm or greater

25085 Capsulotomy, wrist (eg, contracture)

25100 Arthrotomy, wrist joint; with biopsy

25101 with joint exploration, with or without biopsy, with or without removal of loose or foreign body

25105 with synovectomy

25107 Arthrotomy, distal radioulnar joint including repair of triangular cartilage, complex

25109 Excision of tendon, forearm and/or wrist, flexor or extensor, each

25110 Excision, lesion of tendon sheath, forearm and/or wrist

25111 Excision of ganglion, wrist (dorsal or volar); primary

25112 recurrent

(For hand or finger, use 26160)

25115 Radical excision of bursa, synovia of wrist, or forearm tendon sheaths (eg, tenosynovitis, fungus, Tbc, or other granulomas, rheumatoid arthritis); flexors

25116 extensors, with or without transposition of dorsal retinaculum

(For finger synovectomies, use 26145)

25118 Synovectomy, extensor tendon sheath, wrist, single compartment;

25119 with resection of distal ulna

429

	Separate Procedure		Unlisted Procedure		CCI Comp. Code		Non-specific Procedure

25120 Excision or curettage of bone cyst or benign tumor of radius or ulna (excluding head or neck of radius and olecranon process);

(For head or neck of radius or olecranon process, see 24120-24126)

25125 with autograft (includes obtaining graft)

25126 with allograft

25130 Excision or curettage of bone cyst or benign tumor of carpal bones;

25135 with autograft (includes obtaining graft)

25136 with allograft

25145 Sequestrectomy (eg, for osteomyelitis or bone abscess), forearm and/or wrist

25150 Partial excision (craterization, saucerization, or diaphysectomy) of bone (eg, for osteomyelitis); ulna

25151 radius

(For head or neck of radius or olecranon process, see 24145, 24147)

25170 Radical resection of tumor, radius or ulna

25210 Carpectomy; 1 bone

(For carpectomy with implant, see 25441-25445)

25215 all bones of proximal row

25230 Radial styloidectomy (separate procedure)

25240 Excision distal ulna partial or complete (eg, Darrach type or matched resection)

(For implant replacement, distal ulna, use 25442)

(For obtaining fascia for interposition, see 20920, 20922)

● New Code   ▲ Revised Code   + Add-On Code   ⊘ Modifier -51 Exempt   ⊙ Moderate Sedation

INTRODUCTION OR REMOVAL

(For K-wire, pin or rod insertion or removal, see 20650, 20670, 20680)

25246 Injection procedure for wrist arthrography

(For radiological supervision and interpretation, use 73115. Do not report 77002 in addition to 73115)

(For foreign body removal, superficial use 20520)

25248 Exploration with removal of deep foreign body, forearm or wrist

25250 Removal of wrist prosthesis; (separate procedure)

25251 complicated, including total wrist

25259 Manipulation, wrist, under anesthesia

(For application of external fixation, see 20690 or 20692)

REPAIR, REVISION, AND/OR RECONSTRUCTION

25260 Repair, tendon or muscle, flexor, forearm and/or wrist; primary, single, each tendon or muscle

25263 secondary, single, each tendon or muscle

25265 secondary, with free graft (includes obtaining graft), each tendon or muscle

25270 Repair, tendon or muscle, extensor, forearm and/or wrist; primary, single, each tendon or muscle

25272 secondary, single, each tendon or muscle

25274 secondary, with free graft (includes obtaining graft), each tendon or muscle

25275 Repair, tendon sheath, extensor, forearm and/or wrist, with free graft (includes obtaining graft) (eg, for extensor carpi ulnaris subluxation)

25280 Lengthening or shortening of flexor or extensor tendon, forearm and/or wrist, single, each tendon

---

431

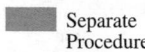 Separate Procedure

Unlisted Procedure

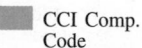 CCI Comp. Code

Non-specific Procedure

25290 Tenotomy, open, flexor or extensor tendon, forearm and/or wrist, single, each tendon

25295 Tenolysis, flexor or extensor tendon, forearm and/or wrist, single, each tendon

25300 Tenodesis at wrist; flexors of fingers

25301 extensors of fingers

25310 Tendon transplantation or transfer, flexor or extensor, forearm and/or wrist, single; each tendon

25312 with tendon graft(s) (includes obtaining graft), each tendon

25315 Flexor origin slide (eg, for cerebral palsy, Volkmann contracture), forearm and/or wrist;

25316 with tendon(s) transfer

25320 Capsulorrhaphy or reconstruction, wrist, open (eg, capsulodesis, ligament repair, tendon transfer or graft) (includes synovectomy, capsulotomy and open reduction) for carpal instability

25332 Arthroplasty, wrist, with or without interposition, with or without external or internal fixation

(For obtaining fascia for interposition, see 20920, 20922)

(For prosthetic replacement arthroplasty, see 25441-25446)

25335 Centralization of wrist on ulna (eg, radial club hand)

25337 Reconstruction for stabilization of unstable distal ulna or distal radioulnar joint, secondary by soft tissue stabilization (eg, tendon transfer, tendon graft or weave, or tenodesis) with or without open reduction of distal radioulnar joint

(For harvesting of fascia lata graft, see 20920, 20922)

25350 Osteotomy, radius; distal third

25355 middle or proximal third

25360 Osteotomy; ulna

25365 radius AND ulna

432 ● New Code ▲ Revised Code + Add-On Code ⊘ Modifier -51 Exempt ⊙ Moderate Sedation

25370	Multiple osteotomies, with realignment on intramedullary rod (Sofield type procedure); radius OR ulna
25375	radius AND ulna
25390	Osteoplasty, radius OR ulna; shortening
25391	lengthening with autograft
25392	Osteoplasty, radius AND ulna; shortening (excluding 64876)
25393	lengthening with autograft
25394	Osteoplasty, carpal bone, shortening
25400	Repair of nonunion or malunion, radius OR ulna; without graft (eg, compression technique)
25405	with autograft (includes obtaining graft)
25415	Repair of nonunion or malunion, radius AND ulna; without graft (eg, compression technique)
25420	with autograft (includes obtaining graft)
25425	Repair of defect with autograft; radius OR ulna
25426	radius AND ulna
25430	Insertion of vascular pedicle into carpal bone (eg, Hori procedure)
25431	Repair of nonunion of carpal bone (excluding carpal scaphoid (navicular) (includes obtaining graft and necessary fixation), each bone
25440	Repair of nonunion, scaphoid carpal (navicular) bone, with or without radial styloidectomy (includes obtaining graft and necessary fixation)
25441	Arthroplasty with prosthetic replacement; distal radius
25442	distal ulna
25443	scaphoid carpal (navicular)

								433
	Separate Procedure		Unlisted Procedure		CCI Comp. Code		Non-specific Procedure	

25444	lunate
25445	trapezium
25446	distal radius and partial or entire carpus (total wrist)
25447	Arthroplasty, interposition, intercarpal or carpometacarpal joints

(For wrist arthroplasty, use 25332)

25449	Revision of arthroplasty, including removal of implant, wrist joint
25450	Epiphyseal arrest by epiphysiodesis or stapling; distal radius OR ulna
25455	distal radius AND ulna
25490	Prophylactic treatment (nailing, pinning, plating or wiring) with or without methylmethacrylate; radius
25491	ulna
25492	radius AND ulna

FRACTURE AND/OR DISLOCATION

(For application of external fixation in addition to internal fixation, use 20690 and the appropriate internal fixation code)

25500	Closed treatment of radial shaft fracture; without manipulation
25505	with manipulation
25515	Open treatment of radial shaft fracture, includes internal fixation, when performed
25520	Closed treatment of radial shaft fracture and closed treatment of dislocation of distal radioulnar joint (Galeazzi fracture/dislocation)
25525	Open treatment of radial shaft fracture, includes internal fixation, when performed, and closed treatment of distal radioulnar joint dislocation (Galeazzi fracture/dislocation), includes percutaneous skeletal fixation, when performed

● New Code	▲ Revised Code	+ Add-On Code	⊘ Modifier -51 Exempt	⊙ Moderate Sedation

25526 Open treatment of radial shaft fracture, includes internal fixation, when performed, and open treatment, of distal radioulnar joint dislocation (Galeazzi fracture/dislocation), includes internal fixation, when performed, includes repair of triangular fibrocartilage complex

25530 Closed treatment of ulnar shaft fracture; without manipulation

25535 with manipulation

25545 Open treatment of ulnar shaft fracture, includes internal fixation, when performed

25560 Closed treatment of radial and ulnar shaft fractures; without manipulation

25565 with manipulation

25574 Open treatment of radial AND ulnar shaft fractures, with internal fixation, when performed; of radius OR ulna

25575 of radius AND ulna

25600 Closed treatment of distal radial fracture (eg, Colles or Smith type) or epiphyseal separation, includes closed treatment of fracture of ulnar styloid, when performed; without manipulation

25605 with manipulation

(Do not report 25600, 25605 in conjunction with 25650)

25606 Percutaneous skeletal fixation of distal radial fracture or epiphyseal separation

(Do not report 25606 in conjunction with 25650)

(For percutaneous treatment of ulnar styloid fracture, use 25651)

(For open treatment of ulnar styloid fracture, use 25652)

25607 Open treatment of distal radial extra-articular fracture or epiphyseal separation, with internal fixation

(Do not report 25607 in conjunction with 25650)

(For percutaneous treatment of ulnar styloid fracture, use 25651)

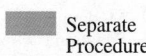 Separate Procedure   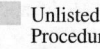 Unlisted Procedure   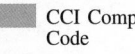 CCI Comp. Code   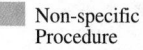 Non-specific Procedure   **435**

(For open treatment of ulnar styloid fracture, use 25652)

25608 Open treatment of distal radial intra-articular fracture or epiphyseal separation; with internal fixation of 2 fragments

(Do not report 25608 in conjunction with 25609)

25609 with internal fixation of 3 or more fragments

(Do not report 25608, 25609 in conjunction with 25650)

(For percutaneous treatment of ulnar styloid fracture, use 25651)

(For open treatment of ulnar styloid fracture, use 25652)

25622 Closed treatment of carpal scaphoid (navicular) fracture; without manipulation

25624 with manipulation

25628 Open treatment of carpal scaphoid (navicular) fracture, includes internal fixation, when performed

25630 Closed treatment of carpal bone fracture (excluding carpal scaphoid [navicular]); without manipulation, each bone

25635 with manipulation, each bone

25645 Open treatment of carpal bone fracture (other than carpal scaphoid [navicular]), each bone

25650 Closed treatment of ulnar styloid fracture

(Do not report 25650 in conjunction with 25600, 25605, 25607-25609)

25651 Percutaneous skeletal fixation of ulnar styloid fracture

25652 Open treatment of ulnar styloid fracture

25660 Closed treatment of radiocarpal or intercarpal dislocation, 1 or more bones, with manipulation

25670 Open treatment of radiocarpal or intercarpal dislocation, 1 or more bones

25671 Percutaneous skeletal fixation of distal radioulnar dislocation

● New Code ▲ Revised Code + Add-On Code ⊘ Modifier -51 Exempt ⊙ Moderate Sedation

25675 Closed treatment of distal radioulnar dislocation with manipulation

25676 Open treatment of distal radioulnar dislocation, acute or chronic

25680 Closed treatment of trans-scaphoperilunar type of fracture dislocation, with manipulation

25685 Open treatment of trans-scaphoperilunar type of fracture dislocation

25690 Closed treatment of lunate dislocation, with manipulation

25695 Open treatment of lunate dislocation

ARTHRODESIS

25800 Arthrodesis, wrist; complete, without bone graft (includes radiocarpal and/or intercarpal and/or carpometacarpal joints)

25805   with sliding graft

25810   with iliac or other autograft (includes obtaining graft)

25820 Arthrodesis, wrist; limited, without bone graft (eg, intercarpal or radiocarpal)

25825   with autograft (includes obtaining graft)

25830 Arthrodesis, distal radioulnar joint with segmental resection of ulna, with or without bone graft (eg, Sauve-Kapandji procedure)

AMPUTATION

25900 Amputation, forearm, through radius and ulna;

25905   open, circular (guillotine)

25907   secondary closure or scar revision

25909   re-amputation

25915 Krukenberg procedure

25920 Disarticulation through wrist;

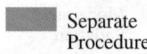 Separate Procedure   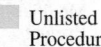 Unlisted Procedure   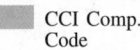 CCI Comp. Code   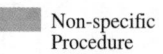 Non-specific Procedure

25922 secondary closure or scar revision

25924 re-amputation

25927 Transmetacarpal amputation;

25929 secondary closure or scar revision

25931 re-amputation

OTHER PROCEDURES

25999 Unlisted procedure, forearm or wrist

HAND AND FINGERS

INCISION

26010 Drainage of finger abscess; simple

26011 complicated (eg, felon)

26020 Drainage of tendon sheath, digit and/or palm, each

26025 Drainage of palmar bursa; single, bursa

26030 multiple bursa

26034 Incision, bone cortex, hand or finger (eg, osteomyelitis or bone abscess)

26035 Decompression fingers and/or hand, injection injury (eg, grease gun)

26037 Decompressive fasciotomy, hand (excludes 26035)

(For injection injury, use 26035)

26040 Fasciotomy, palmar (eg, Dupuytren's contracture); percutaneous

26045 open, partial

(For palmar fasciotomy by enzyme injection (eg, collagenase), see 20527, 26341)

(For fasciectomy, see 26121-26125)

● New Code   ▲ Revised Code   ✚ Add-On Code   ⊘ Modifier -51 Exempt   ☉ Moderate Sedation

26055 Tendon sheath incision (eg, for trigger finger)

26060 Tenotomy, percutaneous, single, each digit

26070 Arthrotomy, with exploration, drainage, or removal of loose or foreign body; carpometacarpal joint

26075 metacarpophalangeal joint, each

26080 interphalangeal joint, each

EXCISION

26100 Arthrotomy with biopsy; carpometacarpal joint, each

26105 metacarpophalangeal joint, each

26110 interphalangeal joint, each

26111 This code is out of order. See page 439

26113 This code is out of order. See page 439

26115 Excision, tumor or vascular malformation, soft tissue of hand or finger, subcutaneous; less than 1.5 cm

26111 1.5 cm or greater

26116 Excision, tumor or vascular malformation, soft tissue of hand or finger, subfascial (eg, intramuscular); less than 1.5 cm

26113 1.5 cm or greater

26117 Radical resection of tumor (eg, malignant neoplasm), soft tissue of hand or finger; less than 3 cm

26118 3 cm or greater

26121 Fasciectomy, palm only, with or without Z-plasty, other local tissue rearrangement, or skin grafting (includes obtaining graft)

26123 Fasciectomy, partial palmar with release of single digit including proximal interphalangeal joint, with or without Z-plasty, other local tissue rearrangement, or skin grafting (includes obtaining graft);

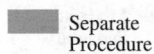 Separate Procedure   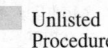 Unlisted Procedure   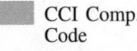 CCI Comp. Code   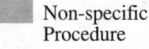 Non-specific Procedure

+ 26125   each additional digit (List separately in addition to code for primary procedure)

(Use 26125 in conjunction with code 26123)

(For palmar fasciotomy by enzyme injection (eg, collagenase), see 20527, 26341)

(For fasciotomy, see 26040, 26045)

26130   Synovectomy, carpometacarpal joint

26135   Synovectomy, metacarpophalangeal joint including intrinsic release and extensor hood reconstruction, each digit

26140   Synovectomy, proximal interphalangeal joint, including extensor reconstruction, each interphalangeal joint

26145   Synovectomy, tendon sheath, radical (tenosynovectomy), flexor tendon, palm and/or finger, each tendon

(For tendon sheath synovectomies at wrist, see 25115, 25116)

26160   Excision of lesion of tendon sheath or joint capsule (eg, cyst, mucous cyst, or ganglion), hand or finger

(For wrist ganglion, see 25111, 25112)

(For trigger digit, use 26055)

26170   Excision of tendon, palm, flexor or extensor, single, each tendon

(Do not report 26170 in conjunction with 26390, 26415)

26180   Excision of tendon, finger, flexor or extensor, each tendon

(Do not report 26180 in conjunction with 26390, 26415)

26185   Sesamoidectomy, thumb or finger (separate procedure)

26200   Excision or curettage of bone cyst or benign tumor of metacarpal;

26205   with autograft (includes obtaining graft)

26210   Excision or curettage of bone cyst or benign tumor of proximal, middle, or distal phalanx of finger;

440

● New Code	▲ Revised Code	+ Add-On Code	⊘ Modifier -51 Exempt	⊙ Moderate Sedation

26215 with autograft (includes obtaining graft)

26230 Partial excision (craterization, saucerization, or diaphysectomy) bone (eg, osteomyelitis); metacarpal

26235 proximal or middle phalanx of finger

26236 distal phalanx of finger

26250 Radical resection of tumor, metacarpal

(26255 Deleted 2009 [2010 edition])

26260 Radical resection of tumor, proximal or middle phalanx of finger

(26261 Deleted 2009 [2010 edition])

26262 Radical resection of tumor, distal phalanx of finger

INTRODUCTION OR REMOVAL

26320 Removal of implant from finger or hand

(For removal of foreign body in hand or finger, see 20520, 20525)

REPAIR, REVISION, AND/OR RECONSTRUCTION

26340 Manipulation, finger joint, under anesthesia, each joint

(For application of external fixation, see 20690 or 20692)

26341 Manipulation, palmar fascial cord (ie, Dupuytren's cord), post enzyme injection (eg, collagenase), single cord

(For enzyme injection (eg, collagenase), palmar fascial cord (eg., Dupuytren's contracture), use 20527)

(Report custom orthotic fabrication/application separately)

26350 Repair or advancement, flexor tendon, not in zone 2 digital flexor tendon sheath (eg, no man's land); primary or secondary without free graft, each tendon

26352 secondary with free graft (includes obtaining graft), each tendon

---

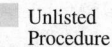 Separate Procedure

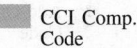 Unlisted Procedure

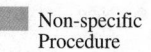 CCI Comp. Code

Non-specific Procedure

441

26356 Repair or advancement, flexor tendon, in zone 2 digital flexor tendon sheath (eg, no man's land); primary, without free graft, each tendon

26357 secondary, without free graft, each tendon

26358 secondary with free graft (includes obtaining graft), each tendon

26370 Repair or advancement of profundus tendon, with intact superficialis tendon; primary, each tendon

26372 secondary with free graft (includes obtaining graft), each tendon

26373 secondary without free graft, each tendon

26390 Excision flexor tendon, with implantation of synthetic rod for delayed tendon graft, hand or finger, each rod

26392 Removal of synthetic rod and insertion of flexor tendon graft, hand or finger (includes obtaining graft), each rod

26410 Repair, extensor tendon, hand, primary or secondary; without free graft, each tendon

26412 with free graft (includes obtaining graft), each tendon

26415 Excision of extensor tendon, with implantation of synthetic rod for delayed tendon graft, hand or finger, each rod

26416 Removal of synthetic rod and insertion of extensor tendon graft (includes obtaining graft), hand or finger, each rod

26418 Repair, extensor tendon, finger, primary or secondary; without free graft, each tendon

26420 with free graft (includes obtaining graft) each tendon

26426 Repair of extensor tendon, central slip, secondary (eg, boutonniere deformity); using local tissue(s), including lateral band(s), each finger

26428 with free graft (includes obtaining graft), each finger

● New Code ▲ Revised Code + Add-On Code ⊘ Modifier -51 Exempt ⊙ Moderate Sedation

26432 Closed treatment of distal extensor tendon insertion, with or without percutaneous pinning (eg, mallet finger)

26433 Repair of extensor tendon, distal insertion, primary or secondary; without graft (eg, mallet finger)

26434 with free graft (includes obtaining graft)

(For tenovaginotomy for trigger finger, use 26055)

26437 Realignment of extensor tendon, hand, each tendon

26440 Tenolysis, flexor tendon; palm OR finger, each tendon

26442 palm AND finger, each tendon

26445 Tenolysis, extensor tendon, hand or finger; each tendon

26449 Tenolysis, complex, extensor tendon, finger, including forearm, each tendon

26450 Tenotomy, flexor, palm, open, each tendon

26455 Tenotomy, flexor, finger, open, each tendon

26460 Tenotomy, extensor, hand or finger, open, each tendon

26471 Tenodesis; of proximal interphalangeal joint, each joint

26474 of distal joint, each joint

26476 Lengthening of tendon, extensor, hand or finger, each tendon

26477 Shortening of tendon, extensor, hand or finger, each tendon

26478 Lengthening of tendon, flexor, hand or finger, each tendon

26479 Shortening of tendon, flexor, hand or finger, each tendon

26480 Transfer or transplant of tendon, carpometacarpal area or dorsum of hand; without free graft, each tendon

26483 with free tendon graft (includes obtaining graft), each tendon

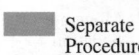 Separate Procedure 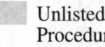 Unlisted Procedure 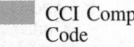 CCI Comp. Code 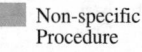 Non-specific Procedure

26485 Transfer or transplant of tendon, palmar; without free tendon graft, each tendon

26489 with free tendon graft (includes obtaining graft), each tendon

26490 Opponensplasty; superficialis tendon transfer type, each tendon

26492 tendon transfer with graft (includes obtaining graft), each tendon

26494 hypothenar muscle transfer

26496 other methods

(For thumb fusion in opposition, use 26820)

26497 Transfer of tendon to restore intrinsic function; ring and small finger

26498 all 4 fingers

26499 Correction claw finger, other methods

26500 Reconstruction of tendon pulley, each tendon; with local tissues (separate procedure)

26502 with tendon or fascial graft (includes obtaining graft) (separate procedure)

26508 Release of thenar muscle(s) (eg, thumb contracture)

26510 Cross intrinsic transfer, each tendon

26516 Capsulodesis, metacarpophalangeal joint; single digit

26517 2 digits

26518 3 or 4 digits

26520 Capsulectomy or capsulotomy; metacarpophalangeal joint, each joint

26525 interphalangeal joint, each joint

(To report carpometacarpal joint arthroplasty, use 25447)

● New Code   ▲ Revised Code   ✚ Add-On Code   ⊘ Modifier -51 Exempt   ⊙ Moderate Sedation

26530 Arthroplasty, metacarpophalangeal joint; each joint

26531 with prosthetic implant, each joint

26535 Arthroplasty, interphalangeal joint; each joint

26536 with prosthetic implant, each joint

26540 Repair of collateral ligament, metacarpophalangeal or interphalangeal joint

26541 Reconstruction, collateral ligament, metacarpophalangeal joint, single; with tendon or fascial graft (includes obtaining graft)

26542 with local tissue (eg, adductor advancement)

26545 Reconstruction, collateral ligament, interphalangeal joint, single, including graft, each joint

26546 Repair non-union, metacarpal or phalanx, (includes obtaining bone graft with or without external or internal fixation)

26548 Repair and reconstruction, finger, volar plate, interphalangeal joint

26550 Pollicization of a digit

26551 Transfer, toe-to-hand with microvascular anastomosis; great toe wrap-around with bone graft

(For great toe with web space, use 20973)

26553 other than great toe, single

26554 other than great toe, double

(Do not report code 69990 in addition to codes 26551-26554)

26555 Transfer, finger to another position without microvascular anastomosis

26556 Transfer, free toe joint, with microvascular anastomosis

(Do not report code 69990 in addition to code 26556)

(To report great toe-to-hand transfer, use 20973)

445

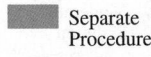 Separate
Procedure

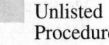 Unlisted
Procedure

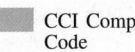 CCI Comp.
Code

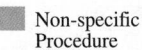 Non-specific
Procedure

26560 Repair of syndactyly (web finger) each web space; with skin flaps

26561 with skin flaps and grafts

26562 complex (eg, involving bone, nails)

26565 Osteotomy; metacarpal, each

26567 phalanx of finger, each

26568 Osteoplasty, lengthening, metacarpal or phalanx

26580 Repair cleft hand

26587 Reconstruction of polydactylous digit, soft tissue and bone

(For excision of polydactylous digit, soft tissue only, use 11200)

26590 Repair macrodactylia, each digit

26591 Repair, intrinsic muscles of hand, each muscle

26593 Release, intrinsic muscles of hand, each muscle

26596 Excision of constricting ring of finger, with multiple Z-plasties

(To report release of scar contracture or graft repairs, see 11042, 14040-14041, or 15120, 15240)

FRACTURE AND/OR DISLOCATION

26600 Closed treatment of metacarpal fracture, single; without manipulation, each bone

26605 with manipulation, each bone

26607 Closed treatment of metacarpal fracture, with manipulation, with external fixation, each bone

26608 Percutaneous skeletal fixation of metacarpal fracture, each bone

26615 Open treatment of metacarpal fracture, single, includes internal fixation, when performed, each bone

● New Code ▲ Revised Code + Add-On Code ⊘ Modifier -51 Exempt ⊙ Moderate Sedation

26641 Closed treatment of carpometacarpal dislocation, thumb, with manipulation

26645 Closed treatment of carpometacarpal fracture dislocation, thumb (Bennett fracture), with manipulation

26650 Percutaneous skeletal fixation of carpometacarpal fracture dislocation, thumb (Bennett fracture), with manipulation

26665 Open treatment of carpometacarpal fracture dislocation, thumb (Bennett fracture), includes internal fixation, when performed

26670 Closed treatment of carpometacarpal dislocation, other than thumb, with manipulation, each joint; without anesthesia

26675 requiring anesthesia

26676 Percutaneous skeletal fixation of carpometacarpal dislocation, other than thumb, with manipulation, each joint

26685 Open treatment of carpometacarpal dislocation, other than thumb; includes internal fixation, when performed, each joint

26686 complex, multiple or delayed reduction

26700 Closed treatment of metacarpophalangeal dislocation, single, with manipulation; without anesthesia

26705 requiring anesthesia

26706 Percutaneous skeletal fixation of metacarpophalangeal dislocation, single, with manipulation

26715 Open treatment of metacarpophalangeal dislocation, single, includes internal fixation, when performed

26720 Closed treatment of phalangeal shaft fracture, proximal or middle phalanx, finger or thumb; without manipulation, each

26725 with manipulation, with or without skin or skeletal traction, each

26727 Percutaneous skeletal fixation of unstable phalangeal shaft fracture, proximal or middle phalanx, finger or thumb, with manipulation, each

---

447

	Separate Procedure		Unlisted Procedure		CCI Comp. Code		Non-specific Procedure

26735   Open treatment of phalangeal shaft fracture, proximal or middle phalanx, finger or thumb, includes internal fixation, when performed, each

26740   Closed treatment of articular fracture, involving metacarpophalangeal or interphalangeal joint; without manipulation, each

26742   with manipulation, each

26746   Open treatment of articular fracture, involving metacarpophalangeal or interphalangeal joint, includes internal fixation, when performed, each

26750   Closed treatment of distal phalangeal fracture, finger or thumb; without manipulation, each

26755   with manipulation, each

26756   Percutaneous skeletal fixation of distal phalangeal fracture, finger or thumb, each

26765   Open treatment of distal phalangeal fracture, finger or thumb, includes internal fixation, when performed, each

26770   Closed treatment of interphalangeal joint dislocation, single, with manipulation; without anesthesia

26775   requiring anesthesia

26776   Percutaneous skeletal fixation of interphalangeal joint dislocation, single, with manipulation

26785   Open treatment of interphalangeal joint dislocation, includes internal fixation, when performed, single

ARTHRODESIS

26820   Fusion in opposition, thumb, with autogenous graft (includes obtaining graft)

26841   Arthrodesis, carpometacarpal joint, thumb, with or without internal fixation;

26842   with autograft (includes obtaining graft)

● New Code   ▲ Revised Code   ✚ Add-On Code   ⊘ Modifier -51 Exempt   ⊙ Moderate Sedation

26843   Arthrodesis, carpometacarpal joint, digit, other than thumb, each;

26844   with autograft (includes obtaining graft)

26850   Arthrodesis, metacarpophalangeal joint, with or without internal fixation;

26852   with autograft (includes obtaining graft)

26860   Arthrodesis, interphalangeal joint, with or without internal fixation;

+ 26861   each additional interphalangeal joint (List separately in addition to code for primary procedure)

(Use 26861 in conjunction with code 26860)

26862   with autograft (includes obtaining graft)

+ 26863   with autograft (includes obtaining graft), each additional joint (List separately in addition to code for primary procedure)

(Use 26863 in conjunction with code 26862)

AMPUTATION

(For hand through metacarpal bones, use 25927)

26910   Amputation, metacarpal, with finger or thumb (ray amputation), single, with or without interosseous transfer

(For repositioning see 26550, 26555)

26951   Amputation, finger or thumb, primary or secondary, any joint or phalanx, single, including neurectomies; with direct closure

26952   with local advancement flaps (V-Y, hood)

(For repair of soft tissue defect requiring split or full thickness graft or other pedicle flaps, see 15050-15758)

OTHER PROCEDURES

26989   Unlisted procedure, hands or fingers

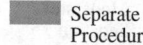 Separate Procedure   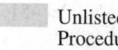 Unlisted Procedure   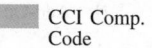 CCI Comp. Code   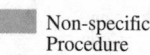 Non-specific Procedure   **449**

PELVIS AND HIP JOINT

INCISION

(For incision and drainage procedures, superficial, see 10040-10160)

26990 Incision and drainage, pelvis or hip joint area; deep abscess or hematoma

26991 infected bursa

26992 Incision, bone cortex, pelvis and/or hip joint (eg, osteomyelitis or bone abscess)

27000 Tenotomy, adductor of hip, percutaneous (separate procedure)

27001 Tenotomy, adductor of hip, open

(To report bilateral procedures, report 27001 with modifier -50)

27003 Tenotomy, adductor, subcutaneous, open, with obturator neurectomy

(To report bilateral procedures, report 27003 with modifier -50)

27005 Tenotomy, hip flexor(s), open (separate procedure)

27006 Tenotomy, abductors and/or extensor(s) of hip, open (separate procedure)

27025 Fasciotomy, hip or thigh, any type

(To report bilateral procedures, report 27025 with modifier -50)

27027 Decompression fasciotomy(ies), pelvic (buttock) compartment(s) (eg, gluteus medius-minimus, gluteus maximus, iliopsoas, and/or tensor fascia lata muscle), unilateral

(To report bilateral procedure, report 27027 with modifier 50)

27030 Arthrotomy, hip, with drainage (eg, infection)

27033 Arthrotomy, hip, including exploration or removal of loose or foreign body

27035 Denervation, hip joint, intrapelvic or extrapelvic intra-articular branches of sciatic, femoral, or obturator nerves

---

450

● New Code	▲ Revised Code	✚ Add-On Code	⊘ Modifier -51 Exempt	⊙ Moderate Sedation

(For obturator neurectomy, see 64763, 64766)

27036 Capsulectomy or capsulotomy, hip, with or without excision of heterotopic bone, with release of hip flexor muscles (ie, gluteus medius, gluteus minimus, tensor fascia latae, rectus femoris, sartorius, iliopsoas)

EXCISION

27040 Biopsy, soft tissue of pelvis and hip area; superficial

27041   deep, subfascial or intramuscular

    (For needle biopsy of soft tissue, use 20206)

27043   This code is out of order. See page 451

27045   This code is out of order. See page 451

27047 Excision, tumor, soft tissue of pelvis and hip area, subcutaneous; less than 3 cm

27043   3 cm or greater

27048 Excision, tumor, soft tissue of pelvis and hip area, subfascial (eg, intramuscular); less than 5 cm

27045   5 cm or greater

27049 Radical resection of tumor (eg, malignant neoplasm), soft tissue of pelvis and hip area; less than 5 cm

27059   5 cm or greater

27050 Arthrotomy, with biopsy; sacroiliac joint

27052   hip joint

27054 Arthrotomy with synovectomy, hip joint

27057 Decompression fasciotomy(ies), pelvic (buttock) compartment(s) (eg, gluteus medius-minimus, gluteus maximus, iliopsoas, and/or tensor fascia lata muscle) with debridement of nonviable muscle, unilateral

    (To report bilateral procedure, report 27057 with modifier 50)

451

	Separate Procedure		Unlisted Procedure		CCI Comp. Code		Non-specific Procedure

27059   This code is out of order. See page 451.

27060   Excision; ischial bursa

27062   trochanteric bursa or calcification

(For arthrocentesis or needling of bursa, use 20610)

27065   Excision of bone cyst or benign tumor, wing of ilium, symphysis pubis, or greater trochanter of femur; superficial, includes autograft when performed

27066   deep (subfascial), includes autograft when performed

27067   with autograft requiring separate incision

27070   Partial excision, wing of ilium, symphysis pubis, or greater trochanter of femur, (craterization, saucerization) (eg, osteomyelitis or bone abscess); superficial

27071   deep (subfascial or intramuscular)

27075   Radical resection of tumor; wing of ilium, one pubic or ischial ramus or symphysis pubis

27076   ilium, including acetabulum, both pubic rami, or ischium and acetabulum

27077   innominate bone, total

27078   ischial tuberosity and greater trochanter of femur

(27079   Deleted 2009 [2010 edition])

27080   Coccygectomy, primary

(For pressure (decubitus) ulcer, see 15920, 15922 and 15931-15958)

INTRODUCTION OR REMOVAL

27086   Removal of foreign body, pelvis or hip; subcutaneous tissue

27087   deep (subfascial or intramuscular)

27090   Removal of hip prosthesis; (separate procedure)

27091 complicated, including total hip prosthesis, methylmethacrylate with or without insertion of spacer

27093 Injection procedure for hip arthrography; without anesthesia

(For radiological supervision and interpretation, use 73525. Do not report 77002 in conjunction with 73525)

27095 with anesthesia

(For radiological supervision and interpretation, use 73525. Do not report 77002 in conjunction with 73525)

27096 Injection procedure for sacroiliac joint, anesthetic/steroid, with image guidance (fluoroscopy or CT) including arthrography when performed

(27096 is to be used only with CT or fluoroscopic imaging confirmation of intra-articular needle positioning)

(If CT or fluoroscopic imaging is not performed, use 20552)

(Code 27096 is a unilateral procedure. For bilateral procedure, use modifier -50)

REPAIR, REVISION, AND/OR RECONSTRUCTION

27097 Release or recession, hamstring, proximal

27098 Transfer, adductor to ischium

27100 Transfer external oblique muscle to greater trochanter including fascial or tendon extension (graft)

27105 Transfer paraspinal muscle to hip (includes fascial or tendon extension graft)

27110 Transfer iliopsoas; to greater trochanter of femur

27111 to femoral neck

27120 Acetabuloplasty; (eg, Whitman, Colonna, Haygroves, or cup type)

27122 resection, femoral head (eg, Girdlestone procedure)

27125 Hemiarthroplasty, hip, partial (eg, femoral stem prosthesis, bipolar arthroplasty)

 Separate Procedure   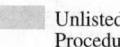 Unlisted Procedure   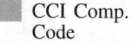 CCI Comp. Code   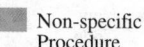 Non-specific Procedure   **453**

(For prosthetic replacement following fracture of the hip, use 27236)

27130 Arthroplasty, acetabular and proximal femoral prosthetic replacement (total hip arthroplasty), with or without autograft or allograft

27132 Conversion of previous hip surgery to total hip arthroplasty, with or without autograft or allograft

27134 Revision of total hip arthroplasty; both components, with or without autograft or allograft

27137 acetabular component only, with or without autograft or allograft

27138 femoral component only, with or without allograft

27140 Osteotomy and transfer of greater trochanter of femur (separate procedure)

27146 Osteotomy, iliac, acetabular or innominate bone;

27147 with open reduction of hip

27151 with femoral osteotomy

27156 with femoral osteotomy and with open reduction of hip

27158 Osteotomy, pelvis, bilateral (eg, congenital malformation)

27161 Osteotomy, femoral neck (separate procedure)

27165 Osteotomy, intertrochanteric or subtrochanteric including internal or external fixation and/or cast

27170 Bone graft, femoral head, neck, intertrochanteric or subtrochanteric area (includes obtaining bone graft)

27175 Treatment of slipped femoral epiphysis; by traction, without reduction

27176 by single or multiple pinning, in situ

27177 Open treatment of slipped femoral epiphysis; single or multiple pinning or bone graft (includes obtaining graft)

● New Code ▲ Revised Code + Add-On Code ⊘ Modifier -51 Exempt ⊙ Moderate Sedation

27178   closed manipulation with single or multiple pinning

27179   osteoplasty of femoral neck (Heyman type procedure)

27181   osteotomy and internal fixation

27185   Epiphyseal arrest by epiphysiodesis or stapling, greater trochanter of femur

27187   Prophylactic treatment (nailing, pinning, plating or wiring) with or without methylmethacrylate, femoral neck and proximal femur

FRACTURE AND/OR DISLOCATION

27193   Closed treatment of pelvic ring fracture, dislocation, diastasis or subluxation; without manipulation

27194   with manipulation, requiring more than local anesthesia

27200   Closed treatment of coccygeal fracture

27202   Open treatment of coccygeal fracture

27215   Open treatment of iliac spine(s), tuberosity avulsion, or iliac wing fracture(s), unilateral for pelvic bone fracture patterns that do not disrupt the pelvic ring, includes internal fixation, when performed

(To report bilateral procedure, report 27215 with modifier 50)

27216   Percutaneous skeletal fixation of posterior pelvic bone fracture and/or dislocation, for fracture patterns that disrupt the pelvic ring, unilateral (includes ipsilateral ilium, sacroiliac joint and/or sacrum)

(To report bilateral procedure, report 27216 with modifier 50)

27217   Open treatment of anterior pelvic bone fracture and/or dislocation for fracture patterns that disrupt the pelvic ring, unilateral, includes internal fixation, when performed (includes pubic symphysis and/or ipsilateral superior/inferior rami)

(To report bilateral procedure, report 27217 with modifier 50)

27218   Open treatment of posterior pelvic bone fracture and/or dislocation for fracture patterns that disrupt the pelvic ring,

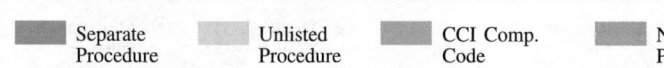

| | Separate Procedure | | Unlisted Procedure | | CCI Comp. Code | | Non-specific Procedure |

455

unilateral, includes internal fixation, when performed (includes ipsilateral ilium, sacroiliac joint and/or sacrum)

(To report bilateral procedure, report 27218 with modifier 50)

27220 Closed treatment of acetabulum (hip socket) fracture(s); without manipulation

27222 with manipulation, with or without skeletal traction

27226 Open treatment of posterior or anterior acetabular wall fracture, with internal fixation

27227 Open treatment of acetabular fracture(s) involving anterior or posterior (one) column, or a fracture running transversely across the acetabulum, with internal fixation

27228 Open treatment of acetabular fracture(s) involving anterior and posterior (two) columns, includes T-fracture and both column fracture with complete articular detachment, or single column or transverse fracture with associated acetabular wall fracture, with internal fixation

27230 Closed treatment of femoral fracture, proximal end, neck; without manipulation

27232 with manipulation, with or without skeletal traction

27235 Percutaneous skeletal fixation of femoral fracture, proximal end, neck

27236 Open treatment of femoral fracture, proximal end, neck, internal fixation or prosthetic replacement

27238 Closed treatment of intertrochanteric, pertrochanteric, or subtrochanteric femoral fracture; without manipulation

27240 with manipulation, with or without skin or skeletal traction

27244 Treatment of intertrochanteric, pertrochanteric or subtrochanteric femoral fracture; with plate/screw type implant, with or without cerclage

27245 with intramedullary implant, with or without interlocking screws and/or cerclage

● New Code   ▲ Revised Code   + Add-On Code   ⊘ Modifier -51 Exempt   ⊙ Moderate Sedation

27246 Closed treatment of greater trochanteric fracture, without manipulation

27248 Open treatment of greater trochanteric fracture, includes internal fixation, when performed

27250 Closed treatment of hip dislocation, traumatic; without anesthesia

27252 requiring anesthesia

27253 Open treatment of hip dislocation, traumatic, without internal fixation

27254 Open treatment of hip dislocation, traumatic, with acetabular wall and femoral head fracture, with or without internal or external fixation

(For treatment of acetabular fracture with fixation, see 27226, 27227)

27256 Treatment of spontaneous hip dislocation (developmental, including congenital or pathological), by abduction, splint or traction; without anesthesia, without manipulation

27257 with manipulation, requiring anesthesia

27258 Open treatment of spontaneous hip dislocation (developmental, including congenital or pathological), replacement of femoral head in acetabulum (including tenotomy, etc);

27259 with femoral shaft shortening

27265 Closed treatment of post hip arthroplasty dislocation; without anesthesia

27266 requiring regional or general anesthesia

27267 Closed treatment of femoral fracture, proximal end, head; without manipulation

27268 with manipulation

27269 Open treatment of femoral fracture, proximal end, head, includes internal fixation, when performed

(Do not report 27269 in conjunction with 27033, 27253)

| | Separate Procedure | | Unlisted Procedure | | CCI Comp. Code | | Non-specific Procedure | **457** |

MANIPULATION

27275 Manipulation, hip joint, requiring general anesthesia

ARTHRODESIS

27280 Arthrodesis, sacroiliac joint (including obtaining graft)

(To report bilateral procedures, report 27280 with modifier -50)

27282 Arthrodesis, symphysis pubis (including obtaining graft)

27284 Arthrodesis, hip joint (including obtaining graft);

27286 with subtrochanteric osteotomy

AMPUTATION

27290 Interpelviabdominal amputation (hindquarter amputation)

27295 Disarticulation of hip

OTHER PROCEDURES

27299 Unlisted procedure, pelvis or hip joint

FEMUR (THIGH REGION) AND KNEE JOINT

INCISION

(For incision and drainage of abscess or hematoma, superficial, see 10040-10160)

27301 Incision and drainage, deep abscess, bursa, or hematoma, thigh or knee region

27303 Incision, deep, with opening of bone cortex, femur or knee (eg, osteomyelitis or bone abscess)

27305 Fasciotomy, iliotibial (tenotomy), open

(For combined Ober-Yount fasciotomy, use 27025)

27306 Tenotomy, percutaneous, adductor or hamstring; single tendon (separate procedure)

27307 multiple tendons

458

27310 Arthrotomy, knee, with exploration, drainage, or removal of foreign body(eg, infection)

EXCISION

27323 Biopsy, soft tissue of thigh or knee area; superficial

27324 deep (subfascial or intramuscular)

(For needle biopsy of soft tissue, use 20206)

27325 Neurectomy, hamstring muscle

27326 Neurectomy, popliteal (gastrocnemius)

27327 Excision, tumor, soft tissue of thigh or knee area, subcutaneous; less than 3 cm

27337 3 cm or greater

27328 Excision, tumor, soft tissue of thigh or knee area, subfascial (eg, intramuscular); less than 5 cm

27339 5 cm or greater

27329 This code is out of order. See page 460

27330 Arthrotomy, knee; with synovial biopsy only

27331 including joint exploration, biopsy, or removal of loose or foreign bodies

27332 Arthrotomy, with excision of semilunar cartilage (meniscectomy) knee; medial OR lateral

27333 medial AND lateral

27334 Arthrotomy, with synovectomy, knee; anterior OR posterior

27335 anterior AND posterior including popliteal area

27337 This code is out of order. See page 459

27339 This code is out of order. See page 459

27340 Excision, prepatellar bursa

	Separate Procedure		Unlisted Procedure		CCI Comp. Code		Non-specific Procedure

459

27345   Excision of synovial cyst of popliteal space (eg, Baker's cyst)

27347   Excision of lesion of meniscus or capsule (eg, cyst, ganglion), knee

27350   Patellectomy or hemipatellectomy

27355   Excision or curettage of bone cyst or benign tumor of femur;

27356   with allograft

27357   with autograft (includes obtaining graft)

+ 27358   with internal fixation (List in addition to code for primary procedure)

     (Use 27358 in conjunction with codes 27355, 27356 or 27357)

27360   Partial excision (craterization, saucerization, or diaphysectomy) bone, femur, proximal tibia and/or fibula (eg, osteomyelitis or bone abscess)

27329   Radical resection of tumor (eg, malignant neoplasm), soft tissue of thigh or knee area; less than 5 cm

27364   5 cm or greater

27365   Radical resection of tumor, femur or knee

     (For radical resection of tumor, soft tissue of thigh or knee area, use 27329, 27364)

INTRODUCTION OR REMOVAL

27370   Injection procedure for knee arthrography

     (For radiological supervision and interpretation, use 73580. Do not report 77002 in conjunction with 73580)

27372   Removal of foreign body, deep, thigh region or knee area

     (For removal of knee prosthesis including "total knee," use 27488)

     (For surgical arthroscopic knee procedures, see 29870-29887)

   ● New Code   ▲ Revised Code   + Add-On Code   ⊘ Modifier -51 Exempt   ⊙ Moderate Sedation

REPAIR, REVISION, AND/OR RECONSTRUCTION

27380 Suture of infrapatellar tendon; primary

27381 secondary reconstruction, including fascial or tendon graft

27385 Suture of quadriceps or hamstring muscle rupture; primary

27386 secondary reconstruction, including fascial or tendon graft

27390 Tenotomy, open, hamstring, knee to hip; single tendon

27391 multiple tendons, 1 leg

27392 multiple tendons, bilateral

27393 Lengthening of hamstring tendon; single tendon

27394 multiple tendons, 1 leg

27395 multiple tendons, bilateral

27396 Transplant or transfer (with muscle redirection or rerouting), thigh (eg., extensor to flexor); single tendon

27397 multiple tendons

27400 Transfer, tendon or muscle, hamstrings to femur (eg, Egger's type procedure)

27403 Arthrotomy with meniscus repair, knee

(For arthroscopic repair, use 29882)

27405 Repair, primary, torn ligament and/or capsule, knee; collateral

27407 cruciate

(For cruciate ligament reconstruction, use 27427)

27409 collateral and cruciate ligaments

(For ligament reconstruction, see 27427-27429)

27412 Autologous chondrocyte implantation, knee

(Do not report 27412 in conjunction with 20926, 27331, 27570)

461

	Separate Procedure		Unlisted Procedure		CCI Comp. Code		Non-specific Procedure

(For harvesting of chondrocytes, use 29870)

27415 Osteochondral allograft, knee, open

(For arthroscopic implant of osteochondral allograft, use 29867)

(Do not report 27415 in conjunction with 27416)

27416 Osteochondral autograf(s), knee, open (eg, mosaicplasty) (includes harvesting of autograft[s])

(Do not report 27416 in conjunction with 27415, 29870, 29871, 29875, 29884 when performed at the same session and/or 29874, 29877, 29879, 29885-29887 when performed in the same compartment)

(For arthroscopic osteochondral autograft of knee, use 29866)

27418 Anterior tibial tubercleplasty (eg, Maquet type procedure)

27420 Reconstruction of dislocating patella; (eg, Hauser type procedure)

27422 with extensor realignment and/or muscle advancement or release (eg, Campbell, Goldwaite type procedure)

27424 with patellectomy

27425 Lateral retinacular release open

(For arthroscopic lateral release, use 29873)

27427 Ligamentous reconstruction (augmentation), knee; extra-articular

27428 intra-articular (open)

27429 intra-articular (open) and extra-articular

(For primary repair of ligament(s) performed in addition to reconstruction, report 27405, 27407 or 27409 in addition to code 27427, 27428 or 27429)

27430 Quadricepsplasty (eg, Bennett or Thompson type)

27435 Capsulotomy, posterior capsular release, knee

27437 Arthroplasty, patella; without prosthesis

● New Code   ▲ Revised Code   + Add-On Code   ⊘ Modifier -51 Exempt   ⊙ Moderate Sedation

27438   with prosthesis

27440   Arthroplasty, knee, tibial plateau;

27441   with debridement and partial synovectomy

27442   Arthroplasty, femoral condyles or tibial plateau(s), knee;

27443   with debridement and partial synovectomy

27445   Arthroplasty, knee, hinge prosthesis (eg, Walldius type)

27446   Arthroplasty, knee, condyle and plateau; medial OR lateral compartment

27447   medial AND lateral compartments with or without patella resurfacing (total knee arthroplasty)

(For revision of total knee arthroplasty, use 27487)

(For removal of total knee prosthesis, use 27488)

27448   Osteotomy, femur, shaft or supracondylar; without fixation

(To report bilateral procedures, report 27448 with modifier -50)

27450   with fixation

(To report bilateral procedures, report 27450 with modifier -50)

27454   Osteotomy, multiple, with realignment on intramedullary rod, femoral shaft (eg, Sofield type procedure)

27455   Osteotomy, proximal tibia, including fibular excision or osteotomy (includes correction of genu varus [bowleg] or genu valgus [knock-knee]); before epiphyseal closure

(To report bilateral procedures, report 27455 with modifier -50)

27457   after epiphyseal closure

(To report bilateral procedures, report 27457 with modifier -50)

27465   Osteoplasty, femur; shortening (excluding 64876)

27466   lengthening

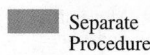 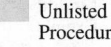

27468 combined, lengthening and shortening with femoral segment transfer

27470 Repair, nonunion or malunion, femur, distal to head and neck; without graft (eg, compression technique)

27472 with iliac or other autogenous bone graft (includes obtaining graft)

27475 Arrest, epiphyseal, any method (eg, epiphysiodesis); distal femur

27477 tibia and fibula, proximal

27479 combined distal femur, proximal tibia and fibula

27485 Arrest, hemiepiphyseal, distal femur or proximal tibia or fibula (eg, genu varus or valgus)

27486 Revision of total knee arthroplasty, with or without allograft; 1 component

27487 femoral and entire tibial component

27488 Removal of prosthesis, including total knee prosthesis, methylmethacrylate with or without insertion of spacer, knee

27495 Prophylactic treatment (nailing, pinning, plating or wiring) with or without methylmethacrylate, femur

27496 Decompression fasciotomy, thigh and/or knee, 1 compartment (flexor or extensor or adductor);

27497 with debridement of nonviable muscle and/or nerve

27498 Decompression fasciotomy, thigh and/or knee, multiple compartments;

27499 with debridement of nonviable muscle and/or nerve

● New Code ▲ Revised Code + Add-On Code ⊘ Modifier -51 Exempt 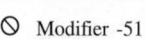 Moderate Sedation

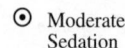

FRACTURE AND/OR DISLOCATION

(For arthroscopic treatment of intercondylar spine(s) and tuberosity fracture(s) of the knee, see 29850, 29851)

(For arthroscopic treatment of tibial fracture, see 29855, 29856)

27500 Closed treatment of femoral shaft fracture, without manipulation

27501 Closed treatment of supracondylar or transcondylar femoral fracture with or without intercondylar extension, without manipulation

27502 Closed treatment of femoral shaft fracture, with manipulation, with or without skin or skeletal traction

27503 Closed treatment of supracondylar or transcondylar femoral fracture with or without intercondylar extension, with manipulation, with or without skin or skeletal traction

27506 Open treatment of femoral shaft fracture, with or without external fixation, with insertion of intramedullary implant, with or without cerclage and/or locking screws

27507 Open treatment of femoral shaft fracture with plate/screws, with or without cerclage

27508 Closed treatment of femoral fracture, distal end, medial or lateral condyle, without manipulation

27509 Percutaneous skeletal fixation of femoral fracture, distal end, medial or lateral condyle, or supracondylar or transcondylar, with or without intercondylar extension, or distal femoral epiphyseal separation

27510 Closed treatment of femoral fracture, distal end, medial or lateral condyle, with manipulation

27511 Open treatment of femoral supracondylar or transcondylar fracture without intercondylar extension, includes internal fixation, when performed

27513 Open treatment of femoral supracondylar or transcondylar fracture with intercondylar extension, includes internal fixation, when performed

27514 Open treatment of femoral fracture, distal end, medial or lateral condyle, includes internal fixation, when performed

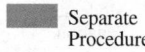 Separate Procedure 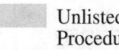 Unlisted Procedure 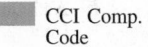 CCI Comp. Code Non-specific Procedure

465

27516 Closed treatment of distal femoral epiphyseal separation; without manipulation

27517   with manipulation, with or without skin or skeletal traction

27519 Open treatment of distal femoral epiphyseal separation, includes internal fixation, when performed

27520 Closed treatment of patellar fracture, without manipulation

27524 Open treatment of patellar fracture, with internal fixation and/or partial or complete patellectomy and soft tissue repair

27530 Closed treatment of tibial fracture, proximal (plateau); without manipulation

27532   with or without manipulation, with skeletal traction

(For arthroscopic treatment, see 29855, 29856)

27535 Open treatment of tibial fracture, proximal (plateau); unicondylar, includes internal fixation, when performed

27536   bicondylar, with or without internal fixation

(For arthroscopic treatment, see 29855, 29856)

27538 Closed treatment of intercondylar spine(s) and/or tuberosity fracture(s) of knee, with or without manipulation

(For arthroscopic treatment, see 29850, 29851)

27540 Open treatment of intercondylar spine(s) and/or tuberosity fracture(s) of the knee, includes internal fixation, when performed

27550 Closed treatment of knee dislocation; without anesthesia

27552   requiring anesthesia

27556 Open treatment of knee dislocation, includes internal fixation, when performed; without primary ligamentous repair or augmentation/reconstruction

27557   with primary ligamentous repair

● New Code   ▲ Revised Code   ✛ Add-On Code   ⊘ Modifier -51 Exempt   ⊙ Moderate Sedation

27558   with primary ligamentous repair, with augmentation/ reconstruction

27560   Closed treatment of patellar dislocation; without anesthesia

           (For recurrent dislocation, see 27420-27424)

27562   requiring anesthesia

27566   Open treatment of patellar dislocation, with or without partial or total patellectomy

MANIPULATION

27570   Manipulation of knee joint under general anesthesia (includes application of traction or other fixation devices)

ARTHRODESIS

27580   Arthrodesis, knee, any technique

AMPUTATION

27590   Amputation, thigh, through femur, any level;

27591   immediate fitting technique including first cast

27592   open, circular (guillotine)

27594   secondary closure or scar revision

27596   re-amputation

27598   Disarticulation at knee

OTHER PROCEDURES

27599   Unlisted procedure, femur or knee

LEG (TIBIA AND FIBULA) AND ANKLE JOINT

INCISION

27600   Decompression fasciotomy, leg; anterior and/or lateral compartments only

27601   posterior compartment(s) only

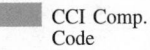

	Separate Procedure		Unlisted Procedure		CCI Comp. Code		Non-specific Procedure

467

27602   anterior and/or lateral, and posterior compartment(s)

(For incision and drainage procedures, superficial, see 10040-10160)

(For decompression fasciotomy with debridement, see 27892-27894)

27603 Incision and drainage, leg or ankle; deep abscess or hematoma

27604   infected bursa

27605 Tenotomy, percutaneous, Achilles tendon (separate procedure); local anesthesia

27606   general anesthesia

27607 Incision (eg, osteomyelitis or bone abscess), leg or ankle

27610 Arthrotomy, ankle, including exploration, drainage, or removal of foreign body

27612 Arthrotomy, posterior capsular release, ankle, with or without Achilles tendon lengthening

(See also 27685)

EXCISION

27613 Biopsy, soft tissue of leg or ankle area; superficial

27614   deep (subfascial or intramuscular)

(For needle biopsy of soft tissue, use 20206)

27615 Radical resection of tumor (eg, malignant neoplasm), soft tissue of leg or ankle area; less than 5 cm

27616   5 cm or greater

27618 Excision, tumor, soft tissue of leg or ankle area, subcutaneous; less than 3 cm

27632   3 cm or greater

27619 Excision, tumor, soft tissue of leg or ankle area, subfascial (eg, intramuscular); less than 5 cm

468   ● New Code   ▲ Revised Code   ✛ Add-On Code   ⊘ Modifier -51 Exempt   ⊙ Moderate Sedation

27634   5 cm or greater

27620   Arthrotomy, ankle, with joint exploration, with or without biopsy, with or without removal of loose or foreign body

27625   Arthrotomy, with synovectomy, ankle;

27626   including tenosynovectomy

27630   Excision of lesion of tendon sheath or capsule (eg, cyst or ganglion), leg and/or ankle

27632   This code is out of order. See page 468

27634   This code is out of order. See page 469

27635   Excision or curettage of bone cyst or benign tumor, tibia or fibula;

27637   with autograft (includes obtaining graft)

27638   with allograft

27640   Partial excision (craterization, saucerization, or diaphysectomy) bone (eg, osteomyelitis); tibia

(For exostosis excision, use 27635)

27641   fibula

(For exostosis excision, use 27635)

27645   Radical resection of tumor; tibia

27646   fibula

27647   talus or calcaneus

INTRODUCTION OR REMOVAL

27648   Injection procedure for ankle arthrography

(For radiological supervision and interpretation use 73615. Do not report 77002 in addition to 73615)

(For ankle arthroscopy, see 29894-29898)

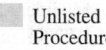 Separate
Procedure

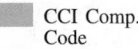 Unlisted
Procedure

CCI Comp.
Code

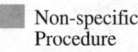 Non-specific
Procedure

469

CPT PLUS! 2013

REPAIR, REVISION, AND/OR RECONSTRUCTION

27650 Repair, primary, open or percutaneous, ruptured Achilles tendon;

27652 with graft (includes obtaining graft)

27654 Repair, secondary, Achilles tendon, with or without graft

27656 Repair, fascial defect of leg

27658 Repair, flexor tendon, leg; primary, without graft, each tendon

27659 secondary, with or without graft, each tendon

27664 Repair, extensor tendon, leg; primary, without graft, each tendon

27665 secondary, with or without graft, each tendon

27675 Repair, dislocating peroneal tendons; without fibular osteotomy

27676 with fibular osteotomy

27680 Tenolysis, flexor or extensor tendon, leg and/or ankle; single, each tendon

27681 multiple tendons (through separate incision(s))

27685 Lengthening or shortening of tendon, leg or ankle; single tendon (separate procedure)

27686 multiple tendons (through same incision), each

27687 Gastrocnemius recession (eg, Strayer procedure)

(Toe extensors are considered as a group to be single tendon when transplanted into midfoot)

27690 Transfer or transplant of single tendon (with muscle redirection or rerouting); superficial (eg, anterior tibial extensors into midfoot)

27691 deep (eg, anterior tibial or posterior tibial through interosseous space, flexor digitorum longus, flexor hallucis longus, or peroneal tendon to midfoot or hind foot)

● New Code   ▲ Revised Code   + Add-On Code   ⊘ Modifier -51 Exempt   ⊙ Moderate Sedation

CPT codes and descriptions only ©2012 American Medical Association. All rights reserved.

+ 27692   each additional tendon (List separately in addition to code for primary procedure)

(Use 27692 in conjunction with codes 27690, 27691)

27695   Repair, primary, disrupted ligament, ankle; collateral

27696   both collateral ligaments

27698   Repair, secondary disrupted ligament, ankle, collateral (eg, Watson-Jones procedure)

27700   Arthroplasty, ankle;

27702   with implant (total ankle)

27703   revision, total ankle

27704   Removal of ankle implant

27705   Osteotomy; tibia

27707   fibula

27709   tibia and fibula

27712   multiple, with realignment on intramedullary rod (eg, Sofield type procedure)

(For osteotomy to correct genu varus (bowleg) or genu valgus (knock-knee), see 27455-27457)

27715   Osteoplasty, tibia and fibula, lengthening or shortening

27720   Repair of nonunion or malunion, tibia; without graft, (eg, compression technique)

27722   with sliding graft

27724   with iliac or other autograft (includes obtaining graft)

27725   by synostosis, with fibula, any method

27726   Repair of fibula nonunion and/or malunion with internal fixation

(Do not reprt 27726 in conjunction with 27707)

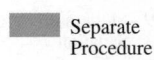 Separate Procedure   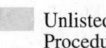 Unlisted Procedure   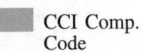 CCI Comp. Code   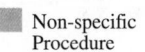 Non-specific Procedure   **471**

27727 Repair of congenital pseudarthrosis, tibia

27730 Arrest, epiphyseal (epiphysiodesis), open; distal tibia

27732 distal fibula

27734 distal tibia and fibula

27740 Arrest, epiphyseal (epiphysiodesis), any method, combined, proximal and distal tibia and fibula;

27742 and distal femur

(For epiphyseal arrest of proximal tibia and fibula, use 27477)

27745 Prophylactic treatment (nailing, pinning, plating or wiring) with or without methylmethacrylate, tibia

FRACTURE AND/OR DISLOCATION

27750 Closed treatment of tibial shaft fracture (with or without fibular fracture); without manipulation

27752 with manipulation, with or without skeletal traction

27756 Percutaneous skeletal fixation of tibial shaft fracture (with or without fibular fracture) (eg, pins or screws)

27758 Open treatment of tibial shaft fracture, (with or without fibular fracture) with plate/screws, with or without cerclage

27759 Treatment of tibial shaft fracture (with or without fibular fracture) by intramedullary implant, with or without interlocking screws and/or cerclage

27760 Closed treatment of medial malleolus fracture; without manipulation

27762 with manipulation, with or without skin or skeletal traction

27766 Open treatment of medial malleolus fracture, includes internal fixation, when performed

27767 Closed treatment of posterior malleolus fracture; without manipulation

27768 with manipulation

● New Code ▲ Revised Code + Add-On Code ⊘ Modifier -51 Exempt ⊙ Moderate Sedation

27769 Open treatment of posterior malleolus fracture, includes internal fixation, when performed

(Do not report 27767-27769 in conjunction with 27808-27823)

27780 Closed treatment of proximal fibula or shaft fracture; without manipulation

27781 with manipulation

27784 Open treatment of proximal fibula or shaft fracture, includes internal fixation, when performed

27786 Closed treatment of distal fibular fracture (lateral malleolus); without manipulation

27788 with manipulation

27792 Open treatment of distal fibular fracture (lateral malleolus), includes internal fixation, when performed

(For treatment of tibia and fibula shaft fractures, see 27750-27759)

27808 Closed treatment of bimalleolar ankle fracture, (eg, lateral and medial malleoli, or lateral and posterior malleoli or medial and posterior malleoli); without manipulation

27810 with manipulation

27814 Open treatment of bimalleolar ankle fracture (eg, lateral and medial malleoli, or lateral and posterior malleoli, or medial and posterior malleoli), includes internal fixation, when performed

27816 Closed treatment of trimalleolar ankle fracture; without manipulation

27818 with manipulation

27822 Open treatment of trimalleolar ankle fracture, includes internal fixation, when performed, medial and/or lateral malleolus; without fixation of posterior lip

27823 with fixation of posterior lip

	Separate Procedure		Unlisted Procedure		CCI Comp. Code		Non-specific Procedure

27824 Closed treatment of fracture of weight bearing articular portion of distal tibia (eg, pilon or tibial plafond), with or without anesthesia; without manipulation

27825 with skeletal traction and/or requiring manipulation

27826 Open treatment of fracture of weight bearing articular surface/portion of distal tibia (eg, pilon or tibial plafond), with internal fixation, when performed; of fibula only

27827 of tibia only

27828 of both tibia and fibula

27829 Open treatment of distal tibiofibular joint (syndesmosis) disruption, includes internal fixation, when performed

27830 Closed treatment of proximal tibiofibular joint dislocation; without anesthesia

27831 requiring anesthesia

27832 Open treatment of proximal tibiofibular joint dislocation, includes internal fixation, when performed, or with excision of proximal fibula

27840 Closed treatment of ankle dislocation; without anesthesia

27842 requiring anesthesia, with or without percutaneous skeletal fixation

27846 Open treatment of ankle dislocation, with or without percutaneous skeletal fixation; without repair or internal fixation

27848 with repair or internal or external fixation

(For surgical diagnostic arthroscopic procedures, see 29894-29898)

MANIPULATION

27860 Manipulation of ankle under general anesthesia (includes application of traction or other fixation apparatus)

ARTHRODESIS

27870 Arthrodesis, ankle, open

● New Code ▲ Revised Code + Add-On Code ⊘ Modifier -51 Exempt ⊙ Moderate Sedation

(For arthroscopic ankle arthrodesis, use 29899)

27871 Arthrodesis, tibiofibular joint, proximal or distal

AMPUTATION

27880 Amputation, leg, through tibia and fibula;

27881   with immediate fitting technique including application of first cast

27882   open, circular (guillotine)

27884   secondary closure or scar revision

27886   re-amputation

27888 Amputation, ankle, through malleoli of tibia and fibula (eg, Syme, Pirogoff type procedures), with plastic closure and resection of nerves

27889 Ankle disarticulation

OTHER PROCEDURES

27892 Decompression fasciotomy, leg; anterior and/or lateral compartments only, with debridement of nonviable muscle and/or nerve

(For decompression fasciotomy of the leg without debridement, use 27600)

27893   posterior compartment(s) only, with debridement of nonviable muscle and/or nerve

(For decompession fasciotomy of the leg without debridement, use 27601)

27894   anterior and/or lateral, and posterior compartment(s), with debridement of nonviable muscle and/or nerve

(For decompression fasciotomy of the leg without debridement, use 27602)

27899 Unlisted procedure, leg or ankle

	Separate Procedure		Unlisted Procedure		CCI Comp. Code		Non-specific Procedure

475

FOOT AND TOES

INCISION

(For incision and drainage procedures, superficial, see 10040-10160)

28001 Incision and drainage, bursa, foot

28002 Incision and drainage below fascia, with or without tendon sheath involvement, foot; single bursal space

28003   multiple areas

28005 Incision, bone cortex (eg, osteomyelitis or bone abscess), foot

28008 Fasciotomy, foot and/or toe

(See also 28060, 28062, 28250)

28010 Tenotomy, percutaneous, toe; single tendon

28011   multiple tendons

(For open tenotomy, see 28230-28234)

28020 Arthrotomy, including exploration, drainage, or removal of loose or foreign body; intertarsal or tarsometatarsal joint

28022   metatarsophalangeal joint

28024   interphalangeal joint

28035 Release, tarsal tunnel (posterior tibial nerve decompression)

(For other nerve entrapments, see 64704, 64722)

EXCISION

28039 This code is out of order. See page 476

28041 This code is out of order. See page 477

28043 Excision, tumor, soft tissue of foot or toe, subcutaneous; less than 1.5 cm

28039   1.5 cm or greater

● New Code   ▲ Revised Code   + Add-On Code   ⊘ Modifier -51 Exempt   ⊙ Moderate Sedation

28045 Excision, tumor, soft tissue of foot or toe, subfascial (eg, intramuscular); less than 1.5 cm

28041   1.5 cm or greater

28046 Radical resection of tumor (eg, malignant neoplasm), soft tissue of foot or toe; less than 3 cm

28047   3 cm or greater

28050 Arthrotomy with biopsy; intertarsal or tarsometatarsal joint

28052   metatarsophalangeal joint

28054   interphalangeal joint

28055 Neurectomy, intrinsic musculature of foot

28060 Fasciectomy, plantar fascia; partial (separate procedure)

28062   radical (separate procedure)

    (For plantar fasciotomy, see 28008, 28250)

28070 Synovectomy; intertarsal or tarsometatarsal joint, each

28072   metatarsophalangeal joint, each

28080 Excision, interdigital (Morton) neuroma, single, each

28086 Synovectomy, tendon sheath, foot; flexor

28088   extensor

28090 Excision of lesion, tendon, tendon sheath, or capsule (including synovectomy) (eg, cyst or ganglion); foot

28092   toe(s), each

28100 Excision or curettage of bone cyst or benign tumor, talus or calcaneus;

28102   with iliac or other autograft (includes obtaining graft)

28103   with allograft

477

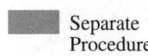 Separate Procedure   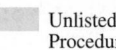 Unlisted Procedure   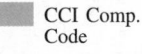 CCI Comp. Code   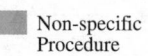 Non-specific Procedure

28104 Excision or curettage of bone cyst or benign tumor, tarsal or metatarsal, except talus or calcaneus;

28106   with iliac or other autograft (includes obtaining graft)

28107   with allograft

28108 Excision or curettage of bone cyst or benign tumor, phalanges of foot

   (For ostectomy, partial (eg, hallux valgus, Silver type procedure), use 28290)

28110 Ostectomy, partial excision, fifth metatarsal head (bunionette) (separate procedure)

28111 Ostectomy, complete excision; first metatarsal head

28112   other metatarsal head (second, third or fourth)

28113   fifth metatarsal head

28114   all metatarsal heads, with partial proximal phalangectomy, excluding first metatarsal (eg, Clayton type procedure)

28116 Ostectomy, excision of tarsal coalition

28118 Ostectomy, calcaneus;

28119   for spur, with or without plantar fascial release

28120 Partial excision (craterization, saucerization, sequestrectomy, or diaphysectomy) bone (eg, osteomyelitis or bossing); talus or calcaneus

28122   tarsal or metatarsal bone, except talus or calcaneus

   (For partial excision of talus or calcaneus, use 28120)

   (For cheilectomy for hallux rigidus, use 28289)

28124   phalanx of toe

28126 Resection, partial or complete, phalangeal base, each toe

28130 Talectomy (astragalectomy)

● New Code   ▲ Revised Code   + Add-On Code   ⊘ Modifier -51 Exempt   ⊙ Moderate Sedation

(For calcanectomy, use 28118)

28140 Metatarsectomy

28150 Phalangectomy, toe, each toe

28153 Resection, condyle(s), distal end of phalanx, each toe

28160 Hemiphalangectomy or interphalangeal joint excision, toe, proximal end of phalanx, each

28171 Radical resection of tumor; tarsal (except talus or calcaneus)

28173 metatarsal

28175 phalanx of toe

(For talus or calcaneus, use 27647)

INTRODUCTION OR REMOVAL

28190 Removal of foreign body, foot; subcutaneous

28192 deep

28193 complicated

REPAIR, REVISION, AND/OR RECONSTRUCTION

28200 Repair, tendon, flexor, foot; primary or secondary, without free graft, each tendon

28202 secondary with free graft, each tendon (includes obtaining graft)

28208 Repair, tendon, extensor, foot; primary or secondary, each tendon

28210 secondary with free graft, each tendon (includes obtaining graft)

28220 Tenolysis, flexor, foot; single tendon

28222 multiple tendons

28225 Tenolysis, extensor, foot; single tendon

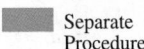 Separate Procedure
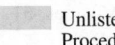 Unlisted Procedure
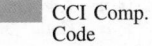 CCI Comp. Code
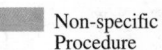 Non-specific Procedure

479

28226	multiple tendons
28230	Tenotomy, open, tendon flexor; foot, single or multiple tendon(s) (separate procedure)
28232	toe, single tendon (separate procedure)
28234	Tenotomy, open, extensor, foot or toe, each tendon

(For tendon transfer to midfoot or hindfoot, see 27690, 27691)

28238	Reconstruction (advancement), posterior tibial tendon with excision of accessory tarsal navicular bone (eg, Kidner type procedure)

(For subcutaneous tenotomy, see 28010, 28011)

(For transfer or transplant of tendon with muscle redirection or rerouting, see 27690-27692)

(For extensor hallucis longus transfer with great toe IP fusion (Jones procedure), use 28760)

28240	Tenotomy, lengthening, or release, abductor hallucis muscle
28250	Division of plantar fascia and muscle (eg, Steindler stripping) (separate procedure)
28260	Capsulotomy, midfoot; medial release only (separate procedure)
28261	with tendon lengthening
28262	extensive, including posterior talotibial capsulotomy and tendon(s) lengthening (eg, resistant clubfoot deformity)
28264	Capsulotomy, midtarsal (eg, Heyman type procedure)
28270	Capsulotomy; metatarsophalangeal joint, with or without tenorrhaphy, each joint (separate procedure)
28272	interphalangeal joint, each joint (separate procedure)
28280	Syndactylization, toes (eg, webbing or Kelikian type procedure)
28285	Correction, hammertoe (eg, interphalangeal fusion, partial or total phalangectomy)

● New Code ▲ Revised Code ✛ Add-On Code ⊘ Modifier -51 Exempt ⊙ Moderate Sedation

28286 Correction, cock-up fifth toe, with plastic skin closure (eg, Ruiz-Mora type procedure)

28288 Ostectomy, partial, exostectomy or condylectomy, metatarsal head, each metatarsal head

28289 Hallux rigidus correction with cheilectomy, debridement and capsular release of the first metatarsophalangeal joint

28290 Correction, hallux valgus (bunion), with or without sesamoidectomy; simple exostectomy (eg, Silver type procedure)

28292 Keller, McBride, or Mayo type procedure

28293 resection of joint with implant

28294 with tendon transplants (eg, Joplin type procedure)

28296 with metatarsal osteotomy (eg, Mitchell, Chevron, or concentric type procedures)

28297 Lapidus type procedure

28298 by phalanx osteotomy

28299 by double osteotomy

28300 Osteotomy; calcaneus (eg, Dwyer or Chambers type procedure), with or without internal fixation

28302 talus

28304 Osteotomy, tarsal bones, other than calcaneus or talus;

28305 with autograft (includes obtaining graft) (eg, Fowler type)

28306 Osteotomy, with or without lengthening, shortening or angular correction, metatarsal; first metatarsal

28307 first metatarsal with autograft (other than first toe)

28308 other than first metatarsal, each

28309 multiple (eg, Swanson type cavus foot procedure)

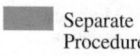 Separate Procedure   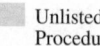 Unlisted Procedure   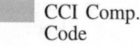 CCI Comp. Code   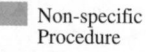 Non-specific Procedure

28310 Osteotomy, shortening, angular or rotational correction; proximal phalanx, first toe (separate procedure)

28312 other phalanges, any toe

28313 Reconstruction, angular deformity of toe, soft tissue procedures only (eg, overlapping second toe, fifth toe, curly toes)

28315 Sesamoidectomy, first toe (separate procedure)

28320 Repair, nonunion or malunion; tarsal bones

28322 metatarsal, with or without bone graft (includes obtaining graft)

28340 Reconstruction, toe, macrodactyly; soft tissue resection

28341 requiring bone resection

28344 Reconstruction, toe(s); polydactyly

28345 syndactyly, with or without skin graft(s), each web

28360 Reconstruction, cleft foot

FRACTURE AND/OR DISLOCATION

28400 Closed treatment of calcaneal fracture; without manipulation

28405 with manipulation

28406 Percutaneous skeletal fixation of calcaneal fracture, with manipulation

28415 Open treatment of calcaneal fracture, includes internal fixation, when performed;

28420 with primary iliac or other autogenous bone graft (includes obtaining graft)

28430 Closed treatment of talus fracture; without manipulation

28435 with manipulation

28436 Percutaneous skeletal fixation of talus fracture, with manipulation

● New Code ▲ Revised Code + Add-On Code ⊘ Modifier -51 Exempt ⊙ Moderate Sedation

28445 Open treatment of talus fracture, includes internal fixation, when performed

28446 Open osteochondral autograft, talus (includes obtaining graft[s])

(Do not report 28446 in conjunction with 27705, 27707)

(For arthroscopic osteochondral talus graft, use 29892)

(For open osteochondral allograft or repairs with industrial grafts, use 28899)

28450 Treatment of tarsal bone fracture (except talus and calcaneus); without manipulation, each

28455 with manipulation, each

28456 Percutaneous skeletal fixation of tarsal bone fracture (except talus and calcaneus), with manipulation, each

28465 Open treatment of tarsal bone fracture (except talus and calcaneus), includes internal fixation, when performed, each

28470 Closed treatment of metatarsal fracture; without manipulation, each

28475 with manipulation, each

28476 Percutaneous skeletal fixation of metatarsal fracture, with manipulation, each

28485 Open treatment of metatarsal fracture, includes internal fixation, when performed, each

28490 Closed treatment of fracture great toe, phalanx or phalanges; without manipulation

28495 with manipulation

28496 Percutaneous skeletal fixation of fracture great toe, phalanx or phalanges, with manipulation

28505 Open treatment of fracture great toe, phalanx or phalanges, includes internal fixation, when performed

28510 Closed treatment of fracture, phalanx or phalanges, other than great toe; without manipulation, each

Separate Procedure   Unlisted Procedure   CCI Comp. Code   Non-specific Procedure

483

28515   with manipulation, each

28525   Open treatment of fracture, phalanx or phalanges, other than great toe, includes internal fixation, when performed, each

28530   Closed treatment of sesamoid fracture

28531   Open treatment of sesamoid fracture, with or without internal fixation

28540   Closed treatment of tarsal bone dislocation, other than talotarsal; without anesthesia

28545   requiring anesthesia

28546   Percutaneous skeletal fixation of tarsal bone dislocation, other than talotarsal, with manipulation

28555   Open treatment of tarsal bone dislocation, includes internal fixation, when performed

28570   Closed treatment of talotarsal joint dislocation; without anesthesia

28575   requiring anesthesia

28576   Percutaneous skeletal fixation of talotarsal joint dislocation, with manipulation

28585   Open treatment of talotarsal joint dislocation, includes internal fixation, when performed

28600   Closed treatment of tarsometatarsal joint dislocation; without anesthesia

28605   requiring anesthesia

28606   Percutaneous skeletal fixation of tarsometatarsal joint dislocation, with manipulation

28615   Open treatment of tarsometatarsal joint dislocation, includes internal fixation, when performed

28630   Closed treatment of metatarsophalangeal joint dislocation; without anesthesia

484   New Code   Revised Code   Add-On Code   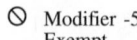 Modifier -51 Exempt   Moderate Sedation

28635   requiring anesthesia

28636   Percutaneous skeletal fixation of metatarsophalangeal joint dislocation, with manipulation

28645   Open treatment of metatarsophalangeal joint dislocation, includes internal fixation, when performed

28660   Closed treatment of interphalangeal joint dislocation; without anesthesia

28665   requiring anesthesia

28666   Percutaneous skeletal fixation of interphalangeal joint dislocation, with manipulation

28675   Open treatment of interphalangeal joint dislocation, includes internal fixation, when performed

ARTHRODESIS

28705   Arthrodesis; pantalar

28715   triple

28725   subtalar

28730   Arthrodesis, midtarsal or tarsometatarsal, multiple or transverse;

28735   with osteotomy (eg, flatfoot correction)

28737   Arthrodesis, with tendon lengthening and advancement, midtarsal, tarsal navicular-cuneiform (eg, Miller type procedure)

28740   Arthrodesis, midtarsal or tarsometatarsal, single joint

28750   Arthrodesis, great toe; metatarsophalangeal joint

28755   interphalangeal joint

28760   Arthrodesis, with extensor hallucis longus transfer to first metatarsal neck, great toe, interphalangeal joint (eg, Jones type procedure)

        (For hammertoe operation or interphalangeal fusion, use 28285)

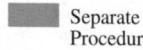 Separate Procedure
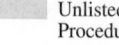 Unlisted Procedure
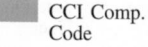 CCI Comp. Code
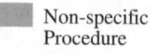 Non-specific Procedure

485

AMPUTATION

28800   Amputation, foot; midtarsal (eg, Chopart type procedure)

28805   transmetatarsal

28810   Amputation, metatarsal, with toe, single

28820   Amputation, toe; metatarsophalangeal joint

28825   interphalangeal joint

(For amputation of tuft of distal phalanx, use 11752)

OTHER PROCEDURES

28890   Extracorporeal shock wave, high energy, performed by a physician or other qualified health care professional, requiring anesthesia other than local, including ultrasound guidance, involving the plantar fascia

(For extracorporeal shock wave therapy involving musculoskeletal system, not otherwise specified, see Category III codes 0019T, 0101T, 0102T)

(For extracorporeal shock wave therapy involving integumentary system not otherwise specified, see 0299T, 0300T)

(Do not report 28890 in conjunction with 0299T, 0300T when treating in the same area)

28899   Unlisted procedure, foot or toes

APPLICATION OF CASTS AND STRAPPING

CPT codes in this section are used only when the cast application or strapping is a replacement procedure performed during or after the period of follow-up care. An additional evaluation and management service code, dependent on location, is reportable only if significant identifiable other services are provided at the time of the cast application or strapping.

For coding cast or strap application in situations not involving surgery, for example, casting of a sprained ankle or knee, use the appropriate level of evaluation and management services code plus code 99070 or equivalent HCPCS Level II code to report casting materials.

(For orthotics management and training, see 97760-97762)

● New Code   ▲ Revised Code   + Add-On Code   ⊘ Modifier -51 Exempt   ⊙ Moderate Sedation

BODY AND UPPER EXTREMITY

Casts

29000 Application of halo type body cast (see 20661-20663 for insertion)

29010 Application of Risser jacket, localizer, body; only

29015   including head

29020 Application of turnbuckle jacket, body; only

29025   including head

29035 Application of body cast, shoulder to hips;

29040   including head, Minerva type

29044   including 1 thigh

29046   including both thighs

29049 Application, cast; figure-of-eight

29055   shoulder spica

29058   plaster Velpeau

29065   shoulder to hand (long arm)

29075   elbow to finger (short arm)

29085   hand and lower forearm (gauntlet)

29086   finger (eg, contracture)

Splints

29105 Application of long arm splint (shoulder to hand)

29125 Application of short arm splint (forearm to hand); static

29126   dynamic

29130 Application of finger splint; static

487

Separate Procedure   Unlisted Procedure   CCI Comp. Code   Non-specific Procedure

29131   dynamic

Strapping - Any Age

29200 Strapping; thorax

(29220 Deleted 2009 [2010 edition])

    (To report low back strapping, use 29799)

29240   shoulder (eg, Velpeau)

29260   elbow or wrist

29280   hand or finger

LOWER EXTREMITY

Casts

29305 Application of hip spica cast; 1 leg

29325   1 and one-half spica or both legs

    (For hip spica (body) cast, including thighs only, use 29046)

29345 Application of long leg cast (thigh to toes);

29355   walker or ambulatory type

29358 Application of long leg cast brace

29365 Application of cylinder cast (thigh to ankle)

29405 Application of short leg cast (below knee to toes);

29425   walking or ambulatory type

29435 Application of patellar tendon bearing (PTB) cast

29440 Adding walker to previously applied cast

29445 Application of rigid total contact leg cast

29450 Application of clubfoot cast with molding or manipulation, long or short leg

 ● New ▲ Revised + Add-On ⊘ Modifier -51 ⊙ Moderate
   Code   Code   Code   Exempt   Sedation

(To report bilateral procedures, use 29450 with modifier -50)

Splints

29505 Application of long leg splint (thigh to ankle or toes)

29515 Application of short leg splint (calf to foot)

Strapping - Any Age

29520 Strapping; hip

29530 knee

29540 ankle and/or foot

(Do not report 29540 in conjunction with 29581, 29582)

29550 toes

29580 Unna boot

(Do not report 29580 in conjunction with 29581, 29582)

29581 Application of multi-layer compression system; leg (below knee), including ankle and foot

(Do not report 29581 in conjunction with 29540, 29580, 29582, 36475, 36478)

29582 thigh and leg, including ankle and foot, when performed

(Do not report 29582 in conjunction with 29540, 29580, 29581, 36475, 36478)

29583 upper arm and forearm

(Do not report 29583 in conjunction with 29584)

29584 upper arm, forearm, hand and fingers

(Do not report 29584 in conjunction with 29583)

(29590 deleted 2012 [2013 edition])

REMOVAL OR REPAIR

29700 Removal or bivalving; gauntlet, boot or body cast

489

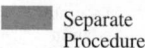 Separate Procedure   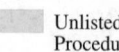 Unlisted Procedure   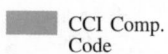 CCI Comp. Code   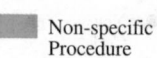 Non-specific Procedure

| 29705 | full arm or full leg cast |

| 29710 | shoulder or hip spica, Minerva, or Risser jacket, etc. |

| 29715 | turnbuckle jacket |

| 29720 | Repair of spica, body cast or jacket |

| 29730 | Windowing of cast |

| 29740 | Wedging of cast (except clubfoot casts) |

| 29750 | Wedging of clubfoot cast |

(To report bilateral procedures, use 29750 with modifier -50)

OTHER PROCEDURES

| 29799 | Unlisted procedure, casting or strapping |

ENDOSCOPY/ARTHROSCOPY

Surgical endoscopy/arthroscopy always includes a diagnostic endoscopy/ arthroscopy and is therefore never reported in addition to the surgical procedure. However, there are several arthroscopy procedures defined as separate procedures, indicating that the codes may be reported if the diagnostic arthroscopy is the only procedure performed.

When arthroscopy is performed in conjunction with arthrotomy, add modifier 51.

| 29800 | Arthroscopy, temporomandibular joint, diagnostic, with or without synovial biopsy (separate procedure) |

| 29804 | Arthroscopy, temporomandibular joint, surgical |

(For open procedure, use 21010)

| 29805 | Arthroscopy, shoulder, diagnostic, with or without synovial biopsy (separate procedure) |

(For open procedure, see 23065-23066, 23100-23101)

| 29806 | Arthroscopy, shoulder, surgical; capsulorrhaphy |

(For open procedure, see 23450-23466)

(To report thermal capsulorrhaphy, use 29999)

490

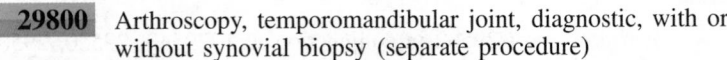

| ● New Code | ▲ Revised Code | ✛ Add-On Code | ⊘ Modifier -51 Exempt | ⊙ Moderate Sedation |

29807   repair of slap lesion

29819   with removal of loose body or foreign body

(For open procedure, see 23040-23044, 23107)

29820   synovectomy, partial

(For open procedure, see 23105)

29821   synovectomy, complete

(For open procedure, see 23105)

29822   debridement, limited

(For open procedure, see specific open shoulder procedure performed)

29823   debridement, extensive

(For open procedure, see specific open shoulder procedure performed)

29824   distal claviculectomy including distal articular surface (Mumford procedure)

(For open procedure, use 23120)

29825   with lysis and resection of adhesions, with or without manipulation

(For open procedure, see specific open shoulder procedure performed)

+ **29826**   decompression of subacromial space with partial acromioplasty, with coracoacromial ligament (ie, arch) release, when performed (List separately in addition to code for primary procedure

(For open procedure, use 23130 or 23415)

(Use 29826 in conjunction with 29806-29825, 29827, 29828)

29827   with rotator cuff repair

(For open or mini-open rotator cuff repair, use 23412)

(When arthroscopic distal clavicle resection is performed at the same setting, use 29824 and append modifier '-51')

Separate Procedure	Unlisted Procedure	CCI Comp. Code	Non-specific Procedure

491

29828   biceps tenodesis

(Do not report 29828 in conjunction with 29805, 29820, 29822)

(For open biceps tenodesis, use 23430)

29830   Arthroscopy, elbow, diagnostic, with or without synovial biopsy (separate procedure)

29834   Arthroscopy, elbow, surgical; with removal of loose body or foreign body

29835   synovectomy, partial

29836   synovectomy, complete

29837   debridement, limited

29838   debridement, extensive

29840   Arthroscopy, wrist, diagnostic, with or without synovial biopsy (separate procedure)

29843   Arthroscopy, wrist, surgical; for infection, lavage and drainage

29844   synovectomy, partial

29845   synovectomy, complete

29846   excision and/or repair of triangular fibrocartilage and/or joint debridement

29847   internal fixation for fracture or instability

29848   Endoscopy, wrist, surgical, with release of transverse carpal ligament

(For open procedure, use 64721)

29850   Arthroscopically aided treatment of intercondylar spine(s) and/or tuberosity fracture(s) of the knee, with or without manipulation; without internal or external fixation (includes arthroscopy)

29851   with internal or external fixation (includes arthroscopy)

(For bone graft, use 20900, 20902)

● New Code   ▲ Revised Code   + Add-On Code   ⊘ Modifier -51 Exempt   ⊙ Moderate Sedation

29855 Arthroscopically aided treatment of tibial fracture, proximal (plateau); nicondylar, includes internal fixation, when performed (includes arthroscopy)

29856 bicondylar, includes internal fixation, when performed (includes arthroscopy)

(For bone graft, use 20900, 20902)

29860 Arthroscopy, hip, diagnostic with or without synovial biopsy (separate procedure)

29861 Arthroscopy, hip, surgical; with removal of loose body or foreign body

29862 with debridement/shaving of articular cartilage (chondroplasty), abrasion arthroplasty, and/or resection of labrum

29863 with synovectomy

29914 with femoroplasty (ie, treatment of cam lesion)

29915 with acetabuloplasty (ie, treatment of pincer lesion)

(Do not report 29914, 29915 in conjunction with 29862, 29863)

29916 with labral repair

(Do not report 29916 in conjunction with 29915, 29862, 29863)

29866 Arthroscopy, knee, surgical; osteochondral autograft(s) (eg, mosaicplasty) (includes harvesting of the autograft[s])

(Do not report 29866 in conjunction with 29870, 29871, 29875, 29884 when performed at the same session and/or 29874, 29877, 29879, 29885-29887 when performed in the same compartment)

(For open osteochondral autograft of knee, use 27416)

29867 osteochondral allograft (eg, mosaicplasty)

(Do not report 29867 in conjunction with 27570, 29870, 29871, 29875, 29884 when performed at the same session and/or 29874, 29877, 29879, 29885-29887 when performed in the same compartment)

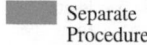 Separate Procedure   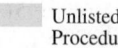 Unlisted Procedure   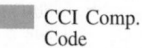 CCI Comp. Code   Non-specific Procedure   **493**

(Do not report 29867 in conjunction with 27415)

29868 meniscal transplantation (includes arthrotomy for meniscal insertion), medial or lateral

(Do not report 29868 in conjunction with 29870, 29871, 29875, 29880, 29883, 29884 when performed at the same session or 29874, 29877, 29881, 29882 when performed in the same compartment)

29870 Arthroscopy, knee, diagnostic, with or without synovial biopsy (separate procedure)

(For open autologous chondrocyte implantation of the knee, use 27412)

29871 Arthroscopy, knee, surgical; for infection, lavage and drainage

(For implantation of osteochondral graft for treatment of articular surface defect, see 27412, 27415, 29866, 29867)

29873 with lateral release

(For open lateral release, use 27425)

29874 for removal of loose body or foreign body (eg, osteochondritis dissecans fragmentation, chondral fragmentation)

29875 synovectomy, limited (eg, plica or shelf resection) (separate procedure)

29876 synovectomy, major, 2 or more compartments (eg, medial or lateral)

29877 debridement/shaving of articular cartilage (chondroplasty)

(When performed with arthroscopic meniscectomy, see 29880 or 29881)

29879 abrasion arthroplasty (includes chondroplasty where necessary) or multiple drilling or microfracture

29880 with meniscectomy (medial AND lateral, including any meniscal shaving) including debridement/shaving of articular cartilage (chondroplasty), same or separate compartment(s), when performed

---

● New Code   ▲ Revised Code   + Add-On Code   ⊘ Modifier -51 Exempt   ⊙ Moderate Sedation

29881 with meniscectomy (medial OR lateral, including any meniscal shaving) including debridement/shaving of articular cartilage (chondroplasty), same or separate compartment(s), when performed

29882 with meniscus repair (medial OR lateral)

29883 with meniscus repair (medial AND lateral)

(For meniscal transplantation, medial or lateral, knee, use 29868)

29884 with lysis of adhesions, with or without manipulation (separate procedure)

29885 drilling for osteochondritis dissecans with bone grafting, with or without internal fixation (including debridement of base of lesion)

29886 drilling for intact osteochondritis dissecans lesion

29887 drilling for intact osteochondritis dissecans lesion with internal fixation

29888 Arthroscopically aided anterior cruciate ligament repair/augmentation or reconstruction

29889 Arthroscopically aided posterior cruciate ligament repair/augmentation or reconstruction

(Procedures 29888 and 29889 should not be used with reconstruction procedures 27427-27429)

29891 Arthroscopy, ankle, surgical, excision of osteochondral defect of talus and/or tibia, including drilling of the defect

29892 Arthroscopically aided repair of large osteochondritis dissecans lesion, talar dome fracture, or tibial plafond fracture, with or without internal fixation (includes arthroscopy)

29893 Endoscopic plantar fasciotomy

29894 Arthroscopy, ankle (tibiotalar and fibulotalar joints), surgical; with removal of loose body or foreign body

29895 synovectomy, partial

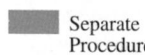 Separate Procedure   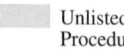 Unlisted Procedure   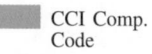 CCI Comp. Code   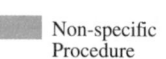 Non-specific Procedure **495**

29897 debridement, limited

29898 debridement, extensive

29899 with ankle arthrodesis

(For open ankle arthrodesis, use 27870)

29900 Arthroscopy, metacarpophalangeal joint, diagnostic, includes synovial biopsy

(Do not report 29900 with 29901, 29902)

29901 Arthroscopy, metacarpophalangeal joint, surgical; with debridement

29902 with reduction of displaced ulnar collateral ligament (eg, Stenar lesion)

29904 Arthroscropy, subtalar joint, surgical; with removal of loose body or foreign body

29905 with synovectomy

29906 with debridement

29907 with subtalar arthrodesis

29914 This code is out of order. See page 493

29915 This code is out of order. See page 493

29916 This code is out of order. See page 493

29999 Unlisted procedure, arthroscopy

● New Code ▲ Revised Code + Add-On Code ⊘ Modifier -51 Exempt ⊙ Moderate Sedation

RESPIRATORY SYSTEM

CPT codes from this section of the CPT coding system are used to report invasive and surgical procedures performed on the nose, sinuses, larynx, trachea and bronchi, and the lungs and pleura.

MISCELLANEOUS CODING RULES

Functional Endoscopic Sinus Surgery (FESS) codes are coded based on the procedures described in the operative report or on the nasal sinus endoscopy report. Each FESS code represents a unilateral procedure. To express that a procedure was performed bilaterally requires the application of the modifier -50, bilateral procedure.

Indirect laryngoscopy involves the visualization of the larynx using a warm laryngeal mirror positioned at the back of the throat. Direct laryngoscopy involves the visualization using a rigid or fiberoptic endoscope. Operative direct laryngoscopy involves an endoscopic examination under general anesthesia.

To code nasal hemorrhages appropriately, documentation needs to substantiate whether the hemorrhage is anterior or posterior and how the hemorrhage is controlled. Control of anterior nasal hemorrhage typically involves the insertion of gauze packing, or anterior packing or performance of cauterization. Control of posterior nasal hemorrhage most likely requires the insertion of nasal stents, tampons, balloon catheters, or posterior packing.

NOSE

INCISION

30000 Drainage abscess or hematoma, nasal, internal approach

(For external approach, see 10060, 10140)

30020 Drainage abscess or hematoma, nasal septum

(For lateral rhinotomy, see specific application (eg, 30118, 30320))

RESP
CVS
30000

EXCISION

30100 Biopsy, intranasal

(For biopsy skin of nose, see 11100, 11101)

30110 Excision, nasal polyp(s), simple

497

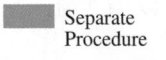 Separate Procedure   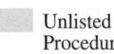 Unlisted Procedure   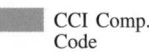 CCI Comp. Code   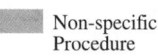 Non-specific Procedure

(30110 would normally be completed in an office setting)

(To report bilateral procedure, use 30110 with modifier -50)

30115 Excision, nasal polyp(s), extensive

(30115 would normally require the facilities available in a hospital setting)

(To report bilateral procedure, use 30115 with modifier -50)

30117 Excision or destruction (eg, laser), intranasal lesion; internal approach

30118 external approach (lateral rhinotomy)

30120 Excision or surgical planing of skin of nose for rhinophyma

30124 Excision dermoid cyst, nose; simple, skin, subcutaneous

30125 complex, under bone or cartilage

30130 Excision inferior turbinate, partial or complete, any method

(For excision of superior or middle turbinate, use 30999)

30140 Submucous resection inferior turbinate, partial or complete, any method

(Do not report 30130 or 30140 in conjunction with 30801, 30802, 30930)

(For submucous resection of superior or middle turbinate, use 30999)

(For endoscopic resection of concha bullosa of middle turbinate, use 31240)

(For submucous resection of nasal septum, use 30520)

30150 Rhinectomy; partial

30160 total

(For closure and/or reconstruction, primary or delayed, see Integumentary System, 13150-13160, 14060-14302, 15120, 15121, 15260, 15261, 15760, 20900-20912)

● New Code ▲ Revised Code + Add-On Code ⊘ Modifier -51 Exempt ⊙ Moderate Sedation

INTRODUCTION

30200 Injection into turbinate(s), therapeutic

30210 Displacement therapy (Proetz type)

30220 Insertion, nasal septal prosthesis (button)

REMOVAL OF FOREIGN BODY

30300 Removal foreign body, intranasal; office type procedure

30310 requiring general anesthesia

30320 by lateral rhinotomy

REPAIR

(For obtaining tissues for graft, see 20900-20926, 21210)

30400 Rhinoplasty, primary; lateral and alar cartilages and/or elevation of nasal tip

(For columellar reconstruction, see 13150 et seq)

30410 complete, external parts including bony pyramid, lateral and alar cartilages, and/or elevation of nasal tip

30420 including major septal repair

30430 Rhinoplasty, secondary; minor revision (small amount of nasal tip work)

30435 intermediate revision (bony work with osteotomies)

30450 major revision (nasal tip work and osteotomies)

30460 Rhinoplasty for nasal deformity secondary to congenital cleft lip and/or palate, including columellar lengthening; tip only

30462 tip, septum, osteotomies

30465 Repair of nasal vestibular stenosis (eg, spreader grafting, lateral nasal wall reconstruction)

(30465 excludes obtaining graft. For graft procedure, see 20900-20926, 21210)

499

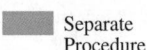 Separate Procedure   Unlisted Procedure   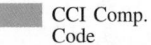 CCI Comp. Code   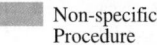 Non-specific Procedure

(30465 is used to report a bilateral procedure. For unilateral procedure, use modifier -52)

30520 Septoplasty or submucous resection, with or without cartilage scoring, contouring or replacement with graft

(For submucous resection of turbinates, use 30140)

30540 Repair choanal atresia; intranasal

30545　　transpalatine

(Do not report modifier '-63' in conjunction with 30540, 30545)

30560 Lysis intranasal synechia

30580 Repair fistula; oromaxillary (combine with 31030 if antrotomy is included)

30600　　oronasal

30620 Septal or other intranasal dermatoplasty (does not include obtaining graft)

30630 Repair nasal septal perforations

DESTRUCTION

30801 Ablation, soft tissue of inferior turbinates, unilateral or bilateral, any method (eg, electrocautery, radiofrequency ablation, or tissue volume reduction); superficial

(For ablation of superior or middle turbinates, use 30999)

30802　　intramural (ie, submucosal)

(Do not report 30801 in conjunction with 30802)

(Do not report 30801, 30802, 30930 in conjunction with 30130 or 30140)

(For cautery performed for control of nasal hemorrhage, see 30901-30906)

OTHER PROCEDURES

30901 Control nasal hemorrhage, anterior, simple (limited cautery and/or packing) any method

● New Code　　▲ Revised Code　　+ Add-On Code　　⊘ Modifier -51 Exempt　　⊙ Moderate Sedation

(To report bilateral procedure, use 30901 with modifier -50)

30903 Control nasal hemorrhage, anterior, complex (extensive cautery and/or packing) any method

(To report bilateral procedure, use 30903 with modifier -50)

30905 Control nasal hemorrhage, posterior, with posterior nasal packs and/or cautery, any method; initial

30906 subsequent

30915 Ligation arteries; ethmoidal

30920 internal maxillary artery, transantral

(For ligation external carotid artery, use 37600)

30930 Fracture nasal inferior turbinate(s), therapeutic

(Do not report 30801, 30802, 30930 in conjunction with 30130 or 30140)

(For fracture of superior or middle turbinate(s), use 30999)

30999 Unlisted procedure, nose

ACCESSORY SINUSES

INCISION

31000 Lavage by cannulation; maxillary sinus (antrum puncture or natural ostium)

(To report bilateral procedure, use 31000 with modifier -50)

31002 sphenoid sinus

31020 Sinusotomy, maxillary (antrotomy); intranasal

(To report bilateral procedure, use 31020 with modifier -50)

31030 radical (Caldwell-Luc) without removal of antrochoanal polyps

(To report bilateral procedure, use 31030 with modifier -50)

31032 radical (Caldwell-Luc) with removal of antrochoanal polyps

---

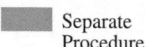 Separate Procedure   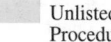 Unlisted Procedure   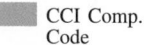 CCI Comp. Code   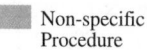 Non-specific Procedure   **501**

(To report bilateral procedure, use 31032 with modifier -50)

31040 Pterygomaxillary fossa surgery, any approach

(For transantral ligation of internal maxillary artery, use 30920)

31050 Sinusotomy, sphenoid, with or without biopsy;

31051   with mucosal stripping or removal of polyp(s)

31070 Sinusotomy frontal; external, simple (trephine operation)

(For frontal intranasal sinusotomy, use 31276)

31075   transorbital, unilateral (for mucocele or osteoma, Lynch type)

31080   obliterative without osteoplastic flap, brow incision (includes ablation)

31081   obliterative, without osteoplastic flap, coronal incision (includes ablation)

31084   obliterative, with osteoplastic flap, brow incision

31085   obliterative, with osteoplastic flap, coronal incision

31086   nonobliterative, with osteoplastic flap, brow incision

31087   nonobliterative, with osteoplastic flap, coronal incision

31090 Sinusotomy, unilateral, 3 or more paranasal sinuses (frontal, maxillary, ethmoid, sphenoid)

EXCISION

31200 Ethmoidectomy; intranasal, anterior

31201   intranasal, total

31205   extranasal, total

31225 Maxillectomy; without orbital exenteration

31230   with orbital exenteration (en bloc)

(For orbital exenteration only, see 65110 et seq)

● New Code   ▲ Revised Code   ✚ Add-On Code   ⊘ Modifier -51 Exempt   ⊙ Moderate Sedation

(For skin graft, see 15120 et seq)

ENDOSCOPY

A surgical sinus endoscopy includes a sinusotomy (when appropriate) and diagnostic endoscopy.

Codes 31295-31297 describe dilation of sinus ostia by displacement of tissue, any method, and include fluoroscopy if performed.

Codes 31233-31297 are used to report unilateral procedures unless otherwise specified.

The codes 31231-31235 for diagnostic evaluation refer to employing a nasal/sinus endoscope to inspect the interior of the nasal cavity and the middle and superior meatus, the turbinates, and the spheno-ethmoid recess. Any time a diagnostic evaluation is performed, all these areas would be inspected and a separate code is not reported for each area.

31231 Nasal endoscopy, diagnostic, unilateral or bilateral (separate procedure)

31233 Nasal/sinus endoscopy, diagnostic with maxillary sinusoscopy (via inferior meatus or canine fossa puncture)

(Do not report 31233 in conjunction with 31295 when performed on the same sinus)

31235 Nasal/sinus endoscopy, diagnostic with sphenoid sinusoscopy (via puncture of sphenoidal face or cannulation of ostium)

(Do not report 31235 in conjunction with 31297 when performed on the same sinus)

31237 Nasal/sinus endoscopy, surgical; with biopsy, polypectomy or debridement (separate procedure)

31238 with control of nasal hemorrhage

31239 with dacryocystorhinostomy

31240 with concha bullosa resection

(For endoscopic osteomeatal complex (OMC) resection with antrostomy and/or anterior ethmoidectomy, with or without removal of polyp(s), use 31254 and 31256)

(For endoscopic osteomeatal complex (OMC) resection with antrostomy, removal of antral mucosal disease, and/or anterior

503

ethmoidectomy, with or without removal of polyp(s), use 31254 and 31257)

(For endoscopic frontal sinus exploration, osteomeatal complex (OMC) resection and./or anterior ethmoidecomy, with or without removal of polyp(s), use 31254 and 31276)

(For endoscopic frontal sinus exploration, osteomeatal complex (OMC) resection, antrostomy, and./or anterior ethmoidecomy, with or without removal of polyp(s), use 31254, 31256 and 31276)

(For endoscopic nasal diagnostic endoscopy, see 31231-31235)

(For endoscopic osteomeatal complex (OMC) resection, frontal sinus exploration, antrostomy, removal of antral mucosal disease, and/or anterior ethmoidecomy, with or without removal of polyp(s), use 31254, 31267, and 31276)

31254 Nasal/sinus endoscopy, surgical; with ethmoidectomy, partial (anterior)

31255 with ethmoidectomy, total (anterior andposterior)

31256 Nasal/sinus endoscopy, surgical, with maxillary antrostomy;

(For endoscopic anterior and posterior ethmoidectomy (APE) and antrostomy, with or without removal of polyp(s), use 31255 and 31256)

(For endoscopic anterior and posterior ethmoidectomy (APE), antrostomy and removal of antral mucosal disease, with or without removal of polyp(s), use 31255 and 31267)

(For endoscopic anterior and posterior ethmoidectomy (APE) and frontal sinus exploration, with or without removal of polyp(s), use 31255 and 31276)

31267 with removal of tissue from maxillary sinus

(Do not report 31256, 31267 in conjunction with 31295 when performed on the same sinus)

(For endoscopic anterior and posterior ethmoidectomy (APE) and frontal sinus exploration and antrostomy, with or without removal of polyp(s), use 31255, 31256, and 31276)

(For endoscopic anterior and posterior ethmoidectomy (APE), frontal sinus exploration, antrostomy, and removal of antral mucosal disease, with or without removal of polyp(s), use 31255, 31267, and 31276)

● New Code   ▲ Revised Code   ✛ Add-On Code   ⃠ Modifier -51 Exempt   ⊙ Moderate Sedation

31276 Nasal/sinus endoscopy, surgical with frontal sinus exploration, with or without removal of tissue from frontal sinus

(Do not report 31276 in conjunction with 31296 when performed on the same sinus)

(For endoscopic anterior and posterior ethmoidectomy and sphenoidotomy (APS), with or without removal of polyp(s), use 31255, 31287 or 31288)

(For endoscopic anterior and posterior ethmoidectomy and sphenoidotomy (APS), and antrostomy, with or without removal of polyp(s), use 31255, 31256, and 31287 or 31288)

(For endoscopic anterior and posterior ethmoidectomy and sphenoidotomy (APS), antrostomy and removal of antral mucosal disease, with or without removal of polyp(s), use 31255, 31267, and 31287 or 31288)

(For endoscopic anterior and posterior ethmoidectomy and sphenoidotomy (APS), and frontal sinus exploration, with or without removal of polyp(s), use 31255, 31287 or 31288, and 31276)

(For endoscopic anterior and posterior ethmoidectomy and sphenoidotomy (APS), with or without removal of polyp(s), with frontal sinus exploration and antrostomy, use 31255, 31256, 31287 or 31288, and 31276)

(For unilateral endoscopy of two or more sinuses, see 31231-31235)

(For endoscopic anterior and posterior ethmoidectomy and sphenoidotomy (APS), frontal sinus exploration, antrostomy and removal of antral mucosal disease, with or without the removal of polyp(s), see 31255, 31267, 31287 or 31288, and 31276)

31287 Nasal/sinus endoscopy, surgical, with sphenoidotomy;

31288   with removal of tissue from the sphenoid sinus

(Do not report 31287, 31288 in conjunction with 31297 when performed on the same sinus)

31290 Nasal/sinus endoscopy, surgical, with repair of cerebrospinal fluid leak; ethmoid region

31291   sphenoid region

31292 Nasal/sinus endoscopy, surgical; with medial or inferior orbital wall decompression

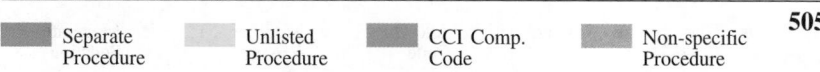

	Separate Procedure		Unlisted Procedure		CCI Comp. Code		Non-specific Procedure

505

31293   with medial orbital wall and inferior orbital wall decompression

31294   with optic nerve decompression

31295   Nasal/sinus endoscopy, surgical; with dilation of maxillary sinus ostium (eg, balloon dilation), transnasal or via canine fossa

(Do not report 31295 in conjunction with 31233, 31256, 31267 when performed on the same sinus)

31296   with dilation of frontal sinua ostium (eg, balloon dilation)

(Do not report 31296 in conjunction with 31276 when performed on the same sinus)

31297   with dilation of sphenoid sinus ostium (eg, balloon dilation)

(Do not report 31297 in conjunction with 31235, 31287, 31288 when performed on the same sinus)

OTHER PROCEDURES

(For hypophysectomy, transantral or transeptal approach, use 61548)

(For transcranial hypophysectomy, use 61546)

31299   Unlisted procedure, accessory sinuses

LARYNX

EXCISION

31300   Laryngotomy (thyrotomy, laryngofissure); with removal of tumor or laryngocele, cordectomy

31320   diagnostic

31360   Laryngectomy; total, without radical neck dissection

31365   total, with radical neck dissection

31367   subtotal supraglottic, without radical neck dissection

31368   subtotal supraglottic, with radical neck dissection

31370   Partial laryngectomy (hemilaryngectomy); horizontal

● New Code   ▲ Revised Code   ＋ Add-On Code   ⊘ Modifier -51 Exempt   ⊙ Moderate Sedation

31375	laterovertical
31380	anterovertical
31382	antero-latero-vertical
31390	Pharyngolaryngectomy, with radical neck dissection; without reconstruction
31395	with reconstruction
31400	Arytenoidectomy or arytenoidopexy, external approach

(For endoscopic arytenoidecomy, use 31560)

31420	Epiglottidectomy

INTRODUCTION

⊘ **31500**	Intubation, endotracheal, emergency procedure
31502	Tracheotomy tube change prior to establishment of fistula tract

ENDOSCOPY

For endoscopic procedures, code appropriate endoscopy of each anatomic site examined. If using operating microscope, telescope, or both, use the applicable code only once per operative session.

31505	Laryngoscopy, indirect; diagnostic (separate procedure)
31510	with biopsy
31511	with removal of foreign body
31512	with removal of lesion
31513	with vocal cord injection
31515	Laryngoscopy direct, with or without tracheoscopy; for aspiration
31520	diagnostic, newborn

(Do not report modifier -63 in conjunction with 31520)

31525	diagnostic, except newborn

Separate Procedure	Unlisted Procedure	CCI Comp. Code	Non-specific Procedure

507

31526   diagnostic, with operating microscope or telescope

(Do not report code 69990 in addition to code 31526)

31527   with insertion of obturator

31528   with dilation, initial

31529   with dilation, subsequent

31530   Laryngoscopy, direct, operative, with foreign body removal;

31531   with operating microscope or telescope

(Do not report code 69990 in addition to code 31531)

31535   Laryngoscopy, direct, operative, with biopsy;

31536   with operating microscope or telescope

(Do not report code 69990 in addition to code 31536)

31540   Laryngoscopy, direct, operative, with excision of tumor and/or stripping of vocal cords or epiglottis;

31541   with operating microscope or telescope

(Do not report code 69990 in addition to code 31541)

31545   Laryngoscopy, direct, operative, with operating microscope or telescope, with submucosal removal of non-neoplastic lesion(s) of vocal cord; reconstruction with local tissue flap(s)

31546   reconstruction with graft(s) (includes obtaining autograft)

(Do not report 31546 in addition to 20926 for graft harvest)

(For reconstruction of vocal cord with allograft, use 31599)

(Do not report 31545 or 31546 in conjunction with 31540, 31541, 69990)

31560   Laryngoscopy, direct, operative, with arytenoidectomy;

31561   with operating microscope or telescope

(Do not report code 69990 in addition to code 31561)

---

508 ● New Code ▲ Revised Code + Add-On Code ⊘ Modifier -51 Exempt ⊙ Moderate Sedation

31570 Laryngoscopy, direct, with injection into vocal cord(s), therapeutic;

31571 with operating microscope or telescope

(Do not report code 69990 in addition to code 31571)

31575 Laryngoscopy, flexible fiberoptic; diagnostic

31576 with biopsy

31577 with removal of foreign body

31578 with removal of lesion

(To report flexible fiberoptic endoscopic evaluation of swallowing, see 92612-92613)

(To report flexible fiberoptic endoscopic evaluation with sensory testing, see 92614-92615)

(To report flexible fiberoptic endoscopic evaluation of swallowing with sensory testing, see 92616-92617)

(For flexible fiberoptic laryngoscopy as part of flexible fiberoptic endoscopic evaluation of swallowing and/or laryngeal sensory testing by cine or video recording, see 92612-92617)

31579 Laryngoscopy, flexible or rigid fiberoptic, with stroboscopy

REPAIR

31580 Laryngoplasty; for laryngeal web, 2 stage, with keel insertion and removal

31582 for laryngeal stenosis, with graft or core mold, including tracheotomy

31584 with open reduction of fracture

31587 Laryngoplasty, cricoid split

31588 Laryngoplasty, not otherwise specified (eg, for burns, reconstruction after partial laryngectomy)

31590 Laryngeal reinnervation by neuromuscular pedicle

509

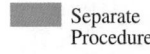 Separate Procedure   Unlisted Procedure 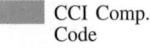 CCI Comp. Code 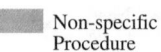 Non-specific Procedure

DESTRUCTION

31595 Section recurrent laryngeal nerve, therapeutic (separate procedure), unilateral

OTHER PROCEDURES

31599 Unlisted procedure, larynx

TRACHEA AND BRONCHI

INCISION

31600 Tracheostomy, planned (separate procedure);

31601 under 2 years

31603 Tracheostomy, emergency procedure; transtracheal

31605 cricothyroid membrane

31610 Tracheostomy, fenestration procedure with skin flaps

(For endotracheal intubation, use 31500)

(For tracheal aspiration under direct vision, use 31515)

31611 Construction of tracheoesophageal fistula and subsequent insertion of an alaryngeal speech prosthesis (eg, voice button, Blom-Singer prosthesis)

31612 Tracheal puncture, percutaneous with transtracheal aspiration and/or injection

31613 Tracheostoma revision; simple, without flap rotation

31614 complex, with flap rotation

ENDOSCOPY

For endoscopy procedures, code appropriate endoscopy of each anatomic site examined. Surgical bronchoscopy always includes diagnostic bronchoscopy when performed by the same physician. Codes 31622-31651, 31660, 31661 include fluoroscopic guidance, when performed.

(For tracheoscopy, see laryngoscopy codes 31515-31578)

⊙ **31615** Tracheobronchoscopy through established tracheostomy incision

● New Code   ▲ Revised Code   + Add-On Code   ⊘ Modifier -51 Exempt   ⊙ Moderate Sedation

⊙+31620 Endobronchial ultrasound (EBUS) during bronchoscopic diagnostic or therapeutic intervention(s) (List separately in addition to code for primary procedure[s])

(Use 31620 in conjunction with 31622-31646)

⊙ 31622 Bronchoscopy, rigid or flexible, including fluoroscopic guidance, when performed; diagnostic, with cell washing, when performed (separate procedure)

⊙ 31623 with brushing or protected brushings

⊙ 31624 with bronchial alveolar lavage

⊙ 31625 with bronchial or endobronchial biopsy(s), single or multiple sites

⊙ 31626 with placement of fiducial markers, single or multiple

(Report supply of device separately)

⊙+31627 with computer-assisted, image-guided navigation (List separately in addition to code for primary procedure[s])

(31627 includes 3D reconstruction. Do not report 31627 in conjunction with 76376, 76377)

(Use 31627 in conjunction with 31615, 31622-31626, 31628-31631, 31635, 31636, 31638-31643)

⊙ 31628 with transbronchial lung biopsy(s), single lobe

(31628 should be reported only once regardless of how many transbronchial lung biopsies are performed in a lobe)

(To report transbronchial lung biopsies performed on additional lobe, use 31632)

⊙ 31629 with transbronchial needle aspiration biopsy(s), trachea, main stem and/or lobar bronchus(i)

(31629 should be reported only once for upper airway biopsies regardless of how many transbronchial needle aspiration biopsies are performed in the upper airway or in a lobe)

(To report transbronchial needle aspiration biopsies performed on additional lobe(s), use 31633)

31630 with tracheal/bronchial dilation or closed reduction of fracture

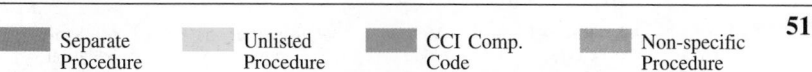

Separate Procedure Unlisted Procedure CCI Comp. Code Non-specific Procedure **511**

31631 with placement of tracheal stent(s) (includes tracheal/bronchial dilation as required)

(For placement of bronchial stent, see 31636, 31637)

(For revision of tracheal/bronchial stent, use 31638)

+ **31632** with transbronchial lung biopsy(s), each additional lobe (List separately in addition to code for primary procedure)

(Use 31632 in conjunction with 31628)

(31632 should be reported only once regardless of how many transbronchial lung biopsies are performed in a lobe)

+ **31633** with transbronchial needle aspiration biopsy(s), each additional lobe (List separately in addition to code for primary procedure)

(Use 31633 in conjunction with 31629)

(31633 should be reported only once regardless of how many transbronchial needle aspiration biopsies are performed in the trachea or the additional lobe)

⊙ **31634** with balloon occlusion, with assessment of air leak, with administration of occlusive substance (eg, fibrin glue), if performed

(Do not report 31534 in conjunction with 31647, 31651 at the same session)

⊙ **31635** with removal of foreign body

(For removal of implanted bronchial valves, see 31648-31649)

31636 with placement of bronchial stent(s) (includes tracheal/bronchial dilation as required), initial bronchus

+ **31637** each additional major bronchus stented (List separately in addition to code for primary procedure)

(Use 31637 in conjunction with 31636)

31638 with revision of tracheal or bronchial stent inserted at previous session (includes tracheal/bronchial dilation as required)

31640 with excision of tumor

● New Code   ▲ Revised Code   + Add-On Code   ⊘ Modifier -51 Exempt   ⊙ Moderate Sedation

| 31641 | with destruction of tumor or relief of stenosis by any method other than excision (eg, laser therapy, cryotherapy) |

(For bronchoscopic photodynamic therapy, report 31641 in addition to 96570, 96571 as appropriate)

| 31643 | with placement of catheter(s) for intracavitary radioelement application |

(For intracavitary radioelement application, see 77761-77763, 77785-77787)

⊙ 31645   with therapeutic aspiration of tracheobronchial tree, initial (eg, drainage of lung abscess)

⊙ 31646   with therapeutic aspiration of tracheobronchial tree, subsequent

(For catheter aspiration of tracheobronchial tree at bedside, use 31725)

●⊙31647   with balloon occlusion, when performed assessment of air leak, airway sizing, and insertion of bronchial valve(s), initial lobe

●⊙31648   with removal of bronchial valve(s), initial lobe

(For removal and insertion of a bronchial valve at the same session, see 31647, 31648, and 31651)

●⊙+31649   with removal of bronchial valve(s), each additional lobe (List separately in addition to code for primary procedure)

(Use 31649 in conjunction with 31648)

●⊙+31651   with balloon occlusion, when performed, assessment of air leak, airway sizing, and insertion of bronchial valve(s), each additional lobe (List separately in addition to code for primary procedure[s])

(Use 31651 in conjunction with 31647)

(31656   deleted 2012 [2013 edition]. To report, use 31899)

■ Separate Procedure   ■ Unlisted Procedure   ■ CCI Comp. Code   ■ Non-specific Procedure   **513**

BRONCHIAL THERMOPLASTY

●⊙ **31660** Bronchoscopy, rigid or flexible, including fluoroscopic guidance, when performed; with bronchial thermoplasty, 1 lobe

●⊙ **31661** with bronchial thermoplasty, 2 or more lobes

INTRODUCTION

(For endotracheal intubation, use 31500)

(For tracheal aspiration under direct vision, see 31515)

(31715 deleted 2012 [2013 edition]. To report, use 31899)

31717 Catheterization with bronchial brush biopsy

31720 Catheter aspiration (separate procedure); nasotracheal

⊙ **31725** tracheobronchial with fiberscope, bedside

31730 Transtracheal (percutaneous) introduction of needle wire dilator/stent or indwelling tube for oxygen therapy

EXCISION, REPAIR

31750 Tracheoplasty; cervical

31755 tracheopharyngeal fistulization, each stage

31760 intrathoracic

31766 Carinal reconstruction

31770 Bronchoplasty; graft repair

31775 excision stenosis and anastomosis

(For lobectomy and bronchoplasty, use 32501)

31780 Excision tracheal stenosis and anastomosis; cervical

31781 cervicothoracic

31785 Excision of tracheal tumor or carcinoma; cervical

31786 thoracic

514 ● New Code ▲ Revised Code + Add-On Code ⊘ Modifier -51 Exempt ⊙ Moderate Sedation

31800 Suture of tracheal wound or injury; cervical

31805   intrathoracic

31820 Surgical closure tracheostomy or fistula; without plastic repair

31825   with plastic repair

(For repair tracheoesophageal fistula, see 43305, 43312)

31830 Revision of tracheostomy scar

OTHER PROCEDURES

31899 Unlisted procedure, trachea, bronchi

LUNGS AND PLEURA

Pleural cavity or lung biopsy procedures may be accomplished using a percutaneous, thorascopic (Video-Assisted Thoracoscopic Surgery [VATS]), or thoracotomy approach. They involve the removal of differing amounts of tissue for diagnosis. A biopsy may be performed using different techniques such as incision or wedge. Lung resection procedures include diagnostic and therapeutic procedures, including the removal of blebs, bullae, cysts, and benign or malignant tumors or lesions. These procedures may involve the removal of small portions of the lung or even an entire lung. Additionally, lung resection procedures may require the removal of adjacent structures. Both diagnostic lung biopsies and therapeutic lung resections can be performed utilizing a wedge technique. However, a diagnostic biopsy of a lung nodule using a wedge technique requires only that a tissue sample be obtained without particular attention to resection margins. A therapeutic wedge resection requires attention to margins and complete resection even when the wedge resection is ultimately followed by a more extensive resection. In the case of a wedge resection where intraoperative pathology consultation determines that a more extensive resection is required in the same anatomic location, it becomes classified as a diagnostic wedge resection (32507, 32668). When no more extensive resection is required, the same procedure is a therapeutic wedge resection (32505, 32666).

Pleural or lung biopsies or diagnostic wedge resections should be reported using codes 32096, 32097, 32098, 32400, 32405, 32507, 32607, 32608, 32609 or 32668. The open or thorasoscopic (VATS) therapeutic resection of lung mass or nodules via a wedge resection is reported using codes 32505, 32506, 32666 and 32667. More extensive anatomic lung resection procedures, which can be performed with either thoracotomy or thoracoscopic (VATS) approaches, include: segmentectomy, lobectomy, bilobectomy, and pneumonectomy.

| | Separate Procedure | | Unlisted Procedure | | CCI Comp. Code | | Non-specific Procedure |

When diagnostic biopsy(ies) of the lung are performed, regardless of the approach (ie, open or thoracoscopic [VATS]), or technique (eg, incisional resection, cautery resection, or stapled wedge), and the specimen is sent for intraoperative pathology consultation, and during that same operative session the surgeon uses these results to determine the extent of the necessary surgical resection that includes the anatomical location biopsied, only the most extensive procedure performed (eg, segmentectomy, lobectomy, thoracoscopic [VATS] lobectomy) should be reported.

The therapeutic wedge resection codes (32505, 32506, 32666, or 32667) should not be reported in addition to the more extensive lung procedure (eg, lobectomy) unless the therapeutic wedge resection was performed on a different lobe or on the contralateral lung, whether or not an intraoperative pathology consultation is used to determine the extent of lung resection. When a diagnostic wedge resection is followed by a more extensive procedure in the same anatomical location, report add-on codes 32507 or 32668 with the more extensive procedure(s). When a therapeutic wedge resection (32505, 32506, 32666 or 32667) is performed in a different lobe than the more extensive lung resection (eg, lobectomy), report the therapeutic wedge resection with modifier 59.

INCISION

(32000   deleted 2008 edition, see 32421)

(32002   deleted 2008 edition, see 32422)

(32005   deleted 2008 edition, see 32560)

(32019   deleted 2008 edition, see 32550)

(32020   deleted 2008 edition, see 32551)

32035   Thoracostomy; with rib resection for empyema

32036   with open flap drainage for empyema

(To report wound exploration due to penetrating trauma without thoracotomy, use 20101)

(32095   deleted 2011 [2012 edition]. To report, see 32096, 32097, 32098 for thoracotomy with biopsy of the lung or pleura)

32096   Thoracotomy, with diagnostic biopsy(ies) of lung infiltrate(s) (eg, wedge, incisional), unilateral

(Do not report 32096 more than once per lung)

(Do not report 32096 in conjunction with 32440, 32442, 32445, 32488)

● New Code ▲ Revised Code + Add-On Code ⊘ Modifier -51 Exempt ⊙ Moderate Sedation

32097 Thoracotomy, with diagnostic biopsy(ies) of lung nodule(s) or mass(es) (eg, wedge, incisional), unilateral

(Do not report 32097 more than once per lung)

(Do not report 32097 in conjunction with 32440, 32442, 32445, 32488)

32098 Thoracotomy, with biopsy(ies) of pleura

32100 Thoracotomy; with exploration

(Do not report 32100 in conjunction with 19260, 19271, 19272, 32503, 32504)

32110 with control of traumatic hemorrhage and/or repair of lung tear

32120 for postoperative complications

32124 with open intrapleural pneumonolysis

32140 with cyst(s) removal, includes pleural procedure when performed

32141 with resection-plication of bullae, includes any pleural procedure when performed

(For lung volume reduction, use 32491)

32150 with removal of intrapleural foreign body or fibrin deposit

32151 with removal of intrapulmonary foreign body

32160 with cardiac massage

(For segmental or other resections of lung, see 32480-32504)

32200 Pneumonostomy; with open drainage of abscess or cyst

⊙ **32201** with percutaneous drainage of abscess or cyst

(For radiological supervision and interpretation, use 75989)

32215 Pleural scarification for repeat pneumothorax

32220 Decortication, pulmonary (separate procedure); total

 Separate Procedure   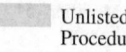 Unlisted Procedure   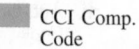 CCI Comp. Code   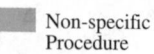 Non-specific Procedure   **517**

32225   partial

EXCISION/RESECTION

32310   Pleurectomy, parietal (separate procedure)

32320   Decortication and parietal pleurectomy

32400   Biopsy, pleura; percutaneous needle

(If imaging guidance is performed, see 76942, 77002, 77012, 77021)

(For fine needle aspiration, use 10021 or 10022)

(32402   deleted 2011 [2012 edition]. To report open biopsy of pleura, use 32098)

⊙ 32405   Biopsy, lung or mediastinum, percutaneous needle

(For open biopsy of lung, see 32096, 32097. For open biopsy of mediastinum, see 39000 or 39010. For thoracoscopic [VATS] biopsy of lung, pleura, pericardium or mediastinal space structure, see 32604, 32606, 32607, 32608, 32609)

(For radiological supervision and interpretation, see 76942, 77002, 77012, 77021)

(For fine needle aspiration, use 10022)

REMOVAL

(32420   deleted 2012 [2013 edition]. To report, use 32405)

(32421   deleted 2012 [2013 edition]. To report, see 32554, 32555)

(32422   deleted 2012 [2013 edition]. To report, see 32554, 32555)

32440   Removal of lung, pneumonectomy;

32442   with resection of segment of trachea followed by broncho-tracheal anastomosis (sleeve pneumonectomy)

32445   extrapleural

(For extrapleural pneumonectomy, with empyemectomy, use 32445 and 32540)

● New Code   ▲ Revised Code   ＋ Add-On Code   ⊘ Modifier -51 Exempt   ⊙ Moderate Sedation

(If lung resection is performed with chest wall tumor resection, report the appropriate chest wall tumor resection 19260-19272, in addition to lung resection 32440-32445)

32480 Removal of lung, other than pneumonectomy; single lobe (lobectomy)

32482 2 lobes (bilobectomy)

32484 single segment (segmentectomy)

(For removal of lung with bronchoplasty, use 32501)

32486 with circumferential resection of segment of bronchus followed by broncho-bronchial anastomosis (sleeve lobectomy)

32488 with all remaining lung following previous removal of a portion of lung (completion pneumonectomy)

(For lobectomy or segmentectomy, with concomitant decortication, use 32320 and the appropriate removal of lung code)

32491 with resection-plication of emphysematous lung(s) (bullous or non-bullous) for lung volume reduction, sternal split or transthoracic approach, includes any pleural procedure, when performed

(32500 deleted 2011 [2012 edition]. To report open wedge resection of lung, see 32505, 32506, 32507)

(If lung resection is performed with chest wall tumor resection, report the appropriate chest wall tumor resection 19260-19272, in addition to lung resection 32480, 32482, 32484, 32486, 32488, 32505, 32506, 32507)

+ **32501** Resection and repair of portion of bronchus (bronchoplasty) when performed at time of lobectomy or segmentectomy (List separately in addition to code for primary procedure)

(Use 32501 in conjunction with codes 32480, 32482, 32484)

(32501 is to be used when a portion of the bronchus to preserved lung is removed and requires plastic closure to preserve function of that preserved lung. It is not to be used for closure for the proximal end of a resected bronchus.)

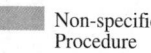

519

Separate Procedure   Unlisted Procedure   CCI Comp. Code   Non-specific Procedure

32503 Resection of apical lung tumor (eg, Pancoast tumor), including chest wall resection, rib(s) resection(s), neurovascular dissection, when performed; without chest wall reconstruction(s)

32504 with chest wall reconstruction

(Do not report 32503, 32504 in conjunction with 19260, 19271, 19272, 32100, 32551, 32554, 32555)

32505 Thoracotomy; with therapeutic wedge resection (eg, mass, nodule), initial

(Do not report 32505 in conjunction with 32440, 32442, 32445, 32488)

+ 32506 with therapeutic wedge resection (eg, mass or nodule), each additional resection, ipsilateral (List separately in addition to code for primary procedure)

(Report 32506 only in conjunction with 32505)

(If lung resection is performed with chest wall tumor resection, report the appropriate chest wall tumor resection 19260-19272, in addition to lung resection 32480, 32482, 32484, 32486, 32488, 32505, 32506, 32507)

+ 32507 with diagnostic wedge resection followed by anatomic lung resection (List separately in addition to code for primary procedure)

(Report 32507 in conjunction with 32440, 32442, 32445, 32480, 32482, 32484, 32486, 32488, 32503, 32504)

32540 Extrapleural enucleation of empyema (empyemectomy)

(For extrapleural enucleation of empyema (empyemectomy) with lobectomy, use 32540 and the appropriate removal of lung code)

INTRODUCTION AND REMOVAL

⊙ **32550** Insertion of indwelling tunneled pleural catheter with cuff

(Do not report 32550 in conjunction with 32554, 32555)

(If imaging guidance is performed, use 75989)

▲⊙**32551** Tube thoracostomy, includes connection to drainage system (eg, water seal), when performed, open (separate procedure)

● New Code ▲ Revised Code + Add-On Code ⊘ Modifier -51 Exempt ⊙ Moderate Sedation

32552 Removal of indwelling tunneled pleural catheter with cuff

⊙ **32553** Placement of interstitial device(s) for radiation therapy guidance (eg, fiducial markers, dosimeter), percutaneous, intra thoracic, single or multiple

(Report supply of device separately)

(For imaging guidance, see 76942, 77002, 77012, 77021)

(For percutaneous placement of interstitial device[s] for intra-abdominal, intrapelvic, and/or retroperitoneal radiation therapy guidance, use 49411)

● **32554** Thoraqcentesis, needle or catheter, aspiration of the pleural space; without imaging guidance

● **32555** with imaging guidance

● **32556** Pleural drainage, percutaneous, with insertion of indwelling catheter; without imaging guidance

● **32557** with imaging guidance

(For insertion of indwelling tunneled pleural catheter with cuff, use 32550)

(For open procedure, use 32551)

(Do not report 32554-32557 in conjunction with 32550, 32551, 76942, 77002, 77012, 77021, 75989)

DESTRUCTION

The instillation of a fibrinolytic agent may be performed multiple times per day over the course of several days. Code 32561 should be reported only once on the initial day treatment. Code 32562 should be reported only once on each subsequent day of treatment.

32560 Instillation, via chest tube/catheter, agent for pleurodesis (eg, talc for recurrent or persistent pneumothorax)

(For chest tube insertion, use 32551)

32561 Instillation(s), via chest tube/catheter, agent for fibrinolysis (eg, fibrinolytic agent for break up of multiloculated effusion); initial day

(For chest tube insertion, use 32551)

32562 subsequent day

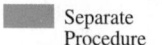 Separate Procedure	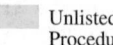 Unlisted Procedure	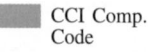 CCI Comp. Code	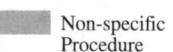 Non-specific Procedure

521

(For chest tube insertion, use 32551)

THORACOSCOPY (VIDEO-ASSISTED THORACIC SURGERY [VATS])

Surgical thoracoscopy (video-assisted thoracic surgery [VATS]) always includes diagnostic thoracoscopy.

32601 Thoracoscopy, diagnostic (separate procedure); lungs, pericardial sac, mediastinal or pleural space, without biopsy

(32602 deleted 2011 [2012 edition]. To report lung or pleural space biopsy(ies), see 32607, 32608, 32609)

(32603 deleted 2011 [2012 edition]. To report diagnostic thoracoscopy, pericardial sac, without biopsy, use 32601)

32604 pericardial sac, with biopsy

(32605 deleted 2011 [2012 edition]. To report diagnostic thoracoscopy within the mediastinal space, use 32601)

(For open pericardial biopsy, use 39010)

32606 mediastinal space, with biopsy

32607 Thoracoscopy; with diagnostic biopsy(ies) of lung infiltrate(s) (eg, wedge, incisional), unilateral

(Do not report 32607 more than once per lung)

(Do not report 32607 in conjunction with 32440, 32442, 32445, 32488, 32671)

32608 with diagnostic biopsy(ies) of lung nodule(s) or mass(es) (eg, wedge, incisional), unilateral

(Do not report 32608 more than once per lung)

(Do not report 32608 in conjunction with 32440, 32442, 32445, 32488, 32671)

32609 with biopsy(ies) of pleura

32650 Thoracoscopy, surgical; with pleurodesis (eg, mechanical or chemical)

32651 with partial pulmonary decortication

● New Code ▲ Revised Code + Add-On Code ⊘ Modifier -51 Exempt ⊙ Moderate Sedation

32652   with total pulmonary decortication, including intrapleural pneumonolysis

32653   with removal of intrapleural foreign body or fibrin deposit

32654   with control of traumatic hemorrhage

32655   with resection-plication of bullae, including any pleural procedure when performed

(For thoracoscopic [VATS] lung volume reduction surgery, use 32672)

32656   with parietal pleurectomy

(32657   deleted 2011 [2012 edition]. To report thoracoscopic [VATS] wedge resection of lung, see 32666, 32667, 32668)

32658   with removal of clot or foreign body from pericardial sac

32659   with creation of pericardial window or partial resection of pericardial sac for drainage

(32660   deleted 2011 [2012 edition])

32661   with excision of pericardial cyst, tumor, or mass

32662   with excision of mediastinal cyst, tumor, or mass

32663   with lobectomy (single lobe)

(For thoracoscopic [VATS] segmentectomy, use 32669)

32664   with thoracic sympathectomy

32665   with esophagomyotomy (Heller type)

(For exploratory thoracoscopy, and exploratory throacoscopy with biopsy, see 32601-32609)

32666   with therapeutic wedge resection (eg, mass, nodule), initial unilateral

(To report bilateral procedure, report 32666 with modifier 50)

(Do not report 32666 in conjunction with 32440, 32442, 32445, 32488, 32671)

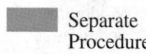 Separate Procedure   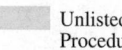 Unlisted Procedure   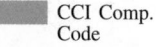 CCI Comp. Code   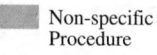 Non-specific Procedure   **523**

+ 32667   with therapeutic wedge resection (eg, mass or nodule), each additional resection, ipsilateral (List separately in addition to code for primary procedure)

(Report 32667 only in conjunction with 32666)

(Do not report 32667 in conjunction with 32440, 32442, 32445, 32488, 32671)

+ 32668   with diagnostic wedge resection followed by anatomic lung resection (List separately in addition to code for primary procedure)

(Report 32668 in conjunction with 32440, 32442, 32445, 32480, 32482, 32484, 32486, 32488, 32503, 32504, 32663, 32669, 32670, 32671)

32669   with removal of a single lung segment (segmentectomy)

32670   with removal of two lobes (bilobectomy)

32671   with removal of lung (pneumonectomy)

32672   with resection-plication for emphysematous lung (bullous or non-bullous) for lung volume reduction (LVRS), unilateral includes any pleural procedure, when performed

32673   with resection of thymus, unilateral or bilateral

(For open thymectomy, see 60520, 60521, 60522)

(For open excision mediastinal cyst, see 39200. For open excision mediastinal tumor, use 39220)

(For exploratory thoracoscopy, and exploratory thoracoscopy with biopsy, see 32601-32609)

+ 32674   with mediastinal and regional lymphadenectomy (List separately in addition to code for primary procedure)

(On the right, mediastinal lymph nodes include the paratracheal, subcarinal, paraesophageal, and inferior pulmonary ligament)

(On the left, mediastinal lymph nodes include the aortopulmonary window, subcarinal, paraesophageal, and inferior pulmonary ligament)

(Report 32674 in conjunction with 32440, 32442, 32445, 32480, 32482, 32484, 32486, 32488, , 332503, 32504, 32505, 32663, 32666, 32667, 32669, 32670, 32671)

---

524   ● New Code   ▲ Revised Code   + Add-On Code   ⊘ Modifier -51 Exempt   ⊙ Moderate Sedation

(To report mediastinal and regional lymphadenectomy via thoracotomy, use 38746)

STEREOTACTIC RADIATION THERAPY

Thoracic stereotactic body radiation therapy (SRS/SBRT) is a distinct procedure which may involve collaboration between a surgeon and radiation oncologist. The surgeon identifies and delineates the target for therapy. The radiation oncologist reports the appropriate code(s) for clinical treatment planning, physics and dosimetry, treatment delivery and management from the Radiation Oncology section (see 77295, 77331, 77370, 77373, 77435). The same physicican should not report target delineation services with radiation treatment management codes (77427-77499).

Target delineation involves specific determination of tumor borders to identify tumor volume and relationship with adjacent structures (eg, chest wall, intraparenchymal vasculature and atelectatic lung) and previously placed fiducial markers, when present. Target delineation also includes availability to identify and validate the thoracic target prior to treatment delivery when a difucial-less tracking system is utilized.

Do not report target delineation more than once per entire course of treatment when the treatment requires greater than one session.

● **32701**   Thoracic target(s) delineation for stereotactic body radiation therapy (SRS/SBRT), (photon or particle beam), entire course of treatment

((Do not report 32701 in conjunction with 77261-77799)

(For placement of fiducial markers, see 31626, 32553)

REPAIR

32800   Repair lung hernia through chest wall

32810   Closure of chest wall following open flap drainage for empyema (Clagett type procedure)

32815   Open closure of major bronchial fistula

32820   Major reconstruction, chest wall (posttraumatic)

LUNG TRANSPLANTATION

Lung allotransplantation involves three distinct components of physician work:

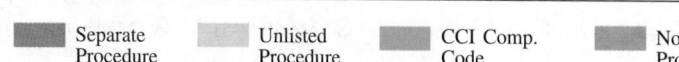

	Separate Procedure		Unlisted Procedure		CCI Comp. Code		Non-specific Procedure

525

1) **Cadaver donor pneumonectomy(s)**, which include(s) harvesting the allograft and cold preservation of the allograft (perfusing with cold preservation solution and cold maintenance) (use 32850).

2) **Backbench work:**

Preparation of a cadaver donor single lung allograft prior to transplantation, including dissection of the allograft from surrounding soft tissues to prepare the pulmonary venous/atrial cuff, pulmonary artery, and bronchus unilaterally (use 32855).

Preparation of a cadaver donor double lung allograft prior to transplantation, including dissection of the allograft from surrounding soft tissues to prepare the pulmonary venous/atrial cuff, pulmonary artery, and bronchus bilaterally (use 32856).

3) **Recipient lung allotransplantation**, which includes transplantation of a single or double lung allograft and care of the recipient (see 32851-32854).

32850 Donor pneumonectomy (including cold preservation), from cadaver donor

32851 Lung transplant, single; without cardiopulmonary bypass

32852 with cardiopulmonary bypass

32853 Lung transplant, double (bilateral sequential or en bloc); without cardiopulmonary bypass

32854 with cardiopulmonary bypass

32855 Backbench standard preparation of cadaver donor lung allograft prior to transplantation, including dissection of allograft from surrounding soft tissues to prepare pulmonary venous/atrial cuff, pulmonary artery, and bronchus; unilateral

32856 bilateral

(For repair or resection procedures on the donor lung, see 32491, 32505, 32506, 32507, 35216, 35276)

SURGICAL COLLAPSE THERAPY; THORACOPLASTY

(See also 32503, 32504)

32900 Resection of ribs, extrapleural, all stages

32905 Thoracoplasty, Schede type or extrapleural (all stages);

32906   with closure of bronchopleural fistula

(For open closure of major bronchial fistula, use 32815)

(For resection of first rib for thoracic outlet compression, see 21615, 21616)

32940   Pneumonolysis, extraperiosteal, including filling or packing procedures

32960   Pneumothorax, therapeutic, intrapleural injection of air

OTHER PROCEDURES

32997   Total lung lavage (unilateral)

(For bronchoscopic bronchial alveolar lavage, use 31624)

32998   Ablation therapy for reduction or eradication of 1 or more pulmonary tumor(s) including pleura or chest wall when involved by tumor extension, percutaneous, radiofrequency, unilateral

(For imaging guidance and monitoring, see 76940, 77013, 77022)

32999   Unlisted procedure, lungs and pleura

| | Separate Procedure | | Unlisted Procedure | | CCI Comp. Code | | Non-specific Procedure | 527 |

This page intentionally left blank.

● New
Code

▲ Revised
Code

✛ Add-On
Code

⊘ Modifier -51
Exempt

⊙ Moderate
Sedation

CARDIOVASCULAR SYSTEM

CPT codes from this section of the CPT coding system are used to report invasive and surgical procedures performed on the heart and pericardium, including pacemakers or defibrillators; cardiac valves; coronary arteries; aorta; and arteries and veins.

For coding services such as monitoring, operation of pump and other non-surgical services performed during cardiovascular surgery, see the Special Services CPT codes 99150, 99151, 99160-99162 or CPT codes 99291-99292 and 99190-99192 from the evaluation and management section of the CPT coding system.

MISCELLANEOUS CODING RULES

A pacemaker system includes a pulse generator containing electronics, a battery, and one or more electrodes (leads) inserted one of several ways. Pulse generators may be placed in a subcutaneous "pocket" created in either a subclavicular or intra-abdominal site. Electrodes may be inserted through a vein (transvenous) or on the surface of the heart (epicardial). A single chamber system includes a pulse generator, one electrode inserted into either the atrium or ventricle. A dual chamber system includes a pulse generator, one electrode inserted in the atrium, and one electrode inserted in the ventricle.

Assign two CPT codes when a pacemaker or cardioverter-defibrillator "battery"/pulse generator is replaced. One code should describe the removal of the old pulse generator and the other should describe the insertion of the new pulse generator.

Cardiac catheterization codes are classified in the Medicine Section of the CPT coding system. Insertion of a dilator into a vein prior to the placement of a catheter should not be separately coded.

Selective vascular catheterization should be coded to include introduction and all lesser order selective catheterization used in the approach (eg., the description for a selective right middle cerebral artery catheterization includes the introduction and placement catheterization of the right common and internal carotid arteries).

Additional second and/or third order arterial catheterizations within the same family of arteries supplied by a single first order artery should be expressed by 36218 or 36248. Additional first order or higher catheterizations in vascular families supplied by a first order vessel different from a previously selected and coded family should be separately coded using the conventions described above.

(For monitoring, operation of pump and other nonsurgical services, see 99190-99192, 99291, 99292, 99354-99360)

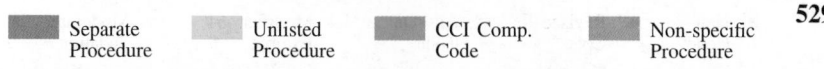

	Separate Procedure		Unlisted Procedure		CCI Comp. Code		Non-specific Procedure

529

> (For other medical or laboratory related services, see appropriate section)
>
> (For radiological supervision and interpretation, see 75600-75978)

HEART AND PERICARDIUM

PERICARDIUM

> (For thoracoscopic [VATS] pericardial procedures, see 32601, 32604, 32658, 32659, 32661)

⊙ **33010** Pericardiocentesis; initial

> (For radiological supervision and interpretation, use 76930)

⊙ **33011**   subsequent

> (For radiological supervision and interpretation, use 76930)

33015 Tube pericardiostomy

33020 Pericardiotomy for removal of clot or foreign body (primary procedure)

33025 Creation of pericardial window or partial resection for drainage

> (For thoracoscopic [VATS] pericardial window, use 32659)

33030 Pericardiectomy, subtotal or complete; without cardiopulmonary bypass

33031   with cardiopulmonary bypass

33050 Resection of pericardial cyst or tumor electrode(s); atrial

> (For open pericardial biopsy, use 39010)
>
> (For thoracoscopic [VATS] resection of pericardial cyst, tumor or mass, use 32661)

CARDIAC TUMOR

33120 Excision of intracardiac tumor, resection with cardiopulmonary bypass

33130 Resection of external cardiac tumor

● New Code   ▲ Revised Code   + Add-On Code   ⊘ Modifier -51 Exempt   ⊙ Moderate Sedation

TRANSMYOCARDIAL REVASCULARIZATION

33140 Transmyocardial laser revascularization, by thoracotomy (separate procedure)

+ 33141 performed at the time of other open cardiac procedure(s) (List separately in addition to code for primary procedure)

(Use 33141 in conjunction with codes 33400-33496, 33510-33536, 33542)

PACEMAKER OR PACING CARDIOVERTER-DEFIBRILLATOR

A pacemaker generally has two parts; a generator and the leads. The generator is where the battery and the information to regulate the heartbeat are stored. The leads are wires that go from the generator through a large vein to the heart, where the wires are anchored. The leads send the electrical impulses to the heart to tell it to beat. The battery can last anywhere from 7-8 years on average and will be routinely monitored by your health care professional and replaced when necessary.

A pacemaker can usually sense if the heartbeat is above a certain level, at which point it will automatically turn off. Likewise, the pacemaker can sense when the heartbeat slows down too much, and will automatically turn back on in order to start pacing again. A pacemaker is often the treatment of choice for bradycardia. Less commonly, pacemakers may also be used to terminate tachycardia. The pacemaker can sense the abnormally fast heart rate and take control of it by first speeding up, then slowing down to normal.

In most cases, the procedure for inserting a pacemaker takes about one hour. The patient is awake for the procedure, and pain medication is given throughout the procedure. A small incision is made traditionally in the left side of the chest, and a small "pocket" is created underneath the skin. After the leads have been positioned in the heart under X-ray guidance, they are then connected to the generator. The generator is then placed into the pocket, and the pocket is closed with sutures. Most patients are able to go home within 1 day of the procedure, if there are no other medical issues requiring further hospitalization.

A single chamber pacemaker system includes a pulse generator and one electrode inserted in either the atrium or ventricle. A dual chamber pacemaker system includes a pulse generator and one electrode inserted in the right atrium and one electrode inserted in the right ventricle. In certain circumstances, an additional electrode may be required to achieve pacing of the left ventricle (bi-ventricular pacing). In this event, transvenous (cardiac vein) placement of the electrode should be separately reported using code 33224 or 33225. Epicardial placement of the electrode should be separately reported using 33202-33203.

531

Separate Procedure · Unlisted Procedure · CCI Comp. Code · Non-specific Procedure

IMPLANTABLE CARDIOVERTER DEFIBRILLATOR

An implantable cardioverter defibrillator is used in patients at risk for recurrent, sustained ventricular tachycardia or fibrillation.

The device is connected to leads positioned inside the heart or on its surface. These leads are used to deliver electrical shocks, sense the cardiac rhythm and sometimes pace the heart, as needed. The various leads are tunneled to a pulse generator, which is implanted in a pouch beneath the skin of the chest or abdomen. These generators are typically a little larger than a wallet and have electronics that automatically monitor and treat heart rhythms recognized as abnormal. Newer devices are smaller and have simpler lead systems. They can be installed through blood vessels, eliminating the need for open chest surgery.

When an implantable cardioverter defibrillator detects ventricular tachycardia or fibrillation, it shocks the heart to restore the normal rhythm. New devices also provide overdrive pacing to electrically convert a sustained ventricular tachycardia, and "backup" pacing if bradycardia occurs. They also offer a host of other sophisticated functions (such as storage of detected arrhythmic events and the ability to do "noninvasive" electrophysiologic testing).

The electrodes (leads) of a pacing cardioverter-defibrillator system are positioned in the heart via the venous system (transvenously), in most circumstances. In certain circumstances, an additional electrode may be required to achieve pacing of the left ventricle (bi-ventricular pacing). In this event, transvenous (cardiac vein) placement of the electrode should be separately reported using code 33224 or 33225. Epicardial placement of the electrode should be separately reported using 33202-33203.

Electrode positioning on the epicardial surface of the heart requires thoracotomy, or thoracoscopic placement of the leads. Removal of electrode(s) may first be attempted by transvenous extraction (33234, 33235, or 33244). However, if transvenous extraction is unsuccessful, a thoracotomy may be required to remove the electrodes (33238 or 33243). Use 33212, 33213, 33221, 33230, 33231, 33240 as appropriate in addition to the thoracotomy or endoscopic epicardial lead placement codes (33202 or 33203) to report the insertion of the generator if done by the same physician during the same session.

When the "battery" of a pacemaker or pacing cardioverty-defibrillator is changed, it is actually the pulse generator that is changed. Removal of pacemaker or pacing cardioverter-defibrillator pulse generator only is reported with 33233 or 33241. Removal of a pacemaker or pacing cardioverter-defibrillator pulse generator with insertion of a new pulse generator without any replacement or insertion of lead(s) is reported with 33227-33229 and 33262-33264. Insertion of a new pulse generator, when existing leads are already in place and when no prior pulse generator is removed, is reported with 33212, 33213, 33221, 33230, 33231, 33240. When a pulse generator insertion involves the insertion or replacement of one or more lead(s), use the system codes 33206-33208 for pacemaker or 33249 for

● New Code   ▲ Revised Code   + Add-On Code   ⊘ Modifier -51 Exempt   ⊙ Moderate Sedation

pacing cardioverter-defibrillator. Removal of a pulse generator (33233 or 33241) or extraction of transvenous leads (33234, 33235 or 33244) should be reported separately. An exception involves a pacemaker upgrade from single to dual system which includes removal of pulse generator, replacement of new pulse generator and insertion of new lead, reported with 33214.

Repositioning of a pacemaker electrode, pacing cardioverter-defibrillator electrode(s), or a left ventricular pacing electrode is reported using 33215 or 33226, as appropriate.

The pacemaker and pacing cardioverter-defibrillator device evaluation codes 93279-93299 may not be reported in conjunction with pulse generator and lead insertion or revision codes 33206-33249. Defibrillator threshold testing (DFT) during pacing cardioverter-defibrillator insertion or replacement may be separately reported using 93640, 93641.

Radiological supervision and interpretation related to the pacemaker or pacing cardioverter-defibrillator procedure is included in 33206-33249. To report fluoroscopic guidance for diagnostic lead evaluatin without lead insertion, replacement, or revision procedures, use 76000.

The following definitions apply to 33206-33249:

Single lead: a pacemaker or pacing cardioverter-defibrillator with pacing and sensing function in only one chamber of the heart

Dual lead: a pacemaker or pacing cardiovertee-defibrillator with pacing and sensing function in only two chambers of the heart.

Multiple lead: a pacemaker or pacing cardioverter-defibrillator with pacing and sensing function in three or more chambers of the heart.

33202	Insertion of epicardial electrode(s); open incision (eg, thoracotomy, median sternotomy, subxiphoid approach)
33203	endoscopic approach (eg, thoracoscopy, pericardioscopy)

(When epicardial lead placement is performed with insertion of the generator, report 33202, 33203 in conjunction with 33212, 33213, 33221, 33230, 33231, 33240)

⊙ **33206**	Insertion of new or replacement of permanent pacemaker with transvenous electrode(s); atrial
⊙ **33207**	ventricular
⊙ **33208**	atrial and ventricular

533

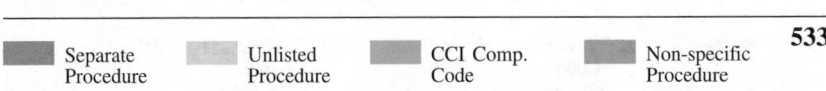

Transvenous Procedures	System	
	Pacemaker	Implantable Cardioverter-Defibrillator
Insert transvenous single lead only w/o pulse generator	33216	33216
Insert transvenous dual leads w/o pulse generator	33217	33217
Insert transvenous multiple leads w/o pulse generator	33217 + 33224	33217 + 33224
Initial pulse generator insertion only w/ existing single lead	33212	33240
Initial pulse generator insertion only w/ existing dual leads	33213	33230
Initial pulse generator insertion only w/ existing multiple leads	33221	33231
Initial pulse generator insertion or replacement plus insertion of transvenous single lead	33206 (atrial) or 33207 (ventricular)	33249
Initial pulse generator insertion or replacement plus insertion of transvenous dual leads	33208	33249
Initial pulse generator insertion or replacement plus insertion of transvenous multiple leads	33208 + 33225	33249 + 33225
Upgrade single chamber system to dual chamber system	33214 (incl. removal of existing pulse generator)	33241 + 33249
Removal pulse generator only (w/o replacement)	33233	33241
Removal pulse generator with replacement pulse generator only single lead system (transvenous)	33227	33262
Removal pulse generator with replacement pulse generator only dual lead system (transvenous)	33228	33263
Removal pulse generator with replacement pulse generator only multiple lead system (transvenous)	33229	33264
Removal transvenous electrode only single lead system	33234	33244
Removal transvenous electrode only dual lead system	33235	33244
Removal and replacement of pulse generator and transvenous electrodes	33233 + (33234 or 33235) + (33206 or 33207 or 33208) and 33225, when appropriate	33241 + 33244 + 33249 and 33225, when appropriate
Conversion of existing system to bi-ventricular system (addition of LV lead and removal of current pulse generator with insertion of new pulse generator with bi-ventricular pacing capabilities)	33225 + 33228 or 33229	33225 + 33263 or 33264

(Codes 33206-33208 include subcutaneous insertion of the pulse generator and transvenous placement of electrode(s))

(For removal and replacement of pacemaker pulse generator and transvenous electrode(s), use 33233 in conjunction with either 33234 or 33235 and 33206-33208)

534 ● New Code   ▲ Revised Code   + Add-On Code   ⊘ Modifier -51 Exempt   ⊙ Moderate Sedation

(Do not report 33206-33208 in conjunction with 33227-33229)

⊙ **33210** Insertion or replacement of temporary transvenous single chamber cardiac electrode or pacemaker catheter (separate procedure)

⊙ **33211** Insertion or replacement of temporary transvenous dual chamber pacing electrodes (separate procedure)

⊙ **33212** Insertion of pacemaker pulse generator only; with existing single lead

⊙ **33213**   with existing dual leads

⊙ **33221**   with existing multiple leads

(Do not report 33212, 33213, 33221 in conjunction with 33233 for removal and replacement of the pacemaker pulse generator. Use 33227-33229, as appropriate, when pulse generator replacment is indicated.)

(When epicardial lead placement is performed with insertion of generator, report 33202, 33203 in conjunction with 33212, 33213, 33221)

⊙ **33214** Upgrade of implanted pacemaker system, conversion of single chamber system to dual chamber system (includes removal of previously placed pulse generator, testing of existing lead, insertion of new lead, insertion of new pulse generator)

(Do not report 33214 in conjunction with 33227-33229)

33215 Repositioning of previously implanted transvenous pacemaker or pacing cardioverter-defibillator (right atrial or right ventricular) electrode

⊙ **33216** Insertion of a single transvenous electrode, permanent pacemaker or cardioverter-defibrillator

⊙ **33217** Insertion of 2 transvenous electrodes, permanent pacemaker or cardioverter-defibrillator

(Do not report 33216-33217 in conjunction with code 33214)

(For insertion or replacement of cardiac venous system lead, see 33224, 33225)

⊙ **33218** Repair of single transvenous electrode, permanent pacemaker or pacing cardioverter-defibrillator

535

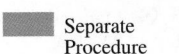 Separate Procedure   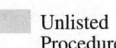 Unlisted Procedure   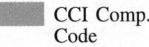 CCI Comp. Code   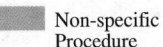 Non-specific Procedure

(For repair of single permanent pacemaker or pacing cardioverter-defibrillator electrode with replacement of pulse generator, see 33227-33229 or 33262-33264 and 33218)

⊙ **33220**   Repair of 2 transvenous electrodes for permanent pacemaker or pacing cardioverter-defibrillator

(For repair of 2 tranvenous electrodes for permanent pacemaker or pacing cardioverter-defibrillator with replacement of pulse generator, use 33220 in conjunction with 33228, 33229, 33263, 33264)

33221   Code out of order. See page 535

⊙ **33222**   Revision or relocation of skin pocket for pacemaker

⊙ **33223**   Revision of skin pocket for cardioverter-defibrillator

33224   Insertion of pacing electrode, cardiac venous system, for left ventricular pacing, with attachment to previously placed pacemaker or pacing cardioverter-defibrillator pulse generator (including revision of pocket, removal, insertion and/or replacement of existing generator)

(When epicardial electrode placement is performed, report 33224 in conjunction with 33202, 33203)

▲⊙**33225**   Insertion of pacing electrode, cardiac venous system, for left ventricular pacing, at time of insertion of pacing cardioverter-defibrillator or pacemaker pulse generator (eg, for upgrade to dual chamber system) (List separately in addition to code for primary procedure)

(Use 33225 in conjunction with 33206, 33207, 33208, 33212, 33213, 33214, 33216, 33217, 33221, 33228, 33229, 33230, 33231, 33233, 33234, 33235, 33240, 33249, 33263, 33264)

(Use 33225 in conjunction with 33222 only with pacemaker pulse generator pocket relocation and with 33223 only with pacing cardioverter-defibrillator [ICD] pocket relocation)

33226   Repositioning of previously implanted cardiac venous system (left ventricular) electrode (including removal, insertion and/or replacement of existing generator)

33227   Code out of order. See page 537

33228   Code out of order. See page 537

● New Code   ▲ Revised Code   + Add-On Code   ⊘ Modifier -51 Exempt   ⊙ Moderate Sedation

33229 Code out of order. See page 537

33230 Code out of order. See page 537

33231 Code out of order. See page 537

⊙ **33233** Removal of permanent pacemaker pulse generator only

⊙ **33227** Removal of permanent pacemaker pulse generator with replacement of pacemaker pulse generator; single lead system

⊙ **33228**   dual lead system

⊙ **33229**   multiple lead system

(Do not report 33227-33229 in conjunction with 33233)

(For removal and replacement of pacemaker pulse generator and transvenous electrode[s], use 33233 in conjunction with either 33234 or 33235 and 33206-33208)

⊙ **33234** Removal of transvenous pacemaker electrode(s); single lead system, atrial or ventricular

⊙ **33235**   dual lead system

33236 Removal of permanent epicardial pacemaker and electrodes by thoracotomy; single lead system, atrial or ventricular

33237   dual lead system

33238 Removal of permanent transvenous electrode(s) by thoracotomy

⊙ **33240** Insertion of pacing cardioverter-defibrillator pulse generator only; with existing single lead

(Use 33240, as appropriate, in addition to the epicardial lead placement codes to report the insertion of the generator when done by the same physician during the same session)

⊙ **33230**   with existing dual leads

⊙ **33231**   with existing multiple leads

(Do not report 33230, 33231, 33240 in conjunction with 33241 for removal and replacement of the pacing cardioverter-defibrillator pulse generator. Use 33262-33264, as appropriate, when pulse generator replacement is indicated)

Separate Procedure	Unlisted Procedure	CCI Comp. Code	Non-specific Procedure

537

(When epicardial lead placement if performed with insertion of generator, report 33202, 33203 in conjunction with 33230, 33231, 33240)

⊙ **33241** Removal of pacing cardioverter-defibrillator pulse generator only

(For removal and replacement of a pacing cardioverter-defibrillator pulse generator and electrode(s), use 33241 in conjunction with either 33243 or 33244 and 33249)

⊙ **33262** Removal of pacing cardioverter-defibrillator pulse generator with replacement of pacing cardioverter-defibrillator pulse generator; single lead system

⊙ **33263**   dual lead system

⊙ **33264**   multiple lead system

(Do not report 33262-33264 in conjunction with 33241)

(For removal of electrode[s] by thoracotomy in conjunction with pulse generator removal or replacement, use 33243 in conjunction with 33241, 33262-33264)

(For removal of electrode[s] by tranvenous extraction in conjunction with pulse generator removal or replacement, use 33244 in conjunction with 33241, 33262-33264)

(For repair of implantable cardioverter-defibrillator pulse generator and/or leads, see 33218, 33220)

33243 Removal of single or dual chamber pacing cardioverter-defibrillator electrode(s); by thoracotomy

⊙ **33244**   by transvenous extraction

⊙ **33249** Insertion or replacement of permanent pacing cardioverter-defibrillator system with transvenous lead(s), single or dual chamber

(For removal and replacement of a pacing cardioverter-defibrillator system (pulse generator and electrodes), report 33241 in conjunction with either 33243 or 33244 and 33249)

(For insertion of implantable cardioverter-defibrillator lead(s), without thoracotomy, use 33216 or 33217)

● New Code   ▲ Revised Code   ✛ Add-On Code   ⊘ Modifier -51 Exempt   ⊙ Moderate Sedation

ELECTROPHYSIOLOGIC OPERATIVE PROCEDURES

If excision or isolation of the left atrial appendage by any method, including stapling, oversewing, ligation, or plication, is performed in conjunction with any of the atrial tissue ablation and reconstruction (maze) procedures (33254-33259, 33265-33266), it is considered part of the procedure. Codes 33254-33256 are only to be reported when there is no concurrently performed procedure that requires median sternotomy or cardiopulmonary bypass. The appropriate atrial tissue ablation add-on code, 33257, 33258, 33259 should be reported in addition to an open cardiac procedure requiring sternotomy or cardiopulmonary bypass if performed concurrently.

Incision

33250 Operative ablation of supraventricular arrhythmogenic focus or pathway (eg, Wolff-Parkinson-White, atrioventricular node re-entry), tract(s) and/or focus (foci); without cardiopulmonary bypass

(For intraoperative pacing and mapping by a separate provider, use 93631)

33251 with cardiopulmonary bypass

33254 Operative tissue ablation and reconstruction of atria, limited (eg, modified maze procedure)

33255 Operative tissue ablation and reconstruction of atria, extensive (eg, maze procedure); without cardiopulmonary bypass

33256 with cardiopulmonary bypass

(Do not report 33254-33256 in conjunction with 32100, 32551, 33120, 33130, 33210, 33211, 33400-33507, 33510-33523, 33533-33548, 33600-33853, 33860-33864, 33910-33920)

+ 33257 Operative tissue ablation and reconstruction of atria, performed at the time of other cardiac procedure(s), limited (eg, modified maze procedure) (List separately in addition ot code for primary procedure)

(Use 33257 in conjunction with 33120-33130, 33250-33251, 33261, 33300-33335, 33400-33496, 33500-33507, 33510-33516, 33533-33548, 33600-33619, 33641-33697, 33702-33732, 33735-33767, 33770-33814, 33840-33877, 33910-33922, 33925-33926, 33935, 33945, 33975-33980)

+ 33258 Operative tissue ablation and reconstruction of atria, performed at the time of other cardiac procedure(s), extensive (eg, maze

| | Separate Procedure | | Unlisted Procedure | | CCI Comp. Code | | Non-specific Procedure | **539** |

procedure), without cardiopulmonary bypass (List separately in addition to code for primary procedure)

(Use 33258 in conjunction with 33130, 33250, 33300, 33310, 33320, 33321, 33330, 33332, 33401, 33414-33417, 33420, 33470-33472, 33501-33503, 33510-33516, 33533-33536, 33690, 33735, 33737, 33800-33813, 33840-33852, 33915, 33925 when the procedure is performed without cardiopulmonary bypass)

+ 33259 Operative tissue ablation and reconstruction of atria, performed at the time of other cardiac procedure(s), extensive (eg, maze procedure), with cardiopulmonary bypass (List separately in addition to code for primary procedure)

(Use 33259 in conjunction with 33120, 33251, 33261, 33305, 33315, 33322, 33335, 33400, 33403-33413, 33422-33468, 33474-33478, 33496, 33500, 33504-33507, 33510-33516, 33533-33548, 33600-33688, 33692-33722, 33730, 33732, 33736, 33750-33767, 33770-33781, 33786-33788, 33814, 33853, 33860-33877, 33910, 33916-33922, 33926, 33935, 33945, 33975-33980 when the procedure is performed with cardiopulmonary bypass)

(Do not report 33257, 33258 and 33259 inconjunction with 32551, 33210, 33211, 33254-33256, 33265, 33266)

33261 Operative ablation of ventricular arrhythmogenic focus with cardiopulmonary bypass

33262 Code out of order. See page 538

33263 Code out of order. See page 538

33264 Code out of order. See page 538

Endoscopy

33265 Endoscopy, surgical; operative tissue ablation and reconstruction of atria, limited (eg, modified maze procedure), without cardiopulmonary bypass

33266 operative tissue ablation and reconstruction of atria, extensive (eg, maze procedure), without cardiopulmonary bypass

(Do not report 33265-33266 in conjunction with 32551, 33210, 33211)

● New Code   ▲ Revised Code   + Add-On Code   ⊘ Modifier -51 Exempt   ⊙ Moderate Sedation

PATIENT-ACTIVATED EVENT RECORDER

33282   Implantation of patient-activated cardiac event recorder

(Initial implantation includes programming. For subsequent electronic analysis and/or reprogramming, use 93285, 93291, 93298, 93299)

33284   Removal of an implantable, patient-activated cardiac event recorder

HEART (INCLUDING VALVES) AND GREAT VESSELS

Patients receiving major cardiac procedures may require simultaneous cardiopulmonary bypass insertion of cannulae into the venous and arterial vasculatures with support of circulation and oxygenation by a heart-lung machine. Most services are described by codes in dyad arrangements to allow distinct reporting of procedures with or without cardiopulmonary bypass. Cardiopulmonary bypass is distinct from support of cardiac output using devices (eg, ventricular assist or intra-aortic balloon). For cardiac assist services see 33960-33983, 33990-33993.

33300   Repair of cardiac wound; without bypass

33305   with cardiopulmonary bypass

33310   Cardiotomy, exploratory (includes removal of foreign body, atrial or ventricular thrombus); without bypass

33315   with cardiopulmonary bypass

(Do not report removal of thrombus (33310-33315) in conjunction with other cardiac procedures unless a separate incision in the heart is required to remove the atrial or ventricular thrombus)

(If removal of thrombus with coronary bypass (33315) is reported in conjunction with 33120, 33130, 33420-33430, 33460-33468, 33496, 33542, 33545, 33641-33647, 33670, 33681, 33975-33980 which requires a separate heart incision, report 33315 with modifier '-59')

33320   Suture repair of aorta or great vessels; without shunt or cardiopulmonary bypass

33321   with shunt bypass

33322   with cardiopulmonary bypass

Separate Procedure | Unlisted Procedure | CCI Comp. Code | Non-specific Procedure

541

33330	Insertion of graft, aorta or great vessels; without shunt, or cardiopulmonary bypass
33332	with shunt bypass
33335	with cardiopulmonary bypass

CARDIAC VALVES

(For multiple valve procedures, see 33400-33478 and add modifier -51 to the secondary valve procedure code)

Aortic Valve

Codes 33361-33365, 0318T are used to report transcatheter aortic valve replacement (TAVR)/transcatheter aortic valve implantation (TAVI). TAVR/TAVI requires two physician operators and all components of the procedure are reported using modifier 62.

Codes 33361-33365, 0318T include the work, when performed, of percutaneous access, placing the access sheath, balloon aortic valvuloplasty, advancing the valve delivery system into position, repositioning the valve as needed, deploying the valve, temporary pacemaker insertion for rapid pacing (33210), and closure of the arteriotomy when performed. Codes 33361-33365, 0318T include open arterial or cardiac approach.

Angiography, radiological supervision, and interpretation performed to guide TAVR/TAVI (eg, guiding valve placement, documenting completion of the intervention, assessing the vascular access site for closure) are included in these codes.

Diagnostic left heart catheterization codes (93452, 93453, 93458-93461) and the supravalvular aortography code (93567) should **not** be used with TAVR/TAVI services (33361-33365, 0318T) to report:

1. Contrast injections, angiography, roadmapping, and/or fluoroscopic guidance for the TAVR/TAVI,

2. Aorta/left ventricular outflow tract measurement for the TAVR/TAVI, or

3. Post-TAVR/TAVI aortic or left ventricular angiography, as this work is captured in the TAVR/TAVI services codes (33361-33365, 0318T).

Diagnostic coronary angiography performed at the time of TAVR/TAVI may be separately reportable if:

1. No prior catheter-based coronary angiography study is available and a full diagnostic study is performed, or

---

542

| ● New Code | ▲ Revised Code | + Add-On Code | ⊘ Modifier -51 Exempt | ⊙ Moderate Sedation |

2. A prior study is available, but as documented in the medical record:

    a. The patient's condition with respect to the clinical indication has changed since the prior study, or

    b. There is inadequate visualization of the anatomy and/or pathology, or

    c There is a clinical change during the procedure that requires new evaluation.

    d. For same session/same day diagnostic coronary angiography services, report the appropriate diagnostic cardac catheterization code(s) appended with modifier 59 indicating separate and distance procedural service from TAVR/TAVI.

Diagnostic coronary angiography performed at a separate session from an interventional procedure may be separately reportable.

Other cardiac catheterization services are reported separately when performed for diagnostic purposes not intrinsic to TAVR/TAVI.

Percutaneous coronary interventional procedures are reported separately, when performed.

When transcatheter ventricular support is required in conjunction with TAVR/TAVI, the appropriate code should be reported with the appropriate ventricular assist device (VAD) procedure code (33990-33993, 33975, 33976, 33999), or balloon pump insertion code (33967, 33970, 33973).

The TAVR/TAVI cardiovascular access and delivery procedures are reported with 33361-33365, 0318T. When cardiopulmonary bypass is performed in conjunction with TAVR/TAVI, codes 33361-33365, 0318T should be reported with the appropriate add-on code for percutaneous peripheral bypass (33367), open peripheral bypass (33368), or central bypass (33369)

- **33361**   Transcatheter aortic valve replacement (TAVR/TAVI) with prosthetic valve; percutaneous femoral artery approach

- **33362**   open femoral artery approach

- **33363**   open axillary artery approach

- **33364**   open iliac artery approach

- **33365**   transaortic approach (eg, median sternotomy, mediastinotomy)

    (Use 0318T for transapical approach [eg, left thoracotomy])

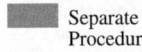 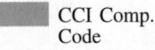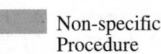

●+33367   cardiopulmonary bypass support with percutaneous peripheral arterial and venous cannulation (eg, femoral vessels) (List separately in addition to code for primary procedure)

(Use 33367 in conjunction with 33361-33365, 0318T)

(Do not report 33367 in conjunction with 33368, 33369)

●+33368   cardiopulmonary bypass support with open peripheral arterial and venous cannulation (eg, femoral, iliac, axillary vessels) (List separately in addition to code for primary procedure)

(Use 33368 in conjunction with 33361-33365, 0318T)

(Do not report 33368 in conjunction with 33367, 33369)

●+33369   cardiopulmonary bypass support with central arterial and venous cannulation (eg, aorta, right atrium, pulmonary artery) (List separately in addition to code for primary procedure)

(Use 33369 in conjunction with 33361-33365, 0318T)

(Do not report 33369 in conjunction with 33367, 33368)

33400 Valvuloplasty, aortic valve; open, with cardiopulmonary bypass

33401   open, with inflow occlusion

33403   using transventricular dilation, with cardiopulmonary bypass

(Do not report modifier '-63' in conjunction with 33401, 33403)

33404 Construction of apical-aortic conduit

33405 Replacement, aortic valve, with cardiopulmonary bypass; with prosthetic valve other than homograft or stentless valve

33406   with allograft valve (freehand)

(For aortic valve valvotomy, (commissurotomy) with inflow occlusion, use 33401)

(For aortic valve valvotomy, (commissurotomy) with cardiopulmonary bypass, use 33403)

33410   with stentless tissue valve

● New Code ▲ Revised Code + Add-On Code ⊘ Modifier -51 Exempt ⊙ Moderate Sedation

33411 Replacement, aortic valve; with aortic annulus enlargement, noncoronary sinus

33412 with transventricular aortic annulus enlargement (Konno procedure)

33413 by translocation of autologous pulmonary valve with allograft replacement of pulmonary valve (Ross procedure)

33414 Repair of left ventricular outflow tract obstruction by patch enlargement of the outflow tract

33415 Resection or incision of subvalvular tissue for discrete subvalvular aortic stenosis

33416 Ventriculomyotomy (-myectomy) for idiopathic hypertrophic subaortic stenosis (eg, asymmetric septal hypertrophy)

33417 Aortoplasty (gusset) for supravalvular stenosis

Mitral Valve

33420 Valvotomy, mitral valve; closed heart

33422 open heart, with cardiopulmonary bypass

33425 Valvuloplasty, mitral valve, with cardiopulmonary bypass;

33426 with prosthetic ring

33427 radical reconstruction, with or without ring

33430 Replacement, mitral valve, with cardiopulmonary bypass

Tricuspid Valve

33460 Valvectomy, tricuspid valve, with cardiopulmonary bypass

33463 Valvuloplasty, tricuspid valve; without ring insertion

33464 with ring insertion

33465 Replacement, tricuspid valve, with cardiopulmonary bypass

33468 Tricuspid valve repositioning and plication for Ebstein anomaly

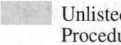 Separate Procedure

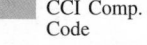 Unlisted Procedure

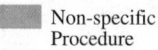 CCI Comp. Code

Non-specific Procedure

545

Pulmonary Valve

33470 Valvotomy, pulmonary valve, closed heart; transventricular

(Do not report modifier '-63' in conjunction with 33470)

33471 via pulmonary artery

(To report percutaneous valvuloplasty of pulmonary valve, use 92990)

33472 Valvotomy, pulmonary valve, open heart; with inflow occlusion

(Do not report modifier '-63' in conjunction with 33472)

33474 with cardiopulmonary bypass

33475 Replacement, pulmonary valve

33476 Right ventricular resection for infundibular stenosis, with or without commissurotomy

33478 Outflow tract augmentation (gusset), with or without commissurotomy or infundibular resection

(Use 33478 in conjunction with 33768 when a cavopulmonary anastomosis to a second superior vena cava is performed)

OTHER VALVULAR PROCEDURES

33496 Repair of non-structural prosthetic valve dysfunction with cardiopulmonary bypass (separate procedure)

(For reoperation, use 33530 in addition to 33496)

CORONARY ARTERY ANOMALIES

Basic procedures include endarterectomy or angioplasty.

33500 Repair of coronary arteriovenous or arteriocardiac chamber fistula; with cardiopulmonary bypass

33501 without cardiopulmonary bypass

33502 Repair of anomalous coronary artery from pulmonary artery origin; by ligation

33503 by graft, without cardiopulmonary bypass

● New Code ▲ Revised Code ＋ Add-On Code ⊘ Modifier -51 Exempt ⊙ Moderate Sedation

(Do not report modifier '-63' in conjunction with 33502, 33503)

33504   by graft, with cardiopulmonary bypass

33505   with construction of intrapulmonary artery tunnel (Takeuchi procedure)

33506   by translocation from pulmonary artery to aorta

(Do not report modifier '-63' in conjunction with 33505, 33506)

33507   Repair of anomalous (eg, intramural) aortic origin of coronary artery by unroofing or translocation

ENDOSCOPY

Surgical vascular endoscopy always includes diagnostic endoscopy

+ 33508   Endoscopy, surgical, including video-assisted harvest of vein(s) for coronary artery bypass procedure (List separately in addition to code for primary procedure)

(Use 33508 in conjunction with code 33510-33523)

(For open harvest of upper extremity vein procedure, use 35500)

VENOUS GRAFTING ONLY FOR CORONARY ARTERY BYPASS

The following codes are used to report coronary artery bypass procedures using venous grafts only. These codes should NOT be used to report the performance of coronary artery bypass procedures using arterial grafts and venous grafts during the same procedure. See 33517-33523 and 33533-33536 for reporting combined arterial-venous grafts.

Procurement of the saphenous vein graft is included in the description of the work for 33510-33516 and should not be reported as a separate service or co-surgery. To report harvesting of an upper extremity vein, use 35500 in addition to the bypass procedure. To report harvesting of a femoropopliteal vein segment, report 35572 in addition to the bypass procedure. When surgical assistant performs graft procurement, add modifier 80 to 33510-33516. For percutaneous ventricular assist device insertion, removal, repositioning, see 33990-33993.

33510   Coronary artery bypass, vein only; single coronary venous graft

33511   2 coronary venous grafts

33512	3 coronary venous grafts
33513	4 coronary venous grafts
33514	5 coronary venous grafts
33516	6 or more coronary venous grafts

COMBINED ARTERIAL-VENOUS GRAFTING FOR CORONARY BYPASS

The following codes are used to report coronary artery bypass procedures using venous grafts and arterial grafts during the same procedure. These codes may NOT be reported alone.

To report combined arterial-venous grafts it is necessary to report two codes: 1) the appropriate combined arterial venous graft code (33517-33523); and 2) the appropriate arterial graft code (33533-33536).

Procurement of the saphenous vein graft is included in the description of the work for 33517-33523 and should not be reported as a separate service or co-surgery. Procurement of the artery for grafting is included in the description of the work for 33533-33536 and should not be reported as a separate service or co-surgery, except when an upper extremity artery (eg., radial artery) is procured. To report harvesting of an upper extremity artery, use 35600 in addition to the bypass procedure. To report harvesting of an upper extremity vein, use 35500 in addition to the bypass procedure. To report harvesting of a femoropopliteal vein segment, report 35572 in addition to the bypass procedure. When surgical assistant performs arterial and/or venous graft procurement, add modifier 80 to 33517-33523, 33533-33536 as appropriate. For percutaneous ventricular assist device insertion, removal, repositioning, see 33990-33993.

+ 33517   Coronary artery bypass, using venous graft(s) and arterial graft(s); single vein graft (List separately in addition to code for primary procedure)

(Use 33517 in conjunction with 33533-33536)

+ 33518   2 venous grafts (List separately in addition to code for primary procedure)

(Use 33518 in conjunction with 33533-33536)

+ 33519   3 venous grafts (List separately in addition to code for primary procedure)

(Use 33519 in conjunction with 33533-33536)

548

● New Code	▲ Revised Code	+ Add-On Code	⊘ Modifier -51 Exempt	⊙ Moderate Sedation

+ 33521   4 venous grafts (List separately in addition to code for primary procedure)

(Use 33521 in conjunction with 33533-33536)

+ 33522   5 venous grafts (List separately in addition to code for primary procedure)

(Use 33522 in conjunction with 33533-33536)

+ 33523   6 or more venous grafts (List separately in addition to code for primary procedure)

(Use 33523 in conjunction with 33533-33536)

+ 33530   Reoperation, coronary artery bypass procedure or valve procedure, more than 1 month after original operation (List separately in addition to code for primary procedure)

(Use 33530 in conjunction with codes 33400-33496; 33510-33536, 33863)

ARTERIAL GRAFTING FOR CORONARY ARTERY BYPASS

The following codes are used to report coronary artery bypass procedures using either arterial grafts only or a combination of arterial-venous grafts. The codes include the use of the internal mammary artery, gastroepiploic artery, epigastric artery, radial artery, and arterial conduits procured from other sites.

To report combined arterial-venous grafts it is necessary to report two codes: 1) the appropriate arterial graft code (33533-33536); and 2) the appropriate combined arterial-venous graft code (33517-33523).

Procurement of the artery for grafting is included in the description of the work for 33533-33536 and should not be reported as a separate service or co-surgery, except when an upper extremity artery (eg., radial artery) is procured. To report harvesting of upper extremity artery, report 35600 in addition to the bypass procedure. To report harvesting of a an upper extremity vein, report 35500 in addition to the bypass procedure. To report harvesting of a femoropopiliteal vein segment, report 35572 in addition to the bypass procedure. When the surgical assistant performs arterial and/or venous graft procurement, add modifier -80 to 33517-33523, 33533-33536, as appropriate. For percutaneous ventricular assist device insertion, removal, repositioning, see 33990-33993.

33533   Coronary artery bypass, using arterial graft(s); single arterial graft

33534   2 coronary arterial grafts

| | Separate Procedure | | Unlisted Procedure | | CCI Comp. Code | | Non-specific Procedure |

549

| 33535 | 3 coronary arterial grafts |

| 33536 | 4 or more coronary arterial grafts |

| 33542 | Myocardial resection (eg, ventricular aneurysmectomy) |

| 33545 | Repair of postinfarction ventricular septal defect, with or without myocardial resection |

| 33548 | Surgical ventricular restoration procedure, includes prosthetic patch, when performed (eg, ventricular remodeling, SVR, SAVER, DOR procedures) |

(Do not report 33548 in conjunction with 32551, 33210, 33211, 33310, 33315)

(For Batista procedure or pachopexy, use 33999)

CORONARY ENDARTERECTOMY

+ 33572 Coronary endarterectomy, open, any method, of left anterior descending, circumflex, or right coronary artery performed in conjunction with coronary artery bypass graft procedure, each vessel (List separately in addition to primary procedure)

(Use 33572 in conjunction with 33510-33516, 33533-33536)

SINGLE VENTRICLE AND OTHER COMPLEX CARDIAC ANOMALIES

| 33600 | Closure of atrioventricular valve (mitral or tricuspid) by suture or patch |

| 33602 | Closure of semilunar valve (aortic or pulmonary) by suture or patch |

| 33606 | Anastomosis of pulmonary artery to aorta (Damus-Kaye-Stansel procedure) |

| 33608 | Repair of complex cardiac anomaly other than pulmonary atresia with ventricular septal defect by construction or replacement of conduit from right or left ventricle to pulmonary artery |

(For repair of pulmonary artery arborization anomalies by unifocalization, see 33925-33926)

● New Code   ▲ Revised Code   **+** Add-On Code   ⊘ Modifier -51 Exempt   ⊙ Moderate Sedation

33610 Repair of complex cardiac anomalies (eg, single ventricle with subaortic obstruction) by surgical enlargement of ventricular septal defect

(Do not report modifier '-63' in conjunction with 33610)

33611 Repair of double outlet right ventricle with intraventricular tunnel repair;

(Do not report modifier '-63' in conjunction with 33611)

33612 with repair of right ventricular outflow tract obstruction

33615 Repair of complex cardiac anomalies (eg, tricuspid atresia) by closure of atrial septal defect and anastomosis of atria or vena cava to pulmonary artery (simple Fontan procedure)

33617 Repair of complex cardiac anomalies (eg, single ventricle) by modified Fontan procedure

(Use 33617 in conjunction with 33768 when a cavopulmonary anastomosis to a second superior vena cava is performed)

33619 Repair of single ventricle with aortic outflow obstruction and aortic arch hypoplasia (hypoplastic left heart syndrome) (eg, Norwood procedure)

(Do not report modifier '-63' in conjunction with 33619)

33620 Application of right and left pulmonary artery bands (eg, hybrid approach stage 1)

(For banding of the main pulmonary artery related to septal defect, use 33690)

33621 Transthoracic insertion of catheter for stent placement with catheter removal and closure (eg, hybrid approach stage 1)

(For placement of stent, use 37207)

(Report both 33620, 33621 if performed in same session)

33622 Reconstruction of complex cardiac anomaly (eg, single ventricle or hypoplastic left heart) with palliation of single ventricle with aortic outflow obstruction and aortic arch hypoplasia, creation of cavopulmonary anastomosis, and removal of right and left pulmonary bands (eg, hybrid approach stage 2, Norwood, bidirectional Glenn, pulmonary artery debanding)

551

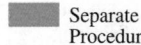 Separate Procedure

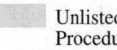 Unlisted Procedure

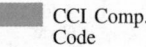 CCI Comp. Code

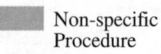 Non-specific Procedure

(Do not report 33622 in conjunction with 33619, 33767, 33822, 33840, 33845, 33851, 33853, 33917)

(For bilateral, bidirectional Glenn procedure, use 33622 in conjunction with 33768)

SEPTAL DEFECT

33641 Repair atrial septal defect, secundum, with cardiopulmonary bypass, with or without patch

33645 Direct or patch closure, sinus venosus, with or without anomalous pulmonary venous drainage

(Do not report 33645 in conjunction with 33724, 33726)

33647 Repair of atrial septal defect and ventricular septal defect, with direct or patch closure

(Do not report modifier -63 in conjunction with 33647)

(For repair of tricuspid atresia (eg., Fontan, Gago procedures), use 33615)

33660 Repair of incomplete or partial atrioventricular canal (ostium primum atrial septal defect), with or without atrioventricular valve repair

33665 Repair of intermediate or transitional atrioventricular canal, with or without atrioventricular valve repair

33670 Repair of complete atrioventricular canal, with or without prosthetic valve

(Do not report modifier -63 in conjunction with 33670)

33675 Closure of multiple ventricular septal defects;

33676 with pulmonary valvotomy or infundibular resection (acyanotic)

33677 with removal of pulmonary artery band, with or without gusset

(Do not report 33675-33677 in conjunction with 32100, 32551, 32554, 32555, 33210, 33681, 33684, 33688)

(For percutaneous closure, use 93581)

● New Code ▲ Revised Code + Add-On Code ⊘ Modifier -51 Exempt ⊙ Moderate Sedation

33681 Closure of single ventricular septal defect, with or without patch;

33684 with pulmonary valvotomy or infundibular resection (acyanotic)

33688 with removal of pulmonary artery band, with or without gusset

(For pulmonary vein repair requiring creation of atrial septal defect, use 33724)

33690 Banding of pulmonary artery

(For right and left pulmonary artery banding in a single ventricle [eg, hybrid approach stage 1], use 33620)

(Do not report modifier 63 in conjunction with 33690)

33692 Complete repair tetralogy of Fallot without pulmonary atresia;

33694 with transannular patch

(Do not report modifier 63 in conjunction with 33694)

(For ligation and takedown of a systematic-to-pulmonary artery shunt, performed in conjunction with a congenital heart procedure, see 33924)

33697 Complete repair tetralogy of Fallot with pulmonary atresia including construction of conduit from right ventricle to pulmonary artery and closure of ventricular septal defect

(For ligation and takedown of a systemic-to-pulmonary artery shunt, performed in conjunction with a congenital heart procedure, see 33924)

SINUS OF VALSALVA

33702 Repair sinus of Valsalva fistula, with cardiopulmonary bypass;

33710 with repair of ventricular septal defect

33720 Repair sinus of Valsalva aneurysm, with cardiopulmonary bypass

33722 Closure of aortico-left ventricular tunnel

553

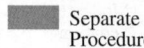 Separate Procedure   Unlisted Procedure   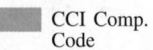 CCI Comp. Code   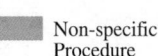 Non-specific Procedure

VENOUS ANOMALIES

33724 Repair of isolated partial anomalous pulmonary venous return (eg, Scimitar Syndrome)

(Do not report 33724 in conjunction with 32551, 33210, 33211)

33726 Repair of pulmonary venous stenosis

(Do not report 33726 in conjunction with 32551, 33210, 33211)

33730 Complete repair of anomalous venous return (supracardiac, intracardiac, or infracardiac types)

(Do not report modifier '-63' in conjunction with 33730)

(For partial anomalous pulmonary venous return, use 33724; for repair of pulmonary venous stenosis, use 33726)

33732 Repair of cor triatriatum or supravalvular mitral ring by resection of left atrial membrane

(Do not report modifier -63 in conjunction with 33732)

SHUNTING PROCEDURES

33735 Atrial septectomy or septostomy; closed heart (Blalock-Hanlon type operation)

33736 open heart with cardiopulmonary bypass

(Do not report modifier '-63' in conjunction with 33735, 33736)

33737 open heart, with inflow occlusion

(For transvenous method cadiac catheterization balloon atrial septectomy or septostomy (Rashkind type), use 92992)

(For blade method cardiac catheterization atrial septectomy or septostomy (Sang-Park septostomy), use 92993)

33750 Shunt; subclavian to pulmonary artery (Blalock-Taussig type operation)

33755 ascending aorta to pulmonary artery (Waterston type operation)

33762 descending aorta to pulmonary artery (Potts-Smith type operation)

● New Code   ▲ Revised Code   + Add-On Code   ⊘ Modifier -51 Exempt   ⊙ Moderate Sedation

(Do not report modifier -63 in conjunction with 33750, 33755, 33762)

33764   central, with prosthetic graft

33766   superior vena cava to pulmonary artery for flow to 1 lung (classical Glenn procedure)

33767   superior vena cava to pulmonary artery for flow to both lungs (bidirectional Glenn procedure)

+ 33768   Anastomosis, cavopulmonary, second superior vena cava (List separately in addition to primary procedure)

(Use 33768 in conjunction with 33478, 33617, 33622, 33767)

(Do not report 33768 in conjunction with 32551, 33210, 33211)

TRANSPOSITION OF THE GREAT VESSELS

33770   Repair of transposition of the great arteries with ventricular septal defect and subpulmonary stenosis; without surgical enlargement of ventricular septal defect

33771   with surgical enlargement of ventricular septal defect

33774   Repair of transposition of the great arteries, atrial baffle procedure (eg, Mustard or Senning type) with cardiopulmonary bypass;

33775   with removal of pulmonary band

33776   with closure of ventricular septal defect

33777   with repair of subpulmonic obstruction

33778   Repair of transposition of the great arteries, aortic pulmonary artery reconstruction (eg, Jatene type);

(Do not report modifier '-63' in conjunction with 33778)

33779   with removal of pulmonary band

33780   with closure of ventricular septal defect

33781   with repair of subpulmonic obstruction

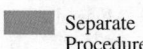 Separate Procedure   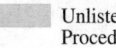 Unlisted Procedure   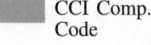 CCI Comp. Code   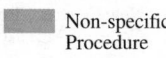 Non-specific Procedure

555

33782 Aortic root translocation with ventricular septal defect and pulmonary stenosis repair (ie, Nikaidoh procedure); without coronary ostium reimplantation

(Do not report 33782 in conjunction with 33412, 33413, 33608, 33681, 33770, 33771, 33778, 33780, 33920)

33783 with reimplantation of 1 or both coronary ostia

TRUNCUS ARTERIOSUS

33786 Total repair, truncus arteriosus (Rastelli type operation)

(Do not report modifier '-63' in conjunction with 33786)

33788 Reimplantation of an anomalous pulmonary artery

(For pulmonary artery band, use 33690)

AORTIC ANOMALIES

33800 Aortic suspension (aortopexy) for tracheal decompression (eg, for tracheomalacia) (separate procedure)

33802 Division of aberrant vessel (vascular ring);

33803 with reanastomosis

33813 Obliteration of aortopulmonary septal defect; without cardiopulmonary bypass

33814 with cardiopulmonary bypass

33820 Repair of patent ductus arteriosus; by ligation

33822 by division, under 18 years

33824 by division, 18 years and older

33840 Excision of coarctation of aorta, with or without associated patent ductus arteriosus; with direct anastomosis

33845 with graft

33851 repair using either left subclavian artery or prosthetic material as gusset for enlargement

---

556 ● New Code   ▲ Revised Code   **+** Add-On Code   ⊘ Modifier -51 Exempt   ⊙ Moderate Sedation

33852 Repair of hypoplastic or interrupted aortic arch using autogenous or prosthetic material; without cardiopulmonary bypass

33853 with cardiopulmonary bypass

(For repair of hypoplastic left heart syndrome (eg., Norwood type), via excision of coarctation of aorta, use 33619)

THORACIC AORTIC ANEURYSM

33860 Ascending aorta graft, with cardiopulmonary bypass, includes valve suspension when performed

(33861 deleted 2010 [2011 edition]; see 33864)

33863 Ascending aorta graft, with cardiopulmonary bypass, with aortic root replacement using valved conduit and coronary reconstruction (eg., Bentall)

(Do not report 33863 in conjunction with 33405, 33406, 33410, 33411, 33412, 33413, 33860)

33864 Ascending aorta graft, with cardiopulmonary bypass with valve suspension, with coronary reconstruction and valve sparing aortic root remodeling (eg, David Procedure, Yacoub Procedure)

(Do not report 33864 in conjunction with 33400, 33860-33863)

33870 Transverse arch graft, with cardiopulmonary bypass

33875 Descending thoracic aorta graft, with or without bypass

33877 Repair of thoracoabdominal aortic aneurysm with graft, with or without cardiopulmonary bypass

ENDOVASCULAR REPAIR OF DESCENDING THORACIC AORTA

Codes 33880-33891 represent a family of procedures to report placement of an endovascular graft for repair of the descending thoracic aorta. These codes include all device introduction, manipulation, positioning, and deployment. All balloon angioplasty and/or stent deployment within the target treatment zone for the endoprosthesis, either before or after endograft deployment, are not separately reportable. Open arterial exposure and associated closure of the arteriotomy sites (eg., 34812, 34820, 34833, 34834), introduction of guidewires and catheters (eg., 36140, 36200-36218), and extensive repair or replacement of an artery (eg., 35226, 35286) should be additionally reported. Transposition of subclavian artery to carotid, and carotid-carotid bypass performed in conjunction with endovascular

557

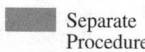 Separate Procedure   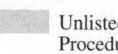 Unlisted Procedure   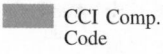 CCI Comp. Code   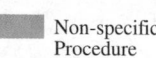 Non-specific Procedure

repair of the descending thoracic aorta (eg., 33889, 33891)should be separately reported. The primary codes, 33880 and 33881, include placement of all distal extensions, if required, in the distal thoracic aorta, while proximal extensions, if needed, are reported separately.

For fluoroscopic guidance in conjunction with endovascular repair of the thoracic aorta, see codes 75956-75959 as appropriate. Codes 75956 and 75957 include all angiography of the thoracic aorta and its branches for diagnostic imaging prior to deployment of the primary endovascular devices (including all routine components of modular devices), fluoroscopic guidance in the delivery of the endovascular components and intraprocedural arterial angiography (eg., confirm position, detect endoleak, evaluate runoff). Code 75958 includes the analogous services for placement of each proximal thoracic endovascular extension. Code 75959 includes the analogous services for placement of a distal thoracic endovascular extension(s) placed during a procedure after the primary repair.

Other interventional procedures performed at the time of endovascular repair of the descending thoracic aorta should be additionally reported (eg., innominate, carotid, subclavian, visceral, or iliac artery transluminal angioplasty or stenting, arterial embolization, intravascular ultrasound) when performed before or after deployment of the aortic prostheses.

(For transcatheter placement of wireless physiologic sensor in aneurysmal sac, use 34806)

(For analysis, interpretation, and report of implanted wireless pressure sensor in aneurysmal sac, use 93982)

33880 Endovascular repair of descending thoracic aorta (eg, aneurysm, pseudoaneurysm, dissection, penetrating ulcer, intramural hematoma, or traumatic disruption); involving coverage of left subclavian artery origin, initial endoprosthesis plus descending thoracic aortic extension(s), if required, to level of celiac artery origin

(For radiological supervision and interpretation, use 75956 in conjunction with 33880)

33881 not involving coverage of left subclavian artery origin, initial endoprosthesis plus descending thoracic aortic extension(s), if required, to level of celiac artery origin

(For radiological supervision and interpretation, use 75957 in conjunction with 33881)

33883 Placement of proximal extension prosthesis for endovascular repair of descending thoracic aorta (eg, aneurysm, pseudoaneurysm, dissection, penetrating ulcer, intramural hematoma, or traumatic disruption); initial extension

● New Code ▲ Revised Code + Add-On Code ⊘ Modifier -51 Exempt ⊙ Moderate Sedation

(For radiological supervision and interpretation, use 75958 in conjunction with 33883)

(Do not report 33881, 33883 when extension placement converts repair to cover left subclavian origin. Use only 33880)

+ 33884   each additional proximal extension (List separately in addition to code for primary procedure)

(Use 33884 in conjunction with 33883)

(For radiological supervision and interpretation, use 75958 in conjunction with 33884)

33886   Placement of distal extension prosthesis(es) delayed after endovascular repair of descending thoracic aorta

(Do not report 33886 in conjunction with 33880, 33881)

(Report 33886 once, regardless of number of modules deployed)

(For radiological supervision and interpretation, use 75959 in conjunction with 33886)

33889   Open subclavian to carotid artery transposition performed in conjunction with endovascular repair of descending thoracic aorta, by neck incision, unilateral

(Do not report 33889 in conjunction with 35694)

33891   Bypass graft, with other than vein, transcervical retropharyngeal carotid-carotid, performed in conjunction with endovascular repair of descending thoracic aorta, by neck incision

(Do not report 33891 in conjunction with 35509, 35601)

PULMONARY ARTERY

33910   Pulmonary artery embolectomy; with cardiopulmonary bypass

33915   without cardiopulmonary bypass

33916   Pulmonary endarterectomy, with or without embolectomy, with cardiopulmonary bypass

33917   Repair of pulmonary artery stenosis by reconstruction with patch or graft

---

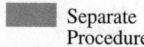 Separate Procedure   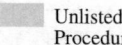 Unlisted Procedure   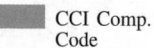 CCI Comp. Code   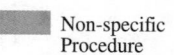 Non-specific Procedure

559

33920 Repair of pulmonary atresia with ventricular septal defect, by construction or replacement of conduit from right or left ventricle to pulmonary artery

(For repair of other complex cardiac anomalies by construction or replacement of right or left ventricle to pulmonary artery conduit, use 33608)

33922 Transection of pulmonary artery with cardiopulmonary bypass

(Do not report modifier '-63' in conjunction with 33922)

+ **33924** Ligation and takedown of a systemic-to-pulmonary artery shunt, performed in conjunction with a congenital heart procedure (List separately in addition to code for primary procedure)

(Use 33924 in conjunction with 33470-33475, 33600-33619, 33684-33688, 33692-33697, 33735-33767, 33770-33781, 33786, 33920-33922)

33925 Repair of pulmonary artery arborization anomalies by unifocalization; without cardiopulmonary bypass

33926   with cardiopulmonary bypass

HEART/LUNG TRANSPLANTATION

Heart with or without lung allotransplantation involves three distinct components of physician work:

1) **Cadaver donor cardiectomy with or without pneumonectomy**, which includes harvesting the allograft and cold preservation of the allograft (perfusing with cold preservation solution and cold maintenance) (see 33930, 33940).

2) **Backbench work**:

Preparation of a cadaver donor heart and lung allograft prior to transplantation, including dissection of the allograft from surrounding soft tissues to prepare the aorta, superior vena cava, inferior vena cava, and trachea for implantation (use 33933).

Preparation of a cadaver donor heart allograft prior to transplantation, including dissection of the allograft from surrounding soft tissues to prepare aorta, superior vena cava, inferior vena cava, pulmonary artery, and left atrium for implantation (use 33944).

3) **Recipient heart with or without lung allotransplantation**, which includes transplantation of allograft and care of the recipient (see 33935, 33945).

● New Code ▲ Revised Code + Add-On Code ⊘ Modifier -51 Exempt ⊙ Moderate Sedation

(For implantation of a total replacement heart system (artificial heart) with recipient cardiectomy or heart replacement system components, see Category III codes 0051T-0053T)

33930 Donor cardiectomy-pneumonectomy (including cold preservation)

33933 Backbench standard preparation of cadaver donor heart/lung allograft prior to transplantation, including dissection of allograft from surrounding soft tissues to prepare aorta, superior vena cava, inferior vena cava, and trachea for implantation

33935 Heart-lung transplant with recipient cardiectomy-pneumonectomy

33940 Donor cardiectomy (including cold preservation)

33944 Backbench standard preparation of cadaver donor heart allograft prior to transplantation, including dissection of allograft from surrounding soft tissues to prepare aorta, superior vena cava, inferior vena cava, pulmonary artery, and left atrium for implantation

(For repair or resection procedures on the donor heart, see 33300, 33310, 33320, 33400, 33463, 33464, 33510, 33641, 35216, 35276 or 35685)

33945 Heart transplant, with or without recipient cardiectomy

CARDIAC ASSIST

The insertion of a ventricular assist device (VAD) can be performed via percutaneous (33990, 33991) or transthoracic (33975, 33976, 33979) approach. The location of the ventricular assist device may be intracorporeal or extracorporeal.

For surgical insertion of cannula(e) for prolonged extracorporeal circulation for cardiopulmonary insufficiency (ECMO), use 36822.

Open arterial exposure when necessary to facilitate percutaneous ventricular assist device insertion (33990, 33991) may be reported separately (34812). Extensive repair or replacement of an artery may be additionally reported (eg, 35226 or 35286).

Removal of a ventricular assist device (33977, 33978, 33980, 33992) includes removal of the entire device, including the cannulas. Removal of a percutaneous ventricular assist device at the same session as insertion is not separately reportable. For removal of a percutaneous ventricular assist device at a separate and

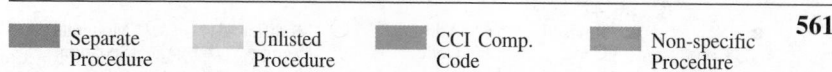

| Separate Procedure | Unlisted Procedure | CCI Comp. Code | Non-specific Procedure | **561** |

distinct session, but on the same day as insertion, report 33992 appended with modifier 59 indicating a distinct procedural service.

Repositioning of a percutaneous ventricular assist device at the same session as insertion is not separately reportable. Repositioning of percutaneous ventricular assist device not necessitating imaging guidance is not a reportable service. For repositioning of a percutaneous ventricular assist device necessitating imaging guidance at a separate and distinct session, but on the same day as insertion, report 33993 with modifier 59 indicating a distinct procedural service.

Replacement of a ventricular assist device pump (ie, 33981-33983) includes the removal of the pump and insertion of a new pump, connection, de-airing, and initiation of the new pump.

Replacement of the entire implantable ventricular assist device system, ie., pump(s) and cannulas, is reported using the insertion codes (ie, 33975, 33976, 33979). Removal (ie, 33977, 33978, 33980) of the ventricular assist device system being replaced is not separately reported. Replacement of a percutaneous ventricular assist device is reported using implantation codes (ie, 33990, 33991). Removal (ie, 33992) is not reported separately.

(For implantation or removal of ventricular assist device, extracorporeal, percutaneous transseptal access, see 0048T, 0050T. For replacement of a ventricular assist device, extracorporeal, percutaneous transseptal access, use 33999)

33960 Prolonged extracorporeal circulation for cardiopulmonary insufficiency; initial day

⊘ **33961** each subsequent day

(Do not report modifier 63 in conjunction with 33960, 33961)

(For insertion of cannula for prolonged extracorporeal circulation, use 36822)

33967 Insertion of intra-aortic balloon assist device, percutaneous

33968 Removal of intra-aortic balloon assist device, percutaneous

33970 Insertion of intra-aortic balloon assist device through the femoral artery, open approach

33971 Removal of intra-aortic balloon assist device including repair of femoral artery, with or without graft

33973 Insertion of intra-aortic balloon assist device through the ascending aorta

● New Code ▲ Revised Code ✚ Add-On Code ⊘ Modifier -51 Exempt ⊙ Moderate Sedation

33974 Removal of intra-aortic balloon assist device from the ascending aorta, including repair of the ascending aorta, with or without graft

33975 Insertion of ventricular assist device; extracorporeal, single ventricle

33976   extracorporeal, biventricular

33977 Removal of ventricular assist device; extracorporeal, single ventricle

33978   extracorporeal, biventricular

33979 Insertion of ventricular assist device, implantable intracorporeal, single ventricle

33980 Removal of ventricular assist device, implantable intracorporeal, single ventricle

33981 Replacement of extracorporeal ventricular assist device, single or biventricular, pump(s), single or each pump

33982 Replacement of ventricular assist device pump(s); implantable intracorporeal, single ventricle, without cardiopulmonary bypass

33983   implantable intracorporeal, single ventricle, with cardiopulmonary bypass

●⊙**33990** Insertion of ventricular assist device, percutaneous including radiological supervision and interpretation; arterial access only

●⊙**33991**   both arterial and venous access, with transseptal puncture

●⊙**33992** Removal of percutaneous ventricular assist device at separate and distinct session from insertion

●⊙**33993** Repositioning of percutaneous ventricular assist device with imaging guidance at separate and distinct session from insertion

OTHER PROCEDURES, CARDIAC SURGERY

33999 Unlisted procedure, cardiac surgery

 Separate Procedure   Unlisted Procedure   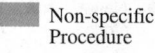 CCI Comp. Code   Non-specific Procedure   **563**

ARTERIES AND VEINS

Primary vascular procedure listings include establishing both inflow and outflow by whatever procedures necessary. Also included is that portion of the operative arteriogram performed by the surgeon, as indicated. Sympathectomy, when done, is included in the listed aortic procedures. For unlisted vascular procedures, use 37799.

EMBOLECTOMY/THROMBECTOMY

Arterial, With or Without Catheter

34001 Embolectomy or thrombectomy, with or without catheter; carotid, subclavian or innominate artery, by neck incision

34051 innominate, subclavian artery, by thoracic incision

34101 axillary, brachial, innominate, subclavian artery, by arm incision

34111 radial or ulnar artery, by arm incision

34151 renal, celiac, mesentery, aortoiliac artery, by abdominal incision

34201 femoropopliteal, aortoiliac artery, by leg incision

34203 popliteal-tibio-peroneal artery, by leg incision

Venous, Direct or With Catheter

34401 Thrombectomy, direct or with catheter; vena cava, iliac vein, by abdominal incision

34421 vena cava, iliac, femoropopliteal vein, by leg incision

34451 vena cava, iliac, femoropopliteal vein, by abdominal and leg incision

34471 subclavian vein, by neck incision

34490 axillary and subclavian vein, by arm incision

VENOUS RECONSTRUCTION

34501 Valvuloplasty, femoral vein

● New Code   ▲ Revised Code   + Add-On Code   ⊘ Modifier -51 Exempt   ⊙ Moderate Sedation

34502 Reconstruction of vena cava, any method

34510 Venous valve transposition, any vein donor

34520 Cross-over vein graft to venous system

34530 Saphenopopliteal vein anastomosis

ENDOVASCULAR REPAIR OF ABDOMINAL AORTIC ANEURYSM

Codes 34800-34826 represent a family of component procedures to report placement of an endovascular graft for abdominal aortic aneurysm repair. These codes describe open femoral or iliac artery exposure, device manipulation and deployment, and closure of the arteriotomy sites. Balloon angioplasty and/or stent deployment within the target treatment zone for the endoprosthesis, either before or after endograft deployment, are not separately reportable. Introduction of guidewires and catheters should be reported separately (eg., 36200, 36245-36248, 36140). Extensive repair or replacement of an artery should be additionally reported (eg., 35226 or 35286).

For fluoroscopic guidance in conjunction with endovascular aneurysm repair, see code 75952 or 75953, as appropriate. Code 75952 includes angiography of the aorta and its branches for diagnostic imaging prior to deployment of the endovascular device (including all routine components of modular devices), fluoroscopic guidance in the delivery of the endovascular components, and intraprocedural arterial angiography (eg., confirm position, detect endoleak, evaluate runoff). Code 75953 includes the analogous services for placement of additional extension prostheses (not for routine components of modular devices).

Other interventional procedures performed at the time of endovascular abdominal aortic aneurysm repair should be additionally reported (eg., renal transluminal angioplasty, arterial embolization, intravascular ultrasound, balloon angioplasty or stenting of native artery[s] outside the endoprosthesis target zone, when done before or after deployment of graft).

(For transcatheter placement of wireless physiologic sensor in aneurysmal sac, use 34806)

(For analysis, interpretation, and report of implanted wireless pressure sensor in aneurysmal sac, use 93982)

34800 Endovascular repair of infrarenal abdominal aortic aneurysm or dissection; using aorto-aortic tube prosthesis

34802 using modular bifurcated prosthesis (1 docking limb)

34803 using modular bifurcated prosthesis (2 docking limbs)

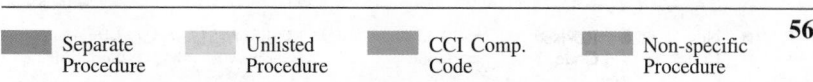

| Separate Procedure | Unlisted Procedure | CCI Comp. Code | Non-specific Procedure |

(For endovascular repair of abdominal aortic aneurysm or dissection involving visceral vessels using a fenestrated modular bifurcated prosthesis (two docking limbs), use Category III codes 0078T, 0079T)

34804   using unibody bifurcated prosthesis

34805   using aorto-uniiliac or aorto-unifemoral prosthesis

(For radiological supervision and interpretation, use 75952 in conjunction with 34800-34805)

+ **34806**   Transcatheter placement of wireless physiologic sensor in aneurysmal sac during endovascular repair, including radiological supervision and interpretation, instrument calibration, and collection of pressure data (List separately in addition to code for primary procedure)

(Use 34806 in conjunction with 33880, 33881, 33886, 34800-34805, 34825, 34900)

(Do not report 34806 in conjunction with 93982)

+ **34808**   Endovascular placement of iliac artery occlusion device (List separately in addition to code for primary procedure)

(Use 34808 in conjunction with codes 34800, 34805, 34813, 34825, 34826)

(For open arterial exposure, report codes 34812, 34820, 34833, 34834 as appropriate, in addition to codes 34800-34808)

34812   Open femoral artery exposure for delivery of endovascular prosthesis, by groin incision, unilateral

(For bilateral procedure, use modifier -50)

+ **34813**   Placement of femoral-femoral prosthetic graft during endovascular aortic aneurysm repair (List separately in addition to code for primary procedure)

(Use 34813 in conjunction with code 34812)

(For femoral artery grafting, see 35521, 35533, 35539, 35540, 35556, 35558, 35566, 35621, 35646, 35654-35661, 35666, 35700)

34820   Open iliac artery exposure for delivery of endovascular prosthesis or iliac occlusion during endovascular therapy, by abdominal or retroperitoneal incision, unilateral

● New Code   ▲ Revised Code   + Add-On Code   ⊘ Modifier -51 Exempt   ⊙ Moderate Sedation

(For bilateral procedure, use modifier -50)

34825 Placement of proximal or distal extension prosthesis for endovascular repair of infrarenal abdominal aortic or iliac aneurysm, false aneurysm, or dissection; initial vessel

+ 34826 each additional vessel (List separately in addition to code for primary procedure)

(Use 34826 in conjunction with code 34825)

(Use 34825, 34826 in addition to 34800-34805, 34900 as appropriate)

(For radiological supervision and interpretation, use 75953)

34830 Open repair of infrarenal aortic aneurysm or dissection, plus repair of associated arterial trauma, following unsuccessful endovascular repair; tube prosthesis

34831 aorto-bi-iliac prosthesis

34832 aorto-bifemoral prosthesis

34833 Open iliac artery exposure with creation of conduit for delivery of aortic or iliac endovascular prosthesis, by abdominal or retroperitoneal incision, unilateral

(Do not report 34833 in addition to 34820)

(For bilateral procedure, use modifier 50)

34834 Open brachial artery exposure to assist in the deployment of aortic or iliac endovascular prosthesis by arm incision, unilateral

(For bilateral procedure, use modifier 50)

ENDOVASCULAR REPAIR OF ILIAC ANEURYSM

Code 34900 represents a procedure to report introduction, positioning, and deployment of an endovascular graft for treatment of aneurysm, pseudoaneurysm, or arteriovenous malformation or trauma of the iliac artery (common, hypogastric, external). All balloon angioplasty and/or stent deployments within the target treatment zone for the endoprosthesis, either before or after endograft deployment, are included in the work of 34900 and are not separately reportable. Open femoral or iliac artery exposure (eg, 34812, 34820), introduction of guidewires and catheters (eg, 36200, 36245-36248), and extensive repair or replacement of an artery (eg, 35206-35286) should be additionally reported.

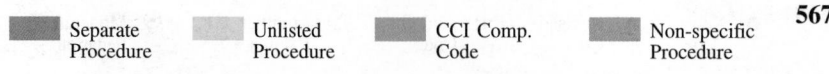

Separate Procedure	Unlisted Procedure	CCI Comp. Code	Non-specific Procedure

567

For fluoroscopic guidance in conjunction with endovascular iliac aneurysm repair, see code 75954. Code 75954 includes angiography of the aorta and iliac arteries for diagnostic imaging prior to deployment of the endovascular device (including all routine components), fluoroscopic guidance in the delivery of the endovascular components, and intraprocedural arterial angiography to confirm appropriate position of the graft, detect endoleaks and evaluate the status of the runoff vessels (eg., evaluation for dissection, stenosis, thrombosis, distal embolization, or iatrogenic injury).

Other interventional procedures performed at the time of endovascular iliac aneurysm repair should be additionally reported (eg., transluminal angioplasty outside the aneurysm target zone, arterial embolization, intravascular ultrasound).

34900   Endovascular repair of iliac artery (eg, aneurysm, pseudoaneurysm, arteriovenous malformation, trauma) using ilio-iliac tube endoprosthesis

(For endovascular repair of iliac artery bifurcation [eg, aneurysm, pseudoaneurysm, arteriovenous malformation, trauma] using bifurcated endoprosthesis, use 0254T)

(For radiological supervision and interpretation, use 75954)

(For placement of extension prosthesis during endovascular iliac artery repair, use 34825)

(For bilateral procedure, use modifier '-50')

DIRECT REPAIR OF ANEURYSM OR EXCISION (PARTIAL OR TOTAL) AND GRAFT INSERTION FOR ANEURYSM, PSEUDOANEURYSM, RUPTURED ANEURYSM, AND ASSOCIATED OCCLUSIVE DISEASE

Procedures 35001-35152 include preparation of artery for anastomosis including endarterectomy.

(For direct repairs associated with occlusive disease only, see 35201-35286)

(For intracranial aneurysm, see 61700 et seq)

(For endovascular repair of abdominal aortic aneurysm, see 34800-34826)

(For endovascular repair of iliac artery aneurysm, see 34900)

(For thoracic aortic aneurysm, see 33860-33875)

(For endovascular repair of descending thoracic aorta, involving coverage of left subclavian artery origin, use 33880)

568   ● New   ▲ Revised   + Add-On   ⊘ Modifier -51   ⊙ Moderate
            Code   Code   Code   Exempt   Sedation

35001 Direct repair of aneurysm, pseudoaneurysm, or excision (partial or total) and graft insertion, with or without patch graft; for aneurysm and associated occlusive disease, carotid, subclavian artery, by neck incision

35002 for ruptured aneurysm, carotid, subclavian artery, by neck incision

35005 for aneurysm, pseudoaneurysm, and associated occlusive disease, vertebral artery

35011 for aneurysm and associated occlusive disease, axillary-brachial artery, by arm incision

35013 for ruptured aneurysm, axillary-brachial artery, by arm incision

35021 for aneurysm, pseudoaneurysm, and associated occlusive disease, innominate, subclavian artery, by thoracic incision

35022 for ruptured aneurysm, innominate, subclavian artery, by thoracic incision

35045 for aneurysm, pseudoaneurysm, and associated occlusive disease, radial or ulnar artery

35081 for aneurysm, pseudoaneurysm, and associated occlusive disease, abdominal aorta

35082 for ruptured aneurysm, abdominal aorta

35091 for aneurysm, pseudoaneurysm, and associated occlusive disease, abdominal aorta involving visceral vessels (mesenteric, celiac, renal)

35092 for ruptured aneurysm, abdominal aorta involving visceral vessels (mesenteric, celiac, renal)

35102 for aneurysm, pseudoaneurysm, and associated occlusive disease, abdominal aorta involving iliac vessels (common, hypogastric, external)

35103 for ruptured aneurysm, abdominal aorta involving iliac vessels (common, hypogastric, external)

35111 for aneurysm, pseudoaneurysm, and associated occlusive disease, splenic artery

Separate Procedure	Unlisted Procedure	CCI Comp. Code	Non-specific Procedure	**569**

| 35112 | for ruptured aneurysm, splenic artery |

| 35121 | for aneurysm, pseudoaneurysm, and associated occlusive disease, hepatic, celiac, renal, or mesenteric artery |

| 35122 | for ruptured aneurysm, hepatic, celiac, renal, or mesenteric artery |

| 35131 | for aneurysm, pseudoaneurysm, and associated occlusive disease, iliac artery (common, hypogastric, external) |

| 35132 | for ruptured aneurysm, iliac artery (common, hypogastric, external) |

| 35141 | for aneurysm, pseudoaneurysm, and associated occlusive disease, common femoral artery (profunda femoris, superficial femoral) |

| 35142 | for ruptured aneurysm, common femoral artery (profunda femoris, superficial femoral) |

| 35151 | for aneurysm, pseudoaneurysm, and associated occlusive disease, popliteal artery |

| 35152 | for ruptured aneurysm, popliteal artery |

REPAIR ARTERIOVENOUS FISTULA

| 35180 | Repair, congenital arteriovenous fistula; head and neck |

| 35182 | thorax and abdomen |

| 35184 | extremities |

| 35188 | Repair, acquired or traumatic arteriovenous fistula; head and neck |

| 35189 | thorax and abdomen |

| 35190 | extremities |

REPAIR BLOOD VESSEL OTHER THAN FOR FISTULA, WITH OR WITHOUT PATCH ANGIOPLASTY

(For AV fistula repair, see 35180-35190)

| 35201 | Repair blood vessel, direct; neck |

● New Code ▲ Revised Code ✚ Add-On Code ⊘ Modifier -51 Exempt ⊙ Moderate Sedation

35206	upper extremity
35207	hand, finger
35211	intrathoracic, with bypass
35216	intrathoracic, without bypass
35221	intra-abdominal
35226	lower extremity
35231	Repair blood vessel with vein graft; neck
35236	upper extremity
35241	intrathoracic, with bypass
35246	intrathoracic, without bypass
35251	intra-abdominal
35256	lower extremity
35261	Repair blood vessel with graft other than vein; neck
35266	upper extremity
35271	intrathoracic, with bypass
35276	intrathoracic, without bypass
35281	intra-abdominal
35286	lower extremity

THROMBOENDARTERECTOMY

(For coronary artery, see 33510-33536 and 33572)

(35301-35372 include harvest of saphenous or upper extremity vein when performed)

35301   Thromboendarterectomy, including patch graft, if performed; carotid, vertebral, subclavian, by neck incision

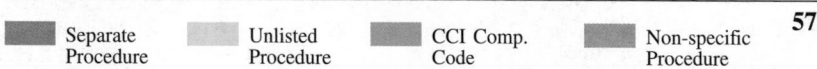

| Separate Procedure | Unlisted Procedure | CCI Comp. Code | Non-specific Procedure | **571** |

35302   superficial femoral artery

35303   popliteal artery

(Do not report 35302, 35303 in conjunction with 35500, 37225, 37227)

35304   tibioperoneal trunk artery

35305   tibial or peroneal artery, initial vessel

+ 35306   each additional tibial or peroneal artery (List separately in addition to code for primary procedure)

(Use 35306 in conjunction with 35305)

(Do not report 35304, 35305, 35306 in conjunction with 35500, 37229, 37231, 37233, 37235)

35311   subclavian, innominate, by thoracic incision

35321   axillary-brachial

35331   abdominal aorta

35341   mesenteric, celiac, or renal

35351   iliac

35355   iliofemoral

35361   combined aortoiliac

35363   combined aortoiliofemoral

35371   common femoral

35372   deep (profunda) femoral

+ 35390   Reoperation, carotid, thromboendarterectomy, more than 1 month after original operation (List separately in addition to code for primary procedure)

(Use 35390 in conjunction with code 35301)

● New Code   ▲ Revised Code   + Add-On Code   ⊘ Modifier -51 Exempt   ⊙ Moderate Sedation

ANGIOSCOPY

+ **35400**   Angioscopy (non-coronary vessels or grafts) during therapeutic intervention (List separately in addition to code for primary procedure)

TRANSLUMINAL ANGIOPLASTY

If done as part of another operation, use modifier 51 or use modifier 52.

(For radiological supervision and interpretation, see 75962-75968 and 75978)

Open

35450   Transluminal balloon angioplasty, open; renal or other visceral artery

35452   aortic

(35454   deleted 2010 [2011 edition]; see 37220-37227)

(35456   deleted 2010 [2011 edition]; see 37220-37227)

35458   brachiocephalic trunk or branches, each vessel

(35459   deleted 2010 [2011 edition]; see 37228-37235)

35460   venous

Percutaneous

Codes for catheter placement and the radiologic supervision and interpretation should also be reported, in addition to the code(s) for the therapeutic aspect of the procedure.

(35470   deleted 2010 [2011 edition]; see 37228-37235)

⊙ **35471**   Transluminal balloon angioplasty, percutaneous; renal or visceral artery

⊙ **35472**   aortic

(35473   deleted 2010 [2011 edition]; see 37220-37227)

(35474   deleted 2010 [2011 edition]; see 37220-37227)

⊙ **35475**   brachiocephalic trunk or branches, each vessel

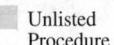 Separate Procedure   Unlisted Procedure   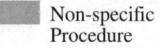 CCI Comp. Code   Non-specific Procedure

573

⊙ 35476   venous

(For radiological supervision and interpretation, use 75978)

TRANSLUMINAL ATHERECTOMY

Open

(35480   deleted 2010 [2011 edition]; see 0234T, 0235T)

(35481   deleted 2010 [2011 edition]; see 0236T)

(35482   deleted 2010 [2011 edition]; see 0238T)

(35483   deleted 2010 [2011 edition]; see 37225, 37227)

(35484   deleted 2010 [2011 edition]; see 0237T)

(35485   deleted 2010 [2011 edition]; see 37229, 37231, 37233, 37235)

Percutaneous

(35490   deleted 2010 [2011 edition]; see 0234T, 0235T)

(35491   deleted 2010 [2011 edition]; see 0236T)

(35492   deleted 2010 [2011 edition]; see 0238T)

(35493   deleted 2010 [2011 edition]; see 37225, 37227)

(35494   deleted 2010 [2011 edition]; see 0237T)

(35495   deleted 2010 [2011 edition]; see 37229, 37231, 37233, 37235)

BYPASS GRAFT

Peripheral vascular bypass CPT codes describe bypass procedures using venous grafts (CPT codes 35500-35587) and using other types of bypass procedures (arterial reconstruction, composite). Because, at a given site of obstruction, only one type of bypass is performed, these groups of codes are mutually exclusive. When different sites are treated with different bypass procedures in the same operative session, the different bypass procedures may be separately reported, using an anatomic modifier or modifier -59.

Procurement of the saphenous vein graft is included in the description of the work for 35501-35587 and should not be reported as a separate service or co-surgery. To report harvesting of an upper extremity vein, use 35500 in addition to the bypass

● New Code   ▲ Revised Code   + Add-On Code   ⊘ Modifier -51 Exempt   ⊙ Moderate Sedation

procedure. To report harvesting of a femoropopliteal vein segment, use 35572 in addition to the bypass procedure. To report harvesting and construction of an autogenous composite graft of two segments from two distant locations, report 35682 in addition to the bypass procedure, for autogenous composite of three or more segments from distant sites, report 35683.

Vein

+ 35500   Harvest of upper extremity vein, 1 segment, for lower extremity or coronary artery bypass procedure (List separately in addition to code for primary procedure)

(Use 35500 in conjunction with 33510-33536, 35556, 35566, 35570, 35571, 35583-35587)

(For harvest of more than one vein segment, see 35682, 35683)

(For endoscopic procedure, use 33508)

35501   Bypass graft, with vein; common carotid-ipsilateral internal carotid

35506   carotid-subclavian or subclavian-carotid

35508   carotid-vertebral

35509   carotid-contralateral carotid

35510   carotid-brachial

35511   subclavian-subclavian

35512   subclavian-brachial

35515   subclavian-vertebral

35516   subclavian-axillary

35518   axillary-axillary

35521   axillary-femoral

(For bypass graft performed with synthetic graft, use 35621)

35522   axillary-brachial

35523   brachial-ulnar or -radial

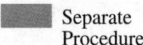 Separate Procedure   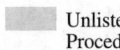 Unlisted Procedure   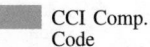 CCI Comp. Code   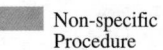 Non-specific Procedure

575

(Do not report 35523 in conjunction with 35206, 35500, 35525, 36838)

(For bypass graft performed with synthetic conduit, use 37799)

35525   brachial-brachial

35526   aortosubclavian, aortoinnominate, or aortocarotid

(For bypass graft performed with synthetic graft, use 35626)

35531   aortoceliac or aortomesenteric

35533   axillary-femoral-femoral

(For bypass graft performed with synthetic graft, use 35654)

35535   hepatorenal

(Do not report 35535 in conjunction with 35221, 35251, 35281, 35500, 35536, 35560, 35631, 35636)

35536   splenorenal

35537   aortoiliac

(For bypass graft performed with synthetic graft, use 35637)

(Do not report 35537 in conjunction with 35538)

35538   aortobi-iliac

(For bypass graft performed with synthetic graft, use 35638)

(Do not report 35538 in conjunction with 35537)

35539   aortofemoral

(For bypass graft performed with synthetic graft, use 35647)

(Do not report 35539 in conjunction with 35540)

35540   aortobifemoral

(For bypass graft performed with synthetic graft, use 35646)

(Do not report 35540 in conjunction with 35539)

(35548   deleted 2011 [2012 edition]. To report, see 35537, 35539, 35565)

● New Code   ▲ Revised Code   ✚ Add-On Code   ⊘ Modifier -51 Exempt   ⊙ Moderate Sedation

(35549   deleted 2011 [2012 edition]. To report, see 35537, 35538, 35539, 35540, 35565)

(35551   deleted 2011 [2012 edition]. To report, see 35539, 35540, 35556, 35583)

35556   femoral-popliteal

35558   femoral-femoral

35560   aortorenal

35563   ilioiliac

35565   iliofemoral

35566   femoral-anterior tibial, posterior tibial, peroneal artery or other distal vessels

35570   tibial-tibial, peroneal-tibial, or tibial/peroneal trunk-tibial

(Do not report 35570 in conjunction with 35256, 35286)

35571   popliteal-tibial, -peroneal artery or other distal vessels

+ 35572 Harvest of femoropopliteal vein, 1 segment, for vascular reconstruction procedure (eg, aortic, vena caval, coronary, peripheral artery) (List separately in addition to code for primary procedure)

(Use 35572 in conjunction with codes 33510-33516, 33517-33523, 33533-33536, 34502, 34520, 35001, 35002, 35011-35022, 35102, 35103, 35121-35152, 35231-35256, 35501-35587, 35879-35907)

(For bilateral procedure, use modifier '-50')

In-Situ Vein

(To report aortobifemoral bypass using synthetic conduit, and femoral-popliteal bypass with vein conduit in situ, use 35646 and 35583. To report aorto(uni)femoral bypass with synthetic conduit, and femoral-popliteal bypass with vein conduit in-situ, use 35647 and 35583. To report aortofemoral bypass using vein conduit, and femoral-popliteal bypass with vein conduit in situ, use 35539 and 35583)

35583 In-situ vein bypass; femoral-popliteal

| | Separate Procedure | | Unlisted Procedure | | CCI Comp. Code | | Non-specific Procedure |

577

| 35585 | femoral-anterior tibial, posterior tibial, or peroneal artery |

| 35587 | popliteal-tibial, peroneal |

Other Than Vein

(For aterial transposition and/or reimplantation, see 35691-35695)

+ 35600 Harvest of upper extremity artery, 1 segment, for coronary artery bypass procedure (List separately in addition to code for primary procedure)

(Use 35600 in conjunction with 33533-33536)

| 35601 | Bypass graft, with other than vein; common carotid-ipsilateral internal carotid |

| 35606 | carotid-subclavian |

(For open transcervical common carotid-common carotid bypass performed in conjunction with endovascular repair of descending thoracic aorta, use 33891)

(For open subclavian to carotid artery transposition performed in conjunction with endovascular thoracic aneurysm repair by neck incision, use 33889)

| 35612 | subclavian-subclavian |

| 35616 | subclavian-axillary |

| 35621 | axillary-femoral |

| 35623 | axillary-popliteal or -tibial |

| 35626 | aortosubclavian, aortoinnominate, or aortocarotid |

| 35631 | aortoceliac, aortomesenteric, aortorenal |

| 35632 | ilio-celiac |

(Do not report 35632 in conjunction with 35221, 35251, 35281, 35531, 35631)

| 35633 | ilio-mesenteric |

(Do not report 35633 in conjunction with 35221, 35251, 35281, 35531, 35631)

● New Code   ▲ Revised Code   + Add-On Code   ⊘ Modifier -51 Exempt   ⊙ Moderate Sedation

35634   iliorenal

(Do not report 35634 in conjunction with 35221, 35251, 35281, 35560, 35536, 35631)

35636   splenorenal (splenic to renal arterial anastomosis)

35637   aortoiliac

(Do not report 35637 in conjunction with 35638, 35646)

35638   aortobi-iliac

(Do not report 35638 in conjunction with 35637, 35646)

(For open placement of aorto-bi-iliac prosthesis following unsuccessful endovascular repair, use 34831)

35642   carotid-vertebral

35645   subclavian-vertebral

35646   aortobifemoral

(For bypass graft performed with vein graft, use 35540)

(For open placement of aortobifemoral prosthesis following unsuccessful endovascular repair, use 34832)

35647   aortofemoral

(For bypass graft performed with vein graft, use 35539)

35650   axillary-axillary

(35651   deleted 2011 [2012 edition]. To report, see 35646, 35647, 35656)

35654   axillary-femoral-femoral

35656   femoral-popliteal

35661   femoral-femoral

35663   ilioiliac

35665   iliofemoral

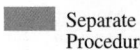 Separate
Procedure

Unlisted
Procedure

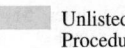 CCI Comp.
Code

Non-specific
Procedure

579

| 35666 | femoral-anterior tibial, posterior tibial, or peroneal artery |

| 35671 | popliteal-tibial or -peroneal artery |

COMPOSITE GRAFTS

Codes 35682, 35683 are used to report harvest and anastomosis of multiple vein segments from distant sites for use as arterial bypass graft conduits. These codes are intended for use when the two or more vein segments are harvested from a limb other than that undergoing bypass.

+ **35681** Bypass graft; composite, prosthetic and vein (List separately in addition to code for primary procedure)

(Do not report 35681 in addition to 35682, 35683)

+ **35682** autogenous composite, 2 segments of veins from 2 locations (List separately in addition to code for primary procedure)

(Use 35682 in conjunction with 35556, 35566, 35570, 35571, 35583-35587)

(Do not report 35682 in addition to 35681, 35683)

+ **35683** autogenous composite, 3 or more segments of vein from 2 or more locations (List separately in addition to code for primary procedure)

(Use 35683 in conjunction with 35556, 35566, 35570, 35571, 35583-35587)

(Do not report 35683 in addition to 35681, 35682)

ADJUVANT TECHNIQUES

Adjuvant (additional) technique(s) may be required at the time a bypass graft is created to improve patency of the lower extremity autogenous or synthetic bypass graft (eg., femoral-popliteal, femoral-tibial, or popliteal-tibial arteries). Code 35685 should be reported in addition to the primary synthetic bypass graft procedure, when an interposition of venous tissue (vein patch or cuff) is placed at the anastomosis between the synthetic bypass conduit and the involved artery (includes harvest).

Code 35686 should be reported in addition to the primary bypass graft procedure, when autogenous vein is used to create a fistula between the tibial or peroneal artery and vein at or beyond the distal bypass anastomosis site of the involved artery.

(For composite graft(s), see 35681-35683)

---

580 ● New Code   ▲ Revised Code   + Add-On Code   ⊘ Modifier -51 Exempt   ⊙ Moderate Sedation

+ 35685 Placement of vein patch or cuff at distal anastomosis of bypass graft, synthetic conduit (List separately in addition to code for primary procedure)

(Use 35685 in conjunction with codes 35656, 35666 or 35671)

+ 35686 Creation of distal arteriovenous fistula during lower extremity bypass surgery (non-hemodialysis) (List separately in addition to code for primary procedure)

(Use 35686 in conjunction with 35556, 35566, 35570, 35571, 35583-35587, 35623, 35656, 35666, 35671)

ARTERIAL TRANSPOSITION

35691 Transposition and/or reimplantation; vertebral to carotid artery

35693 vertebral to subclavian artery

35694 subclavian to carotid artery

(For open subclavian to carotid artery transposition performed in conjunction with endovascular repair of descending thoracic aorta, use 33889)

35695 carotid to subclavian artery

+ 35697 Reimplantation, visceral artery to infrarenal aortic prosthesis, each artery (List separately in addition to code for primary procedure)

(Do not report 35697 in conjunction with 33877)

EXCISION, EXPLORATION, REPAIR, REVISION

+ 35700 Reoperation, femoral-popliteal or femoral (popliteal)-anterior tibial, posterior tibial, peroneal artery or other distal vessels, more than 1 month after original operation (List separately in addition to code for primary procedure)

(Use 35700 in conjunction with codes 35556, 35566, 35570, 35571, 35583, 35585, 35587, 35656, 35666, 35671)

35701 Exploration (not followed by surgical repair), with or without lysis of artery; carotid artery

35721 femoral artery

35741 popliteal artery

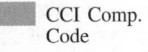

	Separate Procedure		Unlisted Procedure		CCI Comp. Code		Non-specific Procedure

581

35761	other vessels
35800	Exploration for postoperative hemorrhage, thrombosis or infection; neck
35820	chest
35840	abdomen
35860	extremity
35870	Repair of graft-enteric fistula
35875	Thrombectomy of arterial or venous graft (other than hemodialysis graft or fistula);
35876	with revision of arterial or venous graft

(For thrombectomy of hemodialysis graft or fistula, see 36831, 36833)

Codes 35879 and 35881 describe open revision of graft-threatening stenoses of lower extremity arterial bypass graft(s) (previously constructed with autogenous vein conduit) using vein patch angioplasty or segmental vein interposition techniques. For thrombectomy with revision of any non-coronary arterial or venous graft, including those of the lower extremity, (other than hemodialysis graft or fistula), use 35876. For direct repair (other than for fistula) of a lower extremity blood vessel (with or without patch angioplasty), use 35226. For repair (other than for fistula) of a lower extremity blood vessel using a vein graft, use 35256.

35879	Revision, lower extremity arterial bypass, without thrombectomy, open; with vein patch angioplasty
35881	with segmental vein interposition

(For revision or femoral anastomosis of sythetic arterial bypass graft, see 35883, 35884)

(For excision of infected graft, see 35901-35907 and appropriate revascularization code)

35883	Revision, femoral anastomosis of synthetic arterial bypass graft in groin, open; with nonautogenous patch graft (eg, Dacron, ePTFE, bovine pericardium)

(For bilateral procedure, use modifier 50)

● New Code   ▲ Revised Code   + Add-On Code   ⊘ Modifier -51 Exempt   ⊙ Moderate Sedation

(Do not report 35883 in conjunction with 35700, 35875, 35876, 35884)

35884 with autogenous vein patch graft

(For bilateral procedure, use modifier -50)

(Do not report 35884 in conjunction with 35700, 35875, 35876, 35883)

35901 Excision of infected graft; neck

35903 extremity

35905 thorax

35907 abdomen

VASCULAR INJECTION PROCEDURES

Listed services for injection procedures include necessary local anesthesia, introduction of needles or catheter, injection of contrast media with or without automatic power injection, and/or necessary pre- and post-injection care specifically related to the injection procedure.

Catheters, drugs, and contrast media are not included in the listed service for the injection procedures.

Selective vascular catheterization should be coded to include introduction and all lesser order selective catheterization used in the approach (eg., the description for a selective right middle cerebral artery catheterization includes the introduction and placement catheterization of the right common and internal carotid arteries).

Additional second and/or third order arterial catheterization within the same family of arteries or veins supplied by a single first order vessel should be expressed by 36012, 36218, or 36248.

Additional first order or higher catheterization in vascular families supplied by a first order vessel different from a previously selected and coded family should be separately coded using the conventions described above.

(For radiological supervision and interpretation, see RADIOLOGY)

(For injection procedures in conjunction with cardiac catheterization, see 93452-93461, 93563-93568)

(For chemotherapy of malignant disease, see 96400-96549)

Separate Procedure   Unlisted Procedure   CCI Comp. Code   Non-specific Procedure   **583**

Intravenous

36000 Introduction of needle or intracatheter, vein

36002 Injection procedures (eg, thrombin) for percutaneous treatment of extremity pseudoaneurysm

(For imaging guidance, see 76942, 77002, 77012, 77021)

(For ultrasound guided compression repair of pseudoaneurysms, use 76936)

(Do not report 36002 for vascular sealant of an arteriotomy site)

36005 Injection procedure for extremity venography (including introduction of needle or intracatheter)

(For radiological supervision and interpretation, see 75820, 75822)

▲⊙**36010** Introduction of catheter, superior or inferior vena cava

36011 Selective catheter placement, venous system; first order branch (eg, renal vein, jugular vein)

36012 second order, or more selective, branch (eg, left adrenal vein, petrosal sinus)

36013 Introduction of catheter, right heart or main pulmonary artery

36014 Selective catheter placement, left or right pulmonary artery

36015 Selective catheter placement, segmental or subsegmental pulmonary artery

(For insertion of flow directed catheter (eg, Swan-Ganz), use 93503)

(For venous catheterization for selective organ blood sampling, use 36500)

Intra-Arterial/Intra-Aortic

(For radiological supervision and interpretation, see RADIOLOGY)

36100 Introduction of needle or intracatheter, carotid or vertebral artery

---

584 ● New Code   ▲ Revised Code   + Add-On Code   ⊘ Modifier -51 Exempt   ⊙ Moderate Sedation

(For bilateral procedure, report 36100 with modifier -50)

36120 Introduction of needle or intracatheter; retrograde brachial artery

▲⊙**36140** extremity artery

(For insertion of arteriovenous cannula, see 36810-36821)

(36145 Deleted 2009 [2010 edition]. To report, see 36147, 36148)

Diagnostic Studies of Arteriovenous (AV) Shunts for Dialysis

For diagnostic studies, the arteriovenous (AV) dialysis shunt (AV shunt) is defined as beginning with the arterial anasomosis and extending to the right atrium. This definition includes all upper and lower extremity AV shunts (arteriovenous fistulae [AVF] and arteriovenous grafts [AVG]). Code 36147 includes the work of directly accessing and imaging the entire AV shunt. Antegrade and/or retrograde puncutres of the AV shunt are typically used for imaging, and contrast may be injected directly through a needle or through a catheter placed into the AV shunt. Occasionally the catheter needs to be advanced further into the shunt to adequately visualize the arterial anastomosis or the central veins, and all manipulation of the catheter for diagnostic imaging of the AV shunt is included in 36147. Advancement of the catheter to the vena cava to adequately image that segment of the AV shunt is included in 36147 and is not separately reported. Advancement of the catheter tip through the arterial anastomosis to adequately visualize the anastomosis is also considered integral to the work of 36147 and is not separately reported.

Ultrasound guidance for puncture of the AV shunt is not included in 36147. Particularly in the case of new or failing AVF, ultrasound may be necessary to safely and effectively puncture the AV access for evaluation and this may be reported separately with 76937 if all the appropriate elements for reporting 76937 are performed.

Evaluation of the peri-anastomotic portion of the inflow is considered an integral part of the dialysis fistulagram and is included in the work of 36147. The peri-anastomotic portion of the vessel at the arterial anastomosis includes the short segment of the artery immediately adjacent to the anastomosis, the anastomosis itself, and the portion of the vessel or graft immediately distal to the anastomosis.

The arterial inflow to the AV access is considered a separate vessel. If a more proximal inflow problem separate from the peri-anastomotic segment is suspected and additional catheter work and imaging must be done for adequate evaluation, this work is not included in 36147. If a catheter is selectively advanced from the AV shunt puncture into the inflow artery, an additional catheterization code may be reported. In the typical case of an upper extremity AV shunt, 36215 is used to report this work, and includes placement of the catheter retrograde into the inflow

■ Separate Procedure　　■ Unlisted Procedure　　■ CCI Comp. Code　　■ Non-specific Procedure

artery and into the aorta if necessary (ie, 36200 may not be also reported since that work is included in the work defined by 36215).

Interventions for Arteriovenous (AV) Shunts Created for Dialysis (AV Grafts and AV Fistulae)

For the purposes of coding interventional procedures in arteriovenous (AV) shunts created for dialysis (both arteriovenous fistulae [AVF] and arteriovenous grafts [AVG]), the AV shunt is artificially divided into two vessel segments. The first segment is peripheral and extends from the peri-arterial anastomosis through the axillary vein (or entire cephalic vein in the case of cephalic venous outflow). The second segment includes the veins central to the axillary and cephalic veins, including the subclavian and innominate veins through the vena cava. Interventions performed in a single segment, regardless of the number of lesions treated, are coded as a single intervention.

The AV shunt is considered to be venous and most interventions are coded with the venous intervention codes (ie, angioplasty is reported with venous angioplasty codes 35476, 75978). Codes 35476 and 75978 would be reported once to describe all angioplasty work performed in one segment of the AV dialysis shunt, regardless of the number of distinct lesions treated within that segment, the number of times the balloon is inflated, or the number of balloon catheters required to open all lesions.

There is an exception to the use of venous interventional codes. When there is a stenosis at the arterial anastomosis, it typically extends across the anastomosis and involves the artery just proximal to and at the anastomosis as well as the outflow vessel or graft. This segment is called the peri-anastomotic (or juxta-anastomotic) region, and even though the stenosis can involve multiple vessels, it is typically a single lesion with a single etiology crossing the anastomosis, and treatment to open this lesion crosses from the artery into the vein or venous graft. An intervention treated in this peri-anastomotic segment is coded as an arterial intervention (35475, 75962). Since the entire segment of the AV shunt from the peri-arterial anastomosis through the axillary vein is considered a single vessel for coding of interventions, the arterial angioplasty codes include the work of opening the peri-anastomotic stenosis, as well as all other stenoses treated within this segment of the vessel. Codes 35475 and 75962 are reported once to describe all work done to angioplasty any lesion from the peri-arterial anastomosis through the axillary vein in procedures that involve angioplasty of the peri-arterial anastomosis of the AV shunt. In these special instances, venous angioplasty codes would not be reported additionally for this first or most peripheral shunt segment, even if balloon angioplasty is performed on segments of the AV dialysis shunt that are purely venous anatomy within this specific vessel segment.

It is never appropriate to report removal of the arterial plug during a declot/thrombectomy procedure as an arterial or venous angioplasty (35475, 35476). Removal of the arterial plug is included in the work of a fistula

● New Code ▲ Revised Code ✛ Add-On Code ⊘ Modifier -51 Exempt ⊙ Moderate Sedation

thrombectomy (36870) even if a balloon catheter is used to mechanically dislodge the resistant thrombus.

The central veins (eg, subclavian, innominate, and cava) are considered an additional, separate venous vessel segment for purposes of interventional coding for AV dialysis shunt interventions. If one or more central venous stenoses are treated with angioplasty, this is reported as a single venous angioplasty (35476, 75978), regardless of the number of discrete lesions treated within this segment, and also independent of the number of balloon inflations or number of balloon catheters or sizes required. This additional work should be clearly documented in the patient record and in the recorded images.

The codes for stents placed in AV dialysis accesses are generic for intravascular work and not specific for arterial or venous anatomy. However, the same rules used for angioplasty apply to stent placements for AV dialysis shunts with respect to the number of intervention reported for each patient. Stent codes (37205, 75960) are reported once to describe all work of stenting lesions within the defined AV dialysis shunt segment from the peri-arterial anastomosis through the axillary and cephalic veins, regardless of the number of stents placed or the number of discrete lesions treated within that vessel segment. If additional stenting is required for central venous stenosis, this may be reported as an additional stent placement (37206, 75960), describing all the work of stent placement within the central venous segment.

The work of catheterizing all the veins in the dialysis AV shunt is included in 36147 (and, if appropriate, 36148). Selective catheterization of the inferior/superior vena cava and central veins cannot be separately reported when performed from a direct puncture of the AVF/AVG.

However, if additional venous side branches off of the conduit, known as accessory veins, are separately catheterized for intervention such as embolization of a large competing accessory vein, this additional work may be separately reported using the appropriate selective venous catheterization codes (36011 and 36012). The embolization may be reported using 37204, 75894.

⊙ **36147** Introduction of needle and/or catheter, arteriovenous shunt created for dialysis (graft/fistula); initial access with complete radiological evaluation of dialysis access, including fluoroscopy, image documentation and report (includes access of shunt, injection[s] of contrast, and all necessary imaging from the arterial anastomosis and adjacent artery through entire venous outflow including the inferior or superior vena cava)

(If 36147 indicates the need for a therapeutic intervention requiring a second catheterization of the shunt, use 36148)

(Do not report 36147 in conjunction with 75791)

| Separate Procedure | Unlisted Procedure | CCI Comp. Code | Non-specific Procedure |

⊙+36148   additional access for therapeutic intervention (List separately in addition to code for primary procedure)

(Use 36148 in conjunction with 36147)

36160   Introduction of needle or intracatheter, aortic, translumbar

Diagnostic Studies of Cervicocerebral Arteries

Codes 36221-36228 describe non-selective and selective arterial catheter placement and diagnostic imaging of the aortic arch, carotid, and vertebral arterial. Codes 36221-36226 include the work of accessing the vessel, placement of catheter(s), contrast injection(s), fluoroscopy, radiological supervision and interpretation, and closure of the arteriotomy by pressure, or application of an arterial closure device. Codes 36221-36228 describe arterial contrast injections with arterial, capillary, and venous phase imaging, when performed.

Code 36227 is an add-on code to report unilateral selective arterial catheter placement and diagnostic imaging of the ipsilateral external carotid circulation and includes all the work of accessing the additional vessel, placement of catheter(s), contrast injection(s), fluoroscopy, radiological supervision and interpretation. Code 36227 is reported in conjunction with 36222, 36223, or 36224.

Code 36228 is an add-on code to report unilateral selective arterial catheter placement and diagnostic imaging of the initial and each additional intracranial branch of the internal carotid or vertebral arteries. Code 36228 is reported in conjunction with 36224 or 36226. This includes any additional second or third order catheter selective placement in the same primary branch of the internal carotid, vertebral, or basilar artery and includes all the work of accessing the additional vessel, placement of catheter(s), contrast injection(s), fluoroscopy, radiological supervision and interpretation. It is not reported more than twice per side regardless of the number of additional branches selectively catheterized.

Codes 36221-36226 are built on progressive hierarchies with more intensive services inclusive of less intensive services. The code inclusive of all the services provided for that vessel should be reported (ie, use the code inclusive of the most intensive services provided). Only one code in the range 36222-36224 may be reported for each ipsilateral carotid territory. Only one code in the range 36225-36226 may be reported for each ipsilateral vertebral territory.

Code 36221 is reported for non-selective arterial catheter placement in the thoracic aorta and diagnostic imaging of the aortic arch and great vessel origins. Codes 36222-36228 are reported for unilateral artery catheterization. Do not report 36221 in conjunction with 36222-36226 as these selective codes include the work of 36221 when performed.

Do not report 36222, 36223, or 36224 together for ipsilateral angiography. Instead, select the code that represents the most comprehensive service using the following

● New Code   ▲ Revised Code   + Add-On Code   ⊘ Modifier -51 Exempt   ⊙ Moderate Sedation

hierarchy of complexity (listed in descending order of complexity): 36224>36223>36222.

Do not report 36225 and 36226 together for ipsilateral angiography. Select the code that represents the more comprehensive service using the following hierarchy of complexity (listed in descending order of complexity): 36226>36225.

When bilateral carotid and/or vertebral arterial catheterization and imaging is performed, add modifier 50 to codes 36222-36228 if the same procedure is performed on both sides. For example, bilateral extracranial carotid angiography with selective catheterization of each common carotid artery would be reported with 36222 and modifier 50. However, when different territory(ies) is studied in the same session on both sides of the body, modifiers may be required to report the imaging performed. use modifier 59 to denote that different carotid and/or vertebral arteries are being studied. For example, when selective right internal carotid artery catheterization accompanied by right extracranial and intracranial carotid angiography is followed by selective left common carotid artery catheterization with left extracranial carotid angiography, use 36224 to report the right side and 36222-59 to report the left side.

Diagnostic angiography of the cervicocerebral vessels may be followed by an interventional procedure at the same session. Interventional procedure may be separately reportable using standard coding conventions.

Do not report 75774 as part of diagnostic angiography of the extracranial and intracranial cervicocerebral vessels. It may be appropriate to report 75774 for diagnostic angiography of upper extremities and other vascular beds performed in the same session.

Report 76376 or 76377 for 3D rendering when performed in conjunction with 36221-36228.

Report 76937 for ultrasound guidance for vascular access, when performed in conjunction with 36221-36228.

⊙ **36200** Introduction of catheter, aorta

(For non-selective angiography of the extracranial carotid and/or cerebral vessels adn cervicocerebral arch, when performed, use 36221)

36215 Selective catheter placement, arterial system; each first order thoracic or brachiocephalic branch, within a vascular family

(For catheter placement for coronary angiography, see 93454-93961)

36216 initial second order thoracic or brachiocephalic branch, within a vascular family

■ Separate Procedure	■ Unlisted Procedure	■ CCI Comp. Code	■ Non-specific Procedure

589

36217   initial third order or more selective thoracic or brachiocephalic branch, within a vascular family

+ 36218   additional second order, third order, and beyond, thoracic or brachiocephalic branch, within a vascular family (List in addition to code for initial second or third order vessel as appropriate)

(Use 36218 in conjunction with codes 36216, 36217)

(For angiography, see 36147, 36222-36228, 75600-75774, 75791)

(For angioplasty, see 35471, 35472, 35475)

(For transcatheter therapies, see 37200-37208, 61624, 61626)

(When coronary artery, arterial conduit [eg., internal mammary, inferior epigastric or free radical artery] or venous bypass graft angiography is performed in conjunction with cardiac catheterization, see the appropriate cardiac catheterization, injection procedure, and imaging supervision code(s) [93455, 93457, 93459, 93461, 93530-93533, 93564] in the **Medicine** section of CPT. When internal mammary artery angiography only is performed without a concomitant cardiac catheterization, use 36216 or 36217 as appropriate.)

●⊙**36221**   Non-selective catheter placement, thoracic aorta, with angiography of the extracranial carotid, vertebral, and/or intracranial vessels, unilateral or bilateral, and all associated radiological supervision and interpretation, includes angiography of the cervicocerebral arch, when performed

(Do not report 36221 with 36222-36226)

●⊙**36222**   Selective catheter placement, common carotid or innominate artery, unilateral, any approach, with angiography of the ipsilateral extracranial carotid circulation and all associated radiological supervision and interpretation, includes angiography of the cervicocerebral arch, when performed

●⊙**36223**   Selective catheter placement, common carotid or innominate artery, unilateral, any approach, with angiography of the ipsilateral intracranial carotid circulation and all associated radiological supervision and interpretation, includes angiography of the extracranial carotid and cervicocerebral arch, when performed

●⊙**36224**   Selective catheter placement, internal carotid artery, unilateral, with angiography of the ipsilateral intracranial carotid

590   ● New   ▲ Revised   + Add-On   ⊘ Modifier -51   ⊙ Moderate
          Code   Code   Code   Exempt   Sedation

circulation and all associated radiological supervision and interpretation, includes angiography of the extracranial carotid and cervicocerebral arch, when performed

●⊙**36225** Selective catheter placement, subclavian or innominate artery, unilateal with angiography of the ipsilateral vertebral circulation and allassociated radiological supervision and interpretation, includes angiography of the cervicocerebral arch, when performed

●⊙**36226** Selective catheter placement, vertebral artery, unilateral, with angiography of the ipsilateral vertebral circulation and all associated radiological supervision and interpretation, includes angiography of the cervicocerebral arch, when performed

●⊙**+36227** Selective catheter placement, external carotid artery, unilateral, with angiography of the ipsilateral external carotid circulation and all associated radiological supervision and interpretation (List separately in addition to code for primary procedure)

(Use 36227 in conjunction with 36222, 36223 or 36224)

●⊙**+36228** Selective catheter placement, each intracranial branch of the internal carotid or vertebral arteries, unilateral, with angiography of the selected vessel circulation and all associated radiological supervision adn interpretation (eg, middle cerebral artery, posterior inferior cerebellar artery) (List separately in addition to code for primary procedure)

(Use 36228 in conjunction with 36224 or 36226)

(Do not report 36228 more than twice per side)

⊙ **36245** Selective catheter placement, arterial system; each first order abdominal, pelvic, or lower extremity artery branch, within a vascular family

⊙ **36246** initial second order abdominal, pelvic, or lower extremity artery branch, within a vascular family

⊙ **36247** initial third order or more selective abdominal, pelvic, or lower extremity artery branch, within a vascular family

⊙**+36248** additional second order, third order, and beyond, abdominal, pelvic, or lower extremity artery branch, within a vascular family (List in addition to code for initial second or third order vessel as appropriate)

(Use 36248 in conjunction with codes 36246, 36247)

591

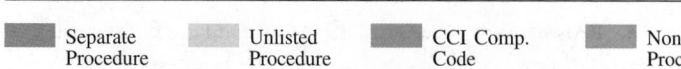

| Separate Procedure | Unlisted Procedure | CCI Comp. Code | Non-specific Procedure |

⊙ **36251** Selective catheter placement (first-order), main renal artery and any accessory renal artery(s) for renal angiography, including arterial puncture and catheter placement(s), fluoroscopy, contrast injection(s), image postprocessing, permanent recording of images, and radiological supervision and interpretation, including pressure gradient measurements when performed, and flush aortogram when performed; unilateral

⊙ **36252** bilateral

⊙ **36253** Superselective catheter placement (one or more second order or higher renal artery branches) renal artery and any accessory renal artery(s) for renal angiography, including arterial puncture, catheterization, fluoroscopy, contrast injection(s), image postprocessing, permanent recording of images, and radiological supervision and interpretation, including pressure gradient measurements when performed, and flush aortogram when performed; unilateral

(Do not report 36253 in conjunction with 36251 when performed for the same kidney)

⊙ **36254** bilateral

(Do not report 36254 in conjunction with 36252)

(Placement of closure device at the vascular access site is not separately reported with 36251-36254)

36260 Insertion of implantable intra-arterial infusion pump (eg, for chemotherapy of liver)

36261 Revision of implanted intra-arterial infusion pump

36262 Removal of implanted intra-arterial infusion pump

36299 Unlisted procedure, vascular injection

Venous

Venipuncture, needle or catheter for diagnostic study or intravenous therapy, percutaneous. These codes are also used to report the therapy as specified. For collection of a specimen from an established catheter, use 36592. For collection of a specimen from a completely implantable venous access device, use 36591.

▲ **36400** Venipuncture, younger than age 3 years, necessitating the skill of a physician or other qualified health care professional, not to be used for routine venipuncture; femoral or jugular vein

● New Code	▲ Revised Code	+ Add-On Code	⊘ Modifier -51 Exempt	⊙ Moderate Sedation

▲ 36405   scalp vein

▲ 36406   other vein

▲ 36410   Venipuncture, age 3 years or older, necessitating the skill of a physician or other qualified health care professional (separate procedure), for diagnostic or therapeutic purposes (not to be used for routine venipuncture)

36415   Collection of venous blood by venipuncture

(Do not report modifier 63 in conjunction with 36415)

36416   Collection of capillary blood specimen (eg, finger, heel, ear stick)

36420   Venipuncture, cutdown; under age 1 year

(Do not report modifier 63 in conjunction with 36420)

36425   age 1 or over

36430   Transfusion, blood or blood components

36440   Push transfusion, blood, 2 years or under

36450   Exchange transfusion, blood; newborn

(Do not report modifier 63 in conjunction with 36450)

36455   other than newborn

36460   Transfusion, intrauterine, fetal

(Do not report modifier 63 in conjunction with 36460)

(For radiological supervision and interpretation, use 76941)

36468   Single or multiple injections of sclerosing solutions, spider veins (telangiectasia); limb or trunk

36469   face

36470   Injection of sclerosing solution; single vein

36471   multiple veins, same leg

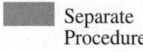 Separate Procedure   Unlisted Procedure   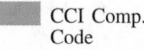 CCI Comp. Code   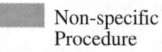 Non-specific Procedure   **593**

36475 Endovenous ablation therapy of incompetent vein, extremity, inclusive of all imaging guidance and monitoring, percutaneous, radiofrequency; first vein treated

+ 36476 second and subsequent veins treated in a single extremity, each through separate access sites (list separately in addition to code for primary procedure)

(Use 36476 in conjunction with 36475)

(Do not report 36475, 36476 in conjunction with 29581, 29582, 36000-36005, 36410, 36425, 36478, 36479, 37204, 75894, 76000, 76001, 76937, 76942, 76998, 77022, 93970, 93971)

36478 Endovenous ablation therapy of incompetent vein, extremity, inclusive of all imaging guidance and monitoring, percutaneous, laser; first vein treated

+ 36479 second and subsequent veins treated in a single extremity, each through separate access sites (List separately in addition to code for primary procedure)

(Use 36479 in conjunction with 36478)

(Do not report 36478, 36479 in conjunction with 29581, 29582, 36000-36005, 36410, 36425, 36475, 36476, 37204, 75894, 76000, 76001, 76937, 76942, 76998, 77022, 93970, 93971)

⊙ **36481** Percutaneous portal vein catheterization by any method

(For radiological supervision and interpretation, see 75885, 75887)

36500 Venous catheterization for selective organ blood sampling

(For catheterization in superior or inferior vena cava, use 36010)

(For radiological supervision and interpretation, use 75893)

36510 Catheterization of umbilical vein for diagnosis or therapy, newborn

(Do not report modifier '-63' in conjunction with 36510)

36511 Therapeutic apheresis; for white blood cells

36512 for red blood cells

36513 for platelets

● New Code ▲ Revised Code + Add-On Code ⊘ Modifier -51 Exempt ⊙ Moderate Sedation

36514   for plasma pheresis

36515   with extracorporeal immunoadsorption and plasma reinfusion

36516   with extracorporeal selective adsorption or selective filtration and plasma reinfusion

(For professional evaluation, use modifier -26)

36522   Photopheresis, extracorporeal

Central Venous Access Procedures

(For refilling and maintenance of an implantable pump or reservoir for intravenous or intra-arterial drug delivery, use 96530)

Insertion of Central Venous Access Device

⊙ **36555**   Insertion of non-tunneled centrally inserted central venous catheter; under 5 years of age

(For peripherally inserted non-tunneled central venous catheter, under 5 years of age, use 36568)

36556   age 5 years or older

(For peripherally inserted non-tunneled central venous catheter, age 5 years or older, use 36569)

⊙ **36557**   Insertion of tunneled centrally inserted central venous catheter, without subcutaneous port or pump; under 5 years of age

⊙ **36558**   age 5 years or older

(For peripherally inserted central venous catheter with port, age 5 years or older, use 36571)

⊙ **36560**   Insertion of tunneled centrally inserted central venous access device, with subcutaneous port; under 5 years of age

(For peripherally inserted central venous access device with subcutaneous port, under 5 years of age, use 36570)

⊙ **36561**   age 5 years or older

(For peripherally inserted central venous catheter with subcutaneous port, 5 years or older, use 36571)

595

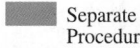 Separate Procedure   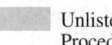 Unlisted Procedure   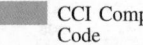 CCI Comp. Code   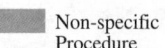 Non-specific Procedure

The Central Venous Access Procedures Table									
	Non-Tunneled	Tunneled w/o port or pump	Central Tunneled	Tunneled with port	Tunneled with pump	Peripheral	<5 years	≥5 years	Any Age
Insertion									
Catheter	36555						36555		
	36556							36556	
		36557	36557				36557		
		36558	36558					36558	
	36568 (w/o port or pump)					36568 (w/o port or pump)	36568 (w/o port or pump)		
	36569 (w/o port or pump)					36569 (w/o port or pump)		36569 (w/o port or pump)	
Device			36560	36560		36560			
			36561	36561				36561	
			36563		36563				36563
		36565	36565						36565
			36566	36566					
	36570 (w port0			36570 (w port)		36570 (w port)	36570 (w port)		
	36571 (w port)			36571 (w port)		36571 (w port)		36571 (w port)	
Repair									
Catheter	36575 (w/o port or pump)	36575 (w/o port or pump)	36575 (w/o port or pump)			36575 (w/o port or pump)			36575
Device	36576 (w port or pump)					36576 (w port or pump)			36576
Partial Replacement - Central Venous Access Device (Catheter only)									
			36578	36578	36578	36578			36578
Complete Replacement - Central Venous Access Device (through same venous access site)									
Catheter	36580 (w/o port or pump)								36580
		36581	36581						36581
	36584 (w/o port or pump)					36584 (w/o port or pump)			36584
Device			36582	36582					36582
			36583		36583				36583
				36585 (w port)		36585 (w port)			36585
Removal									
Catheter		36589							36589
Device			36590	36590	36590	36590			36590
Removal of Obstructive Material from Device									
	36595 peri-catheter	36595 peri-catheter	36595 peri-catheter	36595 peri-catheter	36595 peri-catheter	36595 peri-catheter			36595 peri-catheter
	36596 intra-luminal	36596 intra-luminal	36596 intra-luminal	36596 intra-luminal	36596 intra-luminal	36596 intra-luminal			36596 intra-luminal
Repositioning of Catheter									
	36597	36597	36597	36597	36597	36597	36597	36597	36597

596 ● New Code ▲ Revised Code + Add-On Code ⊘ Modifier -51 Exempt ⊙ Moderate Sedation

⊙ 36563   Insertion of tunneled centrally inserted central venous access device with subcutaneous pump

⊙ 36565   Insertion of tunneled centrally inserted central venous access device, requiring 2 catheters via 2 separate venous access sites; without subcutaneous port or pump (eg, Tesio type catheter)

⊙ 36566   with subcutaneous port(s)

⊙ 36568   Insertion of peripherally inserted central venous catheter (PICC), without subcutaneous port or pump; under 5 years of age

(For placement of centrally inserted non-tunneled central venous catheter, without subcutaneous port or pump, under 5 years of age, use 36555)

36569   age 5 years or older

(For placement of centrally inserted non-tunneled central venous catheter, without subcutaneous port or pump, age 5 years or older, use 36556)

⊙ 36570   Insertion of peripherally inserted central venous access device, with subcutaneous port; under 5 years of age

(For insertion of tunneled centrally inserted central venous access device with subcutaneous port, under 5 years of age, use 36560)

⊙ 36571   age 5 years or older

(For insertion of tunneled centrally inserted central venous access device with subcutaneous port, age 5 years or older, use 36561)

Repair of Central Venous Access Device

(For mechanical removal of pericatheter obstructive material, use 36595)

(For mechanical removal of intracatheter obstructive material, use 36596)

36575   Repair of tunneled or non-tunneled central venous access catheter, without subcutaneous port or pump, central or peripheral insertion site

⊙ 36576   Repair of central venous access device, with subcutaneous port or pump, central or peripheral insertion site

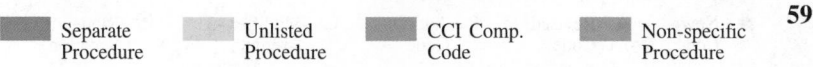

597

| Separate Procedure | Unlisted Procedure | CCI Comp. Code | Non-specific Procedure |

Partial Replacement of Central Venous Access Device (Catheter Only)

⊙ **36578**   Replacement, catheter only, of central venous access device, with subcutaneous port or pump, central or peripheral insertion site

(For complete replacement of entire device through same venous access, use 36582 or 36583)

Complete Replacement of Central Venous Access Device Through Same Venous Access Site

36580   Replacement, complete, of a non-tunneled centrally inserted central venous catheter, without subcutaneous port or pump, through same venous access

⊙ **36581**   Replacement, complete, of a tunneled centrally inserted central venous catheter, without subcutaneous port or pump, through same venous access

⊙ **36582**   Replacement, complete, of a tunneled centrally inserted central venous access device, with subcutaneous port, through same venous access

⊙ **36583**   Replacement, complete, of a tunneled centrally inserted central venous access device, with subcutaneous pump, through same venous access

36584   Replacement, complete, of a peripherally inserted central venous catheter (PICC), without subcutaneous port or pump, through same venous access

⊙ **36585**   Replacement, complete, of a peripherally inserted central venous access device, with subcutaneous port, through same venous access

Removal of Central Venous Access Device

36589   Removal of tunneled central venous catheter, without subcutaneous port or pump

⊙ **36590**   Removal of tunneled central venous access device, with subcutaneous port or pump, central or peripheral insertion

(Do not report 36589 or 36590 for removal of non-tunneled central venous catheters)

● New Code   ▲ Revised Code   **+** Add-On Code   ⊘ Modifier -51 Exempt   ⊙ Moderate Sedation

Other Central Venous Access Procedures

36591   Collection of blood specimen from a completely implantable venous access device

(Do not report 36591 in conjunction with other service except a laboratory service)

(For collection of venous blood specimen by venipuncture, use 36415)

(For collection of capillary blood specimen, use 36416)

36592   Collection of blood specimen using established central or peripheral catheter, venous, not otherwise specified

(For blood collection from an established arterial catheter, use 37799)

(Do not report 36592 in conjunction with other services except a laboratory service)

36593   Declotting by thrombolytic agent of implanted vascular access device or catheter

36595   Mechanical removal of pericatheter obstructive material (eg, fibrin sheath) from central venous device via separate venous access

(Do not report 36595 in conjunction with 36593)

(For venous catheterization, see 36010-36012)

(For radiological supervision and interpretation, use 75901)

36596   Mechanical removal of intraluminal (intracatheter) obstructive material from central venous device through device lumen

(Do not report 365596 in conjunction with 36593)

(For venous catheterization, see 36010-36012)

(For radiological supervision and interpretation, use 75902)

36597   Repositioning of previously placed central venous catheter under fluoroscopic guidance

(For fluoroscopic guidance, use 76000)

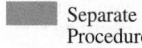 Separate Procedure   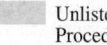 Unlisted Procedure   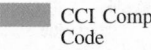 CCI Comp. Code   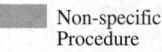 Non-specific Procedure

36598 Contrast injection(s) for radiologic evaluation of existing central venous access device, including fluoroscopy, image documentation and report

(Do not report 36598 in conjunction with 76000)

(Do not report 36598 in conjunction with 36595, 36596)

(For complete diagnostic studies, see 75820, 75825, 75827)

ARTERIAL

36600 Arterial puncture, withdrawal of blood for diagnosis

⊘ **36620** Arterial catheterization or cannulation for sampling, monitoring or transfusion (separate procedure); percutaneous

36625 cutdown

36640 Arterial catheterization for prolonged infusion therapy (chemotherapy), cutdown

(See also 96420-96425)

(For arterial catheterization for occlusion therapy, see 75894)

36660 Catheterization, umbilical artery, newborn, for diagnosis or therapy

(Do not report modifier '-63' in conjunction with 36660)

INTRAOSSEOUS

36680 Placement of needle for intraosseous infusion

HEMODIALYSIS ACCESS, INTERVASCULAR CANNULIZATION FOR EXTRACORPOREAL CIRCULATION, OR SHUNT INSERTION

36800 Insertion of cannula for hemodialysis, other purpose (separate procedure); vein to vein

36810 arteriovenous, external (Scribner type)

36815 arteriovenous, external revision, or closure

36818 Arteriovenous anastomosis, open; by upper arm cephalic vein transposition

(Do not report 36818 in conjunction with 36819, 36820, 36821, 36830 during a unilateral upper extremity procedure. For

● New Code ▲ Revised Code + Add-On Code ⊘ Modifier -51 Exempt ⊙ Moderate Sedation

bilateral upper extremity open arteriovenous anastomoses performed at the same operative session, use modifier 50 or 59 as appropriate)

36819   by upper arm basilic vein transposition

(Do not report 36819 in conjunction with 36818, 36820, 36821, 36830 during a unilateral upper extremity procedure. For bilateral upper extremity open arteriovenous anastomoses performed at the same operative session, use modifier 50 or 59 as appropriate)

36820   by forearm vein transposition

36821   direct, any site (eg, Cimino type) (separate procedure)

36822 Insertion of cannula(s) for prolonged extracorporeal circulation for cardiopulmonary insufficiency (ECMO) (separate procedure)

(For maintenance of prolonged extracorporeal circulation, use 33960, 33961)

36823 Insertion of arterial and venous cannula(s) for isolated extracorporeal circulation including regional chemotherapy perfusion to an extremity, with or without hyperthermia, with removal of cannula(s) and repair of arteriotomy and venotomy sites

(36823 includes chemotherapy perfusion supported by a membrane oxygenator/perfusion pump. Do not report 96408-96425 in conjunction with 36823)

36825 Creation of arteriovenous fistula by other than direct arteriovenous anastomosis (separate procedure); autogenous graft

(For direct arteriovenous anastomosis, use 36821)

36830   nonautogenous graft (eg, biological collagen, thermoplastic graft)

(For direct arteriovenous anastomosis, use 36821)

36831 Thrombectomy, open, arteriovenous fistula without revision, autogenous or nonautogenous dialysis graft (separate procedure)

36832 Revision, open, arteriovenous fistula; without thrombectomy, autogenous or nonautogenous dialysis graft (separate procedure)

36833   with thrombectomy, autogenous or nonautogenous dialysis graft (separate procedure)

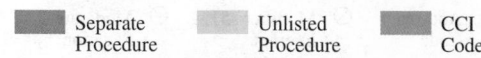

| Separate Procedure | Unlisted Procedure | CCI Comp. Code | Non-specific Procedure |

601

(36834   Deleted 2009 [2010 edition]. To report anarteriovenous access fistula or graft revision, use 36832)

36835   Insertion of Thomas shunt (separate procedure)

36838   Distal revascularization and interval ligation (DRIL), upper extremity hemodialysis access (steal syndrome)

       (Do not report 36838 in conjunction with 35512, 35522, 35523, 36832, 37607, 37618)

36860   External cannula declotting (separate procedure); without balloon catheter

36861   with balloon catheter

       (If imaging guidance is performed, use 76000)

⊙ **36870**   Thrombectomy, percutaneous, arteriovenous fistula, autogenous or nonautogenous graft (includes mechanical thrombus extraction and intra-graft thrombolysis)

       (Do not report 36870 in conjunction with 36593)

       (For catheterization, use 36147, 36148)

       (For radiological supervision and interpretation, use 36147, 75791)

PORTAL DECOMPRESSION PROCEDURES

37140   Venous anastomosis, open; portocaval

       (For peritoneal-venous shunt, use 49425)

37145   renoportal

37160   caval-mesenteric

37180   splenorenal, proximal

37181   splenorenal, distal (selective decompression of esophagogastric varices, any technique)

       (For percutaneous procedure, use 37182)

37182   Insertion of transvenous intrahepatic portosystemic shunt(s) (TIPS) (includes venous access, hepatic and portal vein catheterization, portography with hemodynamic evaluation,

---

602   ● New Code   ▲ Revised Code   ✚ Add-On Code   ⊘ Modifier -51 Exempt   ⊙ Moderate Sedation

intrahepatic tract formation/dilatation, stent placement and all associated imaging guidance and documentation)

(Do not report 75885 or 75887 in conjunction with code 37182)

(For open procedure, use 37140)

⊙ **37183** Revision of transvenous intrahepatic portosystemic shunt(s) (TIPS) (includes venous access, hepatic and portal vein catheterization, portography with hemodynamic evaluation, intrahepatic tract recanulization/dilatation, stent placement and all associated imaging guidance and documentation)

(Do not report 75885 or 75887 in conjunction with code 37183)

(For repair of arteriovenous aneurysm, use 36832)

TRANSCATHETER PROCEDURES

Codes for catheter placement and the radiologic supervision and interpretation should also be reported, in addition to the code(s) for the therapeutic aspect of the procedure.

Mechanical Thrombectomy

Code(s) for catheter placement(s), diagnostic studies, and other percutaneous interventions (eg., transluminal balloon angioplasty, stent placement) provided are separately reportable.

Codes 37184-37188 specifically include intraprocedural fluoroscopic radiological supervision and interpretation services for guidance of the procedure.

Intraprocedural injection(s) of a thrombolytic agent is an included service and not separately reportable in conjunction with mechanical thrombectomy. However, subsequent or prior continuous infusion of a thrombolytic is not an included service and is separately reportable (see 37211-37214).

For coronary mechanical thrombectomy, use 92973.

For mechanical thrombectomy for dialysis fistula, use 36870.

Transcatheter Thrombolytic Infusion

Codes 37211 or 37212 are used to report the initial day of transcatheter thrombolytic infusion(s) including follow-up arteriography/venography, and catheter position change or exchange, when performed. To report bilateral thrombolytic infusion through a separate access site(s), use modifier 50 in conjunction with 37211, 37212. Code 37213 is used to report continued

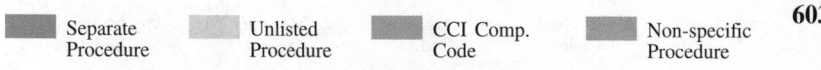

| Separate Procedure | Unlisted Procedure | CCI Comp. Code | Non-specific Procedure |

603

transcatheter thrombolytic infusion(s) on subsequent day(s), other than initial day and final day of treatment. Code 37214 is used to report final day of transcatheter thrombolytic infusion(s). When initiation and completion of thrombolysis occur on the same day, report only 37211 or 37212.

Code(s) for catheter placement(s), diagnostic studies, and other percutaneous interventions (eg, transluminal balloon angioplasty, stent placement) provided may be separately reportable.

Codes 37211-37214 include fluoroscopic guidance and associated radiological supervision and interpretation.

Ongoing E/M services on the day of the procedure related to thrombolysis are included in 37211-37214. If a significant, separately identifiable E/M service is performed by the same physician on the same day of the procedure, report the appropriate level of E/M service and append modifier 25.

Ultrasound guidance for vascular access is not included in 37211-37214. Code 76937 may be reported separately when performed if all the required elements are performed.

Arterial Mechanical Thrombectomy

Primary mechanical thrombectomy is reported per vascular family using 37184 for the initial vessel treated and 37185 for second or all subsequent vessel(s) within the same vascular family. To report mechanical thrombectomy of an additional vascular family treated through a separate access site, use modifier 51 in conjunction with 37184-37185.

Do NOT report 37184-37185 for mechanical thrombectomy performed for the retrieval of short segments of thrombus or embolus evident during other percutaneous interventional procedures. See 37186 for these procedures.

Secondary mechanical thrombectomy is reported using 37186. Do NOT report 37186 in conjunction with 37184-37185.

Venous Mechanical Thrombectomy

Use 37187 to report the initial application of venous mechanical thrombectomy. To report bilateral venous mechanical thrombectomy performed through a separate access site(s), use modifier 50 in conjunction with 37187. For repeat treatment on a subsequent day during a course of thrombolytic therapy, use 37188.

Arterial Mechanical Thrombectomy

⊙ **37184** Primary percutaneous transluminal mechanical thrombectomy, noncoronary, arterial or arterial bypass graft, including fluoroscopic guidance and intraprocedural pharmacological thrombolytic injection(s); initial vessel

● New Code   ▲ Revised Code   + Add-On Code   ⊘ Modifier -51 Exempt   ⊙ Moderate Sedation

(Do not report 37184 in conjunction with 76000, 76001, 96374, 99143-99150)

⊙+**37185**   second and all subsequent vessel(s) within the same vascular family (List separately in addition to code for primary mechanical thrombectomy procedure)

(Do not report 37185 in conjunction with 76000, 76001, 96375)

⊙+**37186**   Secondary percutaneous transluminal thrombectomy (eg, nonprimary mechanical, snare basket, suction technique), noncoronary, arterial or arterial bypass graft, including fluoroscopic guidance and intraprocedural pharmacological thrombolytic injections, provided in conjunction with another percutaneous intervention other than primary mechanical thrombectomy (List separately in addition to code for primary procedure)

(Do not report 37186 in conjunction with 76000, 76001, 96375)

Venous Mechanical Thrombectomy

⊙ **37187**   Percutaneous transluminal mechanical thrombectomy, vein(s), including intraprocedural pharmacological thrombolytic injections and fluoroscopic guidance

(Do not report 37187 in conjunction with 76000, 76001, 96375)

⊙ **37188**   Percutaneous transluminal mechanical thrombectomy, vein(s), including intraprocedural pharmacological thrombolytic injections and fluoroscopic guidance, repeat treatment on subsequent day during course of thrombolytic therapy

(Do not report 37188 in conjunction with 76000, 76001, 96375)

Other Procedures

⊙ **37191**   Insertion of intravascular vena cava filter, endovascular approach including vascular access, vessel selection, and radiological supervision and interpretation, intraprocedural roadmapping, and imaging guidance (ultrasound and fluoroscopy), when performed

(for open surgical interruption of the inferior vena cava through a laparotomy or retroperitoneal exposure, use 37619)

⊙ **37192**   Repositioning of intravascular vena cava filter, endovascular approach including vascular access, vessel selection, and radiological supervision and interpretation, intraprocedural

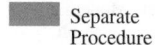 Separate Procedure   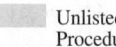 Unlisted Procedure   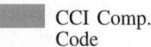 CCI Comp. Code   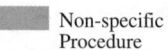 Non-specific Procedure

605

roadmapping, and imaging guidance (ultrasound and fluoroscopy), when performed

(Do not report 37192 in conjunction with 37191)

⊙ **37193** Retrieval (removal) of intravascular vena cava filter, endovascular approach including vascular access, vessel selection, and radiological supervision and interpretation, intraprocedural roadmapping, and imaging guidance (ultrasound and fluoroscopy), when performed

(Do not report 37193 in conjunction with 37197)

37195 Thrombolysis, cerebral, by intravenous infusion

●⊙**37197** Transcatheter retrieval, percutaneous, of intravascular foreign body (eg, fractured venous or arterial catheter), includes radiological supervision and interpretation, and imaging guidance (ultrasound or fluoroscopy), when performed

(For percutaneous retrieval of a vena cava filter, use 37193)

37200 Transcatheter biopsy

(For radiological supervision and interpretation, use 75970)

(37201 deleted 2012 [2013 edition]. To report, see 37211-37214)

●⊙**37211** Transcatheter therapy, arterial infusion for thrombolysis other than coronary, any method, including radiological supervision and interpretation, initial treatment day

●⊙**37212** Transcatheter therapy, venous infusion for thrombolysis, any method, including radiological supervision and interpretation, initial treatment day

●⊙**37213** Transcatheter therapy, arterial or venous infusion for thrombolysis other than coronary, any method, including radiological supervision and interpretation, continued treatment on subsequent day during course of thrombolytic therapy, including follow-up catheter contrast injection, position change, or exchange, when performed;

●⊙**37214** cessation of thrombolysis including removal of catheter and vessel closure by any method

(Report 37211-37214 once per date of treatment)

● New Code	▲ Revised Code	+ Add-On Code	⊘ Modifier -51 Exempt	⊙ Moderate Sedation

(For declotting by thrombolytic agent of implanted vascular access device or catheter, use 36593)

37202 Transcatheter therapy, infusion other than for thrombolysis, any type (eg, spasmolytic, vasoconstrictive)

(For thrombolysis of coronary vessels, see 92975, 92977)

(For radiological supervision and interpretation, use 75896)

(37203 deleted 2012 [2013 edition]. To report, use 37197)

(For removal of a vena cava filter, use 37193)

37204 Transcatheter occlusion or embolization (eg, for tumor destruction, to achieve hemostasis, to occlude a vascular malformation), percutaneous, any method, non-central nervous system, non-head or neck

(See also 61624, 61626)

(For radiological supervision and interpretation, use 75894)

(For uterine fibroid embolization [uterine artery embolization performed to treat uterine fibroids], use 37210)

(For obstetrical and gynecological embolization procedures other than uterine fibroid embolization (eg., embolization to treat obstetrical or postpartum hemorrhage), use 37204)

37205 Transcatheter placement of an intravascular stent(s), (except coronary, carotid, vertebral, iliac, and lower extremity arteries), percutaneous; initial vessel

(For radiological supervision and interpretation, use 75960)

(For transcatheter placement of intravascular cervical carotid artery stent(s), see 37215, 37216)

(For transcatheter placement of intracranial stents, use 61635)

(For transcatheter coronary stent placement, see 92928-92944)

(For transcatheter stent placement of extracranial vertebral or intrathoracic carotid artery stent(s), see Category III codes 0075T, 0076T)

(For stent placement in iliac, femoral, popliteal, and tibial/peroneal arteries, see 37221, 37223, 37226, 37227, 37230, 37231, 37234, 37235)

607

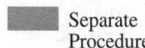 Separate Procedure	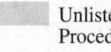 Unlisted Procedure	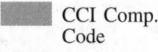 CCI Comp. Code	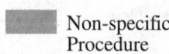 Non-specific Procedure

+ 37206   each additional vessel (List separately in addition to code for primary procedure)

(Use 37206 in conjunction with 37205)

(For radiological supervision and interpretation, use 75960)

37207   Transcatheter placement of an intravascular stent(s), (except coronary, carotid, vertebral, iliac and lower extremity arteries), open; initial vessel

(For stent placement in iliac, femoral, popliteal, and tibial/peroneal arteries, see 37221, 37223, 37226, 37227, 37230, 37231, 37234, 37235)

+ 37208   each additional vessel (List separately in addition to code for primary procedure)

(Use 37208 in conjunction with 37207)

(For radiological supervision and interpretation, use 75960)

(For catheterizations, see 36215-36248)

(For transcatheter placement of intracoronary stent(s), see 92928-92944)

(37209   deleted 2012 [2013 edition]. For exchange of a previously placed intravascular catheter during thrombolytic therapy, see 37211-37214)

(For radiological supervision and interpretation, use 75900)

⊙ **37210**   Uterine fibroid embolization (UFE, embolization of the uterine arteries to treat uterine fibroids, leiomyomata), percutaneous approach inclusive of vascular access, vessel selection, embolization, and all radiological supervision and interpretation, intraprocedural roadmapping, and imaging guidance necessary to complete the procedure

(37210 includes all catheterization and intraprocedural imaging required for a UFE procedure to confirm the presence of previously known fibroids and to roadmap vascular anatomy to enable appropriate therapy)

(Do not report 37210 in conjunction with 36200, 36245-36248, 37204, 75894, 75898)

(For all othre non-central nervous system (CNS) embolization procedures, use 37204)

37211 Code out of order. See page 606

37212 Code out of order. See page 606

37213 Code out of order. See page 606

37214 Code out of order. See page 606

⊙ **37215** Transcatheter placement of intravascular stent(s), cervical carotid artery, percutaneous; with distal embolic protection

⊙ **37216** without distal embolic protection

(37215 and 37216 include all ipsilateral selective carotid catheterization, all diagnostic imaging for ipsilateral, cervical and cerebral carotid arteriography, and all related radiological supervision and interpretation. When ipsilateral carotid arteriogram (including imaging and selective catheterization) confirms the need for carotid stenting, 37215 and 37216 are inclusive of these services. If carotid stenting is not indicated, then the appropriate codes for carotid catheterization and imaging should be reported in lieu of 37215 and 37216)

(Do not report 37215, 37216 in conjunction with 36222-36224 for the treated carotid artery)

(For transcatheter placement of extracranial vertebral or intrathoracic carotid artery stent(s), see Category III codes 0075T, 0076T)

(For percutaneous transcatheter placement of intravascular stents other than coronary, carotid, or vertebral, see 37205, 37206)

ENDOVASCULAR REVASCULARIZATION (OPEN OR PERCUTANEOUS, TRANSCATHETER)

Codes 37220-37235 are to be used to describe lower extremity endovascular revascularization services performed for occlusive disease. These lower extremity codes are built on progressive hierarchies with more intensive services inclusive of lesser intensive services. The code inclusive of all of the services provided for that vessel should be reported (ie, use the code inclusive of the most intensive services provided). Only one code from this family (37220-37235) should be reported for each lower extremity vessel treated.

These lower extremity endovascular revascularization codes all include the work of accessing and selectively catheterizing the vessel, traversing the lesion, radiological supervision and interpretation directly related to the intervention(s) performed, embolic protection if used, closure of the arteriotomy by pressureand application of an arterial closure device or standard closure of the puncture by suture, and

| ■ Separate Procedure | ■ Unlisted Procedure | ■ CCI Comp. Code | ■ Non-specific Procedure | **609** |

imaging performed to document completion of the intervention in addition to the intervention(s) performed. Extensive repair or replacement of an artery may be additionally reported (eg, 35226, or 35286). These codes describe endovascular procedures performed percutaneously and/or through an open surgical exposure. These codes include balloon angioplasty (eg, low-profile, cutting balloon, cryoplasty), atherectomy (eg, directional, rotational, laser), and stentin (eg, balloon-expandable, self-expanding, bare metal, covered, drug-eluting). Each code in this family (37220-37235) includes balloon angioplasty, when performed.

These codes describe revascularization therapies (ie, transluminal angioplasty, atherectomy, and stent placement) provided in three arterial vascular territories: iliac, femoral/popliteal, and tibial/peroneal.

When treating multiple vessels within a territory, report each additional vessel using an add-on code, as applicable. Select the base code that represents the most complex service using the following hierarchy of complexity (in descending order of complexity): atherectomy and stent>atherectomy>stent>angioplasty. When treating multiple lesions within the same vessel, report one service that reflects the combined procedures, whether done on one lesion or different lesions, using the same hierarchy.

1. **Iliac Vascular Territory** — The iliac territory is divided into 3 vessels: common iliac, internal iliac, and external iliac.

2. **Femoral/Popliteal Vascular Territory** — The entire femoral/popliteal territory of 1 lower extremity is considered a single vessel for CPT reporting specifically for the endovascular lower extremity revascularization codes 37224-37227.

3. **Tibial/Peroneal Territory** — The tibial/peroneal territory is divided into 3 vessels: anterior, tibial, posterial tibial, and peroneal arteries.

There are specific coding guidelines for each of the 3 vascular territories.

1. **Iliac Vascular Territory** — A single primary code is used for the initial iliac artery treated in each leg (37220 or 37221). If other iliac vessels are also treated in that leg, these interventions are reported with th appropriate add-on code(s) (37222, 37223). Up to 2 add-on codes can be used in a unilateral iliac vascular territory since there are 3 vessels which could be treated. Add-on codes are used for different vessels, not distinct lesions within the same vessel.

2. **Femoral/Popliteal Territory** — A single interventional code is used no matter what combination of angioplasty/stent/atherectomy is applied to all segments, including the common, deep and superficial femoral arteries as well as the popliteal artery (37224, 37225, 37226 or 37227). There are no add-on codes for additional vessels treated within the femoral/popliteal territory. Because only 1 service is reported when 2 lesions are treated in this territory, report the most complex service (eg, use 37227 if a stent is placed for 1 lesion and an atherectomy is performed on a second lesion).

● New Code	▲ Revised Code	＋ Add-On Code	⊘ Modifier -51 Exempt	⊙ Moderate Sedation

3. **Tibial/Peroneal Territory** — A single primary code is used for the initial tibial/peroneal artery treated in each leg (37228, 37229, 37230, or 37231). If other tibial/peroneal vessels are also treated in the same leg, these interventions are reported with the appropriate add-on code(s) (37232-37235). Up to 2 add-on codes could be used to describe services provided in a single leg since there are 3 tibial/peroneal vessels which could be treated. Add-on codes are used for different vessels, not distinct lesions within the same vessel. The common tibio-peroneal trunk is considered part of the tibial/peroneal territory, but is not considered a separate, fourth segment of vessel in the tibio-peroneal family for CPT reporting of endovascular lower extremity interventions. For instance, if lesions in the common tibio-peroneal trunk are treated in conjunction with lesions in the posterior tibial artery, a single code would be reported for treatment of this segment.

When treating multiple territories in the same leg, one primary lower extremity revascularization code is used for each territory treated. When second or third vessel(s) are treated in the iliac and/or tibial/peroneal territories, add-on codes are used to report the additional services. When more than one stent is placed in the same vessel, the code should be reported only once.

When multiple vessels in multiple territories in a single leg are treated at the same setting, the primary code for the treatment in the initial vessel in each vascular territory is reported. Add-on code(s) are reported when second and third iliac or tibial/peroneal arteries are treated in addition to the initial vessel in that vascular territory.

If a lesion extends across the margins of one vessel vascular territory into another, but can be opened with a single therapy, this intervention should be reported with a single code despite treating more than one vessel and/or vascular territory. For instance, if a stenosis extends from the common iliac artery into the proximal external iliac artery, and a single stent is placed to open the entire lesion, this therapy should be coded as a single stent placement in the iliac artery (37221). In this example, a code for an additional vessel treatment would not be used (do not report both 37221 and 37223).

For bifurcation lesions distal to the common iliac origins which require therapy of 2 distinct branches of the iliac or tibial/peroneal vascular territories, a primary code and an add-on code would be used to describe the intervention. In the femoral/popliteal territory, all branches are included in the primary code, so treatment of a bifurcation lesion would be reported as a single code.

When the same territor(ies) of both legs are treated in the same session, modifiers may be required to describe the interventions. Use modifier 59 to denote that different legs are being treated, even if the mode of therapy is different.

Mechanical thrombectomy and/or thrombolysis in the lower extremity vessels are sometimes necessary to aid in restoring flow to areas of occlusive disease, and are reported separately.

⊙ **37220** Revascularization, endovascular, open or percutaneous, iliac artery, unilateral, initial vessel, with transluminal angioplasty

⊙ **37221** with transluminal stent placement(s), includes angioplasty within the same vessel, when performed

⊙+**37222** Revascularization, endovascular, open or percutaneous, iliac artery, each additional ipsilateral iliac vessel, with transluminal angioplasty (list separately in addition to code for primary procedure)

(Use 37222 in conjunction with 37220, 37221)

⊙+**37223** with transluminal stent placement(s), includes angioplasty within the same vessel, when performed (list separately in addition to code for primary procedure)

(Use 37223 in conjunction with 37221)

⊙ **37224** Revascularization, endovascular, open or percutaneous, femoral, popliteal artery(s), unilateral, with transluminal angioplasty

⊙ **37225** with atherectomy, includes angioplasty within the same vessel, when performed

⊙ **37226** with transluminal stent placement(s), includes angioplasty within the same vessel, when performed

⊙ **37227** with transluminal stent placement(s) and atherectomy, includes angioplasty within the same vessel when performed

⊙ **37228** Revascularization, endovascular, open or percutaneous, tibial, peroneal artery, unilateral, initial vessel, with transluminal angioplasty

⊙ **37229** with atherectomy, includes angioplasty within the same vessel, when performed

⊙ **37230** with transluminal stent placement(s), includes angioplasty within the same vessel, when performed

⊙ **37231** with transluminal stent placement(s) and atherectomy, includes angioplasty within the same vessel, when performed

⊙+**37232** Revascularization, endovascular, open or percutaneous, tibial/peroneal artery, unilateral, each additional vessel, with

● New   ▲ Revised   ✚ Add-On   ⊘ Modifier -51   ⊙ Moderate
        Code   Code   Code   Exempt   Sedation

transluminal angioplasty (list separately in addition to code for primary procedure)

(Use 37232 in conjunction with 37228-37231)

⊙+37233   with atherectomy, includes angioplasty within the same vessel, when performed (list separately in addition to code for primary procedure)

(Use 37233 in conjunction with 37229, 37231)

⊙+37234   with transluminal stent placement(s), includes angioplasty within the same vessel, when performed (list separately in addition to code for primary procedure)

(Use 37234 in conjunction with 37229, 37230, 37231)

⊙+37235   with transluminal stent placement(s) and atherectomy, includes angioplasty within the same vessel, when performed (list separately in addition to code for primary procedure)

(Use 37235 in conjunction with 37231)

INTRAVASCULAR ULTRASOUND SERVICES

Intravascular ultrasound services include all transducer manipulations and repositioning within the specific vessel being examined, both before and after therapeutic intervention (eg, stent placement).

Vascular access for intravascular ultrasound performed during a therapeutic intervention is not reported separately.

+ 37250   Intravascular ultrasound (non-coronary vessel) during diagnostic evaluation and/or therapeutic intervention; initial vessel (List separately in addition to code for primary procedure)

+ 37251   each additional vessel (List separately in addition to code for primary procedure)

(Use 37251 in conjunction with 37250)

(For catheterizations, see 36215-36248)

(For transcatheter therapies, see 37200-37208, 61624, 61626)

(For radiological supervision and interpretation, see 75945, 75946)

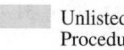 Separate Procedure   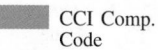 Unlisted Procedure   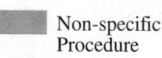 CCI Comp. Code   Non-specific Procedure

ENDOSCOPY

Surgical vascular endoscopy always includes diagnostic endoscopy.

37500 Vascular endoscopy, surgical, with ligation or perforator veins, subfascial (SEPS)

(For open procedure, use 37760)

37501 Unlisted vascular endoscopy procedure

LIGATION

(For phleborraphy and arteriorraphy, see 35201-35286)

37565 Ligation, internal jugular vein

37600 Ligation; external carotid artery

37605 internal or common carotid artery

37606 internal or common carotid artery, with gradual occlusion, as with Selverstone or Crutchfield clamp

(For transcatheter permanent arterial occlusion or embolization, see 61624-61626)

(For endovascular temporary arterial balloon occlusion, use 61623)

(For ligation treatment of intracranial aneurysm, use 61703)

37607 Ligation or banding of angioaccess arteriovenous fistula

37609 Ligation or biopsy, temporal artery

37615 Ligation, major artery (eg, post-traumatic, rupture); neck

37616 chest

37617 abdomen

37618 extremity

37619 Ligation of inferior vena cava

(For endovascular delivery of an inferior vena cava filter, use 37191)

---

614 • New Code ▲ Revised Code + Add-On Code ⊘ Modifier -51 Exempt ⊙ Moderate Sedation

(37620 deleted 2011 [2012 edition]. To report, see 37191 for endovascular placement of intravascular filter or 37619 for open surgical ligation of the inferior vena cava)

37650 Ligation of femoral vein

(For bilateral procedure, report 37650 with modifier -50)

37660 Ligation of common iliac vein

37700 Ligation and division of long saphenous vein at saphenofemoral junction, or distal interruptions

(Do not report 37700 in conjunction with 37718, 37722)

(For bilateral procedure, report 37700 with modifier -50)

37718 Ligation, division, and stripping, short saphenous vein

(For bilateral procedure, use modifier 50)

(Do not report 37718 in conjunction with 37735, 37780)

37722 Ligation, division, and stripping, long (greater) saphenous veins from saphenofemoral junction to knee or below

(For ligation and stripping of the short saphenous vein, use 37718)

(For bilateral procedure, report 37722 with modifier 50)

(Do not report 37722 in conjunction with 37700, 37735)

(For ligation, division, and stripping of the greater saphenous vein, use 37722. For ligation, division, and stripping of the short saphenous vein, use 37718)

37735 Ligation and division and complete stripping of long or short saphenous veins with radical excision of ulcer and skin graft and/or interruption of communicating veins of lower leg, with excision of deep fascia

(Do not report 37735 in conjunction with 37700, 37718, 37722, 37780)

(For bilateral procedure, report 37735 with modifier -50)

37760 Ligation of perforator veins, subfascial, radical (Linton type), including skin graft, when performed, open, 1 leg

(For endoscopic procedure, use 37500)

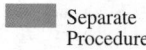 Separate Procedure   Unlisted Procedure   CCI Comp. Code   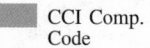 Non-specific Procedure

37761 Ligation of perforator vein(s), subfascial, open, including ultrasound guidance, when performed, 1 leg

(For bilateral procedure, report 37761 with modifier -50)

(Do not report 37760, 37761 in conjunction with 76937, 76942, 76998, 93971)

(For endoscopic ligation of subfascial perforator veins, use 37500)

37765 Stab phlebectomy of varicose veins, 1 extremity; 10-20 stab incisions

(For less than 10 incisions, use 37799)

(For more than 20 incisions, use 37766)

37766 more than 20 incisions

37780 Ligation and division of short saphenous vein at saphenopopliteal junction (separate procedure)

(For bilateral procedure, report 37780 with modifier -50)

37785 Ligation, division, and/or excision of varicose vein cluster(s), 1 leg

(For bilateral procedure, report 37785 with modifier -50)

OTHER PROCEDURES

37788 Penile revascularization, artery, with or without vein graft

37790 Penile venous occlusive procedure

37799 Unlisted procedure, vascular surgery

● New Code   ▲ Revised Code   + Add-On Code   ⊘ Modifier -51 Exempt   ☉ Moderate Sedation

HEMIC AND LYMPHATIC SYSTEMS

CPT codes from this section of CPT are used to report invasive and surgical procedures performed on the spleen and lymph nodes. Bone marrow transplants are reported using CPT codes 38230-38241 from this section.

When bone marrow aspiration is performed alone, the appropriate code to report is CPT code 38220. When a bone marrow biopsy is performed, the appropriate code is CPT code 38221 (bone marrow biopsy). This code cannot be reported with CPT code 20220 (bone biopsy). CPT codes 38220 and 38221 may only be reported together if the two procedures are performed at separate sites or at separate patient encounters. Separate sites include bone marrow aspiration and biopsy in different bones or two separate skin incisions over the same bone.

When both a bone marrow biopsy (CPT code 38221) and bone marrow aspiration (CPT code 38220) are performed at the same site through the same skin incision, do not report the bone marrow aspiration, CPT code 38220, in addition to the bone marrow biopsy (CPT code 38221). HCPCS/CPT code G0364 may be reported to describe the bone marrow aspiration performed with bone marrow biopsy through the same skin incision on the same date of service.

SPLEEN

EXCISION

38100 Splenectomy; total (separate procedure)

38101 partial (separate procedure)

+ **38102** total, en bloc for extensive disease, in conjunction with other procedure (List in addition to code for primary procedure)

REPAIR

38115 Repair of ruptured spleen (splenorrhaphy) with or without partial splenectomy

LAPAROSCOPY

Surgical laparoscopy always includes diagnostic laparoscopy. To report a diagnostic laparoscopy (peritoneoscopy) (separate procedure), use 49320.

38120 Laparoscopy, surgical, splenectomy

| | Separate Procedure | | Unlisted Procedure | | CCI Comp. Code | | Non-specific Procedure | **617** |

38129 Unlisted laparoscopy procedure, spleen

INTRODUCTION

38200 Injection procedure for splenoportography

(For radiological supervision and interpretation, use 75810)

GENERAL

BONE MARROW OR STEM CELL SERVICES/PROCEDURES

Codes 38207-38215 describe various steps used to preserve, prepare and purify bone marrow/stem cells prior to transplantation or reinfusion. Each code may be reported only once per day regardless of the quantity of bone marrow/stem cells manipulated.

38204 Management of recipient hematopoietic progenitor cell donor search and cell acquisition

38205 Blood-derived hematopoietic progenitor cell harvesting for transplantation, per collection; allogeneic

38206 autologous

38207 Transplant preparation of hematopoietic progenitor cells; cryopreservation and storage

(For diagnostic cryopreservation and storage, see 88240)

38208 thawing of previously frozen harvest, without washing, per donor

(For diagnostic thawing and expansion of frozen cells, see 88241)

38209 thawing of previously frozen harvest, with washing, per donor

38210 specific cell depletion within harvest, T-cell depletion

38211 tumor cell depletion

38212 red blood cell removal

38213 platelet depletion

38214 plasma (volume) depletion

618

● New Code	▲ Revised Code	✚ Add-On Code	⊘ Modifier -51 Exempt	⊙ Moderate Sedation

38215   cell concentration in plasma, mononuclear, or buffy coat layer

(Do not report 38207-38215 in conjunction with 88182, 88184-88189)

38220   Bone marrow; aspiration only

(For needle aspiration of bone marrow for the purpose of bone grafting, use 38220)

(Do not report 38220-38230 for bone marrow aspiration for platelet rich stem cell injection. For bone marrow aspiration for platelet rich stem cell injection, use 0232T)

38221   biopsy, needle or trocar

(For bone marrow biopsy interpretation, use 88305)

38230   Bone marrow harvesting for transplantation; allogenic

38232   autologous

(For autologous and allogenic blood-derived peripheral stem cell harvesting for transplantation, see 38205-38206)

(For bone marrow aspiration, use 38220)

TRANSPLANTATION AND POST-TRANSPLANTATION CELLULAR INFUSIONS

Hematopoietic cell transplantation (HCT) refers to the infusion of hematopoietic progenitor cells (HPC) obtained from bone marrow, peripheral blood apheresis, and/or umbilical cord blood. These procedure codes (38240-38243) include physician monitoring of multiple physiologic parameters, physician verification of cell processing, evaluation of the patient during as well as immediately before and after the HPC/lymphocyte infusion, physician presence during the HPC/lymphocyte infusion with associated direct physician supervision of clinical staff, and management of uncomplicated adverse events (eg, nausea, urticaria) during the infusion, which is not separately reportable.

HOT may be autologous (when the HPV donor and recipient are the same person) or allogenic (when the HPV donor and recipient are not the same person). Code 38241 is used to report any autologous transplant while 38240 is used to report an allogenic transplant. In some cases allogenic transplants involve more than one donor and cells from each donor are infused sequentially whereby one unit of 38240 is reported for each donor infused. code 38242 is used to report a donor lymphocyte infusion. Code 38243 is used to report a HPC boost from the original allogenic HPC donor. A lymphocyte infusion or HPC boost can occur days, months or even years after the initial hematopoietic cell transplant. The lymphocyte

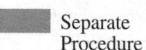 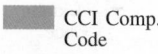

infusion is used to treat relapse, infection, or post-transplant lymphoproliferative syndrome. HPC boost represents an infusion of hematopoietic progenitor cells from the original donor that is being used to treat a relapse or or post-transplant cytopenia(s). Codes 38240, 38242, and 38243 should not be reported together on the same date of service.

If a separately identifiable E/M service is performed on the same date of service, the appropriate E/M service code, including office or other outpatient services, established (99211-99215), hospital observation services (99217-99220, 99224-99226), hospital inpatient services (99221-99223, 99231-99239), and inpatient neonatal and pediatric critical care (99471, 99472, 99475, 99476) may be reported, using modifier 25, in addition to 38240, 38242, or 38243. Post transplant infusion management of adverse reactions is reported separately using the appropriate E/M, prolonged service or critical care code(s). In accordance with place of service and facility reporting guideline, the fluid used to administer the cells and other infusions for incidental hydration (eg, 96360, 96361) are not separately reportable. Similarly, infusions of any medication(s) concurrently with the transplant infusion are not separately reportable. However, hydration or administration of medication (eg, antibiotics, narcotics) unrelated to the transplant are separately reportable using modifier 59.

▲ 38240   Hematopoietic progenitor cell (HPC); allogeneic transplantation per donor

▲ 38241   autologous transplantation

● 38243   HPC boost

▲ 38242   Allogeneic lymphocyte infusions

(For bone marrow aspiration, use 38220)

(For modification, treatment, and processing of hematopoietic progenitor cell specimens for transplantation, see 38210-38215)

(For cryopreservation, freezing and storage of hematopoietic progenitor cells for transplantation, use 38207)

(For thawing and expansion of hematopoietic progenitor cells for transplantation, use 38208, 38209)

(For compatibility studies, see 81379-81383, 86812-86822)

38243   Code out of order. See page 620

● New Code   ▲ Revised Code   + Add-On Code   ⊘ Modifier -51 Exempt   ⊙ Moderate Sedation

LYMPH NODES AND LYMPHATIC CHANNELS

INCISION

38300 Drainage of lymph node abscess or lymphadenitis; simple

38305   extensive

38308 Lymphangiotomy or other operations on lymphatic channels

38380 Suture and/or ligation of thoracic duct; cervical approach

38381   thoracic approach

38382   abdominal approach

EXCISION

(For injection for sentinel node identification, use 38792)

38500 Biopsy or excision of lymph node(s); open, superficial

(Do not report 38500 with 38700-38780)

38505   by needle, superficial (eg, cervical, inguinal, axillary)

(If imaging guidance is performed, see 76942, 77012, 77021)

(For fine needle aspiration, use 10021 or 10022)

(For evaluation of fine needle aspirate, see 88172, 88173)

38510   open, deep cervical node(s)

38520   open, deep cervical node(s) with excision scalene fat pad

38525   open, deep axillary node(s)

38530   open, internal mammary node(s)

(Do not report 38530 with 38720-38746)

(For percutaneous needle biopsy, retroperitoneal lymph node or mass, use 49180. For fine needle aspiration, use 10022)

38542 Dissection, deep jugular node(s)

(For radical cervical neck dissection, use 38720)

621

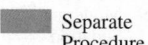 Separate Procedure   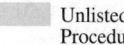 Unlisted Procedure   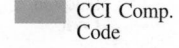 CCI Comp. Code   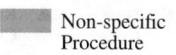 Non-specific Procedure

38550　Excision of cystic hygroma, axillary or cervical; without deep neurovascular dissection

38555　　with deep neurovascular dissection

LIMITED LYMPHADENECTOMY FOR STAGING

38562　Limited lymphadenectomy for staging (separate procedure); pelvic and para-aortic

(When combined with prostatectomy, use 55812 or 55842)

(When combined with insertion of radioactive substance into prostate, use 55862)

38564　　retroperitoneal (aortic and/or splenic)

LAPAROSCOPY

Surgical laparoscopy always includes diagnostic laparoscopy. To report a diagnostic laparoscopy (peritoneoscopy), (separate procedure), use 49320.

38570　Laparoscopy, surgical; with retroperitoneal lymph node sampling (biopsy), single or multiple

38571　　with bilateral total pelvic lymphadenectomy

38572　　with bilateral total pelvic lymphadenectomy and peri-aortic lymph node sampling (biopsy), single or multiple

(For drainage of lymphocele to peritoneal cavity, use 49323)

38589　Unlisted laparoscopy procedure, lymphatic system

RADICAL LYMPHADENECTOMY (RADICAL RESECTION OF LYMPH NODES)

(For limited pelvic and retroperitoneal lymphadenectomies, see 38562, 38564)

38700　Suprahyoid lymphadenectomy

(For bilateral procedure, report 38700 with modifier -50)

38720　Cervical lymphadenectomy (complete)

(For bilateral procedure, report 38720 with modifier -50)

38724　Cervical lymphadenectomy (modified radical neck dissection)

　● New Code　▲ Revised Code　+ Add-On Code　⊘ Modifier -51 Exempt　⊙ Moderate Sedation

38740 Axillary lymphadenectomy; superficial

38745 complete

+ 38746 Thoracic lymphadenectomy by thoracotomy, mediastinal and regional lymphadenectomy (List separately in addition to code for primary procedure)

(On the right, mediastinal lymph nodes include the paratracheal, subcarinal, paraesophageal, and inferior pulmonary ligament)

(On the left, mediastinal lymph nodes include the aortopulmonary window, subcarinal, paraesophageal, and inferior pulmonary ligament)

(Report 38746 in conjunction with 32440, 32442, 32445, 32480, 32482, 32484, 32486, 32488, 32503, 32504, 32505)

(To report mediastinal and regional lymphadenectomy via thoracoscopy [VATS], see 32674)

+ 38747 Abdominal lymphadenectomy, regional, including celiac, gastric, portal, peripancreatic, with or without para-aortic and vena caval nodes (List separately in addition to code for primary procedure)

38760 Inguinofemoral lymphadenectomy, superficial, including Cloquets node (separate procedure)

(For bilateral procedure, report 38760 with modifier -50)

38765 Inguinofemoral lymphadenectomy, superficial, in continuity with pelvic lymphadenectomy, including external iliac, hypogastric, and obturator nodes (separate procedure)

(For bilateral procedure, report 38765 with modifier -50)

38770 Pelvic lymphadenectomy, including external iliac, hypogastric, and obturator nodes (separate procedure)

(For bilateral procedure, report 38770 with modifier -50)

38780 Retroperitoneal transabdominal lymphadenectomy, extensive, including pelvic, aortic, and renal nodes (separate procedure)

(For excision and repair of lymphedematous skin and subcutaneous tissue, see 15004-15005, 15570-15650)

623

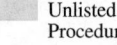 Separate Procedure   Unlisted Procedure   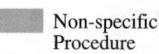 CCI Comp. Code   Non-specific Procedure

INTRODUCTION

38790 Injection procedure; lymphangiography

(For bilateral procedure, report 38790 with modifier -50)

(For radiological supervision and interpretation, see 75801-75807)

38792 radioactive tracer for identification of sentinel node

(For excision of sentinel node, see 38500-38542)

(For nuclear medicine lymphatics and lymph gland imaging, use 78195)

(For intraoperative identification (eg, mapping) of sentinel lymph node(s) including injection of non-radioactive dye, see 38900)

38794 Cannulation, thoracic duct

OTHER PROCEDURES

+ 38900 Intraoperative identification (eg, mapping) of sentinel lymph node(s) includes injection of non-radioactive dye, when performed (list separately in addition to code for primary procedure)

(Use 38900 in conjunction with 19302, 19307, 38500, 38510, 38520, 38525, 38530, 38542, 38740, 38745)

(For injection of radioactive tracer for identification of sentinel node, use 38792)

38999 Unlisted procedure, hemic or lymphatic system

● New Code   ▲ Revised Code   + Add-On Code   ⊘ Modifier -51 Exempt   ⊙ Moderate Sedation

MEDIASTINUM AND DIAPHRAGM

MEDIASTINUM

INCISION

39000   Mediastinotomy with exploration, drainage, removal of foreign body, or biopsy; cervical approach

39010   transthoracic approach, including either transthoracic or median sternotomy

(For VATS pericardial biopsy, use 32604)

EXCISION/RESECTION

39200   Resection of mediastinal cyst

39220   Resection of mediastinal tumor

(For substernal thyroidectomy, use 60270)

(For thymectomy, use 60520)

(For thoracoscopic [VATS] resection of mediastinal cyst, tumor or mass, use 32662)

ENDOSCOPY

39400   Mediastinoscopy, includes biopsy(ies), when performed

OTHER PROCEDURES

39499   Unlisted procedure, mediastinum

DIAPHRAGM

REPAIR

(For transabdominal repair of diaphragmatic [esophageal hiatal] hernia, use 43325)

(For laparoscopic repair of diaphragmatic [esophageal hiatal] hernias and fundoplication, see 43280, 43281, 43282)

39501   Repair, laceration of diaphragm, any approach

	Separate Procedure		Unlisted Procedure		CCI Comp. Code		Non-specific Procedure

625

(39502 deleted 2010 [2011 edition]. To report transabdominal paraesophageal hiatal hernia repair with fundoplasty, vagotomy, and/or pyloroplasty, when performed, see 43332, 43333, 43335, 43337)

(For laparoscopic paraesophageal hernia repair, see 43281, 43282)

39503 Repair, neonatal diaphragmatic hernia, with or without chest tube insertion and with or without creation of ventral hernia

(Do not report modifier 63 in conjunction with 39503)

(39520 deleted 2010 [2011 edition]. To report transthoracic diaphragmatic [esophageal hiatal] hernia repair, see 43334, 43335)

(For laparoscopic paraesophageal hernia repair, see 43281, 43282)

(39530 deleted 2010 [2011 edition]. To report thoracoabdominal diaphragmatic [esophageal hiatal] hernia repair, see 43336, 43337)

(39531 deleted 2010 [2011 edition]. To report thoracoabdominal diaphragmatic [esophageal hiatal] hernia repair, see 43336, 43337)

39540 Repair, diaphragmatic hernia (other than neonatal), traumatic; acute

39541 chronic

39545 Imbrication of diaphragm for eventration, transthoracic or transabdominal, paralytic or nonparalytic

39560 Resection, diaphragm; with simple repair (eg, primary suture)

39561 with complex repair (eg, prosthetic material, local muscle flap)

OTHER PROCEDURES

39599 Unlisted procedure, diaphragm

● New Code ▲ Revised Code + Add-On Code ⊘ Modifier -51 Exempt ⊙ Moderate Sedation

DIGESTIVE SYSTEM

MISCELLANEOUS CODING RULES

Gastrointestinal endoscopy codes should be assigned based on the extent of visualization performed. CMS's official guidelines for excision or destruction of a lesion are:

1. *use only the biopsy code if a single lesion is biopsied but not excised;*

2. *code only for the excision if a lesion is biopsied and the remaining portion is excised;*

3. *use the biopsy code once even if multiple biopsies are performed and none are excised; and*

4. *use both a biopsy and excision code if each lesion is taken from different sites.*

If the phrase "with or without biopsy" appears in the excision code's narrative, do not use a separate biopsy code. Diagnostic endoscopies are included in surgical endoscopies.

For upper gastrointestinal endoscopies, choose the appropriate code from documentation indicating whether the procedure was a simple exam, a diagnostic procedure or surgical procedure. Remember that code selection is based on the procedure(s) performed and the anatomical sites through which the scope passes. For example, if the scope is passed to the esophagus only, the code would be chosen from endoscopy codes beginning with 43200. If the scope is passed through the esophagus to the stomach, duodenum and/or the jejunum, the code selection would begin at 43235.

HERNIA REPAIR

Review the patient's age, the kind of hernia, the clinical presentation of the hernia, and method of repair documented in the medical record before assigning a hernia repair code.

APPENDECTOMY

To code appendectomies appropriately, review the documentation for an indicated purpose for the removal. If there is none, then it is probably incidental to a more serious surgery and should not be coded.

DIGEST
40000

	Separate Procedure		Unlisted Procedure		CCI Comp. Code		Non-specific Procedure

LIPS

(For procedures on skin of lips, see 10040 et seq)

EXCISION

40490   Biopsy of lip

40500   Vermilionectomy (lip shave), with mucosal advancement

40510   Excision of lip; transverse wedge excision with primary closure

40520   V-excision with primary direct linear closure

(For excision of mucous lesions, see 40810-40816)

40525   full thickness, reconstruction with local flap (eg, Estlander or fan)

40527   full thickness, reconstruction with cross lip flap (Abbe-Estlander)

40530   Resection of lip, more than one-fourth, without reconstruction

(For reconstruction, see 13131 et seq)

REPAIR (CHEILOPLASTY)

40650   Repair lip, full thickness; vermilion only

40652   up to half vertical height

40654   over one-half vertical height, or complex

40700   Plastic repair of cleft lip/nasal deformity; primary, partial or complete, unilateral

40701   primary bilateral, 1 stage procedure

40702   primary bilateral, 1 of 2 stages

40720   secondary, by recreation of defect and reclosure

(For bilateral procedure, report 40720 with modifier -50)

(To report rhinoplasty only for nasal deformity secondary to congenital cleft lip, see 30460, 30462)

● New Code   ▲ Revised Code   + Add-On Code   ⊘ Modifier -51 Exempt   ⊙ Moderate Sedation

(For repair of cleft lip, with cross lip pedicle flap (Abbe-Estlander type), use 40527)

40761   with cross lip pedicle flap (Abbe-Estlander type), including sectioning and inserting of pedicle

(For repair cleft palate, see 42200 et seq)

(For other reconstructive procedures, see 14060, 14061, 15120-15261, 15574, 15576, 15630)

OTHER PROCEDURES

40799 Unlisted procedure, lips

VESTIBULE OF MOUTH

INCISION

40800 Drainage of abscess, cyst, hematoma, vestibule of mouth; simple

40801   complicated

40804 Removal of embedded foreign body, vestibule of mouth; simple

40805   complicated

40806 Incision of labial frenum (frenotomy)

EXCISION, DESTRUCTION

40808 Biopsy, vestibule of mouth

40810 Excision of lesion of mucosa and submucosa, vestibule of mouth; without repair

40812   with simple repair

40814   with complex repair

40816   complex, with excision of underlying muscle

40818 Excision of mucosa of vestibule of mouth as donor graft

40819 Excision of frenum, labial or buccal (frenumectomy, frenulectomy, frenectomy)

629

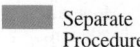 Separate Procedure
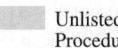 Unlisted Procedure
CCI Comp. Code
Non-specific Procedure

40820 Destruction of lesion or scar of vestibule of mouth by physical methods (eg, laser, thermal, cryo, chemical)

REPAIR

40830 Closure of laceration, vestibule of mouth; 2.5 cm or less

40831 over 2.5 cm or complex

40840 Vestibuloplasty; anterior

40842 posterior, unilateral

40843 posterior, bilateral

40844 entire arch

40845 complex (including ridge extension, muscle repositioning)

(For skin grafts, see 15002 et seq)

OTHER PROCEDURES

40899 Unlisted procedure, vestibule of mouth

TONGUE AND FLOOR OF MOUTH

INCISION

41000 Intraoral incision and drainage of abscess, cyst, or hematoma of tongue or floor of mouth; lingual

41005 sublingual, superficial

41006 sublingual, deep, supramylohyoid

41007 submental space

41008 submandibular space

41009 masticator space

41010 Incision of lingual frenum (frenotomy)

41015 Extraoral incision and drainage of abscess, cyst, or hematoma of floor of mouth; sublingual

● New Code ▲ Revised Code + Add-On Code ⊘ Modifier -51 Exempt ⊙ Moderate Sedation

41016	submental
41017	submandibular
41018	masticator space

(For frenoplasty, use 41520)

41019 Placement of needles, catheters, or other device(s) into the head and/or neck region (percutaneous, transoral, or transnasal) for subsequent interstitial radioelement application

(For imaging guidance, see 76942, 77002, 77012, 77021)

(For stereotactic insertion of intracranial brachytherapy radiation sources, use 61770)

(For interstitial radioelement application, see 77776-77787)

EXCISION

41100	Biopsy of tongue; anterior two-thirds
41105	posterior one-third
41108	Biopsy of floor of mouth
41110	Excision of lesion of tongue without closure
41112	Excision of lesion of tongue with closure; anterior two-thirds
41113	posterior one-third
41114	with local tongue flap

(Do not report 41114 in conjunction with 41112, 41113)

41115	Excision of lingual frenum (frenectomy)
41116	Excision, lesion of floor of mouth
41120	Glossectomy; less than one-half tongue
41130	hemiglossectomy
41135	partial, with unilateral radical neck dissection

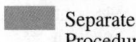 Separate Procedure 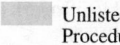 Unlisted Procedure 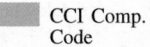 CCI Comp. Code 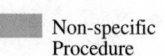 Non-specific Procedure

631

| 41140 | complete or total, with or without tracheostomy, without radical neck dissection |

| 41145 | complete or total, with or without tracheostomy, with unilateral radical neck dissection |

| 41150 | composite procedure with resection floor of mouth and mandibular resection, without radical neck dissection |

| 41153 | composite procedure with resection floor of mouth, with suprahyoid neck dissection |

| 41155 | composite procedure with resection floor of mouth, mandibular resection, and radical neck dissection (Commando type) |

REPAIR

| 41250 | Repair of laceration 2.5 cm or less; floor of mouth and/or anterior two-thirds of tongue |

| 41251 | posterior one-third of tongue |

| 41252 | Repair of laceration of tongue, floor of mouth, over 2.6 cm or complex |

OTHER PROCEDURES

| 41500 | Fixation of tongue, mechanical, other than suture (eg, K-wire) |

| 41510 | Suture of tongue to lip for micrognathia (Douglas type procedure) |

| 41512 | Tongue base suspension, permanent suture technique |

(For fixation of tongue, mechanical, other than suture, use 41500)

(For suture of tongue to lip for micrognathia, use 41510)

| 41520 | Frenoplasty (surgical revision of frenum, eg, with Z-plasty) |

(For frenotomy, see 40806, 41010)

| 41530 | Submucosal ablation of the tongue base, radiofrequency, 1 or more sites, per session |

| 41599 | Unlisted procedure, tongue, floor of mouth |

● New Code   ▲ Revised Code   + Add-On Code   ⊘ Modifier -51 Exempt   ⊙ Moderate Sedation

DENTOALVEOLAR STRUCTURES

INCISION

41800 Drainage of abscess, cyst, hematoma from dentoalveolar structures

41805 Removal of embedded foreign body from dentoalveolar structures; soft tissues

41806 bone

EXCISION, DESTRUCTION

41820 Gingivectomy, excision gingiva, each quadrant

41821 Operculectomy, excision pericoronal tissues

41822 Excision of fibrous tuberosities, dentoalveolar structures

41823 Excision of osseous tuberosities, dentoalveolar structures

41825 Excision of lesion or tumor (except listed above), dentoalveolar structures; without repair

41826 with simple repair

41827 with complex repair

(For nonexcisional destruction, use 41850)

41828 Excision of hyperplastic alveolar mucosa, each quadrant (specify)

41830 Alveolectomy, including curettage of osteitis or sequestrectomy

41850 Destruction of lesion (except excision), dentoalveolar structures

OTHER PROCEDURES

41870 Periodontal mucosal grafting

41872 Gingivoplasty, each quadrant (specify)

41874 Alveoloplasty, each quadrant (specify)

(For closure of lacerations, see 40830, 40831)

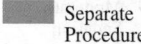 Separate Procedure   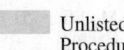 Unlisted Procedure   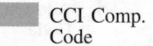 CCI Comp. Code   Non-specific Procedure

633

(For segmental osteotomy, use 21206)

(For reduction of fractures, see 21421-21490)

41899 Unlisted procedure, dentoalveolar structures

PALATE AND UVULA

INCISION

42000 Drainage of abscess of palate, uvula

EXCISION, DESTRUCTION

42100 Biopsy of palate, uvula

42104 Excision, lesion of palate, uvula; without closure

42106 with simple primary closure

42107 with local flap closure

(For skin graft, see 14040-14302)

(For mucosal graft, use 40818)

42120 Resection of palate or extensive resection of lesion

(For reconstruction of palate with extraoral tissue, see 14040-14302, 15050, 15120, 15240, 15576)

42140 Uvulectomy, excision of uvula

42145 Palatopharyngoplasty (eg, uvulopalatopharyngoplasty, uvulopharyngoplasty)

(For removal of exostosis of the bony palate, see 21031, 21032)

42160 Destruction of lesion, palate or uvula (thermal, cryo or chemical)

REPAIR

42180 Repair, laceration of palate; up to 2 cm

42182 over 2 cm or complex

42200 Palatoplasty for cleft palate, soft and/or hard palate only

● New Code   ▲ Revised Code   + Add-On Code   ⊘ Modifier -51 Exempt   ⊙ Moderate Sedation

42205 Palatoplasty for cleft palate, with closure of alveolar ridge; soft tissue only

42210 with bone graft to alveolar ridge (includes obtaining graft)

42215 Palatoplasty for cleft palate; major revision

42220 secondary lengthening procedure

42225 attachment pharyngeal flap

42226 Lengthening of palate, and pharyngeal flap

42227 Lengthening of palate, with island flap

42235 Repair of anterior palate, including vomer flap

(For repair of oronasal fistula, use 30600)

42260 Repair of nasolabial fistula

(For repair of cleft lip, see 40700 et seq)

42280 Maxillary impression for palatal prosthesis

42281 Insertion of pin-retained palatal prosthesis

OTHER PROCEDURES

42299 Unlisted procedure, palate, uvula

SALIVARY GLAND AND DUCTS

INCISION

42300 Drainage of abscess; parotid, simple

42305 parotid, complicated

42310 submaxillary or sublingual, intraoral

42320 submaxillary, external

42330 Sialolithotomy; submandibular (submaxillary), sublingual or parotid, uncomplicated, intraoral

Separate Procedure	Unlisted Procedure	CCI Comp. Code	Non-specific Procedure	**635**

42335   submandibular (submaxillary), complicated, intraoral

42340   parotid, extraoral or complicated intraoral

EXCISION

42400 Biopsy of salivary gland; needle

(For fine needle aspiration, see 10021, 10022)

(For evaluation of fine needle aspirate, see 88172, 88173)

(If imaging guidance, is performed, see 76942, 77002, 77012, 77021)

42405   incisional

(If imaging guidance is performed, see 76942, 77002, 77012, 77021)

42408 Excision of sublingual salivary cyst (ranula)

42409 Marsupialization of sublingual salivary cyst (ranula)

42410 Excision of parotid tumor or parotid gland; lateral lobe, without nerve dissection

42415   lateral lobe, with dissection and preservation of facial nerve

42420   total, with dissection and preservation of facial nerve

42425   total, en bloc removal with sacrifice of facial nerve

42426   total, with unilateral radical neck dissection

(For suture or grafting of facial nerve, see 64864, 64865, 69740, 69745)

42440 Excision of submandibular (submaxillary) gland

42450 Excision of sublingual gland

REPAIR

42500 Plastic repair of salivary duct, sialodochoplasty; primary or simple

42505   secondary or complicated

● New Code ▲ Revised Code + Add-On Code ⊘ Modifier -51 Exempt ⊙ Moderate Sedation

| 42507 | Parotid duct diversion, bilateral (Wilke type procedure); |

42508   with excision of 1 submandibular gland

42509   with excision of both submandibular glands

42510   with ligation of both submandibular (Wharton's) ducts

OTHER PROCEDURES

42550   Injection procedure for sialography

(For radiological supervision and interpretation, use 70390)

42600   Closure salivary fistula

42650   Dilation salivary duct

42660   Dilation and catheterization of salivary duct, with or without injection

42665   Ligation salivary duct, intraoral

42699   Unlisted procedure, salivary glands or ducts

PHARYNX, ADENOIDS, AND TONSILS

INCISION

42700   Incision and drainage abscess; peritonsillar

42720   retropharyngeal or parapharyngeal, intraoral approach

42725   retropharyngeal or parapharyngeal, external approach

EXCISION, DESTRUCTION

42800   Biopsy; oropharynx

42802   hypopharynx

42804   nasopharynx, visible lesion, simple

42806   nasopharynx, survey for unknown primary lesion

(For laryngoscopic biopsy, see 31510, 31535, 31536)

637

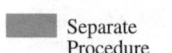 Separate Procedure   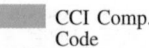 Unlisted Procedure   CCI Comp. Code   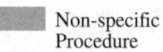 Non-specific Procedure

42808 Excision or destruction of lesion of pharynx, any method

42809 Removal of foreign body from pharynx

42810 Excision branchial cleft cyst or vestige, confined to skin and subcutaneous tissues

42815 Excision branchial cleft cyst, vestige, or fistula, extending beneath subcutaneous tissues and/or into pharynx

42820 Tonsillectomy and adenoidectomy; under age 12

42821   age 12 or over

42825 Tonsillectomy, primary or secondary; under age 12

42826   age 12 or over

42830 Adenoidectomy, primary; under age 12

42831   age 12 or over

42835 Adenoidectomy, secondary; under age 12

42836   age 12 or over

42842 Radical resection of tonsil, tonsillar pillars, and/or retromolar trigone; without closure

42844   closure with local flap (eg, tongue, buccal)

42845   closure with other flap

(For closure with other flap(s), use appropriate number for flap(s))

(When combined with radical neck dissection, use also 38720)

42860 Excision of tonsil tags

42870 Excision or destruction lingual tonsil, any method (separate procedure)

(For resection of the nasopharynx (eg., juvenile angiofibroma) by bicoronal and/or transzygomatic approach, see 61586 and 61600)

● New Code   ▲ Revised Code   ✚ Add-On Code   ⊘ Modifier -51 Exempt   ⊙ Moderate Sedation

42890 Limited pharyngectomy

42892 Resection of lateral pharyngeal wall or pyriform sinus, direct closure by advancement of lateral and posterior pharyngeal walls

(When combined with radical neck dissection, use also 38720)

42894 Resection of pharyngeal wall requiring closure with myocutaneous or fasciocutaneous flap or free muscle, skin, or fascial flap with microvascular anastamosis

(When combined with radical neck dissection, use also 38720)

(For limited pharyngectomy with radical neck dissection, use 38720 with 42890)

(For flap used for reconstruction, see 15732, 15734, 15756, 15757, 15758)

REPAIR

42900 Suture pharynx for wound or injury

42950 Pharyngoplasty (plastic or reconstructive operation on pharynx)

(For pharyngeal flap, use 42225)

42953 Pharyngoesophageal repair

(For closure with myocutaneous or other flap, use appropriate number in addition)

OTHER PROCEDURES

42955 Pharyngostomy (fistulization of pharynx, external for feeding)

42960 Control oropharyngeal hemorrhage, primary or secondary (eg, post-tonsillectomy); simple

42961 complicated, requiring hospitalization

42962 with secondary surgical intervention

42970 Control of nasopharyngeal hemorrhage, primary or secondary (eg, postadenoidectomy); simple, with posterior nasal packs, with or without anterior packs and/or cautery

42971 complicated, requiring hospitalization

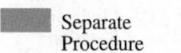 Separate Procedure 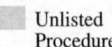 Unlisted Procedure 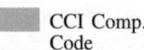 CCI Comp. Code 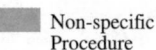 Non-specific Procedure

639

42972   with secondary surgical intervention

42999   Unlisted procedure, pharynx, adenoids, or tonsils

ESOPHAGUS

INCISION

(For esophageal intubation with laparotomy, use 43510)

43020   Esophagotomy, cervical approach, with removal of foreign body

43030   Cricopharyngeal myotomy

43045   Esophagotomy, thoracic approach, with removal of foreign body

EXCISION

(For gastrointestinal reconstruction for previous esophagectomy, see 43360, 43361)

43100   Excision of lesion, esophagus, with primary repair; cervical approach

43101   thoracic or abdominal approach

(For wide excision of malignant lesion of cervical esophagus, with total laryngectomy without radical neck dissection, see 43107, 43116, 43124 and 31360)

(For wide excision of malignant lesion of cervical esophagus, with total laryngectomy with radical neck dissection, see 43107, 43116, 43124, and 31365)

43107   Total or near total esophagectomy, without thoracotomy; with pharyngogastrostomy or cervical esophagogastrostomy, with or without pyloroplasty (transhiatal)

43108   with colon interposition or small intestine reconstruction, including intestine mobilization, preparation and anastomosis(es)

43112   Total or near total esophagectomy, with thoracotomy; with pharyngogastrostomy or cervical esophagogastrostomy, with or without pyloroplasty

● New Code   ▲ Revised Code   + Add-On Code   ⊘ Modifier -51 Exempt   ⊙ Moderate Sedation

43113   with colon interposition or small intestine reconstruction, including intestine mobilization, preparation, and anastomosis(es)

43116   Partial esophagectomy, cervical, with free intestinal graft, including microvascular anastomosis, obtaining the graft and intestinal reconstruction

(Do not report 43116 in conjunction with 69990)

(Report 43116 with the modifier -52 appended if intestinal or free jejunal graft with microvascular anastomosis is performed by another physician)

(For free jejunal graft with microvascular anastomosis performed by another physician, use 43496)

43117   Partial esophagectomy, distal two-thirds, with thoracotomy and separate abdominal incision, with or without proximal gastrectomy; with thoracic esophagogastrostomy, with or without pyloroplasty (Ivor Lewis)

43118   with colon interposition or small intestine reconstruction, including intestine mobilization, preparation, and anastomosis(es)

(For total esophagectomy with gastropharyngostomy, see 43107, 43124)

(For esophagogastrectomy (lower third) and vagotomy, use 43122)

43121   Partial esophagectomy, distal two-thirds, with thoracotomy only, with or without proximal gastrectomy, with thoracic esophagogastrostomy, with or without pyloroplasty

43122   Partial esophagectomy, thoracoabdominal or abdominal approach, with or without proximal gastrectomy; with esophagogastrostomy, with or without pyloroplasty

43123   with colon interposition or small intestine reconstruction, including intestine mobilization, preparation, and anastomosis(es)

43124   Total or partial esophagectomy, without reconstruction (any approach), with cervical esophagostomy

43130   Diverticulectomy of hypopharynx or esophagus, with or without myotomy; cervical approach

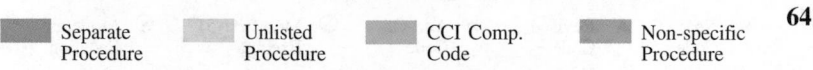

	Separate Procedure		Unlisted Procedure		CCI Comp. Code		Non-specific Procedure

641

43135	thoracic approach

ENDOSCOPY

For endoscopic procdures, code appropriate endoscopy of each anatomic site examined. Surgical endoscopy always includes diagnostic endoscopy.

⊙ **43200**   Esophagoscopy, rigid or flexible; diagnostic, with or without collection of specimen(s) by brushing or washing (separate procedure)

⊙ **43201**   with directed submucosal injection(s), any substance

(For injection sclerosis of esophageal varices, use 43204)

⊙ **43202**   with biopsy, single or multiple

⊙ **43204**   with injection sclerosis of esophageal varices

⊙ **43205**   with band ligation of esophageal varices

●⊙**43206**   with optial endomicroscopy

(Report supply of contrast agent separately)

(Do not report 43206 in conjunction with 88375)

⊙ **43215**   with removal of foreign body

(For radiological supervision and interpretation, use 74235)

⊙ **43216**   with removal of tumor(s), polyp(s), or other lesion(s) by hot biopsy forceps or bipolar cautery

⊙ **43217**   with removal of tumor(s), polyp(s), or other lesion(s) by snare technique

⊙ **43219**   with insertion of plastic tube or stent

⊙ **43220**   with balloon dilation (less than 30 mm diameter)

(If imaging guidance is performed, use 74360)

(For endoscopic dilation with balloon 30 mm diameter or larger, use 43458)

(For dilation without visualization, see 43450-43453)

(For diagnostic fiberoptic esophagogastroscopy, use 43200, 43235)

● New Code   ▲ Revised Code   ＋ Add-On Code   ⊘ Modifier -51 Exempt   ⊙ Moderate Sedation

(For fiberoptic esophagogastroscopy with biopsy or collection of specimen, use 43200, 43202, 43235, 43239)

(For fiberoptic esophagogastroscopy with removal of foreign body, use 43215, 43247)

(For fiberoptic esophagogastroscopy with removal of polyp(s), use 43217, 43251)

⊙ **43226**   with insertion of guide wire followed by dilation over guide wire

(For radiological supervision and interpretation, use 74360)

⊙ **43227**   with control of bleeding (eg, injection, bipolar cautery, unipolar cautery, laser, heater probe, stapler, plasma coagulator)

⊙ **43228**   with ablation of tumor(s), polyp(s), or other lesion(s), not amenable to removal by hot biopsy forceps, bipolar cautery or snare technique

(For esophagoscopic photodynamic therapy, report 43228 in addition to 96570, 96571 as appropriate)

⊙ **43231**   with endoscopic ultrasound examination

(Do not report 43231 in conjunction with 76975)

⊙ **43232**   with transendoscopic ultrasound-guided intramural or transmural fine needle aspiration/biopsy(s)

(Do not report 43232 in conjunction with 76942, 76975)

(For interpretation of specimen, see 88172-88173)

(43234   deleted 2012 [2013 edition] To report, use 43235)

⊙ **43235**   Upper gastrointestinal endoscopy including esophagus, stomach, and either the duodenum and/or jejunum as appropriate; diagnostic, with or without collection of specimen(s) by brushing or washing (separate procedure)

⊙ **43236**   with directed submucosal injection(s), any substance

(For injection sclerosis of esophageal and/or gastric varices, use 43243)

⊙ **43237**   with endoscopic ultrasound examination limited to the esophagus

643

| Separate Procedure | Unlisted Procedure | CCI Comp. Code | Non-specific Procedure |

(Do not report 43237 in conjunction with 76975)

⊙ **43238** with transendoscopic ultrasound-guided intramural or transmural fine needle aspiration/biopsy(s), esophagus (includes endoscopic ultrasound examination limited to the esophagus)

(Do not report 43238 in conjunction with 76942 or 76975)

⊙ **43239** with biopsy, single or multiple

⊙ **43240** with transmural drainage of pseudocyst

⊙ **43241** with transendoscopic intraluminal tube or catheter placement

⊙ **43242** with transendoscopic ultrasound-guided intramural or transmural fine needle aspiration/biopsy(s) (includes endoscopic ultrasound examination of the esophagus, stomach, and either the duodenum and/or jejunum as appropriate

(Do not report 43242 in conjunction with 76942 or 76975)

(For transendoscopic fine needle aspiration/biopsy limited to esophagus, use 43238)

(For interpretation of specimen, see 88172-88173)

⊙ **43243** with injection sclerosis of esophageal and/or gastric varices

⊙ **43244** with band ligation of esophageal and/or gastric varices

⊙ **43245** with dilation of gastric outlet for obstruction (eg, balloon, guide wire, bougie)

(Do not report 43245 in conjunction with 43256)

⊙ **43246** with directed placement of percutaneous gastrostomy tube

(For nonendoscopic percutaneous placement of gastrostomy tube, see 49440)

⊙ **43247** with removal of foreign body

(For radiological supervision and interpretation, use 74235)

⊙ **43248** with insertion of guide wire followed by dilation of esophagus over guide wire

● New Code ▲ Revised Code ✛ Add-On Code ⊘ Modifier -51 Exempt ⊙ Moderate Sedation

⊙ **43249**   with balloon dilation of esophagus (less than 30 mm diameter)

⊙ **43250**   with removal of tumor(s), polyp(s), or other lesion(s) by hot biopsy forceps or bipolar cautery

⊙ **43251**   with removal of tumor(s), polyp(s), or other lesion(s) by snare technique

●⊙**43252**   with optical endomicroscopy

(Report supply of contrast agent separately)

(Do not report 43252 in conjunction with 88375)

(For biopsy specimen pathology, use 88305)

⊙ **43255**   with control of bleeding, any method

⊙ **43256**   with transendoscopic stent placement (includes predilation)

⊙ **43257**   with delivery of thermal energy to the muscle of lower esophageal sphincter and/or gastric cardia, for treatment of gastroesophageal reflux disease

⊙ **43258**   with ablation of tumor(s), polyp(s), or other lesion(s) not amenable to removal by hot biopsy forceps, bipolar cautery or snare technique

(For injection sclerosis of esophageal varices, use 43204 or 43243)

⊙ **43259**   with endoscopic ultrasound examination, including the esophagus, stomach, and either the duodenum and/or jejunum as appropriate

(Do not report 43259 in conjunction with 76975)

⊙ **43260**   Endoscopic retrograde cholangiopancreatography (ERCP); diagnostic, with or without collection of specimen(s) by brushing or washing (separate procedure)

(For radiological supervision and interpretation, see 74328, 74329, 74330)

⊙ **43261**   with biopsy, single or multiple

(For radiological supervision and interpretation, see 74328, 74329, 74330)

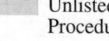 Separate Procedure   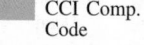 Unlisted Procedure   CCI Comp. Code   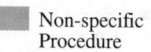 Non-specific Procedure

⊙ **43262**   with sphincterotomy/papillotomy

(For radiological supervision and interpretation, see 74328, 74329, 74330)

⊙ **43263**   with pressure measurement of sphincter of Oddi (pancreatic duct or common bile duct)

(For radiological supervision and interpretation, see 74328, 74329, 74330)

⊙ **43264**   with endoscopic retrograde removal of calculus/calculi from biliary and/or pancreatic ducts

(When done with sphincterotomy, also use 43262)

(For radiological supervision and interpretation, see 74328, 74329, 74330)

⊙ **43265**   with endoscopic retrograde destruction, lithotripsy of calculus/calculi, any method

(When done with sphincterotomy, also use 43262)

(For radiological supervision and interpretation, see 74328, 74329, 74330)

⊙ **43267**   with endoscopic retrograde insertion of nasobiliary or nasopancreatic drainage tube

(When done with sphincterotomy, also use 43262)

(For radiological supervision and interpretation, see 74328, 74329, 74330)

⊙ **43268**   with endoscopic retrograde insertion of tube or stent into bile or pancreatic duct

(When done with sphincterotomy, also use 43262)

(For radiological supervision and interpretation, see 74328, 74329, 74330)

⊙ **43269**   with endoscopic retrograde removal of foreign body and/or change of tube or stent

(When done with sphincterotomy, also use 43262)

(For radiological supervision and interpretation, see 74328, 74329, 74330)

● New Code   ▲ Revised Code   + Add-On Code   ⊘ Modifier -51 Exempt   ⊙ Moderate Sedation

⊙ **43271**   with endoscopic retrograde balloon dilation of ampulla, biliary and/or pancreatic duct(s)

(When done with sphincterotomy, also use 43262)

(For radiological supervision and interpretation, see 74328, 74329, 74330)

⊙ **43272**   with ablation of tumor(s), polyp(s), or other lesion(s) not amenable to removal by hot biopsy forceps, bipolar cautery or snare technique

(For radiological supervision and interpretation, see 74328, 74329, 74330)

⊙+**43273** Endoscopic cannulation of papilla with direct visualization of common bile duct(s) and/or pancreatic duct(s) (list separately in addition to code(s) for primary procedure)

(Use 43273 in conjunction with 43260-43265, 43267-43272)

LAPAROSCOPY

Surgical laparoscopy always includes diagnostic laparoscopy. To report a diagnostic laparoscopy (peritoneoscopy) (separate procedure), use 49320.

43279 Laparoscopy, surgical, esophagomyotomy (Heller type), with fundoplasty, when performed

(For open approach, see 43330, 43331)

(Do not report 43279 in conjunction with 43280)

43280 Laparoscopy, surgical, esophagogastric fundoplasty (eg, Nissen, Toupet procedures)

(Do not report 43280 in conjunction with 43279)

(For open approach, see 43327, 43328)

43281 Laparoscopy, surgical, repair of paraesophageal hernia, includes fundoplasty, when performed; without implantation of mesh

43282   with implantation of mesh

(To report transabdominal paraesophageal hiatal hernia repair, see 43332, 43333. To report transthoracic diaphragmatic hernia repair, see 43334, 43335)

(Do not report 43281, 43282 in conjunction with 43280, 43450, 43453, 43456, 43458, 43568)

647

| Separate Procedure | Unlisted Procedure | CCI Comp. Code | Non-specific Procedure |

+ 43283   Laparoscopy, surgical, esophageal lengthening procedure (eg, Collis gastroplasty or wedge gastroplasty) (list separately in addition to code for primary procedure)

(Use 43283 in conjunction with 43280, 43281, 43282)

43289   Unlisted laparoscopy procedure, esophagus

REPAIR

43300   Esophagoplasty, (plastic repair or reconstruction), cervical approach; without repair of tracheoesophageal fistula

43305   with repair of tracheoesophageal fistula

43310   Esophagoplasty, (plastic repair or reconstruction), thoracic approach; without repair of tracheoesophageal fistula

43312   with repair of tracheoesophageal fistula

43313   Esophagoplasty for congenital defect, (plastic repair or reconstruction), thoracic approach; without repair of congenital tracheoesophageal fistula

43314   with repair of congenital tracheoesophageal fistula

(Do not report modifier '-63' in conjunction with 43313, 43314)

43320   Esophagogastrostomy (cardioplasty), with or without vagotomy and pyloroplasty, transabdominal or transthoracic approach

(43324   deleted 2010 [2011 edition]. To report esophagogastric fundoplasty, see 43327, 43328)

(For laparoscopic procedure, use 43280)

43325   Esophagogastric fundoplasty; with fundic patch (Thal-Nissen procedure)

(For cricopharyngeal myotomy, use 43030)

(43326   deleted 2010 [2011 edition]. To report esophagogastric fundoplasty with gastroplasty, see 43327, 43328, 43332-43338)

43327   Esophagogastric fundoplasty, partial or complete; laparotomy

43328   thoracotomy

● New Code   ▲ Revised Code   + Add-On Code   ⊘ Modifier -51 Exempt   ⊙ Moderate Sedation

43330   Esophagomyotomy (Heller type); abdominal approach

(For laparoscopic esophagomyotomy procedure, use 43279)

43331   thoracic approach

(For thoracoscopic esophagomyotomy, use 32665)

43332   Repair, paraesophageal hiatal hernia (including fundoplication), via laparotomy, except neonatal; without implantation of mesh or other prosthesis

43333   with implantation of mesh or other prosthesis

(For neonatal diaphragmatic hernia repair, use 39503)

43334   Repair, paraesophageal hiatal hernia (including fundoplication), via thoracotomy, except neonatal; without implantation of mesh or other prosthesis

43335   with implantation of mesh or other prosthesis

(For neonatal diaphragmatic hernia repair, use 39503)

43336   Repair, paraesophageal hiatal hernia (including fundoplication), via thoracoabdominal incision, except neonatal; without implantation of mesh or other prosthesis

43337   with implantation of mesh or other prosthesis

(For neonatal diaphragmatic hernia repair, use 39503)

+ 43338   Esophageal lengthening procedure (eg, Collis gastroplasty or wedge gastroplasty) (List separately in addition to code for primary procedure)

(Use 43338 in conjunction with 43280, 43327-43337)

43340   Esophagojejunostomy (without total gastrectomy); abdominal approach

43341   thoracic approach

43350   Esophagostomy, fistulization of esophagus, external; abdominal approach

43351   thoracic approach

| | Separate Procedure | | Unlisted Procedure | | CCI Comp. Code | | Non-specific Procedure | **649** |

43352   cervical approach

43360   Gastrointestinal reconstruction for previous esophagectomy, for obstructing esophageal lesion or fistula, or for previous esophageal exclusion; with stomach, with or without pyloroplasty

43361   with colon interposition or small intestine reconstruction, including intestine mobilization, preparation, and anastomosis(es)

43400   Ligation, direct, esophageal varices

43401   Transection of esophagus with repair, for esophageal varices

43405   Ligation or stapling at gastroesophageal junction for pre-existing esophageal perforation

43410   Suture of esophageal wound or injury; cervical approach

43415   transthoracic or transabdominal approach

43420   Closure of esophagostomy or fistula; cervical approach

43425   transthoracic or transabdominal approach

(To report transabdominal paraesophageal hiatal hernia repair, see 43332, 43333. To report transthoracic diaphragmatic hernia repair, see 43334, 43335.)

MANIPULATION

(For associated esophagogram, use 74220)

43450   Dilation of esophagus, by unguided sound or bougie, single or multiple passes

(For radiological supervision and interpretation, use 74360)

⊙ **43453**   Dilation of esophagus, over guide wire

(For dilation with direct visualization, use 43220)

(For dilation of esophagus, by balloon or dilator, see 43220, 43458, and 74360)

(For radiological supervision and interpretation, use 74360)

⊙ **43456**   Dilation of esophagus, by balloon or dilator, retrograde

650
   ● New Code   ▲ Revised Code   ✚ Add-On Code   ⊘ Modifier -51 Exempt   ⊙ Moderate Sedation

(For radiological supervision and interpretation, use 74360)

⊙ **43458** Dilation of esophagus with balloon (30 mm diameter or larger) for achalasia

(For dilation with balloon less than 30 mm diameter, use 43220)

(For radiological supervision and interpretation, use 74360)

43460 Esophagogastric tamponade, with balloon (Sengstaken type)

(For removal of esophageal foreign body by balloon catheter, see 43215, 43247, 74235)

OTHER PROCEDURES

43496 Free jejunum transfer with microvascular anastomosis

(Do not report code 69990 in addition to code 43496)

43499 Unlisted procedure, esophagus

STOMACH

INCISION

43500 Gastrotomy; with exploration or foreign body removal

43501   with suture repair of bleeding ulcer

43502   with suture repair of pre-existing esophagogastric laceration (eg, Mallory-Weiss)

43510   with esophageal dilation and insertion of permanent intraluminal tube (eg, Celestin or Mousseaux-Barbin)

43520 Pyloromyotomy, cutting of pyloric muscle (Fredet-Ramstedt type operation)

(Do not report modifier '-63' in conjunction with 43520)

EXCISION

(43600   deleted 2010 [2011 edition])

43605 Biopsy of stomach by laparotomy

43610 Excision, local; ulcer or benign tumor of stomach

| 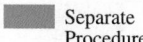 Separate Procedure | 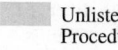 Unlisted Procedure | 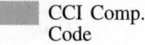 CCI Comp. Code | 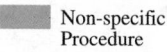 Non-specific Procedure | **651** |

43611	malignant tumor of stomach
43620	Gastrectomy, total; with esophagoenterostomy
43621	with Roux-en-Y reconstruction
43622	with formation of intestinal pouch, any type
43631	Gastrectomy, partial, distal; with gastroduodenostomy
43632	with gastrojejunostomy
43633	with Roux-en-Y reconstruction
43634	with formation of intestinal pouch

+ **43635** Vagotomy when performed with partial distal gastrectomy (List separately in addition to code(s) for primary procedure)

(Use 43635 in conjunction with codes 43631, 43632, 43633, 43634)

43640 Vagotomy including pyloroplasty, with or without gastrostomy; truncal or selective

(For pyloroplasty, use 43800)

(For vagotomy, see 64752-64760)

43641 parietal cell (highly selective)

(For upper gastrointestinal endoscopy, see 43235-43259)

LAPAROSCOPY

Surgical laparoscopy always includes diagnostic laparoscopy. To report a diagnostic laparoscopy (peritoneoscopy) (separate procedure), use 49320.

(For upper gastrointestinal endoscopy including esophagus, stomach, and either the duodenum and/or jejunum, see 43235-43259)

43644 Laparoscopy, surgical, gastric restrictive procedure; with gastric bypass and Roux-en-Y gastroenterostomy (Roux limb 150 cm or less)

(Do not report 43644 in conjunction with 43846, 49320)

(Esophagogastroduodenoscopy (EGD) performed for a separate condition should be reported with modifier 59)

● New Code ▲ Revised Code + Add-On Code ⊘ Modifier -51 Exempt ⊙ Moderate Sedation

(For greater than 150 cm, use 43645)

(For open procedure, use 43846)

43645   with gastric bypass and small intestine reconstruction to limit absorption

(Do not report 43645 in conjunction with 49320, 43847)

43647   Laparoscopy, surgical; implantation or replacement of gastric neurostimulator electrodes, antrum

43648   revision or removal of gastric neurostimulator electrodes, antrum

(For open approach, see 43881, 43882)

(For insertion of gastric neruostimulator pulse generator, use 64590)

(For revision or removal of gastric neurostimulator pulse generator, use 64595)

(For electronic analaysis and programming of gastric neurostimulator pulse generator, see 95980-95982)

(For laparoscopic implantation, revision, or removal of gastric neurostimulator electrodes, lesser curvature [morbid obesity], use 43659)

(For laparoscopic implantation, revision, replacement, or removal of vagus nerve blocking neurostimulator electrode array and/or pulse generator at the esophagogastric junction, see 0312T-0317T)

43651   Laparoscopy, surgical; transection of vagus nerves, truncal

43652   transection of vagus nerves, selective or highly selective

43653   gastrostomy, without construction of gastric tube (eg, Stamm procedure) (separate procedure)

43659   Unlisted laparoscopy procedure, stomach

INTRODUCTION

43752   Naso- or oro-gastric tube placement, requiring physician's skill and fluoroscopic guidance (includes fluoroscopy, image documentation and report)

653

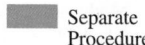 Separate Procedure   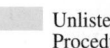 Unlisted Procedure   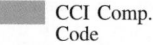 CCI Comp. Code   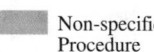 Non-specific Procedure

(Do not report 43752 in conjunction with critical care codes 99291-99292, neonatal critical care codes 99468, pediatric critical care codes 99471, 99472 or low birth weight intensive care service codes 99478, 99479)

(For percutaneous placement of gastrostomy tube, use 49440)

(For enteric tube placement, see 44500, 74340)

43753 Gastric intubation and aspiration(s), therapeutic, necessitating physician's skill (eg, for gastrointestinal hemorrhage), including lavage if performed

43754 Gastric intubation and aspiration, diagnostic; single specimen (eg, acid analysis)

43755 collection of multiple fractional specimens with gastric stimulation, single or double lumen tube (gastric secretory study) (eg, histamine, insulin, pentagastrin, calcium, secretin), includes drug administration

(For gastric acid analysis, use 82930)

(For naso- or oro-gastric tube placement by physician with fluoroscopic guidance, use 43752)

(Report the drug(s) or substance(s) administered. The fluid used to administer the drug(s) is not separately reported)

43756 Duodenal intubation and aspiration, diagnostic, includes image guidance; single specimen (eg, bile study for crystals or afferent loop culture)

43757 collection of multiple fractional specimens with pancreatic or gallbladder stimulation, single or double lumen tube, includes drug administration

(For appropriate chemical analysis procedures, see 89049-89240)

(Report the substance(s) or drug(s) administered. The fluid used to administer the drug(s) is not separately reported)

43760 Change of gastrostomy tube, percutaneous, without imaging or endoscopic guidance

(To report fluoroscopically guided replacement of gastrostomy tube, use 49450)

(For endoscopic placement of gastrostomy tube, use 43246)

● New Code   ▲ Revised Code   ＋ Add-On Code   ⊘ Modifier -51 Exempt   ⊙ Moderate Sedation

43761 Repositioning of a naso- or oro-gastric feeding tube, through the duodenum for enteric nutrition

(Do not report 43761 in conjunction with 44500, 49446)

(If imaging guidance is performed, use 76000)

(For endoscopic conversion of a gastrostomy tube to jejunostomy tube, use 44373)

(For placement of a long gastrointestinal tube into the duodenum, use 44500)

BARIATRIC SURGERY

Laparoscopy

Surgical laparoscopy always includes diagnostic laparoscopy. To report a diagnostic laparoscopy (separate procedure), use 49320.

43770 Laparoscopy, surgical, gastric restrictive procedure; placement of adjustable gastric restrictive device (eg, gastric band and subcutaneous port components)

(For individual component placement, report 43770 with modifier 52)

43771 revision of adjustable gastric restrictive device component only

43772 removal of adjustable gastric restrictive device component only

43773 removal and replacement of adjustable gastric restrictive device component only

(Do not report 43773 in conjunction with 43772)

43774 removal of adjustable gastric restrictive device and subcutaneous port components

(For removal and replacement of both gastric band and subcutaneous port components, use 43659)

43775 longitudinal gastrectomy (ie, sleeve gastrectomy)

(For open gastric restrictive procedure, without gastric bypass, for morbid obesity, other than vertical-banded gastroplasty, use 43843)

655

	Separate Procedure		Unlisted Procedure		CCI Comp. Code		Non-specific Procedure

(For laparoscopic implantation, revision, replacement, removal or reprogramming of vagus nerve blocking neurostimulator electrode array and/or pulse generator at the esophagogastric junction, see 0312T-0317T)

OTHER PROCEDURES

43800 Pyloroplasty

(For pyloroplasty and vagotomy, use 43640)

43810 Gastroduodenostomy

43820 Gastrojejunostomy; without vagotomy

43825 with vagotomy, any type

43830 Gastrostomy, open; without construction of gastric tube (eg, Stamm procedure) (separate procedure)

43831 neonatal, for feeding

(For change of gastrostomy tube, use 43760)

(Do not report modifier '-63' in conjunction with 43831)

43832 with construction of gastric tube (eg, Janeway procedure)

(For percutaneous endoscopic gastrostomy, use 43246)

43840 Gastrorrhaphy, suture of perforated duodenal or gastric ulcer, wound, or injury

43842 Gastric restrictive procedure, without gastric bypass, for morbid obesity; vertical-banded gastroplasty

43843 other than vertical-banded gastroplasty

(For laparoscopic longitudinal gastrectomy [ie, sleeve gastrectomy], use 43775)

43845 Gastric restrictive procedure with partial gastrectomy, pylorus-preserving duodenoileostomy and ileoileostomy (50 to 100 cm common channel) to limit absorption (biliopancreatic diversion with duodenal switch)

(Do not report 43845 in conjunction with 43633, 43847, 44130, 49000)

● New Code   ▲ Revised Code   + Add-On Code   ⊘ Modifier -51 Exempt   ⊙ Moderate Sedation

43846 Gastric restrictive procedure, with gastric bypass for morbid obesity; with short limb (150 cm or less) Roux-en-Y gastroenterostomy

(For greater than 150 cm, use 43847)

(For laparoscopic procedure, use 43644)

43847 with small intestine reconstruction to limit absorption

43848 Revision, open, of gastric restrictive procedure for morbid obesity, other than adjustable gastric restrictive device (separate procedure)

(For laparoscopic adjustable gastric restrictive procedures, see 43770-43774)

(For gastric restrictive port procedures, see 43886-43888)

43850 Revision of gastroduodenal anastomosis (gastroduodenostomy) with reconstruction; without vagotomy

43855 with vagotomy

43860 Revision of gastrojejunal anastomosis (gastrojejunostomy) with reconstruction, with or without partial gastrectomy or intestine resection; without vagotomy

43865 with vagotomy

43870 Closure of gastrostomy, surgical

43880 Closure of gastrocolic fistula

43881 Implantation or replacement of gastric neurostimulator electrodes, antrum, open

43882 Revision or removal of gastric neurostimulator electrodes, antrum, open

(For laparoscopic approach, see 43647, 43648)

(For insertion of gastric neurostimulator pulse generator, use 64590)

(For revision or removal of gastric neurostimulator pulse generator, use 64595)

657

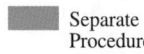 Separate Procedure Unlisted Procedure 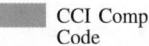 CCI Comp. Code 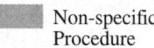 Non-specific Procedure

(For electronic analysis and programming of gastric neurostimulator pulse generator, use 95980-95982)

(For open implantation, revision, or removal of gastric neurostimulator electrodes, lesser curvature [morbid obesity], use 43999)

(For laparaoscopic implantation, revision, replacement, removal or reprogramming of vagus nerve blocking neurostimulator electrode array and/or pulse generator at the esophagogastric junction, see 0312T-0317T)

(For open implantation, revision, or removal of gastric lesser curvature or vagal trunk (EGJ) neurostimulator electrodes, [morbid obesity], use 43999)

43886 Gastric restrictive procedure, open; revision of subcutaneous port component only

43887 removal of subcutaneous port component only

43888 removal and replacement of subcutaneous port component only

(Do not report 43888 in conjunction with 43774, 43887)

(For laparoscopic removal of both gastric restrictive device and subcutaneous port components, use 43774)

(For removal and replacement of both gastric restrictive device and subcutaneous port components, use 43659)

43999 Unlisted procedure, stomach

INTESTINES (EXCEPT RECTUM)

INCISION

44005 Enterolysis (freeing of intestinal adhesion) (separate procedure)

(Do not report 44005 in addition to 45136)

(For laparoscopic approach, use 44180)

44010 Duodenotomy, for exploration, biopsy(s), or foreign body removal

+ **44015** Tube or needle catheter jejunostomy for enteral alimentation, intraoperative, any method (List separately in addition to primary procedure)

| ● New Code | ▲ Revised Code | + Add-On Code | ⊘ Modifier -51 Exempt | ⊙ Moderate Sedation |

44020 Enterotomy, small intestine, other than duodenum; for exploration, biopsy(s), or foreign body removal

44021 for decompression (eg, Baker tube)

44025 Colotomy, for exploration, biopsy(s), or foreign body removal

(For exteriorization of intestine (Mikulicz resection with crushing of spur), see 44602-44605)

44050 Reduction of volvulus, intussusception, internal hernia, by laparotomy

44055 Correction of malrotation by lysis of duodenal bands and/or reduction of midgut volvulus (eg, Ladd procedure)

(Do not report modifier '-63' in conjunction with 44055)

EXCISION

Intestinal allotransplantation involves three distinct components of physician work:

1) **Cadaver donor enterectomy**, which includes harvesting the intestine graft and cold preservation of the graft (perfusing with cold preservation solution and cold maintenance) (use 44132). **Living donor enterectomy**, which includes harvesting the intestine graft, cold preservation of the graft (perfusing with cold preservation solution and cold maintenance), and care of the donor (use 44133).

2) **Backbench work**:

Standard preparation of an intestine allograft prior to transplantation includes mobilization and fashioning of the superior mesenteric artery and vein (see 44715).

Additional reconstruction of an intestine allograft prior to transplantation may include venous and/or arterial anastomosis(es) (see 44720-44721).

3) **Recipient intestinal allotransplantation with or without recipient enterectomy**, which includes transplantation of allograft and care of the recipient (see 44135, 44136)

44100 Biopsy of intestine by capsule, tube, peroral (1 or more specimens)

44110 Excision of 1 or more lesions of small or large intestine not requiring anastomosis, exteriorization, or fistulization; single enterotomy

44111 multiple enterotomies

			659
Separate Procedure	Unlisted Procedure	CCI Comp. Code	Non-specific Procedure

44120 Enterectomy, resection of small intestine; single resection and anastomosis

(Do not report 44120 in addition to 45136)

+ 44121 each additional resection and anastomosis (List separately in addition to code for primary procedure)

(Use 44121 in conjunction with code 44120)

44125 with enterostomy

44126 Enterectomy, resection of small intestine for congenital atresia, single resection and anastomosis of proximal segment of intestine; without tapering

44127 with tapering

+ 44128 each additional resection and anastomosis (List separately in addition to code for primary procedure)

(Use 44128 in conjunction with codes 44126, 44127)

(Do not report modifier '-63' in conjunction with 44126, 44127, 44128)

44130 Enteroenterostomy, anastomosis of intestine, with or without cutaneous enterostomy (separate procedure)

44132 Donor enterectomy (including cold preservation), open; from cadaver donor

44133 partial, from living donor

(For backbench intestinal graft preparation or reconstruction, see 44715, 44720, 44721)

44135 Intestinal allotransplantation; from cadaver donor

44136 from living donor

44137 Removal of transplanted intestinal allograft, complete

(For partial removal of transplant allograft, see 44120, 44121, 44140)

+ 44139 Mobilization (take-down) of splenic flexure performed in conjunction with partial colectomy (List separately in addition to primary procedure)

● New Code ▲ Revised Code + Add-On Code ⊘ Modifier -51 Exempt ⊙ Moderate Sedation

(Use 44139 in conjunction with codes 44140-44147)

44140 Colectomy, partial; with anastomosis

(For laparoscopic procedure, use 44204)

44141 with skin level cecostomy or colostomy

44143 with end colostomy and closure of distal segment (Hartmann type procedure)

(For laparoscopic procedure, use 44206)

44144 with resection, with colostomy or ileostomy and creation of mucofistula

44145 with coloproctostomy (low pelvic anastomosis)

(For laparoscopic procedure, use 44207)

44146 with coloproctostomy (low pelvic anastomosis), with colostomy

(For laparoscopic procedure, use 44208)

44147 abdominal and transanal approach

44150 Colectomy, total, abdominal, without proctectomy; with ileostomy or ileoproctostomy

(For laparoscopic procedure, use 44210)

44151 with continent ileostomy

44155 Colectomy, total, abdominal, with proctectomy; with ileostomy

(For laparoscopic procedure, use 44212)

44156 with continent ileostomy

44157 with ileoanal anastomosis, includes loop ileostomy, and rectal mucosectomy, when performed

44158 with ileoanal anastomosis, creation of ileal reservoir (S or J), includes loop ileostomy, and rectal mucosectomy, when performed

(For laparoscopic procedure, use 44211)

 Separate Procedure   Unlisted Procedure   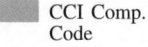 CCI Comp. Code   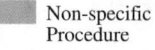 Non-specific Procedure

44160　Colectomy, partial, with removal of terminal ileum and ileocolostomy

(For laparoscopic procedure, use 44205)

LAPAROSCOPY

Surgical laparoscopy always includes diagnostic laparoscopy. To report a diagnostic laparoscopy (peritoneoscopy) (separate procedure), use 49320.

Incision

44180　Laparoscopy, surgical, enterolysis (freeing of intestinal adhesion) (separate procedure)

(For laparoscopy with salpingolysis, ovariolysis, use 58660)

Enterostomy—External Fistulization of Intestines

44186　Laparoscopy, surgical; jejunostomy (eg, for decompression or feeding)

44187　ileostomy or jejunostomy, non-tube

(For open procedure, use 44310)

44188　Laparoscopy, surgical, colostomy or skin level cecostomy

(For open procedure, use 44320)

(Do not report 44188 in conjunction with 44970)

Excision

44202　Laparoscopy, surgical; enterectomy, resection of small intestine, single resection and anastomosis

+ 44203　each additional small intestine resection and anastomosis (List separately in addition to code for primary procedure)

(Use 44203 in conjunction with code 44202)

(For open procedure, see 44120, 44121)

44204　colectomy, partial, with anastomosis

(For open procedure, use 44140)

44205　colectomy, partial, with removal of terminal ileum with ileocolostomy

662　● New　▲ Revised　+ Add-On　⊘ Modifier -51　⊙ Moderate
　　　　Code　　Code　　Code　　Exempt　　Sedation

(For open procedure, use 44160)

44206 colectomy, partial, with end colostomy and closure of distal segment (Hartmann type procedure)

(For open procedure, use 44143)

44207 colectomy, partial, with anastomosis, with coloproctostomy (low pelvic anastomosis)

(For open procedure, use 44145)

44208 colectomy, partial, with anastomosis, with coloproctostomy (low pelvic anastomosis) with colostomy

(For open procedure, use 44146)

44210 colectomy, total, abdominal, without proctectomy, with ileostomy or ileoproctostomy

(For open procedure, use 44150)

44211 colectomy, total, abdominal, with proctectomy, with ileoanal anastomosis, creation of ileal reservoir (S or J), with loop ileostomy, includes rectal mucosectomy, when performed

(For open procedure, see 44157, 44158)

44212 colectomy, total, abdominal, with proctectomy, with ileostomy

(For open procedure, use 44155)

+ 44213 Laparoscopy, surgical, mobilization (take-down) of splenic flexure performed in conjunction with partial colectomy (List separately in addition to primary procedure)

(Use 44213 in conjunction with 44204-44208)

(For open procedure, use 44139)

Repair

44227 Laparoscopy, surgical, closure of enterostomy, large or small intestine, with resection and anastomosis

(For open procedure, see 44625, 44626)

663

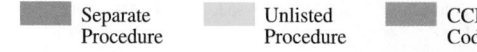 Separate Procedure   Unlisted Procedure   CCI Comp. Code   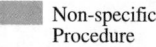 Non-specific Procedure

Other Procedures

44238 Unlisted laparoscopy procedure, intestine (except rectum)

ENTEROSTOMY—EXTERNAL FISTULIZATION OF INTESTINES

44300 Placement, enterostomy or cecostomy, tube open (eg, for feeding or decompression) (separate procedure)

(For percutaneous placement of duodenostomy, jejunostomy, gastro-jejunostomy or cecostomy [or other colonic] tube including fluoroscopic imaging guidance, see 49441-49442)

44310 Ileostomy or jejunostomy, non-tube

(For laparoscopic procedure, use 44187)

(Do not report 44310 in conjunction with 44144, 44150-44153, 44155, 44156, 45113, 45119, 45136)

44312 Revision of ileostomy; simple (release of superficial scar) (separate procedure)

44314 complicated (reconstruction in-depth) (separate procedure)

44316 Continent ileostomy (Kock procedure) (separate procedure)

(For fiberoptic evaluation, use 44385)

44320 Colostomy or skin level cecostomy

(For laparoscopic procedure, use 44188)

(Do not report 44320 in conjunction with 44141, 44144, 44146, 44605, 45110, 45119, 45126, 45563, 45805, 45825, 50810, 51597, 57307, or 58240)

44322 with multiple biopsies (eg, for congenital megacolon) (separate procedure)

44340 Revision of colostomy; simple (release of superficial scar) (separate procedure)

44345 complicated (reconstruction in-depth) (separate procedure)

44346 with repair of paracolostomy hernia (separate procedure)

● New Code   ▲ Revised Code   ✚ Add-On Code   ⦰ Modifier -51 Exempt   ⊙ Moderate Sedation

ENDOSCOPY, SMALL INTESTINE AND STOMAL

Surgical endoscopy always includes diagnostic endoscopy.

(For upper gastrointestinal endoscopy, see 43235-43258)

⊙ **44360** Small intestinal endoscopy, enteroscopy beyond second portion of duodenum, not including ileum; diagnostic, with or without collection of specimen(s) by brushing or washing (separate procedure)

⊙ **44361** with biopsy, single or multiple

⊙ **44363** with removal of foreign body

⊙ **44364** with removal of tumor(s), polyp(s), or other lesion(s) by snare technique

⊙ **44365** with removal of tumor(s), polyp(s), or other lesion(s) by hot biopsy forceps or bipolar cautery

⊙ **44366** with control of bleeding (eg, injection, bipolar cautery, unipolar cautery, laser, heater probe, stapler, plasma coagulator)

⊙ **44369** with ablation of tumor(s), polyp(s), or other lesion(s) not amenable to removal by hot biopsy forceps, bipolar cautery or snare technique

⊙ **44370** with transendoscopic stent placement (includes predilation)

⊙ **44372** with placement of percutaneous jejunostomy tube

⊙ **44373** with conversion of percutaneous gastrostomy tube to percutaneous jejunostomy tube

(For fiberoptic jejunostomy through stoma, use 43235)

⊙ **44376** Small intestinal endoscopy, enteroscopy beyond second portion of duodenum, including ileum; diagnostic, with or without collection of specimen(s) by brushing or washing (separate procedure)

⊙ **44377** with biopsy, single or multiple

⊙ **44378** with control of bleeding (eg, injection, bipolar cautery, unipolar cautery, laser, heater probe, stapler, plasma coagulator)

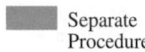

	Separate Procedure		Unlisted Procedure		CCI Comp. Code		Non-specific Procedure

665

⊙ **44379**   with transendoscopic stent placement (includes predilation)

⊙ **44380**   Ileoscopy, through stoma; diagnostic, with or without collection of specimen(s) by brushing or washing (separate procedure)

⊙ **44382**   with biopsy, single or multiple

⊙ **44383**   with transendoscopic stent placement (includes predilation)

⊙ **44385**   Endoscopic evaluation of small intestinal (abdominal or pelvic) pouch; diagnostic, with or without collection of specimen(s) by brushing or washing (separate procedure)

⊙ **44386**   with biopsy, single or multiple

⊙ **44388**   Colonoscopy through stoma; diagnostic, with or without collection of specimen(s) by brushing or washing (separate procedure)

⊙ **44389**   with biopsy, single or multiple

⊙ **44390**   with removal of foreign body

⊙ **44391**   with control of bleeding (eg, injection, bipolar cautery, unipolar cautery, laser, heater probe, stapler, plasma coagulator)

⊙ **44392**   with removal of tumor(s), polyp(s), or other lesion(s) by hot biopsy forceps or bipolar cautery

⊙ **44393**   with ablation of tumor(s), polyp(s), or other lesion(s) not amenable to removal by hot biopsy forceps, bipolar cautery or snare technique

⊙ **44394**   with removal of tumor(s), polyp(s), or other lesion(s) by snare technique

(For colonoscopy per rectum, see 45330-45385)

⊙ **44397**   with transendoscopic stent placement (includes predilation)

INTRODUCTION

⊘ ⊙**44500**   Introduction of long gastrointestinal tube (eg, Miller-Abbott) (separate procedure)

(For radiological supervision and interpretation, use 74340)

---

666   ● New Code   ▲ Revised Code   ✚ Add-On Code   ⊘ Modifier -51 Exempt   ⊙ Moderate Sedation

(For naso- or oro-gastric tube placement, use 43752)

REPAIR

44602 Suture of small intestine (enterorrhaphy) for perforated ulcer, diverticulum, wound, injury or rupture; single perforation

44603 multiple perforations

44604 Suture of large intestine (colorrhaphy) for perforated ulcer, diverticulum, wound, injury, or rupture (single or multiple perforations); without colostomy

44605 with colostomy

44615 Intestinal stricturoplasty (enterotomy and enterorrhaphy) with or without dilation, for intestinal obstruction

44620 Closure of enterostomy, large or small intestine;

44625 with resection and anastomosis other than colorectal

44626 with resection and colorectal anastomosis (eg, closure of Hartmann type procedure)

(For laparoscopic procedure, use 44227)

44640 Closure of intestinal cutaneous fistula

44650 Closure of enteroenteric or enterocolic fistula

44660 Closure of enterovesical fistula; without intestinal or bladder resection

44661 with intestine and/or bladder resection

(For closure of renocolic fistula, see 50525, 50526)

(For closure of gastrocolic fistula, use 43880)

(For closure of rectovesical fistula, see 45800, 45805)

44680 Intestinal plication (separate procedure)

OTHER PROCEDURES

44700 Exclusion of small intestine from pelvis by mesh or other prosthesis, or native tissue (eg, bladder or omentum)

(For therapeutic radiation clinical treatment, see Radiation Oncology section)

+ 44701 Intraoperative colonic lavage (List separately in addition to code for primary procedure)

(Use 44701 in conjunction with codes 44140, 44145, 44150, or 44604 as appropriate)

(Do not report 44701 in conjunction with 44300, 44950-44960)

● 44705 Preparation of fecal microbiota for instillation, including assessment of donor specimen

(Do not report 44705 in conjunction with 74283)

(For fecal instillation by oro-nasogastric tube or enema, use 44799)

44715 Backbench standard preparation of cadaver or living donor intestine allograft prior to transplantation, including mobilization and fashioning of the superior mesenteric artery and vein

44720 Backbench reconstruction of cadaver or living donor intestine allograft prior to transplantation; venous anastomosis, each

44721 arterial anastomosis, each

44799 Unlisted procedure, intestine

(For unlisted laparoscopic procedure, intestine except rectum, use 44238)

MECKEL'S DIVERTICULUM AND THE MESENTERY

EXCISION

44800 Excision of Meckel's diverticulum (diverticulectomy) or omphalomesenteric duct

44820 Excision of lesion of mesentery (separate procedure)

(With intestine resection, see 44120 or 44140 et seq)

SUTURE

44850 Suture of mesentery (separate procedure)

(For reduction and repair of internal hernia, use 44050)

668

● New Code	▲ Revised Code	+ Add-On Code	⊘ Modifier -51 Exempt	⊙ Moderate Sedation

OTHER PROCEDURES

44899 Unlisted procedure, Meckel's diverticulum and the mesentery

APPENDIX

INCISION

44900 Incision and drainage of appendiceal abscess; open

⊙ **44901** percutaneous

(For radiological supervision and interpretation, use 75989)

EXCISION

44950 Appendectomy;

(Incidental appendectomy during intra-abdominal surgery does not usually warrant a separate identification. If necessary to report, add modifier -52)

+ **44955** when done for indicated purpose at time of other major procedure (not as separate procedure) (List separately in addition to code for primary procedure)

44960 for ruptured appendix with abscess or generalized peritonitis

LAPAROSCOPY

Surgical laparoscopy always includes diagnostic laparoscopy. To report a diagnostic laparoscopy (peritoneoscopy) (separate procedure), use 49320.

44970 Laparoscopy, surgical, appendectomy

44979 Unlisted laparoscopy procedure, appendix

RECTUM

INCISION

45000 Transrectal drainage of pelvic abscess

45005 Incision and drainage of submucosal abscess, rectum

45020 Incision and drainage of deep supralevator, pelvirectal, or retrorectal abscess

---

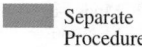 Separate Procedure   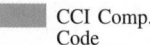 Unlisted Procedure   CCI Comp. Code   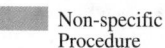 Non-specific Procedure

669

(See also 46050, 46060)

EXCISION

45100   Biopsy of anorectal wall, anal approach (eg, congenital megacolon)

(For endoscopic biopsy, use 45305)

45108   Anorectal myomectomy

45110   Proctectomy; complete, combined abdominoperineal, with colostomy

(For laparoscopic procedure, use 45395)

45111   partial resection of rectum, transabdominal approach

45112   Proctectomy, combined abdominoperineal, pull-through procedure (eg, colo-anal anastomosis)

(For colo-anal anastomosis with colonic reservoir or pouch, use 45119)

45113   Proctectomy, partial, with rectal mucosectomy, ileoanal anastomosis, creation of ileal reservoir (S or J), with or without loop ileostomy

45114   Proctectomy, partial, with anastomosis; abdominal and transsacral approach

45116   transsacral approach only (Kraske type)

45119   Proctectomy, combined abdominoperineal pull-through procedure (eg, colo-anal anastomosis), with creation of colonic reservoir (eg, J-pouch), with diverting enterostomy when performed

(For laparoscopic procedure, use 45397)

45120   Proctectomy, complete (for congenital megacolon), abdominal and perineal approach; with pull-through procedure and anastomosis (eg, Swenson, Duhamel, or Soave type operation)

45121   with subtotal or total colectomy, with multiple biopsies

45123   Proctectomy, partial, without anastomosis, perineal approach

---

● New   ▲ Revised   + Add-On   ⊘ Modifier -51   ⊙ Moderate
       Code   Code   Code   Exempt   Sedation

45126 Pelvic exenteration for colorectal malignancy, with proctectomy (with or without colostomy), with removal of bladder and ureteral transplantations, and/or hysterectomy, or cervicectomy, with or without removal of tube(s), with or without removal of ovary(s), or any combination thereof

45130 Excision of rectal procidentia, with anastomosis; perineal approach

45135   abdominal and perineal approach

45136 Excision of ileoanal reservoir with ileostomy

(Do not report 45136 in addition to 44005, 44120, 44310)

45150 Division of stricture of rectum

45160 Excision of rectal tumor by proctotomy, transsacral or transcoccygeal approach

(45170 Deleted 2009 [2010 edition]. To report excision of rectal tumor, transanal approach, see 45171, 45172)

45171 Excision of rectal tumor, transanal approach; not including muscularis propria (ie, partial thickness)

45172   including muscularis propria (ie, full thickness)

(For destruction of rectal tumor, transanal approach, use 45190)

(For transanal endoscopic microsurgical [ie, TEMS] excision of rectal tumor, including muscularis propria [ie., full thickness], use 0184T)

DESTRUCTION

45190 Destruction of rectal tumor (eg, electrodesiccation, electrosurgery, laser ablation, laser resection, cryosurgery) transanal approach

(For excision of rectal tumor, transanal approach, see 45171, 45172)

(For transanal endoscopic microsurgical [ie, TEMS] excision of rectal tumor, including muscularis propria [ie., full thickness], use 0184T)

| | Separate Procedure | | Unlisted Procedure | | CCI Comp. Code | | Non-specific Procedure | **671** |

ENDOSCOPY

When performing an endoscopy on a patient who is scheduled and prepared for a total colonoscopy, if the physician is unable to advance the colonoscope beyond the splenic flexure, due to unforseen circumstances, report the colonoscopy code with modifier 53 and appropriate documentation.

Surgical endoscopy always includes diagnostic endoscopy.

For computed tomographic colonography, see 74261-74263.

45300 Proctosigmoidoscopy, rigid; diagnostic, with or without collection of specimen(s) by brushing or washing (separate procedure)

⊙ **45303** with dilation (eg, balloon, guide wire, bougie)

(For radiological supervision and interpretation, use 74360)

⊙ **45305** with biopsy, single or multiple

⊙ **45307** with removal of foreign body

⊙ **45308** with removal of single tumor, polyp, or other lesion by hot biopsy forceps or bipolar cautery

⊙ **45309** with removal of single tumor, polyp, or other lesion by snare technique

⊙ **45315** with removal of multiple tumors, polyps, or other lesions by hot biopsy forceps, bipolar cautery or snare technique

⊙ **45317** with control of bleeding (eg, injection, bipolar cautery, unipolar cautery, laser, heater probe, stapler, plasma coagulator)

⊙ **45320** with ablation of tumor(s), polyp(s), or other lesion(s) not amenable to removal by hot biopsy forceps, bipolar cautery or snare technique (eg, laser)

⊙ **45321** with decompression of volvulus

⊙ **45327** with transendoscopic stent placement (includes predilation)

45330 Sigmoidoscopy, flexible; diagnostic, with or without collection of specimen(s) by brushing or washing (separate procedure)

45331 with biopsy, single or multiple

672   ● New   ▲ Revised   + Add-On   ⊘ Modifier -51   ⊙ Moderate
         Code   Code   Code   Exempt   Sedation

⊙ **45332**   with removal of foreign body

⊙ **45333**   with removal of tumor(s), polyp(s), or other lesion(s) by hot biopsy forceps or bipolar cautery

⊙ **45334**   with control of bleeding (eg, injection, bipolar cautery, unipolar cautery, laser, heater probe, stapler, plasma coagulator)

⊙ **45335**   with directed submucosal injection(s), any substance

⊙ **45337**   with decompression of volvulus, any method

⊙ **45338**   with removal of tumor(s), polyp(s), or other lesion(s) by snare technique

⊙ **45339**   with ablation of tumor(s), polyp(s), or other lesion(s) not amenable to removal by hot biopsy forceps, bipolar cautery or snare technique

⊙ **45340**   with dilation by balloon, 1 or more strictures

(Do not report 45340 in conjunction with 45345)

⊙ **45341**   with endoscopic ultrasound examination

⊙ **45342**   with transendoscopic ultrasound guided intramural or transmural fine needle aspiration/biopsy(s)

(Do not report 45341, 45342 in conjunction with 76942, 76975)

(For interpretation of specimen, see 88172-88173)

(For transrectal ultrasound utilizing rigid probe device, use 76872)

⊙ **45345**   with transendoscopic stent placement (includes predilation)

⊙ **45355**   Colonoscopy, rigid or flexible, transabdominal via colotomy, single or multiple

(For fiberoptic colonoscopy beyond 25 cm to splenic flexure, see 45330-45345)

⊙ **45378**   Colonoscopy, flexible, proximal to splenic flexure; diagnostic, with or without collection of specimen(s) by brushing or washing, with or without colon decompression (separate procedure)

	Separate Procedure		Unlisted Procedure		CCI Comp. Code		Non-specific Procedure

673

⊙ **45379**   with removal of foreign body

⊙ **45380**   with biopsy, single or multiple

⊙ **45381**   with directed submucosal injection(s), any substance

⊙ **45382**   with control of bleeding (eg, injection, bipolar cautery, unipolar cautery, laser, heater probe, stapler, plasma coagulator)

⊙ **45383**   with ablation of tumor(s), polyp(s), or other lesion(s) not amenable to removal by hot biopsy forceps, bipolar cautery or snare technique

⊙ **45384**   with removal of tumor(s), polyp(s), or other lesion(s) by hot biopsy forceps or bipolar cautery

⊙ **45385**   with removal of tumor(s), polyp(s), or other lesion(s) by snare technique

(For small intestine and stomal endoscopy, see 44360-44393)

⊙ **45386**   with dilation by balloon, 1 or more strictures

(Do not report 45386 in conjunction with 45387)

⊙ **45387**   with transendoscopic stent placement (includes predilation)

⊙ **45391**   with endoscopic ultrasound examination

(Do not report 45391 in conjunction with 45330, 45341, 45342, 45378, 76872)

⊙ **45392**   with transendoscopic ultrasound guided intramural or transmural fine needle aspiration/biopsy(s)

(Do not report 45392 in conjunction with 45330, 45341, 45342, 45378, 76872)

LAPAROSCOPY

Surgical laparoscopy always includes diagnostic laparoscopy. To report a diagnostic laparoscopy (peritoneoscopy) (separate procedure), use 49320.

Excision

45395   Laparoscopy, surgical; proctectomy, complete, combined abdominoperineal, with colostomy

(For open procedure, use 45110)

674   ● New Code   ▲ Revised Code   ✚ Add-On Code   ⊘ Modifier -51 Exempt   ⊙ Moderate Sedation

45397   proctectomy, combined abdominoperineal pull-through procedure (eg, colo-anal anastomosis), with creation of colonic reservoir (eg, J-pouch), with diverting enterostomy, when performed

(For open procedure, use 45119)

Repair

45400 Laparoscopy, surgical; proctopexy (for prolapse)

(For open procedure, use 45540, 45541)

45402   proctopexy (for prolapse), with sigmoid resection

(For open procedure, use 45550)

45499 Unlisted laparoscopy procedure, rectum

REPAIR

45500 Proctoplasty; for stenosis

45505   for prolapse of mucous membrane

45520 Perirectal injection of sclerosing solution for prolapse

45540 Proctopexy (eg, for prolapse); abdominal approach

(For laparoscopic procedure, use 45400)

45541   perineal approach

45550   with sigmoid resection, abdominal approach

(For laparoscopic procedure, use 45402)

45560 Repair of rectocele (separate procedure)

(For repair of rectocele with posterior colporrhaphy, use 57250)

45562 Exploration, repair, and presacral drainage for rectal injury;

45563   with colostomy

45800 Closure of rectovesical fistula;

45805   with colostomy

675

	Separate Procedure		Unlisted Procedure		CCI Comp. Code		Non-specific Procedure

45820   Closure of rectourethral fistula;

45825   with colostomy

(For rectovaginal fistula closure, see 57300-57308)

MANIPULATION

45900   Reduction of procidentia (separate procedure) under anesthesia

45905   Dilation of anal sphincter (separate procedure) under anesthesia other than local

45910   Dilation of rectal stricture (separate procedure) under anesthesia other than local

45915   Removal of fecal impaction or foreign body (separate procedure) under anesthesia

OTHER PROCEDURES

Surgical diagnostic anorectal exam (45990) includes the following elements: external perineal exam, digital rectal exam, pelvic exam (when performed), diagnostic anoscopy, and diagnostic rigid proctoscopy.

45990   Anorectal exam, surgical, requiring anesthesia (general, spinal, or epidural), diagnostic

(Do not report 45990 in conjunction with 45300-45327, 46600, 57410, 99170)

45999   Unlisted procedure, rectum

(For unlisted laparoscopic procedure, rectum, use 45499)

ANUS

For incision of thrombosed external hemorrhoid, use 46083. For ligation of internal hemorrhoid, see 46221, 46945, 46946. For excision of internal and/or external hemorrhoid, see 46250-46262, 46320. For injection of hemorrhoid, use 46500. For destruction of internal hemorrhoids by thermal energy, use 46930. For destruction of hemorrhoid by cryosurgery, use 46999. For hemorrhoidopexy, use 46947.

INCISION

(For subcutaneous fistulotomy, use 46270)

46020   Placement of seton

● New Code   ▲ Revised Code   + Add-On Code   ⊘ Modifier -51 Exempt   ⊙ Moderate Sedation

(Do not report 46020 in addition to 46060, 46280, 46600, 0249T)

46030 Removal of anal seton, other marker

46040 Incision and drainage of ischiorectal and/or perirectal abscess (separate procedure)

46045 Incision and drainage of intramural, intramuscular, or submucosal abscess, transanal, under anesthesia

46050 Incision and drainage, perianal abscess, superficial

(See also 45020, 46060)

46060 Incision and drainage of ischiorectal or intramural abscess, with fistulectomy or fistulotomy, submuscular, with or without placement of seton

(Do not report 46060 in addition to 46020)

(See also 45020)

46070 Incision, anal septum (infant)

(For anoplasty, see 46700-46705)

(Do not report modifier '-63' in conjunction with 46070)

46080 Sphincterotomy, anal, division of sphincter (separate procedure)

46083 Incision of thrombosed hemorrhoid, external

EXCISION

46200 Fissurectomy, including sphincterotomy when performed

(46210 Deleted 2009 [2010 edition]; see 46999)

(46211 Deleted 2009 [2010 edition]; see 46999)

46220 This code is out of order. See page 678

46221 Hemorrhoidectomy, internal, by rubber band ligation(s)

(For ligation, hemorrhoidal vascular bundle(s), including ultrasound guidance, use 0249T)

677

| Separate Procedure | Unlisted Procedure | CCI Comp. Code | Non-specific Procedure |

46945 Hemorrhoidectomy, internal, by ligation other than rubber band; single hemorrhoid column/group

46946 2 or more hemorrhoid columns/groups

(Do not report 46221, 46945, and 46946 in conjunction with 0249T)

46220 Excision of single external papilla or tag, anus

46230 Excision of multiple external papillae or tags, anus

46320 Excision of thrombosed hemorrhoid, external

46250 Hemorrhoidectomy, external, 2 or more columns/groups

(For hemorrhoidectomy, external, single column/group, use 46999)

46255 Hemorrhoidectomy, internal and external, single column/group;

46257 with fissurectomy

46258 with fistulectomy, including fissurectomy, when performed

46260 Hemorrhoidectomy, internal and external, 2 or more columns/groups;

46261 with fissurectomy

46262 with fistulectomy, including fissurectomy, when performed

(Do not report 46250-46262 in conjunction with 0249T)

46270 Surgical treatment of anal fistula (fistulectomy/fistulotomy); subcutaneous

46275 intersphincteric

46280 transsphincteric, suprasphincteric, extrasphincteric or multiple, including placement of seton, when performed

(Do not report 46280 in addition to 46020)

46285 second stage

46288 Closure of anal fistula with rectal advancement flap

678 ● New Code ▲ Revised Code ✛ Add-On Code ⊘ Modifier -51 Exempt ⊙ Moderate Sedation

46320   This code is out of order. See page 678

INTRODUCTION

46500   Injection of sclerosing solution, hemorrhoids

46505   Chemodenervation of internal anal sphincter

(For chemodenervation of other muscles, see 64612-64614. For destruction of nerve by neurolytic agent, see 64630, 64640)

(Report the specific service in conjunction with the specific substance(s) or drug(s) provided)

ENDOSCOPY

Surgical endoscopy always includes diagnostic endoscopy.

46600   Anoscopy; diagnostic, with or without collection of specimen(s) by brushing or washing (separate procedure)

(Do not report 46600 in conjunction with 46020, 0249T)

(For diagnostic high resolution anoscopy [HRA], use 0226T)

46604   with dilation (eg, balloon, guide wire, bougie)

46606   with biopsy, single or multiple

(For high resolution anoscopy [HRA] with biopsy, use 0227T)

46608   with removal of foreign body

46610   with removal of single tumor, polyp, or other lesion by hot biopsy forceps or bipolar cautery

46611   with removal of single tumor, polyp, or other lesion by snare technique

46612   with removal of multiple tumors, polyps, or other lesions by hot biopsy forceps, bipolar cautery or snare technique

46614   with control of bleeding (eg, injection, bipolar cautery, unipolar cautery, laser, heater probe, stapler, plasma coagulator)

46615   with ablation of tumor(s), polyp(s), or other lesion(s) not amenable to removal by hot biopsy forceps, bipolar cautery or snare technique

	Separate Procedure		Unlisted Procedure		CCI Comp. Code		Non-specific Procedure

679

(For delivery of thermal energy to the muscle of the anal canal, use 0288T)

REPAIR

46700 Anoplasty, plastic operation for stricture; adult

46705 infant

(Do not report modifier '-63' in conjunction with 46705)

(For simple incision of anal septum, use 46070)

46706 Repair of anal fistula with fibrin glue

46707 Repair of anorectal fistula with plug (eg, porcine small intestine submucosa [SIS])

46710 Repair of ileoanal pouch fistula/sinus (eg, perineal or vaginal), pouch advancement; transperineal approach

46712 combined transperineal and transabdominal approach

46715 Repair of low imperforate anus; with anoperineal fistula (cut-back procedure)

46716 with transposition of anoperineal or anovestibular fistula

(Do not report modifier 63 in conjunction with 46715, 46716)

46730 Repair of high imperforate anus without fistula; perineal or sacroperineal approach

46735 combined transabdominal and sacroperineal approaches

(Do not report modifier 63 in conjunction with 46730, 46735)

46740 Repair of high imperforate anus with rectourethral or rectovaginal fistula; perineal or sacroperineal approach

46742 combined transabdominal and sacroperineal approaches

(Do not report modifier 63 in conjunction with 46740, 46742)

46744 Repair of cloacal anomaly by anorectovaginoplasty and urethroplasty, sacroperineal approach

(Do not report modifier 63 in conjunction with 46744)

● New Code ▲ Revised Code + Add-On Code ⊘ Modifier -51 Exempt ⊙ Moderate Sedation

46746 Repair of cloacal anomaly by anorectovaginoplasty and urethroplasty, combined abdominal and sacroperineal approach;

46748 with vaginal lengthening by intestinal graft or pedicle flaps

46750 Sphincteroplasty, anal, for incontinence or prolapse; adult

46751 child

46753 Graft (Thiersch operation) for rectal incontinence and/or prolapse

46754 Removal of Thiersch wire or suture, anal canal

46760 Sphincteroplasty, anal, for incontinence, adult; muscle transplant

46761 levator muscle imbrication (Park posterior anal repair)

46762 implantation artificial sphincter

46947 Hemorrhoidopexy (eg, for prolapsing internal hemorrhoids) by stapling

DESTRUCTION

46900 Destruction of lesion(s), anus (eg, condyloma, papilloma, molluscum contagiosum, herpetic vesicle), simple; chemical

46910 electrodesiccation

46916 cryosurgery

46917 laser surgery

46922 surgical excision

46924 Destruction of lesion(s), anus (eg, condyloma, papilloma, molluscum contagiosum, herpetic vesicle), extensive (eg, laser surgery, electrosurgery, cryosurgery, chemosurgery)

46930 Destruction of internal hemorrhoid(s) by thermal energy (eg, infrared coagulation, cautery, radiofrequency)

(46934 deleted 2009 edition)

(46935 deleted 2009 edition)

	Separate Procedure		Unlisted Procedure		CCI Comp. Code		Non-specific Procedure

681

(46936   deleted 2009 edition)

(46937   Deleted 2009 [2010 edition]; use 45190)

(46938   Deleted 2009 [2010 edition]; use 45190)

46940   Curettage or cautery of anal fissure, including dilation of anal sphincter (separate procedure); initial

46942   subsequent

46945   This code is out of order. See page 678

46946   This code is out of order. See page 678

46947   This code is out of order. See page 681

OTHER PROCEDURES

46999   Unlisted procedure, anus

LIVER

INCISION

47000   Biopsy of liver, needle; percutaneous

(If imaging guidance is performed, see 76942, 77002, 77012, 77021)

+ **47001**   when done for indicated purpose at time of other major procedure (List separately in addition to code for primary procedure)

(If imaging guidance is performed, see 76942, 77002)

(For fine needle aspiration in conjunction with 47000, 47001, see 10021, 10022)

(For evaluation of fine needle aspirate in conjunction with 47000, 47001, see 88172, 88173)

47010   Hepatotomy; for open drainage of abscess or cyst, 1 or 2 stages

⊙ **47011**   for percutaneous drainage of abscess or cyst, 1 or 2 stages

(For radiological supervision and interpretation, use 75989)

---

682   ● New   ▲ Revised   + Add-On   ⊘ Modifier -51   ⊙ Moderate
              Code   Code   Code   Exempt   Sedation

47015 Laparotomy, with aspiration and/or injection of hepatic parasitic (eg, amoebic or echinococcal) cyst(s) or abscess(es)

EXCISION

47100 Biopsy of liver, wedge

47120 Hepatectomy, resection of liver; partial lobectomy

47122 trisegmentectomy

47125 total left lobectomy

47130 total right lobectomy

LIVER TRANSPLANTATION

Liver allotransplantation involves three distinct components of physician work:

1) **Cadaver donor hepatectomy**, which includes harvesting the graft and cold preservation of the graft (perfusing with cold preservation solution and cold maintenance) (use 47133). **Living donor hepatectomy**, which includes harvesting the graft, cold preservation of the graft (perfusing with cold preservation solution and cold maintenance), and care of the donor (see 47140-47142).

2) **Backbench work**:

Standard preparation of the whole liver graft will include one of the following:

Preparation of whole liver graft (including cholecystectomy, if necessary, and dissection and removal of surrounding soft tissues to prepare vena cava, portal vein, hepatic artery, and common bile duct for implantation) (use 47143).

Preparation as described for whole liver graft, plus trisegment split into two partial grafts (use 47144).

Preparation as described for whole liver graft, plus lobe split into two partial grafts (use 47145).

Additional reconstruction of the liver graft may include venous and/or arterial anastomosis(es) (see 47146, 47147).

3) **Recipient liver allotransplantation**, which includes recipient hepatectomy (partial or whole), transplantation of the allograft (partial or whole), and care of the recipient (see 47135, 47136).

47133 Donor hepatectomy (including cold preservation), from cadaver donor

| | Separate Procedure | | Unlisted Procedure | | CCI Comp. Code | | Non-specific Procedure | **683** |

47135 Liver allotransplantation; orthotopic, partial or whole, from cadaver or living donor, any age

47136 heterotopic, partial or whole, from cadaver or living donor, any age

47140 Donor hepatectomy (including cold preservation), from living donor; left lateral segment only (segments II and III)

47141 total left lobectomy (segments II, III, and IV)

47142 total right lobectomy (segments V, VI, VII, and VIII)

47143 Backbench standard preparation of cadaver donor whole liver graft prior to allotransplantation, including cholecystectomy, if necessary, and dissection and removal of surrounding soft tissues to prepare the vena cava, portal vein, hepatic artery, and common bile duct for implantation; without trisegment or lobe split

47144 with trisegment split of whole liver graft into 2 partial liver grafts (ie, left lateral segment [segments II and III] and right trisegment [segments I and IV through VIII])

47145 with lobe split of whole liver graft into 2 partial liver grafts (ie, left lobe (segments II, III, and IV) and right lobe (segments I and V through VIII))

47146 Backbench reconstruction of cadaver or living donor liver graft prior to allotransplantation; venous anastomosis, each

47147 arterial anastomosis, each

(Do not report 47143-47147 in conjunction with 47120-47125, 47600, 47610)

REPAIR

47300 Marsupialization of cyst or abscess of liver

47350 Management of liver hemorrhage; simple suture of liver wound or injury

47360 complex suture of liver wound or injury, with or without hepatic artery ligation

● New Code   ▲ Revised Code   + Add-On Code   ⊘ Modifier -51 Exempt   ⊙ Moderate Sedation

47361   exploration of hepatic wound, extensive debridement, coagulation and/or suture, with or without packing of liver

47362   re-exploration of hepatic wound for removal of packing

LAPAROSCOPY

Surgical laparoscopy always include diagnostic laparoscopy. To report a diagnostic laparoscopy (peritneoscopy) (separate procedure), use 49320.

47370   Laparoscopy, surgical, ablation of 1 or more liver tumor(s); radiofrequency

(For imaging guidance, use 76490)

47371   cryosurgical

(For imaging guidance, use 76490)

47379   Unlisted laparoscopic procedure, liver

OTHER PROCEDURES

47380   Ablation, open, of 1 or more liver tumor(s); radiofrequency

(For imaging guidance, use 76490)

47381   cryosurgical

(For imaging guidance, use 76490)

⊙ **47382**   Ablation, 1 or more liver tumor(s), percutaneous, radiofrequency

(For imaging guidance and monitoring, see 76490, 77013, 77022)

47399   Unlisted procedure, liver

BILIARY TRACT

INCISION

47400   Hepaticotomy or hepaticostomy with exploration, drainage, or removal of calculus

47420   Choledochotomy or choledochostomy with exploration, drainage, or removal of calculus, with or without cholecystotomy; without transduodenal sphincterotomy or sphincteroplasty

| 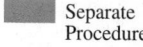 Separate Procedure | 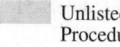 Unlisted Procedure | CCI Comp. Code | Non-specific Procedure | **685** |

47425   with transduodenal sphincterotomy or sphincteroplasty

47460   Transduodenal sphincterotomy or sphincteroplasty, with or without transduodenal extraction of calculus (separate procedure)

47480   Cholecystotomy or cholecystostomy, open, with exploration, drainage, or removal of calculus (separate procedure)

(For percutaneous cholecystostomy, use 47490)

INTRODUCTION

47490   Cholecystostomy, percutaneous, complete procedure, including imaging guidance, catheter placement, cholecystogram when performed, and radiological supervision and interpretation

(Do not report 47490 in conjunction with 47505, 74305, 75989, 76942, 77002, 77012, 77021)

47500   Injection procedure for percutaneous transhepatic cholangiography

(For radiological supervision and interpretation, use 74320)

47505   Injection procedure for cholangiography through an existing catheter (eg, percutaneous transhepatic or T-tube)

(For radiological supervision and interpretation, use 74305)

47510   Introduction of percutaneous transhepatic catheter for biliary drainage

(For radiological supervision and interpretation, use 75980)

47511   Introduction of percutaneous transhepatic stent for internal and external biliary drainage

(For radiological supervision and interpretation, use 75982)

⊙ **47525**   Change of percutaneous biliary drainage catheter

(For radiological supervision and interpretation, use 75984)

47530   Revision and/or reinsertion of transhepatic tube

(For radiological supervision and interpretation, use 75984)

ENDOSCOPY

Surgical endoscopy always includes diagnostic endoscopy.

+ 47550 Biliary endoscopy, intraoperative (choledochoscopy) (List separately in addition to code for primary procedure)

47552 Biliary endoscopy, percutaneous via T-tube or other tract; diagnostic, with or without collection of specimen(s) by brushing and/or washing (separate procedure)

47553 with biopsy, single or multiple

47554 with removal of calculus/calculi

47555 with dilation of biliary duct stricture(s) without stent

47556 with dilation of biliary duct stricture(s) with stent

(For ERCP, see 43260-43272, 74363)

(If imaging guidance is performed, see 74363, 75982)

LAPAROSCOPY

Surgical laparoscopy always include diagnostic laparoscopy. To report a diagnostic laparoscopy (peritneoscopy) (separate procedure), use 49320.

47560 Laparoscopy, surgical; with guided transhepatic cholangiography, without biopsy

47561 with guided transhepatic cholangiography with biopsy

47562 cholecystectomy

47563 cholecystectomy with cholangiography

47564 cholecystectomy with exploration of common duct

47570 cholecystoenterostomy

47579 Unlisted laparoscopy procedure, biliary tract

EXCISION

47600 Cholecystectomy;

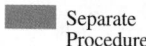 Separate Procedure   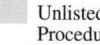 Unlisted Procedure   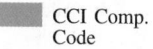 CCI Comp. Code   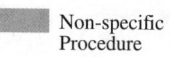 Non-specific Procedure   **687**

47605   with cholangiography

(For laparoscopic approach, see 47562-47564)

47610   Cholecystectomy with exploration of common duct;

(For cholecystectomy with exploration of common duct with biliary endoscopy, use 47610 with 47550)

47612   with choledochoenterostomy

47620   with transduodenal sphincterotomy or sphincteroplasty, with or without cholangiography

47630   Biliary duct stone extraction, percutaneous via T-tube tract, basket, or snare (eg, Burhenne technique)

(For radiological supervision and interpretation, use 74327)

47700   Exploration for congenital atresia of bile ducts, without repair, with or without liver biopsy, with or without cholangiography

(Do not report modifier 63 in conjunction with 47700)

47701   Portoenterostomy (eg, Kasai procedure)

(Do not report modifier 63 in conjunction with 47701)

47711   Excision of bile duct tumor, with or without primary repair of bile duct; extrahepatic

47712   intrahepatic

(For anastomosis, see 47760-47800)

47715   Excision of choledochal cyst

REPAIR

47720   Cholecystoenterostomy; direct

(For laparoscopic approach, use 47570)

47721   with gastroenterostomy

47740   Roux-en-Y

47741   Roux-en-Y with gastroenterostomy

● New Code   ▲ Revised Code   + Add-On Code   ⊘ Modifier -51 Exempt   ⊙ Moderate Sedation

47760 Anastomosis, of extrahepatic biliary ducts and gastrointestinal tract

47765 Anastomosis, of intrahepatic ducts and gastrointestinal tract

47780 Anastomosis, Roux-en-Y, of extrahepatic biliary ducts and gastrointestinal tract

47785 Anastomosis, Roux-en-Y, of intrahepatic biliary ducts and gastrointestinal tract

47800 Reconstruction, plastic, of extrahepatic biliary ducts with end-to-end anastomosis

47801 Placement of choledochal stent

47802 U-tube hepaticoenterostomy

47900 Suture of extrahepatic biliary duct for pre-existing injury (separate procedure)

OTHER PROCEDURES

47999 Unlisted procedure, biliary tract

PANCREAS

(For peroral pancreatic endoscopic procedures, see 43260-43272)

INCISION

48000 Placement of drains, peripancreatic, for acute pancreatitis;

48001   with cholecystostomy, gastrostomy, and jejunostomy

48020 Removal of pancreatic calculus

EXCISION

48100 Biopsy of pancreas, open (eg, fine needle aspiration, needle core biopsy, wedge biopsy)

48102 Biopsy of pancreas, percutaneous needle

(For radiological supervision and interpretation, see 76942, 77002, 77012, 77021)

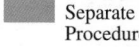 Separate Procedure   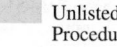 Unlisted Procedure   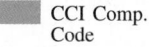 CCI Comp. Code   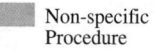 Non-specific Procedure

(For fine needle aspiration, use 10022)

(For evaluation of fine needle aspirate, see 88172, 88173)

48105 Resection or debridement of pancreas and peripancreatic tissue for acute necrotizing pancreatitis

48120 Excision of lesion of pancreas (eg, cyst, adenoma)

48140 Pancreatectomy, distal subtotal, with or without splenectomy; without pancreaticojejunostomy

48145 with pancreaticojejunostomy

48146 Pancreatectomy, distal, near-total with preservation of duodenum (Child-type procedure)

48148 Excision of ampulla of Vater

48150 Pancreatectomy, proximal subtotal with total duodenectomy, partial gastrectomy, choledochoenterostomy and gastrojejunostomy (Whipple-type procedure); with pancreatojejunostomy

48152 without pancreatojejunostomy

48153 Pancreatectomy, proximal subtotal with near-total duodenectomy, choledochoenterostomy, and duodenojejunostomy (pylorus-sparing, whipple-type procedure); with pancreatojejunostomy

48154 without pancreatojejunostomy

48155 Pancreatectomy, total

48160 Pancreatectomy, total or subtotal, with autologous transplantation of pancreas or pancreatic islet cells

INTRODUCTION

+ 48400 Injection procedure for intraoperative pancreatography (List separately in addition to code for primary procedure)

(For radiological supervision and interpretation, see 74300-74305)

● New Code ▲ Revised Code + Add-On Code ⊘ Modifier -51 Exempt ⊙ Moderate Sedation

REPAIR

48500 Marsupialization of pancreatic cyst

48510 External drainage, pseudocyst of pancreas; open

⊙ **48511** percutaneous

(For radiological supervision and interpretation, use 75989)

48520 Internal anastomosis of pancreatic cyst to gastrointestinal tract; direct

48540 Roux-en-Y

48545 Pancreatorrhaphy for injury

48547 Duodenal exclusion with gastrojejunostomy for pancreatic injury

48548 Pancreaticojejunostomy, side-to-side anastomosis (Puestow-type operation)

PANCREAS TRANSPLANTATION

Pancreas allotransplantation involves three distinct components of physician work:

1) **Cadaver donor pancreatectomy**, which includes harvesting the pancreas graft, with or without duodenal segment, and cold preservation of the graft (perfusing with cold preservation solution and cold maintenance) (use 48550).

2) **Backbench work**:

Standard preparation of a cadaver donor pancreas allograft prior to transplantation includes dissection of the allograft from surrounding soft tissues, splenectomy, duodenotomy, ligation of bile duct, ligation of mesenteric vessels, and Y-graft arterial anastomoses from the iliac artery to the superior mesenteric artery and to the splenic artery (use 48551).

Additional reconstruction of a cadaver donor pancreas allograft prior to transplantation may include venous anastomosis(es) (use 48552).

3) **Recipient pancreas allotransplantation**, which includes transplantation of allograft, and care of the recipient (use 48554).

48550 Donor pancreatectomy (including cold preservation), with or without duodenal segment for transplantation

---

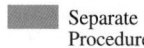 Separate Procedure

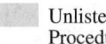 Unlisted Procedure

CCI Comp. Code

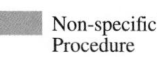 Non-specific Procedure

691

48551 Backbench standard preparation of cadaver donor pancreas allograft prior to transplantation, including dissection of allograft from surrounding soft tissues, splenectomy, duodenotomy, ligation of bile duct, ligation of mesenteric vessels, and Y-graft arterial anastomoses from iliac artery to superior mesenteric artery and to splenic artery

48552 Backbench reconstruction of cadaver donor pancreas allograft prior to transplantation, venous anastomosis, each

(Do not report 48551 and 48552 in conjunction with 35531, 35563, 35685, 38100-38102, 44010, 44820, 44850, 47460, 47505-47525, 47550-47556, 48100-48120, 48545)

48554 Transplantation of pancreatic allograft

48556 Removal of transplanted pancreatic allograft

OTHER PROCEDURES

48999 Unlisted procedure, pancreas

ABDOMEN, PERITONEUM, AND OMENTUM

INCISION

49000 Exploratory laparotomy, exploratory celiotomy with or without biopsy(s) (separate procedure)

(To report wound exploration due to penetrating trauma without laparatomy, use 20102)

49002 Reopening of recent laparotomy

(To report re-exploration of hepatic wound for removal of packing, use 47362)

49010 Exploration, retroperitoneal area with or without biopsy(s) (separate procedure)

(To report wound exploration due to penetrating trauma without laparatomy, use 20102)

49020 Drainage of peritoneal abscess or localized peritonitis, exclusive of appendiceal abscess; open

(For appendiceal abscess, use 44900)

⊙ **49021**   percutaneous

(For radiological supervision and interpretation, use 75989)

49040 Drainage of subdiaphragmatic or subphrenic abscess; open

⊙ **49041**   percutaneous

(For radiological supervision and interpretation, use 75989)

49060 Drainage of retroperitoneal abscess; open

⊙ **49061**   percutaneous

(For laparoscopic drainage, use 49323)

(For radiological supervision and interpretation, use 75989)

49062 Drainage of extraperitoneal lymphocele to peritoneal cavity, open

(49080   deleted 2011 [2012 edition]. See 49082-49084)

(49081   deleted 2011 [2012 edition]. See 49082-49084)

49082 Abdominal paracentesis (diagnostic or therapeutic); without imaging guidance

49083   with imaging guidance

(Do not report 49083 in conjunction with 76942, 77002, 77012, 77021)

49084 Peritoneal lavage, including imaging guidance, when performed

(Do not report 49084 in conjunction with 76942, 77002, 77012, 77021)

EXCISION, DESTRUCTION

(For lysis of intestinal adhesions, use 44005)

49180 Biopsy, abdominal or retroperitoneal mass, percutaneous needle

(If imaging guidance is performed, see 76942, 77002, 77012, 77021)

(For fine needle aspiration, use 10021 or 10022)

(For evaluation of fine needle aspirate, see 88172, 88173)

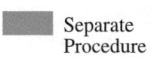 Separate Procedure   Unlisted Procedure   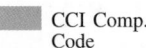 CCI Comp. Code   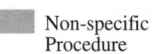 Non-specific Procedure

693

49203   Excision or destruction, open, intra-abdominal tumors, cysts or endometriomas, 1 or more peritoneal, mesenteric, or retroperitoneal primary or secondary tumors; largest tumor 5 cm diameter or less

49204   largest tumor 5.1-10.0 cm diameter

49205   largest tumor greater than 10.0 cm diameter

(Do not report 49203-49205 in conjunction with 38770, 38780, 49000, 49010, 49215, 50010, 50205, 50225, 50236, 50250, 50290, 58900-58960)

(For partial or total nephrectomy, use 50220 or 50240 in conjunction with 49203-49205)

(For colectomy, use 44140 in conjunction with 49203-49205)

(For small bowel resection, use 44120 in conjunction with 49203-49205)

(For vena caval resection with reconstruction, use 49203-49205 in conjunction with 37799)

(For resection of recurrent ovarian, tubal, primary peritoneal, or uterine malignancy, see 58957, 58958)

(For cryoablation of renal tumors, see 50250, 50593)

49215   Excision of presacral or sacrococcygeal tumor

(Do not report modifier '-63' in conjunction with 49215)

49220   Staging laparotomy for Hodgkins disease or lymphoma (includes splenectomy, needle or open biopsies of both liver lobes, possibly also removal of abdominal nodes, abdominal node and/or bone marrow biopsies, ovarian repositioning)

49250   Umbilectomy, omphalectomy, excision of umbilicus (separate procedure)

49255   Omentectomy, epiploectomy, resection of omentum (separate procedure)

LAPAROSCOPY

Surgical laparoscopy always includes diagnostic laparoscopy. To report a diagnostic laparoscopy (peritneoscopy) (separate procedure), use 49320.

  ● New Code   ▲ Revised Code   + Add-On Code   ⊘ Modifier -51 Exempt   ⊙ Moderate Sedation

For laparoscopic fulguration or excision of lesions of the ovary, pelvic viscera, or peritoneal surface, use 58662.

49320 Laparoscopy, abdomen, peritoneum, and omentum; diagnostic, with or without collection of specimen(s) by brushing or washing (separate procedure)

49321 Laparoscopy, surgical; with biopsy (single or multiple)

49322 with aspiration of cavity or cyst (eg, ovarian cyst) (single or multiple)

49323 with drainage of lymphocele to peritoneal cavity

(For percutaneous or open drainage, see 49060, 49061)

49324 with insertion of tunneled intraperitoneal catheter

(For subcutaneous extension of intraperitoneal catheter with remote chest exit site, use 49435 in conjunction with 49324)

(For open insertion of tunneled intraperitoneal catheter, use 49421)

49325 with revision of previously placed intraperitoneal cannula or catheter, with removal of intraluminal obstructive material if performed

+ 49326 with omentopexy (omental tacking procedure) (List separately in addition to code for primary procedure)

(Use 49326 in conjunction with 49324, 49325)

+ 49327 Laparoscopy, surgical, with placement of interstitial device(s) for radiation therapy guidance (eg, fiducial markers, dosimeter), intra-abdominal, intrapelvic, and/or retroperitoneum, including imaging guidance, if performed, single or multiple (List separately in addition to code for primary procedure)

(Use 49327 in conjunction with laparoscopic abdominal, pelvic, or retroperitoneal procedure[s] performed concurrently)

(For placement of interstitial device[s] for intra-abdominal, intrapelvic, and/or retroperitoneal radiation therapy guidance concurrent with open procedure, use 49412)

(For percutaneous placement of interstitial device[s] for intra-abdominal, intrapelvic, and/or retroperitoneal radiation therapy guidance, use 49411)

	Separate Procedure		Unlisted Procedure		CCI Comp. Code		Non-specific Procedure

695

49329 Unlisted laparoscopy procedure, abdomen, peritoneum and omentum

INTRODUCTION, REVISION, REMOVAL

49400 Injection of air or contrast into peritoneal cavity (separate procedure)

(For radiological supervision and interpretation, use 74190)

49402 Removal of peritoneal foreign body from peritoneal cavity

(For lysis of intestinal adhesions, use 44005)

49411 Placement of interstitial device(s) for radiation therapy guidance (eg, fiducial markers, dosimeter), percutaneous, intra abdominal, intra pelvic (except prostate), and/or retroperitoneum, single or multiple

(Report supply of device separately)

(For imaging guidance, see 76942, 77002, 77012, 77021)

(For percutaneous placement of interstitial device[s] for intra-thoracic radiation therapy guidance, use 32553)

+ 49412 Placement of interstitial device(s) for radiation therapy guidance (eg, fiducial markers, dosimeter), open, intra-abdominal, intrapelvic and/or retroperitoneum, including imaging guidance, if performed, single or multiple (List separately in addition to code for primary procedure)

(Use 49412 in conjunction with open abdominal, pelvic, or retroperitoneal procedure[s] performed concurrently)

(For placement of interstitial device[s] for intra-abdominal, intrapelvic, and/or retroperitoneal radiation therapy guidance concurrent with laparoscopic procedure, use 49327)

(For percutaneous placement of interstitial device[s] for intra-abdominal, intrapelvic, and/or retroperitoneal radiation therapy guidance, use 49411)

⊙ 49418 Insertion of tunneled intraperitoneal catheter (eg, dialysis, intraperitoneal chemotherapy instillation, management of ascites), complete procedure, including imaging guidance, catheter placement, contrast injection when performed, and radiological supervision and interpretation, percutaneous

49419 Insertion of tunneled intraperitoneal catheter, with subcutaneous port (ie, totally implantable)

696 ● New Code ▲ Revised Code + Add-On Code ⊘ Modifier -51 Exempt ⊙ Moderate Sedation

(For removal, use 49422)

(49420   deleted 2010 [2011 edition]. To report open placement of a
tunneled intraperitoneal catheter for dialysis, use 49421. To
report open or percutaneous peritoneal drainage or lavage, see
49020, 49021, 49040, 49041, 49082-49084, as appropriate. To
report percutaneous insertion of a tunneled intraperitoneal
catheter without subcutaneous port, use 49418.)

49421   Insertion of tunneled intraperitoneal catheter for dialysis, open

(For laparoscopic insertion of tunneled intraperitoneal catheter,
use 49324)

(For subcutaneous extension of intraperitoneal catheter with
remote chest exit site, use 49435 in conjunction with 49421)

49422   Removal of tunneled intraperitoneal catheter

(For removal of a non-tunneled catheter, use appropriate E/M
code)

49423   Exchange of previously placed abscess or cyst drainage catheter
under radiological guidance (separate procedure)

(For radiological supervision and interpretation, use 75984)

49424   Contrast injection for assessment of abscess or cyst via
previously placed drainage catheter or tube (separate procedure)

(For radiological supervision and interpretation, use 76080)

49425   Insertion of peritoneal-venous shunt

49426   Revision of peritoneal-venous shunt

(For shunt patency test, use 78291)

49427   Injection procedure (eg, contrast media) for evaluation of
previously placed peritoneal-venous shunt

(For radiological supervision and interpretation, see 75809,
78291)

49428   Ligation of peritoneal-venous shunt

49429   Removal of peritoneal-venous shunt

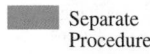 Separate
Procedure   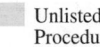 Unlisted
Procedure   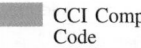 CCI Comp.
Code   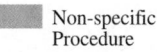 Non-specific
Procedure

697

+ 49435   Insertion of subcutaneous extension to intraperitoneal cannula or catheter with remote chest exit site (List separately in addition to code for primary procedure)

(Use 49435 in conjunction with 49324, 49421)

49436   Delayed creation of exit site from embedded subcutaneous segment of intraperitoneal cannula or catheter

Initial Placement

Do not additionally report 43752 for placement of a nasogastric (NG) or orogastric (OG) tube to insufflate the stomach prior to percutaneous gastrointestinal tube placement. NG or OG tube placement is considered part of the procedure in this family of codes.

⊙ **49440**   Insertion of gastrostomy tube, percutaneous, under fluoroscopic guidance including contrast injection(s), image documentation and report

(For conversion to a gastro-jejunostomy tube at the time of initial gastrostomy tube placement, use 49440 in conjunction with 49446)

⊙ **49441**   Insertion of duodenostomy or jejunostomy tube, percutaneous, under fluoroscopic guidance including contrast injection(s), image documentation and report

(For conversion of gastrostomy tube to gastro-jejunostomry tube, use 49446)

⊙ **49442**   Insertion of cecostomy or other colonic, tube, percutaneous, under fluoroscopic guidance including contrast injection(s), image documentation and report

Conversion

⊙ **49446**   Conversion of gastrostomy tube to gastro-jejunostomy tube, percutaneous, under fluoroscopic guidance including contrast injection(s), image documentation and report

(For conversion to a gastro-jejunostomy tube at the time of initial gastrostomy tube placement, use 49446 in conjunction with 49440)

Replacement

If an existing gastrostomy, duodenostomy, jejunostomy, gastro-jejunostomy, or cecostomy (or other colonic) tube is removed and a new tube is placed via a separate percutaneous access site, the placement of the new tube is not considered a replacement and would be reported using the appropriate initial placement codes 49440-49442.

49450 Replacement of gastrostomy or cecostomy (or other colonic) tube, percutaneous, under fluoroscopic guidance including contrast injection(s), image documentation and report

(To report a percutaneous change of a gastrostomy tube without imaging or endoscopic guidance, use 43760)

49451 Replacement of duodenostomy or jejunostormy tube, percutaneous, under fluoroscopic guidance including contrast injection(s), image documentation and report

49452 Replacement of gastro-jejunostomy tube, percutaneous, under fluoroscopic guidance including contrast injection(s), image documentation and report

Mechanical Removal Of Obstructive Material

49460 Mechanical removal of obstructive material from gastrostomy, duodenostomy, jejunostomy, gastro-jejunostomy, or cecostomy (or other colonic) tube, any method, under fluoroscopic guidance including contrast injection(s), if performed, image documentation and report

(Do not report 49460 in conjunction with 49450-49452, 49465)

Other

49465 Contrast injection(s) for radiological evaluation of existing gastrostomy, duodenostomy, jejunostomy, gastro-jejunostomy, or cecostomy (or other colonic) tube, from a percutaneous approach including image documentation and report

(Do not report 49465 in conjunction with 49450-49460)

REPAIR

Hernioplasty, Herniorrhaphy, Herniotomy

With the exception of the incisional hernia repairs (see 49560-49566) the use of mesh or other prostheses is not separately reported.

The excision/repair of strangulated organs or structures such as testicle(s), intestine, ovaries are reported by using the appropriate code for the excision/repair (eg., 44120, 54520, and 58940) in addition to the appropriate code for the repair of the strangulated hernia.

(For reduction and repair of intra-abdominal hernia, use 44050)

699

Separate Procedure   Unlisted Procedure   CCI Comp. Code   Non-specific Procedure

(For debridement of abdominal wall, see 11042, 11043)

(Codes 49491-49651 are unilateral procedures. To report bilateral procedures, report modifier -50 with the appropriate procedure code)

49491   Repair, initial inguinal hernia, preterm infant (less than 37 weeks gestation at birth), performed from birth up to 50 weeks postconception age, with or without hydrocelectomy; reducible

49492   incarcerated or strangulated

(Do not report modifier -63 in conjunction with 49491, 49492)

(Post-conception age equals gestational age at birth plus age of infant in weeks at the time of the hernia repair. Initial inguinal hernia repairs that are performed on preterm infants who are over 50 weeks postconceptual age and under age 6 months at the time of surgery, should be reported using codes 49495, 49496)

49495   Repair, initial inguinal hernia, full term infant under age 6 months, or preterm infant over 50 weeks postconception age and under age 6 months at the time of surgery, with or without hydrocelectomy; reducible

49496   incarcerated or strangulated

(Do not report modifier -63 in conjunction with 49491, 49492)

(Post-conception age equals gestational age at birth plus age in weeks at the time of the hernia repair. Initial inguinal hernia repairs that are performed on preterm infants who are under or up to 50 weeks postconceptual age but under 6 months of age since birth, should be reported using codes 49491, 49492. Inguinal hernia repairs on infants age 6 months to under 5 years should be reported using codes 49500-49501)

49500   Repair initial inguinal hernia, age 6 months to under 5 years, with or without hydrocelectomy; reducible

49501   incarcerated or strangulated

49505   Repair initial inguinal hernia, age 5 years or over; reducible

49507   incarcerated or strangulated

(For inguinal hernia repair, with simple orchiectomy, see 49505 or 49507 and 54520)

● New Code   ▲ Revised Code   + Add-On Code   ⊘ Modifier -51 Exempt   ⊙ Moderate Sedation

(For inguinal hernia repair, with excision of hydrocele or spermatocele, see 49505 or 49507 and 54840 or 55040)

49520 Repair recurrent inguinal hernia, any age; reducible

49521 incarcerated or strangulated

49525 Repair inguinal hernia, sliding, any age

(For incarcerated or strangulated inguinal hernia repair, see 49496, 49501, 49507, 49521)

49540 Repair lumbar hernia

49550 Repair initial femoral hernia, any age; reducible

49553 incarcerated or strangulated

49555 Repair recurrent femoral hernia; reducible

49557 incarcerated or strangulated

49560 Repair initial incisional or ventral hernia; reducible

49561 incarcerated or strangulated

49565 Repair recurrent incisional or ventral hernia; reducible

49566 incarcerated or strangulated

+ **49568** Implantation of mesh or other prosthesis for open incisional or ventral hernia repair or mesh for closure of debridement for necrotizing soft tissue infection (List separately in addition to code for the incisional or ventral hernia repair)

(Use 49568 in conjunction with 11004-11006, 49560-49566)

49570 Repair epigastric hernia (eg, preperitoneal fat); reducible (separate procedure)

49572 incarcerated or strangulated

49580 Repair umbilical hernia, under age 5 years; reducible

49582 incarcerated or strangulated

49585 Repair umbilical hernia, age 5 years or over; reducible

| | Separate Procedure | | Unlisted Procedure | | CCI Comp. Code | | Non-specific Procedure | **701** |

49587   incarcerated or strangulated

49590 Repair spigelian hernia

49600 Repair of small omphalocele, with primary closure

(Do not report modifier -63 in conjunction with 49600)

49605 Repair of large omphalocele or gastroschisis; with or without prosthesis

49606   with removal of prosthesis, final reduction and closure, in operating room

(Do not report modifier -63 in conjunction with 49605, 49606)

49610 Repair of omphalocele (Gross type operation); first stage

49611   second stage

(Do not report modifier -63 in conjunction with 49610, 49611)

(For diaphragmatic or hiatal hernia repair, see 39503, 43332)

(For surgical repair of omentum, use 49999)

LAPAROSCOPY

Surgical laparoscopy always includes diagnostic laparoscopy. To report a diagnostic laparoscopy (peritoneoscopy) (separate procedure), use 49320.

49650 Laparoscopy, surgical; repair initial inguinal hernia

49651   repair recurrent inguinal hernia

49652 Laparoscopy, surgical, repair, ventral, umbilical, spigelian or epigastric hernia (includes mesh insertion, when performed); reducible

(Do not report 49652 in conjunction with 44180, 49568)

49653   incarcerated or strangulated

(Do not report 49653 in conjunction with 44180, 49568)

49654 Laparoscopy, surgical, repair, incisional hernia (includes mesh insertion, when performed); reducible

(Do not report 49654 in conjunction with 44180, 49568)

● New Code   ▲ Revised Code   ✛ Add-On Code   ⊘ Modifier -51 Exempt   ⊙ Moderate Sedation

49655   incarcerated or strangulated

(Do not report 49655 in conjunction with 44180, 49568)

49656 Laparoscopy, surgical, repair, recurrent incisional hernia (includes mesh insertion, when performed); reducible

(Do not report 49656 in conjunction with 44180, 49568)

49657   incarcerated or strangulated

(Do not report 49657 in conjunction with 44180, 49568)

49659 Unlisted laparoscopy procedure, hernioplasty, herniorrhaphy, herniotomy

SUTURE

49900 Suture, secondary, of abdominal wall for evisceration or dehiscence

(For suture of ruptured diaphragm, see 39540, 39541)

(For debridement of abdominal wall, see 11042, 11043)

OTHER PROCEDURES

49904 Omental flap, extra-abdominal (eg, for reconstruction of sternal and chest wall defects)

(Code 49904 includes harvest and transfer. If a second surgeon harvests the omental flap, then the two surgeons should code 49904 as co-surgeons, using modifier -62)

+ **49905** Omental flap, intra-abdominal (List separately in addition to code for primary procedure)

(Do not report 49905 in conjunction with 44700)

49906 Free omental flap with microvascular anastomosis

(Do not report code 69990 in addition to code 49906)

49999 Unlisted procedure, abdomen, peritoneum and omentum

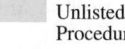

| Separate Procedure | Unlisted Procedure | CCI Comp. Code | Non-specific Procedure |

URINARY SYSTEM

CPT codes from this section are used to report invasive and surgical procedures performed on the kidney; ureter; bladder; prostate (resection); and urethra.

URODYNAMICS

CPT codes in this section may be used separately or in various combinations.When multiple procedures are performed in the same session, modifier -51 should be added .to the second and all subsequent CPT codes. Procedures in this section are performed by, or under the direct supervision of, a physician.

In addition, all materials and supplies, used in the provision of these services, such as instruments, equipment, fluids, gases, probes, catheters, technician's fees, medications, gloves, trays, tubing and other sterile supplies are considered to be included in the base code. Use modifier -26 to code and report interpretation of results or operation of equipment only.

CYSTOSCOPY, URETHROSCOPY, and CYSTOURETHROSCOPY

The descriptions of CPT codes in this section are listed so that the main procedure can be identified without having to list all of the minor related procedures performed at the same time. For example:

52601 Transurethral electrosurgical resection of prostate, including control of postoperative bleeding, complete (vasectomy, meatotomy, cystourethroscopy, urethral calibration and/or dilation, and internal urethrotomy are included)

All of the secondary procedures are included in the single code 52601. If any of the secondary procedures requires significant additional time and effort, to the point of making the procedure "unusual", modifier -22 should be added with an appropriate increase in fee and a report explaining what made the procedure unusual.

(For provision of chemotherapeutic agents, report both the specific service in addition to code(s) for the specific substance(s) or drug(s) provided)

KIDNEY

INCISION

(For retroperitoneal exploration, abscess, tumor, or cyst, see 49010, 49060, 49203-49205)

50010 Renal exploration, not necessitating other specific procedures

(For laparoscopic ablation of renal mass lesion(s), use 50542)

● New Code	▲ Revised Code	✚ Add-On Code	⊘ Modifier -51 Exempt	⊙ Moderate Sedation

50020 Drainage of perirenal or renal abscess; open

⊙ **50021**   percutaneous

     (For radiological supervision and interpretation, use 75989)

50040 Nephrostomy, nephrotomy with drainage

50045 Nephrotomy, with exploration

     (For renal endoscopy performed in conjunction with this procedure, see 50570-50580)

50060 Nephrolithotomy; removal of calculus

50065   secondary surgical operation for calculus

50070   complicated by congenital kidney abnormality

50075   removal of large staghorn calculus filling renal pelvis and calyces (including anatrophic pyelolithotomy)

50080 Percutaneous nephrostolithotomy or pyelostolithotomy, with or without dilation, endoscopy, lithotripsy, stenting, or basket extraction; up to 2 cm

50081   over 2cm

     (For establishment of nephrostomy without nephrostolithotomy, see 50040, 50395, 52334)

     (For fluoroscopic guidance, see 76000, 76001)

50100 Transection or repositioning of aberrant renal vessels (separate procedure)

50120 Pyelotomy; with exploration

     (For renal endoscopy performed in conjunction with this procedure, see 50570-50580)

50125   with drainage, pyelostomy

50130   with removal of calculus (pyelolithotomy, pelviolithotomy, including coagulum pyelolithotomy)

705

 Separate Procedure   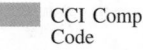 Unlisted Procedure   CCI Comp. Code   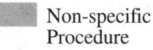 Non-specific Procedure

| 50135 | complicated (eg, secondary operation, congenital kidney abnormality) |

(For supply of anticarcinogenic agents, use 99070 in addition to code for primary procedure)

EXCISION

(For excision of retroperitoneal tumor or cyst, see 49203-49205)

(For laparoscopic ablation of renal mass lesion(s), use 50542)

⊙ **50200** Renal biopsy; percutaneous, by trocar or needle

(For radiological supervision and interpretation, see 76942, 77002, 77012, 77021)

(For fine needle aspiration, use 10022)

(For evaluation of fine needle aspirate, see 88172, 88173)

50205 by surgical exposure of kidney

50220 Nephrectomy, including partial ureterectomy, any open approach including rib resection;

50225 complicated because of previous surgery on same kidney

50230 radical, with regional lymphadenectomy and/or vena caval thrombectomy

(When vena caval resection with reconstruction is necessary, use 37799)

50234 Nephrectomy with total ureterectomy and bladder cuff; through same incision

50236 through separate incision

50240 Nephrectomy, partial

(For laparoscopic partial nephrectomy, use 50543)

50250 Ablation, open, 1 or more renal mass lesion(s), cryosurgical, including intraoperative ultrasound guidance and monitoring, if performed

(For laparoscopic ablation of renal mass lesions, use 50542)

(For percutaneous ablation of renal tumors, see 50592, 50593)

● New Code ▲ Revised Code ＋ Add-On Code ⊘ Modifier -51 Exempt ⊙ Moderate Sedation

50280 Excision or unroofing of cyst(s) of kidney

(For laparoscopic ablation of renal cysts, use 50541)

50290 Excision of perinephric cyst

RENAL TRANSPLANTATION

Renal *auto*transplantation includes reimplantation of the autograft as the primary procedure, along with secondary extra-corporeal procedure(s) (eg., partial nephrectomy, nephrolithotomy) reported with modifier 51 (see 50380 and applicable secondary procedure[s]).

Renal *allo*transplantation involves three distinct components of physician work:

1. **Cadaver donor nephrectomy, unilateral or bilateral**, which includes harvesting the graft(s) and cols preservation of the graft(s) (perfusing with cold preservation solution and cold maintenance) (use 50300). **Living donor nephrectomy**, which includes harvesting the graft, cold preservation of the graft (perfusing with cold preservation solution and cold maintenance), and care of the donor (see 50320, 50547).

2. **Backbench work:**

Standard preparation of a cadaver donor renal allograft prior to transplantation including dissection and removal of perinephric fat, diaphragmatic and retroperitoneal attachments; excision of adrenal gland; and preparation of ureter(s), renal vein(s), and renal artery(s), ligating branches as necessary (use 50325).

Standard preparation of a living donor renal allograft (open or laparoscopic) prior to transplantation including dissection and removal of perinephric fat and preparation of ureter(s), renal vein(s), and renal artery(s), ligating branches as necessary (use 50325).

Additional reconstruction of a cadaver or living donor renal allograft prior to transplantation may include venous, arterial, and/or ureteral anastomosis(es) necessary for implantation (see 50327-50329)

3. **Recipient renal allotransplantation,** which includes transplantation of the allograft (with or without recipient nephrectomy) and care of the recipient (see 50360, 50365).

(For dialysis, see 90935-90999)

(For laparoscopic donor nephrectomy, use 50547)

(For laparoscopic drainage of lymphocele to peritoneal cavity, use 49323)

707

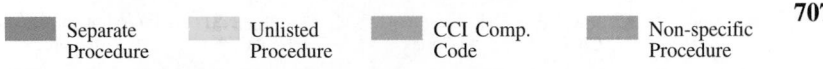

| Separate | Unlisted | CCI Comp. | Non-specific |
| Procedure | Procedure | Code | Procedure |

50300   Donor nephrectomy (including cold preservation); from cadaver donor, unilateral or bilateral

50320   open, from living donor

50323   Backbench standard preparation of cadaver donor renal allograft prior to transplantation, including dissection and removal of perinephric fat, diaphragmatic and retroperitoneal attachments, excision of adrenal gland, and preparation of ureter(s), renal vein(s), and renal artery(s), ligating branches, as necessary

(Do not report 50323 in conjunction with 60540, 60545)

50325   Backbench standard preparation of living donor renal allograft (open or laparoscopic) prior to transplantation, including dissection and removal of perinephric fat and preparation of ureter(s), renal vein(s), and renal artery(s), ligating branches, as necessary

50327   Backbench reconstruction of cadaver or living donor renal allograft prior to transplantation; venous anastomosis, each

50328   arterial anastomosis, each

50329   ureteral anastomosis, each

50340   Recipient nephrectomy (separate procedure)

(For bilateral procedure, report 50340 with modifier -50)

50360   Renal allotransplantation, implantation of graft; without recipient nephrectomy

50365   with recipient nephrectomy

(For bilateral procedure, report 50365 with modifier -50)

50370   Removal of transplanted renal allograft

50380   Renal autotransplantation, reimplantation of kidney

(For renal autotransplantation extra-corporeal (bench) surgery, use autotransplantation as the primary procedure and report secondary procedure(s) (eg, partial nephrectomy, nephrolithotomy) with modifier -51)

● New Code   ▲ Revised Code   + Add-On Code   ⊘ Modifier -51 Exempt   ⊙ Moderate Sedation

INTRODUCTION

Renal Pelvis Catheter Procedures

Internally Dwelling

⊙ **50382** Removal (via snare/capture) and replacement of internally dwelling ureteral stent via percutaneous approach, including radiological supervision and interpretation

(For bilateral procedure, use modifier -50)

(For removal and replacement of an internally dwelling ureteral stent via a transurethral approach, use 50385)

⊙ **50384** Removal (via snare/capture) of internally dwelling ureteral stent via percutaneous approach, including radiological supervision and interpretation

(For bilateral procedure, use modifier 50)

(Do not report 50382, 50384 in conjunction with 50395)

(For removal of an internally dwelling ureteral stent via a transurethral approach, use 50386)

⊙ **50385** Removal (via snare/capture) and replacement of internally dwelling ureteral stent via transurethral approach, without use of cystoscopy, including radiological supervision and interpretation

⊙ **50386** Removal (via snare/capture) of internally dwelling ureteral stent via transurethral approach, without use of cystoscopy, including radiological supervision and interpretation

Externally Accessible

⊙ **50387** Removal and replacement of externally accessible transnephric ureteral stent (eg, external/internal stent) requiring fluoroscopic guidance, including radiological supervision and interpretation

(For bilateral procedure, use modifier 50)

(For removal and replacement of externally accessible ureteral stent via ureterostomy or ileal conduit, use 50688)

(For removal without replacement of an externally accessible ureteral stent not requiring fluoroscopic guidance, see Evaluation and Management services codes)

	Separate Procedure		Unlisted Procedure		CCI Comp. Code		Non-specific Procedure

50389   Removal of nephrostomy tube, requiring fluoroscopic guidance (eg, with concurrent indwelling ureteral stent)

(Removal of nephrostomy tube not requiring fluoroscopic guidance is considered inherent to E/M services. Report the appropriate level of E/M service provided)

Other Introduction Procedures

50390   Aspiration and/or injection of renal cyst or pelvis by needle, percutaneous

(For radiological supervision and interpretation, see 74425, 74470, 76942, 77002, 77012, 77021)

(For evaluation of fine needle aspirate, see 88172, 88173)

50391   Instillation(s) of therapeutic agent into renal pelvis and/or ureter through established nephrostomy, pyelostomy or ureterostomy tube (eg, anticarcinogenic or antifungal agent)

50392   Introduction of intracatheter or catheter into renal pelvis for drainage and/or injection, percutaneous

(For radiological supervision and interpretation, see 74475, 76942, 77012)

50393   Introduction of ureteral catheter or stent into ureter through renal pelvis for drainage and/or injection, percutaneous

(For radiological supervision and interpretation, see 74480, 76942, 77002, 77012)

50394   Injection procedure for pyelography (as nephrostogram, pyelostogram, antegrade pyelouretergrams) through nephrostomy or pyelostomy tube, or indwelling ureteral catheter

(For radiological supervision and interpretation, use 74425)

50395   Introduction of guide into renal pelvis and/or ureter with dilation to establish nephrostomy tract, percutaneous

(For radiological supervision and interpretation, see 74475, 74480, 74485)

(For nephrostolithotomy, see 50080, 50081)

(For retrograde percutaneous nephrostomy, use 52334)

(For endoscopic surgery, see 50551-50561)

   ● New Code   ▲ Revised Code   + Add-On Code   ⊘ Modifier -51 Exempt   ⊙ Moderate Sedation

50396 Manometric studies through nephrostomy or pyelostomy tube, or indwelling ureteral catheter

(For radiological supervision and interpretation, see 74425, 74475, 74480)

50398 Change of nephrostomy or pyelostomy tube

(For radiological supervision and interpretation, use 75984)

REPAIR

50400 Pyeloplasty (Foley Y-pyeloplasty), plastic operation on renal pelvis, with or without plastic operation on ureter, nephropexy, nephrostomy, pyelostomy, or ureteral splinting; simple

50405 complicated (congenital kidney abnormality, secondary pyeloplasty, solitary kidney, calycoplasty)

(For laparoscopic approach, use 50544)

50500 Nephrorrhaphy, suture of kidney wound or injury

50520 Closure of nephrocutaneous or pyelocutaneous fistula

50525 Closure of nephrovisceral fistula (eg, renocolic), including visceral repair; abdominal approach

50526 thoracic approach

50540 Symphysiotomy for horseshoe kidney with or without pyeloplasty and/or other plastic procedure, unilateral or bilateral (1 operation)

LAPAROSCOPY

Surgical laparoscopy always includes diagnostic laparoscopy. To report a diagnostic laparoscopy (peritoneoscopy) (separate procedure), use 49320.

50541 Laparoscopy, surgical; ablation of renal cysts

50542 ablation of renal mass lesion(s), including intraoperative ultrasound guidance and monitoring, when performed

(For open procedure, see 50250)

(For percutaneous ablation of renal tumors, see 50592, 50593)

50543 partial nephrectomy

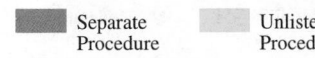 Separate Procedure
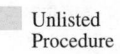 Unlisted Procedure
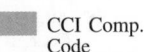 CCI Comp. Code
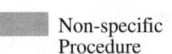 Non-specific Procedure

711

(For open procedure, use 50240)

50544   pyeloplasty

50545   radical nephrectomy (includes removal of Gerota's fascia and surrounding fatty tissue, removal of regional lymph nodes, and adrenalectomy)

(For open procedure, use 50230)

50546   nephrectomy including partial ureterectomy

50547   donor nephrectomy (including cold preservation), from living donor

(For open procedure, use 50320)

(For backbench renal allograft standard preparation prior to transplantation, use 50325)

(For backbench renal allograft reconstruction prior to transplantation, see 50327-50329)

50548   nephrectomy with total ureterectomy

(For open procedure, see 50234, 50236)

50549   Unlisted laparoscopy procedure, renal

(For laparoscopic drainage of lymphocele to peritoneal cavity, use 49323)

ENDOSCOPY

(For supplies and materials, use 99070)

50551   Renal endoscopy through established nephrostomy or pyelostomy, with or without irrigation, instillation, or ureteropyelography, exclusive of radiologic service;

50553   with ureteral catheterization, with or without dilation of ureter

50555   with biopsy

50557   with fulguration and/or incision, with or without biopsy

50561   with removal of foreign body or calculus

50562   with resection of tumor

● New Code   ▲ Revised Code   + Add-On Code   ⊘ Modifier -51 Exempt   ⊙ Moderate Sedation

(When procedures 50570-50580 provide a significant identifiable service, they may be added to 50045 and 50120)

50570 Renal endoscopy through nephrotomy or pyelotomy, with or without irrigation, instillation, or ureteropyelography, exclusive of radiologic service;

(For nephrotomy, use 50045)

(For pyelotomy, use 50120)

50572 with ureteral catheterization, with or without dilation of ureter

50574 with biopsy

50575 with endopyelotomy (includes cystoscopy, ureteroscopy, dilation of ureter and ureteral pelvic junction, incision of ureteral pelvic junction and insertion of endopyelotomy stent)

50576 with fulguration and/or incision, with or without biopsy

50580 with removal of foreign body or calculus

OTHER PROCEDURES

50590 Lithotripsy, extracorporeal shock wave

⊙ **50592** Ablation, one or more renal tumor(s), percutaneous, unilateral, radiofrequency

(50592 is a unilateral procedure. For bilateral procedure, report 50592 with modifier 50)

(For imaging guidance and monitoring, see 76940, 77013, 77022)

⊙ **50593** Ablation, renal tumor(s), unilateral, percutaneous, cryotherapy

(50593 is a unilatral procedure. For bilateral procedure, report 50593 with modifier -50)

(For imaging guidance and monitoring, see codes 76940, 77013, 77022)

713

Separate Procedure	Unlisted Procedure	CCI Comp. Code	Non-specific Procedure

URETER

INCISION

50600 Ureterotomy with exploration or drainage (separate procedure)

(For ureteral endoscopy performed in conjunction with this procedure, see 50970-50980)

50605 Ureterotomy for insertion of indwelling stent, all types

50610 Ureterolithotomy; upper one-third of ureter

50620 middle one-third of ureter

50630 lower one-third of ureter

(For laparoscopic approach, use 50945)

(For transvesical ureterolithotomy, use 51060)

(For cystotomy with stone basket extraction of ureteral calculus, use 51065)

(For endoscopic extraction or manipulation of ureteral calculus, see 50080, 50081, 50561, 50961, 50980, 52320-52330, 52352, 52353)

EXCISION

(For ureterocele, see 51535, 52300)

50650 Ureterectomy, with bladder cuff (separate procedure)

50660 Ureterectomy, total, ectopic ureter, combination abdominal, vaginal and/or perineal approach

INTRODUCTION

50684 Injection procedure for ureterography or ureteropyelography through ureterostomy or indwelling ureteral catheter

(For radiological supervision and interpretation, use 74425)

50686 Manometric studies through ureterostomy or indwelling ureteral catheter

50688 Change of ureterostomy tube or externally accessible ureteral stent via ileal conduit

● New Code ▲ Revised Code + Add-On Code ⊘ Modifier -51 Exempt ⊙ Moderate Sedation

(If imaging guidance is performed, use 75984)

50690 Injection procedure for visualization of ileal conduit and/or ureteropyelography, exclusive of radiologic service

(For radiological supervision and interpretation, use 74425)

REPAIR

50700 Ureteroplasty, plastic operation on ureter (eg, stricture)

50715 Ureterolysis, with or without repositioning of ureter for retroperitoneal fibrosis

(For bilateral procedure, report 50715 with modifier -50)

50722 Ureterolysis for ovarian vein syndrome

50725 Ureterolysis for retrocaval ureter, with reanastomosis of upper urinary tract or vena cava

50727 Revision of urinary-cutaneous anastomosis (any type urostomy);

50728 with repair of fascial defect and hernia

50740 Ureteropyelostomy, anastomosis of ureter and renal pelvis

50750 Ureterocalycostomy, anastomosis of ureter to renal calyx

50760 Ureteroureterostomy

50770 Transureteroureterostomy, anastomosis of ureter to contralateral ureter

(Codes 50780-50785 include minor procedures to prevent vesicoureteral reflux)

50780 Ureteroneocystostomy; anastomosis of single ureter to bladder

(For bilateral procedure, report 50780 with modifier -50)

(When combined with cystourethroplasty or vesical neck revision, use 51820)

50782 anastomosis of duplicated ureter to bladder

50783 with extensive ureteral tailoring

715

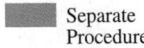 Separate Procedure   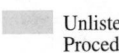 Unlisted Procedure   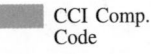 CCI Comp. Code   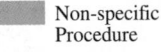 Non-specific Procedure

50785 with vesico-psoas hitch or bladder flap

(For bilateral procedure, report 50785 with modifier -50)

50800 Ureteroenterostomy, direct anastomosis of ureter to intestine

(For bilateral procedure, report 50800 with modifier -50)

50810 Ureterosigmoidostomy, with creation of sigmoid bladder and establishment of abdominal or perineal colostomy, including intestine anastomosis

50815 Ureterocolon conduit, including intestine anastomosis

(For bilateral procedure, report 50815 with modifier -50)

50820 Ureteroileal conduit (ileal bladder), including intestine anastomosis (Bricker operation)

(For bilateral procedure, report 50820 with modifier -50)

(For combination of 50800-50820 with cystectomy, see 51580-51595)

50825 Continent diversion, including intestine anastomosis using any segment of small and/or large intestine (Kock pouch or Camey enterocystoplasty)

50830 Urinary undiversion (eg, taking down of ureteroileal conduit, ureterosigmoidostomy or ureteroenterostomy with ureteroureterostomy or ureteroneocystostomy)

50840 Replacement of all or part of ureter by intestine segment, including intestine anastomosis

(For bilateral procedure, report 50840 with modifier -50)

50845 Cutaneous appendico-vesicostomy

50860 Ureterostomy, transplantation of ureter to skin

(For bilateral procedure, report 50860 with modifier -50)

50900 Ureterorrhaphy, suture of ureter (separate procedure)

50920 Closure of ureterocutaneous fistula

50930 Closure of ureterovisceral fistula (including visceral repair)

● New Code ▲ Revised Code + Add-On Code ⊘ Modifier -51 Exempt ⊙ Moderate Sedation

50940   Deligation of ureter

(For ureteroplasty, ureterolysis, see 50700-50860)

LAPAROSCOPY

Surgical laparoscopy always includes diagnostic laparoscopy. To report a diagnostic laparoscopy (peritoneoscopy) (separate procedure), use 49320.

50945   Laparoscopy, surgical; ureterolithotomy

50947   ureteroneocystostomy with cystoscopy and ureteral stent placement

50948   ureteroneocystostomy without cystoscopy and ureteral stent placement

(For open ureteroneocystostomy, see 50780-50785)

50949   Unlisted laparoscopy procedure, ureter

ENDOSCOPY

50951   Ureteral endoscopy through established ureterostomy, with or without irrigation, instillation, or ureteropyelography, exclusive of radiologic service;

50953   with ureteral catheterization, with or without dilation of ureter

50955   with biopsy

50957   with fulguration and/or incision, with or without biopsy

50961   with removal of foreign body or calculus

(When procedures 50970-50980 provide a significant identifiable service, they may be added to 50600)

50970   Ureteral endoscopy through ureterotomy, with or without irrigation, instillation, or ureteropyelography, exclusive of radiologic service;

(For ureterotomy, use 50600)

50972   with ureteral catheterization, with or without dilation of ureter

---

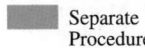 Separate Procedure   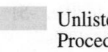 Unlisted Procedure   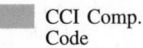 CCI Comp. Code   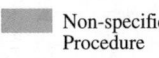 Non-specific Procedure   **717**

50974   with biopsy

50976   with fulguration and/or incision, with or without biopsy

50980   with removal of foreign body or calculus

BLADDER

INCISION

51020   Cystotomy or cystostomy; with fulguration and/or insertion of radioactive material

51030   with cryosurgical destruction of intravesical lesion

51040   Cystostomy, cystotomy with drainage

51045   Cystotomy, with insertion of ureteral catheter or stent (separate procedure)

51050   Cystolithotomy, cystotomy with removal of calculus, without vesical neck resection

51060   Transvesical ureterolithotomy

51065   Cystotomy, with calculus basket extraction and/or ultrasonic or electrohydraulic fragmentation of ureteral calculus

51080   Drainage of perivesical or prevesical space abscess

REMOVAL

51100   Aspiration of bladder; by needle

51101   by trocar or intracatheter

51102   with insertion of suprapubic catheter

(For imaging guidance, see 76942, 77002, 77012)

EXCISION

51500   Excision of urachal cyst or sinus, with or without umbilical hernia repair

51520   Cystotomy; for simple excision of vesical neck (separate procedure)

● New Code   ▲ Revised Code   ✛ Add-On Code   ⊘ Modifier -51 Exempt   ☉ Moderate Sedation

51525   for excision of bladder diverticulum, single or multiple
(separate procedure)

51530   for excision of bladder tumor

(For transurethral resection, see 52234-52240, 52305)

51535 Cystotomy for excision, incision, or repair of ureterocele

(For bilateral procedure, report 51535 with modifier -50)

(For transurethral excision, use 52300)

51550 Cystectomy, partial; simple

51555   complicated (eg, postradiation, previous surgery, difficult
location)

51565 Cystectomy, partial, with reimplantation of ureter(s) into bladder
(ureteroneocystostomy)

51570 Cystectomy, complete; (separate procedure)

51575   with bilateral pelvic lymphadenectomy, including external
iliac, hypogastric, and obturator nodes

51580 Cystectomy, complete, with ureterosigmoidostomy or
ureterocutaneous transplantations;

51585   with bilateral pelvic lymphadenectomy, including external
iliac, hypogastric, and obturator nodes

51590 Cystectomy, complete, with ureteroileal conduit or sigmoid
bladder, including intestine anastomosis;

51595   with bilateral pelvic lymphadenectomy, including external
iliac, hypogastric, and obturator nodes

51596 Cystectomy, complete, with continent diversion, any open
technique, using any segment of small and/or large intestine to
construct neobladder

51597 Pelvic exenteration, complete, for vesical, prostatic or urethral
malignancy, with removal of bladder and ureteral
transplantations, with or without hysterectomy and/or
abdominoperineal resection of rectum and colon and colostomy,
or any combination thereof

	Separate Procedure		Unlisted Procedure		CCI Comp. Code		Non-specific Procedure

719

CPT codes and descriptions only ©2012 American Medical Association. All rights reserved.

(For pelvic exenteration for gynecologic malignancy, use 58240)

INTRODUCTION

51600 Injection procedure for cystography or voiding urethrocystography

(For radiological supervision and interpretation, see 74430, 74455)

51605 Injection procedure and placement of chain for contrast and/or chain urethrocystography

(For radiological supervision and interpretation, use 74430)

51610 Injection procedure for retrograde urethrocystography

(For radiological supervision and interpretation, use 74450)

51700 Bladder irrigation, simple, lavage and/or instillation

(Codes 51701-51702 are reported only when performed independently. Do not report 51701-51702 when catheter insertion is an inclusive component of another procedure.)

51701 Insertion of non-indwelling bladder catheter (eg, straight catheterization of residual urine)

51702 Insertion of temporary indwelling bladder catheter; simple (eg, Foley)

51703 complicated (eg, altered anatomy, fractured catheter/balloon)

51705 Change of cystostomy tube; simple

51710 complicated

(If imaging guidance is performed, use 75984)

51715 Endoscopic injection of implant material into the submucosal tissues of the urethra and/or bladder neck

51720 Bladder instillation of anticarcinogenic agent (including retention time)

● New Code   ▲ Revised Code   ✚ Add-On Code   ⊘ Modifier -51 Exempt   ⊙ Moderate Sedation

URODYNAMICS

The following section (51725-51798) lists procedures that may be used separately or in many and varied combinations.

When multiple procedures are performed in the same investigative session, modifier -51 should be employed.

All procedures in this section imply that these services are performed by, or are under the direct supervision of, a physician or other qualified health care professional and that all instruments, equipment, fluids, gases, probes, catheters, technician's fees, medications, gloves, trays, tubing and other sterile supplies be provided by that individual. When the individual only interprets the results and/or operates the equipment, a professional component, modifier -26 should be used to identify physcians' services.

51725   Simple cystometrogram (CMG) (eg, spinal manometer)

51726   Complex cystometrogram (ie, calibrated electronic equipment)

51727   with urethral pressure profile studies (ie, urethral closure pressure profile), any technique

51728   with voiding pressure studies (ie, bladder voiding pressure), any technique

51729   with voiding pressure studies (ie, bladder voiding pressure) and urethral pressure profile studies (ie, urethral closure pressure profile), any technique

+ **51797**   Voiding pressure studies, intra-abdominal (ie, rectal, gastric, intraperitoneal) (List separately in addition to code for primary procedure)

(Use 51797 in conjunction with 51728, 51729)

51736   Simple uroflowmetry (UFR) (eg, stop-watch flow rate, mechanical uroflowmeter)

51741   Complex uroflowmetry (eg, calibrated electronic equipment)

(51772   Deleted 2009 [2010 edition]. To report urethral pressure profile studies, see 51727, 51729)

51784   Electromyography studies (EMG) of anal or urethral sphincter, other than needle, any technique

---

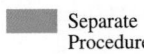 Separate Procedure   Unlisted Procedure   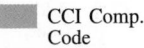 CCI Comp. Code   Non-specific Procedure

721

51785 Needle electromyography studies (EMG) of anal or urethral sphincter, any technique

51792 Stimulus evoked response (eg, measurement of bulbocavernosus reflex latency time)

(51795 Deleted 2009 [2010 edition]. To report bladder pressure voidign studies, see 51728, 51729)

51797 This code is out of order. See page 721

51798 Measurement of post-voiding residual urine and/or bladder capacity by ultrasound, non-imaging

REPAIR

51800 Cystoplasty or cystourethroplasty, plastic operation on bladder and/or vesical neck (anterior Y-plasty, vesical fundus resection), any procedure, with or without wedge resection of posterior vesical neck

51820 Cystourethroplasty with unilateral or bilateral ureteroneocystostomy

51840 Anterior vesicourethropexy, or urethropexy (eg, Marshall-Marchetti-Krantz, Burch); simple

51841   complicated (eg, secondary repair)

(For urethropexy (Pereyra type), use 57289)

51845 Abdomino-vaginal vesical neck suspension, with or without endoscopic control (eg, Stamey, Raz, modified Pereyra)

51860 Cystorrhaphy, suture of bladder wound, injury or rupture; simple

51865   complicated

51880 Closure of cystostomy (separate procedure)

51900 Closure of vesicovaginal fistula, abdominal approach

(For vaginal approach, see 57320-57330)

51920 Closure of vesicouterine fistula;

● New Code   ▲ Revised Code   ✛ Add-On Code   ⊘ Modifier -51 Exempt   ⊙ Moderate Sedation

51925   with hysterectomy

(For closure of vesicoenteric fistula, see 44660, 44661)

(For closure of rectovesical fistula, see 45800-45805)

51940   Closure, exstrophy of bladder

(See also 54390)

51960   Enterocystoplasty, including intestinal anastomosis

51980   Cutaneous vesicostomy

LAPAROSCOPY

Surgical laparoscopy always includes diagnostic laparoscopy. To report a diagnostic laparoscopy (peritoneoscopy) (separate procedure), use 49320.

51990   Laparoscopy, surgical; urethral suspension for stress incontinence

51992   sling operation for stress incontinence (eg, fascia or synthetic)

(For open sling operation for stress incontinence, use 57288)

(For reversal or removal of sling operation for stress incontinence, use 57287)

51999   Unlisted laparoscopy procedure, bladder

ENDOSCOPY—CYSTOSCOPY, URETHROSCOPY, CYSTOURETHROSCOPY

Endoscopic descriptions are listed so that the main procedure can be identified without having to list all the minor related functions performed at the same time. For example, meatotomy, urethral calibration and/or dilation, urethroscopy, and cystoscopy prior to a transurethral resection of prostate; ureteral catheterization following extraction of ureteral calculus; internal urethrotomy and bladder neck fulguration when performing a cystourethroscopy for the female urethral syndrome. When the secondary procedure requires significant additional time and effort, it may be identified by the addition of modifier 22.

For example, urethrotomy performed for a documented pre-existing stricture or bladder neck contracture.

52000   Cystourethroscopy (separate procedure)

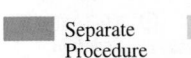 Separate Procedure   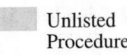 Unlisted Procedure   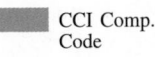 CCI Comp. Code   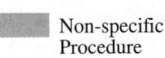 Non-specific Procedure

52001 Cystourethroscopy with irrigation and evacuation of multiple obstructing clots

(Do not report 52001 in addition to 52000)

52005 Cystourethroscopy, with ureteral catheterization, with or without irrigation, instillation, or ureteropyelography, exclusive of radiologic service;

52007 with brush biopsy of ureter and/or renal pelvis

52010 Cystourethroscopy, with ejaculatory duct catheterization, with or without irrigation, instillation, or duct radiography, exclusive of radiologic service

(For radiological supervision and interpretation, use 74440)

TRANSURETHRAL SURGERY

Urethra and Bladder

52204 Cystourethroscopy, with biopsy(s)

52214 Cystourethroscopy, with fulguration (including cryosurgery or laser surgery) of trigone, bladder neck, prostatic fossa, urethra, or periurethral glands

(For transurethral fulguration of prostate tissue performed within the postoperative period of 52601 or 52630 performed by the same physician, append modifier 78)

(For transurethral fulguration of prostate tissue performed within the postoperative period of a related procedure performed by the same physician, append modifier 78)

(For transurethral fulguration of prostate for postoperative bleeding performed by the same physician, append modifier 78)

52224 Cystourethroscopy, with fulguration (including cryosurgery or laser surgery) or treatment of MINOR (less than 0.5 cm) lesion(s) with or without biopsy

52234 Cystourethroscopy, with fulguration (including cryosurgery or laser surgery) and/or resection of; SMALL bladder tumor(s) (0.5 up to 2.0 cm)

52235 MEDIUM bladder tumor(s) (2.0 to 5.0 cm)

52240 LARGE bladder tumor(s)

724

● New Code   ▲ Revised Code   + Add-On Code   ⊘ Modifier -51 Exempt   ⊙ Moderate Sedation

52250 Cystourethroscopy with insertion of radioactive substance, with or without biopsy or fulguration

52260 Cystourethroscopy, with dilation of bladder for interstitial cystitis; general or conduction (spinal) anesthesia

52265 local anesthesia

52270 Cystourethroscopy, with internal urethrotomy; female

52275 male

52276 Cystourethroscopy with direct vision internal urethrotomy

52277 Cystourethroscopy, with resection of external sphincter (sphincterotomy)

52281 Cystourethroscopy, with calibration and/or dilation of urethral stricture or stenosis, with or without meatotomy, with or without injection procedure for cystography, male or female

52282 Cystourethroscopy, with insertion of permanent urethral stent

(For placement of temporary prostatic urethral stent, use 53855)

52283 Cystourethroscopy, with steroid injection into stricture

52285 Cystourethroscopy for treatment of the female urethral syndrome with any or all of the following: urethral meatotomy, urethral dilation, internal urethrotomy, lysis of urethrovaginal septal fibrosis, lateral incisions of the bladder neck, and fulguration of polyp(s) of urethra, bladder neck, and/or trigone

● **52287** Cystourethroscopy, with injection(s) for chemodenervation of the bladder

(The suppy of the chemodenervation agent is reported separately)

52290 Cystourethroscopy; with ureteral meatotomy, unilateral or bilateral

52300 with resection or fulguration of orthotopic ureterocele(s), unilateral or bilateral

52301 with resection or fulguration of ectopic ureterocele(s), unilateral or bilateral

	Separate Procedure		Unlisted Procedure		CCI Comp. Code		Non-specific Procedure

725

52305 with incision or resection of orifice of bladder diverticulum, single or multiple

52310 Cystourethroscopy, with removal of foreign body, calculus, or ureteral stent from urethra or bladder (separate procedure); simple

52315 complicated

52317 Litholapaxy: crushing or fragmentation of calculus by any means in bladder and removal of fragments; simple or small (less than 2.5 cm)

52318 complicated or large (over 2.5 cm)

URETER AND PELVIS

Therapeutic cystourethroscopy always includes diagnostic cystourethroscopy. To report diagnostic cystourethroscopy, use 52000. Therapeutic cystourethroscopy with ureteroscopy and/or pyeloscopy always includes diagnostic cystourethroscopy with ureteroscopy and/or pyeloscopy. To report a diagnostic cystourethroscopy with ureteroscopy and/or pyeloscopy, use 52351.

Do not report 52000 in conjunction with 52320-52343.

Do not report 52351 in conjunction with 52344-52346, 52352-52355.

The insertion and removal of a temporary ureteral catheter (52005) during diagnostic or therapeutic cystourethroscopic with ureteroscopy and/or pyeloscopy is included in 52320-52355 and should not be reported separately.

To report insertion of a self-retaining, indwelling stent performed during diagnostic or therapeutic cystourethroscopy with ureteroscopy and/or pyeloscopy, report 52332 in addition to primary procedure(s) performed (52320-52355) andappend modifier 51. 52332 is used to report a unilateral procedure unless otherwise specified.

For bilateral insertion of self-retaining, indwelling ureteral stents, use code 52332, and append modifier 50.

To report cystourethroscopic removal of a self-retaining indwelling ureteral stent, see 52310, 52315, and append modifier 58 if appropriate

52320 Cystourethroscopy (including ureteral catheterization); with removal of ureteral calculus

52325 with fragmentation of ureteral calculus (eg, ultrasonic or electro-hydraulic technique)

| • New Code | ▲ Revised Code | + Add-On Code | ⊘ Modifier -51 Exempt | ⊙ Moderate Sedation |

52327   with subureteric injection of implant material

52330   with manipulation, without removal of ureteral calculus

52332   Cystourethroscopy, with insertion of indwelling ureteral stent (eg, Gibbons or double-J type)

52334   Cystourethroscopy with insertion of ureteral guide wire through kidney to establish a percutaneous nephrostomy, retrograde

(For percutaneous nephrostolithotomy, see 50080, 50081; for establishment of nephrostomy tract only, use 50395)

(For cystourethroscopy, with ureteroscopy and/or pyeloscopy, see 52351-52355)

(For cystourethroscopy with incision, fulguration, or resection of congential posterior urethral valves or obstructive hypertrophic mucosal folds, use 52400)

52341   Cystourethroscopy; with treatment of ureteral stricture (eg, balloon dilation, laser, electrocautery, and incision)

52342   with treatment of ureteropelvic junction stricture (eg, balloon dilation, laser, electrocautery, and incision)

52343   with treatment of intra-renal stricture (eg, balloon dilation, laser, electrocautery, and incision)

52344   Cystourethroscopy with ureteroscopy; with treatment of ureteral stricture (eg, balloon dilation, laser, electrocautery, and incision)

52345   with treatment of ureteropelvic junction stricture (eg, balloon dilation, laser, electrocautery, and incision)

52346   with treatment of intra-renal stricture (eg, balloon dilation, laser, electrocautery, and incision)

(For transurethral resection or incision of ejaculatory ducts, use 52402)

52351   Cystourethroscopy, with ureteroscopy and/or pyeloscopy; diagnostic

(For radiological supervision and interpretation, use 74485)

(Do not report 52351 in conjunction with 52341-52346, 52352-52355)

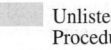 Separate Procedure   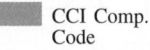 Unlisted Procedure   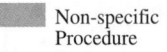 CCI Comp. Code   Non-specific Procedure

727

52352   with removal or manipulation of calculus (ureteral catheterization is included)

52353   with lithotripsy (ureteral catheterization is included)

52354   with biopsy and/or fulguration of ureteral or renal pelvic lesion

52355   with resection of ureteral or renal pelvic tumor

VESICAL NECK AND PROSTATE

52400   Cystourethroscopy with incision, fulguration, or resection of congenital posterior urethral valves, or congenital obstructive hypertrophic mucosal folds

52402   Cystourethroscopy with transurethral resection or incision of ejaculatory ducts

52450   Transurethral incision of prostate

52500   Transurethral resection of bladder neck (separate procedure)

52601   Transurethral electrosurgical resection of prostate, including control of postoperative bleeding, complete (vasectomy, meatotomy, cystourethroscopy, urethral calibration and/or dilation, and internal urethrotomy are included)

(For other approaches, see 55801-55845)

(52606   deleted 2009 edition. For transurethral fulguration of prostate, use 52214)

(52612   deleted 2009 edition. For first stage transurethral partial resection of prostate, use 52601. For second stage partial resection of prostate, use 52601 with modifier -58. For transurethral resection of residual or regrowth of obstructive prostate tissue, use 52630)

(52614   deleted 2009 edition. For first stage transurethral partial resection of prostate, use 52601. For second stage partial resection of prostate, use 52601 with modifier -58. For transurethral resection of residual or regrowth of obstructive prostate tissue, use 52630)

(52620   deleted 2009 edition. For first stage transurethral partial resection of prostate, use 52601. For second stage partial resection of prostate, use 52601 with modifier -58. For

● New Code   ▲ Revised Code   + Add-On Code   ⊘ Modifier -51 Exempt   ⊙ Moderate Sedation

transurethral resection of residual or regrowth of obstructive prostate tissue, use 52630)

52630 Transurethral resection; residual or regrowth of obstructive prostate tissue including control of postoperative bleeding, complete (vasectomy, meatotomy, cystourethroscopy, urethral calibration and/or dilation, and internal urethrotomy are included)

(For resection of residual prostate tissue performed within the postoperative period of a related procedure performed by the same physician, append modifier 78)

52640 of postoperative bladder neck contracture

52647 Laser coagulation of prostate, including control of postoperative bleeding, complete (vasectomy, meatotomy, cystourethroscopy, urethral calibration and/or dilation, and internal urethrotomy are included if performed)

52648 Laser vaporization of prostate, including control of postoperative bleeding, complete (vasectomy, meatotomy, cystourethroscopy, urethral calibration and/or dilation, internal urethrotomy and transurethral resection of prostate are included if performed)

52649 Laser enucleation of the prostate with morcellation, including control of postoperative bleeding, complete (vasectomy, meatotomy, cystourethroscopy, urethral calibration and/or dilation, internal urethrotomy and transurethral resection of prostate are included if performed)

(Do not report 52649 in conjunction with 52000, 52276, 52281, 52601, 52647, 52648, 53020, 55250)

52700 Transurethral drainage of prostatic abscess

(For litholapaxy, use 52317, 52318)

URETHRA

(For endoscopy, see cystoscopy, urethroscopy, cystourethroscopy, 52000-52700)

(For injection procedure for urethrocystography, see 51600-51610)

 Separate Procedure   Unlisted Procedure   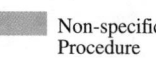 CCI Comp. Code   Non-specific Procedure

INCISION

53000 Urethrotomy or urethrostomy, external (separate procedure); pendulous urethra

53010 perineal urethra, external

53020 Meatotomy, cutting of meatus (separate procedure); except infant

53025 infant

(Do not report modifier '-63' in conjunction with 53025)

53040 Drainage of deep periurethral abscess

(For subcutaneous abscess, see 10060, 10061)

53060 Drainage of Skene's gland abscess or cyst

53080 Drainage of perineal urinary extravasation; uncomplicated (separate procedure)

53085 complicated

EXCISION

53200 Biopsy of urethra

53210 Urethrectomy, total, including cystostomy; female

53215 male

53220 Excision or fulguration of carcinoma of urethra

53230 Excision of urethral diverticulum (separate procedure); female

53235 male

53240 Marsupialization of urethral diverticulum, male or female

53250 Excision of bulbourethral gland (Cowper's gland)

53260 Excision or fulguration; urethral polyp(s), distal urethra

(For endoscopic approach, see 52214, 52224)

● New Code ▲ Revised Code + Add-On Code ⊘ Modifier -51 Exempt ⊙ Moderate Sedation

| 53265 | urethral caruncle |

| 53270 | Skene's glands |

| 53275 | urethral prolapse |

REPAIR

(For hypospadias, see 54300-54352)

| 53400 | Urethroplasty; first stage, for fistula, diverticulum, or stricture (eg, Johannsen type) |

| 53405 | second stage (formation of urethra), including urinary diversion |

| 53410 | Urethroplasty, 1-stage reconstruction of male anterior urethra |

| 53415 | Urethroplasty, transpubic or perineal, one stage, for reconstruction or repair of prostatic or membranous urethra |

| 53420 | Urethroplasty, 2-stage reconstruction or repair of prostatic or membranous urethra; first stage |

| 53425 | second stage |

| 53430 | Urethroplasty, reconstruction of female urethra |

| 53431 | Urethroplasty with tubularization of posterior urethra and/or lower bladder for incontinence (eg, Tenago, Leadbetter procedure) |

| 53440 | Sling operation for correction of male urinary incontinence (eg, fascia or synthetic) |

| 53442 | Removal or revision of sling for male urinary incontinence (eg, fascia or synthetic) |

| 53444 | Insertion of tandem cuff (dual cuff) |

| 53445 | Insertion of inflatable urethral/bladder neck sphincter, including placement of pump, reservoir, and cuff |

| 53446 | Removal of inflatable urethral/bladder neck sphincter, including pump, reservoir, and cuff |

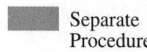 Separate Procedure   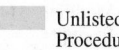 Unlisted Procedure   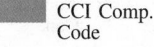 CCI Comp. Code   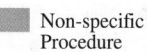 Non-specific Procedure

53447 Removal and replacement of inflatable urethral/bladder neck sphincter including pump, reservoir, and cuff at the same operative session

53448 Removal and replacement of inflatable urethral/bladder neck sphincter including pump, reservoir, and cuff through an infected field at the same operative session including irrigation and debridement of infected tissue

(Do not report 11042, 11043 in addition to 53448)

53449 Repair of inflatable urethral/bladder neck sphincter, including pump, reservoir, and cuff

53450 Urethromeatoplasty, with mucosal advancement

(For meatotomy, see 53020, 53025)

53460 Urethromeatoplasty, with partial excision of distal urethral segment (Richardson type procedure)

53500 Urethrolysis, transvaginal, secondary, open, including cystourethroscopy (eg, postsurgical obstruction, scarring)

(For urethrolysis by retropubic approach, use 53899)

(Do not report 53500 in conjunction with 52000)

53502 Urethrorrhaphy, suture of urethral wound or injury; female

53505 penile

53510 perineal

53515 prostatomembranous

53520 Closure of urethrostomy or urethrocutaneous fistula, male (separate procedure)

(For closure of urethrovaginal fistula, use 57310)

(For closure of urethrorectal fistula, see 45820, 45825)

MANIPULATION

(For radiological supervision and interpretation, use 74485)

53600 Dilation of urethral stricture by passage of sound or urethral dilator, male; initial

● New Code	▲ Revised Code	+ Add-On Code	⊘ Modifier -51 Exempt	⊙ Moderate Sedation

53601   subsequent

53605   Dilation of urethral stricture or vesical neck by passage of sound or urethral dilator, male, general or conduction (spinal) anesthesia

(For dilation of urethral stricture, male, performed under local anesthesia, see 53600, 53601, 53620, 53621)

53620   Dilation of urethral stricture by passage of filiform and follower, male; initial

53621   subsequent

53660   Dilation of female urethra including suppository and/or instillation; initial

53661   subsequent

53665   Dilation of female urethra, general or conduction (spinal) anesthesia

(For urethral catheterization, see 51701-51703)

(For dilation of urethra performed under local anesthesia, female, see 53660, 53661)

OTHER PROCEDURES

(For two or three glass urinalysis, use 81020)

53850   Transurethral destruction of prostate tissue; by microwave thermotherapy

53852   by radiofrequency thermotherapy

(53853   deleted 2009 edition; use 55899)

53855   Insertion of a temporary prostatic urethral stent, including urethral measurement

(For insertion of permanent urethral stent, use 52282)

53860   Transurethral radiofrequency micro-remodeling of the female bladder neck and proximal urethra for stress urinary incontinence

53899   Unlisted procedure, urinary system

733

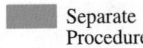 Separate Procedure   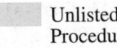 Unlisted Procedure   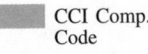 CCI Comp. Code   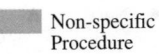 Non-specific Procedure

This page intentionally left blank.

● New
Code

▲ Revised
Code

+ Add-On
Code

⊘ Modifier -51
Exempt

⊙ Moderate
Sedation

MALE GENITAL SYSTEM

CPT codes from this section of CPT are used to report invasive and surgical procedures performed on the penis; testis; epididymis; scrotum; spermatic cord and prostate.

Transurethral drainage of a prostatic abscess (e.g. CPT code 52700) is included in male transurethral prostatic procedures and is not reported separately.

Urethral catheterization (e.g. CPT codes 51701, 51702, and 51703), when medically necessary to successfully accomplish a procedure, should not be separately reported.

The puncture aspiration of a hydrocele (e.g. CPT code 55000) is included in services involving the tunica vaginalis and proximate anatomy (scrotum, vas deferens) and in inguinal hernia repairs.

A number of codes describe surgical procedures of a progressively more comprehensive nature or with different approaches to accomplish similar services. In general, these groups of codes are not to be reported together (see mutually exclusive policy). While a number of these groups of codes exist in CPT, a specific example includes the series of codes describing prostate procedures (CPT codes 55801-55845). In addition, all prostatectomy procedures (e.g. CPT codes 52601-52648 and 55801- 55845) are also mutually exclusive of one another.

PENIS

INCISION

(For abdominal perineal gangrene debridement, see 11004-11006)

54000   Slitting of prepuce, dorsal or lateral (separate procedure); newborn

(Do not report modifier '-63' in conjunction with 54000)

54001   except newborn

54015   Incision and drainage of penis, deep

(For skin and subcutaneous abscess, see 10060-10160)

DESTRUCTION

54050   Destruction of lesion(s), penis (eg, condyloma, papilloma, molluscum contagiosum, herpetic vesicle), simple; chemical

735

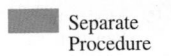 Separate Procedure   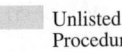 Unlisted Procedure   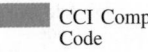 CCI Comp. Code   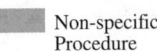 Non-specific Procedure

54055   electrodesiccation

54056   cryosurgery

54057   laser surgery

54060   surgical excision

54065   Destruction of lesion(s), penis (eg, condyloma, papilloma, molluscum contagiosum, herpetic vesicle), extensive (eg, laser surgery, electosurgery, cryosurgery, chemosurgery)

(For destruction or excision of other lesions, see Integumentary System)

EXCISION

54100   Biopsy of penis; (separate procedure)

54105   deep structures

54110   Excision of penile plaque (Peyronie disease);

54111   with graft to 5 cm in length

54112   with graft greater than 5 cm in length

54115   Removal foreign body from deep penile tissue (eg, plastic implant)

54120   Amputation of penis; partial

54125   complete

54130   Amputation of penis, radical; with bilateral inguinofemoral lymphadenectomy

54135   in continuity with bilateral pelvic lymphadenectomy, including external iliac, hypogastric and obturator nodes

(For lymphadenectomy (separate procedure) see 38760-38770)

54150   Circumcision, using clamp or other device with regional dorsal penile or ring block

(Do not report modifier -63 in conjunction with 54150)

---

736   New
Code   Revised
Code   Add-On
Code   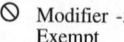 Modifier -51
Exempt   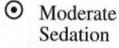 Moderate
Sedation

(Report 54150 with modifier 52 when performed without dorsal penile or ring block)

54160 Circumcision, surgical excision other than clamp, device or dorsal slit; neonate (28 days of age or less)

(Do not report modifier -63 in conjunction with 54160)

54161 older than 28 days of age

54162 Lysis or excision of penile post-circumcision adhesions

54163 Repair incomplete circumcision

54164 Frenulotomy of penis

(Do not report with circumcision codes 54150-54161, 54162, 54163)

INTRODUCTION

54200 Injection procedure for Peyronie disease;

54205 with surgical exposure of plaque

54220 Irrigation of corpora cavernosa for priapism

54230 Injection procedure for corpora cavernosography

(For radiological supervision and interpretation, use 74445)

54231 Dynamic cavernosometry, including intracavernosal injection of vasoactive drugs (eg, papaverine, phentolamine)

54235 Injection of corpora cavernosa with pharmacologic agent(s) (eg, papaverine, phentolamine)

54240 Penile plethysmography

54250 Nocturnal penile tumescence and/or rigidity test

REPAIR

(For other urethroplasties, see 53400-53430)

(For penile revascularization, use 37788)

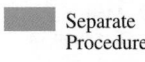 Separate Procedure   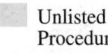 Unlisted Procedure   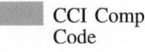 CCI Comp. Code   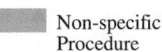 Non-specific Procedure

54300 Plastic operation of penis for straightening of chordee (eg, hypospadias), with or without mobilization of urethra

54304 Plastic operation on penis for correction of chordee or for first stage hypospadias repair with or without transplantation of prepuce and/or skin flaps

54308 Urethroplasty for second stage hypospadias repair (including urinary diversion); less than 3 cm

54312 greater than 3 cm

54316 Urethroplasty for second stage hypospadias repair (including urinary diversion) with free skin graft obtained from site other than genitalia

54318 Urethroplasty for third stage hypospadias repair to release penis from scrotum (eg, third stage Cecil repair)

54322 1 stage distal hypospadias repair (with or without chordee or circumcision); with simple meatal advancement (eg, Magpi, V-flap)

54324 with urethroplasty by local skin flaps (eg, flip-flap, prepucial flap)

54326 with urethroplasty by local skin flaps and mobilization of urethra

54328 with extensive dissection to correct chordee and urethroplasty with local skin flaps, skin graft patch, and/or island flap

(For urethroplasty and straightening of chordee, use 54308)

54332 1 stage proximal penile or penoscrotal hypospadias repair requiring extensive dissection to correct chordee and urethroplasty by use of skin graft tube and/or island flap

54336 1 stage perineal hypospadias repair requiring extensive dissection to correct chordee and urethroplasty by use of skin graft tube and/or island flap

54340 Repair of hypospadias complications (ie, fistula, stricture, diverticula); by closure, incision, or excision, simple

738

● New
Code

▲ Revised
Code

+ Add-On
Code

⊘ Modifier -51
Exempt

⊙ Moderate
Sedation

54344   requiring mobilization of skin flaps and urethroplasty with flap or patch graft

54348   requiring extensive dissection and urethroplasty with flap, patch or tubed graft (includes urinary diversion)

54352   Repair of hypospadias cripple requiring extensive dissection and excision of previously constructed structures including re-release of chordee and reconstruction of urethra and penis by use of local skin as grafts and island flaps and skin brought in as flaps or grafts

54360   Plastic operation on penis to correct angulation

54380   Plastic operation on penis for epispadias distal to external sphincter;

54385   with incontinence

54390   with exstrophy of bladder

54400   Insertion of penile prosthesis; non-inflatable (semi-rigid)

54401   inflatable (self-contained)

(For removal or replacement of penile prosthesis, see 54415, 54416)

54405   Insertion of multi-component inflatable penile prosthesis, including placement of pump, cylinders, and reservoir

(For reduced services, report 54405 with modifier -52)

54406   Removal of all components of a multi-component inflatable penile prosthesis without replacement of prosthesis

(For reduced services, report 54406 with modifier -52)

54408   Repair of component(s) of a multi-component, inflatable penile prosthesis

54410   Removal and replacement of all component(s) of a multi-component inflatable penile prosthesis at the same operative session

54411   Removal and replacement of all components of a multi-component inflatable penile prosthesis through an infected

| | Separate Procedure | | Unlisted Procedure | | CCI Comp. Code | | Non-specific Procedure |

739

field at the same operative session, including irrigation and debridement of infected tissue

(For reduced services, report 54411 with modifier -52)

(Do not report 11042, 11043 in addition to 54411)

54415 Removal of non-inflatable (semi-rigid) or inflatable (self-contained) penile prosthesis, without replacement of prosthesis

54416 Removal and replacement of non-inflatable (semi-rigid) or inflatable (self-contained) penile prosthesis at the same operative session

54417 Removal and replacement of non-inflatable (semi-rigid) or inflatable (self-contained) penile prosthesis through an infected field at the same operative session, including irrigation and debridement of infected tissue

(Do not report 11042, 11043 in addition to 54417)

54420 Corpora cavernosa-saphenous vein shunt (priapism operation), unilateral or bilateral

54430 Corpora cavernosa-corpus spongiosum shunt (priapism operation), unilateral or bilateral

54435 Corpora cavernosa-glans penis fistulization (eg, biopsy needle, Winter procedure, rongeur, or punch) for priapism

54440 Plastic operation of penis for injury

MANIPULATION

54450 Foreskin manipulation including lysis of preputial adhesions and stretching

TESTIS

EXCISION

(For abdominal perineal gangrene debridement, see 11004-11006)

54500 Biopsy of testis, needle (separate procedure)

(For fine needle aspiration, see 10021, 10022)

● New Code ▲ Revised Code ✛ Add-On Code ⊘ Modifier -51 Exempt ☉ Moderate Sedation

(For evaluation of fine needle aspirate, see 88172, 88173)

54505 Biopsy of testis, incisional (separate procedure)

(For bilateral procedure, report 54505 with modifier -50)

(When combined with vasogram, seminal vesiculogram, or epididymogram, use 55300)

54512 Excision of extraparenchymal lesion of testis

54520 Orchiectomy, simple (including subcapsular), with or without testicular prosthesis, scrotal or inguinal approach

(For bilateral procedure, report 54520 with modifier -50)

54522 Orchiectomy, partial

54530 Orchiectomy, radical, for tumor; inguinal approach

54535 with abdominal exploration

(For orchiectomy with repair of hernia, see 49505 or 49507 and 54520)

(For radical retroperitoneal lymphadenectomy, use 38780)

EXPLORATION

54550 Exploration for undescended testis (inguinal or scrotal area)

(For bilateral procedure, report 54550 with modifier -50)

54560 Exploration for undescended testis with abdominal exploration

(For bilateral procedure, report 54560 with modifier -50)

REPAIR

54600 Reduction of torsion of testis, surgical, with or without fixation of contralateral testis

54620 Fixation of contralateral testis (separate procedure)

54640 Orchiopexy, inguinal approach, with or without hernia repair

(For bilateral procedure, report 54640 with modifier -50)

(For inguinal hernia repair performed in conjunction with inguinal orchiopexy, see 49495-49525)

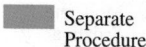 Separate Procedure   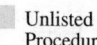 Unlisted Procedure   CCI Comp. Code   Non-specific Procedure

741

54650 Orchiopexy, abdominal approach, for intra-abdominal testis (eg, Fowler-Stephens)

(For laparoscopic approach, use 54692)

54660 Insertion of testicular prosthesis (separate procedure)

(For bilateral procedure, report 54660 with modifier -50)

54670 Suture or repair of testicular injury

54680 Transplantation of testis(es) to thigh (because of scrotal destruction)

LAPAROSCOPY

Surgical laparoscopy always includes diagnostic laparoscopy. To report a diagnostic laparoscopy (peritoneoscopy) (separate procedure), use 49320.

54690 Laparoscopy, surgical; orchiectomy

54692 orchiopexy for intra-abdominal testis

54699 Unlisted laparoscopy procedure, testis

EPIDIDYMIS

INCISION

54700 Incision and drainage of epididymis, testis and/or scrotal space (eg, abscess or hematoma)

(For debridement of necrotizing soft tissue infection of external genitalia, see 11004-11006)

EXCISION

54800 Biopsy of epididymis, needle

(For fine needle aspiration, see 10021, 10022)

(For evaluation of fine needle aspirate, see 88172, 88173)

54830 Excision of local lesion of epididymis

54840 Excision of spermatocele, with or without epididymectomy

54860 Epididymectomy; unilateral

● New Code   ▲ Revised Code   + Add-On Code   ⊘ Modifier -51 Exempt   ⊙ Moderate Sedation

54861 bilateral

EXPLORATION

54865 Exploration of epididymis, with or without biopsy

REPAIR

54900 Epididymovasostomy, anastomosis of epididymis to vas deferens; unilateral

54901 bilateral

(For operating microscope, use 69990)

TUNICA VAGINALIS

INCISION

55000 Puncture aspiration of hydrocele, tunica vaginalis, with or without injection of medication

EXCISION

55040 Excision of hydrocele; unilateral

55041 bilateral

(With hernia repair, see 49495-49501)

REPAIR

55060 Repair of tunica vaginalis hydrocele (Bottle type)

SCROTUM

INCISION

55100 Drainage of scrotal wall abscess

(See also 54700)

(For debridement of necrotizing soft tissue infection of external genitalia, see 11004-11006)

55110 Scrotal exploration

55120 Removal of foreign body in scrotum

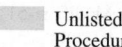 Separate Procedure   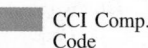 Unlisted Procedure   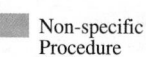 CCI Comp. Code   Non-specific Procedure   **743**

EXCISION

(For excision of local lesion of skin of scrotum, see Integumentary System)

55150 Resection of scrotum

REPAIR

55175 Scrotoplasty; simple

55180 complicated

VAS DEFERENS

INCISION

55200 Vasotomy, cannulization with or without incision of vas, unilateral or bilateral (separate procedure)

EXCISION

55250 Vasectomy, unilateral or bilateral (separate procedure), including postoperative semen examination(s)

INTRODUCTION

55300 Vasotomy for vasograms, seminal vesiculograms, or epididymograms, unilateral or bilateral

(For radiological supervision and interpretation, use 74440)

(When combined with biopsy of testis, see 54505 and use modifier -51)

REPAIR

55400 Vasovasostomy, vasovasorrhaphy

(For bilateral procedure, report 55400 with modifier -50)

(For operating microscope, use 69990)

SUTURE

55450 Ligation (percutaneous) of vas deferens, unilateral or bilateral (separate procedure)

● New Code   ▲ Revised Code   + Add-On Code   ⊘ Modifier -51 Exempt   ⊙ Moderate Sedation

SPERMATIC CORD

EXCISION

55500 Excision of hydrocele of spermatic cord, unilateral (separate procedure)

55520 Excision of lesion of spermatic cord (separate procedure)

55530 Excision of varicocele or ligation of spermatic veins for varicocele; (separate procedure)

55535 abdominal approach

55540 with hernia repair

LAPAROSCOPY

Surgical laparoscopy always includes diagnostic laparoscopy. To report a diagnostic laparoscopy (peritoneoscopy) (separate procedure), use 49320.

55550 Laparoscopy, surgical, with ligation of spermatic veins for varicocele

55559 Unlisted laparoscopy procedure, spermatic cord

SEMINAL VESICLES

INCISION

55600 Vesiculotomy;

(For bilateral procedure, report 55600 with modifier -50)

55605 complicated

EXCISION

55650 Vesiculectomy, any approach

(For bilateral procedure, report 55650 with modifier -50)

55680 Excision of Mullerian duct cyst

(For injection procedure, see 52010, 55300)

745

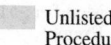 Separate Procedure

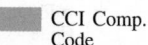 Unlisted Procedure

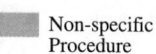 CCI Comp. Code

Non-specific Procedure

PROSTATE

INCISION

55700 Biopsy, prostate; needle or punch, single or multiple, any approach

(If imaging guidance is performed, use 76942)

(For fine needle aspiration, see 10021, 10022)

(For evaluation of fine needle aspirate, see 88172, 88173)

(For transperineal stereotactic template guided saturation prostate biopsies, use 55706)

55705 incisional, any approach

55706 Biopsies, prostate, needle, transperineal, stereotactic template guided saturation sampling, including imaging guidance

(Do not report 55706 in conjunction with 55700)

55720 Prostatotomy, external drainage of prostatic abscess, any approach; simple

55725 complicated

(For transurethral drainage, use 52700)

EXCISION

(For transurethral removal of prostate, see 52601-52640)

(For transurethral destruction of prostate, see 53850-53852)

(For limited pelvic lymphadenectomy for staging (separate procedure), use 38562)

(For independent node dissection, see 38770-38780)

55801 Prostatectomy, perineal, subtotal (including control of postoperative bleeding, vasectomy, meatotomy, urethral calibration and/or dilation, and internal urethrotomy)

55810 Prostatectomy, perineal radical;

55812 with lymph node biopsy(s) (limited pelvic lymphadenectomy)

● New Code   ▲ Revised Code   ✚ Add-On Code   ⊘ Modifier -51 Exempt   ⊙ Moderate Sedation

55815   with bilateral pelvic lymphadenectomy, including external iliac, hypogastric and obturator nodes

(If 55815 is carried out on separate days, use 38770 with modifier -50 and 55810)

55821 Prostatectomy (including control of postoperative bleeding, vasectomy, meatotomy, urethral calibration and/or dilation, and internal urethrotomy); suprapubic, subtotal, one or two stages

55831   retropubic, subtotal

55840 Prostatectomy, retropubic radical, with or without nerve sparing;

55842   with lymph node biopsy(s) (limited pelvic lymphadenectomy)

55845   with bilateral pelvic lymphadenectomy, including external iliac, hypogastric, and obturator nodes

(If 55845 is carried out on separate days, use 38770 with modifier -50 and 55840)

(For laparoscopic retropubic radical prostatectomy, use 55866)

55860 Exposure of prostate, any approach, for insertion of radioactive substance;

(For application of interstitial radioelement, see 77776-77778)

55862   with lymph node biopsy(s) (limited pelvic lymphadenectomy)

55865   with bilateral pelvic lymphadenectomy, including external iliac, hypogastric and obturator nodes

LAPAROSCOPY

Surgical laparoscopy always includes diagnostic laparoscopy. To report a diagnostic laparoscopy (peritoneoscopy) (separate procedure), use 49320.

55866 Laparoscopy, surgical prostatectomy, retropubic radical, including nerve sparing, includes robotic assistance, when performed

(For open procedure, use 55840)

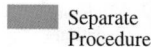 Separate Procedure   Unlisted Procedure   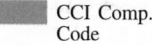 CCI Comp. Code   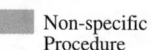 Non-specific Procedure   **747**

OTHER PROCEDURES

(For artificial insemination, see 58321, 58322)

55870   Electroejaculation

55873   Cryosurgical ablation of the prostate (includes ultrasonic guidance and monitoring)

55875   Transperineal placement of needles or catheters into prostate for interstitial radioelement application, with or without cystoscopy

(For placement of needles or catheters into pelvic organs and/or genitalia [except prostate] for interstitial radioelement application, use 55920)

(For interstitial radioelement application, see 77776-77787)

(For ultrasonic guidance for interstitial radioelement application, use 76965)

55876   Placement of interstitial device(s) for radiation therapy guidance (eg, fiducial markers, dosimeter), prostate (via needle, any approach), single or multiple

(Report supply of device separately)

(For imaging guidance, see 76942, 77002, 77012, 77021)

55899   Unlisted procedure, male genital system

● New Code   ▲ Revised Code   + Add-On Code   ⃠ Modifier -51 Exempt   ⊙ Moderate Sedation

REPRODUCTIVE SYSTEM PROCEDURES

55920 Placement of needles or catheters into pelvic organs and/or genitalia (except prostate) for subsequent interstitial radioelement application

(For placement of needles or catheters into prostate, use 55875)

(For insertion of uterine tandems and/or vaginal ovoids for clinical brachytherapy, use 57155)

(For insertion of Heyman capsules for clinical brachytherapy, us 58346)

INTERSEX SURGERY

55970 Intersex surgery; male to female

55980 female to male

| | Separate Procedure | | Unlisted Procedure | | CCI Comp. Code | 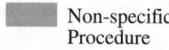 | Non-specific Procedure |

This page intentionally left blank.

● New Code	▲ Revised Code	✚ Add-On Code	⊘ Modifier -51 Exempt	⊙ Moderate Sedation

FEMALE GENITAL SYSTEM

When a pelvic examination is performed in conjunction with a gynecologic procedure, either as a necessary part of the procedure or as a confirmatory examination, the pelvic examination is not separately reported. A diagnostic pelvic examination may be performed for the purposes of deciding to perform a procedure; however, this examination is included in the evaluation and management service at the time the decision to perform the procedure is made.

All surgical laparoscopic, hysteroscopic or peritoneoscopic procedures include diagnostic procedures. Therefore, CPT code 49320 is included in 38120, 38570-38572, 43280, 43651-43653, 44200- 44202, 44970, 47560-47570, 49321- 49323, 49650-49651, 54690-54692, 55550, 58545-58554, 58660-58673, 60650; and 58555 is included in 58558- 58563.

Lysis of adhesions (CPT code 58660) is not to be reported separately when done in conjunction with other surgical laparoscopic procedures.

Pelvic exam under anesthesia indicated by CPT code 57410, is included in all major and most minor gynecological procedures and is not to be reported separately. This procedure represents routine evaluation of the surgical field.

Dilation of vagina or cervix (CPT codes 57400 or 57800), when done in conjunction with vaginal approach procedures, is not to be reported separately unless the CPT code descriptor states "without cervical dilation." 6. Administration of anesthesia, when necessary, is included in every surgical procedure code, when performed by the surgeon.

Colposcopy (CPT codes 56820, 57420, 57452) should not be reported separately when performed as a "scout" procedure to confirm the lesion or to assess the surgical field prior to a surgical procedure. A diagnostic colposcopy resulting in the decision to perform a non-colposcopic procedure may be reported with modifier - 58. Diagnostic colposcopies (56820, 57420, 57452) are not separately reported with other colposcopic procedures.

(For pelvic laparotomy, use 49000)

(For excision or destruction of endometriomas, open method, see 49203-49205, 58957, 58958)

(For paracentesis, see 49082, 49083, 49084)

(For secondary closure of abdominal wall evisceration or disruption, use 49900)

(For fulguration or excision of lesions, laparoscopic approach, use 58662)

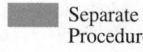 Separate Procedure

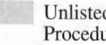 Unlisted Procedure

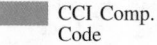 CCI Comp. Code

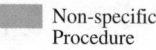 Non-specific Procedure

751

(For chemotherapy, see 96401-96549)

VULVA, PERINEUM AND INTROITUS

The following definitions apply to the vulvectomy codes (56620-56640):

A **simple** procedure is the removal of skin and superficial subcutaneous tissues.

A **radical** procedure is the removal of skin and deep subcutaneous tissues.

A **partial** procedure is the removal of less than 80% of the vulvar area.

A **complete** procedure is the removal of greater than 80% of the vulvar area.

INCISION

(For incision and drainage of sebaceous cyst, furuncle, or abscess, see 10040, 10060, 10061)

56405 Incision and drainage of vulva or perineal abscess

56420 Incision and drainage of Bartholin's gland abscess

(For incision and drainage of Skene's gland abscess or cyst, use 53060)

56440 Marsupialization of Bartholin's gland cyst

56441 Lysis of labial adhesions

56442 Hymenotomy, simple incision

DESTRUCTION

56501 Destruction of lesion(s), vulva; simple (eg, laser surgery, electrosurgery, cryosurgery, chemosurgery)

56515 extensive (eg, laser surgery, electrosurgery, cryosurgery, chemosurgery)

(For destruction of Skene's gland cyst or abscess, use 53270)

(For cautery destruction of urethral caruncle, use 53265)

● New Code   ▲ Revised Code   + Add-On Code   ⊘ Modifier -51 Exempt   ⊙ Moderate Sedation

EXCISION

56605 Biopsy of vulva or perineum (separate procedure); 1 lesion

+ 56606 each separate additional lesion (List separately in addition to code for primary procedure)

(Use 56606 in conjunction with code 56605)

(For excision of local lesion, see 11420-11426, 11620-11626)

56620 Vulvectomy simple; partial

56625 complete

(For skin graft, see 15002 et seq)

56630 Vulvectomy, radical, partial;

(For skin graft, if used, see 15004-15005, 15120, 15121, 15240, 15241)

56631 with unilateral inguinofemoral lymphadenectomy

56632 with bilateral inguinofemoral lymphadenectomy

56633 Vulvectomy, radical, complete;

56634 with unilateral inguinofemoral lymphadenectomy

56637 with bilateral inguinofemoral lymphadenectomy

56640 Vulvectomy, radical, complete, with inguinofemoral, iliac, and pelvic lymphadenectomy

(For bilateral procedure, report 56640 with modifier -50)

(For lymphadenectomy, see 38760-38780)

56700 Partial hymenectomy or revision of hymenal ring

56740 Excision of Bartholin's gland or cyst

(For excision of Skene's gland, use 53270)

(For excision of urethral caruncle, use 53265)

(For excision or fulguration of urethral carcinoma, use 53220)

| | Separate Procedure | | Unlisted Procedure | | CCI Comp. Code | | Non-specific Procedure | **753** |

(For excision or marsupialization of urethral diverticulum, see 53230, 53240)

REPAIR

(For repair of urethra for mucosal prolapse, use 53275)

56800 Plastic repair of introitus

56805 Clitoroplasty for intersex state

56810 Perineoplasty, repair of perineum, nonobstetrical (separate procedure)

(See also 56800)

(For repair of wounds to genitalia, see 12001-12007, 12041-12047, 13131-13133)

(For repair of recent injury of vagina and perineum, nonobstetrical, use 57210)

(For anal sphincteroplasty, see 46750, 46751)

(For episiorrhaphy, episioperineorrhaphy for recent injury of vulva and/or perineum, nonobstetrical, use 57210)

ENDOSCOPY

56820 Colposcopy of the vulva

56821   with biopsy(s)

(For colposcopic examinations/procedures involving the vagina, see 57420, 57421; cervix, see 57452-57461)

VAGINA

INCISION

57000 Colpotomy; with exploration

57010   with drainage of pelvic abscess

57020 Colpocentesis (separate procedure)

57022 Incision and drainage of vaginal hematoma; obstetrical/ postpartum

754 ● New   ▲ Revised   + Add-On   ⊘ Modifier -51   ⊙ Moderate
            Code   Code   Code   Exempt   Sedation

57023   non-obstetrical (eg, post-trauma, spontaneous bleeding)

DESTRUCTION

57061   Destruction of vaginal lesion(s); simple (eg, laser surgery, electrosurgery, cryosurgery, chemosurgery)

57065   extensive (eg, laser surgery, electrosurgery, cryosurgery, chemosurgery)

EXCISION

57100   Biopsy of vaginal mucosa; simple (separate procedure)

57105   extensive, requiring suture (including cysts)

57106   Vaginectomy, partial removal of vaginal wall;

57107   with removal of paravaginal tissue (radical vaginectomy)

57109   with removal of paravaginal tissue (radical vaginectomy) with bilateral total pelvic lymphadenectomy and para-aortic lymph node sampling (biopsy)

57110   Vaginectomy, complete removal of vaginal wall;

57111   with removal of paravaginal tissue (radical vaginectomy)

57112   with removal of paravaginal tissue (radical vaginectomy) with bilateral total pelvic lymphadenectomy and para-aortic lymph node sampling (biopsy)

57120   Colpocleisis (Le Fort type)

57130   Excision of vaginal septum

57135   Excision of vaginal cyst or tumor

INTRODUCTION

57150   Irrigation of vagina and/or application of medicament for treatment of bacterial, parasitic, or fungoid disease

⊙ **57155**   Insertion of uterine tandem and/or vaginal ovoids for clinical brachytherapy

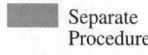 Separate Procedure   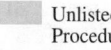 Unlisted Procedure   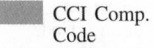 CCI Comp. Code   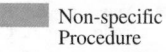 Non-specific Procedure

(For placement of needles or catheters into pelvic organs and/or genitalia [except prostate] for interstitial radioelement application, use 55920)

(For insertion of radioelement sources or ribbons, see 77761-77763, 77785-77787)

57156 Insertion of a vaginal radiation afterloading apparatus for clinical brachytherapy

57160 Fitting and insertion of pessary or other intravaginal support device

57170 Diaphragm or cervical cap fitting with instructions

57180 Introduction of any hemostatic agent or pack for spontaneous or traumatic nonobstetrical vaginal hemorrhage (separate procedure)

REPAIR

(For urethral suspension, Marshall-Marchetti-Krantz type, abdominal approach, see 51840, 51841)

(For laparoscopic suspension, use 51990)

57200 Colporrhaphy, suture of injury of vagina (nonobstetrical)

57210 Colpoperineorrhaphy, suture of injury of vagina and/or perineum (nonobstetrical)

57220 Plastic operation on urethral sphincter, vaginal approach (eg, Kelly urethral plication)

57230 Plastic repair of urethrocele

57240 Anterior colporrhaphy, repair of cystocele with or without repair of urethrocele

57250 Posterior colporrhaphy, repair of rectocele with or without perineorrhaphy

(For repair of rectocele (separate procedure) without posterior colporrhaphy, use 45560)

57260 Combined anteroposterior colporrhaphy;

57265 with enterocele repair

● New Code   ▲ Revised Code   + Add-On Code   ⊘ Modifier -51 Exempt   ⊙ Moderate Sedation

+ 57267 Insertion of mesh or other prosthesis for repair of pelvic floor defect, each site (anterior, posterior compartment), vaginal approach (List separately in addition to code for primary procedure)

(Use 57267 in addition to 45560, 57240-57265, 57285)

57268 Repair of enterocele, vaginal approach (separate procedure)

57270 Repair of enterocele, abdominal approach (separate procedure)

57280 Colpopexy, abdominal approach

57282 Colpopexy, vaginal; extra-peritoneal approach (sacrospinous, iliococcygeus)

57283 intra-peritoneal approach (uterosacral, levator myorrhaphy)

(Do not report 57283 in conjunction with 58263, 57556, 58270, 58280, 58292, 58294)

57284 Paravaginal defect repair (including repair of cystocele, if performed); open abdominal approach

(Do not report 57284 in conjunction with 51840, 51841, 51990, 57240, 57260, 57265, 58152, 58267)

57285 vaginal approach

(Do not report 57285 in conjunction with 51990, 57240, 57260, 57265, 58267)

57287 Removal or revision of sling for stress incontinence (eg, fascia or synthetic)

57288 Sling operation for stress incontinence (eg, fascia or synthetic)

(For laparoscopic approach, use 51992)

57289 Pereyra procedure, including anterior colporrhaphy

57291 Construction of artificial vagina; without graft

57292 with graft

57295 Revision (including removal) of prosthetic vaginal graft, vaginal approach

---

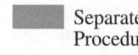 Separate Procedure   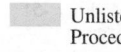 Unlisted Procedure   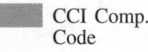 CCI Comp. Code   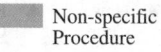 Non-specific Procedure

57296   open abdominal approach

(For laparoscopic approach, use 57426)

57300   Closure of rectovaginal fistula; vaginal or transanal approach

57305   abdominal approach

57307   abdominal approach, with concomitant colostomy

57308   transperineal approach, with perineal body reconstruction, with or without levator plication

57310   Closure of urethrovaginal fistula;

57311   with bulbocavernosus transplant

57320   Closure of vesicovaginal fistula; vaginal approach

(For concomitant cystostomy, see 51020-51040, 51101, 51102)

57330   transvesical and vaginal approach

(For abdominal approach, use 51900)

57335   Vaginoplasty for intersex state

MANIPULATION

57400   Dilation of vagina under anesthesia (other than local)

57410   Pelvic examination under anesthesia (other than local)

57415   Removal of impacted vaginal foreign body (separate procedure) under anesthesia (other than local)

(For removal without anesthesia of an impacted vaginal foreign body, use the appropriate E/M code)

ENDOSCOPY/LAPAROSCOPY

57420   Colposcopy of the entire vagina, with cervix if present;

57421   with biopsy(s) of vagina/cervix

(For colposcopic visualization of cervix and adjacent upper vagina, use 57452)

● New   ▲ Revised   + Add-On   ⊘ Modifier -51   ⊙ Moderate
            Code   Code   Code   Exempt   Sedation

(When reporting colposcopies of multiple sites, use modifier -51 as appropriate. For colposcopic examinations/procedures involving the vulva, see 56820, 56821; cervix, see 57452-57461)

(For endometrial sampling (biopsy) performed in conjunction with colposcopy, use 58110)

57423 Paravaginal defect repair (including repair of cystocele, if performed), laparoscopic approach

(Do not report 57423 in conjunction with 49320, 51840, 51841, 51990, 57240, 57260, 58152, 58267)

57425 Laparoscopy, surgical, colpopexy (suspension of vaginal apex)

57426 Revision (including removal) of prosthetic vaginal graft, laparoscopic approach

(For vaginal approach, see 57295. For open abdominal approach, see 57296)

CERVIX UTERI

(For cervicography, see Category III code 0003T)

ENDOSCOPY

(For colposcopic examinations/procedures involving the vulva, see 56820, 56821; vagina, see 57420, 57421)

57452 Colposcopy of the cervix including upper/adjacent vagina

(Do not report 57452 in addition to 57454-57461)

57454 with biopsy(s) of the cervix and endocervical curettage

57455 with biopsy(s) of the cervix

57456 with endocervical curettage

57460 with loop electrode biopsy(s) of the cervix

57461 with loop electrode conization of the cervix

(Do not report 57456 in addition to 57461)

(For endometrial sampling (biopsy) performed in conjunction with colposcopy, use 58110)

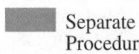 Separate Procedure   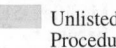 Unlisted Procedure   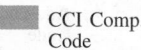 CCI Comp. Code   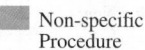 Non-specific Procedure

759

CPT PLUS! 2013

EXCISION

(For radical surgical procedures, see 58200-58240)

57500 Biopsy of cervix, single or multiple, or local excision of lesion, with or without fulguration (separate procedure)

57505 Endocervical curettage (not done as part of a dilation and curettage)

57510 Cautery of cervix; electro or thermal

57511 cryocautery, initial or repeat

57513 laser ablation

57520 Conization of cervix, with or without fulguration, with or without dilation and curettage, with or without repair; cold knife or laser

(See also 58120)

57522 loop electrode excision

57530 Trachelectomy (cervicectomy), amputation of cervix (separate procedure)

57531 Radical trachelectomy, with bilateral total pelvic lymphadenectomy and para-aortic lymph node sampling biopsy, with or without removal of tube(s), with or without removal of ovary(s)

(For radical abdominal hysterectomy, use 58210)

57540 Excision of cervical stump, abdominal approach;

57545 with pelvic floor repair

57550 Excision of cervical stump, vaginal approach;

57555 with anterior and/or posterior repair

57556 with repair of enterocele

(For insertion of intrauterine device, use 58300)

(For insertion of any hemostatic agent or pack for control of spontaneous non-obstetrical hemorrhage, see 57180)

760 ● New Code ▲ Revised Code + Add-On Code ⊘ Modifier -51 Exempt ⊙ Moderate Sedation

CPT codes and descriptions only ©2012 American Medical Association. All rights reserved.

57558 Dilation and curettage of cervical stump

REPAIR

57700 Cerclage of uterine cervix, nonobstetrical

57720 Trachelorrhaphy, plastic repair of uterine cervix, vaginal approach

MANIPULATION

57800 Dilation of cervical canal, instrumental (separate procedure)

CORPUS UTERI

EXCISION

58100 Endometrial sampling (biopsy) with or without endocervical sampling (biopsy), without cervical dilation, any method (separate procedure)

(For endocervical curettage only, use 57505)

(For endometrial sampling (biopsy) performed in conjunction with colposcopy (57420, 57421, 57452-57461), use 58110)

+ **58110** Endometrial sampling (biopsy) performed in conjunction with colposcopy (List separately in addition to code for primary procedure)

(Use 58110 in conjunction with 57420, 57421, 57452-57461)

58120 Dilation and curettage, diagnostic and/or therapeutic (nonobstetrical)

(For postpartum hemorrhage, use 59160)

58140 Myomectomy, excision of fibroid tumor(s) of uterus, 1 to 4 intramural myoma(s) with total weight of 250 grams or less and/or removal of surface myomas; abdominal approach

58145 vaginal approach

58146 Myomectomy, excision of fibroid tumor(s) of uterus, 5 or more intramural myomas and/or intramural myomas with total weight greater than 250 grams, abdominal approach

(Do not report 58146 in addition to 58140-58145, 58150-58240)

761

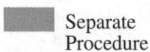 Separate Procedure 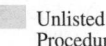 Unlisted Procedure 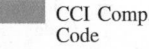 CCI Comp. Code 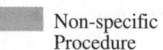 Non-specific Procedure

Hysterectomy Procedures

58150 Total abdominal hysterectomy (corpus and cervix), with or without removal of tube(s), with or without removal of ovary(s);

58152 with colpo-urethrocystopexy (eg, Marshall-Marchetti-Krantz, Burch)

(For urethrocystopexy without hysterectomy, see 51840, 51841)

58180 Supracervical abdominal hysterectomy (subtotal hysterectomy), with or without removal of tube(s), with or without removal of ovary(s)

58200 Total abdominal hysterectomy, including partial vaginectomy, with para-aortic and pelvic lymph node sampling, with or without removal of tube(s), with or without removal of ovary(s)

58210 Radical abdominal hysterectomy, with bilateral total pelvic lymphadenectomy and para-aortic lymph node sampling (biopsy), with or without removal of tube(s), with or without removal of ovary(s)

(For radical hysterectomy with ovarian transposition, use also 58825)

58240 Pelvic exenteration for gynecologic malignancy, with total abdominal hysterectomy or cervicectomy, with or without removal of tube(s), with or without removal of ovary(s), with removal of bladder and ureteral transplantations, and/or abdominoperineal resection of rectum and colon and colostomy, or any combination thereof

(For pelvic exenteration for lower urinary tract or male genital malignancy, use 51597)

58260 Vaginal hysterectomy, for uterus 250 grams or less;

58262 with removal of tube(s), and/or ovary(s)

58263 with removal of tube(s), and/or ovary(s), with repair of enterocele

58267 with colpo-urethrocystopexy (Marshall-Marchetti-Krantz type, Pereyra type) with or without endoscopic control

58270 with repair of enterocele

● New Code ▲ Revised Code + Add-On Code ⊘ Modifier -51 Exempt ⊙ Moderate Sedation

(For repair of enterocele with removal of tubes and/or ovaries, use 58263)

58275 Vaginal hysterectomy, with total or partial vaginectomy;

58280   with repair of enterocele

58285 Vaginal hysterectomy, radical (Schauta type operation)

58290 Vaginal hysterectomy, for uterus greater than 250 grams;

58291   with removal of tube(s) and/or ovary(s)

58292   with removal of tube(s) and/or ovary(s), with repair of enterocele

58293   with colpo-urethrocystopexy (Marshall-Marchetti-Krantz type, Pereyra type) with or without endoscopic control

58294   with repair of enterocele

INTRODUCTION

(To report insertion of non-biodegradable drug delivery implant for contraception, use 11981. To report removal of implantable contraceptive capsules with subsequent insertion of non-biodegradable drug delivery implant, use 11976 and 11981)

58300 Insertion of intrauterine device (IUD)

58301 Removal of intrauterine device (IUD)

58321 Artificial insemination; intra-cervical

58322   intra-uterine

58323 Sperm washing for artificial insemination

58340 Catheterization and introduction of saline or contrast material for saline infusion sonohysterography (SIS) or hysterosalpingography

(For radiological supervision and interpretation of saline infusion sonohysterography, use 76831)

(For radiological supervision and interpretation of hysterosalpingography, use 74740)

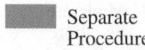 Separate Procedure
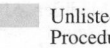 Unlisted Procedure
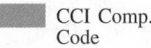 CCI Comp. Code
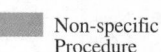 Non-specific Procedure

58345 Transcervical introduction of fallopian tube catheter for diagnosis and/or re-establishing patency (any method), with or without hysterosalpingography

(For radiological supervision and interpretation, use 74742)

58346 Insertion of Heyman capsules for clinical brachytherapy

(For placement of needles or catheters into pelvic organs and/or genitalia [except prostate] for interstitial radioelement application, use 55920)

(For insertion of radioelement sources or ribbons, see 77761-77763, 77785-77787)

58350 Chromotubation of oviduct, including materials

(To report the supply of any materials, use 99070)

58353 Endometrial ablation, thermal, without hysteroscopic guidance

(For hysteroscopic procedure, use 58563)

58356 Endometrial cryoablation with ultrasonic guidance, including endometrial curettage, when performed

(Do not report 58356 in conjunction with 58100, 58120, 58340, 76700, 76856)

REPAIR

58400 Uterine suspension, with or without shortening of round ligaments, with or without shortening of sacrouterine ligaments; (separate procedure)

58410 with presacral sympathectomy

(For anastomosis of tubes to uterus, use 58752)

58520 Hysterorrhaphy, repair of ruptured uterus (nonobstetrical)

58540 Hysteroplasty, repair of uterine anomaly (Strassman type)

(For closure of vesicouterine fistula, use 51920)

● New Code ▲ Revised Code + Add-On Code ⊘ Modifier -51 Exempt ⊙ Moderate Sedation

LAPAROSCOPY/HYSTEROSCOPY

Surgical laparoscopy always includes diagnostic laparoscopy. To report diagnostic laparoscopy (peritoneoscopy) (separate procedure), use 49320. To report a diagnostic hysteroscopy (separate procedure), use 58555.

58541 Laparoscopy, surgical, supracervical hysterectomy, for uterus 250 g or less;

58542 with removal of tube(s) and/or ovary(s)

(Do not report 58541-58542 in conjunction with 49320, 57000, 57180, 57410, 58140-58146, 58545, 58546, 58561, 58661, 58670, 58671)

58543 Laparoscopy, surgical, supracervical hysterectomy, for uterus greater than 250 g;

58544 with removal of tube(s) and/or ovary(s)

(Do not report 58543-58544 in conjunction with 49320, 57000, 57180, 57410, 58140-58146, 58545, 58546, 58561, 58661, 58670, 58671)

58545 Laparoscopy, surgical, myomectomy, excision; 1 to 4 intramural myomas with total weight of 250 g or less and/or removal of surface myomas

58546 5 or more intramural myomas and/or intramural myomas with total weight greater than 250 g

58548 Laparoscopy, surgical, with radical hysterectomy, with bilateral total pelvic lymphadenectomy and para-aortic lymph node sampling (biopsy), with removal of tube(s) and ovary(s), if performed

(Do not report 58548 in conjunction with 38570-38572, 58210 58285, 58550-58554)

58550 Laparoscopy, surgical with vaginal hysterectomy, for uterus 250 grams or less;

58552 with removal of tube(s) and/or ovary(s)

(Do not report 58550-58552 in conjunction with 49320, 57000, 57180, 57410, 58140-58146, 58545, 58546, 58561, 58661, 58670, 58671)

765

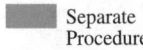 Separate Procedure   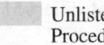 Unlisted Procedure   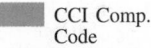 CCI Comp. Code   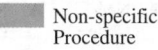 Non-specific Procedure

58553 Laparoscopy, surgical, with vaginal hysterectomy, for uterus greater than 250 grams;

58554 with removal of tube(s) and/or ovary(s)

(Do not report 58553-58554 in conjunction with 49320, 57000, 57180, 57410, 58140-58146, 58545, 58546, 58561, 58661, 58670, 58671)

58555 Hysteroscopy, diagnostic (separate procedure)

58558 Hysteroscopy, surgical; with sampling (biopsy) of endometrium and/or polypectomy, with or without D & C

58559 with lysis of intrauterine adhesions (any method)

58560 with division or resection of intrauterine septum (any method)

58561 with removal of leiomyomata

58562 with removal of impacted foreign body

58563 with endometrial ablation (eg, endometrial resection, electrosurgical ablation, thermoablation)

58565 with bilateral fallopian tube cannulation to induce occlusion by placement of permanent implants

(Do not report 58565 in conjunction with 58555 or 57800)

(For unilateral procedure, use modifier -52)

58570 Laparoscopy, surgical, with total hysterectomy, for uterus 250g or less;

58571 with removal of tube(s) and/or ovary(s)

58572 Laparoscopy, surgical, with total hysterectomy, for uterus greater than 250g;

58573 with removal of tube(s) and/or ovary(s)

(Do not report 58570-58573 in conjunction with 49320, 57000, 57180, 57410, 58140-58146, 58150, 58545, 58546, 58561, 58661, 58670, 58671)

58578 Unlisted laparoscopy procedure, uterus

● New Code	▲ Revised Code	+ Add-On Code	⊘ Modifier -51 Exempt	⊙ Moderate Sedation

58579 Unlisted hysteroscopy procedure, uterus

OVIDUCT/OVARY

INCISION

58600 Ligation or transection of fallopian tube(s), abdominal or vaginal approach, unilateral or bilateral

58605 Ligation or transection of fallopian tube(s), abdominal or vaginal approach, postpartum, unilateral or bilateral, during same hospitalization (separate procedure)

(For laparoscopic procedures, use 58670, 58671)

+ 58611 Ligation or transection of fallopian tube(s) when done at the time of cesarean delivery or intra-abdominal surgery (not a separate procedure) (List separately in addition to code for primary procedure)

58615 Occlusion of fallopian tube(s) by device (eg, band, clip, Falope ring) vaginal or suprapubic approach

(For laparoscopic approach, use 58671)

(For lysis of adnexal adhesions, use 58740)

LAPAROSCOPY

Surgical laparoscopy always includes diagnostic laparoscopy. To report diagnostic laparoscopy (peritoneoscopy) (separate procedure), use 49320.

58660 Laparoscopy, surgical; with lysis of adhesions (salpingolysis, ovariolysis) (separate procedure)

58661 with removal of adnexal structures (partial or total oophorectomy and/or salpingectomy)

58662 with fulguration or excision of lesions of the ovary, pelvic viscera, or peritoneal surface by any method

58670 with fulguration of oviducts (with or without transection)

58671 with occlusion of oviducts by device (eg, band, clip, or Falope ring)

58672 with fimbrioplasty

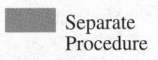 Separate Procedure 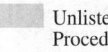 Unlisted Procedure 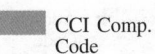 CCI Comp. Code 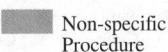 Non-specific Procedure

767

58673   with salpingostomy (salpingoneostomy)

(Codes 58672 and 58673 are used to report unilateral procedures. For bilateral procedure, use modifier -50)

58679   Unlisted laparoscopy procedure, oviduct, ovary

(For laparoscopic aspiration of ovarian cyst, use 49322)

(For laparoscopic biopsy of the ovary or fallopian tube, use 49321)

EXCISION

58700   Salpingectomy, complete or partial, unilateral or bilateral (separate procedure)

58720   Salpingo-oophorectomy, complete or partial, unilateral or bilateral (separate procedure)

REPAIR

58740   Lysis of adhesions (salpingolysis, ovariolysis)

(For laparoscopic approach, use 58660)

(For excision or destruction of endometriomas, open method, see 49203-49205, 58957, 58958)

(For fulguration or excision of lesions, laparscopic approach, use 58662)

58750   Tubotubal anastomosis

58752   Tubouterine implantation

58760   Fimbrioplasty

(For laparoscopic approach, use 58672)

58770   Salpingostomy (salpingoneostomy)

(For laparscopic approach, use 58673)

OVARY

INCISION

58800   Drainage of ovarian cyst(s), unilateral or bilateral, (separate procedure); vaginal approach

768   ● New   ▲ Revised   ✚ Add-On   ⊘ Modifier -51   ⊙ Moderate
          Code   Code   Code   Exempt   Sedation

58805   abdominal approach

58820   Drainage of ovarian abscess; vaginal approach, open

58822   abdominal approach

⊙ **58823**   Drainage of pelvic abscess, transvaginal or transrectal approach, percutaneous (eg, ovarian, pericolic)

(For radiological supervision and interpretation, use 75989)

58825   Transposition, ovary(s)

EXCISION

58900   Biopsy of ovary, unilateral or bilateral (separate procedure)

(For laparoscopic biopsy of the ovary or fallopian tube, use 49321)

58920   Wedge resection or bisection of ovary, unilateral or bilateral

58925   Ovarian cystectomy, unilateral or bilateral

58940   Oophorectomy, partial or total, unilateral or bilateral;

(For oophorectomy with concomitant debulking for ovarian malignancy, use 58592)

58943   for ovarian, tubal or primary peritoneal malignancy, with para-aortic and pelvic lymph node biopsies, peritoneal washings, peritoneal biopsies, diaphragmatic assessments, with or without salpingectomy(s), with or without omentectomy

58950   Resection (initial) of ovarian, tubal or primary peritoneal malignancy with bilateral salpingo-oophorectomy and omentectomy;

58951   with total abdominal hysterectomy, pelvic and limited para-aortic lymphadenectomy

58952   with radical dissection for debulking (ie, radical excision or destruction, intra-abdominal or retroperitoneal tumors)

(For resection of recurrent ovarian, tubal, primary peritoneal, or uterine malignancy, see 58597, 58958)

769

	Separate Procedure		Unlisted Procedure		CCI Comp. Code		Non-specific Procedure

58953 Bilateral salpingo-oophorectomy with omentectomy, total abdominal hysterectomy and radical dissection for debulking;

58954   with pelvic lymphadenectomy and limited para-aortic lymphadenectomy

58956 Bilateral salpingo-oophorectomy with total omentectomy, total abdominal hysterectomy for malignancy

(Do not report 58956 in conjunction with 49255, 58150, 58180, 58262, 58263, 58550, 58661, 58700, 58720, 58900, 58925, 58940, 58957, 58958)

58957 Resection (tumor debulking) of recurrent ovarian, tubal, primary peritoneal, uterine malignancy (intra-abdominal, retroperitoneal tumors), with omentectomy, if performed;

58958   with pelvic lymphadenectomy and limited para-aortic lymphadenectomy

(Do not report 58957, 58958 in conjunction with 38770, 38780, 44005, 49000, 49203-49215, 49255, 58900-58960)

58960 Laparotomy, for staging or restaging of ovarian, tubal or primary peritoneal malignancy (second look), with or without omentectomy, peritoneal washing, biopsy of abdominal and pelvic peritoneum, diaphragmatic assessment with pelvic and limited para-aortic lymphadenectomy

(Do not report 58960 in conjunction with 58957, 58958)

IN VITRO FERTILIZATION

58970 Follicle puncture for oocyte retrieval, any method

(For radiological supervision and interpretation, use 76948)

58974 Embryo transfer, intrauterine

58976 Gamete, zygote, or embryo intrafallopian transfer, any method

(For laparoscopic adnexal procedures, see 58660-58673)

OTHER PROCEDURES

58999 Unlisted procedure, female genital system (nonobstetrical)

● New Code   ▲ Revised Code   + Add-On Code   ⊘ Modifier -51 Exempt   ⊙ Moderate Sedation

MATERNITY CARE AND DELIVERY

CPT codes from this section are used to report routine maternity care and invasive and surgical procedures performed as part of prenatal, delivery and post-partum care. The services normally provided in uncomplicated maternity cases include antepartum care, delivery, and postpartum care.

ANTEPARTUM CARE

The definition of antepartum care for coding purposes includes the initial and subsequent history, physical examinations, recording of weight, blood pressures, fetal heart tones, routine chemical urinalysis, and routine visits. Routine antepartum visits are defined as:

- *Monthly visits up to 28 weeks gestation*

- *Biweekly visits up to 36 weeks gestation, and*

- *Weekly visits until delivery*

Any other visits or services provided within this time period should be coded separately. Using 6 to 8 weeks gestation as the typical starting point, the above definition translates into between 9 and 11 routine visits per patient.

DELIVERY

Delivery services are defined as including hospital admission, the admission history and physical examination, management of uncomplicated labor, and vaginal or cesarean delivery.

- *The definition of delivery services includes the hospital admission, and admission history and physical.*

- *Resuscitation of newborn infants when necessary, defined in previous editions, is not included in the delivery services. If the delivering physician has to resuscitate the newborn infant, he/she may code this service as a separate procedure.*

- *Medical problems "complicating labor and delivery management" may require additional resources and should be reported using evaluation and management service codes.*

POSTPARTUM CARE

Postpartum care is defined as hospital and office visits following vaginal or cesarean delivery. No number of visits is defined by CPT; however, the typical fee for total obstetrical care includes a single office follow-up visit six weeks postpartum.

771

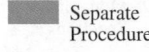 Separate Procedure   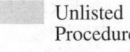 Unlisted Procedure   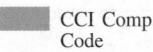 CCI Comp. Code   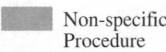 Non-specific Procedure

COMPLICATIONS OF PREGNANCY

The services defined previously are for normal, uncomplicated maternity care. For medical complications of pregnancy, for example, cardiac problems, neurological problems, diabetes, hypertension, toxemia, hyperemesis, pre-term labor and premature rupture of membranes, use evaluation and management service codes.

For surgical complications of pregnancy, such as appendectomy, hernia, ovarian cyst, Bartholin cysts, etc., use CPT codes from the SURGERY section of CPT. Note that in either case, complications are not considered to be part of routine maternity care and should be coded and reported in addition to maternity CPT codes.

PARTIAL MATERNITY SERVICES

Occasionally a physician may provide all or part of the antepartum and/or postpartum care but does not perform the actual delivery due to termination of the pregnancy by abortion, or referral to another physician for delivery. In this circumstance, the physician has the option of using the inclusive CPT codes 59420 or 59430 from the Maternity Care and Delivery section reporting each visit using evaluation and management service codes 99201-99215.

MISCELLANEOUS CODING RULES

The majority of procedures in this section (CPT codes 59000-59899) include only what is described by the code in the CPT definition. Additional procedures performed on the same day would be reported separately.

The few exceptions to this rule consist of: CPT codes 59050 and 59051(fetal monitoring during labor), 59300 (episiotomy) and 59414 (delivery of placenta) are included in CPT codes 59400 (routine obstetric care, vaginal delivery), 59409 (vaginal delivery only), 59410 (vaginal delivery and postpartum care), 59510 (routine obstetric care, cesarean delivery), 59514 (cesarean delivery only), 59515 (cesarean delivery and postpartum care), 59610 (routine obstetric care, vaginal delivery, after previous cesarean delivery), 59612 (vaginal delivery only after previous cesarean delivery), 59614 (vaginal delivery and postpartum care after previous cesarean delivery), 59618 (routine obstetric care, cesarean delivery, after previous cesarean delivery), 59620 (cesarean delivery only after previous cesarean delivery), and 59622 (cesarean delivery and postpartum care after previous cesarean delivery). They are not to be separately reported.

The total obstetrical packages (e.g. CPT codes 59400 and 59510) include antepartum care, the delivery, and postpartum care. They do not include among other services, ultrasound, amniocentesis, special screening tests for genetic conditions, visits for unrelated conditions (incidental to pregnancy) or additional and frequent visits due to high risk conditions.

Obstetric care can be coded as a global package or can be broken down when necessary into antepartum, delivery and postpartum care.

● New Code ▲ Revised Code + Add-On Code ⊘ Modifier -51 Exempt ⊙ Moderate Sedation

Complicated pregnancies and deliveries need to be coded appropriately to indicate the increased work on the physician's part during the patient's care. There are several options for recording these circumstances.

Postpartum care only services (59430) include office or other outpatient visits following vaginal or cesarean section delivery.

Delivery services include admission to the hospital, the admission history and physical examination, management of uncomplicated labor, vaginal delivery (with or without episiotomy, with or without forceps), or cesarean delivery. When reporting delivery only services (59409, 59514, 59612, 59620) report inpatient post delivery management and discharge services using Evaluation and Management Services codes (99217-99239). Delivery and postpartum services (59410, 59515, 59614, 59622) include delivery services and all inpatient and outpatient postpartum services. Medical complications of pregnancy (eg, cardiac problems, neurological problems, diabetes, hypertension, toxemia, hpyeremisis, preterm labor, premature rupture of membraines, trauma) and medical problems complicating labor and delivery management may require additional resources and may be reported separately.

For surgical complications of pregnancy (eg., appendectomy, hernia, ovarian cyst, Bartholin cyst), see services in the Surgery section.

If all or part of the antepartum and/or postpartum patient care is provided except delivery due to termination of pregnancy by abortion or referral to another physician or other qualified health care professional for delivery, see the antepartum and postpartum care codes 59425, 59426 and 59430.

(For circumcision of newborn, see 54150, 54160)

ANTEPARTUM AND FETAL INVASIVE SERVICES

(For fetal intrauterine transfusion, use 36460)

(For unlisted fetal invasive procedure, use 59897)

59000 Amniocentesis, diagnostic

(For radiological supervision and interpretation, use 76946)

59001 therapeutic amniotic fluid reduction (includes ultrasound guidance)

59012 Cordocentesis (intrauterine), any method

(For radiological supervision and interpretation, use 76941)

59015 Chorionic villus sampling, any method

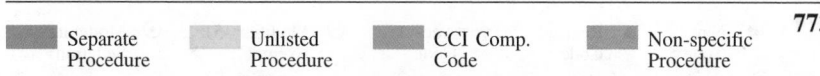

				773
Separate Procedure	Unlisted Procedure	CCI Comp. Code	Non-specific Procedure	

(For radiological supervision and interpretation, use 76945)

59020 Fetal contraction stress test

59025 Fetal non-stress test

59030 Fetal scalp blood sampling

(For repeat fetal scalp blood sampling, use 59030 and see modifiers -76 and -77)

59050 Fetal monitoring during labor by consulting physician (ie, non-attending physician) with written report; supervision and interpretation

59051 interpretation only

59070 Transabdominal amnioinfusion, including ultrasound guidance

59072 Fetal umbilical cord occlusion, including ultrasound guidance

59074 Fetal fluid drainage (eg, vesicocentesis, thoracocentesis, paracentesis), including ultrasound guidance

59076 Fetal shunt placement, including ultrasound guidance

EXCISION

59100 Hysterotomy, abdominal (eg, for hydatidiform mole, abortion)

(When tubal ligation is performed at the same time as hysterotomy, use 58611 in addition to 59100)

59120 Surgical treatment of ectopic pregnancy; tubal or ovarian, requiring salpingectomy and/or oophorectomy, abdominal or vaginal approach

59121 tubal or ovarian, without salpingectomy and/or oophorectomy

59130 abdominal pregnancy

59135 interstitial, uterine pregnancy requiring total hysterectomy

59136 interstitial, uterine pregnancy with partial resection of uterus

59140 cervical, with evacuation

● New Code   ▲ Revised Code   + Add-On Code   ⊘ Modifier -51 Exempt   ⊙ Moderate Sedation

59150 Laparoscopic treatment of ectopic pregnancy; without salpingectomy and/or oophorectomy

59151 with salpingectomy and/or oophorectomy

59160 Curettage, postpartum

INTRODUCTION

(For intrauterine fetal transfusion, use 36460)

(For introduction of hypertonic solution and/or prostaglandins to initiate labor, see 59850-59857)

59200 Insertion of cervical dilator (eg, laminaria, prostaglandin) (separate procedure)

REPAIR

(For tracheoplasty, use 57700)

▲ **59300** Episiotomy or vaginal repair, by other than attending

59320 Cerclage of cervix, during pregnancy; vaginal

59325 abdominal

59350 Hysterorrhaphy of ruptured uterus

VAGINAL DELIVERY, ANTEPARTUM AND POSTPARTUM CARE

59400 Routine obstetric care including antepartum care, vaginal delivery (with or without episiotomy, and/or forceps) and postpartum care

59409 Vaginal delivery only (with or without episiotomy and/or forceps);

59410 including postpartum care

59412 External cephalic version, with or without tocolysis

(Use 59412 in addition to code(s) for delivery)

59414 Delivery of placenta (separate procedure)

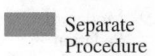 Separate Procedure 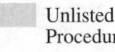 Unlisted Procedure 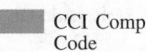 CCI Comp. Code 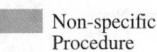 Non-specific Procedure

775

(For antepartum care only, see 59425, 59426 or appropriate E/M code(s))

(For 1-3 antepartum care visits, see appropriate E/M code(s))

59425 Antepartum care only; 4-6 visits

59426 7 or more visits

59430 Postpartum care only (separate procedure)

CESAREAN DELIVERY

(For standby attendance for infant, use 99360)

(For low cervical cesarean section, see 59510, 59515, 59525)

59510 Routine obstetric care including antepartum care, cesarean delivery, and postpartum care

59514 Cesarean delivery only;

59515 including postpartum care

(For classic cesarean section, see 59510, 59515, 59525)

+ 59525 Subtotal or total hysterectomy after cesarean delivery (List separately in addition to code for primary procedure)

(Use 59525 in conjunction with codes 59510, 59514, 59515, 59618, 59620, 59622)

(For extraperitoneal cesarean section, or cesarean section with subtotal or total hysterectomy, see 59510, 59515, 59525)

DELIVERY AFTER PREVIOUS CESAREAN DELIVERY

Patients who have had a previous cesarean delivery and now present with the expectation of a vaginal delivery are coded using codes 59610-59622. If the patient has a successful vaginal delivery after a previous cesarean delivery (VBAC), use codes 59610-59614. If the attempt is unsuccessful and another cesarean delivery is carried out, use codes 59618-59622. To report elective cesarean deliveries use code 59510, 59514 or 59515.

59610 Routine obstetric care including antepartum care, vaginal delivery (with or without episiotomy, and/or forceps) and postpartum care, after previous cesarean delivery

776 ● New Code   ▲ Revised Code   + Add-On Code   ⊘ Modifier -51 Exempt   ⊙ Moderate Sedation

59612 Vaginal delivery only, after previous cesarean delivery (with or without episiotomy and/or forceps);

59614   including postpartum care

59618 Routine obstetric care including antepartum care, cesarean delivery, and postpartum care, following attempted vaginal delivery after previous cesarean delivery

59620 Cesarean delivery only, following attempted vaginal delivery after previous cesarean delivery;

59622   including postpartum care

ABORTION

(For medical treatment of spontaneous complete abortion, any trimester, use E/M codes 99201-99233)

(For surgical treatment of spontaneous abortion, use 59812)

59812 Treatment of incomplete abortion, any trimester, completed surgically

59820 Treatment of missed abortion, completed surgically; first trimester

59821   second trimester

59830 Treatment of septic abortion, completed surgically

59840 Induced abortion, by dilation and curettage

59841 Induced abortion, by dilation and evacuation

59850 Induced abortion, by 1 or more intra-amniotic injections (amniocentesis-injections), including hospital admission and visits, delivery of fetus and secundines;

59851   with dilation and curettage and/or evacuation

59852   with hysterotomy (failed intra-amniotic injection)

(For insertion of cervical dilator, use 59200)

59855 Induced abortion, by 1 or more vaginal suppositories (eg, prostaglandin) with or without cervical dilation (eg, laminaria),

---

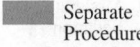 Separate Procedure   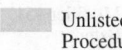 Unlisted Procedure   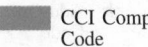 CCI Comp. Code   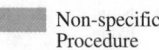 Non-specific Procedure

777

including hospital admission and visits, delivery of fetus and secundines;

59856   with dilation and curettage and/or evacuation

59857   with hysterotomy (failed medical evacuation)

OTHER PROCEDURES

59866 Multifetal pregnancy reduction(s) (MPR)

59870 Uterine evacuation and curettage for hydatidiform mole

59871 Removal of cerclage suture under anesthesia (other than local)

59897 Unlisted fetal invasive procedure, including ultrasound guidance, when performed

59898 Unlisted laparoscopy procedure, maternity care and delivery

59899 Unlisted procedure, maternity care and delivery

 New Code   Revised Code   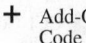 Add-On Code   ⊘ Modifier -51 Exempt   ⊙ Moderate Sedation

ENDOCRINE SYSTEM

(For pituitary and pineal surgery, see Nervous System)

THYROID GLAND

INCISION

60000 Incision and drainage of thyroglossal duct cyst, infected

EXCISION

60100 Biopsy thyroid, percutaneous core needle

(If imaging guidance is performed, see 76942, 77002, 77012, 77021)

(For fine needle aspiration, use 10021 or 10022)

(For evaluation of fine needle aspirate, see 88172, 88173)

60200 Excision of cyst or adenoma of thyroid, or transection of isthmus

60210 Partial thyroid lobectomy, unilateral; with or without isthmusectomy

60212 with contralateral subtotal lobectomy, including isthmusectomy

60220 Total thyroid lobectomy, unilateral; with or without isthmusectomy

60225 with contralateral subtotal lobectomy, including isthmusectomy

60240 Thyroidectomy, total or complete

(For thyroidectomy, subtotal or partial, use 60271)

60252 Thyroidectomy, total or subtotal for malignancy; with limited neck dissection

60254 with radical neck dissection

60260 Thyroidectomy, removal of all remaining thyroid tissue following previous removal of a portion of thyroid

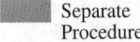 Separate Procedure   Unlisted Procedure   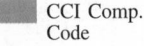 CCI Comp. Code   Non-specific Procedure

779

(For bilateral procedure, report 60260 with modifier -50)

60270 Thyroidectomy, including substernal thyroid; sternal split or transthoracic approach

60271   cervical approach

60280 Excision of thyroglossal duct cyst or sinus;

60281   recurrent

(For thyroid ultrasonography, use 76536)

REMOVAL

60300 Aspiration and/or injection, thyroid cyst

(For fine needle aspiration, see 10021, 10022)

(If imaging guidance is performed, see 76942, 77012)

PARATHYROID, THYMUS, ADRENAL GLANDS, PANCREAS, AND CAROTID BODY

EXCISION

(For pituitary and pineal surgery, see Nervous System)

60500 Parathyroidectomy or exploration of parathyroid(s);

60502   re-exploration

60505   with mediastinal exploration, sternal split or transthoracic approach

+ **60512** Parathyroid autotransplantation (List separately in addition to code for primary procedure)

(Use 60512 in conjunction with codes 60500, 60502, 60505, 60212, 60225, 60240, 60252, 60254, 60260, 60270, 60271)

60520 Thymectomy, partial or total; transcervical approach (separate procedure)

60521   sternal split or transthoracic approach, without radical mediastinal dissection (separate procedure)

60522   sternal split or transthoracic approach, with radical mediastinal dissection (separate procedure)

(For thoracoscopic [VATS] thymectomy, see 32673)

60540   Adrenalectomy, partial or complete, or exploration of adrenal gland with or without biopsy, transabdominal, lumbar or dorsal (separate procedure);

60545   with excision of adjacent retroperitoneal tumor

(Do not report 60540, 60545 in conjunction with 50323)

(For bilateral procedure, report 60540 with modifier 50)

(For excision of remote or disseminated pheochromocytoma, see 49203-49205)

(For laparoscopic approach, use 56321)

60600   Excision of carotid body tumor; without excision of carotid artery

60605   with excision of carotid artery

LAPAROSCOPY

Surgical laparoscopy always includes diagnostic laparoscopy. To report a diagnostic laparoscopy (peritoneoscopy) (separate procedure), use 49320.

60650   Laparoscopy, surgical, with adrenalectomy, partial or complete, or exploration of adrenal gland with or without biopsy, transabdominal, lumbar or dorsal

60659   Unlisted laparoscopy procedure, endocrine system

OTHER PROCEDURES

60699   Unlisted procedure, endocrine system

781

Separate Procedure	Unlisted Procedure	CCI Comp. Code	Non-specific Procedure

This page intentionally left blank.

● New
  Code

▲ Revised
  Code

✚ Add-On
  Code

⊘ Modifier -51
  Exempt

⊙ Moderate
  Sedation

NERVOUS SYSTEM

There are numerous codes for spinal injections found in this section. Review documentation for whether the injection is a single one, differential one or continuous. Also determine the number of levels involved when a regional block is administered.

SKULL, MENINGES, AND BRAIN

(For injection procedure for cerebral angiography, see 36100-36218)

(For injection procedure for ventriculography, see 61026, 61120, 61130)

(For injection procedure for pneumoencephalography, use 61055)

INJECTION, DRAINAGE OR ASPIRATION

61000 Subdural tap through fontanelle, or suture, infant, unilateral or bilateral; initial

61001   subsequent taps

61020 Ventricular puncture through previous burr hole, fontanelle, suture, or implanted ventricular catheter/reservoir; without injection

61026   with injection of medication or other substance for diagnosis or treatment

61050 Cisternal or lateral cervical (C1-C2) puncture; without injection (separate procedure)

61055   with injection of medication or other substance for diagnosis or treatment (eg, C1-C2)

(For radiological supervision and interpretation, see Radiology)

61070 Puncture of shunt tubing or reservoir for aspiration or injection procedure

(For radiological supervision and interpretation, use 75809)

TWIST DRILL, BURR HOLE(S), OR TREPHINE

61105 Twist drill hole(s) for subdural or ventricular puncture;

| | Separate Procedure | | Unlisted Procedure | | CCI Comp. Code | | Non-specific Procedure | **783** |

⊘ **61107** Twist drill hole(s) for subdural, intracerebral or ventricular puncture; for implanting ventricular catheter, pressure recording device, or other intracerebral monitoring device

(For intracranial neuroendoscopic ventricular catheter placement, use 62160)

61108 for evacuation and/or drainage of subdural hematoma

61120 Burr hole(s) for ventricular puncture (including injection of gas, contrast media, dye, or radioactive material)

61140 Burr hole(s) or trephine; with biopsy of brain or intracranial lesion

61150 with drainage of brain abscess or cyst

61151 with subsequent tapping (aspiration) of intracranial abscess or cyst

61154 Burr hole(s) with evacuation and/or drainage of hematoma, extradural or subdural

(For bilateral procedure, report 61154 with modifier -50)

61156 Burr hole(s); with aspiration of hematoma or cyst, intracerebral

61210 for implanting ventricular catheter, reservoir, EEG electrode(s), pressure recording device, or other cerebral monitoring device (separate procedure)

(For intracranial neuroendoscopic ventricular catheter placement, use 62160)

61215 Insertion of subcutaneous reservoir, pump or continuous infusion system for connection to ventricular catheter

(For refilling and maintenance of an implantable infusion pump for spinal or brain drug therapy, use 95990)

(For chemotherapy, use 96450)

61250 Burr hole(s) or trephine, supratentorial, exploratory, not followed by other surgery

(For bilateral procedure, report 61250 with modifier -50)

61253 Burr hole(s) or trephine, infratentorial, unilateral or bilateral

---

784   ● New   ▲ Revised   + Add-On   ⊘ Modifier -51   ⊙ Moderate
        Code   Code   Code   Exempt   Sedation

(If burr hole(s) or trephine are followed by craniotomy at same operative session, use 61304-61321; do not use 61250 or 61253)

CRANIECTOMY OR CRANIOTOMY

61304   Craniectomy or craniotomy, exploratory; supratentorial

61305   infratentorial (posterior fossa)

61312   Craniectomy or craniotomy for evacuation of hematoma, supratentorial; extradural or subdural

61313   intracerebral

61314   Craniectomy or craniotomy for evacuation of hematoma, infratentorial; extradural or subdural

61315   intracerebellar

+ **61316**   Incision and subcutaneous placement of cranial bone graft (List separately in addition to code for primary procedure)

   (Use 61316 in conjunction with codes 61304, 61312, 61313, 61322, 61323, 61340, 61570, 61571, 61680-61705)

61320   Craniectomy or craniotomy, drainage of intracranial abscess; supratentorial

61321   infratentorial

61322   Craniectomy or craniotomy, decompressive, with or without duraplasty, for treatment of intracranial hypertension, without evacuation of associated intraparenchymal hematoma; without lobectomy

   (Do not report 61313 in addition to 61322)

   (For subtemporal decompression, use 61340)

61323   with lobectomy

   (Do not report 61313 in addition to 61323)

   (For subtemporal decompression, use 61340)

61330   Decompression of orbit only, transcranial approach

   (For bilateral procedure, report 61330 with modifier -50)

785

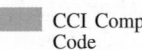

Separate Procedure   Unlisted Procedure   CCI Comp. Code   Non-specific Procedure

61332 Exploration of orbit (transcranial approach); with biopsy

61333   with removal of lesion

61334   with removal of foreign body

61340 Subtemporal cranial decompression (pseudotumor cerebri, slit ventricle syndrome)

(For bilateral procedure, report 61340 with modifier -50)

(For decompressive craniotomy or craniectomy for intracranial hypertension, without hematoma evacuation, see 61322, 61323)

61343 Craniectomy, suboccipital with cervical laminectomy for decompression of medulla and spinal cord, with or without dural graft (eg, Arnold-Chiari malformation)

61345 Other cranial decompression, posterior fossa

(For orbital decompression by lateral wall approach, Kroenlein type, use 67445)

61440 Craniotomy for section of tentorium cerebelli (separate procedure)

61450 Craniectomy, subtemporal, for section, compression, or decompression of sensory root of gasserian ganglion

61458 Craniectomy, suboccipital; for exploration or decompression of cranial nerves

61460   for section of 1 or more cranial nerves

61470   for medullary tractotomy

61480   for mesencephalic tractotomy or pedunculotomy

61490 Craniotomy for lobotomy, including cingulotomy

(For bilateral procedure, report 61490 with modifier -50)

61500 Craniectomy; with excision of tumor or other bone lesion of skull

61501   for osteomyelitis

---

786   ● New   ▲ Revised.   ✚ Add-On   ⊘ Modifier -51   ⊙ Moderate
              Code   Code   Code   Exempt   Sedation

61510 Craniectomy, trephination, bone flap craniotomy; for excision of brain tumor, supratentorial, except meningioma

61512 for excision of meningioma, supratentorial

61514 for excision of brain abscess, supratentorial

61516 for excision or fenestration of cyst, supratentorial

(For excision of pituitary tumor or craniopharyngioma, see 61545, 61546, 61548)

+ 61517 Implantation of brain intracavitary chemotherapy agent (List separately in addition to code for primary procedure)

(Use 61517 only in conjunction with codes 61510 or 61518)

(Do not report 61517 for brachytherapy insertion. For intracavitary insertion of radioelement sources or ribbons, see 77785-77787)

61518 Craniectomy for excision of brain tumor, infratentorial or posterior fossa; except meningioma, cerebellopontine angle tumor, or midline tumor at base of skull

61519 meningioma

61520 cerebellopontine angle tumor

61521 midline tumor at base of skull

61522 Craniectomy, infratentorial or posterior fossa; for excision of brain abscess

61524 for excision or fenestration of cyst

61526 Craniectomy, bone flap craniotomy, transtemporal (mastoid) for excision of cerebellopontine angle tumor;

61530 combined with middle/posterior fossa craniotomy/ craniectomy

61531 Subdural implantation of strip electrodes through 1 or more burr or trephine hole(s) for long term seizure monitoring

(For stereotactic implantation of electrodes, use 61760)

787

| Separate Procedure | Unlisted Procedure | CCI Comp. Code | Non-specific Procedure |

(For craniotomy for excision of intracranial arteriovenous malformation, see 61680-61692)

61533 Craniotomy with elevation of bone flap; for subdural implantation of an electrode array, for long term seizure monitoring

(For continuous EEG monitoring, see 95950-95954)

61534 for excision of epileptogenic focus without electrocorticography during surgery

61535 for removal of epidural or subdural electrode array, without excision of cerebral tissue (separate procedure)

61536 for excision of cerebral epileptogenic focus, with electrocorticography during surgery (includes removal of electrode array)

61537 for lobectomy, temporal lobe, without electrocorticography during surgery

61538 for lobectomy, temporal lobe, with electrocorticography during surgery

61539 for lobectomy, other than temporal lobe, partial or total, with electrocorticography during surgery

61540 for lobectomy, other than temporal lobe, partial or total, without electrocorticography during surgery

61541 for transection of corpus callosum

61542 for total hemispherectomy

61543 for partial or subtotal (functional) hemispherectomy

61544 for excision or coagulation of choroid plexus

61545 for excision of craniopharyngioma

(For craniotomy for selective amygdalohippocampectomy, use 61566)

(For craniotomy for multiple subpial transections during surgery, use 61567)

● New Code   ▲ Revised Code   + Add-On Code   ⊘ Modifier -51 Exempt   ⊙ Moderate Sedation

61546 Craniotomy for hypophysectomy or excision of pituitary tumor, intracranial approach

61548 Hypophysectomy or excision of pituitary tumor, transnasal or transseptal approach, nonstereotactic

(Do not report code 69990 in addition to code 61548)

61550 Craniectomy for craniosynostosis; single cranial suture

61552   multiple cranial sutures

(For cranial reconstruction for orbital hypertelorism, see 21260-21263)

(For reconstruction, see 21172-21180)

61556 Craniotomy for craniosynostosis; frontal or parietal bone flap

61557   bifrontal bone flap

61558 Extensive craniectomy for multiple cranial suture craniosynostosis (eg, cloverleaf skull); not requiring bone grafts

61559   recontouring with multiple osteotomies and bone autografts (eg, barrel-stave procedure) (includes obtaining grafts)

(For reconstruction, see 21172-21180)

61563 Excision, intra and extracranial, benign tumor of cranial bone (eg, fibrous dysplasia); without optic nerve decompression

61564   with optic nerve decompression

(For reconstruction, see 21181-21183)

61566 Craniotomy with elevation of bone flap; for selective amygdalohippocampectomy

61567   for multiple subpial transections, with electrocorticography during surgery

61570 Craniectomy or craniotomy; with excision of foreign body from brain

61571   with treatment of penetrating wound of brain

(For sequestrectomy for osteomyelitis, use 61501)

789

	Separate Procedure		Unlisted Procedure		CCI Comp. Code		Non-specific Procedure

61575 Transoral approach to skull base, brain stem or upper spinal cord for biopsy, decompression or excision of lesion;

61576 requiring splitting of tongue and/or mandible (including tracheostomy)

(For arthrodesis, use 22548)

SURGERY OF SKULL BASE

For primary closure, see the appropriate codes, ie, 15732, 15756-15758.

When one surgeon performs the approach procedure, another surgeon performs the definitive procedure, and another surgeon performs the repair/reconstruction procedure, each surgeon reports only the code for the specific procedure performed.

If one surgeon performs more than one procedure (ie, approach procedure and definitive procedure), then both codes are reported, adding modifier -51 to the seondary, additional procedure(s).

APPROACH PROCEDURES

Anterior Cranial Fossa

61580 Craniofacial approach to anterior cranial fossa; extradural, including lateral rhinotomy, ethmoidectomy, sphenoidectomy, without maxillectomy or orbital exenteration

61581 extradural, including lateral rhinotomy, orbital exenteration, ethmoidectomy, sphenoidectomy and/or maxillectomy

61582 extradural, including unilateral or bifrontal craniotomy, elevation of frontal lobe(s), osteotomy of base of anterior cranial fossa

61583 intradural, including unilateral or bifrontal craniotomy, elevation or resection of frontal lobe, osteotomy of base of anterior cranial fossa

61584 Orbitocranial approach to anterior cranial fossa, extradural, including supraorbital ridge osteotomy and elevation of frontal and/or temporal lobe(s); without orbital exenteration

61585 with orbital exenteration

● New Code	▲ Revised Code	+ Add-On Code	⊘ Modifier -51 Exempt	⊙ Moderate Sedation

61586 Bicoronal, transzygomatic and/or LeFort I osteotomy approach to anterior cranial fossa with or without internal fixation, without bone graft

Middle Cranial Fossa

61590 Infratemporal pre-auricular approach to middle cranial fossa (parapharyngeal space, infratemporal and midline skull base, nasopharynx), with or without disarticulation of the mandible, including parotidectomy, craniotomy, decompression and/or mobilization of the facial nerve and/or petrous carotid artery

61591 Infratemporal post-auricular approach to middle cranial fossa (internal auditory meatus, petrous apex, tentorium, cavernous sinus, parasellar area, infratemporal fossa) including mastoidectomy, resection of sigmoid sinus, with or without decompression and/or mobilization of contents of auditory canal or petrous carotid artery

61592 Orbitocranial zygomatic approach to middle cranial fossa (cavernous sinus and carotid artery, clivus, basilar artery or petrous apex) including osteotomy of zygoma, craniotomy, extra- or intradural elevation of temporal lobe

Posterior Cranial Fossa

61595 Transtemporal approach to posterior cranial fossa, jugular foramen or midline skull base, including mastoidectomy, decompression of sigmoid sinus and/or facial nerve, with or without mobilization

61596 Transcochlear approach to posterior cranial fossa, jugular foramen or midline skull base, including labyrinthectomy, decompression, with or without mobilization of facial nerve and/or petrous carotid artery

61597 Transcondylar (far lateral) approach to posterior cranial fossa, jugular foramen or midline skull base, including occipital condylectomy, mastoidectomy, resection of C1-C3 vertebral body(s), decompression of vertebral artery, with or without mobilization

61598 Transpetrosal approach to posterior cranial fossa, clivus or foramen magnum, including ligation of superior petrosal sinus and/or sigmoid sinus

	Separate Procedure		Unlisted Procedure		CCI Comp. Code		Non-specific Procedure

DEFINITIVE PROCEDURES

Base of Anterior Cranial Fossa

61600 Resection or excision of neoplastic, vascular or infectious lesion of base of anterior cranial fossa; extradural

61601 intradural, including dural repair, with or without graft

Base of Middle Cranial Fossa

61605 Resection or excision of neoplastic, vascular or infectious lesion of infratemporal fossa, parapharyngeal space, petrous apex; extradural

61606 intradural, including dural repair, with or without graft

61607 Resection or excision of neoplastic, vascular or infectious lesion of parasellar area, cavernous sinus, clivus or midline skull base; extradural

61608 intradural, including dural repair, with or without graft

Codes 61609-61612 are reported in addition to code(s) for primary procedure(s) 61605-61608. Report only one transection or ligation of carotid artery code per operative session.

+ 61609 Transection or ligation, carotid artery in cavernous sinus; without repair (List separately in addition to code for primary procedure)

+ 61610 with repair by anastomosis or graft (List separately in addition to code for primary procedure)

+ 61611 Transection or ligation, carotid artery in petrous canal; without repair (List separately in addition to code for primary procedure)

+ 61612 with repair by anastomosis or graft (List separately in addition to code for primary procedure)

61613 Obliteration of carotid aneurysm, arteriovenous malformation, or carotid-cavernous fistula by dissection within cavernous sinus

● New Code   ▲ Revised Code   + Add-On Code   ⊘ Modifier -51 Exempt   ⊙ Moderate Sedation

Base of Posterior Cranial Fossa

61615 Resection or excision of neoplastic, vascular or infectious lesion of base of posterior cranial fossa, jugular foramen, foramen magnum, or C1-C3 vertebral bodies; extradural

61616 intradural, including dural repair, with or without graft

REPAIR AND/OR RECONSTRUCTION OF SURGICAL DEFECTS OF SKULL BASE

61618 Secondary repair of dura for cerebrospinal fluid leak, anterior, middle or posterior cranial fossa following surgery of the skull base; by free tissue graft (eg, pericranium, fascia, tensor fascia lata, adipose tissue, homologous or synthetic grafts)

61619 by local or regionalized vascularized pedicle flap or myocutaneous flap (including galea, temporalis, frontalis or occipitalis muscle)

ENDOVASCULAR THERAPY

61623 Endovascular temporary balloon arterial occlusion, head or neck (extracranial/intracranial) including selective catheterization of vessel to be occluded, positioning and inflation of occlusion balloon, concomitant neurological monitoring, and radiologic supervision and interpretation of all angiography required for balloon occlusion and to exclude vascular injury post occlusion

(If selective catheterization and angiography of arteries other than artery to be occluded is performed, use appropriate catheterization and radiologic supervision and interpretation codes)

(If complete diagnostic angiography of the artery to be occluded is performed immediately prior to temporary occlusion, use appropriate radiologic supervision and interpretation codes only)

61624 Transcatheter permanent occlusion or embolization (eg, for tumor destruction, to achieve hemostasis, to occlude a vascular malformation), percutaneous, any method; central nervous system (intracranial, spinal cord)

(See also 37204)

(For radiological supervision and interpretation, use 75894)

61626 non-central nervous system, head or neck (extracranial, brachiocephalic branch)

	Separate Procedure		Unlisted Procedure		CCI Comp. Code		Non-specific Procedure

793

(See also 37204)

(For radiological supervision and interpretation, use 75894)

61630 Balloon angioplasty, intracranial (eg, atherosclerotic stenosis), percutaneous

61635 Transcatheter placement of intravascular stent(s), intracranial (eg, atherosclerotic stenosis), including balloon angioplasty, if performed

(61630 and 61635 include all selective vascular catheterization of the target vascular family, all diagnostic imaging for arteriography of the target vascular family, and all related radiological supervision and interpretation. When diagnostic arteriogram (including imaging and selective catheterization) confirms the need for angioplasty or stent placement, 61630 and 61635 are inclusive of these services. If angioplasty or stenting are not indicated, then the appropriate codes for selective catheterization and imaging should be reported in lieu of 61630 and 61635)

61640 Balloon dilatation of intracranial vasospasm, percutaneous; initial vessel

+ 61641 each additional vessel in same vascular family (List separately in addition to code for primary procedure)

+ 61642 each additional vessel in different vascular family (List separately in addition to code for primary procedure)

(Use 61641 and 61642 in conjunction with 61640)

(61640, 61641, 61642 include all selective vascular catheterization of the target vessel, contrast injection(s), vessel measurement, roadmapping, postdilatation angiography, and fluoroscopic guidance for the balloon dilatation)

SURGERY FOR ANEURYSM, ARTERIOVENOUS MALFORMATION OR VASCULAR DISEASE

Includes craniotomy when appropriate for procedure.

61680 Surgery of intracranial arteriovenous malformation; supratentorial, simple

61682 supratentorial, complex

61684 infratentorial, simple

● New Code ▲ Revised Code + Add-On Code ⊘ Modifier -51 Exempt ⊙ Moderate Sedation

61686   infratentorial, complex

61690   dural, simple

61692   dural, complex

61697 Surgery of complex intracranial aneurysm, intracranial approach; carotid circulation

61698   vertebrobasilar circulation

(61697, 61698 involve aneurysms that are larger than 15 mm or with calcification of the aneurysm neck, or with incorporation of normal vessels into the aneurysm neck, or a procedure requiring temporary vessel occlusion, trapping or cardiopulmonary bypass to successfully treat the aneurysm)

61700 Surgery of simple intracranial aneurysm, intracranial approach; carotid circulation

61702   vertebrobasilar circulation

61703 Surgery of intracranial aneurysm, cervical approach by application of occluding clamp to cervical carotid artery (Selverstone-Crutchfield type)

(For cervical approach for direct ligation of carotid artery, see 37600-37606)

61705 Surgery of aneurysm, vascular malformation or carotid-cavernous fistula; by intracranial and cervical occlusion of carotid artery

61708   by intracranial electrothrombosis

(For ligation or gradual occlusion of internal/common carotid artery, see 37605, 37606)

61710   by intra-arterial embolization, injection procedure, or balloon catheter

61711 Anastomosis, arterial, extracranial-intracranial (eg, middle cerebral/cortical) arteries

(For carotid or vertebral thromboendarterectomy, use 35301)

795

| Separate Procedure | Unlisted Procedure | CCI Comp. Code | Non-specific Procedure |

(Use 69990 when the surgical microscope is employed for the microsurgical procedure. Do not use 69990 for visualization with magnifying loupes or corrected vision)

STEREOTAXIS

61720 Creation of lesion by stereotactic method, including burr hole(s) and localizing and recording techniques, single or multiple stages; globus pallidus or thalamus

61735 subcortical structure(s) other than globus pallidus or thalamus

61750 Stereotactic biopsy, aspiration, or excision, including burr hole(s), for intracranial lesion;

61751 with computed tomography and/or magnetic resonance guidance

(For radiological supervision and interpretation of computerized tomography, see 70450, 70460, or 70470 as appropriate)

(For radiological supervision and interpretation of magnetic resonance imaging, see 70551, 70552, or 70553 as appropriate)

61760 Stereotactic implantation of depth electrodes into the cerebrum for long term seizure monitoring

61770 Stereotactic localization, including burr hole(s), with insertion of catheter(s) or probe(s) for placement of radiation source

+ **61781** Stereotactic computer-assisted (navigational) procedure; cranial, intradural (list separately in addition to code for primary procedure)

(Do not report 61781 in conjunction with 61720-61791, 61796-61799, 61863-61868, 62201, 77371-77373, 77432)

+ **61782** cranial, extradural (list separately in addition to code for primary procedure)

(Do not report 61781, 61782 by the same individual during the same surgical session)

+ **61783** spinal (list separately in addition to code for primary procedure)

(Do not report 61783 in conjunction with 63620, 63621)

● New Code ▲ Revised Code + Add-On Code ⊘ Modifier -51 Exempt ⊙ Moderate Sedation

61790 Creation of lesion by stereotactic method, percutaneous, by neurolytic agent (eg, alcohol, thermal, electrical, radiofrequency); gasserian ganglion

61791 trigeminal medullary tract

(61793 deleted 2009 edition; see 61796-61800, 63620-63621)

STEREOTACTIC RADIOSURGERY (CRANIAL)

Cranial stereotactic radiosurgery is a distinct procedure that utilizes externally generated ionizing radiation to inactivate or eradicate defined target(s) in the head without the need to make an incision. The target is defined by and the treatment is delivered using high-resolution stereotactic imaging. Stereotactic radiosurgery codes and headframe application procedures are reported by the neurosurgeon. The radiation oncologist reports the appropriate code(s) for clinical treatment planning, physics and dosimetry, treatment delivery, and management from the Radiation Oncology section (77261-77790). Any necessary planning, dosimetry, targeting, positioning, or blocking by the neurosurgeon is included in the stereotactic radiation surgery services. The same individual should not report stereotactic radiosurgery services with radiation treatment management codes (77427-77435).

Do not report stereotactic radiosurgery more than once per lesion per course of treatment when the treatment requires more than one session.

Codes 61796 and 61797 involve stereotactic radiosurgery for simple cranial lesions. Simple cranial lesions are lesions less than 3.5 cm in maximum dimension that do not meet the definition of a complex lesion provided below. Report code 61796 when all lesions are simple.

Codes 61798 and 61799 involve stereotactic radiosurgery for complex cranial lesions and procedures that create therapeutic lesions (eg., thalamotomy or pallidotomy). All lesions 3.5 cm in maximum dimension or greater are complex. When performing therapeutic lesion creation procedures, report code 61798 only once regardless of the number of lesions created. Schwannomas, arterio-venous malformations, pituitary tumors, glomus tumors, pineal region tumors and cavernous sinus/parasellar/petroclival tumors are complex. Any lesion that is adjacent (5 mm or less) to the optic nerve/optic chasm/optic tract or within the brainstem is complex. If treating multiple lesions, and any single lesion treated is complex, use 61798.

Do not report 61796-61800 in conjunction with code 20660.

Codes 61796-61799 include computer-assisted planning. Do not report codes 61796-61799 in conjunction with 61795.

	Separate Procedure		Unlisted Procedure		CCI Comp. Code		Non-specific Procedure

(For intensity modulated beam delivery plan and treatment, see 77301, 77418. For stereotactic body radiation therapy, see 77373, 77435)

(61795   deleted 2010 [2011 edition]. To report, see 61781, 61782, 61783)

61796   Stereotactic radiosurgery (particle beam, gamma ray, or linear accelerator); 1 simple cranial lesion

(Do not report 61796 more than once per course of treatment)

(Do not report 61796 in conjunction with 61798)

+ 61797   each additional cranial lesion, simple (list separately in addition to code for primary procedure)

(Use 61797 in conjunction with 61796, 61798)

(For each course of treatment, 61797 and 61799 may be reported no more than once per lesion. Do not report any combination of 61797 and 61799 more than 4 times for entire course of treatment regardless of number of lesions treated)

61798   1 complex cranial lesion

(Do not report 61798 more than once per course of treatment)

(Do not report 61798 in conjunction with 61796)

+ 61799   each additional cranial lesion, complex (list separately in addition to code for primary procedure)

(Use 61799 in conjunction with 61798)

(For each course of treatment, 61797 and 61799 may be reported no more than once per lesion. Do not report any combination of 61797 and 61799 more than 4 times for entire course of treatment regardless of number of lesions treated)

+ 61800   Application of stereotactic headframe for stereotactic radiosurgery (list separately in addition to code for primary procedure)

(Use 61800 in conjunction with 61796, 61798)

NEUROSTIMULATORS (INTRACRANIAL)

Codes 61850-61888 apply to both simple and complex neurostimulators. For initial or subsequent electronic analysis and programming of neurostimulator pulse generators, see codes 95970-95975.

  ● New Code   ▲ Revised Code   + Add-On Code   ⊘ Modifier -51 Exempt   ⊙ Moderate Sedation

Microelectrode recording, when performed by the operating surgeon in association with implantation of neurostimulator electrode arrays, is an inclusive service and should not be reported separately. If another individual participates in neurophysiological mapping during a deep brain stimulator implantation procedure, this service may be reported by the second individual with codes 95961-95962.

61850 Twist drill or burr hole(s) for implantation of neurostimulator electrodes, cortical

61860 Craniectomy or craniotomy for implantation of neurostimulator electrodes, cerebral, cortical

61863 Twist drill, burr hole, craniotomy, or craniectomy with stereotactic implantation of neurostimulator electrode array in subcortical site (eg, thalamus, globus pallidus, subthalamic nucleus, periventricular, periaqueductal gray), without use of intraoperative microelectrode recording; first array

+ 61864 each additional array (List separately in addition to primary procedure)

(Use 61864 in conjunction with 61863)

61867 Twist drill, burr hole, craniotomy, or craniectomy with stereotactic implantation of neurostimulator electrode array in subcortical site (eg, thalamus, globus pallidus, subthalamic nucleus, periventricular, periaqueductal gray), with use of intraoperative microelectrode recording; first array

+ 61868 each additional array (List separately in addition to primary procedure)

(Use 61868 in conjunction with 61867)

61870 Craniectomy for implantation of neurostimulator electrodes, cerebellar; cortical

61875 subcortical

61880 Revision or removal of intracranial neurostimulator electrodes

61885 Insertion or replacement of cranial neurostimulator pulse generator or receiver, direct or inductive coupling; with connection to a single electrode array

61886 with connection to 2 or more electrode arrays

799

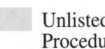 Separate Procedure   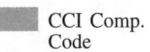 Unlisted Procedure   CCI Comp. Code   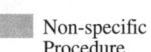 Non-specific Procedure

(For percutaneous placement of cranial nerve (eg, vagus, trigeminal) neurostimulator electrode(s), use 64553)

(For revision or removal of cranial nerve (eg, vagus, trigeminal) neurostimulator electrode array, use 64569)

61888 Revision or removal of cranial neurostimulator pulse generator or receiver

(Do not report 61888 in conjunction with 61885 or 61886 for the same pulse generator)

REPAIR

62000 Elevation of depressed skull fracture; simple, extradural

62005 compound or comminuted, extradural

62010 with repair of dura and/or debridement of brain

62100 Craniotomy for repair of dural/cerebrospinal fluid leak, including surgery for rhinorrhea/otorrhea

(For repair of spinal dural/CSF leak, see 63707, 63709)

62115 Reduction of craniomegalic skull (eg, treated hydrocephalus); not requiring bone grafts or cranioplasty

62116 with simple cranioplasty

62117 requiring craniotomy and reconstruction with or without bone graft (includes obtaining grafts)

62120 Repair of encephalocele, skull vault, including cranioplasty

62121 Craniotomy for repair of encephalocele, skull base

62140 Cranioplasty for skull defect; up to 5 cm diameter

62141 larger than 5 cm diameter

62142 Removal of bone flap or prosthetic plate of skull

62143 Replacement of bone flap or prosthetic plate of skull

62145 Cranioplasty for skull defect with reparative brain surgery

● New Code ▲ Revised Code ✛ Add-On Code ⊘ Modifier -51 Exempt ⊙ Moderate Sedation

62146 Cranioplasty with autograft (includes obtaining bone grafts); up to 5 cm diameter

62147 larger than 5 cm diameter

+ **62148** Incision and retrieval of subcutaneous cranial bone graft for cranioplasty (List separately in addition to code for primary procedure)

(Use 62148 in conjunction with codes 62140-62147)

NEUROENDOSCOPY

Surgical endoscopy always includes diagnostic endoscopy

+ **62160** Neuroendoscopy, intracranial, for placement or replacement of ventricular catheter and attachment to shunt system or external drainage (List separately in addition to code for primary procedure)

(Use 62160 only in conjunction with codes 61107, 61210, 62220-62230, 62258)

62161 Neuroendoscopy, intracranial; with dissection of adhesions, fenestration of septum pellucidum or intraventricular cysts (including placement, replacement, or removal of ventricular catheter)

62162 with fenestration or excision of colloid cyst, including placement of external ventricular catheter for drainage

62163 with retrieval of foreign body

62164 with excision of brain tumor, including placement of external ventricular catheter for drainage

62165 with excision of pituitary tumor, transnasal or transsphenoidal approach

CEREBROSPINAL FLUID (CSF) SHUNT

62180 Ventriculocisternostomy (Torkildsen type operation)

62190 Creation of shunt; subarachnoid/subdural-atrial, -jugular, -auricular

62192 subarachnoid/subdural-peritoneal, -pleural, other terminus

---

801

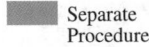 Separate Procedure

 Unlisted Procedure

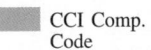 CCI Comp. Code

Non-specific Procedure

62194 Replacement or irrigation, subarachnoid/subdural catheter

62200 Ventriculocisternostomy, third ventricle;

62201 stereotactic, neuroendoscopic method

(For intracranial neuroendoscopic procedures, see 62161-62165)

62220 Creation of shunt; ventriculo-atrial, -jugular, -auricular

(For intracranial neuroendoscopic ventricular catheter placement, use 62160)

62223 ventriculo-peritoneal, -pleural, other terminus

(For intracranial neuroendoscopic ventricular catheter placement, use 62160)

62225 Replacement or irrigation, ventricular catheter

(For intracranial neuroendoscopic ventricular catheter placement, use 62160)

62230 Replacement or revision of cerebrospinal fluid shunt, obstructed valve, or distal catheter in shunt system

(For intracranial neuroendoscopic ventricular catheter placement, use 62160)

62252 Reprogramming of programmable cerebrospinal shunt

62256 Removal of complete cerebrospinal fluid shunt system; without replacement

62258 with replacement by similar or other shunt at same operation

(For percutaneous irrigation or aspiration of shunt reservoir, use 61070)

(For reprogramming of programmable CSF shunt, use 62252)

(For intracranial neuroendoscopic ventricular catheter placement, use 62160)

● New Code ▲ Revised Code ✚ Add-On Code ⊘ Modifier -51 Exempt ⊙ Moderate Sedation

SPINE AND SPINAL CORD

(For application of caliper or tongs, use 20660)

(For treatment of fracture or dislocation of spine, see 22305-22327)

INJECTION, DRAINAGE, OR ASPIRATION

Injection of contract during fluoroscopic guidance and localization is an inclusive component of codes 62263, 62264, 62267, 62270-62273, 62280-62282, 62310-62319. Fluoroscopic guidance and localization is reported with code 77003, unless a formal contrast study (myelography, epidurography, or arthrography) is performed, in which case the use of fluoroscopy is included in the supervision and interpretation codes.

For radiologic supervision and interpretation of epidurography, use 72275. Code 72275 is only to be used when an epidurogram is performed, images documented, and a formal radiologic report is issued.

Code 62263 describes a catheter-based treatment involving targeted injection of various substances (eg., hypertonic saline, steroid, anesthetic) via an indwelling epidural catheter. Code 62263 includes percutaneous insertion and removal of an epidural catheter (remaining in place over a several-day period), for the administration of multiple injections of a neurolytic agent(s) performed during serial treatment sessions (ie., spanning two or more treatment days). If required, adhesions or scarring may also be lysed by mechanical means. Code 62263 is NOT reported for each adhesiolysis treatment, but should be reported ONCE to describe the entire series of injections/infusions spanning two or more treatment days.

Code 62264 describes multiple adhesiolysis treatment sessions performed on the same day. Adhesions or scarring may be lysed by injections of neurolytic agent(s). If required, adhesions or scarring may also be lysed mechanically using a percutaneously-deployed catheter.

Codes 62263 and 62264 include the procedure of injections of contrast for epidurography (72275) and fluoroscopic guidance and localization (77003) during initial or subsequent sessions.

Fluoroscopy (for localization) may be used in the placement of injections reported with 62310-62319, but is not required. If used, fluoroscopy should be reported with 77003. For epidurography, use 72275.

The placement and use of a catheter to administer one or more epidural or subarachnoid injectiions on a single calendar day should be reported in the same manner as if a needle had been used, ie, as a single injection using either 62310 or 62311. Such injections should not be reported with 62318 or 62319.

803

	Separate Procedure		Unlisted Procedure		CCI Comp. Code		Non-specific Procedure

Threading a catheter into the epidural space, injecting substances at one or more levels and then removing the catheter should be treated as a single injection (62310, 62311). If the catheter is left in place to deliver substance(s) over a prolonged period (ie, more than a single calendar day) either continuously or via intermittent bolus, use 62318, 62319 as appropriate.

When reporting 62310-62319, code choice is based on the region at which the needle or catheter entered the body (eg, lumbar). Codes 62310-62319 should be reported only once, when the substance injected spreads or catheter tip insertion moves into another spinal region (eg, 62311 is reported only once for injection or catheter insertion at L3-4 with spread of the substance or placement of the catheter tip to the thoracic region).

Percutaneous spinal procedures are done with indirect visualization (eg, image guidance or endoscopic approaches) and without direct visualization (including through a microscope). Endoscopic assistance during an open procedure with direct visualization is reported using excision codes (eg, 63020-63035).

(Report 01996 for daily hospital management of continuous epidural or subarachnoid drug administration performed in conjunction with 62318-62319)

62263 Percutaneous lysis of epidural adhesions using solution injection (eg, hypertonic saline, enzyme) or mechanical means (eg, catheter) including radiologic localization (includes contrast when administered), multiple adhesiolysis sessions; 2 or more days

(62263 includes codes 72275 and 77003)

62264 1 day

(Do not report 62264 with 62263)

(62264 includes codes 72275 and 77003)

62267 Percutaneous aspiration within the nucleus pulposus, intervertebral, disc, or paravertebral tissue for diagnostic purposes

(For imaging, use 77003)

(Do not report 62267 in conjunction with 10022, 20225, 62287, 62290, 62291)

62268 Percutaneous aspiration, spinal cord cyst or syrinx

(For radiological supervision and interpretation, see 76942, 77002, 77012)

● New Code ▲ Revised Code + Add-On Code ⊘ Modifier -51 Exempt ⊙ Moderate Sedation

62269 Biopsy of spinal cord, percutaneous needle

(For radiological supervision and interpretation, see 76942, 77002, 77012)

(For fine needle aspiration, see 10021, 10022)

(For evaluation of fine needle aspirate, see 88172, 88173)

62270 Spinal puncture, lumbar, diagnostic

62272 Spinal puncture, therapeutic, for drainage of cerebrospinal fluid (by needle or catheter)

62273 Injection, epidural, of blood or clot patch

(For injection of diagnostic or therapeutic substance(s), see 62310, 62311, 62318, 62319)

62280 Injection/infusion of neurolytic substance (eg, alcohol, phenol, iced saline solutions), with or without other therapeutic substance; subarachnoid

62281 epidural, cervical or thoracic

62282 epidural, lumbar, sacral (caudal)

62284 Injection procedure for myelography and/or computed tomography, spinal (other than C1-C2 and posterior fossa)

(For injection procedure at C1-C2, use 61055)

(For radiological supervision and interpretation, see Radiology)

62287 Decompression procedure, percutaneous, of nucleus pulposus of intervertebral disc, any method utilizing needle based technique to remove disc material under fluoroscopic imaging or other form of indirect visualization, with the use of an endoscope, with discography and/or epidural injection(s) at the treated level(s), when performed, single or multiple levels, lumbar

(This includes endoscopic approach)

(Do not report 62287 in conjunction with 62267, 62290, 62311, 77003, 77012, 72295, when performed at same level)

(For non-needle based technique for percutaneous decompression of nucleus pulposus of intervertebral disc, see codes 0274T, 0275T)

805

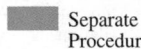 Separate Procedure   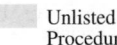 Unlisted Procedure   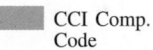 CCI Comp. Code   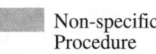 Non-specific Procedure

62290 Injection procedure for diskography, each level; lumbar

62291   cervical or thoracic

(For radiological supervision or interpretation, see 72285, 72295)

62292 Injection procedure for chemonucleolysis, including diskography, intervertebral disk, single or multiple levels, lumbar

62294 Injection procedure, arterial, for occlusion of arteriovenous malformation, spinal

62310 Injection(s), of diagnostic or therapeutic substance(s) (including anesthetic, antispasmodic, opioid, steroid, other solution), not including neurolytic substances, including needle or catheter placement, includes contrast for localization when performed, epidural or subarachnoid; cervical or thoracic

62311   lumbar or sacral (caudal)

62318 Injection(s), including indwelling catheter placement, continuous infusion or intermittent bolus, of diagnostic or therapeutic substance(s) (including anesthetic, antispasmodic, opioid, steroid, other solution), not including neurolytic substances, includes contrast for localization when performed, epidural or subarachnoid; cervical or thoracic

62319   lumbar or sacral (caudal)

(For transforaminal epidural injection, see 64479-64484)

(Report 01996 for daily hospital management of continuous epidural or subarachnoid drug administration performed in conjunction with codes 62318-62319)

CATHETER IMPLANTATION

(For percutaneous placement of intrathecal or epidural catheter, see codes 62270-62273, 62280-62284, 62310-62319)

62350 Implantation, revision or repositioning of tunneled intrathecal or epidural catheter, for long-term medication administration via an external pump or implantable reservoir/infusion pump; without laminectomy

62351   with laminectomy

● New Code   ▲ Revised Code   + Add-On Code   ⊘ Modifier -51 Exempt   ⊙ Moderate Sedation

(For refilling and maintenance of an implantable infusion pump for spinal or brain drug therapy, use 95990)

62355 Removal of previously implanted intrathecal or epidural catheter

RESERVOIR/PUMP IMPLANTATION

62360 Implantation or replacement of device for intrathecal or epidural drug infusion; subcutaneous reservoir

62361 non-programmable pump

62362 programmable pump, including preparation of pump, with or without programming

62365 Removal of subcutaneous reservoir or pump, previously implanted for intrathecal or epidural infusion

62367 Electronic analysis of programmable, implanted pump for intrathecal or epidural drug infusion (includes evaluation of reservoir status, alarm status, drug prescription status); without reprogramming or refill

62368 with reprogramming

(For refilling and maintenance of an implantable infusion pump for spinal or brain drug therapy, use 95990)

62369 with reprogramming and refill

▲ **62370** with reprogramming and refill (requiring skill of a physician or other qualified health care professional)

(Do not report 62367-62370 in conjunction with 95990, 95991. For refilling and maintenance of a reservoir or an implantable infusion pump for spinal or brain drug delivery without reprogramming, see 95990, 95991)

POSTERIOR EXTRADURAL LAMINOTOMY OR LAMINECTOMY FOR EXPLORATION/DECOMPRESSION OF NEURAL ELEMENTS OR EXCISION OF HERNIATED INTERVERTEBRAL DISKS

Endoscopically assisted laminotomy (hemilaminectomy) requires open and direct visualization. When visualization is only endoscopic and/or image guidance, the procedure is percutaneous and reported using 0274T, 0275T

(When 63001-63048 are followed by arthrodesis, see 22590-22614)

807

	Separate Procedure		Unlisted Procedure		CCI Comp. Code		Non-specific Procedure

63001 Laminectomy with exploration and/or decompression of spinal cord and/or cauda equina, without facetectomy, foraminotomy or diskectomy, (eg, spinal stenosis), one or two vertebral segments; cervical

63003 thoracic

63005 lumbar, except for spondylolisthesis

63011 sacral

63012 Laminectomy with removal of abnormal facets and/or pars inter-articularis with decompression of cauda equina and nerve roots for spondylolisthesis, lumbar (Gill type procedure)

63015 Laminectomy with exploration and/or decompression of spinal cord and/or cauda equina, without facetectomy, foraminotomy or diskectomy, (eg, spinal stenosis), more than 2 vertebral segments; cervical

63016 thoracic

63017 lumbar

63020 Laminotomy (hemilaminectomy), with decompression of nerve root(s), including partial facetectomy, foraminotomy and/or excision of herniated intervertebral disc; 1 interspace, cervical

(For bilateral procedure, report 63020 with modifier -50)

63030 1 interspace, lumbar

(For bilateral procedure, report 63030 with modifier -50)

+ 63035 each additional interspace, cervical or lumbar (List separately in addition to code for primary procedure)

(Use 63035 in conjunction with codes 63020-63030)

(For bilateral procedures, report 63035 with modifier -50)

(For percutaneous endoscopic approach, see 0274T, 0275T)

63040 Laminotomy (hemilaminectomy), with decompression of nerve root(s), including partial facetectomy, foraminotomy and/or excision of herniated intervertebral disk, reexploration, single interspace; cervical

(For bilateral procedure, report 63040 with modifier -50)

● New Code   ▲ Revised Code   + Add-On Code   ⊘ Modifier -51 Exempt   ⊙ Moderate Sedation

63042   lumbar

(For bilateral procedure, report 63042 with modifier -50)

+ 63043   each additional cervical interspace (List separately in addition to code for primary procedure)

(Use 63043 in conjunction with code 63040)

(For bilateral procedure, report 63043 with modifier -50)

+ 63044   each additional lumbar interspace (List separately in addition to code for primary procedure)

(Use 63044 in conjunction with code 63042)

(For bilateral procedure, report 63044 with modifier -50)

63045 Laminectomy, facetectomy and foraminotomy (unilateral or bilateral with decompression of spinal cord, cauda equina and/or nerve root(s), (eg, spinal or lateral recess stenosis)), single vertebral segment; cervical

63046   thoracic

63047   lumbar

+ 63048   each additional segment, cervical, thoracic, or lumbar (List separately in addition to code for primary procedure)

(Use 63048 in conjunction with codes 63045-63047)

63050 Laminoplasty, cervical, with decompression of the spinal cord, 2 or more vertebral segments;

63051   with reconstruction of the posterior bony elements (including the application of bridging bone graft and non-segmental fixation devices (eg, wire, suture, mini-plates), when performed)

(Do not report 63050 or 63051 in conjunction with 22600, 22614, 22840-22842, 63001, 63015, 63045, 63048, 63295 for the same vertebral segment(s))

Separate Procedure   Unlisted Procedure   CCI Comp. Code   Non-specific Procedure

TRANSPEDICULAR OR COSTOVERTEBRAL APPROACH FOR POSTEROLATERAL EXTRADURAL EXPLORATION/ DECOMPRESSION

63055 Transpedicular approach with decompression of spinal cord, equina and/or nerve root(s) (eg, herniated intervertebral disk), single segment; thoracic

63056 lumbar (including transfacet, or lateral extraforaminal approach) (eg, far lateral herniated intervertebral disk)

+ 63057 each additional segment, thoracic or lumbar (List separately in addition to code for primary procedure)

(Use 63057 in conjunction with codes 63055, 63056)

63064 Costovertebral approach with decompression of spinal cord or nerve root(s), (eg, herniated intervertebral disk), thoracic; single segment

+ 63066 each additional segment (List separately in addition to code for primary procedure)

(Use 63066 in conjunction with code 63064)

(For excision of thoracic intraspinal lesions by laminectomy, see 63266, 63271, 63276, 63281, 63286)

ANTERIOR OR ANTEROLATERAL APPROACH FOR EXTRADURAL EXPLORATION/DECOMPRESSION

For the following codes, when two surgeons work together as primary surgeons performing distinct part(s) of spinal cord exploration/decompression operation, each surgeon should report his/her distinct operative work by appending modifier 62 to the procedure code (and any associated add-on codes for that procedure code as long as both surgeons continue to work together as primary surgeons). In this situation, modifier 62 may be appended to the definitive procedure code(s) 63075, 63077, 63081, 63085, 63087, 63090 and, as appropriate, to associated additional interspace add-on code(s) 63076, 63078 or additional segment add-on codes 63082, 63086, 63088, 63091 as long as both surgeons continue to work together as primary surgeons.

63075 Diskectomy, anterior, with decompression of spinal cord and/or nerve root(s), including osteophytectomy; cervical, single interspace

(Do not report 63075 in conjunction with 22554, even if performed by separate individuals. To report anterior cervical discectomy and interbody fusion at the same level during the same session, use 22551)

● New Code ▲ Revised Code + Add-On Code ⊘ Modifier -51 Exempt ⊙ Moderate Sedation

+ 63076   cervical, each additional interspace (List separately in addition to code for primary procedure)

(Do not report 63076 in conjunction with 22554, even if performed by separate individuals. To report anterior cervical discectomy and interbody fusion at the same level during the same session, use 22552)

(Use 63076 in conjunction with code 63075)

63077   thoracic, single interspace

+ 63078   thoracic, each additional interspace (List separately in addition to code for primary procedure)

(Use 63078 in conjunction with code 63077)

(Do not report code 69990 in addition to codes 63075-63078)

63081   Vertebral corpectomy (vertebral body resection), partial or complete, anterior approach with decompression of spinal cord and/or nerve root(s); cervical, single segment

+ 63082   cervical, each additional segment (List separately in addition to code for primary procedure)

(Use 63082 in conjunction with code 63081)

(For transoral approach, see 61575, 61576)

63085   Vertebral corpectomy (vertebral body resection), partial or complete, transthoracic approach with decompression of spinal cord and/or nerve root(s); thoracic, single segment

+ 63086   thoracic, each additional segment (List separately in addition to code for primary procedure)

(Use 63086 in conjunction with code 63085)

63087   Vertebral corpectomy (vertebral body resection), partial or complete, combined thoracolumbar approach with decompression of spinal cord, cauda equina or nerve root(s), lower thoracic or lumbar; single segment

+ 63088   each additional segment (List separately in addition to code for primary procedure)

(Use 63088 in conjunction with code 63087)

811

| | Separate Procedure | | Unlisted Procedure | | CCI Comp. Code | | Non-specific Procedure |

63090 Vertebral corpectomy (vertebral body resection), partial or complete, transperitoneal or retroperitoneal approach with decompression of spinal cord, cauda equina or nerve root(s), lower thoracic, lumbar, or sacral; single segment

+ 63091 each additional segment (List separately in addition to code for primary procedure)

(Use 63091 in conjunction with code 63090)

(Procedures 63081-63091 include diskectomy above and/or below vertebral segment)

(If followed by arthrodesis, see 22548-22812)

(For reconstruction of spine, use appropriate vertebral corpectomy codes 63081-63091, bone graft codes 20930-20938, arthrodesis codes 22548-22812, and spinal instrumentation codes 22840-22855)

LATERAL EXTRACAVITARY APPROACH FOR EXTRADURAL EXPLORATION/DECOMPRESSION

63101 Vertebral corpectomy (vertebral body resection), partial or complete, lateral extracavitary approach with decompression of spinal cord and/or nerve root(s) (eg, for tumor or retropulsed bone fragments); thoracic, single segment

63102 lumbar, single segment

+ 63103 thoracic or lumbar, each additional segment (List separately in addition to code for primary procedure)

(Use 63103 in conjunction with 63101 and 63102)

INCISION

63170 Laminectomy with myelotomy (eg, Bischof or DREZ type), cervical, thoracic, or thoracolumbar

63172 Laminectomy with drainage of intramedullary cyst/syrinx; to subarachnoid space

63173 to peritoneal or pleural space

63180 Laminectomy and section of dentate ligaments, with or without dural graft, cervical; 1 or 2 segments

63182 more than 2 segments

812

● New Code	▲ Revised Code	+ Add-On Code	⊘ Modifier -51 Exempt	⊙ Moderate Sedation

63185 Laminectomy with rhizotomy; 1 or 2 segments

63190   more than 2 segments

63191 Laminectomy with section of spinal accessory nerve

(For bilateral procedure, report 63191 with modifier -50)

(For resection of sternocleidomastoid muscle, use 21720)

63194 Laminectomy with cordotomy, with section of one spinothalamic tract, 1 stage; cervical

63195   thoracic

63196 Laminectomy with cordotomy, with section of both spinothalamic tracts, 1 stage; cervical

63197   thoracic

63198 Laminectomy with cordotomy with section of both spinothalamic tracts, 2 stages within 14 days; cervical

63199   thoracic

63200 Laminectomy, with release of tethered spinal cord, lumbar

EXCISION BY LAMINECTOMY OF LESION OTHER THAN HERNIATED DISC

63250 Laminectomy for excision or occlusion of arteriovenous malformation of spinal cord; cervical

63251   thoracic

63252   thoracolumbar

63265 Laminectomy for excision or evacuation of intraspinal lesion other than neoplasm, extradural; cervical

63266   thoracic

63267   lumbar

63268   sacral

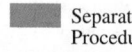 Separate Procedure   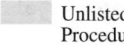 Unlisted Procedure   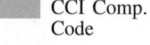 CCI Comp. Code   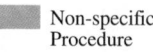 Non-specific Procedure

813

63270	Laminectomy for excision of intraspinal lesion other than neoplasm, intradural; cervical
63271	thoracic
63272	lumbar
63273	sacral
63275	Laminectomy for biopsy/excision of intraspinal neoplasm; extradural, cervical
63276	extradural, thoracic
63277	extradural, lumbar
63278	extradural, sacral
63280	intradural, extramedullary, cervical
63281	intradural, extramedullary, thoracic
63282	intradural, extramedullary, lumbar
63283	intradural, sacral
63285	intradural, intramedullary, cervical
63286	intradural, intramedullary, thoracic
63287	intradural, intramedullary, thoracolumbar
63290	combined extradural-intradural lesion, any level

(For drainage of intramedullary cyst/syrinx, use 63172, 63173)

+ **63295** Osteoplastic reconstruction of dorsal spinal elements, following primary intraspinal procedure (List separately in addition to code for primary procedure)

(Use 63295 in conjunction with 63172, 63173, 63185, 63190, 63200-63290)

(Do not report 63295 in conjunction with 22590-22614, 22840-22844, 63050, 63051 for the same vertebral segment(s))

● New Code ▲ Revised Code + Add-On Code ⊘ Modifier -51 Exempt ⊙ Moderate Sedation

EXCISION, ANTERIOR OR ANTEROLATERAL APPROACH, INTRASPINAL LESION

For the following codes, when two surgeons work together as primary surgeons performing distinct part(s) of an anterior approach for an intraspinal excision, each surgeon should report his/her distinct operative work by appending modifier 62 to the single definitive procedure code. In this situation, modifier 62 may be appended to the definitive procedure code(s) 63300-63307 and, as appropriate, to the associated additional segment add-on code 63308 as long as both surgeons continue to work together as primary surgeons.

(For arthrodesis, see 22548-22585)

(For reconstruction of spine, see 20930-20938)

63300 Vertebral corpectomy (vertebral body resection), partial or complete, for excision of intraspinal lesion, single segment; extradural, cervical

63301 extradural, thoracic by transthoracic approach

63302 extradural, thoracic by thoracolumbar approach

63303 extradural, lumbar or sacral by transperitoneal or retroperitoneal approach

63304 intradural, cervical

63305 intradural, thoracic by transthoracic approach

63306 intradural, thoracic by thoracolumbar approach

63307 intradural, lumbar or sacral by transperitoneal or retroperitoneal approach

+ 63308 each additional segment (List separately in addition to codes for single segment)

(Use 63308 in conjunction with codes 63300-63307)

STEREOTAXIS

63600 Creation of lesion of spinal cord by stereotactic method, percutaneous, any modality (including stimulation and/or recording)

63610 Stereotactic stimulation of spinal cord, percutaneous, separate procedure not followed by other surgery

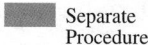 Separate Procedure   Unlisted Procedure   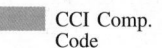 CCI Comp. Code   Non-specific Procedure

815

63615 Stereotactic biopsy, aspiration, or excision of lesion, spinal cord

STEREOTACTIC RADIOSURGERY (SPINAL)

These codes are reported by the surgeon. The radiation oncologist reports the appropriate code(s) for clinical treatment planning, physics and dosimetry, treatment delivery and management from the Radiation Oncology section (77261-77790). Any necessary planning, dosimetry, targeting, positioning, or blocking by the neurosurgeon is included in the stereotactic radiation surgery services. The same individual should not report stereotactic radiosurgery services with radiation treatment management codes (77427-77432).

Do not report stereotactic radiosurgery more than once per lesion per course of treatment when the treatment requires greater than one session.

For other radiation services of the spine, see Radiation Oncology services.

Codes 63620, 63621 include computer-assisted planning. Do not report 63620, 63621 in conjunction with 61781-61783.

(For intensity modulated beam delivery plan and treatment, see 77301, 77418. For stereotactic body radiation therapy, see 77373, 77435)

63620 Stereotactic radiosurgery (particle beam, gamma ray, or linear accelerator); 1 spinal lesion

(Do not report 63620 more than once per course of treatment)

+ 63621 each additional spinal lesion (list separately in addition to code for primary procedure)

(Report 63621 in conjunction with 63620)

(For each course of treatment, 63621 may be reported no more than once per lesion. Do not report 63621 more than 2 times for entire course of treatment regardless of number of lesions treated)

NEUROSTIMULATORS (SPINAL)

Codes 63650-63688 apply to both simple and complex neurostimulators. For initial or subsequent electronic analysis and programming of neurostimulator pulse generators, see codes 95970-95975.

Codes 63650, 63655, and 63661-63664 describe the operative placement, revision, replacement, or removal of the spinal neurostimulator system components to provide spinal electrical stimulation. A neurostimulator system includes an implanted neurostimulator, external controller, extension, and collection of

● New Code   ▲ Revised Code   + Add-On Code   ⊘ Modifier -51 Exempt   ⊙ Moderate Sedation

contacts. Multiple contacts or electrodes (4 or more) provide the actual electrical stimulation in the epidural space.

For percutaneously placed neurostimulator systems (63650, 63661, 63663), the contacts are on a catheter-like lead. An array defines the collection of contacts that are on one catheter.

For systems placed via an open surgical exposure (63655, 63662, 63664), the contacts are on a plate or paddle-shaped surface.

Do not report 63661 or 63663 when removing or replacing a temporary percutaneously placed array for an external generator.

63650 Percutaneous implantation of neurostimulator electrode array, epidural

63655 Laminectomy for implantation of neurostimulator electrodes, plate/paddle, epidural

(63660 Deleted 2009 [2010 edition]; see 63661-63664)

63661 Removal of spinal neurostimulator electrode percutaneous array(s), including fluoroscopy, when performed

63662 Removal of spinal neurostimulator electrode plate/paddle(s) placed via laminotomy or laminectomy, including fluoroscopy, when performed

63663 Revision including replacement, when performed, of spinal neurostimulator electrode percutaneous array(s), including fluoroscopy, when performed

(Do not report 63663 in conjunction with 63661, 63662 for the same spinal level)

63664 Revision including replacement, when performed, of spinal neurostimulator electrode plate/paddle(s) placed via laminotomy or laminectomy, including fluoroscopy, when performed

(Do not report 63664 in conjunction with 63661, 63662 for the same spinal level)

63685 Insertion or replacement of spinal neurostimulator pulse generator or receiver, direct or inductive coupling

(Do not report 63685 in conjunction with 63688 for the same pulse generator or receiver)

	Separate Procedure		Unlisted Procedure		CCI Comp. Code		Non-specific Procedure

817

63688 Revision or removal of implanted spinal neurostimulator pulse generator or receiver

(For electronic analysis of implanted neurostimulator pulse generator system, see 95970-95975)

REPAIR

63700 Repair of meningocele; less than 5 cm diameter

63702 larger than 5 cm diameter

(Do not use modifier -63 in conjunction with 63700, 63702)

63704 Repair of myelomeningocele; less than 5 cm diameter

63706 larger than 5 cm diameter

(Do not use modifier -63 in conjunction with 63704, 63706)

(For complex skin closure, see Integumentary System)

63707 Repair of dural/cerebrospinal fluid leak, not requiring laminectomy

63709 Repair of dural/cerebrospinal fluid leak or pseudomeningocele, with laminectomy

63710 Dural graft, spinal

(For laminectomy and section of dentate ligaments, with or without dural graft, cervical, see 63180, 63182)

SHUNT, SPINAL CSF

63740 Creation of shunt, lumbar, subarachnoid-peritoneal, -pleural, or other; including laminectomy

63741 percutaneous, not requiring laminectomy

63744 Replacement, irrigation or revision of lumbosubarachnoid shunt

63746 Removal of entire lumbosubarachnoid shunt system without replacement

(For insertion of subarachnoid catheter with reservoir and/or pump for intermittent or continuous infusion of drug including laminectomy, see 62351 and 62360, 62361 or 62362)

● New Code   ▲ Revised Code   + Add-On Code   ⊘ Modifier -51 Exempt   ⊙ Moderate Sedation

(For insertion or replacement of subarachnoid or epidural catheter, with reservoir and/or pump for drug infusion without laminectomy, see 62350 and 62360, 62361 or 62362)

EXTRACRANIAL NERVES, PERIPHERAL NERVES, AND AUTONOMIC NERVOUS SYSTEM

(For intracranial surgery on cranial nerves, see 61450, 61460, 61790)

INTRODUCTION/INJECTION OF ANESTHETIC AGENT (NERVE BLOCK), DIAGNOSTIC OR THERAPEUTIC

(For destruction by neurolytic agent or chemodenervation, see 62280-62282, 64600-64681)

(For epidural or subarachnoid injection, see 62310-62319)

(64479-64495 are unilateral procedures. For bilateral procedures, use modifier -50)

Somatic Nerves

64400 Injection, anesthetic agent; trigeminal nerve, any division or branch

64402 facial nerve

64405 greater occipital nerve

64408 vagus nerve

64410 phrenic nerve

64412 spinal accessory nerve

64413 cervical plexus

64415 brachial plexus, single

64416 brachial plexus, continuous infusion by catheter (including catheter placement)

(Do not report 64416 in conjunction with 01996)

64417 axillary nerve

64418 suprascapular nerve

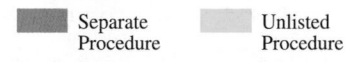 Separate Procedure

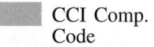 Unlisted Procedure

CCI Comp. Code

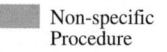 Non-specific Procedure

819

64420   intercostal nerve, single

64421   intercostal nerves, multiple, regional block

64425   ilioinguinal, iliohypogastric nerves

64430   pudendal nerve

64435   paracervical (uterine) nerve

64445   sciatic nerve, single

64446   sciatic nerve, continuous infusion by catheter, (including catheter placement)

(Do not report 64446 in conjuction with 01996)

64447   femoral nerve, single

(Do not report 64447 in conjunction with 01996)

64448   femoral nerve, continuous infusion by catheter (including catheter placement)

(Do not report 64448 in conjunction with 01996)

64449   lumbar plexus, posterior approach, continuous infusion by catheter (including catheter placement)

(Do not report 64449 in conjunction with 01996)

64450   other peripheral nerve or branch

64455   Injection(s), anesthetic agent and/or steroid, plantar common digital nerve(s) (eg, morton's neuroma)

(Do note report 64455 in conjunction with 64632)

(Imaging guidance (fluoroscopy or CT) and any injection of contrast are inclusive components of 64479-64484. Imaging guidance and localization are required for the performance of 64479-64484.)

(Codes 64470-64476 have been deleted. To report, see 64490-64495)

64479   Injection(s), anesthetic agent and/or steroid, transforaminal epidural, with imaging guidance (fluoroscopy or CT); cervical or thoracic, single level

● New Code   ▲ Revised Code   + Add-On Code   ⊘ Modifier -51 Exempt   ⊙ Moderate Sedation

(For transforaminal epidural injection under ultrasound guidance, use 0228T)

+ 64480   cervical or thoracic, each additional level (List separately in addition to code for primary procedure)

(Use 64480 in conjunction with code 64479)

(For transforaminal epidural injection under ultrasound guidance, use 0229T)

(For transforaminal epidural injection at the T12-L1 level, use 64479)

64483   lumbar or sacral, single level

(For transforaminal epidural injection under ultrasound guidance, use 0230T)

+ 64484   lumbar or sacral, each additional level (List separately in addition to code for primary procedure)

(Use 64484 in conjunction with code 64483)

(For transforaminal epidural injection under ultrasound guidance, use 0231T)

(64479-64484 are unilateral procedures. For bilateral procedures, use modifier 50.)

Paravertebral Spinal Nerves and Branches

(Image guidance [fluoroscopy or CT] and any injection of contrast are inclusive components of 64490-64495. Imaging guidance and localization are required for the performance of paravertebral facet joint injections described by codes 64490-64495. If imaging is not used, report 20552-20553. If ultrasound guidance is used, report 0213T-0218T)

(For bilateral paravertebral facet injection procedure, use modifier 50)

(For paravertebral facet injection of the T12-L1 joint, or nerves innervating that joint, use 64490)

64490   Injection(s), diagnostic or therapeutic agent, paravertebral facet (zygapophyseal) joint (or nerves innervating that joint) with image guidance (fluoroscopy or CT), cervical or thoracic; single level

821

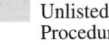 Separate Procedure   Unlisted Procedure   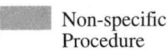 CCI Comp. Code   Non-specific Procedure

+ **64491**   second level (List separately in addition to code for primary procedure)

+ **64492**   third and any additional level(s) (List separately in addition to code for primary procedure)

(Do not report 64492 more than once per day)

(Use 64491, 64492 in conjunction with 64490)

64493   Injection(s), diagnostic or therapeutic agent, paravertebral facet (zygapophyseal) joint (or nerves innervating that joint) with image guidance (fluoroscopy or CT), lumbar or sacral; single level

+ **64494**   second level (List separately in addition to code for primary procedure)

+ **64495**   third and any additional level(s) (List separately in addition to code for primary procedure)

(Do not report 64495 more than once per day)

(Use 64494, 64495 in conjunction with 64493)

Autonomic Nerves

64505   Injection, anesthetic agent; sphenopalatine ganglion

64508   carotid sinus (separate procedure)

64510   stellate ganglion (cervical sympathetic)

64517   superior hypogastric plexus

64520   lumbar or thoracic (paravertebral sympathetic)

64530   celiac plexus, with or without radiologic monitoring

NEUROSTIMULATORS (PERIPHERAL NERVE)

Codes 64553-64595 apply to both simple and complex neurostimulators. For initial or subsequent electronic analysis and programming of neurostimulator pulse generators, see codes 95970-95975. An electrode array is a catheter or other device with more than one contact. The function of each contact may be capable of being adjusted during programming services.

  ● New Code   ▲ Revised Code   + Add-On Code   ⊘ Modifier -51 Exempt   ⊙ Moderate Sedation

(For implantation of trial or permanent electrode arrays or pulse generators for peripheral subcutaneous filed stimulation, see 0282T-0284T)

64550 Application of surface (transcutaneous) neurostimulator

64553 Percutaneous implantation of neurostimulator electrode array; cranial nerve

(For open placement of cranial nerve (eg, vagus, trigeminal) neurostimulator pulse generator or receiver, see 61885, 61886, as appropriate)

64555 peripheral nerve (excludes sacral nerve)

(Do not report 64555 in conjunction with 64566)

(64560 deleted 2011 [2012 edition])

▲ **64561** sacral nerve (transforaminal placement) including image guidance, if performed

64565 neuromuscular

64566 Posterior tibial neurostimulation, percutaneous needle electrode, single treatment, includes programming

(Do not report 64566 in conjunction with 64555, 95970-95972)

64568 Incision for implantation of cranial nerve (eg, vagus nerve) neurostimulator electrode array and pulse generator

(Do not report 64568 in conjunction with 61885, 61886, 64570)

64569 Revision or replacement of cranial nerve (eg, vagus nerve) neurostimulator electrode array, including connection to existing pulse generator

(Do not report 64569 in conjunction with 64570 or 61888)

(For replacement of pulse generator, use 61885)

64570 Removal of cranial nerve (eg, vagus nerve) neurostimulator electrode array and pulse generator

(Do not report 64570 in conjunction with 61888)

(For laparoscopic implantation, revision, replacement, or removal of vagus nerve blocking neurostimulator electrode array

823

 Separate Procedure   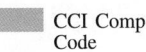 Unlisted Procedure   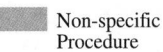 CCI Comp. Code   Non-specific Procedure

and/or pulse generator at the esophagogastric junction, see 0312T-0317T)

(64573   deleted 2010 [2011 edition])

64575   Incision for implantation of neurostimulator electrode array; peripheral nerve (excludes sacral nerve)

(64577   deleted 2011 [2012 edition])

64580   neuromuscular

64581   sacral nerve (transforaminal placement)

64585   Revision or removal of peripheral neurostimulator electrode array

64590   Insertion or replacement of peripheral or gastric neurostimulator pulse generator or receiver, direct or inductive coupling

(Do not report 64590 in conjunction with 64595)

64595   Revision or removal of peripheral or gastric neurostimulator pulse generator or receiver

DESTRUCTION BY NEUROLYTIC AGENT (eg, CHEMICAL, THERMAL, ELECTRICAL, OR RADIOFREQUENCY), CHEMODENERVATION

Codes 64600-64681 include the injection of other therapeutic agents (eg., corticosteroids). Do not report diagnostic/therapeutic injections separately. Do not report a code labeled as destruction when using theraies that are not destructive of the target nerve (eg, pulsed radiofrequency), use 64999. For codes labeled as chemodenervation, the supply of the chemodenervation agent is reported separately.

(For chemodenervation of internal anal sphincter, use 46505)

(For chemodenervation of the bladder, use 52287)

(For chemodenervation for strabismus involving the extraocular muscles, use 67345)

(For chemodenervation guided by needle electromyography or muscle electrical stimulation, see 95873, 95874)

● New Code	▲ Revised Code	＋ Add-On Code	⊘ Modifier -51 Exempt	⊙ Moderate Sedation

Somatic Nerves

64600 Destruction by neurolytic agent, trigeminal nerve; supraorbital, infraorbital, mental, or inferior alveolar branch

64605 second and third division branches at foramen ovale

64610 second and third division branches at foramen ovale under radiologic monitoring

64611 Chemodenervation of parotid and submandibular salivary glands, bilateral

(Report 64611 with modifier 52 if fewer than four salivary glands are injected)

▲ **64612** Chemodenervation of muscle(s); muscle(s) innervated by facial nerve, unilateral (eg, for blepharospasm, hemifacial spasm)

(To report a bilateral procedure, use modifier 50)

64613 neck muscle(s) (eg, for spasmodic torticollis, spasmodic dysphonia)

(Report 64613 only once per session)

(Do not report 64613 with modifier 50)

▲ **64614** extremity and/or trunk muscle(s) (eg, for dystonia, cerebral palsy, multiple sclerosis)

(Report 64614 only once per session)

● **64615** muscle(s) innervated by facial, trigeminal, cervical spinal and accessory nerves, bilateral (eg, for chronic migraine)

(Report 64615 only once per session)

(Do not report 64615 in conjunction with 64612, 64613, 64614)

64620 Destruction by neurolytic agent, intercostal nerve

(64622 deleted 2011 [2012 edition]. For image guided neurolysis of facet joint nerve(s), see 64633-64636)

(64623 deleted 2011 [2012 edition]. For image guided neurolysis of facet joint nerve(s), see 64633-64636)

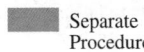 Separate Procedure
 Unlisted Procedure
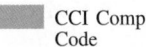 CCI Comp. Code
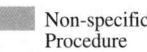 Non-specific Procedure

(64626   deleted 2011 [2012 edition]. For image guided neurolysis of
          facet joint nerve(s), see 64633-64636)

(64627   deleted 2011 [2012 edition]. For image guided neurolysis of
          facet joint nerve(s), see 64633-64636)

          (Imaging guidance [fluoroscopy, CT] are inclusive components
          of 64633-64636)

          (Imaging guidance [fluoroscopy, CT] and any injection of
          contrast are inclusive components of 64633-64636. Image
          guidance and localization are required for the performance of
          paravertebral facet joint nerve destruction by neurolytic agent
          described by 64633-64636. If CT or fluoroscopic imaging is not
          used, report 64999)

          (For paravertebral facet destruction by neurolysis of the T12-L1
          joint, or nerves innervating that joint, use 64633)

64633   Destruction by neurolytic agent, paravertebral facet joint
          nerve(s), with imaging guidance (fluoroscopy or CT); cervical
          or thoracic, single facet joint

          (For bilateral procedure, report 64633 with modifier 50)

+ 64634   cervical or thoracic, each additional facet joint (List
              separately in addition to code for primary procedure)

          (Use 64634 in conjunction with 64633)

          (For bilateral procedure, report 64634 with modifier 50)

64635   Destruction by neurolytic agent, paravertebral facet joint
          nerve(s), with imaging guidance (fluoroscopy or CT); lumbar or
          sacral, single facet joint

          (For bilateral procedure, report 64635 with modifier 50)

+ 64636   lumbar or sacral, each additional facet joint (List separately
              in addition to code for primary procedure)

          (Use 64636 in conjunction with 64635)

          (For bilateral procedure, report 64636 with modifier 50)

          (Do not report 64633-64636 in conjunction with 77003, 77012)

64630   Destruction by neurolytic agent; pudendal nerve

64632   plantar common digital nerve

● New   ▲ Revised   + Add-On   ⊘ Modifier -51   ⊙ Moderate
       Code   Code   Code   Exempt   Sedation

(Do not report 64632 in conjunction with 64455)

64633 Code out of order. See page 826

64634 Code out of order. See page 826

64635 Code out of order. See page 826

64636 Code out of order. See page 826

64640 other peripheral nerve or branch

Sympathetic Nerves

64650 Chemodenervation of eccrine glands; both axillae

64653 other area(s) (eg, scalp, face, neck), per day

(Report the specific service in conjunction with code(s) for the specific substance(s) or drug(s) provided)

(For chemodenervation of extremities (eg, hands or feet), use 64999)

(For chemodenervation of bladder, use 52287)

64680 Destruction by neurolytic agent, with or without radiologic monitoring; celiac plexus

64681 superior hypogastric plexus

NEUROPLASTY (EXPLORATION, NEUROLYSIS OR NERVE DECOMPRESSION)

(For percutaneous neurolysis, see 62263, 62264, 62280-62282)

(For internal neurolysis requiring use of operating microscope, use 64727)

(For facial nerve decompression, use 69720)

(For neuroplasty with nerve wrapping, see 64702-64727, 64999)

64702 Neuroplasty; digital, 1 or both, same digit

64704 nerve of hand or foot

64708 Neuroplasty, major peripheral nerve, arm or leg, open; other than specified

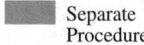 Separate Procedure   Unlisted Procedure   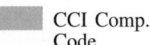 CCI Comp. Code   Non-specific Procedure

| 64712 | sciatic nerve |

| 64713 | brachial plexus |

| 64714 | lumbar plexus |

| 64716 | Neuroplasty and/or transposition; cranial nerve (specify) |

| 64718 | ulnar nerve at elbow |

| 64719 | ulnar nerve at wrist |

| 64721 | median nerve at carpal tunnel |

(For arthroscopic procedure, use 29848)

| 64722 | Decompression; unspecified nerve(s) (specify) |

| 64726 | plantar digital nerve |

+ | 64727 | Internal neurolysis, requiring use of operating microscope (List separately in addition to code for neuroplasty) (Neuroplasty includes external neurolysis) |

(Do not report code 69990 in addition to code 64727)

TRANSECTION OR AVULSION

(For stereotactic lesion of gasserian ganglion, use 61790)

| 64732 | Transection or avulsion of; supraorbital nerve |

| 64734 | infraorbital nerve |

| 64736 | mental nerve |

| 64738 | inferior alveolar nerve by osteotomy |

| 64740 | lingual nerve |

| 64742 | facial nerve, differential or complete |

| 64744 | greater occipital nerve |

| 64746 | phrenic nerve |

(For section of recurrent laryngeal nerve, use 31595)

● New Code   ▲ Revised Code   + Add-On Code   ⊘ Modifier -51 Exempt   ⊙ Moderate Sedation

64752   vagus nerve (vagotomy), transthoracic

64755   vagus nerves limited to proximal stomach (selective proximal vagotomy, proximal gastric vagotomy, parietal cell vagotomy, supra- or highly selective vagotomy)

(For laparoscopic approach, use 43652)

64760   vagus nerve (vagotomy), abdominal

(For laparoscopic approach, use 43651)

64761   pudendal nerve

(For bilateral procedure, report 64761 with modifier -50)

64763   Transection or avulsion of obturator nerve, extrapelvic, with or without adductor tenotomy

(For bilateral procedure, report 64763 with modifier -50)

64766   Transection or avulsion of obturator nerve, intrapelvic, with or without adductor tenotomy

(For bilateral procedure, report 64766 with modifier -50)

64771   Transection or avulsion of other cranial nerve, extradural

64772   Transection or avulsion of other spinal nerve, extradural

(For excision of tender scar, skin and subcutaneous tissue, with or without tiny neuroma, see 11400-11446, 13100-13153)

EXCISION

Somatic Nerves

(For Morton neurectomy, use 28080)

64774   Excision of neuroma; cutaneous nerve, surgically identifiable

64776   digital nerve, 1 or both, same digit

+ **64778**   digital nerve, each additional digit (List separately in addition to code for primary procedure)

(Use 64778 in conjunction with code 64776)

64782   hand or foot, except digital nerve

+ 64783   hand or foot, each additional nerve, except same digit (List separately in addition to code for primary procedure)

(Use 64783 in conjunction with code 64782)

64784   major peripheral nerve, except sciatic

64786   sciatic nerve

+ 64787 Implantation of nerve end into bone or muscle (List separately in addition to neuroma excision)

(Use 64787 in conjunction with codes 64774-64786)

64788 Excision of neurofibroma or neurolemmoma; cutaneous nerve

64790   major peripheral nerve

64792   extensive (including malignant type)

64795 Biopsy of nerve

Sympathetic Nerves

64802 Sympathectomy, cervical

(For bilateral procedure, report 64802 with modifier -50)

64804 Sympathectomy, cervicothoracic

(For bilateral procedure, report 64804 with modifier -50)

64809 Sympathectomy, thoracolumbar

(For bilateral procedure, report 64809 with modifier -50)

64818 Sympathectomy, lumbar

(For bilateral procedure, report 64818 with modifier -50)

64820 Sympathectomy; digital arteries, each digit

(Do not report 69990 in addition to code 64820)

64821   radial artery

(Do not report 69990 in addition to code 64821)

64822   ulnar artery

● New Code   ▲ Revised Code   + Add-On Code   ⊘ Modifier -51 Exempt   ⊙ Moderate Sedation

(Do not report 69990 in addition to code 64822)

64823   superficial palmar arch

(Do not report 69990 in addition to code 64823)

NEURORRHAPHY

64831   Suture of digital nerve, hand or foot; 1 nerve

+ **64832**   each additional digital nerve (List separately in addition to code for primary procedure)

(Use 64832 in conjunction with code 64831)

64834   Suture of 1 nerve; hand or foot, common sensory nerve

64835   median motor thenar

64836   ulnar motor

+ **64837**   Suture of each additional nerve, hand or foot (List separately in addition to code for primary procedure)

(Use 64837 in conjunction with codes 64834-64836)

64840   Suture of posterior tibial nerve

64856   Suture of major peripheral nerve, arm or leg, except sciatic; including transposition

64857   without transposition

64858   Suture of sciatic nerve

+ **64859**   Suture of each additional major peripheral nerve (List separately in addition to code for primary procedure)

(Use 64859 in conjunction with codes 64856, 64857)

64861   Suture of; brachial plexus

64862   lumbar plexus

64864   Suture of facial nerve; extracranial

64865   infratemporal, with or without grafting

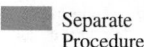 Separate Procedure

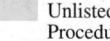 Unlisted Procedure

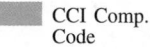 CCI Comp. Code

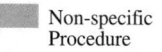 Non-specific Procedure

831

| 64866 | Anastomosis; facial-spinal accessory |

| 64868 | facial-hypoglossal |

| 64870 | facial-phrenic |

| + 64872 | Suture of nerve; requiring secondary or delayed suture (List separately in addition to code for primary neurorrhaphy) |

(Use 64872 in conjunction with codes 64831-64865)

| + 64874 | requiring extensive mobilization, or transposition of nerve (List separately in addition to code for nerve suture) |

(Use 64874 in conjunction with codes 64831-64865)

| + 64876 | requiring shortening of bone of extremity (List separately in addition to code for nerve suture) |

(Use 64876 in conjunction with codes 64831-64865)

NEURORRHAPHY WITH NERVE GRAFT, VEIN GRAFT, OR CONDUIT

| 64885 | Nerve graft (includes obtaining graft), head or neck; up to 4 cm in length |

| 64886 | more than 4 cm length |

| 64890 | Nerve graft (includes obtaining graft), single strand, hand or foot; up to 4 cm length |

| 64891 | more than 4 cm length |

| 64892 | Nerve graft (includes obtaining graft), single strand, arm or leg; up to 4 cm length |

| 64893 | more than 4 cm length |

| 64895 | Nerve graft (includes obtaining graft), multiple strands (cable), hand or foot; up to 4 cm length |

| 64896 | more than 4 cm length |

| 64897 | Nerve graft (includes obtaining graft), multiple strands (cable), arm or leg; up to 4 cm length |

| 64898 | more than 4 cm length |

● New Code ▲ Revised Code + Add-On Code ⊘ Modifier -51 Exempt ⊙ Moderate Sedation

+ 64901   Nerve graft, each additional nerve; single strand (List separately in addition to code for primary procedure)

(Use 64901 in conjunction with codes 64885-64893)

+ 64902   multiple strands (cable) (List separately in addition to code for primary procedure)

(Use 64902 in conjunction with codes 64885, 64886, 64895-64898)

64905   Nerve pedicle transfer; first stage

64907   second stage

64910   Nerve repair; with synthetic conduit or vein allograft (eg, nerve tube), each nerve

64911   with autogenous vein graft (includes harvest of vein graft), each nerve

(Do not report 69990 in addition to 64910, 64911)

OTHER PROCEDURES

64999   Unlisted procedure, nervous system

	Separate Procedure		Unlisted Procedure		CCI Comp. Code		Non-specific Procedure

This page intentionally left blank.

● New
Code

▲ Revised
Code

＋ Add-On
Code

⊘ Modifier -51
Exempt

⊙ Moderate
Sedation

EYE AND OCULAR ADNEXA

CPT codes from this section of the CPT coding system are used to report surgical procedures on the eye and ocular adnexa. Diagnostic services and medical treatment of the eye are defined in the Medicine Section of the CPT manual.

If surgical procedures are performed only on the eyelid, code from the Integumentary System subsection of the CPT coding system. Cataract codes are selected on the type of procedure performed. Whenever injections are performed during cataract surgery, do not report them separately.

When a subconjunctival injection (e.g. CPT code 68200) with a local anesthetic is performed as part of a more extensive anesthetic procedure (e.g. peribulbar or retrobulbar block), a separate service for this procedure is not to be reported. This is a routine part of the anesthetic procedure and does not represent a separate service.

Iridectomy, trabeculectomy, and anterior vitrectomy may be performed in conjunction with cataract removal. When an iridectomy is performed in order to accomplish the cataract extraction, it is an integral part of the procedure; it does not represent a separate service, and is not separately reported. Similarly, the minimal vitreous loss occurring during routine cataract extraction does not represent a vitrectomy and is not to be separately reported unless it is medically necessary for a different diagnosis.

While a trabeculectomy is not performed as a part of a cataract extraction, it may be performed to control glaucoma at the same time as a cataract extraction. If the procedure is medically necessary at the same time as a cataract extraction, it can be reported under a different diagnosis (e.g. glaucoma). The codes describing iridectomies, trabeculectomies, and anterior vitrectomies, when performed with a cataract extraction under a separate diagnosis, must be reported with modifier -59. This indicates that the procedure was performed as a different service for a separate situation. The medical record should reflect the medical necessity of the service if separately reported.

For example, if a patient presents with a cataract and has evidence of glaucoma, (i.e. elevated intraocular pressure preoperatively) and a trabeculectomy represents the appropriate treatment for the glaucoma, a separate service for the trabeculectomy would be separately reported. Performance of a trabeculectomy as a preventative service for an expected transient increase in intraocular pressure postoperatively, without other evidence for glaucoma, is not to be separately reported.

The various approaches to removing a cataract are mutually exclusive of one another when performed on the same eye.

835

	Separate Procedure		Unlisted Procedure		CCI Comp. Code		Non-specific Procedure

Some retinal detachment repair procedures include some vitreous procedures (e.g. CPT code 67108 includes 67015, 67025, 67028, 67031, 67036, 67039, and 67040). Certain retinal detachment repairs are mutually exclusive to anterior procedures such as focal endolaser photocoagulation (e.g. CPT codes 67110 and 67112 are mutually exclusive to CPT code 67108).

CPT codes 68020-68200 (incision, drainage, excision of the conjunctiva) are included in all conjunctivoplasties (CPT codes 68320-68362).

CPT code 67950 (canthoplasty) is included in repair procedures such as blepharoplasties (CPT codes 67917, 67924, 67961, 67966).

Correction of lid retraction (CPT code 67911) includes full thickness graft (e.g. CPT code 15260) as part of the total service performed.

In the circumstance that it is medically necessary and reasonable to inject sclerosing agents in the same session as surgery to correct glaucoma, the service is included in the glaucoma surgery. Accordingly, codes such as CPT codes 67500, 67515, and 68200 for injection of sclerosing agents (e.g. 5-FU, HCPCS/CPT code J9190) should not be reported with other pressure- reducing or glaucoma procedures.

(For diagnostic and treatment ophthalmological services, see Medicine, Ophthalmology, and 92002 et seq)

(Do not report code 69990 in addition to codes 65091-68850)

EYEBALL

REMOVAL OF EYE

65091 Evisceration of ocular contents; without implant

65093 with implant

65101 Enucleation of eye; without implant

65103 with implant, muscles not attached to implant

65105 with implant, muscles attached to implant

(For conjunctivoplasty after enucleation, see 68320 et seq)

65110 Exenteration of orbit (does not include skin graft), removal of orbital contents; only

65112 with therapeutic removal of bone

● New Code   ▲ Revised Code   + Add-On Code   ⊘ Modifier -51 Exempt   ⊙ Moderate Sedation

65114   with muscle or myocutaneous flap

(For skin graft to orbit (split skin), see 15120, 15121; free, full thickness, see 15260, 15261)

(For eyelid repair involving more than skin, see 67930 et seq)

SECONDARY IMPLANT(S) PROCEDURES

65125   Modification of ocular implant with placement or replacement of pegs (eg, drilling receptacle for prosthesis appendage) (separate procedure)

65130   Insertion of ocular implant secondary; after evisceration, in scleral shell

65135   after enucleation, muscles not attached to implant

65140   after enucleation, muscles attached to implant

65150   Reinsertion of ocular implant; with or without conjunctival graft

65155   with use of foreign material for reinforcement and/or attachment of muscles to implant

65175   Removal of ocular implant

(For orbital implant (implant outside muscle cone) insertion, use 67550; removal, use 67560)

REMOVAL OF FOREIGN BODY

(For removal of implanted material: ocular implant, use 65175; anterior segment implant, use 65920; posterior segment implant, use 67120; orbital implant, use 67560)

(For diagnostic x-ray for foreign body, use 70030)

(For diagnostic echography for foreign body, use 76529)

(For removal of foreign body from orbit: frontal approach, use 67413; lateral approach, use 67430; transcranial approach, use 61334)

(For removal of foreign body from eyelid, embedded, use 67938)

(For removal of foreign body from lacrimal system, use 68530)

65205   Removal of foreign body, external eye; conjunctival superficial

837

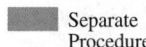 Separate Procedure   Unlisted Procedure   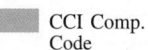 CCI Comp. Code   Non-specific Procedure

| 65210 | conjunctival embedded (includes concretions), subconjunctival, or scleral nonperforating |

65220   corneal, without slit lamp

65222   corneal, with slit lamp

(For repair of corneal laceration with foreign body, use 65275)

65235   Removal of foreign body, intraocular; from anterior chamber of eye or lens

(For removal of implanted material from anterior segment, use 65920)

65260   from posterior segment, magnetic extraction, anterior or posterior route

65265   from posterior segment, nonmagnetic extraction

(For removal of implanted material from posterior segment, use 67120)

REPAIR OF LACERATION

(For fracture of orbit, see 21385 et seq)

(For repair of wound of eyelid, skin, linear, simple, see 12011-12018; intermediate, layered closure, see 12051-12057; linear, complex, see 13150-13160; other, see 67930, 67935)

(For repair of wound of lacrimal system, use 68700)

(For repair of operative wound, use 66250)

65270   Repair of laceration; conjunctiva, with or without nonperforating laceration sclera, direct closure

65272   conjunctiva, by mobilization and rearrangement, without hospitalization

65273   conjunctiva, by mobilization and rearrangement, with hospitalization

65275   cornea, nonperforating, with or without removal foreign body

65280   cornea and/or sclera, perforating, not involving uveal tissue

● New Code   ▲ Revised Code   + Add-On Code   ⃠ Modifier -51 Exempt   ⊙ Moderate Sedation

65285   cornea and/or sclera, perforating, with reposition or resection of uveal tissue

(65280 amd 65285 are not used for repair of a surgical wound)

65286   application of tissue glue, wounds of cornea and/or sclera

(Repair of laceration includes use of conjunctival flap and restoration of anterior chamber, by air or saline injection when indicated)

(For repair of iris or ciliary body, use 66680)

65290   Repair of wound, extraocular muscle, tendon and/or Tenon's capsule

ANTERIOR SEGMENT

CORNEA

Excision

65400   Excision of lesion, cornea (keratectomy, lamellar, partial), except pterygium

65410   Biopsy of cornea

65420   Excision or transposition of pterygium; without graft

65426   with graft

Removal or Destruction

65430   Scraping of cornea, diagnostic, for smear and/or culture

65435   Removal of corneal epithelium; with or without chemocauterization (abrasion, curettage)

65436   with application of chelating agent (eg, EDTA)

65450   Destruction of lesion of cornea by cryotherapy, photocoagulation or thermocauterization

65600   Multiple punctures of anterior cornea (eg, for corneal erosion, tattoo)

839

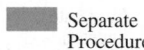 Separate Procedure   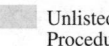 Unlisted Procedure   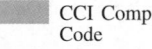 CCI Comp. Code   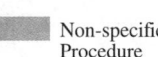 Non-specific Procedure

Keratoplasty

Corneal transplant includes use of fresh or preserved grafts. The preparation of donor material is included for penetrating or anterior lamellar keratoplasty, but reported separately for endothelial keratoplasty. Do not report 65710-65757 in conjunction with 92025.

(Keratoplasty excludes refractive keratoplasty procedures, 65760, 65765, and 65767)

65710   Keratoplasty (corneal transplant); anterior lamellar

65730   penetrating (except in aphakia or pseudoaphakia)

65750   penetrating (in aphakia)

65755   penetrating (in pseudophakia)

65756   endothelial

+ 65757   Backbench preparation of corneal endothelial allograft prior to transplantation (list separately in addition to code for primary procedure)

(Use 65757 in conjunction with 65756)

Other Procedures

Do not report 65760-65771 in conjunction with 92025.

65760   Keratomileusis

65765   Keratophakia

65767   Epikeratoplasty

65770   Keratoprosthesis

65771   Radial keratotomy

65772   Corneal relaxing incision for correction of surgically induced astigmatism

65775   Corneal wedge resection for correction of surgically induced astigmatism

(For fitting of contact lens for treatment of disease, use 92071, 92072)

● New Code   ▲ Revised Code   + Add-On Code   ⊘ Modifier -51 Exempt   ⊙ Moderate Sedation

(For unlisted procedures on cornea, use 66999)

65778 Placement of amniotic membrane on the ocular surface for wound healing; self-retaining

65779 single layer, sutured

(Do not report 65778, 65779 in conjunction with 65430, 65435, 65780)

(For placement of amniotic membrane using tissue glue, use 66999)

65780 Ocular surface reconstruction; amniotic membrane transplantation, multiple layers

(For placement of amniotic membrane without reconstruction using self-retaining or single layer suture technique, see 65778, 65779)

65781 limbal stem cell allograft (eg, cadaveric or living donor)

65782 limbal conjunctival autograft (includes obtaining graft)

(For harvesting conjunctival allograft, living donor, use 68371)

ANTERIOR CHAMBER

Incision

▲ **65800** Paracentesis of anterior chamber of eye (separate procedure); with removal of aqueous

(65805 deleted 2012 [2013 edition]. To report, use 65800)

65810 with removal of vitreous and/or discission of anterior hyaloid membrane, with or without air injection

65815 with removal of blood, with or without irrigation and/or air injection

(For injection, see 66020-66030)

(For removal of blood clot, use 65930)

65820 Goniotomy

(Do not report modifier -63 in conjunction with 65820)

(For use of ophthalmic endoscope with 65820, use 66990)

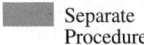

▉ Separate Procedure	▉ Unlisted Procedure	▉ CCI Comp. Code	▉ Non-specific Procedure

841

65850 Trabeculotomy ab externo

65855 Trabeculoplasty by laser surgery, 1 or more sessions (defined treatment series)

(If re-treatment is necessary after several months because of disease progression, a new treatment or treatment series should be reported with a modifier, if necessary, to indicate lesser or greater complexity)

(For trabeculectomy, use 66170)

65860 Severing adhesions of anterior segment, laser technique (separate procedure)

65865 Severing adhesions of anterior segment of eye, incisional technique (with or without injection of air or liquid) (separate procedure); goniosynechiae

(For trabeculoplasty by laser surgery, use 65855)

⊙ **65870** anterior synechiae, except goniosynechiae

⊙ **65875** posterior synechiae

(For use of ophthalmic endoscope with 65875, use 66990)

⊙ **65880** corneovitreal adhesions

(For laser surgery, use 66821)

Removal

65900 Removal of epithelial downgrowth, anterior chamber of eye

65920 Removal of implanted material, anterior segment of eye

(For use of ophthalmic endoscope with 65920, use 66990)

65930 Removal of blood clot, anterior segment of eye

Introduction

⊙ **66020** Injection, anterior chamber of eye (separate procedure); air or liquid

⊙ **66030** medication

(For unlisted procedures on anterior segment, use 66999)

842

| ● New Code | ▲ Revised Code | + Add-On Code | ⊘ Modifier -51 Exempt | ⊙ Moderate Sedation |

ANTERIOR SCLERA

Excision

(For removal of intraocular foreign body, use 65235)

(For operations on posterior sclera, use 67250, 67255)

66130 Excision of lesion, sclera

66150 Fistulization of sclera for glaucoma; trephination with iridectomy

66155 thermocauterization with iridectomy

66160 sclerectomy with punch or scissors, with iridectomy

66165 iridencleisis or iridotasis

66170 trabeculectomy ab externo in absence of previous surgery

(For trabeculotomy ab externo, use 65850)

(For repair of operative wound, use 66250)

66172 trabeculectomy ab externo with scarring from previous ocular surgery or trauma (includes injection of antifibrotic agents)

66174 Transluminal dilation of aqueous outflow canal; without retention of device or stent

66175 with retention of device or stent

Aqueous Shunt

66180 Aqueous shunt to extraocular reservoir (eg, Molteno, Schocket, Denver-Krupin)

66185 Revision of aqueous shunt to extraocular reservoir

(For removal of implanted shunt, use 67120)

Repair or Revision

(For scleral procedures in retinal surgery, see 67101 et seq)

66220 Repair of scleral staphyloma; without graft

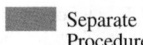 Separate Procedure

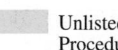 Unlisted Procedure

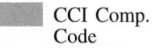 CCI Comp. Code

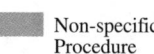 Non-specific Procedure

66225   with graft

(For scleral reinforcement, see 67250, 67255)

66250   Revision or repair of operative wound of anterior segment, any type, early or late, major or minor procedure

(For unlisted procedures on anterior sclera, use 66999)

IRIS, CILIARY BODY

Incision

66500   Iridotomy by stab incision (separate procedure); except transfixion

66505   with transfixion as for iris bombe

(For iridotomy by photocoagulation, use 66761)

Excision

66600   Iridectomy, with corneoscleral or corneal section; for removal of lesion

66605   with cyclectomy

66625   peripheral for glaucoma (separate procedure)

66630   sector for glaucoma (separate procedure)

66635   optical (separate procedure)

(For coreoplasty by photocoagulation, use 66762)

Repair

66680   Repair of iris, ciliary body (as for iridodialysis)

(For reposition or resection of uveal tissue with perforating wound of cornea or sclera, use 65285)

66682   Suture of iris, ciliary body (separate procedure) with retrieval of suture through small incision (eg, McCannel suture)

Destruction

66700   Ciliary body destruction; diathermy

---

844   ● New Code   ▲ Revised Code   + Add-On Code   ⊘ Modifier -51 Exempt   ⊙ Moderate Sedation

66710   cyclophotocoagulation, transscleral

66711   cyclophotocoagulation, endoscopic

(Do not report 66711 in conjunction with 66990)

⊙ **66720**   cryotherapy

66740   cyclodialysis

66761   Iridotomy/iridectomy by laser surgery (eg, for glaucoma) (per session)

66__   Iridoplasty by photocoagulation (1 or more sessions) (eg, for improvement of vision, for widening of anterior chamber angle)

66770   Destruction of cyst or lesion iris or ciliary body (nonexcisional procedure)

(For excision lesion iris, ciliary body, see 66600, 66605; for removal of epithelial downgrowth, use 65900)

(For unlisted procedures on iris, ciliary body, use 66999)

LENS

Incision

66820   Discission of secondary membranous cataract (opacified posterior lens capsule and/or anterior hyaloid); stab incision technique (Ziegler or Wheeler knife)

66821   laser surgery (eg, YAG laser) (1 or more stages)

66825   Repositioning of intraocular lens prosthesis, requiring an incision (separate procedure)

Removal

Lateral canthotomy, iridectomy, iridotomy, anterior capsulotomy, posterior capsulotomy, the use of viscoelastic agents, enzymatic zonulysis, use of other pharmacologic agents, and subconjunctival or sub-tenon injections are included as part of the code for the extraction of lens.

66830   Removal of secondary membranous cataract (opacified posterior lens capsule and/or anterior hyaloid) with corneo-scleral section, with or without iridectomy (iridocapsulotomy, iridocapsulectomy)

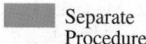 Separate Procedure
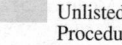 Unlisted Procedure
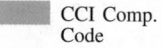 CCI Comp. Code
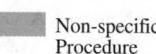 Non-specific Procedure

845

66840   Removal of lens material; aspiration technique, 1 or more stages

66850   phacofragmentation technique (mechanical or ultrasonic) (eg, phacoemulsification), with aspiration

66852   pars plana approach, with or without vitrectomy

66920   intracapsular

66930   intracapsular, for dislocated lens

66940   extracapsular (other than 66840, 66850, 66852)

(For removal of intralenticular foreign body without lens extraction, use 65235)

(For repair of operative wound, use 66250)

INTRAOCULAR LENS PROCEDURES

66982   Extracapsular cataract removal with insertion of intraocular lens prosthesis (1 stage procedure), manual or mechanical technique (eg, irrigation and aspiration or phacoemulsification), complex, requiring devices or techniques not generally used in routine cataract surgery (eg, iris expansion device, suture support for intraocular lens, or primary posterior capsulorrhexis) or performed on patients in the amblyogenic developmental stage

(For insertion of ocular telescope prosthesis including removal of crystalline lens, use 0308T)

66983   Intracapsular cataract extraction with insertion of intraocular lens prosthesis (1 stage procedure)

(Do not report 66983 in conjunction with 0308T)

66984   Extracapsular cataract removal with insertion of intraocular lens prosthesis (1 stage procedure), manual or mechanical technique (eg, irrigation and aspiration or phacoemulsification)

(For complex extracapsular cataract removal, use 66982)

(For insertion of ocular telescope prosthesis including removal of crystalline lens, use 0308T)

66985   Insertion of intraocular lens prosthesis (secondary implant), not associated with concurrent cataract removal

846   ● New Code   ▲ Revised Code   + Add-On Code   ⊘ Modifier -51 Exempt   ⊙ Moderate Sedation

(To code implant at time of concurrent cataract surgery, see 66982, 66983, 66984)

(To report supply of intraocular lens prosthesis, use 99070)

(For ultrasonic determination of intraocular lens power, use 76519)

(For removal of implanted material from anterior segment, use 65920)

(For secondary fixation (separate procedure), use 66682)

(For use of ophthalmic endoscope with 66985, use 66990)

66986 Exchange of intraocular lens

(For use of ophthalmic endoscope with 66986, use 66990)

OTHER PROCEDURES

+ **66990** Use of ophthalmic endoscope (List separately in addition to code for primary procedure)

(66990 may be used only with codes 65820, 65875, 65920, 66985, 66986, 67036, 67039, 67040, 67041, 67042, 67043, 67112, 67113)

66999 Unlisted procedure, anterior segment of eye

POSTERIOR SEGMENT

VITREOUS

67005 Removal of vitreous, anterior approach (open sky technique or limbal incision); partial removal

67010 subtotal removal with mechanical vitrectomy

(For removal of vitreous by paracentesis of anterior chamber, use 65810)

(For removal of corneovitreal adhesions, use 65880)

67015 Aspiration or release of vitreous, subretinal or choroidal fluid, pars plana approach (posterior sclerotomy)

67025 Injection of vitreous substitute, pars plana or limbal approach, (fluid-gas exchange), with or without aspiration (separate procedure)

 Separate Procedure 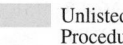 Unlisted Procedure 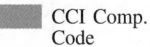 CCI Comp. Code 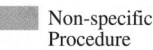 Non-specific Procedure

847

67027 Implantation of intravitreal drug delivery system (eg, ganciclovir implant), includes concomitant removal of vitreous

(For removal, use 67121)

67028 Intravitreal injection of a pharmacologic agent (separate procedure)

67030 Discission of vitreous strands (without removal), pars plana approach

67031 Severing of vitreous strands, vitreous face adhesions, sheets, membranes or opacities, laser surgery (1 or more stages)

67036 Vitrectomy, mechanical, pars plana approach;

(For application of intraocular epiretinal radiation with 67036, use 0190T)

67039 with focal endolaser photocoagulation

67040 with endolaser panretinal photocoagulation

67041 with removal of preretinal cellular membrane (eg, macular pucker)

67042 with removal of internal limiting membrane of retina (eg, for repair of macular hole, diabetic macular edema), includes, if performed, intraocular tamponade (ie, air, gas or silicone oil)

67043 with removal of subretinal membrane (eg, choroidal neovascularization), includes, if performed, intraocular tamponade (ie, air, gas or silicone oil) and laser photocoagulation

(For use of ophthalmic endoscope with 67036, 67039, 67040-67043, use 66990)

(For associated lensectomy, use 66850)

(For use of vitrectomy in retinal detachment surgery, see 67108, 67113)

(For associated removal of foreign body, see 65260, 65265)

(For unlisted procedures on vitreous, use 67299)

● New Code ▲ Revised Code + Add-On Code ⊘ Modifier -51 Exempt ⊙ Moderate Sedation

RETINA OR CHOROID

Repair

(If diathermy, cryotherapy and/or photocoagulation are combined, report under principal modality used)

67101 Repair of retinal detachment, 1 or more sessions; cryotherapy or diathermy, with or without drainage of subretinal fluid

67105 photocoagulation, with or without drainage of subretinal fluid

67107 Repair of retinal detachment; scleral buckling (such as lamellar scleral dissection, imbrication or encircling procedure), with or without implant, with or without cryotherapy, photocoagulation, and drainage of subretinal fluid

67108 with vitrectomy, any method, with or without air or gas tamponade, focal endolaser photocoagulation, cryotherapy, drainage of subretinal fluid, scleral buckling, and/or removal of lens by same technique

67110 by injection of air or other gas (eg, pneumatic retinopexy)

67112 by scleral buckling or vitrectomy, on patient having previous ipsilateral retinal detachment repair(s) using scleral buckling or vitrectomy techniques

(For aspiration of drainage of subretinal or subchoroidal fluid, use 67015)

(For use of ophthalmic endoscope with 67112, use 66990)

67113 Repair of complex retinal detachment (eg, proliferative vitreoretinopathy, stage C-1 or greater, diabetic traction retinal detachment, retinopathy of prematurity, retinaltear of greater than 90 degrees), with vitrectomy and membrane peeling, may include air, gas, or silicone oil tamponade, cryotherapy, endolaser photocoagulation, drainage of subretinal fluid, scleral buckling, and/or removal of lens

(To report vitrectomy, pars plana approach, other than in retinal detachment surgery, see 67036-67043)

(For use of ophthalmic endoscope with 67113, use 66990)

67115 Release of encircling material (posterior segment)

849

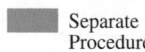 Separate Procedure   Unlisted Procedure   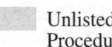 CCI Comp. Code   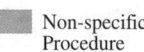 Non-specific Procedure

67120 Removal of implanted material, posterior segment; extraocular

67121 intraocular

(For removal from anterior segment, use 65920)

(For removal of foreign body, see 65260, 65265)

Prophylaxis

Codes 67141, 67145 include treatment at one or more sessions that may occur at different encounters. These codes should be reported once during a defined treatment period.

Repetitive services. The services listed below are often performed in multiple sessions or groups of sessions. The methods of reporting vary. The following descriptors are intended to include all sessions in a defined treatment period.

67141 Prophylaxis of retinal detachment (eg, retinal break, lattice degeneration) without drainage, 1 or more sessions; cryotherapy, diathermy

67145 photocoagulation (laser or xenon arc)

Destruction

Codes 67208, 67210, 67218, 67220, 67227, 67228, 67229 include treatment at one or more sessions that may occur at different encounters. These codes should be reported once during a defined treatment period.

67208 Destruction of localized lesion of retina (eg, macular edema, tumors), 1 or more sessions; cryotherapy, diathermy

67210 photocoagulation

67218 radiation by implantation of source (includes removal of source)

67220 Destruction of localized lesion of choroid (eg, choroidal neovascularization); photocoagulation (eg, laser), 1 or more sessions

67221 photodynamic therapy (includes intravenous infusion)

+ **67225** photodynamic therapy, second eye, at single session (List separately in addition to code for primary eye treatment)

(Use 67225 in conjunction with code 67221)

850 ● New Code   ▲ Revised Code   + Add-On Code   ⊘ Modifier -51 Exempt   ⊙ Moderate Sedation

67227 Destruction of extensive or progressive retinopathy (eg, diabetic retinopathy), 1 or more sessions, cryotherapy, diathermy

67228 Treatment of extensive or progressive retinopathy, 1 or more sessions; (eg, diabetic retinopathy), photocoagulation

67229 preterm infant (less than 37 weeks gestation at birth), performed from birth up to 1 year of age (eg, retinopathy of prematurity), photocoagulation or cryotherapy

(For bilateral procedure, use modifier -50)

(For unlisted procedures on retina, use 67299)

POSTERIOR SCLERA

Repair

(For excision lesion sclera, use 66130)

67250 Scleral reinforcement (separate procedure); without graft

67255 with graft

(For repair scleral staphyloma, see 66220, 66225)

OTHER PROCEDURES

67299 Unlisted procedure, posterior segment

OCULAR ADNEXA

EXTRAOCULAR MUSCLES

67311 Strabismus surgery, recession or resection procedure; 1 horizontal muscle

67312 2 horizontal muscles

67314 1 vertical muscle (excluding superior oblique)

67316 2 or more vertical muscles (excluding superior oblique)

(For adjustable sutures, use 67335 in addition to codes 67311-67334 for primary procedure reflecting number of muscles operated on)

67318 Strabismus surgery, any procedure, superior oblique muscle

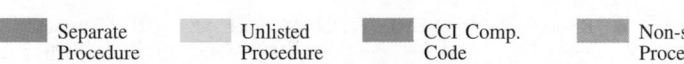

| Separate Procedure | Unlisted Procedure | CCI Comp. Code | Non-specific Procedure |

851

+ **67320** Transposition procedure (eg, for paretic extraocular muscle), any extraocular muscle (specify) (List separately in addition to code for primary procedure)

(Use 67320 in conjunction with codes 67311-67318)

+ **67331** Strabismus surgery on patient with previous eye surgery or injury that did not involve the extraocular muscles (List separately in addition to code for primary procedure)

(Use 67331 in conjunction with codes 67311-67318)

+ **67332** Strabismus surgery on patient with scarring of extraocular muscles (eg, prior ocular injury, strabismus or retinal detachment surgery) or restrictive myopathy (eg, dysthyroid ophthalmopathy) (List separately in addition to code for primary procedure)

(Use 67332 in conjunction with codes 67311-67318)

+ **67334** Strabismus surgery by posterior fixation suture technique, with or without muscle recession (List separately in addition to code for primary procedure)

(Use 67334 in conjunction with codes 67311-67318)

+ **67335** Placement of adjustable suture(s) during strabismus surgery, including postoperative adjustment(s) of suture(s) (List separately in addition to code for specific strabismus surgery)

(Use 67335 in conjunction with codes 67311-67334)

+ **67340** Strabismus surgery involving exploration and/or repair of detached extraocular muscle(s) (List separately in addition to code for primary procedure)

(Use 67340 in conjunction with codes 67311-67334)

67343 Release of extensive scar tissue without detaching extraocular muscle (separate procedure)

(Use 67343 in conjunction with codes 67311-67340, when such procedures are performed other than on the affected muscle)

67345 Chemodenervation of extraocular muscle

(For chemodenervation for blepharospasm and other neurological disorders, see 64612 and 64613)

67346 Biopsy of extraocular muscle

● New Code ▲ Revised Code + Add-On Code ⊘ Modifier -51 Exempt ⊙ Moderate Sedation

(For repair of wound, extraocular muscle, tendon or Tenon's capsule, use 65290)

Other Procedures

67399 Unlisted procedure, ocular muscle

ORBIT

Exploration, Excision, Decompression

67400 Orbitotomy without bone flap (frontal or transconjunctival approach); for exploration, with or without biopsy

67405 with drainage only

67412 with removal of lesion

67413 with removal of foreign body

67414 with removal of bone for decompression

67415 Fine needle aspiration of orbital contents

(For exenteration, enucleation, and repair, see 65101 et seq; for optic nerve decompression, use 67570)

67420 Orbitotomy with bone flap or window, lateral approach (eg, Kroenlein); with removal of lesion

67430 with removal of foreign body

67440 with drainage

67445 with removal of bone for decompression

(For optic nerve sheath decompression, use 67570)

67450 for exploration, with or without biopsy

(For orbitotomy, transcranial approach, see 61330-61334)

(For orbital implant, see 67550, 67560)

(For removal of eyeball or for repair after removal, see 65091-65175)

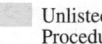 Separate
Procedure

Unlisted
Procedure

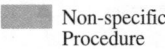 CCI Comp.
Code

Non-specific
Procedure

853

Other Procedures

67500 Retrobulbar injection; medication (separate procedure, does not include supply of medication)

67505 alcohol

67515 Injection of medication or other substance into Tenon's capsule

(For subconjunctival injection, use 68200)

67550 Orbital implant (implant outside muscle cone); insertion

67560 removal or revision

(For ocular implant (implant inside muscle cone), see 65093-65105, 65130-65175)

(For treatment of fractures of malar area, orbit, see 21355 et seq)

67570 Optic nerve decompression (eg, incision or fenestration of optic nerve sheath)

67599 Unlisted procedure, orbit

EYELIDS

Incision

67700 Blepharotomy, drainage of abscess, eyelid

67710 Severing of tarsorrhaphy

67715 Canthotomy (separate procedure)

(For canthoplasty, use 67950)

(For division of symblepharon, use 68340)

▲ **67810** Incisional biopsy of eyelid skin includnig lid margin

(For biopsy of skin of eyelid, see 11100, 11101, 11310-11313)

Excision, Destruction

Codes for removal of lesions include more than skin (ie., involving lid margin, tarsus, and/or palpebral conjunctiva).

● New Code   ▲ Revised Code   + Add-On Code   ⊘ Modifier -51 Exempt   ⊙ Moderate Sedation

(For removal of lesion, involving mainly skin of eyelid, see 11310-11313; 11440-11446, 11640-11646; 17000-17004)

(For repair of wounds, blepharoplasty, grafts, reconstructive surgery, see 67930-67975)

67800 Excision of chalazion; single

67801 multiple, same lid

67805 multiple, different lids

67808 under general anesthesia and/or requiring hospitalization, single or multiple

67810 Code out of order. See page 854

67820 Correction of trichiasis; epilation, by forceps only

67825 epilation by other than forceps (eg, by electrosurgery, cryotherapy, laser surgery)

67830 incision of lid margin

67835 incision of lid margin, with free mucous membrane graft

67840 Excision of lesion of eyelid (except chalazion) without closure or with simple direct closure

(For excision and repair of eyelid by reconstructive surgery, see 67961, 67966)

67850 Destruction of lesion of lid margin (up to 1 cm)

(For Mohs micrographic surgery, see 17311-17315)

(For initiation or follow-up care of topical chemotherapy (eg, 5-FU or similar agents), see appropriate office visits)

Tarsorrhaphy

67875 Temporary closure of eyelids by suture (eg, Frost suture)

67880 Construction of intermarginal adhesions, median tarsorrhaphy, or canthorrhaphy;

67882 with transposition of tarsal plate

855

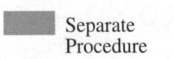 Separate Procedure   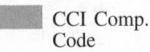 Unlisted Procedure   CCI Comp. Code   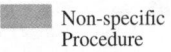 Non-specific Procedure

(For severing of tarsorrhaphy, use 67710)

(For canthoplasty, reconstruction canthus, use 67950)

(For canthotomy, use 67715)

Repair (Brow Ptosis, Blepharoptosis, Lid Retraction, Ectropion, Entropion)

67900 Repair of brow ptosis (supraciliary, mid-forehead or coronal approach)

(For forehead rhytidectomy, use 15824)

67901 Repair of blepharoptosis; frontalis muscle technique with suture or other material (eg, banked fascia)

67902 frontalis muscle technique with autologous fascial sling (includes obtaining fascia)

67903 (tarso) levator resection or advancement, internal approach

67904 (tarso) levator resection or advancement, external approach

67906 superior rectus technique with fascial sling (includes obtaining fascia)

67908 conjunctivo-tarso-Muller's muscle-levator resection (eg, Fasanella-Servat type)

67909 Reduction of overcorrection of ptosis

67911 Correction of lid retraction

(For obtaining autogenous graft materials, see 20920, 20922, or 20926)

(For correction of trichiasis by mucous membrane graft, use 67835)

67912 Correction of lagophthalmos, with implantation of upper eyelid load (eg, gold weight)

67914 Repair of ectropion; suture

67915 thermocauterization

67916 excision tarsal wedge

● New Code   ▲ Revised Code   + Add-On Code   ⊘ Modifier -51 Exempt   ⊙ Moderate Sedation

67917   extensive (eg, tarsal strip operations)

(For correction of everted punctum, use 68705)

67921   Repair of entropion; suture

67922   thermocauterization

67923   excision tarsal wedge

67924   extensive (eg, tarsal strip or capsulopalpebral fascia repairs operation)

(For repair of cicatricial ectropion or entropion requiring scar excision or skin graft, see also 67961 et seq)

Reconstruction

Codes for blepharoplasty involve more than skin (ie., involving lid margin, tarsus, and/or palpebral conjunctiva).

67930   Suture of recent wound, eyelid, involving lid margin, tarsus, and/or palpebral conjunctiva direct closure; partial thickness

67935   full thickness

67938   Removal of embedded foreign body, eyelid

(For repair of skin of eyelid, see 12011-12018; 12051-12057; 13150-13153)

(For tarsorrhaphy, canthorrhaphy, see 67880, 67882)

(For repair of blepharoptosis and lid retraction, see 67901-67911)

(For blepharoplasty for entropion, ectropion, see 67916, 67917, 67923, 67924)

(For correction of blepharochalasis (blepharorhytidectomy), see 15820-15823)

(For repair of skin of eyelid, adjacent tissue transfer, see 14060, 14061; preparation for graft, use 15004; free graft, see 15120, 15121, 15260, 15261)

(For excision of lesion of eyelid, use 67800 et seq)

(For repair of lacrimal canaliculi, use 68700)

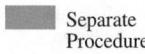 Separate Procedure   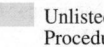 Unlisted Procedure   CCI Comp. Code   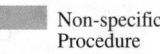 Non-specific Procedure

67950   Canthoplasty (reconstruction of canthus)

67961   Excision and repair of eyelid, involving lid margin, tarsus, conjunctiva, canthus, or full thickness, may include preparation for skin graft or pedicle flap with adjacent tissue transfer or rearrangement; up to one-fourth of lid margin

67966   over one-fourth of lid margin

(For canthoplasty, use 67950)

(For free skin grafts, see 15120, 15121, 15260, 15261)

(For tubed pedicle flap preparation, use 15576; for delay, use 15630; for attachment, use 15650)

67971   Reconstruction of eyelid, full thickness by transfer of tarsoconjunctival flap from opposing eyelid; up to two-thirds of eyelid, 1 stage or first stage

67973   total eyelid, lower, 1 stage or first stage

67974   total eyelid, upper, 1 stage or first stage

67975   second stage

Other Procedures

67999   Unlisted procedure, eyelids

CONJUNCTIVA

(For removal of foreign body, see 65205 et seq)

INCISION AND DRAINAGE

68020   Incision of conjunctiva, drainage of cyst

68040   Expression of conjunctival follicles (eg, for trachoma)

EXCISION AND/OR DESTRUCTION

68100   Biopsy of conjunctiva

68110   Excision of lesion, conjunctiva; up to 1 cm

68115   over 1 cm

   ● New Code   ▲ Revised Code   + Add-On Code   ⊘ Modifier -51 Exempt   ⊙ Moderate Sedation

68130 with adjacent sclera

68135 Destruction of lesion, conjunctiva

INJECTION

(For injection into Tenon's capsule or retrobulbar injection, see 67500-67515)

68200 Subconjunctival injection

CONJUNCTIVOPLASTY

(For wound repair, see 65270-65273)

68320 Conjunctivoplasty; with conjunctival graft or extensive rearrangement

68325 with buccal mucous membrane graft (includes obtaining graft)

68326 Conjunctivoplasty, reconstruction cul-de-sac; with conjunctival graft or extensive rearrangement

68328 with buccal mucous membrane graft (includes obtaining graft)

68330 Repair of symblepharon; conjunctivoplasty, without graft

68335 with free graft conjunctiva or buccal mucous membrane (includes obtaining graft)

68340 division of symblepharon, with or without insertion of conformer or contact lens

OTHER PROCEDURES

68360 Conjunctival flap; bridge or partial (separate procedure)

68362 total (such as Gunderson thin flap or purse string flap)

(For conjunctival flap for perforating injury, see 65280, 65285)

(For repair of operative wound, use 66250)

(For removal of conjunctival foreign body, see 65205, 65210)

68371 Harvesting conjunctival allograft, living donor

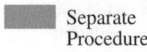 Separate Procedure   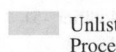 Unlisted Procedure   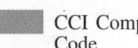 CCI Comp. Code   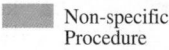 Non-specific Procedure

859

68399   Unlisted procedure, conjunctiva

LACRIMAL SYSTEM

Incision

68400   Incision, drainage of lacrimal gland

68420   Incision, drainage of lacrimal sac (dacryocystotomy or dacryocystostomy)

68440   Snip incision of lacrimal punctum

Excision

68500   Excision of lacrimal gland (dacryoadenectomy), except for tumor; total

68505   partial

68510   Biopsy of lacrimal gland

68520   Excision of lacrimal sac (dacryocystectomy)

68525   Biopsy of lacrimal sac

68530   Removal of foreign body or dacryolith, lacrimal passages

68540   Excision of lacrimal gland tumor; frontal approach

68550   involving osteotomy

Repair

68700   Plastic repair of canaliculi

68705   Correction of everted punctum, cautery

68720   Dacryocystorhinostomy (fistulization of lacrimal sac to nasal cavity)

68745   Conjunctivorhinostomy (fistulization of conjunctiva to nasal cavity); without tube

68750   with insertion of tube or stent

---

860   ● New Code   ▲ Revised Code   ✛ Add-On Code   ⊘ Modifier -51 Exempt   ⊙ Moderate Sedation

68760 Closure of the lacrimal punctum; by thermocauterization, ligation, or laser surgery

68761 by plug, each

68770 Closure of lacrimal fistula (separate procedure)

Probing and/or Related Procedures

68801 Dilation of lacrimal punctum, with or without irrigation

(To report a bilateral procedure, use 68801 with modifier -50)

68810 Probing of nasolacrimal duct, with or without irrigation;

(For bilateral procedure, report 68810 with modifier -50)

68811 requiring general anesthesia

(For bilateral procedure, report 68811 with modifier -50)

68815 with insertion of tube or stent

(See also 92018)

(For bilateral procedure, report 68815 with modifier -50)

68816 with transluminal balloon catheter dilation

(Do not report 68816 in conjunction with 68810, 68811, 68815)

(For bilateral procedure, report 68816 with modifier -50)

68840 Probing of lacrimal canaliculi, with or without irrigation

68850 Injection of contrast medium for dacryocystography

(For radiological supervision and interpretation, see 70170, 78660)

Other Procedures

68899 Unlisted procedure, lacrimal system

 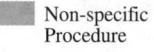

This page intentionally left blank.

● New
Code
▲ Revised
Code
+ Add-On
Code
⊘ Modifier -51
Exempt
⊙ Moderate
Sedation

AUDITORY SYSTEM

CPT codes from this subsection of the CPT coding system are used to report invasive and surgical procedures performed on the external ear; middle ear; inner ear and temporal bone. Includes procedures performed on the inner, outer and middle ear and to the temporal bone.

Diagnostic services, such as otoscopy under general anesthesia, audiometry and vestibular tests, are defined in the Medicine Section of the CPT manual.

Wound repairs to the external ear are located in the Integumentary Subsection of the CPT coding system.

When a mastoidectomy is included in the description of an auditory procedure (e.g. CPT codes 69530, 69910), separate codes describing mastoidectomy are not reported.

Myringotomies (e.g. CPT codes 69420 and 69421) are included in tympanoplasties and tympanostomies.

> (For diagnostic services (eg, audiometry, vestibular tests), see 92502 et seq)

EXTERNAL EAR

INCISION

69000 Drainage external ear, abscess or hematoma; simple

69005 complicated

69020 Drainage external auditory canal, abscess

69090 Ear piercing

EXCISION

69100 Biopsy external ear

69105 Biopsy external auditory canal

69110 Excision external ear; partial, simple repair

69120 complete amputation

> (For reconstruction of ear, see 15120 et seq)

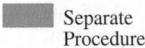 Separate Procedure

Unlisted Procedure

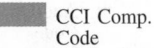 CCI Comp. Code

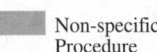 Non-specific Procedure

| 69140 | Excision exostosis(es), external auditory canal |

| 69145 | Excision soft tissue lesion, external auditory canal |

| 69150 | Radical excision external auditory canal lesion; without neck dissection |

| 69155 | with neck dissection |

(For resection of temporal bone, use 69535)

(For skin grafting, see 15004-15261)

REMOVAL

| 69200 | Removal foreign body from external auditory canal; without general anesthesia |

| 69205 | with general anesthesia |

| 69210 | Removal impacted cerumen (separate procedure), 1 or both ears |

| 69220 | Debridement, mastoidectomy cavity, simple (eg, routine cleaning) |

(For bilateral procedure, report 9220 with modifier -50)

| 69222 | Debridement, mastoidectomy cavity, complex (eg, with anesthesia or more than routine cleaning) |

(For bilateral procedure, report 69222 with modifier -50)

REPAIR

(For suture of wound or injury of external ear, see 12011-14302)

⊙ | 69300 | Otoplasty, protruding ear, with or without size reduction |

(For bilateral procedure, report 69300 with modifier -50)

| 69310 | Reconstruction of external auditory canal (meatoplasty) (eg, for stenosis due to injury, infection) (separate procedure) |

| 69320 | Reconstruction external auditory canal for congenital atresia, single stage |

(For combination with middle ear reconstruction, see 69631, 69641)

● New Code   ▲ Revised Code   + Add-On Code   ⃠ Modifier -51 Exempt   ⊙ Moderate Sedation

(For other reconstructive procedures with grafts (eg, skin, cartilage, bone), see 13150-15760, 21230-21235)

OTHER PROCEDURES

(For otoscopy under general anesthesia, use 92502)

69399 Unlisted procedure, external ear

MIDDLE EAR

INTRODUCTION

69400 Eustachian tube inflation, transnasal; with catheterization

69401   without catheterization

69405 Eustachian tube catheterization, transtympanic

INCISION

69420 Myringotomy including aspiration and/or eustachian tube inflation

69421 Myringotomy including aspiration and/or eustachian tube inflation requiring general anesthesia

69424 Ventilating tube removal requiring general anesthesia

(For bilateral procedure, report 69424 with modifier -50)

(Do not report code 69424 in conjunction with codes 69205, 69210, 69420, 69421, 69433-69676, 69710-69745, 69801-69930)

69433 Tympanostomy (requiring insertion of ventilating tube), local or topical anesthesia

(For bilateral procedure, report 69433 with modifier -50)

69436 Tympanostomy (requiring insertion of ventilating tube), general anesthesia

(For bilateral procedure, report 69436 with modifier -50)

69440 Middle ear exploration through postauricular or ear canal incision

(For atticotomy, see 69601 et seq)

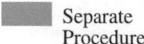 Separate Procedure   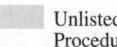 Unlisted Procedure   CCI Comp. Code   Non-specific Procedure

69450 Tympanolysis, transcanal

EXCISION

69501 Transmastoid antrotomy (simple mastoidectomy)

69502 Mastoidectomy; complete

69505   modified radical

69511   radical

(For skin graft, see 15004 et seq)

(For mastoidectomy cavity debridement, see 69220, 69222)

69530 Petrous apicectomy including radical mastoidectomy

69535 Resection temporal bone, external approach

(For middle fossa approach, see 69950-69970)

69540 Excision aural polyp

69550 Excision aural glomus tumor; transcanal

69552   transmastoid

69554   extended (extratemporal)

REPAIR

69601 Revision mastoidectomy; resulting in complete mastoidectomy

69602   resulting in modified radical mastoidectomy

69603   resulting in radical mastoidectomy

69604   resulting in tympanoplasty

(For planned secondary tympanoplasty after mastoidectomy, see 69631, 69632)

69605   with apicectomy

(For skin graft, see 15120, 15121, 15260, 15261)

● New Code	▲ Revised Code	+ Add-On Code	⊘ Modifier -51 Exempt	⊙ Moderate Sedation

69610   Tympanic membrane repair, with or without site preparation or perforation for closure, with or without patch

69620   Myringoplasty (surgery confined to drumhead and donor area)

69631   Tympanoplasty without mastoidectomy (including canalplasty, atticotomy and/or middle ear surgery), initial or revision; without ossicular chain reconstruction

69632   with ossicular chain reconstruction (eg, postfenestration)

69633   with ossicular chain reconstruction and synthetic prosthesis (eg, partial ossicular replacement prosthesis [PORP], total ossicular replacement prosthesis [TORP])

69635   Tympanoplasty with antrotomy or mastoidotomy (including canalplasty, atticotomy, middle ear surgery, and/or tympanic membrane repair); without ossicular chain reconstruction

69636   with ossicular chain reconstruction

69637   with ossicular chain reconstruction and synthetic prosthesis (eg, partial ossicular replacement prosthesis [PORP], total ossicular replacement prosthesis [TORP])

69641   Tympanoplasty with mastoidectomy (including canalplasty, middle ear surgery, tympanic membrane repair); without ossicular chain reconstruction

69642   with ossicular chain reconstruction

69643   with intact or reconstructed wall, without ossicular chain reconstruction

69644   with intact or reconstructed canal wall, with ossicular chain reconstruction

69645   radical or complete, without ossicular chain reconstruction

69646   radical or complete, with ossicular chain reconstruction

69650   Stapes mobilization

69660   Stapedectomy or stapedotomy with reestablishment of ossicular continuity, with or without use of foreign material;

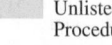 Separate Procedure   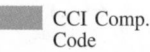 Unlisted Procedure   CCI Comp. Code   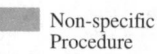 Non-specific Procedure

69661   with footplate drill out

69662   Revision of stapedectomy or stapedotomy

69666   Repair oval window fistula

69667   Repair round window fistula

69670   Mastoid obliteration (separate procedure)

69676   Tympanic neurectomy

(For bilateral procedure, report 69676 with modifier -50)

OTHER PROCEDURES

69700   Closure postauricular fistula, mastoid (separate procedure)

69710   Implantation or replacement of electromagnetic bone conduction hearing device in temporal bone

(Replacement procedure includes removal of old device)

69711   Removal or repair of electromagnetic bone conduction hearing device in temporal bone

69714   Implantation, osseointegrated implant, temporal bone, with percutaneous attachment to external speech processor/cochlear stimulator; without mastoidectomy

69715   with mastoidectomy

69717   Replacement (including removal of existing device), osseointegrated implant, temporal bone, with percutaneous attachment to external speech processor/cochlear stimulator; without mastoidectomy

69718   with mastoidectomy

69720   Decompression facial nerve, intratemporal; lateral to geniculate ganglion

69725   including medial to geniculate ganglion

69740   Suture facial nerve, intratemporal, with or without graft or decompression; lateral to geniculate ganglion

● New Code ▲ Revised Code + Add-On Code ⊘ Modifier -51 Exempt ⊙ Moderate Sedation

69745   including medial to geniculate ganglion

(For extracranial suture of facial nerve, use 64864)

69799 Unlisted procedure, middle ear

INNER EAR

INCISION AND/OR DESTRUCTION

69801 Labyrinthotomy, with perfusion of vestibuloactive drug(s); transcanal

(Do not report 69801 more than once per day)

(Do not report 69801 in conjunction with 69420, 69421, 69433, 69436 when performed on the same ear)

(69802   deleted 2011 [2012 edition])

69805 Endolymphatic sac operation; without shunt

69806   with shunt

69820 Fenestration semicircular canal

69840 Revision fenestration operation

EXCISION

69905 Labyrinthectomy; transcanal

69910   with mastoidectomy

69915 Vestibular nerve section, translabyrinthine approach

(For transcranial approach, use 69950)

INTRODUCTION

69930 Cochlear device implantation, with or without mastoidectomy

OTHER PROCEDURES

69949 Unlisted procedure, inner ear

	Separate Procedure		Unlisted Procedure		CCI Comp. Code		Non-specific Procedure

869

TEMPORAL BONE, MIDDLE FOSSA APPROACH

(For external approach, use 69535)

69950 Vestibular nerve section, transcranial approach

69955 Total facial nerve decompression and/or repair (may include graft)

69960 Decompression internal auditory canal

69970 Removal of tumor, temporal bone

OTHER PROCEDURES

69979 Unlisted procedure, temporal bone, middle fossa approach

● New   ▲ Revised   ＋ Add-On   ⊘ Modifier -51   ⊙ Moderate
   Code   Code   Code   Exempt   Sedation

OPERATING MICROSCOPE

The surgical microscope is employed when the surgical services are performed using the techniques of microsurgery. Code 69990 should be reported (without modifier 51 appended) in addition to the code for the primary procedure performed. Do not use 69990 for visualization with magnifying loupes or corrected vision. Do not report 69990 in addition to procedures where use of the operating microscope is an inclusive component (15756-15758, 15842, 19364, 19368, 20955-20962, 20969-20973, 22551, 22552, 22856-22861, 26551-26554, 26556, 31526, 31531, 31536, 31541, 31545, 31546, 31561, 31571, 43116, 43496, 49906, 61548, 63075-63078, 64727, 64820-64823, 65091-68850, 0184T, 0226T, 0227T, 0308T).

+ 69990   Microsurgical techniques, requiring use of operating microscope (List separately in addition to code for primary procedure)

	Separate Procedure		Unlisted Procedure		CCI Comp. Code		Non-specific Procedure

This page intentionally left blank.

● New
Code

▲ Revised
Code

✚ Add-On
Code

⊘ Modifier -51
Exempt

⊙ Moderate
Sedation

RADIOLOGY

RADIOLOGY SECTION OVERVIEW

The fourth section of the CPT coding system is the radiology section, which includes diagnostic and therapeutic radiology, nuclear medicine and diagnostic ultrasound services. Within each subsection, the CPT codes are arranged by anatomical site.

Diagnostic radiology uses all modalities of radiant energy in medical diagnosis and therapeutic procedures requiring radiologic guidance. This includes imaging techniques and methodologies using radiation emitted by x-ray tubes, radionuclides, ultrasonographic devices, and radiofrequency electromagnetic radiation.

RADIOLOGY SUBSECTIONS

The RADIOLOGY section of the CPT coding system is divided into 7 subsections; namely:

Diagnostic Radiology (Diagnostic Imaging)	70010-76499
Diagnostic Ultrasound	76506-76999
Radiologic Guidance	77001-77032
Breast, Mammography	77051-77059
Bone/Joint Studies	77071-77084
Radiation Oncology	77261-77799
Nuclear Medicine	78012-79999

COMPLETE PROCEDURES

Interventional radiologic procedures or diagnostic studies involving injection of contrast media include all usual preinjection and postinjection services, for example, necessary local anesthesia, placement of needle or catheter, injection of contrast media, supervision of the study, and interpretation of results. When one of these procedures is performed in full by a single physician, it is designated as a "complete procedure."

SUPERVISION AND INTERPRETATION ONLY

When a procedure is performed by a radiologist-clinician team, it is designated as "supervision and interpretation only" and the separate injection procedure is listed in the appropriate section of the SURGERY section of the CPT coding system. These CPT codes are used only when a procedure is performed by more than one physician, for example, a radiologist-clinician team.

873

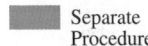 Separate Procedure   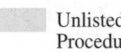 Unlisted Procedure   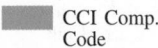 CCI Comp. Code   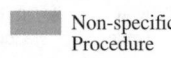 Non-specific Procedure

RADIOLOGY SERVICE MODIFIERS

Listed surgical services and procedures may be modified under certain circumstances. When applicable, the modifying circumstance is identified by adding the appropriate two digit modifier to the base procedure code(s). Modifiers commonly used to report RADIOLOGY services include:

-22 Unusual services

-26 Professional component

-32 Mandated services

-51 Multiple procedures

-52 Reduced services

-62 Two surgeons

-66 Surgical team

-76 Repeat procedure by same physician

-77 Repeat procedure by another physician

-78 Return to the operating room for a related procedure during the postoperative period

-79 Unrelated procedure or service by the same physician during the postoperative period

-80 Assistant surgeon

-90 Reference (outside) laboratory

-99 Multiple modifiers

-LT Left side of body

-RT Right side of body

BILATERAL PROCEDURE CODES

The RADIOLOGY section includes some CPT codes which include the term "bilateral" in the definition. When reporting these services, do not add the modifier -50, because the procedure is already defined as "bilateral."

● New Code   ▲ Revised Code   + Add-On Code   ⊘ Modifier -51 Exempt   ⊙ Moderate Sedation

RADIOLOGY SERVICES MEDICARE CONSIDERATIONS

Most of the CPT codes in this section are subject to Medicare Purchased Diagnostic Services guidelines. Coding and reporting should be as instructed by your local Medicare carrier.

▮ Separate Procedure	▮ Unlisted Procedure	▮ CCI Comp. Code	▮ Non-specific Procedure

This page intentionally left blank.

● New Code	▲ Revised Code	+ Add-On Code	⊘ Modifier -51 Exempt	⊙ Moderate Sedation

RADIOLOGY CODES

DIAGNOSTIC RADIOLOGY (DIAGNOSTIC IMAGING)

HEAD AND NECK

70010 Myelography, posterior fossa, radiological supervision and interpretation

70015 Cisternography, positive contrast, radiological supervision and interpretation

70030 Radiologic examination, eye, for detection of foreign body

70100 Radiologic examination, mandible; partial, less than 4 views

70110 complete, minimum of 4 views

70120 Radiologic examination, mastoids; less than 3 views per side

70130 complete, minimum of 3 views per side

70134 Radiologic examination, internal auditory meati, complete

70140 Radiologic examination, facial bones; less than3e views

70150 complete, minimum of 3 views

70160 Radiologic examination, nasal bones, complete, minimum of 3 views

70170 Dacryocystography, nasolacrimal duct, radiological supervision and interpretation

70190 Radiologic examination; optic foramina

70200 orbits, complete, minimum of 4 views

70210 Radiologic examination, sinuses, paranasal, less than 3 views

70220 Radiologic examination, sinuses, paranasal, complete, minimum of 3 views

	Separate Procedure		Unlisted Procedure		CCI Comp. Code		Non-specific Procedure

877

70240 Radiologic examination, sella turcica

70250 Radiologic examination, skull; less than 4 views

70260   complete, minimum of 4 views

70300 Radiologic examination, teeth; single view

70310   partial examination, less than full mouth

70320   complete, full mouth

70328 Radiologic examination, temporomandibular joint, open and closed mouth; unilateral

70330   bilateral

70332 Temporomandibular joint arthrography, radiological supervision and interpretation

    (Do not report 70332 in conjunction with 77002)

70336 Magnetic resonance (eg, proton) imaging, temporomandibular joint(s)

70350 Cephalogram, orthodontic

70355 Orthopantogram (eg, panoramic x-ray)

70360 Radiologic examination; neck, soft tissue

70370   pharynx or larynx, including fluoroscopy and/or magnification technique

70371 Complex dynamic pharyngeal and speech evaluation by cine or video recording

70373 Laryngography, contrast, radiological supervision and interpretation

70380 Radiologic examination, salivary gland for calculus

70390 Sialography, radiological supervision and interpretation

70450 Computed tomography, head or brain; without contrast material

---

  ● New Code   ▲ Revised Code   + Add-On Code   ⊘ Modifier -51 Exempt   ⊙ Moderate Sedation

70460   with contrast material(s)

70470   without contrast material, followed by contrast material(s) and further sections

(To report 3D rendering, see 76376, 76377)

70480   Computed tomography, orbit, sella, or posterior fossa or outer, middle, or inner ear; without contrast material

70481   with contrast material(s)

70482   without contrast material, followed by contrast material(s) and further sections

(To report 3D rendering, see 76376, 76377)

70486   Computed tomography, maxillofacial area; without contrast material

70487   with contrast material(s)

70488   without contrast material, followed by contrast material(s) and further sections

(To report 3D rendering, see 76376, 76377)

70490   Computed tomography, soft tissue neck; without contrast material

70491   with contrast material(s)

70492   without contrast material followed by contrast material(s) and further sections

(To report 3D rendering, see 76376, 76377)

(For cervical spine, see 72125, 72126)

70496   Computed tomographic angiography, head, with contrast material(s), including noncontrast images, if performed, and image post-processing

70498   Computed tomographic angiography, neck, with contrast material(s), including noncontrast images, if performed, and image post-processing

---

| ▇ | Separate Procedure | � | Unlisted Procedure | ▇ | CCI Comp. Code | ▇ | Non-specific Procedure | **879** |

70540   Magnetic resonance (eg, proton) imaging, orbit, face, and/or neck; without contrast material(s)

(For head or neck magnetic resonance angiography studies, see 70544-70546, 70547-70549)

70542   with contrast material(s)

70543   without contrast material(s), followed by contrast material(s) and further sequences

(Report 70540-70543 once per imaging session)

70544   Magnetic resonance angiography, head; without contrast materials

70545   with contrast materials

70546   without contrast material(s), followed by contrast material(s) and further sequences

70547   Magnetic resonance angiography, neck; without contrast materials

70548   with contrast materials

70549   without contrast material(s), followed by contrast material(s) and further sequences

70551   Magnetic resonance (eg, proton) imaging, brain (including brain stem); without contrast material

70552   with contrast material(s)

70553   without contrast material, followed by contrast material(s) and further sequences

(For magnetic spectroscopy, use 76390)

Functional MRI involves identification and mapping of stimulation of brain function. When neurofunctional tests are administered by a technologist or other non-physician or non-physiologist, use 70554. When neurofunctional tests are entirely administered by a physician or psychologist, use 70555.

70554   Magnetic resonance imaging, brain, functional MRI; including test selection and administration of repetitive body part movement and/or visual stimulation, not requiring physician or psychologist administration

● New Code   ▲ Revised Code   + Add-On Code   ⊘ Modifier -51 Exempt   ⊙ Moderate Sedation

(Do not report 70554 in conjunction with 96020)

70555   requiring physician or psychologist administration of entire neurofunctional testing

(Do not report 70555 unless 96020 is performed)

(Do not report 70554, 70555 in conjunction with 70551-70553 unless a separate diagnostic MRI is performed)

70557 Magnetic resonance (eg, proton) imaging, brain (including brain stem and skull base), during open intracranial procedure (eg, to assess for residual tumor or residual vascular malformation); without contrast material

70558   with contrast material(s)

70559   without contrast material(s), followed by contrast material(s) and further sequences

(For stereotactic biopsy of intracranial lesion with magnetic resonance guidance, use 61751. 70557, 70558 or 70559 may be reported only if a separate report is generated. Report only one of the above codes once per operative session. Do not use these codes in conjunction with 61751, 77021, 77022)

CHEST

(For fluoroscopic or ultrasonic guidance for needle placement procedures (eg., biopsy, aspiration, injection, localization device) of the thorax, see 76942, 77002)

71010 Radiologic examination, chest; single view, frontal

71015   stereo, frontal

71020 Radiologic examination, chest, 2 views, frontal and lateral;

71021   with apical lordotic procedure

71022   with oblique projections

71023   with fluoroscopy

71030 Radiologic examination, chest, complete, minimum of 4 views;

(For concurrent computer-aided detection [CAD] performed in addition to codes 71010, 71020, 71021, 71022, and 71030, use

| Separate Procedure | Unlisted Procedure | CCI Comp. Code | Non-specific Procedure |

0174T. Do not report 71010, 71020, 71021, 71022, and 71030 in conjunction with 0175T for CAD performed remotely from the primary interpretation)

71034   with fluoroscopy

(For separate chest fluoroscopy, use 76000)

71035   Radiologic examination, chest, special views (eg, lateral decubitus, Bucky studies)

(71040   deleted 2012 [2013 edition]. To report, use 76499)

(71060   deleted 2012 [2013 edition]. To report, use 76499)

(71090   deleted 2011 [2012 edition] To report pacemaker or pacing cardioverter-defibrillator lead insertion, replacement, or revision procedures with fluoroscopic guidance, see 33206-33249. To report fluoroscopic guidance for diagnostic lead evaluation without lead insertion, replacement, or revision procedures, use 76000)

71100   Radiologic examination, ribs, unilateral; 2 views

71101   including posteroanterior chest, minimum of 3 views

71110   Radiologic examination, ribs, bilateral; 3 views

71111   including posteroanterior chest, minimum of 4 views

71120   Radiologic examination; sternum, minimum of 2 views

71130   sternoclavicular joint or joints, minimum of 3 views

71250   Computed tomography, thorax; without contrast material

71260   with contrast material(s)

71270   without contrast material, followed by contrast material(s) and further sections

(For cardiac computed tomography of the heart, see 75571-75574)

(To report 3D rendering, see 76376, 76377)

● New Code   ▲ Revised Code   + Add-On Code   ⊘ Modifier -51 Exempt   ⊙ Moderate Sedation

71275 Computed tomographic angiography, chest (noncoronary), with contrast material(s), including noncontrast images, if performed, and image post-processing

(For coronary artery computed tomographic angiography including calcification score and/or cardiac morphology, use 75574)

71550 Magnetic resonance (eg, proton) imaging, chest (eg, for evaluation of hilar and mediastinal lymphadenopathy); without contrast material(s)

71551   with contrast material(s)

71552   without contrast material(s), followed by contrast material(s) and further sequences

(For breast MRI, see 77058, 77059)

71555 Magnetic resonance angiography, chest (excluding myocardium), with or without contrast material(s)

SPINE AND PELVIS

72010 Radiologic examination, spine, entire, survey study, anteroposterior and lateral

72020 Radiologic examination, spine, single view, specify level

▲ **72040** Radiologic examination, spine, cervical; 3 views or less

▲ **72050**   of 4 or 5 views

▲ **72052**   6 or more views

72069 Radiologic examination, spine, thoracolumbar, standing (scoliosis)

72070 Radiologic examination, spine; thoracic, 2 views

72072   thoracic, 3 views

72074   thoracic, minimum of 4 views

72080   thoracolumbar, 2 views

72090   scoliosis study, including supine and erect studies

Separate Procedure	Unlisted Procedure	CCI Comp. Code	Non-specific Procedure

883

72100   Radiologic examination, spine, lumbosacral; 2 or 3 views

72110   minimum of 4 views

72114   complete, including bending views, minimum of 6 views

72120   bending views only, 2 or 3 views

(Contrast material in CT of spine is either by intrathecal or intravenous injection. For intrathecal injection, use also 61055 or 62284. IV injection of contrast material is part of the CT procedure)

72125   Computed tomography, cervical spine; without contrast material

72126   with contrast material

72127   without contrast material, followed by contrast material(s) and further sections

(For intrathecal injection procedure, see 61055, 62284)

72128   Computed tomography, thoracic spine; without contrast material

72129   with contrast material

(For intrathecal injection procedure, see 61055, 62284)

72130   without contrast material, followed by contrast material(s) and further sections

(For intrathecal injection procedure, see 61055, 62284)

72131   Computed tomography, lumbar spine; without contrast material

72132   with contrast material

72133   without contrast material, followed by contrast material(s) and further sections

(For intrathecal injection procedure, see 61055, 62284)

(To report 3D rendering, see 76376, 76377)

72141   Magnetic resonance (eg, proton) imaging, spinal canal and contents, cervical; without contrast material

72142   with contrast material(s)

884   ● New Code   ▲ Revised Code   + Add-On Code   ⊘ Modifier -51 Exempt   ⊙ Moderate Sedation

(For cervical spinal canal imaging without contrast material followed by contrast material, use 72156)

72146 Magnetic resonance (eg, proton) imaging, spinal canal and contents, thoracic; without contrast material

72147 with contrast material(s)

(For thoracic spinal canal imaging without contrast material followed by contrast material, use 72157)

72148 Magnetic resonance (eg, proton) imaging, spinal canal and contents, lumbar; without contrast material

72149 with contrast material(s)

(For lumbar spinal canal imaging without contrast material followed by contrast material, use 72158)

72156 Magnetic resonance (eg, proton) imaging, spinal canal and contents, without contrast material, followed by contrast material(s) and further sequences; cervical

72157 thoracic

72158 lumbar

72159 Magnetic resonance angiography, spinal canal and contents, with or without contrast material(s)

72170 Radiologic examination, pelvis; 1 or 2 views

72190 complete, minimum of 3 views

(For pelvimetry, use 74710)

(For a combined computed tomography (CT) or computed tomographic angiography abdomen and pelvis study, see 74174, 74176-74178)

72191 Computed tomographic angiography, pelvis; with contrast material(s), including noncontrast images, if performed, and image post-processing

(Do not report 72191 in conjunction with 73706 or 75635. For CTA aorto-iliofemoral runoff, use 75635)

885

	Separate Procedure		Unlisted Procedure		CCI Comp. Code		Non-specific Procedure

(Do not report 72191 in conjunction with 74175. For a combined computed tomographic angiography abdomen and pelvis study, use 74174)

72192 Computed tomography, pelvis; without contrast material

72193   with contrast material(s)

72194   without contrast material, followed by contrast material(s) and further sections

(For a combined CT abdomen and pelvis study, see 74176-74178)

(To report 3D rendering, see 76376, 76377)

(For computed tomographic colonography, diagnostic, see 74261-74262. For computed tomographic colonography, screening, use 74263)

(Do not report 72192-72194 in conjunction with 74261-74263)

72195 Magnetic resonance (eg, proton) imaging, pelvis; without contrast material(s)

72196   with contrast material(s)

72197   without contrast material(s), followed by contrast material(s) and further sequences

72198 Magnetic resonance angiography, pelvis, with or without contrast material(s)

72200 Radiologic examination, sacroiliac joints; less than3e views

72202   3 or more views

72220 Radiologic examination, sacrum and coccyx, minimum of 2 views

72240 Myelography, cervical, radiological supervision and interpretation

(For complete cervical myelography, see 61055, 62284, 72240)

72255 Myelography, thoracic, radiological supervision and interpretation

(For complete thoracic myelography, see 61055, 62284, 72255)

● New Code ▲ Revised Code + Add-On Code ⊘ Modifier -51 Exempt ⊙ Moderate Sedation

72265 Myelography, lumbosacral, radiological supervision and interpretation

(For complete lumbosacral myelography, see 61055, 62284, 72265)

72270 Myelography, 2 or more regions (eg, lumbar/thoracic, cervical/thoracic, lumbar/cervical, lumbar/thoracic/cervical), radiological supervision and interpretation

(For complete myelography of entire spinal canal, see 61055, 62284, 72270)

72275 Epidurography, radiological supervision and interpretation

(72275 includes 77003)

(For injection procedure, see 62280-62282, 62310-62319, 64479-64484)

(Use 72275 only when an epidurogram is performed, images documented, and a formal radiologic report is issued)

(Do not report 72275 in conjunction with 22586, 0195T, 0196T, 0309T)

72285 Discography, cervical or thoracic, radiological supervision and interpretation

72291 Radiological supervision and interpretation, percutaneous vertebroplasty, vertebral augmentation, or sacral augmentation (sacroplasty) including cavity creation, per vertebral body or sacrum; under fluoroscopic guidance

72292 under CT guidance

(For procedure, see 22520-22525, 0200T, 0201T)

72295 Discography, lumbar, radiological supervision and interpretation

UPPER EXTREMITIES

(For stress views, any joint, use 77071)

73000 Radiologic examination; clavicle, complete

73010 scapula, complete

73020 Radiologic examination, shoulder; 1 view

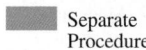 Separate Procedure

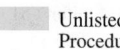 Unlisted Procedure

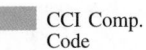 CCI Comp. Code

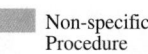 Non-specific Procedure

73030   complete, minimum of 2 views

73040   Radiologic examination, shoulder, arthrography, radiological supervision and interpretation

(Do not report 77002 in conjunction with 73040)

73050   Radiologic examination; acromioclavicular joints, bilateral, with or without weighted distraction

73060   humerus, minimum of 2 views

73070   Radiologic examination, elbow; 2 views

73080   complete, minimum of 3 views

73085   Radiologic examination, elbow, arthrography, radiological supervision and interpretation

(Do not report 77002 in conjunction with 73085)

73090   Radiologic examination; forearm, 2 views

73092   upper extremity, infant, minimum of 2 views

73100   Radiologic examination, wrist; 2 views

73110   complete, minimum of 3 views

73115   Radiologic examination, wrist, arthrography, radiological supervision and interpretation

(Do not report 77002 in conjunction with 73115)

73120   Radiologic examination, hand; 2 views

73130   minimum of 3 views

73140   Radiologic examination, finger(s), minimum of 2 views

73200   Computed tomography, upper extremity; without contrast material

73201   with contrast material(s)

73202   without contrast material, followed by contrast material(s) and further sections

● New Code   ▲ Revised Code   + Add-On Code   ⊘ Modifier -51 Exempt   ⊙ Moderate Sedation

(To report 3D rendering, see 76376, 76377)

73206 Computed tomographic angiography, upper extremity, with contrast material(s), including noncontrast images, if performed, and image post-processing

73218 Magnetic resonance (eg, proton) imaging, upper extremity, other than joint; without contrast material(s)

73219 with contrast material(s)

73220 without contrast material(s), followed by contrast material(s) and further sequences

73221 Magnetic resonance (eg, proton) imaging, any joint of upper extremity; without contrast material(s)

73222 with contrast material(s)

73223 without contrast material(s), followed by contrast material(s) and further sequences

73225 Magnetic resonance angiography, upper extremity, with or without contrast material(s)

LOWER EXTREMITIES

(For stress views, any joint, use 77071)

73500 Radiologic examination, hip, unilateral; 1 view

73510 complete, minimum of 2 views

73520 Radiologic examination, hips, bilateral, minimum of 2 views of each hip, including anteroposterior view of pelvis

73525 Radiologic examination, hip, arthrography, radiological supervision and interpretation

(Do not report 73525 in conjunction with 77002)

73530 Radiologic examination, hip, during operative procedure

73540 Radiologic examination, pelvis and hips, infant or child, minimum of 2 views

(73542 deleted 2011 [2012 edition]. For arthrography, use 27096)

889

	Separate Procedure		Unlisted Procedure		CCI Comp. Code		Non-specific Procedure

73550 Radiologic examination, femur, 2 views

73560 Radiologic examination, knee; 1 or 2 views

73562 3 views

73564 complete, 4 or more views

73565 both knees, standing, anteroposterior

73580 Radiologic examination, knee, arthrography, radiological supervision and interpretation

(Do not report 73580 in conjunction with 77002)

73590 Radiologic examination; tibia and fibula, 2 views

73592 lower extremity, infant, minimum of 2 views

73600 Radiologic examination, ankle; 2 views

73610 complete, minimum of 3 views

73615 Radiologic examination, ankle, arthrography, radiological supervision and interpretation

(Do not report 73615 in conjunction with 77002)

73620 Radiologic examination, foot; 2 views

73630 complete, minimum of 3 views

73650 Radiologic examination; calcaneus, minimum of 2 views

73660 toe(s), minimum of 2 views

73700 Computed tomography, lower extremity; without contrast material

73701 with contrast material(s)

73702 without contrast material, followed by contrast material(s) and further sections

(To report 3D rendering, see 76376, 76377)

● New Code   ▲ Revised Code   + Add-On Code   ⊘ Modifier -51 Exempt   ⊙ Moderate Sedation

73706 Computed tomographic angiography, lower extremity, with contrast material(s), including noncontrast images, if performed, and image post-processing

(For CTA aorto-iliofemoral runoff, use 75635)

73718 Magnetic resonance (eg, proton) imaging, lower extremity, other than joint; without contrast material(s)

73719 with contrast material(s)

73720 without contrast material(s), followed by contrast material(s) and further sequences

73721 Magnetic resonance (eg, proton) imaging, any joint of lower extremity; without contrast material

73722 with contrast material

73723 without contrast material followed by contrast material(s) and further sequences

73725 Magnetic resonance angiography, lower extremity, with or without contrast material(s)

ABDOMEN

74000 Radiologic examination, abdomen; single anteroposterior view

74010 anteroposterior and additional oblique and cone views

74020 complete, including decubitus and/or erect views

74022 complete acute abdomen series, including supine, erect, and/or decubitus views, single view chest

74150 Computed tomography, abdomen; without contrast material

74160 with contrast material(s)

74170 without contrast material, followed by contrast material(s) and further sections

(For a combined CT abdomen and pelvis study, see 74176-74178)

(To report 3D rendering, see 76376, 76377)

Separate Procedure   Unlisted Procedure   CCI Comp. Code   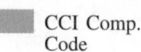 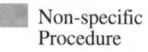 Non-specific Procedure

(For computed tomographic colonography, diagnostic, see 74261-74262. For computed tomographic colonography, screening, use 74263)

(Do not report 74150-74170 in conjunction with 74261-74263)

74174 Computed tomographic angiography, abdomen and pelvis, with contrast material(s), including noncontrast images, if performed, and image postprocessing

(Do not report 74174 in conjunction with 72191, 73706, 74175, 75635, 76376, 76377)

(For CTA aorto-iliofemoral runoff, use 75635)

74175 Computed tomographic angiography, abdomen, with contrast material(s), including noncontrast images, if performed, and image post-processing

(Do not report 74175 in conjunction with 73706 or 75635. For CTA aorto-iliofemoral runoff, use 75635)

(Do not report 74175 in conjunction with 72191. For a combined computed tomographic angiography abdomen and pelvis study, use 74174)

For combinations of CT of the abdomen with CT of the pelvis performed at the same session, use the following table. Do not report more than one CT of the abdomen or CT of the pelvis for any session.

Stand Alone Code	74150 CT Abdomen WO Contrast	74160 CT Abdomen W Contrast	74170 CT Abdomen WO/W Contrast
72192 CT Pelvis WO Contrast	74176	74178	74178
72193 CT Pelvis W Contrast	74178	74177	74178
72194 CT Pelvis WO/W Contrast	74178	74178	74178

74176 Computed tomography, abdomen and pelvis; without contrast material

74177 with contrast material(s)

● New Code   ▲ Revised Code   + Add-On Code   ⊘ Modifier -51 Exempt   ⊙ Moderate Sedation

74178   without contrast material in one or both body regions, followed by contrast material(s) and further sections in one or both body regions

(Do not report 74176-74178 in conjunction with 72192-72194, 74150-74170)

(Report 74176, 74177, or 74178 only once per CT abdomen and pelvis examination)

74181   Magnetic resonance (eg, proton) imaging, abdomen; without contrast material(s)

74182   with contrast material(s)

74183   without contrast material, followed by contrast material(s) and further sequences

74185   Magnetic resonance angiography, abdomen, with or without contrast material(s)

74190   Peritoneogram (eg, after injection of air or contrast), radiological supervision and interpretation

(For procedure, use 49400)

(For computerized axial tomography, see 72192 or 74150)

GASTROINTESTINAL TRACT

(For percutaneous placement of gastrostomy tube, use 43246)

74210   Radiologic examination; pharynx and/or cervical esophagus

74220   esophagus

74230   Swallowing function, with cineradiography/videoradiography

74235   Removal of foreign body(s), esophageal, with use of balloon catheter, radiological supervision and interpretation

(For procedure, see 43215, 43247)

74240   Radiologic examination, gastrointestinal tract, upper; with or without delayed films, without KUB

74241   with or without delayed films, with KUB

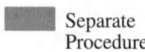 Separate Procedure   Unlisted Procedure   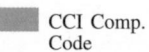 CCI Comp. Code   Non-specific Procedure   **893**

74245   with small intestine, includes multiple serial films

74246   Radiological examination, gastrointestinal tract, upper, air contrast, with specific high density barium, effervescent agent, with or without glucagon; with or without delayed films, without KUB

74247   with or without delayed films, with KUB

74249   with small intestine follow-through

74250   Radiologic examination, small intestine, includes multiple serial films;

74251   via enteroclysis tube

74260   Duodenography, hypotonic

74261   Computed tomographic (CT) colonography, diagnostic, including image postprocessing; without contrast material

74262   with contrast material(s) including non contrast images, if performed

(Do not report 74261, 74262 in conjunction with 72192-72194, 74150-74170, 74263, 76376, 76377)

74263   Computed tomographic (CT) colonography, screening, including image postprocessing

(Do not report 74263 in conjunction with 72192-72194, 74150-74170, 74261, 74262, 76376, 76377)

74270   Radiologic examination, colon; contrast (eg., barium) enema, with or without KUB

74280   air contrast with specific high density barium, with or without glucagon

74283   Therapeutic enema, contrast or air, for reduction of intussusception or other intraluminal obstruction (eg, meconium ileus)

74290   Cholecystography, oral contrast;

74291   additional or repeat examination or multiple day examination

 • New Code   ▲ Revised Code   + Add-On Code   ⊘ Modifier -51 Exempt   ⊙ Moderate Sedation

74300 Cholangiography and/or pancreatography; intraoperative, radiological supervision and interpretation

+ 74301 additional set intraoperative, radiological supervision and interpretation (List separately in addition to code for primary procedure)

(Use 74301 in conjunction with code 74300)

74305 through existing catheter, radiological supervision and interpretation

(For procedure, see 47505, 48400, 47560-47561, 47563)

(For biliary duct stone extraction, percutaneous, see 47630, 74327)

74320 Cholangiography, percutaneous, transhepatic, radiological supervision and interpretation

74327 Postoperative biliary duct calculus removal, percutaneous via T-tube tract, basket, or snare (eg, Burhenne technique), radiological supervision and interpretation

(For procedure, use 47630)

74328 Endoscopic catheterization of the biliary ductal system, radiological supervision and interpretation

(For procedure, see 43260-43272 as appropriate)

74329 Endoscopic catheterization of the pancreatic ductal system, radiological supervision and interpretation

(For procedure, see 43260-43272 as appropriate)

74330 Combined endoscopic catheterization of the biliary and pancreatic ductal systems, radiological supervision and interpretation

(For procedure, see 43260-43272 as appropriate)

74340 Introduction of long gastrointestinal tube (eg, Miller-Abbott), including multiple fluoroscopies and films, radiological supervision and interpretation

(For tube placement, use 44500)

74355 Percutaneous placement of enteroclysis tube, radiological supervision and interpretation

Separate Procedure	Unlisted Procedure	CCI Comp. Code	Non-specific Procedure	**895**

74360   Intraluminal dilation of strictures and/or obstructions (eg, esophagus), radiological supervision and interpretation

74363   Percutaneous transhepatic dilation of biliary duct stricture with or without placement of stent, radiological supervision and interpretation

(For procedure, see 47510, 47511, 47555, 47556)

URINARY TRACT

74400   Urography (pyelography), intravenous, with or without KUB, with or without tomography

74410   Urography, infusion, drip technique and/or bolus technique;

74415   with nephrotomography

74420   Urography, retrograde, with or without KUB

74425   Urography, antegrade, (pyelostogram, nephrostogram, loopogram), radiological supervision and interpretation

74430   Cystography, minimum of three views, radiological supervision and interpretation

74440   Vasography, vesiculography, or epididymography, radiological supervision and interpretation

74445   Corpora cavernosography, radiological supervision and interpretation

74450   Urethrocystography, retrograde, radiological supervision and interpretation

74455   Urethrocystography, voiding, radiological supervision and interpretation

74470   Radiologic examination, renal cyst study, translumbar, contrast visualization, radiological supervision and interpretation

74475   Introduction of intracatheter or catheter into renal pelvis for drainage and/or injection, percutaneous, radiological supervision and interpretation

   ● New Code   ▲ Revised Code   + Add-On Code   ⊘ Modifier -51 Exempt   ⊙ Moderate Sedation

74480 Introduction of ureteral catheter or stent into ureter through renal pelvis for drainage and/or injection, percutaneous, radiological supervision and interpretation

(For transurethral surgery (ureter and pelvis), see 52320-52355)

74485 Dilation of nephrostomy, ureters, or urethra, radiological supervision and interpretation

(For dilation of ureter without radiologic guidance, use 52341, 52344)

(For change of nephrostomy or pyelostomy tube, use 50398)

GYNECOLOGICAL AND OBSTETRICAL

(For abdomen and pelvis, see 72170-72190, 74000-74170)

74710 Pelvimetry, with or without placental localization

74740 Hysterosalpingography, radiological supervision and interpretation

(For introduction of saline or contrast for hysterosalpingography, see 58340)

74742 Transcervical catheterization of fallopian tube, radiological supervision and interpretation

(For procedure, use 58345)

74775 Perineogram (eg, vaginogram, for sex determination or extent of anomalies)

HEART

Flow and velocity assessment for valves and intracardiac shunts is performed in addition to a function and morphologic evaluation. Use 75559 with 75565 to report flow with pharmacologic wall motion stress evaluation without contrast. Use 75563 with 75565 to report flow with pharmacologic perfusion stress with contrast.

Cardiac MRI for velocity flow mapping can be reported in conjunction with 75557, 75559, 75561, or 75563.

Listed procedures may be performed independently or in the course of overall medical care. If the individual providing these services is also responsible for diagnostic workup and/or follow-up care of the patient, see appropriate sections

	Separate Procedure		Unlisted Procedure		CCI Comp. Code		Non-specific Procedure

897

also. Only one procedure in the series 75557-75563 is appropriately reported per session. Only one add-on code for flow velocity can be reported per session.

Cardiac MRI studies may be performed at rest and/or during pharmacologic stress. Therefore, the appropriate stress testing code from the 93015-93018 series should be reported in addition to 75559 or 75563.

Cardiac computed tomography (CT) and coronary computed tomographic angiography (CTA) include the axial source images of the pre-contrast, arterial phase sequence, and venous phase sequence (if performed(, as well as the two-dimensional and three-dimensional reformatted images resulting from the study, including cine review. Contrast enhanced cardiac CT and coronary CTA codes 75571-75574 include any quantitative assessment when performed as part of the same encounter. Report only one computed tomography heart service per encounter.

(For separate injection procedures for vascular radiology, see Surgery section, 36000-36299)

(For cardiac catheterization procedures, see 93451-93572)

(75552-75556 have been deleted. To report, see 75557, 75559, 75561, 75563, 75565)

75557 Cardiac magnetic resonance imaging for morphology and function without contrast material;

75559 with stress imaging

75561 Cardiac magnetic resonance imaging for morphology and function without contrast material(s), followed by contrast material(s) and further sequences;

75563 with stress imaging

(75558, 75560, 75562, 75564 have been deleted. To report flow velocity, use 75565)

+ 75565 Cardiac magnetic resonance imaging for velocity flow mapping (List separately in addition to code for primary procedure)

(Use 75565 in conjunction with 75557, 75559, 75561, 75563)

(Do not report 75557, 75559, 75561, 75563, 75565 in conjunction with 76376, 76377)

75571 Computed tomography, heart, without contrast material, with quantitative evaluation of coronary calcium

---

898

● New Code   ▲ Revised Code   + Add-On Code   ⊘ Modifier -51 Exempt   ⊙ Moderate Sedation

75572 Computed tomography, heart, with contrast material, for evaluation of cardiac structure and morphology (including 3D image postprocessing, assessment of cardiac function, and evaluation of venous structures, if performed)

75573 Computed tomography, heart, with contrast material, for evaluation of cardiac structure and morphology in the setting of congenital heart disease (including 3D image postprocessing, assessment of LV cardiac function, RV structure and function and evaluation of venous structures, if performed)

75574 Computed tomographic angiography, heart, coronary arteries and bypass grafts (when present), with contrast material, including 3D image postprocessing (including evaluation of cardiac structure and morphology, assessment of cardiac function, and evaluation of venous structures, if performed)

VASCULAR PROCEDURES

AORTA AND ARTERIES

Selective vascular catheterizations should be coded to include introduction and all lesser order selective catheterizations used in the approach (eg., the description for a selective right middle cerebral artery catheterization includes the introduction and placement catheterization of the right common and internal carotid arteries).

Additional second and/or third order arterial catheterizations within the same family of arteries supplied by a single first order artery should be expressed by 36218 or 36248. Additional first order or higher catheterizations in vascular families supplied by a first order vessel different from a previously selected and coded family should be separately coded using the conventions described above.

The lower extremity endovascular revascularization codes describing services performed for occlusive disease (37220-37235) include catheterization (36200, 36240, 36245-36248) in the work described by the codes. Catheterization codes are not additionally reported for diagnostic lower extremity angiography when performed through the same access site as the therapy (37220-37235) performed in the same session. However, catheterization for the diagnostic lower extremity angiogram may be reported separately if a different arterial puncture site is necessary.

For angiography performed in conjunction with therapeutic transcatheter radiological supervision and interpretation services, see the Radiology Transcatheter Procedures guidelines.

Diagnostic angiography (radiological supervision and interpretation) codes should NOT be used with interventional procedures for:

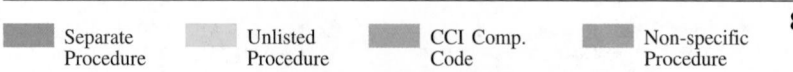

Separate Procedure   Unlisted Procedure   CCI Comp. Code   Non-specific Procedure   **899**

1. Contrast injections, angiography, roadmapping, and/or fluoroscopic guidance for the intervention;

2. Vessel measurement; AND

3. Post-angioplasty/stent/atherectomy angiography, as this work is captured in the radiological supervision and interpretation code(s). In those therapeutic codes that include radiological supervision and interpretation, this work is captured in the therapeutic code.

Diagnostic angiography performed at the time of an interventional procedure is separately reportable if:

1. No prior catheter-based angiographic study is available and a full diagnostic study is performed, and the decision to intervene is based on the diagnostic study, OR

2. A prior study is available, but as documented in the medical record:

a. The patient's condition with respect to the clinical indication has changed since the prior study; OR

b. There is inadequate visualization of the anatomy and/or pathology; OR

c. There is a clinical change during the procedure that requires new evaluation outside the target area of intervention.

Diagnostic angiography performed at a separate session from an interventional procedure is separately reported.

If diagnostic angiography is necessary, is performed at the same session as the interventional procedure, and meets the above criteria, modifier 59 must be appended to the diagnostic radiological supervision and interpretation code(s) to denote that diagnostic work has been done following these guidelines.

Diagnostic angiography performed at the time of an interventional procedure is NOT separately reportable if it is specifically included in the interventional code descriptor.

(For intravenous procedure, see 36000, 36005-36015, and for intra-arterial procedure, see 36100-36248)

(For radiological supervision and interpretation, see 75600-75893)

75600 Aortography, thoracic, without serialography, radiological supervision and interpretation

(For isupravalvular aortography performed at the time of cardiac catheterization, use 93567, which includes imaging supervision, interpretation and report)

● New Code ▲ Revised Code + Add-On Code ⊘ Modifier -51 Exempt ⊙ Moderate Sedation

75605 Aortography, thoracic, by serialography, radiological supervision and interpretation

(For supravalvular aortography performed at the time of cardiac catheterization, use 93567, which includes imaging supervision, interpretation and report)

75625 Aortography, abdominal, by serialography, radiological supervision and interpretation

75630 Aortography, abdominal plus bilateral iliofemoral lower extremity, catheter, by serialography, radiological supervision and interpretation

75635 Computed tomographic angiography, abdominal aorta and bilateral iliofemoral lower extremity runoff, with contrast material(s), including noncontrast images, if performed, and image post-processing

(Do not report 75635 in conjunction with 72191, 73706, 74175, or 74174)

(75650 deleted 2012 [2013 edition]. To report, see 36221-36226)

75658 Angiography, brachial, retrograde, radiological supervision and interpretation

(75660 deleted 2012 [2013 edition]. To report, use 36227)

(75662 deleted 2012 [2013 edition]. To report, use 36227 and append modifier 50)

(75665 deleted 2012 [2013 edition]. To report, see 36223, 36224)

(75671 deleted 2012 [2013 edition]. To report, see 36223 and 36224 and append modifier 50 as appropriate)

(75676 deleted 2012 [2013 edition]. To report, see 36222-36224)

(75680 deleted 2012 [2013 edition]. To report, see 36222-36224 and append modifier 50 as appropriate)

(75685 deleted 2012 [2013 edition]. To report, see 36225, 36226)

75705 Angiography, spinal, selective, radiological supervision and interpretation

---

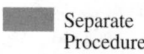 Separate Procedure

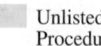 Unlisted Procedure

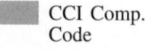 CCI Comp. Code

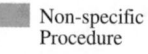 Non-specific Procedure

75710   Angiography, extremity, unilateral, radiological supervision and interpretation

75716   Angiography, extremity, bilateral, radiological supervision and interpretation

(75722   deleted 2011 [2012 edition]. To report, see 36251, 36253))

(75724   deleted 2011 [2012 edition]. To report, see 36252, 36254)

75726   Angiography, visceral, selective or supraselective, (with or without flush aortogram), radiological supervision and interpretation

(For selective angiography, each additional visceral vessel studied after basic examination, use 75774)

75731   Angiography, adrenal, unilateral, selective, radiological supervision and interpretation

75733   Angiography, adrenal, bilateral, selective, radiological supervision and interpretation

75736   Angiography, pelvic, selective or supraselective, radiological supervision and interpretation

75741   Angiography, pulmonary, unilateral, selective, radiological supervision and interpretation

75743   Angiography, pulmonary, bilateral, selective, radiological supervision and interpretation

75746   Angiography, pulmonary, by nonselective catheter or venous injection, radiological supervision and interpretation

(For pulmonary angiography by nonselective catheter or venous injuection performed at the time of cardiac catheterization, use 93568, which includes imaging supervision, interpretation and report)

75756   Angiography, internal mammary, radiological supervision and interpretation

(For internal mammary angiography performed at the time of cardiac catheterization, see 93455, 93457, 93459, 93461, 93564 which include imaging supervision, interpretation and report)

   ● New Code   ▲ Revised Code   + Add-On Code   ⊘ Modifier -51 Exempt   ⊙ Moderate Sedation

+ 75774 Angiography, selective, each additional vessel studied after basic examination, radiological supervision and interpretation (List separately in addition to code for primary procedure)

(Use 75774 in addition to code for specific initial vessel studied)

(Do not report 75774 as part of diagnostic angiography of the extracranial and intracranial cervicocerebral vessels. It may be appropriate to reort 75774 for diagnostic angiography of upper extremities and other vascular beds performed in the same session)

(For angiography, see 36147, 75600-75756, 75791)

(For catheterizations, see codes 36215-36248)

(For cardiac catheterization procedures, see 93452-93462, 93531-93533, 93563-93568)

(75790 Deleted 2009 [2010 edition]; see 36147, 75791)

75791 Angiography, arteriovenous shunt (eg, dialysis patient fistula/graft), complete evaluation of dialysis access, including fluoroscopy, image documentation and report (includes injections of contrast and all necessary imaging from the arterial anastomosis and adjacent artery through entire venous outflow including the inferior or superior vena cava), radiological supervision and interpretation

(Do not report 75791 in conjunction with 36147, 36148)

(For introduction of catheter, if necessary, see 36140, 36215-36217, 36245-36247)

(Use 75791 only if radiological evaluation is performed through an already existing access into the shunt or from an access that is not a direct puncture of the shunt)

(For radiological evaluation with needle/catheter introduction, AV dialysis shunt, complete procedure, use 36147)

VEINS AND LYMPHATICS

For venography performed in conjunction with therapeutic transcatheter radiological supervision and interpretation services, see the Radiology Transcatheter Procedures guidelines.

Diagnostic venography (radiological supervision and interpretation) codes should NOT be used with interventional procedures for:

903

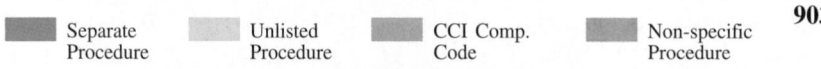

| Separate Procedure | Unlisted Procedure | CCI Comp. Code | Non-specific Procedure |

(1) Contrast injections, venography, roadmapping, and/or fluoroscopic guidance for intervention;

(2) Vessel measurement; and

(3) Post-angioplasty/stent venography, as this work is captured in the radiological supervision and interpretation code(s).

Diagnostic venography performed at the time of an interventional procedure is separately reportable if:

1. No prior catheter-based venographic study is available and a full diagnostic study is performed, and decision to intervene is based on the diagnostic study, OR

2. A prior study is available, but as documented in the medical record:

a. The patient's condition with respect to the clinical indication has changed since the prior study, OR

b. There is inadequate visualization of the anatomy and/or pathology, OR

c. There is a clinical change during the procedure that requires new evaluation outside the target area of intervention.

Diagnostic venography performed at a separate setting from an interventional procedure is separately reported.

Diagnostic venography performed at the time of an interventional procedure is NOT separately reportable if it is specifically included in the interventional code descriptor.

(For injection procedure for venous system, see 36000-36015, 36400-36510)

(For injection procedure for lymphatic system, use 38790)

75801 Lymphangiography, extremity only, unilateral, radiological supervision and interpretation

75803 Lymphangiography, extremity only, bilateral, radiological supervision and interpretation

75805 Lymphangiography, pelvic/abdominal, unilateral, radiological supervision and interpretation

75807 Lymphangiography, pelvic/abdominal, bilateral, radiological supervision and interpretation

● New Code   ▲ Revised Code   + Add-On Code   ⊘ Modifier -51 Exempt   ⊙ Moderate Sedation

75809 Shuntogram for investigation of previously placed indwelling nonvascular shunt (eg, LeVeen shunt, ventriculoperitoneal shunt, indwelling infusion pump), radiological supervision and interpretation

(For procedure, see 49427 or 61070)

75810 Splenoportography, radiological supervision and interpretation

75820 Venography, extremity, unilateral, radiological supervision and interpretation

75822 Venography, extremity, bilateral, radiological supervision and interpretation

75825 Venography, caval, inferior, with serialography, radiological supervision and interpretation

75827 Venography, caval, superior, with serialography, radiological supervision and interpretation

75831 Venography, renal, unilateral, selective, radiological supervision and interpretation

75833 Venography, renal, bilateral, selective, radiological supervision and interpretation

75840 Venography, adrenal, unilateral, selective, radiological supervision and interpretation

75842 Venography, adrenal, bilateral, selective, radiological supervision and interpretation

75860 Venography, venous sinus (eg, petrosal and inferior sagittal) or jugular, catheter, radiological supervision and interpretation

75870 Venography, superior sagittal sinus, radiological supervision and interpretation

75872 Venography, epidural, radiological supervision and interpretation

75880 Venography, orbital, radiological supervision and interpretation

75885 Percutaneous transhepatic portography with hemodynamic evaluation, radiological supervision and interpretation

---

905

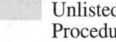 Separate Procedure   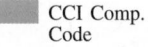 Unlisted Procedure   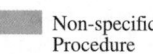 CCI Comp. Code   Non-specific Procedure

75887   Percutaneous transhepatic portography without hemodynamic evaluation, radiological supervision and interpretation

75889   Hepatic venography, wedged or free, with hemodynamic evaluation, radiological supervision and interpretation

75891   Hepatic venography, wedged or free, without hemodynamic evaluation, radiological supervision and interpretation

75893   Venous sampling through catheter, with or without angiography (eg, for parathyroid hormone, renin), radiological supervision and interpretation

       (For procedure, use 36500)

TRANSCATHETER PROCEDURES

Therapeutic transcatheter radiological supervision and interpretation code(s) include the following services associated with that intervention:

    1. Contrast injections, angiography/venography, roadmapping, and fluoroscopic guidance for the intervention;

    2. Vessel measurement; and

    3. Completion angiography/venography (except for those uses permitted by 75898).

Unless specifically included in the code descriptor, diagnostic angiography/venography performed at the time of transcatheter service(s) is separately reportable (eg., no prior catheter-based diagnostic angiography/ venography study of the target vessel is available, prior diagnostic study is inadequate, patient's condition with respect to the clinical indication has changed since the prior study or during the intervention). See 75600-75893.

Codes 75956 and 75957 include all angiography of the thoracic aorta and its branches for diagnostic imaging prior to deployment of the primary endovascular devices (including all routine components of modular devices), fluoroscopic guidance in the delivery of the endovascular components, and intraprocedural arterial angiography (eg., confirm position, detect endoleak, evaluate runoff).

Code 75958 includes the analogous services for placement of each proximal thoracic endovascular extension. Code 75959 includes the analogous services for placement of a distal thoracic endovascular extension(s) placed during a procedure after the primary repair.

75894   Transcatheter therapy, embolization, any method, radiological supervision and interpretation

● New Code	▲ Revised Code	+ Add-On Code	⊘ Modifier -51 Exempt	⊙ Moderate Sedation

(For uterine fibroid embolization [uterine artery embolization performed to treat uterine fibroids], use 37210)

(For obstetrical and gynecological embolization procedures other than uterine fibroid embolization [eg., embolization to treat obstetrical or postpartum hemorrhage], use 37204)

▲ **75896** Transcatheter therapy, infusion, other than for thrombolysis, radiological supervision and interpretation

(For radiological supervision and interpretation for thrombolysis other than coronary, see 37211-37214)

(Do not report 75896 in conjunction with 37211-37214)

(For infusion for coronary disease, see 92975, 92977)

▲ **75898** Angiography through existing catheter for follow-up study for transcatheter therapy, embolization or infusion, other than for thrombolysis

(For thrombolysis infusion management other than coronary, see 37211-37214)

(Do not report 75898 in conjunction with 37211-37214)

(75900 deleted 2012 [2013 edition]. For exchange of a previously placed intravascular catheter during thrombolytic therapy with contrast monitoring, radiological supervision and interpretation, see 37211-37214)

75901 Mechanical removal of pericatheter obstructive material (eg., fibrin sheath) from central venous device via separate venous access, radiologic supervision and interpretation

(For procedure, use 36595)

(For venous catheterization, see 36010-36012)

75902 Mechanical removal of intraluminal (intracatheter) obstructive material from central venous device through device lumen, radiologic supervision and interpretation

(For procedure, use 36596)

(For venous catheterization, see 36010-36012)

(75940 deleted 2011 [2012 edition]. To report, use 37191)

75945 Intravascular ultrasound (non-coronary vessel), radiological supervision and interpretation; initial vessel

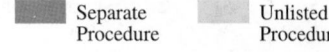 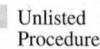 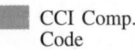

Separate Procedure	Unlisted Procedure	CCI Comp. Code	Non-specific Procedure

+ **75946**   each additional non-coronary vessel (List separately in addition to code for primary procedure)

(Use 75946 in conjunction with code 75945)

(For catheterizations, see codes 36215-36248)

(For transcatheter therapies, see codes 37200-37208, 61624, 61626)

(For procedure, see 37250, 37251)

75952   Endovascular repair of infrarenal abdominal aortic aneurysm or dissection, radiological supervision and interpretation

(For implantation of endovascular grafts, see 34800-34805)

(For radiologic supervision and interpretation of endovascular repair of abdominal aortic aneurysm involving visceral vessels, see Category III codes 0080T-0081T)

75953   Placement of proximal or distal extension prosthesis for endovascular repair of infrarenal aortic or iliac artery aneurysm, pseudoaneurysm, or dissection, radiological supervision and interpretation

(For implantation of endovascular extension prostheses, see 34825, 34826)

75954   Endovascular repair of iliac artery aneurysm, psuedoaneurysm, arteriovenous malformation, or trauma, using ilio-iliac tube endoprosthesis, radiological supervision and interpretation

(For implantation of endovascular graft, see 34900)

(For endovascular repair or iliac artery bifurcation [eg, aneurysm, pseudoaneurysm, arteriovenous malformation, trauma] using bifurcated endoprosthesis, radiological supervision and interpretation, use 0255T)

75956   Endovascular repair of descending thoracic aorta (eg, aneurysm, pseudoaneurysm, dissection, penetrating ulcer, intramural hematoma, or traumatic disruption); involving coverage of left subclavian artery origin, initial endoprosthesis plus descending thoracic aortic extension(s), if required, to level of celiac artery origin, radiological supervision and interpretation

(For implantation of endovascular graft, use 33880)

75957   not involving coverage of left subclavian artery origin, initial endoprosthesis plus descending thoracic aortic

908 ● New Code   ▲ Revised Code   + Add-On Code   ⊘ Modifier -51 Exempt   ⊙ Moderate Sedation

extension(s), if required, to level of celiac artery origin, radiological supervision and interpretation

(For implantation of endovascular graft, use 33881)

75958 Placement of proximal extension prosthesis for endovascular repair of descending thoracic aorta (eg, aneurysm, pseudoaneurysm, dissection, penetrating ulcer, intramural hematoma, or traumatic disruption), radiological supervision and interpretation

(Report 75958 for each proximal extension)

(For implantation of proximal endovascular extension, see 33883, 33884)

75959 Placement of distal extension prosthesis(es) (delayed) after endovascular repair of descending thoracic aorta, as needed, to level of celiac origin, radiological supervision and interpretation

(Do not report 75959 in conjunction with 75956, 75957)

(Report 75959 once, regardless of number of modules deployed)

(For implantation of distal endovascular extension, use 33886)

75960 Transcatheter introduction of intravascular stent(s), (except coronary, carotid, vertebral, iliac, and lower extremity artery), percutaneous and/or open, radiological supervision and interpretation, each vessel

(For stent placement, including radiological supervision and interpretation, in iliac, femoral, popliteal and tibial/peroneal arteries, see 37221, 37223, 37226, 37227, 37230, 27231, 37234, 37235)

(For procedure, see 37205-37208)

(For radiologic supervision and interpretation for transcatheter placement of extracranial vertebral or intrathoracic carotid artery stent(s), see Category III codes 0075T, 0076T)

(75961 deleted 2012 [2013 edition]. To report, use 37197

(For removal of a vena cava filter, use 37193)

75962 Transluminal balloon angioplasty, peripheral artery other than renal, or other visceral artery, iliac or lower extremity, radiological supervision and interpretation

---

Separate Procedure Unlisted Procedure CCI Comp. Code Non-specific Procedure **909**

(For radiological supervision and interpretation for transluminal balloon angioplasty in iliac, femoral, popliteal, and tibial/peroneal arteries, see 37220-37235)

(For procedure, see 35458, 35475)

+ **75964** Transluminal balloon angioplasty, each additional peripheral artery other than renal, or other visceral artery, iliac or lower extremity, radiological supervision and interpretation (List separately in addition to code for primary procedure)

(Use 75964 in conjunction with code 75962)

75966 Transluminal balloon angioplasty, renal or other visceral artery, radiological supervision and interpretation

+ **75968** Transluminal balloon angioplasty, each additional visceral artery, radiological supervision and interpretation (List separately in addition to code for primary procedure)

(Use 75968 in conjunction with code 75966)

(For percutaneous transluminal coronary angioplasty, see 92920-92944)

75970 Transcatheter biopsy, radiological supervision and interpretation

(For injection procedure only for transcatheter therapy or biopsy, see 36100-36299)

(For transcatheter renal and ureteral biopsy, use 52007)

(For percutaneous needle biopsy of pancreas, use 48102; of retroperitoneal lymph node or mass, use 49180)

75978 Transluminal balloon angioplasty, venous (eg, subclavian stenosis), radiological supervision and interpretation

75980 Percutaneous transhepatic biliary drainage with contrast monitoring, radiological supervision and interpretation

75982 Percutaneous placement of drainage catheter for combined internal and external biliary drainage or of a drainage stent for internal biliary drainage in patients with an inoperable mechanical biliary obstruction, radiological supervision and interpretation

75984 Change of percutaneous tube or drainage catheter with contrast monitoring (eg, genitourinary system, abscess), radiological supervision and interpretation

● New Code ▲ Revised Code + Add-On Code ⊘ Modifier -51 Exempt ⊙ Moderate Sedation

(For percutaneous replacement of gastrostomy, duodenostomy, jejunostomy, gastro-jejunostomy, or cecostomy [or other colonic] tube including fluoroscopic imaging guidance, see 49450-49452)

(For change of nephrostomy or pyelostomy tube only, use 50398)

(For introduction procedure only for percutaneous biliary drainage, see 47510, 47511)

(For percutaneous choloecystostomy, use 47490)

(For change of percutaneous biliary drainage catheter only, use 47525)

(For percutaneous nephrostolithotomy or pyelostolithotomy, see 50080, 50081)

(For removal and/or replacement of an internally dwelling ureteral stent via a transurethral approach, see 50385-50386)

75989 Radiological guidance (ie, fluoroscopy, ultrasound, or computed tomography), for percutaneous drainage (eg., abscess, specimen collection), with placement of catheter, radiological supervision and interpretation

(Do not report 75989 in conjunction with 32554, 32555, 32556, 32557, 47490)

TRANSLUMINAL ATHERECTOMY

(75992 deleted 2010 [2011 edition]. To report, see 37225, 37227, 37229, 37231, 0238T)

(75993 deleted 2010 [2011 edition]. To report, see 37233, 37235, 0238T)

(75994 deleted 2010 [2011 edition]. To report, use 0234T)

(75995 deleted 2010 [2011 edition]. To report, use 0235T)

(75996 deleted 2010 [2011 edition]. To report, use 0235T)

OTHER PROCEDURES

(For computed tomography cerebral perfusion analysis, see Category III code 0042T)

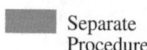 Separate Procedure 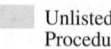 Unlisted Procedure 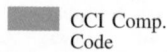 CCI Comp. Code 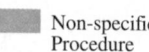 Non-specific Procedure **911**

(For arthrography of shoulder, use 73040; elbow, use 73085; wrist, use 73115; hip, use 73525; knee, use 73580; ankle, use 73615)

▲ **76000** Fluoroscopy (separate procedure), up to 1 hour physician or other qualified health care professional time, other than 71023 or 71034 (eg, cardiac fluoroscopy)

▲ **76001** Fluoroscopy, physician or other qualified health care professional time more than 1 hour, assisting a non-radiologic physician or other qualified health care professional (eg, nephrostolithotomy, ERCP, bronchoscopy, transbronchial biopsy)

76010 Radiologic examination from nose to rectum for foreign body, single view, child

76080 Radiologic examination, abscess, fistula or sinus tract study, radiological supervision and interpretation

(For contrast injection[s] and radiological assessment of gastrostomy, duodenostomy, jejunostomy, gastro-jejunostomy, or cecostomy [or other colonic] tube including fluoroscopic imaging guidance, use 49465)

76098 Radiological examination, surgical specimen

76100 Radiologic examination, single plane body section (eg, tomography), other than with urography

76101 Radiologic examination, complex motion (ie, hypercycloidal) body section (eg, mastoid polytomography), other than with urography; unilateral

76102 bilateral

(Do not report 76101, 76102 more than once per day)

(For panoramic X-ray, use 70355)

(For nephrotomography, use 74415)

76120 Cineradiography/videoradiography, except where specifically included

+ **76125** Cineradiography/videoradiography to complement routine examination (List separately in addition to code for primary procedure)

● New Code ▲ Revised Code + Add-On Code ⊘ Modifier -51 Exempt ☉ Moderate Sedation

76140   Consultation on x-ray examination made elsewhere, written report

(76150   deleted 2010 [2011 edition])

(76350   deleted 2010 [2011 edition])

(2D reformatting is no longer separately reported. To report 3D rendering, see 76376, 76377)

▲ **76376**   3D rendering with interpretation and reporting of computed tomography, magnetic resonance imaging, ultrasound, or other tomographic modality with image post processing under concurrent supervision; not requiring image postprocessing on an independent workstation

(Use 76376 in conjunction with code(s) for base imaging procedure(s))

(Do not report 76376 in conjunction with 31627, 70496, 70498, 70544-70549, 71275, 71555, 72159, 72191, 72198, 73206, 73225, 73706, 73725, 74174, 74175, 74185, 74261-74263, 75557, 75559, 75561, 75563, 75565, 75571-75574, 75635, 76377, 78012-78999, 0159T)

▲ **76377**   requiring image postprocessing on an independent workstation

(Use 76377 in conjunction with code(s) for base imaging procedure(s))

(Do not report 76377 in conjunction with 70496, 70498, 70544-70549, 71275, 71555, 72159, 72191, 72198, 73206, 73225, 73706, 73725, 74174, 74175, 74185, 74261-74263, 75557, 75559, 75561, 75563, 75565, 75571-75574, 75635, 76376, 78012-78999, 0159T)

(To report computer-aided detection, including computer algorithm analysis of MRI data for lesion detection/characterization, pharmacokinetic analysis, breast MRI, use Category III code 0159T)

(76376, 76377 require concurrent supervision of image post processing 3D manipulation of volumetric data set and image rendering)

76380   Computed tomography, limited or localized follow-up study

76390   Magnetic resonance spectroscopy

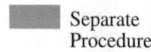 Separate Procedure 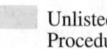 Unlisted Procedure 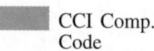 CCI Comp. Code 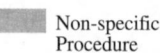 Non-specific Procedure

913

(For magnetic resonance imaging, use appropriate MRI body site code)

76496 Unlisted fluoroscopic procedure (eg., diagnostic, interventional)

76497 Unlisted computed tomography procedure (eg., diagnostic, interventional)

76498 Unlisted magnetic resonance procedure (eg., diagnostic, interventional)

76499 Unlisted diagnostic radiographic procedure

DIAGNOSTIC ULTRASOUND

Diagnostic ultrasound is a non-invasive medical imaging technology that uses high frequency sound waves to form an image of body tissues. Ultrasound, when compared to other imaging modalities like MRI (Magnetic Resonance Imaging) and CT (Computed Tomography), is a relatively low cost non-invasive procedure that does not utilize either magnetic fields or ionizing radiation (x-rays).

All diagnostic ultrasound examinations require permanently recorded images with measurements, when such measurements are clinically indicated. For those codes whose sole diagnostic goal is a biometric measure (ie., 76514, 76516, 76519), permanently recorded images are not required. A final, written report should be issued for inclusion in the patient's medical record. The prescription form for the intraocular lens satisfies the written report requirement for 76519. For those anatomic regions that have "complete" and "limited" ultrasound codes, note the elements that comprise a "complete"exam. The report should contain a description of these elements or the reason that an element could not be visualized (eg., obscured by bowel gas, surgically absent).

If less than the required elements for a "complete" exam are reported (eg., limited number of organs or limited portion of region evaluated), the "limited" code for that anatomic region should be used once per patient exam session. A "limited" exam of an anatomic region should not be reported for the same exam session as a "complete" exam of the same region.

Evaluation of vascular structures using both color and spectral Doppler is separately reportable. To report, see Noninvasive Vascular Diagnostic Studies (93875-93990). However, color Doppler alone, when performed for anatomic structure identification in conjunction with a real-time ultrasound examination, is not reported separately.

Ultrasound guidance procedures also require permanently recorded images of the site to be localized, as well as a documented description of the localization process,

● New Code   ▲ Revised Code   + Add-On Code   ⊘ Modifier -51 Exempt   ⊙ Moderate Sedation

either separately or within the report of the procedure for which the guidance is utilized.

Use of ultrasound, without thorough evaluation of organ(s) or anatomic region, image documentation, and final written report, is not separately reportable.

Ultrasound Modes

A-mode   *Now obsolete in medical imaging. Wave spikes are represented when a single beam passes through objects of different consistency and hardness. The distance between these spikes (for example A and B) can be measured accurately by dividing the speed of sound in tissue (1540 m/sec) by half the sound travel time.*

B-mode   *Same as A-mode, but one-dimensional graphical display, with brightness corresponding to amplitude of reflected sound.*

M-mode   *A single beam in an ultrasound scan can be used to produce an M-mode picture, where movement of a structure such as a heart valve can be depicted in a wave-like manner. Because of its high sampling frequency (up to 1000 pulses per second), this is useful in assessing rates and motion and is still used extensively in cardiac and fetal cardiac imaging.*

Real time   *Most modern ultrasound devices are 2D-real time imaging systems. Multiple crystals (linear, curved or phased-array) or moving crystal. Sequential B-mode pulses sweeping across a plane to display the image in either a linear or 'sector' format. Displayed as real time imaging with up to 100 images per second.*

(To report diagnostic vascular ultrasound studies, see 93880-93990)

(For focused ultrasound ablation treatment of uterine leiomyomata, see Category III codes 0071T, 0072T)

HEAD AND NECK

76506 Echoencephalography, real time with image documentation (gray scale) (for determination of ventricular size, delineation of cerebral contents and detection of fluid masses or other intracranial abnormalities), including A-mode encephalography as secondary component where indicated

76510 Ophthalmic ultrasound, diagnostic; B-scan and quantitative A-scan performed during the same patient encounter

---

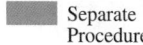 Separate Procedure   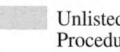 Unlisted Procedure   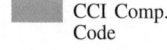 CCI Comp. Code   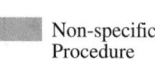 Non-specific Procedure   **915**

| 76511 | quantitative A-scan only |

76512 B-scan (with or without superimposed non-quantitative A-scan)

76513 anterior segment ultrasound, immersion (water bath) B-scan or high resolution biomicroscopy

(For scanning computerized ophthalmic diagnostic imaging of the anterior and posterior segments using technology other than ultrasound, see 92132, 92133, 92134)

76514 corneal pachymetry, unilateral or bilateral (determination of corneal thickness)

76516 Ophthalmic biometry by ultrasound echography, A-scan;

76519 with intraocular lens power calculation

(For partial coherence interferometry, use 92136)

76529 Ophthalmic ultrasonic foreign body localization

76536 Ultrasound, soft tissues of head and neck (eg, thyroid, parathyroid, parotid), real time with image documentation

CHEST

76604 Ultrasound, chest, (includes mediastinum) real time with image documentation

76645 Ultrasound, breast(s) (unilateral or bilateral), real time with image documentation

(Do not report 76645 in conjunction with 0301T)

ABDOMEN AND PERITONEUM

A complete ultrasound examination of the abdomen (76700) consists of real-time scans of the liver, gall bladder, common bile duct, pancreas, spleen, kidneys, and the upper abdominal aorta and inferior vena cava including any demonstrated abdominal abnormality.

A complete ultrasound examination of the retroperitoneum (76770) consists of real-time scans of the kidneys, abdominal aorta, common iliac artery origins, and inferior vena cava, including any demonstrated retroperitoneal abnormality. Alternatively, if clinical history suggests urinary tract pathology, complete

● New Code   ▲ Revised Code   + Add-On Code   ⊘ Modifier -51 Exempt   ⊙ Moderate Sedation

evaluation of the kidneys and urinary bladder also comprises a complete retroperitoneal ultrasound.

Use of ultrasound, without thorough evaluation of organ(s) or anatomic region, image documentation and final, written report, is not separately reportable.

76700 Ultrasound, abdominal, real time with image documentation; complete

76705 limited (eg, single organ, quadrant, follow-up)

76770 Ultrasound, retroperitoneal (eg, renal, aorta, nodes), real time with image documentation; complete

76775 limited

76776 Ultrasound, transplanted kidney, real time and duplex Doppler with image documentation

(For ultrasound or transplanted kidney without duplex Doppler, use 76775)

(For ultrasound and duplex Doppler of a transplanted kidney, do not report 76776 in conjunction with 93975, 93976)

SPINAL CANAL

76800 Ultrasound, spinal canal and contents

PELVIS

OBSTETRICAL

Codes 76801 and 76802 include determination of the number of gestational sacs and fetuses, gestational sac/fetal measurements appropriate for gestation (younger than 14 weeks 0 days), survey of visible fetal and placental anatomic structure, qualitative assessment of amniotic fluid volume/gestational sac shape and examination of the maternal uterus and adnexa.

Codes 76805 and 76810 include determination of number of fetuses and amniotic/chorionic sacs, measurements appropriate for gestational age (older than or equal to 14 weeks 0 days), survey of intracranial/spinal/abdominal anatomy, 4 chambered heart, umbilical cord insertion site, placenta location and amniotic fluid assessment, and when visible, examination of maternal adnexa.

Codes 76811 and 76812 include all elements of codes 76805 and 76810 plus detailed anatomic evaluation of the fetal brain/ventricles, face, heart/outflow tracts and chest anatomy, abdominal organ specific anatomy, number/length/architecture

917

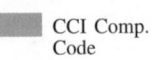

| Separate Procedure | Unlisted Procedure | CCI Comp. Code | Non-specific Procedure |

of limbs and detailed evaluation of the umbilical cord and placenta and other fetal anatomy as clinically indicated.

Report should document the results of the evaluation of each element described above or the reason for non-visualization.

Code 76815 represents a focused "quick look" exam limited to the assessment of one or more of the elements listed in code 76815.

Code 76816 describes an examination designed to reassess fetal size and interval growth or reevaluate one or more anatomic abnormalities of a fetus previously demonstrated on ultrasound, and should be coded once for each fetus requiring reevaluation using modifier 59 for each fetus after the first.

Code 76817 describes a transvaginal obstetric ultrasound performed separately or in addition to one of the transabdominal examinations described above. For transvaginal examinations performed for non-obstetrical purposes, use code 76830

76801 Ultrasound, pregnant uterus, real time with image documentation, fetal and maternal evaluation, first trimester (>14 weeks 0 days), transabdominal approach; single or first gestation

(To report first trimester fetal nuchal translucency measurement, use 76813)

+ 76802 each additional gestation (List separately in addition to code for primary procedure)

(Use 76802 in conjunction with code 76801)

(To report first trimester fetal nuchal translucency measurement, use 76814)

76805 Ultrasound, pregnant uterus, real time with image documentation, fetal and maternal evaluation, after first trimester (>or = 14 weeks 0 days), transabdominal approach; single or first gestation

+ 76810 each additional gestation (List separately in addition to code for primary procedure)

(Use 76810 in conjunction with code 76805)

76811 Ultrasound, pregnant uterus, real time with image documentation, fetal and maternal evaluation plus detailed fetal anatomic examination, transabdominal approach; single or first gestation

● New Code ▲ Revised Code + Add-On Code ⊘ Modifier -51 Exempt ⊙ Moderate Sedation

+ 76812 each additional gestation (List separately in addition to code for primary procedure)

(Use 76812 in conjunction with code 76811)

76813 Ultrasound, pregnant uterus, real time with image documentation, first trimester fetal nuchal translucency measurement, transabdominal or transvaginal approach; single or first gestation

+ 76814 each additional gestation (List separately in addition to code for primary procedure)

(Use 76814 in conjunction with 76813)

76815 Ultrasound, pregnant uterus, real time with image documentation, limited (eg., fetal heart beat, placental location, fetal position, and/or qualitative amniotic fluid volume), 1 or more fetuses

(Use 76815 only once per exam and not per element)

(To report first trimester fetal nuchal translucency measurement, see 76813, 76814)

76816 Ultrasound, pregnant uterus, real time with image documentation, follow-up (eg., re-evaluation of fetal size by measuring standard growth parameters and amniotic fluid volume, re-evaluation of organ system(s) suspected or confirmed to be abnormal on a previous scan), transabdominal approach, per fetus

(Report 76816 with modifier -59 for each additional fetus examined in a multiple pregnancy)

76817 Ultrasound, pregnant uterus, real time with image documentation, transvaginal

(For non-obstetrical transvaginal ultrasound, use 76830)

(If transvaginal examination is done in addition to transabdominal obstetrical ultrasound exam, use 76817 in addition to appropriate transabdominal exam code)

76818 Fetal biophysical profile; with non-stress testing

76819 without non-stress testing

919

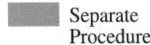 Separate Procedure   Unlisted Procedure   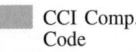 CCI Comp. Code   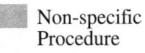 Non-specific Procedure

(Fetal biophysical profile assessments for the second and any additional fetuses, should be reported separately by code 76818 or 76819 with the modifier -59 appended)

(For amniotic fluid index without non-stress test, use 76815)

76820   Doppler velocimetry, fetal; umbilical artery

76821   middle cerebral artery

76825   Echocardiography, fetal, cardiovascular system, real time with image documentation (2D), with or without M-mode recording;

76826   follow-up or repeat study

76827   Doppler echocardiography, fetal, pulsed wave and/or continuous wave with spectral display; complete

76828   follow-up or repeat study

(To report the use of color mapping, use 93325)

NON-OBSTETRICAL

Code 76856 includes the complete evaluation of the female pelvic anatomy. Elements of this examination include a description and measurements of the uterus and adnexal structures, measurement of the endometrium, measurement of the bladder (when applicable) and a description of any pelvic pathology (eg., ovarian cysts, uterine leiomyomata, free pelvic fluid).

Code 76856 is also applicable to a complete evaluation of the male pelvis. Elements of the examination include evaluation and measurement (when applicable) of the urinary bladder, evaluation of the prostate and seminal vesicles to the extent that they are visualized transabdominally, and any pelvic pathology (eg., bladder tumor, enlarged prostate, free pelvic fluid, pelvic abscess).

Code 76857 represents a focused examination limited to the assessment of one or more elements listed in code 76856 and/or the reevaluation of one or more pelvic abnormalities previously demonstrated on ultrasound. Code 76857, rather than 76770, should be utilized if the urinary bladder alone (ie., not including the kidneys) is imaged, whereas code 51798 should be utilized if a bladder volume or post-void residual measurement is obtained without imaging the bladder.

Use of ultrasound, without thorough evaluation of organ(s) or anatomic region, image documentation, and final, written report, is not separately reportable.

76830   Ultrasound, transvaginal

(For obstetrical transvaginal ultrasound, use 76817)

(If transvaginal examination is done in addition to transabdominal non-obstetrical ultrasound exam, use 76830 in addition to appropriate transabdominal exam code)

76831 Saline infusion sonohysterography (SIS), including color flow Doppler, when performed

(For introduction of saline for saline infusion sonohysterography, use 58340)

76856 Ultrasound, pelvic (nonobstetric), real time with image documentation; complete

76857 limited or follow-up (eg, for follicles)

GENITALIA

76870 Ultrasound, scrotum and contents

76872 Ultrasound, transrectal;

(Do not report 76872 in conjunction with 0249T)

76873 prostate volume study for brachytherapy treatment planning (separate procedure)

EXTREMITIES

A complete ultrasound examination of an extremity (76881) consists of real time scans of a specific joint that includes examination of the muscles, tendons, joint, other soft tissue structures, and any identifiable abnormality.

Code 76882 refers to an examination of an extremity that would be performed primarily for evaluation of muscles, tendons, joints, and/or soft tissues. This is a limited examination of the extremity where a specific anatomic structure such as tendon or muscle is assessed. In addition, the code would be used to evaluate a soft-tissue mass that may be present in an extremity where knowledge of its cystic or solid characteristics is needed.

For spectral and color Doppler evaluation of the extremities, use 93925, 93926, 93930, 93931, 93970, or 93971 as appropriate.

(76880 deleted 2010 [2011 edition]. To report ultrasound examination of an extremity, see 76881, 76882)

921

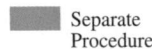 Separate Procedure   Unlisted Procedure 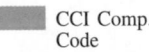 CCI Comp. Code 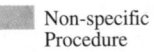 Non-specific Procedure

76881 Ultrasound, extremity, nonvascular, real-time with image documentation; complete

▲ **76882** limited, anatomic specific

▲ **76885** Ultrasound, infant hips, real time with imaging documentation; dynamic (requiring physician or other qualified health care professional manipulation)

▲ **76886** limited, static (not requiring physician or other qualified health care professional manipulation)

ULTRASONIC GUIDANCE PROCEDURES

76930 Ultrasonic guidance for pericardiocentesis, imaging supervision and interpretation

76932 Ultrasonic guidance for endomyocardial biopsy, imaging supervision and interpretation

76936 Ultrasound guided compression repair of arterial pseudoaneurysm or arteriovenous fistulae (includes diagnostic ultrasound evaluation, compression of lesion and imaging)

+ **76937** Ultrasound guidance for vascular access requiring ultrasound evaluation of potential access sites, documentation of selected vessel patency, concurrent realtime ultrasound visualization of vascular needle entry, with permanent recording and reporting (List separately in addition to code for primary procedure)

(Do not report 76937 in conjunction with 37191, 37192, 37193, 37760, 37761, 76942)

(If extremity venous non-invasive vascular diagnostic study is performed separate from venous access guidance, use 93965, 93970, or 93971)

76940 Ultrasound guidance for, and monitoring of, parenchymal tissue ablation

(Do not report 76940 in conjunction with 50250, 50542, 76942, 76998)

(For ablation, see 32998, 47370-47382, 50592, 50593)

76941 Ultrasonic guidance for intrauterine fetal transfusion or cordocentesis, imaging supervision and interpretation

(For procedure, see 36460, 59012)

● New Code	▲ Revised Code	+ Add-On Code	⊘ Modifier -51 Exempt	⊙ Moderate Sedation

76942 Ultrasonic guidance for needle placement (eg, biopsy, aspiration, injection, localization device) imaging supervision and interpretation

(Do not report 76942 in conjunction with 27096, 32554, 32555, 32556, 32557, 37760, 37761, 43232, 43237, 43242, 45341, 45342, 64479-64484, 64490-64495, 76975, 0213T-0218T, 0228T-0231T, 0232T, 0249T, 0301T)

(For injections of platelet rich plasma, use 0232T)

76945 Ultrasonic guidance for chorionic villus sampling, imaging supervision and interpretation

(For procedure, use 59015)

76946 Ultrasonic guidance for amniocentesis, imaging supervision and interpretation

76948 Ultrasonic guidance for aspiration of ova, imaging supervision and interpretation

76950 Ultrasonic guidance for placement of radiation therapy fields

(For placement of interstitial device[s] for radiation therapy guidance, see 31627, 32553, 49411, 55876)

76965 Ultrasonic guidance for interstitial radioelement application

OTHER PROCEDURES

76970 Ultrasound study follow-up (specify)

76975 Gastrointestinal endoscopic ultrasound, imaging supervision and interpretation

(Do not report 76975 in conjunction with 43231, 43232, 43237, 43238, 43242, 43259, 45341, 45342, or 76942)

76977 Ultrasound bone density measurement and interpretation, peripheral site(s), any method

76998 Ultrasonic guidance, intraoperative

(Do not report 76998 in conjunction with 36475-36479, 37760, 37761, 47370-47382, 0249T, 0301T)

(For ultrasound guidance for open and laparoscopic radiofrequency tissue ablation, use 76940)

923

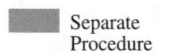 Separate Procedure   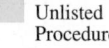 Unlisted Procedure   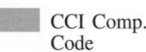 CCI Comp. Code   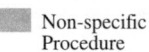 Non-specific Procedure

76999   Unlisted ultrasound procedure (eg., diagnostic, interventional)

RADIOLOGIC GUIDANCE

FLUOROSCOPIC GUIDANCE

(Do not report guidance codes 77001, 77002, 77003 for services in which fluoroscopic guidance is included in the descriptor)

+ 77001 Fluoroscopic guidance for central venous access device placement, replacement (catheter only or complete), or removal (includes fluoroscopic guidance for vascular access and catheter manipulation, any necessary contrast injections through access site or catheter with related venography radiologic supervision and interpretation, and radiographic documentation of final catheter position) (List separately in addition to code for primary procedure)

(Do not use 77001 in conjunction with 77002)

(If formal extremity venography is performed from separate venous access and separately interpreted, use 36005 and 75820, 75822, 75825 or 75827)

77002 Fluoroscopic guidance for needle placement (eg, biopsy, aspiration, injection, localization device)

(See appropriate surgical code for procedure and anatomic location)

(77002 includes all radiographic arthrography with the exception of supervision and interpretation for CT and MR arthrography)

(Do not report 77002 in conjunction with32554, 32555, 32556, 32557, 70332, 73040, 73085, 73115, 73525, 73580, 73615, 0232T)

(For injection of platelet rich plasma, use 0232T)

(77002 is included in the organ/anatomic specific radiological supervision and interpretation procedures 49440, 74320, 74355, 74445, 74470, 74475, 75809, 75810, 75885, 75887, 75980, 75982, 75989)

77003 Fluoroscopic guidance and localization of needle or catheter tip for spine or paraspinous diagnostic or therapeutic injection procedures (epidural or subarachnoid)

● New Code	▲ Revised Code	+ Add-On Code	⊘ Modifier -51 Exempt	⊙ Moderate Sedation

(Injection of contrast during fluoroscopic guidance and localization [77003] is included in 22526, 22527, 27096, 62263, 62264, 62267, 62270-62282, 62310-62319)

(Fluoroscopic guidance for subarachnoid puncture for diagnostic radiographic myelography is included in supervision and interpretation codes 72240-72270)

(For epidural or subarachnoid needle or catheter placement andinjection, see 62270-62282. 62310-62319)

(For sacroiliac joint arthrography, see 27096)

(For paravertebral facet joint injection, see 64490-64495. For paravertebral facet joint nerve destruction by neurolysis, see 64633-64636. For transforaminal epidural needle placement and injection, see 64479-64484)

(Do not report 77002, 77003 in conjunction with 22586, 27096, 64479-64484, 64490-64495, 64633-64636, 0195T, 0196T 0309T)

(For percutaneous or endoscopic lysis of epidural adhesions, 62263, 62264 include fluoroscopic guidance and localization)

COMPUTED TOMOGRAPHY GUIDANCE

77011 Computed tomography guidance for stereotactic localization

77012 Computed tomography guidance for needle placement (eg, biopsy, aspiration, injection, localization device), radiological supervision and interpretation

(Do not report 77011, 77012 in conjunction with 22586, 0195T, 0196T, 0309T)

Do not report 77012 in conjunction with 27096, 32554, 32555, 32556, 32557, 64479-64484, 64490-64495, 64633-64636, 0232T)

(For injection(s) of platelet rich plasma, use 0232T)

77013 Computerized tomography guidance for, and monitoring of, parenchymal tissue ablation

(Do not report 77013 in conjunction with 20982)

(For percutaneous radiofrequency ablation, see 32998, 47382, 50592, 50593)

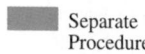 Separate Procedure

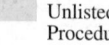 Unlisted Procedure

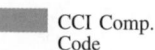 CCI Comp. Code

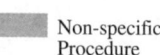 Non-specific Procedure

77014 Computed tomography guidance for placement of radiation therapy fields

(For placement of interstitial device(s) for radiation therapy guidance, see 31627, 32553, 49411, 55876)

MAGNETIC RESONANCE GUIDANCE

77021 Magnetic resonance guidance for needle placement (eg, for biopsy, needle aspiration, injection, or placement of localization device) radiological supervision and interpretation

(For procedure, see appropriate organ or site)

(Do not report 77021 in conjunction with 32554, 32555, 32556, 32557, 0232T)

(For injection of platelet rich plasma, use 0232T)

77022 Magnetic resonance guidance for, and monitoring of, parenchymal tissue ablation

(For percutaneous radiofrequency ablation, see 32998, 47382, 50592, 50593)

(For focused ultrasound ablation treatment of uterine leiomyomata, see Category III codes 0071T, 0072T)

OTHER RADIOLOGIC GUIDANCE

77031 Stereotactic localization guidance for breast biopsy or needle placement (eg, for wire localization or for injection), each lesion, radiological supervision and interpretation

(For procedure, see 10022, 19000-19103, 19290, 19291)

(For injection for sentinel node localization without lymphoscintigraphy, use 38792)

77032 Mammographic guidance for needle placement, breast (eg, for wire localization or for injection), each lesion, radiological supervision and interpretation

(For procedure, see 10022, 19000, 19102, 19103, 19290, 19291)

(For injection for sentinel node localization without lymphoscintigraphy, use 38792)

926 ● New Code   ▲ Revised Code   + Add-On Code   ⊘ Modifier -51 Exempt   ⊙ Moderate Sedation

BREAST, MAMMOGRAPHY

(For mammographic guidance for needle placement of breast lesion, use 77032)

▲+**77051** Computer-aided detection (computer algorithm analysis of digital image data for lesion detection) with further review for interpretation, with or without digitization of film radiographic images; diagnostic mammography (List separately in addition to code for primary procedure)

(Use 77051 in conjunction with 77055, 77056)

▲+**77052** screening mammography (List separately in addition to code for primary procedure)

(Use 77052 in conjunction with 77057)

77053 Mammary ductogram or galactogram, single duct, radiological supervision and interpretation

(For mammary ductogram or galactogram injection, use 19030)

77054 Mammary ductogram or galactogram, multiple ducts, radiological supervision and interpretation

77055 Mammography; unilateral

77056 bilateral

(Use 77055, 77056 in conjunction with 77051 for computer-aided detection applied to a diagnostic mammogram)

77057 Screening mammography, bilateral (2-view film study of each breast)

(Use 77057 in conjunction with 77052 for computer-aided detection applied to a screening mammogram)

(For electrical impedance breast scan, use 76499)

77058 Magnetic resonance imaging, breast, without and/or with contrast material(s); unilateral

77059 bilateral

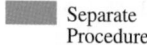 Separate Procedure
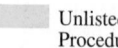 Unlisted Procedure
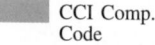 CCI Comp. Code
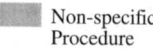 Non-specific Procedure

BONE/JOINT STUDIES

▲ **77071** Manual application of stress performed by physician or other qualified health care professional for joint radiography, including contralateral joint if indicated

(For radiographic interpretation of stressed images, see appropriate anatomic site and number of views)

77072 Bone age studies

77073 Bone length studies (orthoroentgenogram, scanogram)

77074 Radiologic examination, osseous survey; limited (eg, for metastases)

77075 complete (axial and appendicular skeleton)

77076 Radiologic examination, osseous survey, infant

77077 Joint survey, single view, 2 or more joints (specify)

77078 Computed tomography, bone mineral density study, 1 or more sites; axial skeleton (eg, hips, pelvis, spine)

(77079 deleted 2011 [2012 edition])

77080 Dual-energy X-ray absorptiometry (DXA), bone density study, 1 or more sites; axial skeleton (eg, hips, pelvis, spine)

77081 appendicular skeleton (peripheral) (eg, radius, wrist, heel)

77082 vertebral fracture assessment

(For dual-energy X-ray absorptiometry [DEXA] body composition study, use 76499)

(77083 deleted 2011 [2012 edition])

77084 Magnetic resonance (eg, proton) imaging, bone marrow blood supply

● New Code   ▲ Revised Code   + Add-On Code   ⊘ Modifier -51 Exempt   ⊙ Moderate Sedation

RADIATION ONCOLOGY

Radiation therapy is the use of high level radiation to destroy cancer cells. Both tumor cells and healthy cells may be affected by this radiation. The radiation injures the cancer cells so they can no longer continue to divide or multiply. With each treatment, more of the cells die and the tumor shrinks. The dead cells are broken down, carried away by the blood and excreted by the body. Most of the healthy cells are able to recover from this injury. However, the damage to the healthy cells is the reason for the side effects of radiation therapy.

The dose of radiation is determined by the size, extent, type and grade of tumor along with its response to radiation therapy. Complex calculations are done to determine the dose and timing of radiation in treatment planning. Often, the treatment is given over several different angles in order to deliver the maximum amount of radiation to the tumor and the minimum amount to normal tissues.

Services defined in this section of the CPT book coding system teletherapy and brachytherapy. To report Radiation Oncology services, the following must be performed and documented:

- *The initial consultation*

- *Clinical treatment planning with/without simulation*

- *Medical radiation physics, dosimetry, treatment devices and special services*

- *Clinical treatment management procedures*

- *Normal follow-up care during treatment and for three months following completion of treatment*

Continuing medical physics consultation (CPT code 77336) is reported per week of therapy. It may be reported after every five radiation treatments. (It may also be reported if the total number of radiation treatments in a course of radiation therapy is less than five.) Since radiation planning procedures (CPT codes 77261-77334) are generally performed before radiation treatment commences, the NCCI contains edits preventing payment of CPT code 77336 with CPT codes 77261- 77295, 77301-77328, and 77332-77334. Because radiation planning procedures may occasionally be repeated during a course of radiation treatment, the edits allow modifier - 59 to be appended to CPT code 77336 when the radiation planning procedure and continuing medical physics consultation occur on the same date of service.

CONSULTATION OR CLINICAL MANAGEMENT

All consultations, pre-treatment patient evaluations, and/or medical care services are coded using evaluation and management service codes

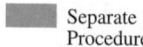 Separate Procedure 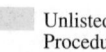 Unlisted Procedure 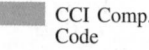 CCI Comp. Code 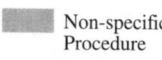 Non-specific Procedure

CLINICAL TREATMENT PLANNING

Clinical treatment planning includes test interpretation, localization of tumor(s), treatment determination, and choice of treatment modality and treatment devices. Clinical treatment planning may be simple, intermediate or complex.

77261 Therapeutic radiology treatment planning; simple

77262 intermediate

77263 complex

77280 Therapeutic radiology simulation-aided field setting; simple

77285 intermediate

77290 complex

77295 three-dimensional

77299 Unlisted procedure, therapeutic radiology clinical treatment planning

MEDICAL RADIATION PHYSICS, DOSIMETRY, TREATMENT DEVICES, AND SPECIAL SERVICES

77300 Basic radiation dosimetry calculation, central axis depth dose calculation, TDF, NSD, gap calculation, off axis factor, tissue inhomogeneity factors, calculation of non-ionizing radiation surface and depth dose, as required during course of treatment, only when prescribed by the treating physician

77301 Intensity modulated radiotherapy plan, including dose-volume histograms for target and critical structure partial tolerance specifications

(Dose plan is optimized using inverse or forward planning technique for modulated beam delivery (eg, binary, dynamic MLC) to create highly conformal dose distribution. Computer plan distribution must be verified for positional accuracy based on dosimetric verification of the intensity map with verification of treatment set up and interpretation of verification methodology)

77305 Teletherapy, isodose plan (whether hand or computer calculated); simple (1 or 2 parallel opposed unmodified ports directed to a single area of interest)

---

930 ● New Code ▲ Revised Code ✛ Add-On Code ⊘ Modifier -51 Exempt ⊙ Moderate Sedation

77310   intermediate (3 or more treatment ports directed to a single area of interest)

77315   complex (mantle or inverted Y, tangential ports, the use of wedges, compensators, complex blocking, rotational beam, or special beam considerations)

(Only one teletherapy isodose plan may be reported for a given course of therapy to a specific treatment area)

77321   Special teletherapy port plan, particles, hemibody, total body

77326   Brachytherapy isodose plan; simple (calculation made from single plane, 1 to 4 sources/ribbon application, remote afterloading brachytherapy, 1 to 8 sources)

(For definition of source/ribbon, see Clinical Brachytherapy)

77327   intermediate (multiplane dosage calculations, application involving 5 to 10 sources/ribbons, remote afterloading brachytherapy, 9 to 12 sources)

77328   complex (multiplane isodose plan, volume implant calculations, over 10 sources/ribbons used, special spatial reconstruction, remote afterloading brachytherapy, over 12 sources)

77331   Special dosimetry (eg, TLD, microdosimetry) (specify), only when prescribed by the treating physician

77332   Treatment devices, design and construction; simple (simple block, simple bolus)

77333   intermediate (multiple blocks, stents, bite blocks, special bolus)

77334   complex (irregular blocks, special shields, compensators, wedges, molds or casts)

77336   Continuing medical physics consultation, including assessment of treatment parameters, quality assurance of dose delivery, and review of patient treatment documentation in support of the radiation oncologist, reported per week of therapy

77338   Multi leaf collimator (MLC) device(s) for intensity modulated radiation therapy (IMRT), design and construction per IMRT plan

931

| Separate Procedure | Unlisted Procedure | CCI Comp. Code | Non-specific Procedure |

(Do not report 77338 more than once per IMRT plan)

(For immobilization in IMRT treatment, see 77332-77334)

(Do not report 77338 in conjunction with 0073T, compensator based IMRT)

77370 Special medical radiation physics consultation

STEREOTACTIC RADIATION TREATMENT DELIVERY

⊙ **77371** Radiation treatment delivery, stereotactic radiosurgery (SRS), complete course of treatment of cranial lesion(s) consisting of 1 session; multi-source Cobalt 60 based

77372 linear accelerator based

(For radiation treatment management, use 77432)

77373 Stereotactic body radiation therapy, treatment delivery, per fraction to 1 or more lesions, including image guidance, entire course not to exceed 5 fractions

(Do not report 77373 in conjunction with 77401-77416, 77418)

(For single fraction cranial lesions(s), see 77371, 77372)

OTHER PROCEDURES

77399 Unlisted procedure, medical radiation physics, dosimetry and treatment devices, and special services

RADIATION TREATMENT DELIVERY

(Radiation treatment delivery (77401-77416) recognizes the technical component and the various energy levels.)

(For intra-fraction localization and tracking of target, use 0197T)

77401 Radiation treatment delivery, superficial and/or ortho voltage

77402 Radiation treatment delivery, single treatment area, single port or parallel opposed ports, simple blocks or no blocks; up to 5 MeV

77403 6-10 MeV

77404 11-19 MeV

● New Code	▲ Revised Code	+ Add-On Code	⊘ Modifier -51 Exempt	⊙ Moderate Sedation

77406   20 MeV or greater

77407   Radiation treatment delivery, 2 separate treatment areas, 3 or more ports on a single treatment area, use of multiple blocks; up to 5 MeV

77408   6-10 MeV

77409   11-19 MeV

77411   20 MeV or greater

77412   Radiation treatment delivery, 3 or more separate treatment areas, custom blocking, tangential ports, wedges, rotational beam, compensators, electron beam; up to 5 MeV

77413   6-10 MeV

77414   11-19 MeV

77416   20 MeV or greater

77417   Therapeutic radiology port film(s)

77418   Intensity modulated treatment delivery, single or multiple fields/arcs, via narrow spatially and temporally modulated beams, binary, dynamic MLC, per treatment session

    (For intensity modulated treatment planning, use 77301)

    (For compensator-based beam modulation treatment delivery, use Category III code 0073T)

77421   Stereoscopic x-ray guidance for localization of target volume for the delivery of radiation therapy

    (Do not report 77421 in conjunction with 77432, 77435)

    (Do not report 77421 more than once per treatment delivery session)

    (For placement of interstitial device(s) for radiation therapy guidance, see 31627, 32553, 49411, 55876)

77424   Intraoperative radiation treatment delivery, x-ray, single treatment session

933

Separate Procedure	Unlisted Procedure	CCI Comp. Code	Non-specific Procedure

77425 Intraoperative radiation treatment delivery, electrons, single treatment session

NEUTRON BEAM TREATMENT DELIVERY

77422 High energy neutron radiation treatment delivery; single treatment area using a single port or parallel-opposed ports with no blocks or simple blocking

77423 1 or more isocenter(s) with coplanar or non-coplanar geometry with blocking and/or wedge, and/or compensator(s)

77424 Code out of order. See page 933

77425 Code out of order. See page 934

RADIATION TREATMENT MANAGEMENT

CPT codes in this section presume treatment on a daily basis (4 or 5 fractions per week) with the use of megavoltage photon or high energy particle sources. Daily and weekly clinical treatment management are mutually exclusive for the same dates. CPT defines three distinct levels of clinical treatment management: simple, intermediate and complex. Review this section of CPT for detailed definitions of these levels of service.

Radiation treatment management is reported in units of five fractions or treatment sessions, regardless of the actual time period in which the services are furnished. The services need not be furnished on consecutive days. Multiple fractions representing two or more treatment sessions furnished on the same day may be counted separately as long as there has been a distinct break in therapy sessions, and the fractions are of the character usually furnished on different days. Code 77427 is also reported if there are three or four fractions beyond a multiple of five at the end of a course of treatment; one or two fractions beyond a multiple of five at the end of a course of treatment are not reported separately.

Radiation treatment management requires **and includes** a minimum of one examination of the patient by the physician for medical evaluation and management (eg., assessment of the patient's response to treatment, coordination of care and treatment, review of imaging and/or lab test results with doumentation) for each reporting of the radiation treatment management service. Code 77469 represents only the intraoperative session management and does not include medical evaluation and management outside of that session.

The professional services furnished during treatment management typically include: review of port films; review of dosimetry, dose delivery and treatment parameters; and review of patient treatment set-up.

● New Code ▲ Revised Code + Add-On Code ⊘ Modifier -51 Exempt ⊙ Moderate Sedation

77427 Radiation treatment management, 5 treatments

77431 Radiation therapy management with complete course of therapy consisting of 1 or 2 fractions only

(77431 is not to be used to fill in the last week of a long course of therapy)

77432 Stereotactic radiation treatment management of cranial lesion(s) (complete course of treatment consisting of 1 session)

(The same physician should not report both stereotactic radiosurgery services [61796-61800] and radiation treatment management [77432 or 77435] for cranial lesions)

(For stereotactic body radiation therapy treatment, use 77435)

77435 Stereotactic body radiation therapy, treatment management, per treatment course, to 1 or more lesions, including image guidance, entire course not to exceed 5 fractions

(Do not report 77435 in conjunction with 77427-77432)

(The same physician should not report both stereotactic radiosurgery services [32701, 63620, 63621] and radiation treatment management [77435])

77469 Intraoperative radiation treatment management

77470 Special treatment procedure (eg, total body irradiation, hemibody irradiation, per oral or endocavitary irradiation)

(77470 assumes that the procedure is performed one or more times during the course of therapy, in addition to daily or weekly patient management)

(For intraoperative radiation treatment delivery and management, see 77424, 77425, 77469

77499 Unlisted procedure, therapeutic radiology treatment management

PROTON BEAM TREATMENT DELIVERY

77520 Proton treatment delivery; simple, without compensation

77522 simple, with compensation

77523 intermediate

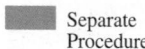 Separate Procedure   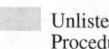 Unlisted Procedure   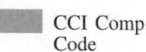 CCI Comp. Code   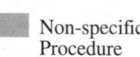 Non-specific Procedure   **935**

| 77525 | complex |

HYPERTHERMIA

Hyperthermia treatments as listed in this section include external (superficial and deep), interstitial, and intracavitary. Radiation therapy when given concurrently is listed separately.

Hyperthermia is used only as an adjunct to radiation therapy or chemotherapy. It may be induced by a variety of sources (eg., microwave, ultrasound, low energy radiofrequency conduction, or by probe).

The listed treatments include management during the course of therapy and follow-up care for three months after completion.

Preliminary consultation is not included (see Evaluation and Management 99241-99255). Physics planning and interstitial insertion of temperature sensors, and use of external or interstitial heat generating sources are included.

The following descriptors are included in the treatment schedule:

⊙ **77600** Hyperthermia, externally generated; superficial (ie, heating to a depth of 4 cm or less)

⊙ **77605** deep (ie, heating to depths greater than 4 cm)

(For focused microwave thermotherapy of the breast, use 0301T)

⊙ **77610** Hyperthermia generated by interstitial probe(s); 5 or fewer interstitial applicators

⊙ **77615** more than 5 interstitial applicators

CLINICAL INTRACAVITARY HYPERTHERMIA

77620 Hyperthermia generated by intracavitary probe(s)

CLINICAL BRACHYTHERAPY

Services 77750-77799 include admission to the hospital and daily visits.

For insertion of ovoids and tandems, use 57155.

For insertion of Heyman capsules, use 58346.

(For high dose rate electronic brachytherapy, per fraction, use Category III code 0182T)

● New Code   ▲ Revised Code   ＋ Add-On Code   ⊘ Modifier -51 Exempt   ⊙ Moderate Sedation

77750   Infusion or instillation of radioelement solution (includes 3 months follow-up care)

(For administration of radiolabeled monoclonal antibodies, use 79403)

(For non-antibody radiopharmaceutical therapy by intravenous administration only, not including three month follow-up care, use 79101)

77761   Intracavitary radiation source application; simple

77762   intermediate

77763   complex

(Do not report 77761-77763 in conjunction with Category III code 0182T)

77776   Interstitial radiation source application; simple

77777   intermediate

77778   complex

(Do not report 77776-77778 in conjunction with Category III code 0182T)

(77781   deleted 2009 edition; see 77785, 77786)

(77782   deleted 2009 edition; see 77785-77787)

(77783   deleted 2009 edition; see 77785-77787)

(77784   deleted 2009 edition; see 77785-77787)

77785   Remote afterloading high dose rate radionuclide brachytherapy; 1 channel

77786   2-12 channels

77787   over 12 channels

(Do not report 77785-77787 in conjunction with Category III code 0182T)

77789   Surface application of radiation source

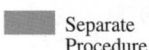 Separate Procedure   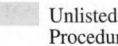 Unlisted Procedure   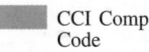 CCI Comp. Code   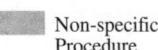 Non-specific Procedure

937

(Do not report 77789 in conjunction with Category III code 0182T)

77790   Supervision, handling, loading of radiation source

77799   Unlisted procedure, clinical brachytherapy

NUCLEAR MEDICINE

Introduction

Nuclear medicine is used in the diagnosis, management, treatment, and prevention of serious disease. Nuclear medicine imaging procedures often identify abnormalities very early in the progression of a disease. This early detection allows a disease to be treated early in its course when there may be a more successful prognosis.

Nuclear medicine uses very small amounts of radioactive materials or radiopharmaceuticals to diagnose and treat disease. Radiopharmaceuticals are substances that are attracted to specific organs, bones, or tissues. The radiopharmaceuticals used in nuclear medicine emit gamma rays that can be detected externally by special types of cameras: gamma or PET cameras. These cameras work in conjunction with computers used to form images that provide data and information about the area of body being imaged. The amount of radiation from a nuclear medicine procedure is comparable to that received during a diagnostic x-ray.

Nuclear medicine procedures may be performed independently or in the course of overall medical care. If the physician providing nuclear medicine services is also responsible for the diagnostic work-up and/or follow-up care of the patient, evaluation and management service codes should be coded in addition to the nuclear medicine procedures.

Radioimmunoassay tests are located in the Clinical Pathology section (codes 82000-84999). These CPT codes can be appropriately used by any specialist performing such tests in a laboratory licensed and/or certified for radioimmunoassays. The reporting of these tests is not confined to clinical pathology laboratories alone.

The injection of a radiopharmaceutical is included as an inherent component of the procedure. Separate vascular access and injection codes (e.g. 36000, 90783 (90773 in 2006), G0345-G0354 (90760-90772, 90774-90775 in 2006) should not be reported. However, the services do not include the actual radiopharmaceutical or drug used. Diagnostic and therapeutic radiopharmaceuticals and drugs supplied by the physician should be reported separately using the appropriate supply code(s), in addition to the procedure code.

● New Code	▲ Revised Code	+ Add-On Code	⊘ Modifier -51 Exempt	⊙ Moderate Sedation

Single photon emission computed tomography (SPECT) studies represent an enhanced methodology over standard planar nuclear imaging. When a limited anatomic area is studied, there is no additional information procured by obtaining both planar and SPECT studies. While both represent medically acceptable imaging studies, when a SPECT study of a limited area is performed, a planar study is not to be separately reported. When vascular flow studies are obtained using planar technology in addition to SPECT studies, the appropriate CPT code for the vascular flow study should be reported, not the flow, planar and SPECT studies. In cases where planar images must be procured because of the extent of the scanned area (e.g. bone imaging), both planar and SPECT scans may be necessary and reported separately.

Myocardial perfusion imaging (CPT codes 78451-78454) are not reportable with cardiac blood pool imaging by gated equilibrium (CPT codes 78472-78473) because the two types of tests utilize different radiopharmaceuticals.

CPT codes 76376, 76377 (3-D rendering) are not separately reportable for nuclear medicine procedures (CPT codes 78000-78999). However, they may be separately reported with modifier - 59 on the same date of service as a nuclear medicine procedure if the 3D rendering procedure is performed in association with a third procedure (other than nuclear medicine) for which 3D rendering is appropriately reported.

Nuclear Medicine Notes

Listed procedures may be performed independently or in the course of overall medical care. If the individual providing these services is also responsible for diagnostic work-up and/or follow-up care of patient, see appropriate sections also.

Radioimmunoassay tests are found in the Clinical Pathology section (codes 82000-84999). These codes can be appropriately used by any specialist performing such tests in a laboratory licensed and/or certified for radioimmunoassays. The reporting of these tests is not confined to clinical pathology laboratories alone.

The services listed do not include the radiopharmaceutical or drug. To separately report supply of diagnostic and therapeutic radiopharmaceuticals and drugs, use the appropriate supply code(s), in addition to the procedure code..

DIAGNOSTIC NUCLEAR MEDICINE

ENDOCRINE SYSTEM

(78000   deleted 2012 [2013 edition]. To report, see 78012-78014)

(78001   deleted 2012 [2013 edition]. To report, see 78012-78014)

(78003   deleted 2012 [2013 edition]. To report, see 78012-78014)

▮ Separate Procedure	▮ Unlisted Procedure	▮ CCI Comp. Code	▮ Non-specific Procedure

(78006   deleted 2012 [2013 edition]. To report, see 78012-78014)

(78007   deleted 2012 [2013 edition]. To report, see 78012-78014)

(78010   deleted 2012 [2013 edition]. To report, see 78012-78014)

(78011   deleted 2012 [2013 edition]. To report, see 78012-78014)

● **78012**   Thyroid uptake, single or multiple quantitative measurement(s) (including stimulation, suppression, or discharge, when performed)

● **78013**   Thyroid imaging (including vascular flow, when performed);

● **78014**   with single or multiple uptake(s) quantitative measurement(s) (including stimulation, suppression, or discharge, when performed)

78015   Thyroid carcinoma metastases imaging; limited area (eg, neck and chest only)

78016   with additional studies (eg, urinary recovery)

78018   whole body

+ **78020**   Thyroid carcinoma metastases uptake (List separately in addition to code for primary procedure)

(Use 78020 in conjunction with code 78018 only)

▲ **78070**   Parathyroid planar imaging (including subtraction, when performed);

● **78071**   with tomographic (SPECT)

● **78072**   with tomographic (SPECT), and concurrently acquired computed tomography (CT) for anatomical localization

78075   Adrenal imaging, cortex and/or medulla

78099   Unlisted endocrine procedure, diagnostic nuclear medicine

(For chemical analysis, see Chemistry section)

HEMATOPOIETIC, RETICULOENDOTHELIAL AND LYMPHATIC SYSTEM

78102 Bone marrow imaging; limited area

78103 multiple areas

78104 whole body

78110 Plasma volume, radiopharmaceutical volume-dilution technique (separate procedure); single sampling

78111 multiple samplings

78120 Red cell volume determination (separate procedure); single sampling

⊙ **78121** multiple samplings

78122 Whole blood volume determination, including separate measurement of plasma volume and red cell volume (radiopharmaceutical volume-dilution technique)

78130 Red cell survival study;

78135 differential organ/tissue kinetics, (eg, splenic and/or hepatic sequestration)

78140 Labeled red cell sequestration, differential organ/tissue, (eg, splenic and/or hepatic)

78185 Spleen imaging only, with or without vascular flow

(If combined with liver study, use procedures 78215 and 78216)

78190 Kinetics, study of platelet survival, with or without differential organ/tissue localization

78191 Platelet survival study

78195 Lymphatics and lymph nodes imaging

(For sentinel node identification without scintigraphy imaging, use 38792)

(For sentinal node excision, see 38500-38542)

| 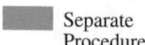 Separate Procedure | 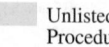 Unlisted Procedure | 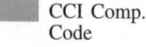 CCI Comp. Code | 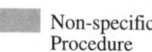 Non-specific Procedure | **941** |

78199 Unlisted hematopoietic, reticuloendothelial and lymphatic procedure, diagnostic nuclear medicine

(For chemical analysis, see Chemistry section)

GASTROINTESTINAL SYSTEM

78201 Liver imaging; static only

78202 with vascular flow

(For spleen imaging only, use 78185)

78205 Liver imaging (SPECT);

78206 with vascular flow

78215 Liver and spleen imaging; static only

78216 with vascular flow

(78220 deleted 2011 [2012 edition])

(78223 deleted 2011 [2012 edition]. To report hepatobiliary system imaging, see 78226, 78227)

78226 Hepatobiliary system imaging, including gallbladder when present;

78227 with pharmacologic intervention, including quantitative measurement(s) when performed.=

78230 Salivary gland imaging;

78231 with serial images

78232 Salivary gland function study

78258 Esophageal motility

78261 Gastric mucosa imaging

78262 Gastroesophageal reflux study

78264 Gastric emptying study

● New Code   ▲ Revised Code   + Add-On Code   ⃠ Modifier -51 Exempt   ⊙ Moderate Sedation

78267 Urea breath test, C-14 (isotopic); acquisition for analysis

78268 analysis

78270 Vitamin B-12 absorption study (eg, Schilling test); without intrinsic factor

78271 with intrinsic factor

78272 Vitamin B-12 absorption studies combined, with and without intrinsic factor

78278 Acute gastrointestinal blood loss imaging

78282 Gastrointestinal protein loss

78290 Intestine imaging (eg, ectopic gastric mucosa, Meckels localization, volvulus)

78291 Peritoneal-venous shunt patency test (eg, for LeVeen, Denver shunt)

(For injection procedure, use 49427)

78299 Unlisted gastrointestinal procedure, diagnostic nuclear medicine

MUSCULOSKELETAL SYSTEM

78300 Bone and/or joint imaging; limited area

78305 multiple areas

78306 whole body

78315 3 phase study

78320 tomographic (SPECT)

78350 Bone density (bone mineral content) study, 1 or more sites; single photon absorptiometry

78351 dual photon absorptiometry, 1 or more sites

(For radiographic bone density (photodensitometry), use 77083)

78399 Unlisted musculoskeletal procedure, diagnostic nuclear medicine

---

	Separate Procedure		Unlisted Procedure		CCI Comp. Code		Non-specific Procedure

943

CARDIOVASCULAR SYSTEM

Myocardial perfusion and cardiac blood pool imaging studies may be performed at rest and/or during stress. When performed during exercise and/or pharmacologic stress, the appropriate stress testing code from the 93015-93018 series should be reported in addition to 78451-78454, 78472-78492.

78414   Determination of central c-v hemodynamics (non-imaging) (eg, ejection fraction with probe technique) with or without pharmacologic intervention or exercise, single or multiple determinations

78428   Cardiac shunt detection

78445   Non-cardiac vascular flow imaging (ie, angiography, venography)

78451   Myocardial perfusion imaging, tomographic (SPECT) (including attenuation correction, qualitative or quantitative wall motion, ejection fraction by first pass or gated technique, additional quantification, when performed); single study, at rest or stress (exercise or pharmacologic)

78452   multiple studies, at rest and/or stress (exercise or pharmacologic) and/or redistribution and/or rest reinjection

78453   Myocardial perfusion imaging, planar (including qualitative or quantitative wall motion, ejection fraction by first pass or gated technique, additional quantification, when performed); single study, at rest or stress (exercise or pharmacologic)

78454   multiple studies, at rest and/or stress (exercise or pharmacologic) and/or redistribution and/or rest reinjection

78456   Acute venous thrombosis imaging, peptide

78457   Venous thrombosis imaging, venogram; unilateral

78458   bilateral

78459   Myocardial imaging, positron emission tomography (PET), metabolic evaluation

(For myocardial perfusion study, see 78491-78492)

(78460   Deleted 2009 [2010 edition]. To report see 78451-78454)

● New Code   ▲ Revised Code   + Add-On Code   ⊘ Modifier -51 Exempt   ⊙ Moderate Sedation

(78461   Deleted 2009 [2010 edition]. To report see 78451-7845)

(78464   Deleted 2009 [2010 edition]. To report see 78451-7845)

(78465   Deleted 2009 [2010 edition]. To report see 78451-7845)

78466   Myocardial imaging, infarct avid, planar; qualitative or quantitative

78468   with ejection fraction by first pass technique

78469   tomographic SPECT with or without quantification

78472   Cardiac blood pool imaging, gated equilibrium; planar, single study at rest or stress (exercise and/or pharmacologic), wall motion study plus ejection fraction, with or without additional quantitative processing

(For assessment of right ventricular ejection fraction by first pass technique, use 78496)

78473   multiple studies, wall motion study plus ejection fraction, at rest and stress (exercise and/or pharmacologic), with or without additional quantification

(Do not report 78472, 78473 in conjunction with 78451-78454, 78481, 78483, 78494)

(78478   Deleted 2009 [2010 edition]; to report see 78451-78454)

(78480   Deleted 2009 [2010 edition]; to report see 78451-78454)

78481   Cardiac blood pool imaging, (planar), first pass technique; single study, at rest or with stress (exercise and/or pharmacologic), wall motion study plus ejection fraction, with or without quantification

78483   multiple studies, at rest and with stress (exercise and/or pharmacologic), wall motion study plus ejection fraction, with or without quantification

(For cerebral blood flow study, use 78610)

(Do not report 78481-78483 in conjunction with 78451-78454)

78491   Myocardial imaging, positron emission tomography (PET), perfusion; single study at rest or stress

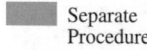 Separate Procedure   Unlisted Procedure   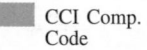 CCI Comp. Code   Non-specific Procedure   **945**

78492   multiple studies at rest and/or stress

78494   Cardiac blood pool imaging, gated equilibrium, SPECT, at rest, wall motion study plus ejection fraction, with or without quantitative processing

+ 78496   Cardiac blood pool imaging, gated equilibrium, single study, at rest, with right ventricular ejection fraction by first pass technique (List separately in addition to code for primary procedure)

(Use 78496 in conjunction with code 78472)

78499   Unlisted cardiovascular procedure, diagnostic nuclear medicine

RESPIRATORY SYSTEM

78579   Pulmonary ventilation imaging (eg, aerosol or gas)

78580   Pulmonary perfusion imaging (eg, particulate)

78582   Pulmonary ventilation (eg, aerosol or gas) and perfusion imaging

(78584   deleted 2011 [2012 edition]. To report, see 78579, 78582-78598)

(78585   deleted 2011 [2012 edition]. To report, see 78579, 78582-78598)

(78586   deleted 2011 [2012 edition]. To report, see 78579, 78582-78598)

(78587   deleted 2011 [2012 edition]. To report, see 78579, 78582-78598)

(78588   deleted 2011 [2012 edition]. To report, see 78579, 78582-78598)

(78591   deleted 2011 [2012 edition]. To report, see 78579, 78582-78598)

(78593   deleted 2011 [2012 edition]. To report, see 78579, 78582-78598)

(78594   deleted 2011 [2012 edition]. To report, see 78579, 78582-78598)

● New Code   ▲ Revised Code   + Add-On Code   ⊘ Modifier -51 Exempt   ⊙ Moderate Sedation

(78596   deleted 2011 [2012 edition]. To report, see 78579, 78582-78598)

78597   Quantitative differential pulmonary perfusion, including imaging when performed

78598   Quantitative differential pulmonary perfusion and ventilation (eg, aerosol or gas), including imaging when performed

(Report 78579, 78580, 78582-78598 only once per imaging session)

(Do not report 78580, 78582-78598 in conjunction with 78451-78454)

78599   Unlisted respiratory procedure, diagnostic nuclear medicine

NERVOUS SYSTEM

78600   Brain imaging, less than 4 static views;

78601   with vascular flow

78605   Brain imaging, minimum 4 static views;

78606   with vascular flow

78607   Brain imaging, tomographic (SPECT)

78608   Brain imaging, positron emission tomography (PET); metabolic evaluation

78609   perfusion evaluation

78610   Brain imaging, vascular flow only

78630   Cerebrospinal fluid flow, imaging (not including introduction of material); cisternography

(For injection procedure, see 61000-61070, 62270-62319)

78635   ventriculography

(For injection procedure, see 61000-61070, 62270-62294)

78645   shunt evaluation

(For injection procedure, see 61000-61070, 62270-62294)

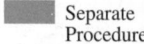 Separate Procedure   Unlisted Procedure   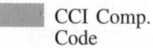 CCI Comp. Code   Non-specific Procedure   947

| 78647 | tomographic (SPECT) |

| 78650 | Cerebrospinal fluid leakage detection and localization |

(For injection procedure, see 61000-61070, 62270-62294)

| 78660 | Radiopharmaceutical dacryocystography |

| 78699 | Unlisted nervous system procedure, diagnostic nuclear medicine |

GENITOURINARY SYSTEM

| 78700 | Kidney imaging morphology; |

| 78701 | with vascular flow |

| 78707 | with vascular flow and function, single study without pharmacological intervention |

| 78708 | with vascular flow and function, single study, with pharmacological intervention (eg, angiotensin converting enzyme inhibitor and/or diuretic) |

| 78709 | with vascular flow and function, multiple studies, with and without pharmacological intervention (eg, angiotensin converting enzyme inhibitor and/or diuretic) |

(For introduction of radioactive substance in association with renal endoscopy, see 77776-77778)

| 78710 | tomographic (SPECT) |

| 78725 | Kidney function study, non-imaging radioisotopic study |

+ 78730 Urinary bladder residual study (List separately in addition to code for primary procedure)

(Use 78730 in conjunction with 78740)

(For measurement of postvoid residual urine and/or bladder capacity by ultrasound, nonimaging, use 51798)

(For ultrasound imaging of the bladder only, with measurement of postvoid residual urine when performed, use 76857)

| 78740 | Ureteral reflux study (radiopharmaceutical voiding cystogram) |

(Use 78740 in conjunction with 78730 for urinary bladder residual study)

| ● New Code | ▲ Revised Code | + Add-On Code | ⊘ Modifier -51 Exempt | ⊙ Moderate Sedation |

(For catheterization, see 51701-51703)

78761 Testicular imaging with vascular flow

78799 Unlisted genitourinary procedure, diagnostic nuclear medicine

(For chemical analysis, see Chemistry section)

OTHER PROCEDURES

(For specific organ, see appropriate heading)

(For radiophosphorus tumor identification, ocular, see 78800)

78800 Radiopharmaceutical localization of tumor or distribution of radiopharmaceutical agent(s); limited area

(For specific organ, see appropriate heading)

78801 multiple areas

78802 whole body, single day imaging

78803 tomographic (SPECT)

78804 whole body, requiring 2 or more days imaging

78805 Radiopharmaceutical localization of inflammatory process; limited area

78806 whole body

78807 tomographic (SPECT)

(For imaging bone infectious or inflammatory disease with a bone imaging radiopharmaceutical, see 78300, 78305, 78306)

78808 Injection procedure for radiopharmaceutical localization by non-imaging probe study, intravenous (eg, parathyroid adenoma)

(For sentinel lymph node identification, use 38792)

(For PET of brain, see 78608, 78609)

(For PET myocardial imaging, see 78459, 78491, 78492)

78811 Positron emission tomography (PET) imaging; limited area (eg, chest, head/neck)

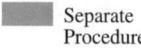 Separate Procedure 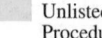 Unlisted Procedure CCI Comp. Code 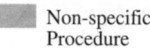 Non-specific Procedure **949**

78812   skull base to mid-thigh

78813   whole body

78814   Positron emission tomography (PET) with concurrently acquired computed tomography (CT) for attenuation correction and anatomical localization imaging; limited area (eg, chest, head/neck)

78815   skull base to mid-thigh

78816   whole body

          (Report 78811-78816 only once per imaging session)

          (Computed tomography (CT) performed for other than attenuation correction and anatomical localization is reported using the appropriate site specific CT code with modifier 59)

(78890   deleted 2009 edition)

(78891   deleted 2009 edition)

78999   Unlisted miscellaneous procedure, diagnostic nuclear medicine

THERAPEUTIC

The oral and intravenous administration codes in this section are inclusive of the mode of administration. For intra-arterial, intra-cavitary, and intra-articular administration, also use the appropriate injection and/or procedure code, as well as imaging guidance and radiological supervision and interpretation codes, when appropriate.

79005   Radiopharmaceutical therapy, by oral administration

          (For monoclonal antibody therapy, use 79403)

79101   Radiopharmaceutical therapy, by intravenous administration

          (Do not report 79101 in conjunction with 36400, 36410, 79403, 96360, 96374 or 96375, 96409)

          (For radiolabeled monoclonal antibody by intravenous infusion, use 79403)

          (For infusion or instillation of non-antibody radioelement solution that includes three months follow-up care, use 77750)

● New Code   ▲ Revised Code   + Add-On Code   ⊘ Modifier -51 Exempt   ⊙ Moderate Sedation

79200 Radiopharmaceutical therapy, by intracavitary administration

79300 Radiopharmaceutical therapy, by interstitial radioactive colloid administration

79403 Radiopharmaceutical therapy, radiolabeled monoclonal antibody by intravenous infusion

(For pre-treatment imaging, see 78802, 78804)

(Do not report 79403 in conjunction with 79101)

79440 Radiopharmaceutical therapy, by intra-articular administration

79445 Radiopharmaceutical therapy, by intra-arterial particulate administration

(Do not report 79445 in conjunction with 96373, 96420)

(Use appropriate procedural and radiological supervision and interpretation codes for the angiographic and interventional procedures provided pre-requisite to intra-arterial radiopharmaceutical therapy)

79999 Radiopharmaceutical therapy, unlisted procedure

Separate Procedure Unlisted Procedure CCI Comp. Code Non-specific Procedure

This page intentionally left blank.

● New Code ▲ Revised Code ✚ Add-On Code ⊘ Modifier -51 Exempt ⊙ Moderate Sedation

PATHOLOGY/ LABORATORY

LABORATORY SECTION OVERVIEW

The fifth section of the CPT coding system is the laboratory section, which includes codes for pathology and laboratory services. Within each subsection, the CPT codes are arranged by the type of testing or service.

LABORATORY SUBSECTIONS

The PATHOLOGY AND LABORATORY section of CPT is divided into the following subsections:

Organ or Disease Oriented Panels	80047-80076
Drug Testing	80100-80104
Therapeutic Drug Assays	80150-80299
Evocative/Suppression Testing	80400-80440
Consultations (Clinical Pathology)	80500-80502
Urinalysis	81000-81099
Molecular Pathology	81200-81479
Multianalyte Assays with Algorithmic Assays	81500-81599
Chemistry	82000-84999
Hematology and Coagulation	85002-85999
Immunology	86000-86849
Transfusion Medicine	86850-86999
Microbiology	87001-87999
Anatomic Pathology	88000-88099
Cytopathology	88104-88199
Cytogenetic Studies	88230-88299
Surgical Pathology	88300-88399
In Vivo (eg. Transcutaneous) Laboratory Procedures	88720-88749
Other Procedures	89049-89240
Reproductive Medicine Procedures	89250-89398

LABORATORY SERVICE MODIFIERS

Pathology and laboratory services and procedures may be modified under certain circumstances. When applicable, the modifying circumstances should be identified by adding the appropriate modifier to the basic service code. The addition of modifier -22 requires a special report. Modifiers commonly used to report PATHOLOGY and LABORATORY procedures include:

-22   unusual services

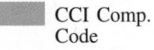

■	Separate Procedure	■	Unlisted Procedure	■	CCI Comp. Code	■	Non-specific Procedure

953

-26 professional component

-32 mandated services

-52 reduced services

-90 reference (outside) laboratory

PATHOLOGY

Pathology is that discipline of the practice of medicine that deals with the causes and nature of disease. It contributes to diagnosis, prognosis, and treatment through knowledge gained by the laboratory application of the biologic, chemical, and physical sciences to man, or materials obtained from man. Pathologists diagnose, exclude, and monitor disease by means of information gathered from the microscopic examination of tissue specimens, cells, and body fluids, and from clinical laboratory tests on body fluids and secretions. Pathologists are involved with the management of laboratories and in data processing and with new developments in high technology.

CLINICAL PATHOLOGY

Clinical Pathology focuses on microbiology (including bacteriology, mycology, parasitology, and virology), immunopathology, blood banking/transfusion medicine, chemical pathology, cytogenetics, hematology, coagulation, toxicology, medical microscopy (including urinalysis), molecular biologic techniques, and other advanced diagnostic techniques as they become available.

● New Code   ▲ Revised Code   ✛ Add-On Code   ⊘ Modifier -51 Exempt   ⊙ Moderate Sedation

Drug Qualitative	Multiple Drug Class Method	Single Drug Class Method	Confirmation	Quantitative
Table of Drugs & the Appropriate Qualitative Screening, Confirmatory, & Quantitative Codes				
Alcohols	80100 (a)	80101 (b)	80102 (c)	82055 or 82075 (d)
Amphetamines	80100 (a)	80101 (b)	80102 (c)	82145
Barbiturates	80100 (a)	80101 (b)	80102 (c)	80184 or 82205 (e)
Benzodiazepines	80100 (a)	80101 (b)	80102 (c)	80154
Cocaine and metabolites	80100 (a)	80101 (b)	80102 (c)	82520
Methadone	80100 (a)	80101 (b)	80102 (c)	83840
Methaqualone	80100 (a)	80101 (b)	80102 (c)	80299 or 82491 (f)
Opiates	80100 (a)	80101 (b)	80102 (c)	83925
Phencyclidine	80100 (a)	80101 (b)	80102 (c)	83992
Phenothiazines	80100 (a)	80101 (b)	80102 (c)	84022
Propoxyphene	80100 (a)	80101 (b)	80102 (c)	80299 or 82491 (f)
Tetrahydrocan-nabinoids	80100 (a)	80101 (b)	80102 (c)	80299 or 82491 (f)
Tricyclic antidepressants	80100 (a)	80101 (b)	80102 (c)	80152, 80160, 80166, 80174, 80182 (g), 80299 or 82491 (f)

(a) Use code 80100 for each combination of mobile phase with stationary phase
(b) Use code 80101 for each single drug class tested and reported
(c) Use code 80102 for each combination of mobile phase with stationary phase used for drug confirmation.
(d) Code 82055 for "Alcohol (ethanol); any specimen except breath," and code 82075 for "Alcohol (ethanol); breath."
(e) Code 80184 for "Phenobarbital," 80188 for "Primidone," and 82205 for "Barbiturates, not elsewhere specified."
(f) If there is no appropriate quantitative code for the drug listed, use code 82491 for chromatographic determination or 80299 for other methods.
(g) Code 80152 "Amitriptyline," 80160 for "Desipramine," 80166 for "Doxepin," 80174 for "Imipramine," or 80182 for "Nortriptyline." 80299 or 82491 (f)

955

Separate Procedure   Unlisted Procedure   CCI Comp. Code   Non-specific Procedure

PATHOLOGY AND LABORATORY CODES

ORGAN OR DISEASE ORIENTED PANELS

CPT codes for organ or disease oriented panels were included in CPT due to the increased use of general screening programs by physicians, clinics, hospitals, and other health care facilities. Other codes in this section define profiles that combine laboratory tests together under a problem oriented classification. There is a list of specific laboratory tests under each of the panel CPT codes which define the components of each panel. However, each laboratory typically establishes its own profile and provides a listing of the components of that panel performed by the laboratory with test results.

The CPT coding system assigns CPT codes to organ or disease oriented panels consisting of a group of specified tests. If all tests of a CPT defined panel are performed, the provider may bill the panel code or the individual component test codes. The panel codes may be used when the tests are ordered as that panel or if the individual component tests of a panel are ordered separately. For example, if the individually ordered tests are cholesterol (CPT code 82465), triglycerides (CPT code 84478), and HDL cholesterol (CPT code 83718), the service could be billed as a lipid panel (CPT code 80061).

These panels were developed for coding purposes only and should not be interpreted as clinical parameters. The tests listed with each panel identify the defined components of that panel.

These panel components are not intended to limit the performance of other tests. If one performs tests in addition to those specifically indicated for a particular panel, those tests should be reported separately in addition to the panel code.

Do not report two or more panel codes that include any of the same constituent tests performed from the same patient collection. If a group of tests overlaps two or more panels, report the panel that incorporates the greater number of tests to fulfill the code definition and report the remaining tests using individual test codes (eg., do not report 80047 in conjunction with 80054).

| **80047** | Basic metabolic panel (Calcium, ionized) |

This panel must include the following:
Calcium, ionized (82330)
Carbon dioxide (82374)
Chloride (82435)
Creatinine (82565)
Glucose (82947)
Potassium (84132)

| | ● New Code | ▲ Revised Code | + Add-On Code | ⊘ Modifier -51 Exempt | ⊙ Moderate Sedation |

Sodium (84295)
Urea Nitrogen (BUN) (84520)

80048 Basic metabolic panel (Calcium, total)

This panel must include the following:
Calcium, total (82310)
Carbon dioxide (82374)
Chloride (82435)
Creatinine (82565)
Glucose (82947)
Potassium (84132)
Sodium (84295)
Urea Nitrogen (BUN) (84520)

80050 General health panel

This panel must include the following:
Comprehensive metabolic panel (80053)
Blood count, complete (CBC), automated and automated
    differential WBC count (85025 or 85027 and 85004)
OR
Blood count, complete (CBC), automated (85027) and
    appropriate manual differential WBC count (85007 or 85009)
Thyroid stimulating hormone (TSH) (84443)

80051 Electrolyte panel

This panel must include the following:
Carbon dioxide (82374)
Chloride (82435)
Potassium (84132)
Sodium (84295)

80053 Comprehensive metabolic panel

This panel must include the following:
Albumin (82040)
Bilirubin, total (82247)
Calcium, total (82310)
Carbon dioxide (bicarbonate) (82374)
Chloride (82435)
Creatinine (82565)
Glucose (82947)
Phosphatase, alkaline (84075)
Potassium (84132)
Protein, total (84155)
Sodium (84295)
Transferase, alanine amino (ALT) (SGPT) (84460)
Transferase, aspartate amino (AST) (SGOT) (84450)

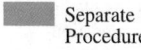 Separate
Procedure

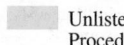 Unlisted
Procedure

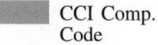 CCI Comp.
Code

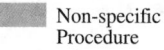 Non-specific
Procedure

957

Urea Nitrogen (BUN) (84520)

80055   Obstetric panel

This panel must include the following:
Blood count, complete (CBC), automated and automated
  differential WBC count (85025 or 85027 and 85004)
OR
Blood count, complete (CBC), automated (85027) and
  appropriate manual differential WBC count (85007 or 85009)
Hepatitis B surface antigen (HBsAg) (87340)
Antibody, rubella (86762)
Syphilis test, non-treponemal antibody; qualitative (eg, VDRL,
  RPR, ART) (86592)
Antibody screen, RBC, each serum technique (86850)
Blood typing, ABO (86900) AND
Blood typing, Rh (D) (86901)

(When syphilis screening is performed using a treponemal
antibody approach [86780], do not use 80055. Use the
individual codes for the tests performed in the obstetric panel)

80061   Lipid panel

This panel must include the following:
Cholesterol, serum, total (82465)
Lipoprotein, direct measurement, high density cholesterol (HDL
  cholesterol) (83718)
Triglycerides (84478)

80069   Renal function panel

This panel must include the following:
Albumin (82040)
Calcium, total (82310)
Carbon dioxide (bicarbonate) (82374)
Chloride (82435)
Creatinine (82565)
Glucose (82947)
Phosphorus inorganic (phosphate) (84100)
Potassium (84132)
Sodium (84295)
Urea nitrogen (BUN) (84520)

80074   Acute hepatitis panel

This panel must include the following:
Hepatitis A antibody (HAAb), IgM antibody (86709)
Hepatitis B core antibody (HbcAb), IgM antibody (86705)
Hepatitis B surface antigen (HbsAg) (87340)

● New Code   ▲ Revised Code   + Add-On Code   ⊘ Modifier -51 Exempt   ⊙ Moderate Sedation

Hepatitis C antibody (86803)

80076 Hepatic function panel

This panel must include the following:
Albumin (82040)
Bilirubin, total (82247)
Bilirubin, direct (82248)
Phosphatase, alkaline (84075)
Protein, total (84155)
Transferase, alanine amino (ALT) (SGPT) (84460)
Transferase, aspartate amino (AST) (SGOT) (84450)

DRUG TESTING

Use 80100 for each multiple drug class chromatographic procedure. Use 80102 for each procedure necessary for confirmation. For chromatography, each combination of stationary and mobile phase is to be counted as one procedure. For example, if detection of three drugs by chromatography requires one stationary phase with three mobile phases, use 80100 three times. However, if multiple drugs can be detected using a single analysis (eg., one stationary phase with one mobile phase), use 80100 only once.

For quantitation of drugs screened, use appropriate code in Chemistry section (82000-84999) or Therapeutic Drug Assay section (80150-80299).

80100 Drug screen, qualitative; multiple drug classes, chromatographic method, each procedure

80101 single drug class method (eg, immunoassay, enzyme assay), each drug class

(For qualitative analysis by multiplexed screening kit for multiple drugs or drug classes, use 80104)

80104 multiple drug classes other than chromatographic method, each procedure

80102 Drug, confirmation, each procedure

80103 Tissue preparation for drug analysis

80104 This code is out of order. See page 959

| | Separate Procedure | | Unlisted Procedure | | CCI Comp. Code | | Non-specific Procedure |

THERAPEUTIC DRUG ASSAYS

The material for examination may be from any source. Examination is quantitative. For nonquantitative testing, see Drug Testing (80100-80103).

80150 Amikacin

80152 Amitriptyline

80154 Benzodiazepines

80156 Carbamazepine; total

80157 free

80158 Cyclosporine

80160 Desipramine

80162 Digoxin

80164 Dipropylacetic acid (valproic acid)

80166 Doxepin

80168 Ethosuximide

80170 Gentamicin

80172 Gold

80173 Haloperidol

80174 Imipramine

80176 Lidocaine

80178 Lithium

80182 Nortriptyline

80184 Phenobarbital

80185 Phenytoin; total

● New Code ▲ Revised Code + Add-On Code ⊘ Modifier -51 Exempt ⊙ Moderate Sedation

80186   free

80188   Primidone

80190   Procainamide;

80192   with metabolites (eg, n-acetyl procainamide)

80194   Quinidine

80195   Sirolimus

80196   Salicylate

80197   Tacrolimus

80198   Theophylline

80200   Tobramycin

80201   Topiramate

80202   Vancomycin

80299   Quantitation of drug, not elsewhere specified

EVOCATIVE/SUPPRESSION TESTING

Evocative/suppression testing involves administration of agents to determine a patient's response to those agents. CPT codes 80400-80440 are to be used for reporting the laboratory components of the testing. When the test requires physician administration of the evocative/suppression agent, see codes 96390, 96361, 96372-96374, 96375. However, when physician attendance is not required, and the agent is administered by ancillary personnel, these codes are not to be separately reported.

In the inpatient setting, these codes are only reported if the physician performs the service personally. In the office setting, the service can be reported when performed by office personnel if the physician is directly supervising the service. While supplies necessary to perform the testing are included in the testing, the appropriate HCPCS J codes for the drugs can be separately reported for the diagnostic agents. Separate evaluation and management services are not to be reported, including prolonged services (in the case of prolonged infusions) unless a significant, separately identifiable service is provided and documented.

Separate Procedure   Unlisted Procedure   CCI Comp. Code   Non-specific Procedure

The following test panels involve the administration of evocative or suppressive agents, and the baseline and subsequent measurement of their effects on chemical constituents. These codes are to be used for the reporting of the laboratory component of the overall testing protocol. For the administration of the evocative or suppressive agents, see Hydration, Therapeutic, Prophylactic, Diagnostic Injections and Infusions, and Chemotherapy and Other Highly Complex drug or Highly Complex Biologic Agent Administration (eg, 96365, 96366, 96367, 96368, 96372, 96374, 96375, 96376). In the code descriptors where reference is made to a particular analyte (eg., Cortisol: 82533 x 2) the "x 2" refers to the number of times the test for that particular analyte is performed.

80400 ACTH stimulation panel; for adrenal insufficiency

This panel must include the following:
Cortisol (82533 x 2)

80402 for 21 hydroxylase deficiency

This panel must include the following:
Cortisol (82533 x 2)
17 hydroxyprogesterone (83498 x 2)

80406 for 3 beta-hydroxydehydrogenase deficiency

This panel must include the following:
Cortisol (82533 x 2)
17 hydroxypregnenolone (84143 x 2)

80408 Aldosterone suppression evaluation panel (eg, saline infusion)

This panel must include the following:
Aldosterone (82088 x 2)
Renin (84244 x 2)

80410 Calcitonin stimulation panel (eg, calcium, pentagastrin)

This panel must include the following:
Calcitonin (82308 x 3)

80412 Corticotropic releasing hormone (CRH) stimulation panel

This panel must include the following:
Cortisol (82533 x 6)
Adrenocorticotropic hormone (ACTH) (82024 x 6)

80414 Chorionic gonadotropin stimulation panel; testosterone response.

This panel must include the following:
Testosterone (84403 x 2 on three pooled blood samples)

● New Code   ▲ Revised Code   + Add-On Code   ⊘ Modifier -51 Exempt   ⊙ Moderate Sedation

80415   estradiol response.

This panel must include the following:
Estradiol (82670 x 2 on three pooled blood samples)

80416 Renal vein renin stimulation panel (eg, captopril)

This panel must include the following:
Renin (84244 x 6)

80417 Peripheral vein renin stimulation panel (eg, captopril)

This panel must include the following:
Renin (84244 x 2)

80418 Combined rapid anterior pituitary evaluation panel

This panel must include the following:
Adrenocorticotropic hormone (ACTH) (82024 x 4)
Luteinizing hormone (LH) (83002 x 4)
Follicle stimulating hormone (FSH) (83001 x 4)
Prolactin (84146 x 4)
Human growth hormone (HGH)(83003 x 4)
Cortisol (82533 x 4)
Thyroid stimulating hormone (TSH) (84443 x 4)

80420 Dexamethasone suppression panel, 48 hour

This panel must include the following:
Free cortisol, urine (82530 x 2)
Cortisol (82533 x 2)
Volume measurement for timed collection (81050 x 2)

(For single dose dexamethasone, use 82533)

80422 Glucagon tolerance panel; for insulinoma

This panel must include the following:
Glucose (82947 x 3)
Insulin (83525 x 3)

80424   for pheochromocytoma.

This panel must include the following:
Catecholamines, fractionated (82384 x 2)

80426 Gonadotropin releasing hormone stimulation panel

This panel must include the following:
Follicle stimulating hormone (FSH) (83001 x 4)
Luteinizing hormone (LH)(83002 x 4)

80428 Growth hormone stimulation panel (eg, arginine infusion, l-dopa administration)

This panel must include the following:
Human growth hormone (HGH)(83003 x 4)

80430 Growth hormone suppression panel (glucose administration)

This panel must include the following:
Glucose (82947 x 3)
Human growth hormone (HGH)(83003 x 4)

80432 Insulin-induced C-peptide suppression panel

This panel must include the following:
Insulin (83525)
C-peptide (84681 x 5)
Glucose (82947 x 5)

80434 Insulin tolerance panel; for ACTH insufficiency

This panel must include the following:
Cortisol (82533 x 5)
Glucose (82947 x 5)

80435 for growth hormone deficiency

This panel must include the following:
Glucose (82947 x 5)
Human growth hormone (HGH) (83003 x 5)

80436 Metyrapone panel

This panel must include the following:
Cortisol (82533 x 2)
11 deoxycortisol (82634 x 2)

80438 Thyrotropin releasing hormone (TRH) stimulation panel; 1 hour

This panel must include the following:
Thyroid stimulating hormone (TSH) (84443 x 3)

---

964 ● New   ▲ Revised   + Add-On   ⊘ Modifier -51   ⊙ Moderate
              Code   Code   Code   Exempt   Sedation

80439   2 hour

This panel must include the following:
Thyroid stimulating hormone (TSH) (84443 x 4)

80440   for hyperprolactinemia

This panel must include the following:
Prolactin (84146 x 3)

CONSULTATIONS (CLINICAL PATHOLOGY)

A clinical pathology consultation is a service, including a written report, rendered by the pathologist in response to a request from a physicia nor qualified health care professional in relation to a test result(s) requiring additional medical interpretive judgment. Reporting of a test result(s) without medical interpretive judgment is not considered a clinical pathology consultation.

80500   Clinical pathology consultation; limited, without review of patients history and medical records

80502   comprehensive, for a complex diagnostic problem, with review of patients history and medical records

(These codes may also be used for pharmacokinetic consultations)

(For consultations involving the examination and evaluation of the patient, see 99241-99275)

URINALYSIS

For specific analyses, see appropriate section.

81000   Urinalysis, by dip stick or tablet reagent for bilirubin, glucose, hemoglobin, ketones, leukocytes, nitrite, pH, protein, specific gravity,urobilinogen, any number of these constituents; non-automated, with microscopy

81001   automated, with microscopy

81002   non-automated, without microscopy

81003   automated, without microscopy

81005   Urinalysis; qualitative or semiquantitative, except immunoassays

965

| ▮ Separate Procedure | ▯ Unlisted Procedure | ▮ CCI Comp. Code | ▮ Non-specific Procedure |

(For non-immunoassay reagent strip urinalysis, see 81000, 81002)

(For immunoassay, qualitative or semiquantitative, use 83518)

(For microalbumin, see 82043, 82044)

81007 bacteriuria screen, except by culture or dipstick

(For culture, see 87086-87088)

(For dipstick, use 81000 or 81002)

81015 microscopic only

(For sperm evaluation for retrograde ejaculation, use 89331)

81020 2 or 3 glass test

81025 Urine pregnancy test, by visual color comparison methods

81050 Volume measurement for timed collection, each

81099 Unlisted urinalysis procedure

MOLECULAR PATHOLOGY

Molecular pathology procedures are medical laboratory procedures involving the analyses of nucleic acid to detect variants in genes that may be indicative of germline (eg, constitutional disorders) or somatic (eg, neoplasia) conditions, or to test for histocompatibility antigens (eg, HLA). Code selection is typically based on the specific gene(s) that is being analyzed. Genes are described using Human Genome Organization (HUGO) approved gene names and are italicized in the code descriptors.

The molecular pathology codes include all analytical services performed in the test (eg, cell lysis, nucleic acid stabilization, extraction, digestion, amplification, and detection). Any procedures required prior to cell lysis (eg, microdissection, codes 88380 and 88381) should be reported separately.

The results of the procedure may require interpretation by a physician or other qualified health care professional. When only the interpretation and report are performed, modifier 26 may be appended to the specific molecular pathology code.

All analyses are qualitative unless otherwise noted.

For microbial identification, see 87149-87153 and 87470-87801, and 87900-87904. For in situ hybridization analyses, see 88271-88275 and 88365-88368.

Molecular pathology procedures that are not specified in 81200-81383 should be reported using either the appropriate Tier 2 code (81400-81408) or the unlisted molecular pathology procedure code, 81479.

TIER 1 MOLECULAR PATHOLOGY PROCEDURES

The following codes represent gene-specific and genomic procedures.

81200   *ASPA (aspartoacylase)* (eg, Canavan disease) gene analysis, common variants (eg, E285A, Y231X)

● **81201**   APC (adenomatous polyposis coli) (eg, familial adenomatosis polyposis [FAP], attenuated FAP) gene analysis; full gene sequence

● **81202**   known familiar variants

● **81203**   duplication/deletion variants

81205   *BCKDHB (branched-chain keto acid dehydrogenase E1, beta polypeptide)* (eg, Maple syrup urine disease) gene analysis, common variants (eg, R183P, G278S, E422X)

81206   *BCR/ABL1 (t(9;22))* (eg, chronic myelogenous leukemia) translocation analysis; major breakpoint, qualitative or quantitative

81207   minor breakpoint, qualitative or quantitative

81208   other breakpoint, qualitative or quantitative

81209   *BLM (Bloom syndrome, RecQ helicase-like)* (eg, Bloom syndrome) gene analysis, 2281del6ins7 variant

81210   *BRAF (v-raf murine sarcoma viral oncogene homolog B1)* (eg, colon cancer), gene analysis, V600E variant

81211   *BRCA1, BRCA2 (breast cancer 1 and 2)* (eg, hereditary breast and ovarian cancer) gene analysis; full sequence analysis and common duplication/deletion variants in BRCA1 (ie, exon 13 del 3.835kb, exon 13 dup 6kb, exon 14-20 del 26kb, exon 22 del 510bp, exon 8-9 del 7.1kb)

81212   185delAG, 5385insC, 6174delT variants

967

Separate Procedure	Unlisted Procedure	CCI Comp. Code	Non-specific Procedure

81213   uncommon duplication/deletion variants

81214   *BRCA1 (breast cancer 1)* (eg, hereditary breast and ovarian cancer) gene analysis; full sequence analysis and common duplication/deletion variants (ie, exon 13 del 3.835kb, exon 13 dup 6kb, exon 14-20 del 26kb, exon 22 del 510bp, exon 8-9 del 7.1kb)

(When performing *BRCA1* full sequence analysis with *BRCA2* full sequence analysis, use 81211)

81215   known familial variant

81216   *BRCA2 (breast cancer 2)* (eg, hereditary breast and ovarian cancer) gene analysis; full sequence analysis

(When performing *BRCA2* full sequence analysis with *BRCA1* full sequence analysis, use 81211)

81217   known familial variant

81220   CFTR (cystic fibrosis transmembrane conductance regulator) (eg, cystic fibrosis) gene analysis; common variants (eg, ACMG/ACOG guidelines)

(When Intron 8 poly-T analysis is performed in conjunction with 81220 in a R117H positive patient, do not report 81224)

81221   known familial variants

81222   duplication/deletion variants

81223   full gene sequence

81224   intron 8 poly-T analysis (eg, male infertility)

81225   *CYP2C19 (cytochrome P450, family 2, subfamily C, polypeptide 19)* (eg, drug metabolism), gene analysis, common variants (eg, *2, *3, *4, *8, *17)

81226   *CYP2D6 (cytochrome P450, family 2, subfamily D, polypeptide 6)* (eg, drug metabolism), gene analysis, common variants (eg, *2, *3, *4, *5, *6, *9, *10, *17, *19, *29, *35, *41, *1XN, *2XN, *4XN)

81227   *CYP2C9 (cytochrome P450, family 2, subfamily C, polypeptide 9)* (eg, drug metabolism), gene analysis, common variants (eg, *2, *3, *5, *6)

81228 Cytogenomic constitutional (genome-wide) microarray analysis; interrogation of genomic regions for copy number variants (eg, Bacterial Artificial Chromosome [BAC] or oligo-based comparative genomic hybridization [CGH] microarray analysis)

81229 interrogation of genomic regions for copy number and single nucleotide polymorphism (SNP) variants for chromosomal abnormalities

(Do not report 81228 in conjunction with 81229)

● **81235** *EGFR (epidermal growth factor receptor)* (eg, non-small cell lunch cancer) gene analysis, common variants (eg, exon 19 LREA deletion, L858R, T790M, G719A, G719S, L861Q)

81240 *F2 (prothrombin, coagulation factor II)* (eg, hereditary hypercoagulability) gene analysis, 20210G>A variant

81241 *F5 (coagulation Factor V)* (eg, hereditary hypercoagulability) gene analysis, Leiden variant

81242 *FANCC (Fanconi anemia, complementation group C)* (eg, Fanconi anemia, type C) gene analysis, common variant (eg, IVS4+4A>T)

81243 *FMR1 (Fragile X mental retardation 1)* (eg, fragile X mental retardation) gene analysis; evaluation to detect abnormal (eg, expanded) alleles

(For evaluation to detect and characterize abnormal alleles, see 81243, 81244)

(For evaluation to detect and characterize abnormal alleles using a single assay [eg, PCR], use 81243)

81244 characterization of alleles (eg, expanded size and methylation status)

81245 *FLT3 (fms-related tyrosine kinase 3)* (eg, acute myeloid leukemia), gene analysis, internal tandem duplication (ITD) variants (ie, exons 14, 15)

81250 *G6PC (glucose-6-phosphatase, catalytic subunit)* (eg, Glycogen storage disease, Type 1a, von Gierke disease) gene analysis, common variants (eg, R83C, Q347X)

81251 *GBA (glucosidase, beta, acid)* (eg, Gaucher disease) gene analysis, common variants (eg, N370S, 84GG, L444P, IVS2+1G>A)

969

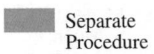 Separate Procedure   Unlisted Procedure   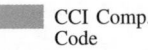 CCI Comp. Code   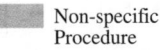 Non-specific Procedure

● **81252** *GJB2 (gap junction protein, beta 2, 26kDa; connexin 26)* (eg, nonsyndromic hearing loss) gene analysis; full gene sequence

● **81253** known familial variants

● **81254** *GJB6 (gap junction protein, beta 6, 30kDa, connexin 30)* (eg, nonsyndromic hearing loss) gene analysis, common variants (eg, 309kb [del(GJB6-D13S1830)] and 232kb [del(GJB6-D13S1854)])

81255 *HEXA (hexosaminidase A [alpha polypeptide])* (eg, Tay-Sachs disease) gene analysis, common variants (eg, 1278insTATC, 1421+1G>C, G269S)

81256 *HFE (hemochromatosis)* (eg, hereditary hemochromatosis) gene analysis, common variants (eg, C282Y, H63D)

81257 *HBA1/HBA2 (alpha globin 1 and alpha globin 2)* (eg, alpha thalassemia, Hb Bart hydrops fetalis syndrome, HbH disease), gene analysis, for common deletions or variant (eg, Southeast Asian, Thai, Filipino, Mediterranean, alpha3.7, alpha4.2, alpha20.5, and Constant Spring)

81260 *IKBKAP (inhibitor of kappa light polypeptide gene enhancer in B-cells, kinase complex-associated protein)* (eg, familial dysautonomia) gene analysis, common variants (eg, 2507+6T>C, R696P)

81261 *IGH@ (Immunoglobulin heavy chain locus)* (eg, leukemias and lymphomas, B-cell), gene rearrangement analysis to detect abnormal clonal population(s); amplified methodology (eg, polymerase chain reaction)

81262 direct probe methodology (eg, Southern blot)

81263 *IGH@ (Immunoglobulin heavy chain locus)* (eg, leukemia and lymphoma, B-cell), variable region somatic mutation analysis

81264 *IGK@ (Immunoglobulin kappa light chain locus)* (eg, leukemia and lymphoma, B-cell), gene rearrangement analysis, evaluation to detect abnormal clonal population(s)

(For immunoglobulin lambda gene [*IGL@*] rearrangement or immunoglobulin kappa deleting element, [*IGKDEL*] analysis, use 81479)

81265 Comparative analysis using Short Tandem Repeat (STR) markers; patient and comparative specimen (eg, pre-transplant

● New Code	▲ Revised Code	+ Add-On Code	○ Modifier -51 Exempt	⊙ Moderate Sedation

recipient and donor germline testing, post-transplant non-hematopoietic recipient germline [eg, buccal swab or other germline tissue sample] and donor testing, twin zygosity testing, or maternal cell contamination of fetal cells)

+ 81266   each additional specimen (eg, additional cord blood donor, additional fetal samples from different cultures, or additional zygosity in multiple birth pregnancies) (List separately in addition to code for primary procedure)

(Use 81266 in conjunction with 81265)

81267   Chimerism (engraftment) analysis, post transplantation specimen (eg, hematopoietic stem cell), includes comparison to previously performed baseline analyses; without cell selection

81268   with cell selection (eg, CD3, CD33), each cell type

(If comparative STR analysis of recipient [using buccal swab or other germline tissue sample] and donor are performed after hematopoietic stem cell transplantation, report 81265, 81266 in conjunction with 81267, 81268 for chimerism testing)

81270   *JAK2 (Janus kinase 2)* (eg, myeloproliferative disorder) gene analysis, p.Val617Phe (V617F) variant

81275   *KRAS (v-Ki-ras2 Kirsten rat sarcoma viral oncogene)* (eg, carcinoma) gene analysis, variants in codons 12 and 13

81280   Long QT syndrome gene analyses (eg, *KCNQ1, KCNH2, SCN5A, KCNE1, KCNE2, KCNJ2, CACNA1C, CAV3, SCN4B, AKAP, SNTA1*, and *ANK2*); full sequence analysis

81281   known familial sequence variant

81282   duplication/deletion variants

81290   *MCOLN1 (mucolipin 1)* (eg, Mucolipidosis, type IV) gene analysis, common variants (eg, IVS3-2A>G, del6.4kb)

81291   *MTHFR (5,10-methylenetetrahydrofolate reductase)* (eg, hereditary hypercoagulability) gene analysis, common variants (eg, 677T, 1298C)

81292   *MLH1 (mutL homolog 1, colon cancer, nonpolyposis type 2)* (eg, hereditary non-polyposis colorectal cancer, Lynch syndrome) gene analysis; full sequence analysis

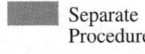 Separate Procedure

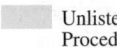 Unlisted Procedure

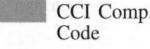 CCI Comp. Code

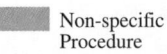 Non-specific Procedure

81293   known familial variants

81294   duplication/deletion variants

81295   *MSH2 (mutS homolog 2, colon cancer, nonpolyposis type 1)* (eg, hereditary non-polyposis colorectal cancer, Lynch syndrome) gene analysis; full sequence analysis

81296   known familial variants

81297   duplication/deletion variants

81298   *MSH6 (mutS homolog 6 [E. coli])* (eg, hereditary non-polyposis colorectal cancer, Lynch syndrome) gene analysis; full sequence analysis

81299   known familial variants

81300   duplication/deletion variants

81301   Microsatellite instability analysis (eg, hereditary non-polyposis colorectal cancer, Lynch syndrome) of markers for mismatch repair deficiency (eg, BAT25, BAT26), includes comparison of neoplastic and normal tissue, if performed

81302   *MECP2 (methyl CpG binding protein 2)* (eg, Rett syndrome) gene analysis; full sequence analysis

81303   known familial variant

81304   duplication/deletion variants

81310   *NPM1 (nucleophosmin)* (eg, acute myeloid leukemia) gene analysis, exon 12 variants

81315   *PML/RAR-alpha, (t(15;17)),* (promyelocytic leukemia/retinoic acid receptor alpha) (eg, promyelocytic leukemia) translocation analysis; common breakpoints (eg, intron 3 and intron 6), qualitative or quantitative

81316   single breakpoint (eg, intron 3, intron 6 or exon 6), qualitative or quantitative

(For intron 3 and intron 6 [including exon 6 if performed] analysis, use 81315)

(If both intron 6 and exon 6 are analyzed, without intron 3, use one unit of 81316)

● New Code   ▲ Revised Code   + Add-On Code   ⊘ Modifier -51 Exempt   ⊙ Moderate Sedation

81317 *PMS2 (postmeiotic segregation increased 2 [S. cerevisiae])* (eg, hereditary non-polyposis colorectal cancer, Lynch syndrome) gene analysis; full sequence analysis

81318 known familial variants

81319 duplication/deletion variants

● **81321** *PTEN (phosphatase and tensin homolog)* (eg, Cowden syndrome, *PTEN* hamartoma tumor syndrome) gene analysis; full sequence analysis

● **81322** known familial variant

● **81323** duplication/deletion variant

● **81324** *PMP22 (peripheral myelin protein 22)* (eg, Charcot-Marie-Tooth, hereditary neuropathy with liability to pressure palsies) gene analysis; duplication/deletion analysis

● **81325** full sequence analysis

● **81326** known familial variant

81330 *SMPD1(sphingomyelin phosphodiesterase 1, acid lysosomal)* (eg, Niemann-Pick disease, Type A) gene analysis, common variants (eg, R496L, L302P, fsP330)

81331 *SNRPN/UBE3A (small nuclear ribonucleoprotein polypeptide N and ubiquitin protein ligase E3A)* (eg, Prader-Willi syndrome and/or Angelman syndrome), methylation analysis

81332 *SERPINA1 (serpin peptidase inhibitor, clade A, alpha-1 antiproteinase, antitrypsin, member 1)* (eg, alpha-1-antitrypsin deficiency), gene analysis, common variants (eg, *S and *Z)

81340 *TRB@ (T cell antigen receptor, beta)* (eg, leukemia and lymphoma), gene rearrangement analysis to detect abnormal clonal population(s); using amplification methodology (eg, polymerase chain reaction)

81341 using direct probe methodology (eg, Southern blot)

81342 *TRG@ (T cell antigen receptor, gamma)* (eg, leukemia and lymphoma), gene rearrangement analysis, evaluation to detect abnormal clonal population(s)

(For T cell antigen alpha [*TRA@*] gene rearrangement analysis, use 81479)

973

■ Separate Procedure	■ Unlisted Procedure	■ CCI Comp. Code	■ Non-specific Procedure

(For T cell antigen delta [*TRD@*] gene rearrangement analysis, report 81402)

81350 *UGT1A1 (UDP glucuronosyltransferase 1 family, polypeptide A1)* (eg, irinotecan metabolism), gene analysis, common variants (eg, *28, *36, *37)

81355 *VKORC1 (vitamin K epoxide reductase complex, subunit 1)* (eg, warfarin metabolism), gene analysis, common variants (eg, -1639/3673)

HUMAN LEUKOCYTE ANTIGEN (HLA) TYPING

Human Leukocyte Antigen (HLA) typing is performed to assess compatibility of recipients and potential donors as a part of solid organ and hematopoietic stem cell pre-transplant testing. HLA testing is also performed to identify HLA alleles and allele groups (antigen equivalents) associated with specific diseases and individualized responses to drug therapy (eg, HLA-B*27 and ankylosing spondylitis and HLA0B*57:01 and abacavir hypersensitivity). as well as other clinical uses. One of more HLA genes may be tested in specific clinical situations (eg, HLA-DQB1 for narcolepsy and HLA-A, -B, -C, -DRB1 and -DQB1 for kidney transplantation). Each HLA gene typically has multiple variant alleles or allele groups that can be identified by typing. For HLA result reporting, a low resolution HLA type is denoted by a two digit HLA name (eg, A*02) and intermediate resolution typing by a string of alleles or an NMDP (National Marrow Donor Program) code (eg, B*14:01/07N/08/12/14, B*39CKGN). Both low and intermediate resolution are considered low resolution for code assignment. High resolution typing resolves the common well defined (CWD) alleles and is usually denoted by at least 4 digits (eg, A*02:02, *03:01:01:01, A*26:01:01G, and C*03:04P), however, high resolution typing may include some ambiguities for rare alleles, which may be reported as a string of alleles or an NMDP code.

If additional testing is required to resolve ambiguous allele combinations for high resolution typing, this is included in the base HLA typing codes below. The gene names have been italicized similar to other molecular pathology codes.

(For HLA antigen typing by non-molecular pathology techniques, see 86812-86822)

81370 HLA Class I and II typing, low resolution (eg, antigen equivalents); *HLA-A, -B, -C, -DRB1/3/4/5*, and *-DQB1*

81371 *HLA-A, -B,* and *-DRB1/3/4/5* (eg, verification typing)

81372 HLA Class I typing, low resolution (eg, antigen equivalents); complete (ie, *HLA-A, -B,* and *-C*)

(When performing both Class I and II low resolution HLA typing for *HLA-A, -B, -C, -DRB1/3/4/5*, and *-DQB1*, use 81370)

81373   one locus (eg, *HLA-A, -B*, or *-C*), each

(When performing a complete Class I [*HLA-A, -B* and *-C*] low resolution HLA typing, use 81372)

(When the presence or absence of a single antigen equivalent is reported using low resolution testing, use 81374)

81374   one antigen equivalent (eg, *B*27*), each

(When testing for presence or absence of more than 2 antigen equivalents at a locus, use 81373 for each locus tested)

81375   HLA Class II typing, low resolution (eg, antigen equivalents); *HLA-DRB1/3/4/5* and *-DQB1*

(When performing both Class I and II low resolution HLA typing for *HLA-A, -B, -C, -DRB1/3/4/5* and *-DQB1*, use 81370)

81376   one locus (eg, *HLA-DRB1/3/4/5, -DQB1, -DQA1, -DPB1*, or *-DPA1*), each

(When low resolution typing is performed for *HLA-DRG1/3/4/5* and *-DQB1*, use 81375)

(For low resolution typing, *HLA-DRB1/3/4/5* should be treated as a single locus)

81377   one antigen equivalent, each

(When testing for presence of absence of more than 2 antigen equivalents at a locus, use 81376 for each locus)

81378   HLA Class I and II typing, high resolution (ie, alleles or allele groups), *HLA-A, -B, -C*, and *-DRB1*

81379   HLA Class I typing, high resolution (ie, alleles or allele groups); complete (ie, *HLA-A, -B*, and *-C*)

81380   one locus (eg, *HLA-A, -B*, or *-C*), each

(When a complete Class I high resolution typing for *HLA-A, -B*, and *-C* is performed, use 81379)

(When the presence of absence of a single allele or allele group is reported using high resolution testing, use 81381)

Separate Procedure   Unlisted Procedure   CCI Comp. Code   Non-specific Procedure

81381   one allele or allele group (eg, *B*57:01P*), each

(When testing for the presence or absence of more than 2 alleles or allele groups at a locus, use 81380 for each locus)

81382 HLA Class II typing, high resolution (ie, alleles or allele groups); one locus (eg, *HLA-DRB1, -DRB3, -DRB4, -DRB5, -DQB1, -DQA1, -DPB1,* or *-DPA1*), each

(When only the presence or absence of a single allele or allele group is reported using high resolution testing, use 81383)

81383   one allele or allele group (eg, *HLA-DQB1*06:02P*), each

(When testing for the presence or absence of more than 2 alleles or allele groups at a locus, use 81382 for each locus)

TIER 2 MOLECULAR PATHOLOGY PROCEDURES

The following molecular pathology procedures (Tier 2) codes are used to report procedures not listed in the Tier 1 molecular pathology codes (81200-81383). They represent medically useful procedures that are generally performed in lower volumes than Tier 1 procedures (eg, the incidence of the disease being tested is rare). They are arranged by level of technical resources and interpretive work by the physician or other qualified health care professional. The individual analyses listed under each code (ie, level of procedure) utilize the definitions and coding principles as described in the introduction preceding the Tier 1 molecular pathology codes. The parenthetical examples of methodologies presented near the beginning of each code provide general guidelines used to group procedures for a given level and are not all-inclusive.

Use the appropriate molecular pathology procedure level code that includes the specific analyte listed after the code descriptor. If the analyte tested is not listed under one of the Tier 2 codes or is not represented by a Tier 1 code, use the unlisted molecular pathology procedure code, 81479.

▲ **81400** Molecular pathology procedure, Level 1 *(eg, identification of single germline variant [eg, SNP] by techniques such as restriction enzyme digestion or melt curve analysis)*

ABCC8 (ATP-binding cassette, sub-family C [CFTR/MRP], member 8) (eg, familial hyperinsulinism), F1388del variant

ACADM (acyl-CoA dehydrogenase, C-4 to C-12 straight chain, MCAD) (eg, medium chain acyl dehydrogenase deficiency), K304E variant

ACE (angiotensin converting enzyme) (eg, hereditary blood pressure regulation), insertion/deletion variant

AGTR1 (angiotensin II receptor, type 1) (eg, essential hypertension), 1166A> variant

CCR5 (chemokine C-C motif receptor 5) (eg, HIV resistance), 32-bp deletion mutation/794 825del32 deletion

CLRN1 (clarin1) (eg, Usher syndrome, type3), N48K variant

DPYD (dihydropyrimidine dehydrogenase) (eg, 5-fluorouracil/5-FU and capecitabine drug metabolism), IVS14+1G>A variant

F2 (coagulation factor 2) (eg, hereditary hypercoagulability), 1199G>A variant

F5 (coagulation factor V) (eg, hereditary hypercoagulability), HR2 variant

F7 (coagulation factor VII [serum prothrombin conversion accelerator]) (eg, hereditary hypercoagulability), R353Q variant

F13B (coagulation factor XIII, B polypeptide) (eg, hereditary hypercoagulability), V34L variant

FGB (fibrinogen beta chain) (eg, hereditary ischemic heart disease), -455G>A variant

FGFR3 (fibroblast growth factor receptor 3) (eg, Muenke syndrome), P250R variant

Human Platelet Antigen 1 genotyping (HPA-1), *ITGB3 (integrin, beta 3 [platelet glycoprotein IIIa], antigen CD61 [GPIIIa])* (eg, neonatal alloimmune thrombocytopenia [NAIT], post-transfusion purpura), HPA-1a/b (L33P)

Human Platelet Antigen 2 genotyping (HPA-2), *GP1BA (glycoprotein Ib [platelet], alpha polypeptide [GPIba])* (eg, neonatal alloimmune thrombocytopenia [NAIT], post-transfusion purpura), HPA-2a/b (T145M)

Human Platelet Antigen 3 genotyping (HPA-3), *ITGA2B (integrin, alpha 2b [platelet glycoprotein IIb of IIb/IIIa complex], antigen CD41 [GPIIb])* (eg, neonatal alloimmune thrombocytopenia [NAIT], post-transfusion purpura), HPA-3a/b (I843S)

Human Platelet Antigen 4 genotyping (HPA-4), *ITGB3 (integrin, beta 3 [platelet glycoprotein IIIa], antigen CD61 [GPIIIa])* (eg, neonatal alloimmune thrombocytopenia [NAIT], post-transfusion purpura), HPA-4a/b (R143Q)

Human Platelet Antigen 5 genotyping (HPA-5), *ITGA2 (integrin, alpha 2 [CD49B, alpha 2 subunit of VLA-2 receptor]*

977

| ■ Separate Procedure | ▨ Unlisted Procedure | ■ CCI Comp. Code | ■ Non-specific Procedure |

[GPIa]) (eg, neonatal alloimmune thrombocytopenia [NAIT], post-transfusion purpura), HPA-5a/b (K505E)

Human Platelet Antigen 6 genotyping (HPA-6w), *ITGB3 (integrin, beta 3 [platelet glycoprotein IIIa, antigen CD61] [GPIIIa])* (eg, neonatal alloimmune thrombocytopenia [NAIT], post-transfusion purpura), HPA-6a/b (R489Q)

Human Platelet Antigen 9 genotyping (HPA-9w), *ITGA2B (integrin, alpha 2b [platelet glycoprotein IIb of IIb/IIIa complex, antigen CD41] [GPIIb])* (eg, neonatal alloimmune thrombocytopenia [NAIT], post-transfusion purpura), HPA-9a/b (V837M)

Human Platelet Antigen 15 genotyping (HPA-15), *CD109 (CD109 molecule)* (eg, neonatal alloimmune thrombocytopenia [NAIT], post-transfusion purpura), HPA-15a/b(S682Y)

IVD (isovaleryl-CoA dehydrogenase) (eg, isovaleric acidemia), A282V variant

SERPINE1 (serpine peptidase inhibitor clade E, member 1, plasminogen activator inhibitor -1, PAI-1) (eg, thrombophilia), 4G variant

SHOC2 (soc-2 suppressor of clear homolog) (eg, Noonan-like syndrome with loose anagen hair), S2G variant

SMN1 (survival of motor neuron 1, telomeric) (eg, spinal muscular atrophy), exon 7 deletion

SRY (sex determining region Y) (eg, 46,XX testicular disorder of sex development, gonadal dysgenesis), gene analysis

TOR1A (torsin family 1, member A [torsin A]) (eg, early-onset primary dystonia [DYT1]), 907_909delGAG (904_906delGAG) variant

▲ **81401** Molecular pathology procedure, Level 2 (eg, 2-10 SNPs, 1 methylated variant, or 1 somatic variant [typically using nonsequencing target variant analysis], or detection of a dynamic mutation disorder/triplet repeat)

ABL (c-abl oncogene 1, receptor tyrosine kinase) (eg, acquired imatinib resistance), T315I variant

ACADM (acyl-CoA dehydrogenase, C-4 to C-12 straight chain, MCAD) (eg, medium chain acyl dehydrogenase deficiency), commons variants (eg, K304E, Y42H)

ADRB2 (adrenergic beta-2 receptor surface) (eg, drug metabolism), common variants (eg, G16R, Q27E)

APOB (apolipoprotein B) (eg, familial hypercholesterolemia type B), common variants (eg, R3500Q, R3500W)

APOE (apolipoprotein E) (eg, hyperlipoproteinemia type III, cardiovascular disease, Alzheimer disease), common variants (eg, *2, *3, *4)

AR (androgen receptor) (eg, spinal and bulbar muscular atrophy, Kennedy disease, X chromosome inactivation), characterization of alleles (eg, expanded size or methylation status)

ATN1 (atrophin 1) (eg, dentatorubral-pallidoluysian atrophy), evaluation to detect abnormal (eg, expanded alleles)

CBFB/MYH11 (inv(16)) (eg, acute myeloid leukemia), qualitative, and quantitative, if performed

CBS (cystathionine-beta-synthase) (eg, homocystinuria, cystathionin beta-synthase deficiency), common variants (eg, I278T, G307S)

CCND1/IGH (BCL1/IgH, t(11;14)) (eg, mantle cell lymphoma) translocation analysis, major breakpoint, qualitative, and quantitative, if performed

CFH/ARMS2 (complement factor H/age-related maculopathy susceptibility 2) (eg, macular degeneration), common variants (eg, Y402H [CFH], A69S [ARMS2])

CYP3A4 (cytochrome P450, family 3, subfamily A, polypeptide 4) (eg, drug metabolism), common variants (eg, *2, *3, *4, *5, *6)

CYP3A5 (cytochrome P450, family 3, subfamily A, polypeptide 5) (eg, drug metabolism), common variants (eg, *2, *3, *4, *5, *6)

DMPK (dystrophia myotonica-protein kinase) (eg, myotonic dystrophy, type 1), evaluation to detect abnormal (eg, expanded) alleles

E2A/PBX1 (t(1;19)) (eg, acute lymphocytic leukemia), translocation analysis, qualitative and quantitative, if performed

EML4/ALK (inv(2)) (eg, non-small cell lunch cancer), translocation or inversion analysis

ETV6/RUNX1 (t(12;21)) (eg, acute lymphocytic leukemia), translocation analysis, qualitative, and quantitative if performed

EWSR1/ERG (t(21;22)) (eg, Ewing sarcoma/peripheral neuroectodermal tumor), translocation analysis, qualitative, and quantitative, if performed

979

| Separate Procedure | Unlisted Procedure | CCI Comp. Code | Non-specific Procedure |

EWSR1/FLI1 (t(21;22)) (eg, Ewing sarcoma/peripheral neuroectodermal tumor), translocation analysis, qualitative, and quantitative, if performed

EWSR/WT1 (t(11;22)) (eg, Ewing sarcoma/peripheral neuroectodermal tumor), translocation analysis, qualitative, and quantitative, if performed

F11 (coagulation factor XI) (eg, coagulation disorder), common variants (eg, E117X [Type II], F283L [Type III], IVS14del14, and IVS14+1G>A [Type I])

FGFR3 (fibroblast growth factor receptor 3) (eg, achondroplasia), common variants (eg, 1138G>A, 1138G>C)

FIP1L1/PDGFRA (del[4q12]) (eg, imatinib-sensitive chronic eosinophilic leukemia), qualitative, and quantitative, if performed

FOXO1/PAX3 (t(1;13)) (eg, Ewing sarcoma/peripheral neuroectodermal tumor), translocation analysis, qualitative, and quantitative, if performed

FOXO1/PAX7 (t(2;13)) (eg, Ewing sarcoma/peripheral neuroectodermal tumor), translocation analysis, qualitative, and quantitative, if performed

FXN (frataxin) (eg, Friedreich ataxia), evaluation to detect abnormal (expanded) alleles

GALT (galactose-1-phosphate uridylyltransferase) (eg, galactosemia), common variants (eg, Q188R, S135L, K285N, T138M, L195P, Y209C, IVS2-2A>G, P171S, del5kb, N314D, L218L/N314D)

H19 (imprinted maternally expressed transcript [non-protein coding]) (eg, Beckwith-Wiedemann syndrome), methylation analysis

HBB (hemoglobin, beta) (eg, sickle cell anemia, hemoglobin C, hemoglobin E), common variants (eg, HbS, HbC, HbE)

HTT (huntingtin) (eg, Huntington disease), evaluation to detect abnormal (eg, expanded) alleles

KCNQ10T1 (KCNQ1 overlapping transcript 1 [non-protein coding]) (eg, Beckwith-Wiedemann syndrome), methylation analysis

MEG3/DLK1 (maternally expressed 3 [non-protein coding]/delta-like 1 homolog [Drosophila]) (eg, intrauterine growth retardation), methylation analysis

MLL/AFF1 (t(4;11)) (eg, acute lymphoblastic leukemia), translocation analysis, qualitative, and quantitative if performed

● New Code   ▲ Revised Code   + Add-On Code   ⊘ Modifier -51 Exempt   ⊙ Moderate Sedation

MLL/MLLT3 (t(9;11)) (eg, acute myeloid leukemia), translocation analysis, qualitative, and quantitative, if performed

MT-RNR1 (mitochondrially encoded 12S RNA) (eg, nonsyndromic hearing loss), common variants (eg, m.1555A>G, m.1494C>T)

MUTYH (mutY homolog [E.coli]) (eg, MYH-associated polyposis), common variants (eg, Y165C, G382D)

MT-ATP6 (mitochondrially encoded ATP synthase 6) (eg, neuropathy with ataxia and retinitis pigmentosa [NARP], Leigh syndrome), common variants (eg, m.8993T>G, m.8993T>C)

MT-ND4, MT-ND6 (mitochondrially encoded NADH dehydrogenase 4, mitochondrially encoded NADH dehydrogenase 6) (eg, Leber hereditary optic neuropathy [LHON]), common variants (eg, m.11778G>A, M.3460G>A, m.14484T>C)

MT-TK (mitochondrially encoded tRNA lysine) (eg, myoclonic epilepsy with ragged-red fibers [MERRF]), common variants (eg, m.8344A>G, m.8356T>C)

MT-TL1 (mitochondrially encoded tRNA leucine 1 [UUA/G]) (eg, diabetes and hearing loss), common variants (eg, M3243A>G, M.14709T>C) MT-TL1,

MT-ND5 (mitochondrially encoded tRNA leucine 1 [UUA/G], mitochondrially encoded NADH dehydrogenase 5) (eg, mitochondrial encephalopathy with lactic acidosis and stroke-like episodes [MELAS]), common variants (eg, m.3243A>G, m.3271T>C, m.3252A>G, m.13513G>A)

MT-TS1, MT-RNR1 (mitochondrially encoded tRNA serine 1 [UCN], mitochondrially encoded 12S RNA) (eg, nonsyndromic sensorineural deafness [including aminoglycoside-induced nonsyndromic deafness]), common variants (eg, m.7445A>G, m.1555A>G)

NPM1/ALK (t(2;5)) (eg, anaplastic large cell lymphoma), transloation analysis

PAX8/PPARG (t(2;3) (q13;p25)) (eg, follicular thyroid carcinoma), translocation analysis

PRSS1 (protease, serine, 1 [trypsin1]) (eg, hereditary pancreatitis), common variants (eg, N29I, A16V, R122H)

PYGM (phosphorylase, glycogen, muscle) (eg, glycogen storage disease type V, McArdle disease), common variants (eg, R50X, G205S)

981

| | Separate Procedure | | Unlisted Procedure | | CCI Comp. Code | | Non-specific Procedure |

RUNX1/RUNX1T1 (t(8;21)) (eg, acute myeloid leukemia) translocation analysis, qualitative, and quantitative, if performed

SEPT9 (Septin 9) (eg, colon cancer), methylation analysis

SMN1/SMN2 (survival of motor neuron 1, telomeric/survival of motor neuron 2, centromeric), (eg, spinal muscular atrophy), dosage analysis (eg, carrier testing)

TPMT (thiopurine S-methyltransferase) (eg, drug metabolism), common variants (eg, *2, *3)

TYMS (thymidylate synthetase) (eg, 5-fluorouracil/5-FU drug metabolism), tandem repeat variant

VWF (von Willebrand factor) (eg, von Willebrand disease type 2N), common variants (eg, T791M, R816W, R854Q)

▲ **81402** Molecular pathology procedure, Level 3 (eg, >10 SNPs, 2-10 methylated variants, or 2-10 somatic variants [typically using non-sequencing target variant analysis], immunoglobulin and T-cell receptor gene rearrangements, duplication/deletion variants of 1 exon, loss of heterozygosity [LOH], uniparental disomy [UPD])

Chromosome 18q- (eg, D18S55, D18S58, D18S61, D18S64, and D18S69) (eg, colon cancer), allelic imbalance assessment (ie, loss of heterozygosity)

CYP21A2 (cytochrome P450, family 21, subfamily A, polypeptide 2) (eg, congenital adrenal hyperplasia, 21-hydroxylase deficiency), common variants (eg, IVS2-13G, P30L, I172N, exon 6 mutation cluster [I235N, V236E, M238K], V281L, L307FfsX6, Q318X, R356W, P453S, G110VfsX21, 30-kb deletion variant)

ESR1/PGR (receptor 1/progesterone receptor) ratio (eg, breast cancer)

KIT (v-kit Hardy-Zuckerman 4 feline sarcoma viral oncogene homolog) (eg, mastocytosis), common variants (eg, D816V, D816Y, D816F)

MEFV (Mediterranean fever) (eg, familial Mediterranean fever), common variants (eg, E148Q, P369S, F479L, M680I, I692del, M694V, M694I, K695R, V726A, A744S, R761H)

MPL (myeloproliferative leukemia virus oncogene, thrombopoietin receptor, TPOR) (eg, myeloproliferative disorder), common variants (eg, W515A, W515K, W515L, W515R)

● New Code   ▲ Revised Code   ＋ Add-On Code   ⊘ Modifier -51 Exempt   ⊙ Moderate Sedation

TRD@ (T cell antigen receptor, delta) (eg, leukemia and lymphoma), gene rearrangement analysis, evaluation to detect abnormal clonal population

Uniparental disomy (UPD) (eg, Russell-Silver syndrome, Prader-Willi/Angelman syndrome), short tandem repeat (STR) analysis

▲ **81403**   Molecular pathology procedure, Level 4 (eg, analysis of single exon by DNA sequence analysis, analysis of >10 amplicons using multiplex PCR in 2 or more independent reactions, mutation scanning or duplication/deletion variants of 2-5 exons)

ABL1 (c-abl oncogene 1, receptor tyrosine kinase) (eg, acquired imatinib tyrosine kinase inhibitor resistance), variants in the kinase domain

ANG (angiogenin, ribonuclease, RNase A family, 5) (eg, amyotrophic lateral sclerosis), full gene sequence

CEBPA (CCAAT/enhancer binding protein [C/EBP], alpha) (eg, acute myeloid leukemia), full gene sequence

CEL (carboxyl ester lipase [bile salt-stimulated lipase]) (eg, maturity-onset diabetes of the young [MODY]), targeted sequence analysis of exon 11 (eg, c.1785delC, c.1686delT)

DAZ/SRY (deleted in azoospermia and sex determining region Y) (eg, male infertility), common deletions (eg, AZFa, AZFb, AZFc, AZFd)

F8 (coagulation factor VIII) (eg, hemophilia A), inversion analysis, intron 1 and intron 22A

FGFR3 (fibroblast growth factor receptor 3) (eg, isolated craniosynostosis), targeted sequence analysis (ex, exon 7)

(For targeted sequence analysis of multiple FGFR3 exons, use 81404)

GJB1 (gap junction protein, beta 1) (eg, Charcot-Marie-Tooth X-linked), full gene sequence

HBB (hemoglobin, beta, beta-globin) (eg, beta thalassemia), duplication/deletion analysis

HRAS (v-Ha-ras Harvey rat sarcoma viral oncogene homolog) (eg, Costello syndrome), exon 2 sequence

IDH1 (isocitrate dehydrogenase 1[NADP+], soluble) (eg, glioma), common exon 4 variants (eg, R132H, R132C)

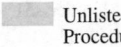 Separate Procedure   Unlisted Procedure   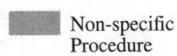 CCI Comp. Code   Non-specific Procedure

IDH2 (isocitrate dehydrogenase 2[NADP+], mitochondrial) (eg, glioma), common exon 4 variants (eg, R140W, R172M)

JAK2 (Janus kinase 2) (eg, myeloproliferative disorder), exon 12 sequence and exon 13 sequence, if performed

KRAS (v-Ki-ras2 Kirsten rat sarcoma viral oncogene) (eg, carcinoma), gene analysis, variant(s) in exon 2

Known familial variant not otherwise specified for gene listed in Tier 1 or Tier 2, DNA sequence analysis, each variant exon

(For a known familial variant that is considered a common variant, use specific common variant Tier 1 or Tier 2 code)

KRAS (v-Ki-ras2 Kirsten rat sarcoma viral oncogene) (eg, carcinoma), gene analysis, variant(s) in exon 3 (eg, codon 61)

MPL (myeloproliferative leukemia virus oncogene, thrombopoietin receptor, TPOR) (eg, myeloproliferative disorder), exon 10 sequence

MT-RNR1 (mitochondrially encoded 12S RNA) (eg, nonsyndromic hearing loss), full gene sequence

MT-TS1 (mitochondrially encoded tRNA serine 1) (eg, nonsyndromic hearing loss), full gene sequence

SMN1 (survival of motor neuron 1, telomeric) (eg, spinal muscular atrophy), known familial sequence variants

VHL (von Hippel-Lindau tumor suppressor) (eg, von Hippel-Lindau familial cancer syndrome), deletion/duplication analysis

VWF (von Willebrand factor) (eg, von Willebrand disease types 2A, 2B, 2M), targeted sequence analysis (eg, exon 28)

▲ **81404**   Molecular pathology procedure, Level 5 (eg, analysis of 2-5 exons by DNA sequence analysis, mutation scanning or duplication/deletion variants of 6-10 exons, or characterization of a dynamic mutation disorder/triplet repeat by Southern blot analysis)

ACADS (acyl-CoA dehydrogenase, C-2 to C-3 short chain) (eg, short chain acyl-CoA dehydrogenase deficiency), targeted sequence analysis (eg, exons 5 and 6)

AQP2 (aquaporin 2 [collecting duct]) (eg, nephrogenic diabetes insipidus), full gene sequence

● New Code   ▲ Revised Code   + Add-On Code   ⊘ Modifier -51 Exempt   ⊙ Moderate Sedation

ARX (aristaless related homeobox) (eg, X-linked lissencephaly with ambiguous genitalia, X-linked mental retardation) full gene sequence

BTD (biotinidase) (eg, biotinidase deficiency), full gene sequence

CAV3 (caveolin 3) (eg, CAV3-related distal myopathy, limb-girdle muscular dystrophy type 1C), full gene sequence

CDKN2A (cyclin-dependent kinase inhibitor 2A) (eg, CDKN2A-related cutaneous malignant melanoma, familiarl atypical mole-malignant melanoma syndrome), full gene sequence

CLRN1 (clarin 1) (eg, Usher syndrome, type 3), full gene sequence

CPT2 (carnitine palmitoyltransferase 2) (eg, carnitine palmitoyltransferase II deficiency), full gene sequence

CYP1B1 (cytochrome P450, family 1, subfamily B, polypeptide 1) (eg, primary congenital glaucoma), full gene sequence

DMPK (dystrophia myotonica-protein kinase) (eg, myotonic dystrophy type 1), characterization of abnormal (eg, expanded) alleles

EGR2 (early growth response 2) (eg, Charcot-Marie-Tooth), full gene sequence

FGFR2 (fibroblast growth factor receptor 2) (eg, craniosynostosis, Apert syndrome, Crouzon syndrome), targeted sequence analysis (eg, exons 8,10)

FGFR3 (fibroblast growth factor receptor 3) (eg, achondroplasia, hypochondroplasia), targeted sequence analysis (eg, exons 8, 11,12,13)

FKRP (Fukutin related protein) (eg, congenital muscular dystrophy type 1C [MDC1C], limb-girdle muscular dystrophy [LGMD] type 2I), full gene sequence

FOXG1 (forkhead box G1) (eg, Rett syndrome), full gene sequence

FSHMD1A (facioscapulohumeral muscular dystrophy 1A) (eg, facioscapulohumeral muscular dystrophy), evaluation to detect abnormal (eg, deleted) alleles

FSHMD1A (facioscapulohumeral muscular dystrophy 1A) (eg, facioscapulohumeral muscular dystrophy), characterization of haplotype(s) (ie, chromosome 4A and 4B haplotypes)

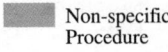

985

| Separate Procedure | Unlisted Procedure | CCI Comp. Code | Non-specific Procedure |

FXN (frataxin) (eg, Friedreich ataxia), full gene sequence

HBA1/HBA2 (alpha globin 1 and alpha globin 2) (eg, alpha thalassemia), duplication/deletion analysis

(For common deletion variants of alpha globin 1 and alpha globin 2 genes, use 81257)

HBB (hemoglobin, beta, Beta-Globin) (eg, thalassemia), full gene sequence

HNF1B (HNF1 homeobox B) (eg, maturity-onset diabetes of the young [MODY]), duplication/deletion analysis

HRAS (v-Ha-ras Harvey rat sarcoma viral oncogene homolog) (eg, Costello syndrome), full gene sequence

KCNJ10 (potassium inwardly-rectifying channel, subfamily J, member 10) (eg, SeSAME syndrome, EAST syndrome, sensorineural hearing loss), full gene sequence

KIT (C-kit) (v-kit Hardy-Zuckerman 4 feline sarcoma viral oncogene homolog) (eg, GIST, acute myeloid leukemia, melanoma), targeted gene analysis (eg, exons 8, 11, 13, 17, 18)

LITAF (lipopolysaccharide-induced TNF factor) (eg, Charcot-Marie-Tooth), full gene sequence

MEFV (Mediterranean fever) (eg, familial Mediterranean fever), full gene sequence

MEN1 (multiple endocrine neoplasia 1) (eg, multiple endocrine neoplasia type 1, Wermer syndrome), duplication/deletion analysis

NRAS (neuroblastoma RAS viral oncogene homolog) (eg, colorectal carcinoma), exon 1 and exon 2 sequences

PDGFRA (platelet-derived growth factor receptor alpha polypeptide) (eg, gastrointestinal stromal tumor), targeted sequence analysis (eg, exons 12, 18)

PDX1 (pancreatic and duodenal homeobox 1) (eg, maturity-onset diabetes of the young [MODY]), full gene sequence

PRNP (prion protein) (eg, genetic prion disease), full gene sequence

PRSS1 (protease, serine, 1[trypsin1]) (eg, hereditary pancreatitis), full gene sequence

● New Code ▲ Revised Code + Add-On Code ⊘ Modifier -51 Exempt ⊙ Moderate Sedation

RAF1 (v-raf-1 murine leukemia viral oncogene homolog 1) (eg, LEOPARD syndrome), targeted sequence analysis (eg, exons 7, 12, 14, 17)

RET (ret proto-oncogene) (eg, multiple endocrine neoplasia, type 2B and familial medullary thyroid carcinoma), common variants (eg, M918T, 2647_2648delinsTT, A883F)

SDHD (succinate dehydrogenase complex, subunit D, integral membrane protein) (eg, hereditary paraganglioma), full gene sequence

SLC25A4 (solute carrier family 25 [mitochondrial carrier; adenine nucleotide translocator], member 4) (eg, progressive external ophthalmoplegia), full gene sequence

TP53 (tumor protein 53) (eg, tumor samples), targeted s equence analysis of 2-5 exons

TTR (transthyretin) (eg, familial transthyretin amyloidosis), full gene sequence

TYR (tyrosinase [oculocutaneous albinism IA]) (eg, oculocutaneous albinism IA), full gene sequence

USH1G (Usher syndrome 1G [autosomal recessive]) (eg, Usher syndrome type 1), full gene sequence

VHL (von Hippel-Lindau tumor suppressor) (eg, von Hippel-Lindau familial cancer syndrome), full gene sequence

VWF (von Willebrand factor) (eg, von Willebrand disease type 1C), targeted sequence analysis (eg, exons 26, 27, 37)

▲ **81405**   Molecular pathology procedure, Level 6 (eg, analysis of 6-10 exons by DNA sequence analysis, mutation scanning or duplication/deletion variants of 11-25 exons)

ABCD1 (ATP-binding cassette, sub-family D [ALD], member 1) (eg, adrenoleukodystrophy), full gene sequence

ACADS (acyl-CoA dehydrogenase, C-2 to C-3 short chain) (eg, short chain acyl-CoA dehydrogenase deficiency) full gene sequence

ACTC1 (actin, alpha, cardiac muscle 1) (eg, familial hypertrophic cardiomyopathy), full gene sequence

APTX (aprataxin) (eg, ataxia with oculomotor apraxia 1), full gene sequence

AR (androgen receptor) (eg, androgen insensitivity syndrome), full gene sequence

 Separate Procedure   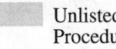 Unlisted Procedure   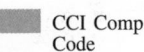 CCI Comp. Code   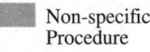 Non-specific Procedure

987

CYP21A2 (cytochrome P450, family 21, subfamily A, polypeptide2) (eg, steroid 21-hydroxylase isoform, congenital adrenal hyperplasia), full gene sequence

DFNB59 (deafness, autosomal recessive 59) (eg, autosomal recessive nonsyndromic hearing impairment), full gene sequence

DHCR7 (7-dehydrocholesterol reductase) (eg, Smith-Lemli-Opitz syndrome), full gene sequence

EYA1 (eyes absent homolog 1 [Drosophila]) (eg, branchio-oto-renal [BOR] spectrum disorders), duplication/deletion analysis

F9 (coagulation factor IX) (eg, hemophilia B), full gene sequence

FH (fumarate hydratase) (eg, fumarate hydratase deficiency, hereditary leiomyomatosis with renal cell cancer), full gene sequence

FKTN (fukutin) (eg, limb-girdle muscular dystrophy [LGMD] type 2M or 2L), full gene sequence

GFAP (glial fibrillary acidic protein) (eg, Alexander disease), full gene sequence

GLA (galactosidase, alpha) (eg, Fabry disease), full gene sequence

HBA1/HBA2 (alpha globin 1 and alpha globin 2) (eg, thalassemia), full gene sequence

HNF1A (HNF1 homeobox A) (eg, maturity-onset diabetes of the young [MODY]), full gene sequence

HNF1B (HNF1 homeobox B) (eg, maturity-onset diabetes of the yound [MODY]), full gene sequence

KRAS (v-Ki-ras2 Kirsten rat sarcoma viral oncogene homolog) (eg, Noonan syndrome), full gene sequence

LAMP2 (lysosomal-associated membrane protein 2) (eg, Danon disease), full gene sequence

MEN1 (multiple endocrine neoplasia 1) (eg, multiple endocrine neoplasia type 1, Wermer syndrome), full gene sequence

MPZ (myelin protein zero) (eg, Charcot-Marie-Tooth), full gene sequence

MYL2 (myosin, light chain 2, regulatory, cardiac, slow) (eg, familial hypertrophic cardiomyopathy), full gene sequence

● New Code ▲ Revised Code + Add-On Code ⊘ Modifier -51 Exempt ⊙ Moderate Sedation

MYL3 (myosin, light chain 3, alkali, ventricular, skeletal, slow) (eg, familial hypertrophic cardiomyopathy), full gene sequence

MYOT (myotilin) (eg, limb-girdle muscular dystrophy), full gene sequenc

NEFL (neurofilament, light polypeptide) (eg, Charcot-Marie-Tooth), full gene sequence

NF2 (neurofibromin 2 [merlin]) (eg, neurofibromatosis, type 2), duplication/deletion analysis

NSD1 (nuclear receptor binding SET domain protein 1) (eg, Sotos syndrome), duplication/deletion analysis

OTC (ornithine carbamoyltransferase) (eg, ornithine transcarbamylase deficiency), full gene sequence

PDHB (pyruvate dehydrogenase [lipoamide] beta) (eg, lactic acidosis), full gene sequence

PSEN1 (presenilin 1) (eg, Alzheimer disease), full gene sequence

RET (ret proto-oncogene) (eg, multiple endocrine neoplasia, type 2A and familial medullary thyroid carcinoma), targeted sequence analysis (eg, exons 10, 11, 13-16)

SDHB (succinate dehydrogenase complex, subunit B, iron sulfur) (eg, hereditary paraganglioma), full gene sequence

SDHC (succinate dehydrogenase complex, submit C, integral membrane protein, 15kDa) (eg, hereditary paraganglioma-pheochromocytoma syndrome), full gene sequence

SGCA (sarcoglycan, alpha [50kDa dystrophin-associated glycoprotein]) (eg, limb-girdle muscular dystrophy), full gene sequence

SGCB (sarcoglycan, beta [43kDa dystrophin-associated glycoprotein]) (eg, limb-girdle muscular dystrophy), full gene sequence

SGCD (sarcoglycanm delta [35kDa dystrophin-associated glycoprotein]) (eg, limb-girdle muscular dystrophy), full gene sequence

SGCG (sarcoglycan, gamma [35kDa dystrophin-associated glycoprotein]) (eg, limb-girdle muscular dystrophy), full gene sequence

	Separate Procedure		Unlisted Procedure		CCI Comp. Code		Non-specific Procedure

SHOC2 (soc-2 suppressor of clear homolog) (eg, Noonan-like syndrome with loose anagen hair), full gene sequence

SMN1 (survival of motor neuron 1, telomeric) (eg, spinal muscular atrophy), full gene sequence

SPRED1 (sprouty-related, EVH1 domain containing 1) (eg, Legius syndrome), full gene sequence

TGFBR1 (transforming growth factor, beta receptor 1) (eg, Marfan syndrome), full gene sequence

TGFBR2 (transforming growth factor, beta receptor 2) (eg, Marfan syndrome), full gene sequence

THRB (thyroid hormone receptor, beta) (eg, thyroid hormone resistance, thyroid hormone beta receptor deficiency), full gene sequence or targeted sequence analysis of >5 exons

TNNI3 (troponin I, type 3 [cardiac]) (eg, familial hypertrophic cardiomyopathy), full gene sequence

TP53 (tumor protein 53) (eg, Li-Fraumeni syndrome, tumor samples), full gene sequence or targeted sequence analysis of >5 exons

TPM1 (tropomyosin 1 [alpha]) (eg, familial hypertrophic cardiomyopathy), full gene sequence

TSC1 (tuberous sclerosis 1) (eg, tuberous sclerosis), duplication/deletion analysis

VWF (von Willebrand factor) (eg, von Willebrand disease type 2N), targeted sequence analysis (eg, exons 18-20, 23-25)

▲ **81406**   Molecular pathology procedure, Level 7 (eg, analysis of 11-25 exons by DNA sequence analysis, mutation scanning or duplication/deletion variants of 26-50 exons, cytogenomic array analysis for neoplasia)

ACADVL (acyl-CoA dehydrogenase, very long chain) (eg, very long chain acyl-coenzyme A dehydrogenase deficiency), full gene sequence

ACTN4 (actinin, alpha 4) (eg, focal segmental glomerulosclerosis), full gene sequence

ANO5 (anoctamin 5) (eg, limb-girdle muscular dystrophy), full gene sequence

APP (amyloid beta [A4] precursor protein) (eg, Alzheimer disease), full gene sequence

● New Code	▲ Revised Code	+ Add-On Code	⊘ Modifier -51 Exempt	⊙ Moderate Sedation

ATP7B (ATPase, Cu++ transporting, beta polypeptide) (eg, Wilson disease), full gene sequence

BRAF (v-raf murine sarcoma viral oncogene homolog B1) (eg, Noonan syndrome), full gene sequence

CAPN3 (Calpain 3) (eg, limb-girdle muscular dystrophy [LGMD] type 2A, calpainopathy), full gene sequence

CBS (cystathionine-beta-synthase) (eg, homocystinuria, cystathionine beta-synthase deficiency), full gene sequence

CDH1 (cadherin 1, type 1, E-cadherin [epithelial]) (eg, hereditary diffuse gastric cancer), full gene sequence

CDKL5 (cyclin-dependent kinase-like 5) (eg, early infantile epileptic encephalopathy), full gene sequence

Cytogenomic microarray analysis, neoplasia (eg, interrogation of copy number, and loss-of-heterozygosity via single nucleotide polymorphism [SNP]-based comparative genomic hybridization [CGH] microarray analysis)

DLAT (dihydrolipoamide S-acetyltransferase) (eg, pyruvate dehydrogenase E2 deficiency), full gene sequence

DLD (dihydrolipoamide dehydrogenase) (eg, maple syrup urine disease, type III), full gene sequence

EYA1 (eyes absent homolog 1 [Drosophila]) (eg, branchio-otorenal [BOR] spectrum disorders), full gene sequence

F8 (coagulation factor VIII) (eg, hemophilia A), duplication/ deletion analysis

GAA (glucosidase, alpha; acid) (eg, glycogen storage disease type II [Pompe disease]), full gene sequence

GALT (galactose-1-phosphate uridylyltransferase) (eg, galactosemia), full gene sequence

GCDH (glutaryl-CoA dehydrogenase) (eg, glutaricacidemia type 1), full gene sequence

GCK (glucokinase [hexokinase 4]) (eg, maturity-onset diabetes of the young [MODY]), full gene sequence

HADHA (hydroxyacyl-CoA dehydrogenase/3-ketoacyl-CoA thiolase/enoyl-CoA hydratase [trifunctional protein] alpha subunit) (eg, long chain acyl-coenzyme A dehydrogenase deficiency), full gene sequence

Separate Procedure · Unlisted Procedure · CCI Comp. Code · Non-specific Procedure

HEXA (hexosaminidase A, alpha polypeptide) (eg, Tay-Sachs disease), full gene sequence

HNF4A (hepatocyte nuclear factor 4, alpha) (eg, maturity-onset diabetes of the young [MODY]), full gene sequence

IVD (isovaleryl-CoA dehydrogenase) (eg, isovaleric acidemia), full gene sequence

JAG1 (jagged 1) (eg, Alagille syndrome), duplication/deletion analysis

LDB3 (LIM domain binding 3) (eg, familial dilated cardiomyopathy, myofibrillar myopathy), full gene sequence

LMNA (lamin A/C) (eg, Emery-Dreifuss muscular dystrophy [EDMD1, 2 and 3] limb-girdle muscular dystrophy [LGMD] type 1B, dilated cardiomyopathy [CMD1A], familial partial lipodystrophy [FPLD2]), full gene sequence

MAP2K1 (mitogen-activated protein kinase 1) (eg, cardiofaciocutaneous syndrome), full gene sequence

MAP2K2 (mitogen-activated protein kinase 2) (eg, cardiofaciocutaneous syndrome), full gene sequence

MCCC2 (methylcrotonoyl-CoA carboxylase 2 [beta]) (eg, 3-methylcrotonyl carboxylase deficiency), full gene sequence

MUTYH (mutY homolog [E. coli]) (eg, MYH-associated polyposis), full gene sequence

NF2 (neurofibromin 2 [merlin]) (eg, neurofibromatosis, type 2), full gene sequence

NOTCH3 (notch 3) (eg, cerebral autosomal dominant arteriopathy with subcortical infarcts and leukoencephalopathy [CADASIL]), targeted sequence analysis (eg, exons 1-23)

NSD1 (nuclear receptor binding SET domain protein 1) (eg, Sotos syndrome), full gene sequence

OPA1 (optic atrophy 1) (eg, optic atrophy), duplication/deletion analysis

PAH (phenylalanine hydroxylase) (eg, phenylketonuria), full gene sequence

PALB2 (partner and localizer of BRCA2) (eg, breast and pancreatic cancer), full gene sequence

PAX2 (paired box 2) (eg, renal coloboma syndrome), full gene sequence

PC (pyruvate carboxylase) (eg, pyruvate carboxylase deficiency), full gene sequence

PCCB (propionyl CoA carboxylase, beta polypeptide) (eg, propionic acidemia), full gene sequence

PDHA1 (pyruvate dehydrogenase [lipoamide] alpha 1) (eg, lactic acidosis), full gene sequence

PDHX (pyruvate dehydrogenase complex, component X) (eg, lactic acidosis), full gene sequence

POLG (polymerase [DNA directed], gamma) (eg, Alpers-Huttenlocher syndrome, autosomal dominant progressive external ophthalmoplegia), full gene sequence

POMGNT1 (protein O-linked mannose beta1,2-N acetylglucosaminyltransferase) (eg, muscle-eye-brain disease, Walker-Warburg syndrome), full gene sequence

POMT1 (protein-O-mannosyltransferase 1) (eg, limb-girdle muscular dystrophy [LGMD] type 2K, Walker-Warburg syndrome), full gene sequence

POMT2 (protein-O-mannosyltransferase 2) (eg, limb-girdle muscular dystrophy [LGMD] type 2N, Walker-Warburg syndrome), full gene sequence

PRKAG2 (protein kinase, AMP-activated, gamma 2 non-catalytic subunit) (eg, familial hypertrophic cardiomyopathy with Wolff-Parkinson-White syndrome, lethal congenital glycogen storagedisease of heart), full gene sequence

PSEN2 (presenilin 2 [Alzheimer disease 4]) (eg, Alzheimer disease), full gene sequence

PTPN11 (protein tyrosine phosphatase, non-receptor type 11) (eg, Noonan syndrome, LEOPARD syndrome), full gene sequence

PYGM (phosphorylase, glycogen, muscle) (eg, glycogen storage disease type V, McArdle disease), full gene sequence

RAF1 (v-raf-1 murine leukemia viral oncogene homolog 1) (eg, LEOPARD syndrome), full gene sequence

RET (ret proto-oncogene) (eg, Hirschsprung disease), full gene sequence

RYR1 (ryanodine receptor 1, skeletal) (eg, malignant hyperthermia), targeted sequence analysis of exons with functionally-confirmed mutations

■ Separate Procedure   ■ Unlisted Procedure   ■ CCI Comp. Code   ■ Non-specific Procedure

SLC9A6 (solute carrier family 9 [sodium/hydrogen exchanger], member 6) (eg, Christianson syndrome), full gene sequence

SLC26A4 (solute carrier family 26, member 4) (eg, Pendred syndrome), full gene sequence

SOS1 (son of sevenless homolog 1) (eg, Noonan syndrome, gingival fibromatosis), full gene sequence

TAZ (tafazzin) (eg, methylglutaconic aciduria type 2, Barth syndrome), full gene sequence

TNNT2 (troponin T, type 2 [cardiac]) (eg, familial hypertrophic cardiomyopathy), full gene sequence

TSC1 (tuberous sclerosis 1) (eg, tuberous sclerosis), full gene sequence

TSC2 (tuberous sclerosis 2) (eg, tuberous sclerosis), duplication/deletion analysis

UBE3A (ubiquitin protein ligase E3A) (eg, Angelman syndrome), full gene sequence

VWF (von Willebrand factor) (von Willebrand disease type 2A), extended targeted sequence analysis (eg, exons 11-16, 24-26, 51, 52)

▲ **81407**   Molecular pathology procedure, Level 8 (eg, analysis of 26-50 exons by DNA sequence analysis, mutation scanning or duplication/deletion variants of >50 exons, sequence analysis of multiple genes on one platform)

ABCC8 (ATP-binding cassette, sub-family C [CFTR/MRP], member 8) (eg, familial hyperinsulinism), full gene sequence

CHD7 (chromodomain helicase DNA binding protein 7) (eg, CHARGE syndrome), full gene sequence

F8 (coagulation factor VIII) (eg, hemophilia A), full gene sequence

JAG1 (jagged 1) (eg, Alagille syndrome), full gene sequence

MYBPC3 (myosin binding protein C, cardiac) (eg, familial hypertrophic cardiomyopathy), full gene sequence

MYH6 (myosin, heavy chain 6, cardiac muscle, alpha) (eg, familial dilated cardiomyopathy), full gene sequence

MYH7 (myosin, heavy chain 7, cardiac muscle, beta) (eg, familial hypertrophic cardiomyopathy, Liang distal myopathy), full gene sequence

MYO7A (myosin VIIA) (eg, Usher syndrome, type 1), full gene sequence

NOTCH1 (notch 1) (eg, aortic valve disease), full gene sequence

OPA1 (optic atrophy 1) (eg, optic atrophy), full gene sequence

PCDH15 (protocadherin-related 15) (eg, Usher syndrome, type 1), full gene sequence

SCN1A (sodium channel, voltage-gated, type 1, alpha subunit) (eg, generalized epilepsy with febrile seizures), full gene sequence

SCN5A (sodium channel, voltage-gated, type V, alpha subunit) (eg, familial dilated cardiomyopathy), full gene sequence

TSC2 (tuberous sclerosis 2) (eg, tuberous sclerosis), full gene sequence

USH1C (Usher syndrome 1C [autosomal recessive, severe]) (eg, Usher syndrome, type 1), full gene sequence

▲ **81408** Molecular pathology procedure, Level 9 (eg, analysis of >50 exons in a single gene by DNA sequence analysis)

ATM (ataxia telangiectasia mutated) (eg, ataxia telangiectasia),full gene sequence

CDH23 (cadherin-related 23) (eg, Usher syndrome, type 1), full gene sequence

COL1A1 (collagen, type I, alpha 1) (eg, osteogenesis imperfecta, type I), full gene sequence

COL1A2 (collagen, type I, alpha 2) (eg, osteogenesis imperfecta, type I), full gene sequence

DYSF (dysferlin, limb girdle muscular dystrophy 2B [autosomal recessive]) (eg, limb-girdle muscular dystrophy), full gene sequence

FBN1 (fibrillin 1) (eg, Marfan syndrome), full gene sequence

NF1 (neurofibromin 1) (eg, neurofibromatosis, type 1), full gene sequence

RYR1 (ryanodine receptor 1, skeletal) (eg, malignant hyperthermia), full gene sequence

USH2A (Usher syndrome 2A [autosomal recessive, mild]) (eg, Usher syndrome, type 2), full gene sequence

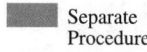 Separate Procedure

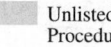 Unlisted Procedure

CCI Comp. Code

Non-specific Procedure

VWF (von Willebrand factor) (eg, von Willebrand disease types 1 and 3), full gene sequence

● **81479**   Unlisted molecular pathology procedure

MULTIANALYTE ASSAYS WITH ALGORITHMIC ANALYSES

Multianalyte Assays with Algorithmic Analyses (MAAAs) are procedures that utilize multiple results derived from assays of various types, including molecular pathology assays, fluorescent in situ hybridization assays and nonnucleic acid-based assays (eg, proteins, polypeptides, lipids, carbohydrates). Algorithmic analysis using the results of these assays as well as other patient information (if used) is then performed, and reported typically as a numeric score(s) or as a probability. MAAAs are typically unique to a single clinical laboratory or manufacturer. The results of individual component procedure(s) that are inputs to the MAAAs may be provided on the associated laboratory report, however these assays are not reported separately using additional codes.

The format for the code descriptors of MAAAs usually include (in order):

Disease type (eg, oncology, autoimmune, tissue rejection),

Material(s) analyzed (eg, DNA, RNA, protein, antibody),

Number of markers (eg, number of genes, number of proteins),

Methodology(ies) (eg, microarray, real-time [RT]-PCR, in situ hybridization [ISH], enzyme linked immunosorbent assays [ELISA],

Number of functional domains (if indicated),

Specimen type (eg, blood, fresh tissue, formalin-fixed paraffin embedded),

Algorithm result type (eg, prognostic, diagnostic),

Report (eg, probability index, risk score)

MAAAs, including those that do not have a Category I code, may be found in Appendix O. MAAAs that do not have a Category I code are identified in Appendix O by a four-digit number followed by the letter "M." The Category 1 MAAA codes that are included in this subsection are also included in Appendix O. All MAAA codes are listed in Appendix O along with the procedure's proprietary name.

When a specific MAAA procedure is not listed below or in Appendix O, the procedure must be reported using the Category 1 MAAA unlisted code (81599).

---

996   ● New   ▲ Revised   + Add-On   ⊘ Modifier -51   ⊙ Moderate
            Code   Code   Code   Exempt   Sedation

These codes encompass all analytical services required (eg, cell lysis, nucleic acid stabilization, extraction, digestion, amplification, hybridization, adn detection) in addition to the algorithmic analysis itself. Procedures that are required prior to cell lysis (eg, microdissection, codes 88380 and 88381) should be reported separately.

● **81500** Oncology (ovarian), biochemical assays of two proteins (CA-125 adn HE4), utilizing serum, with menopausal status, algorithm reported as a risk score

   (Do note report 81500 in conjunction with 86304, 86305)

● **81503** Oncology (ovarian), biochemical assays of five proteins (CA-125, apolipoprotein A1, beta-2 microglobulin, transferrin, and pre-albumin), utilizing serum, algorithm reported as a risk score

   (Do not report 81503 in conjunction with 82172, 82232, 83695, 83700, 84134, 84466, 86304)

● **81506** Endocrinology (type 2 diabetes), biochemical assays of seven analytes (glucose, HbA1c, insulin, hs-CRP, adoponectin, ferritin, interleukin 2-receptor alpha), utilizing serum or plasma, algorithm reporting a risk score

   (Do not report 81506 in conjunction with constituent components [ie, 82728, 82947, 83036, 83525, 86141], 84999 [for adopectin], and 83520 [for interleukin 2-receptor alpha])

● **81508** Fetal congenital abnormalities, biochemical assays of two proteins (PAPP-A, hCG [any form]), utilizing maternal serum, algorithm reported as a risk score

   (Do not report 81508 in conjunction with 84163, 84702)

● **81509** Fetal congenital abnormalities, biochemical assays of three proteins (PAPP-A, hCG [any form], DIA), utilizing maternal serum, algorithm reported as a risk score

   (Do not report 81509 in conjunction with 84163, 84702, 86336)

● **81510** Fetal congenital abnormalities, biochemical assays of three analytes (AFP, uE3, hCG [any form]), utilizing maternal serum, algorithm reported as a risk score

   (Do note report 81510 in conjunction with 82105, 82677, 84702)

● **81511** Fetal congenital abnormalities, biochemical assays of four analytes (AFP, uE3, hCG [any form], DIA) utilizing maternal serum, algorithm reported as a risk score (may include additional results from previous biochemical testing)

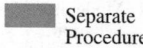 Separate Procedure 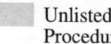 Unlisted Procedure   CCI Comp. Code   Non-specific Procedure

(Do not report 81511 in conjunction with 82105, 82677, 84702,. 86336)

● **81512**   Fetal congenital abnormalities, biochemical assays of five analytes (AFP, uE3, total hCG, hyperglycosylated hCG, DIA) utilizing maternal serum, algorithm reported as a risk score

(Do not report 81512 in conjunction with 82105, 82677, 84702, 86336)

● **81599**   Unlisted multianalyte assay with algorithmic analysis

(Do not report 81599 for multianalyte assays with algorithmic analyses listed in Appendix O)

CHEMISTRY

The material for examination may be from any source unless otherwise specified in the code descriptor. When an analyte is measured in multiple specimens from different sources, or in specimens that are obtained at different times, the analyte is reported separately for each source and for each specimen. The examination is quantitative unless specified. To report an organ or disease oriented panel, see codes 80048-80076.

When a code describes a method where measurement of multiple analytes may require one or several procedures, each procedure is coded separately (eg., 82491-82492, 82541-82544). For example, if two analytes are measured using column chromatography using a single stationary or mobile phase, use 82492. If the same two analytes are measured using different stationary or mobile phase conditions, 82491 would be used twice. If a total of four analytes are measured where two analytes are measured with a single stationary and mobile phase, and the other two analytes are measured using a different stationary and mobile phase, use 82492 twice. If a total of three analytes are measured where two analytes are measured using a single stationary or mobile phase condition, and the third analyte is measured separately using a different stationary or mobile phase procedure, use 82492 once for the two analytes measured under the same condition, and use 82491 once for the third analyte measured separately.

Clinical information or mathematically calculated values, which are not specifically requested by the ordering physician and are derived from the results of other ordered or performed laboratory tests, are considered part of the ordered test procedure(s) and therefore are not separately reportable service(s).

When the requested analyte result is derived using a calculation that requires values from nonrequested laboratory analyses, only the requested analyte code should be reported.

---

998   ● New Code   ▲ Revised Code   + Add-On Code   ⊘ Modifier -51 Exempt   ⊙ Moderate Sedation

When the calculated analyte determination requires values derived from other requested and nonrequested laboratory analyses, the requested analyte codes (including those calculated) should be reported.

An exception to the above is when an analyte (eg, urinary creatinine) is performed to compensate for variations in urine concentration (eg, microalbumin, thromboxane metabolites) in random urine samples; the appropriate CPT code is reported for both the ordered analyte and the additional required analyte. When the calculated result(s) represent an algorithmically derived numeric score or probability, see the appropriate multianalyte assay with algorithmic analyses (MAAA) code or the MAAA unlisted code (81599).

82000	Acetaldehyde, blood
82003	Acetaminophen
▲ **82009**	Ketone body(s) (eg, acetone, acetoacetic acid, beta-hydroxybutyrate); qualitative
▲ **82010**	quantitative
82013	Acetylcholinesterase

(For gastric acid analysis, use 82930)

(Acid phosphatase, see 84060-84066)

82016 Acylcarnitines; qualitative, each specimen

82017 quantitative, each specimen

(For carnitine, use 82379)

82024 Adrenocorticotropic hormone (ACTH)

82030 Adenosine, 5-monophosphate, cyclic (cyclic AMP)

82040 Albumin; serum, plasma or whole blood

82042 urine, quantitative, each specimen

82043 urine, microalbumin, quantitative

82044 urine, microalbumin, semiquantitative (eg, reagent strip assay)

(For prealbumin, use 84134)

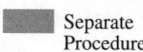 Separate Procedure 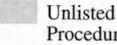 Unlisted Procedure CCI Comp. Code Non-specific Procedure

82045   ischemia modified

82055   Alcohol (ethanol); any specimen except breath

(For other volatiles, alcohol, use 84600)

82075   breath

82085   Aldolase

82088   Aldosterone

(Alkaline phosphatase, see 84075, 84080)

82101   Alkaloids, urine, quantitative

(Alphaketoglutarate, see 82009, 82010)

(Alpha tocopherol (Vitamin E), use 84446)

82103   Alpha-1-antitrypsin; total

82104   phenotype

82105   Alpha-fetoprotein; serum

82106   amniotic fluid

82107   AFP-L3 fraction isoform and total AFP (including ratio)

82108   Aluminum

82120   Amines, vaginal fluid, qualitative

(For combined pH and amines test for vaginitis, use 82120 and 83986)

82127   Amino acids; single, qualitative, each specimen

82128   multiple, qualitative, each specimen

82131   single, quantitative, each specimen

82135   Aminolevulinic acid, delta (ALA)

82136   Amino acids, 2 to 5 amino acids, quantitative, each specimen

● New Code   ▲ Revised Code   + Add-On Code   ⊘ Modifier -51 Exempt   ⊙ Moderate Sedation

82139 Amino acids, 6 or more amino acids, quantitative, each specimen

82140 Ammonia

82143 Amniotic fluid scan (spectrophotometric)

(For L/S ratio, use 83661)

(Amobarbital, see 80100-80103 for qualitative analysis, 82205 for quantitative analysis)

82145 Amphetamine or methamphetamine

(For qualitative analysis, see 80100-80103)

82150 Amylase

82154 Androstanediol glucuronide

82157 Androstenedione

82160 Androsterone

82163 Angiotensin II

82164 Angiotensin I - converting enzyme (ACE)

(Antidiuretic hormone (ADH), use 84588)

(Antimony, use 83015)

(Antitrypsin, alph-1-, see 82103, 82104)

82172 Apolipoprotein, each

82175 Arsenic

(For heavy metal screening, use 83015)

82180 Ascorbic acid (Vitamin C), blood

(Aspirin, see acetylsalicylic acid, 80196)

(Atherogenic index, blood, ultracentrifugation, quantitative, use 83717)

82190 Atomic absorption spectroscopy, each analyte

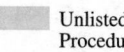 Separate Procedure 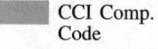 Unlisted Procedure 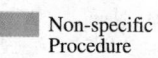 CCI Comp. Code   Non-specific Procedure   **1001**

82205 Barbiturates, not elsewhere specified

(For qualitative analysis, see 80100-80103)

(For B-Natriuretic peptide, use 83880)

82232 Beta-2 microglobulin

(Bicarbonate, use 82374)

82239 Bile acids; total

82240 cholylglycine

(For bile pigments, urine, see 81000-81005)

82247 Bilirubin; total

82248 direct

82252 feces, qualitative

82261 Biotinidase, each specimen

82270 Blood, occult, by peroxidase activity (eg, guaiac), qualitative; feces, consecutive collected specimens with single determination, for colorectal neoplasm screening (ie, patient was provided three cards or single triple card for consecutive collection)

82271 other sources

82272 Blood, occult, by peroxidase activity (eg, guaiac), qualitative, feces, 1-3 simultaneous determinations, performed for other than colorectal neoplasm screening

(Blood urea nitrogen (BUN), see 84520, 84525)

82274 Blood, occult, by fecal hemoglobin determination by immunoassay, qualitative, feces, 1-3 simultaneous determinations

82286 Bradykinin

82300 Cadmium

82306 Vitamin D; 25 hydroxy, includes fraction(s), if performed

82652 1, 25-dihydroxy, includes fraction(s), if performed

● New Code   ▲ Revised Code   + Add-On Code   ⊘ Modifier -51 Exempt   ⊙ Moderate Sedation

(82307 Deleted 2009 [2010 edition]. For 25 hydroxy vitamin D, use 82306)

82308 Calcitonin

82310 Calcium; total

82330   ionized

82331   after calcium infusion test

82340   urine quantitative, timed specimen

82355 Calculus; qualitative analysis

82360   quantitative analysis, chemical

82365   infrared spectroscopy

82370   x-ray diffraction

(Carbamates, see individual listings)

82373 Carbohydrate deficient transferrin

82374 Carbon dioxide (bicarbonate)

(See also 82803)

82375 Carboxyhemoglobin; quantitative

82376   qualitative

(For transcutaneous measurement of carboxyhemoglobin, use 88740)

82378 Carcinoembryonic antigen (CEA)

82379 Carnitine (total and free), quantitative, each specimen

(For acylcarnitine, see 82016, 82017)

82380 Carotene

82382 Catecholamines; total urine

82383   blood

1003

	Separate Procedure		Unlisted Procedure		CCI Comp. Code		Non-specific Procedure

82384   fractionated

(For urine metabolites, see 83835, 84585)

82387 Cathepsin-D

82390 Ceruloplasmin

82397 Chemiluminescent assay

82415 Chloramphenicol

82435 Chloride; blood

82436   urine

82438   other source

(For sweat collection by iontophoresis, use 89230)

82441 Chlorinated hydrocarbons, screen

(Chlorpromazine, use 84022)

(Cholecalciferol [Vitamin D], use 82306)

82465 Cholesterol, serum or whole blood, total

(For high density lipoprotein (HDL), use 83718)

82480 Cholinesterase; serum

82482   RBC

82485 Chondroitin B sulfate, quantitative

(Chorionic gonadotropin, see gonadotropin, 84702, 84703)

82486 Chromatography, qualitative; column (eg, gas liquid or HPLC), analyte not elsewhere specified

82487   paper, 1-dimensional, analyte not elsewhere specified

82488   paper, 2-dimensional, analyte not elsewhere specified

82489   thin layer, analyte not elsewhere specified

● New Code   ▲ Revised Code   ✚ Add-On Code   ⊘ Modifier -51 Exempt   ☉ Moderate Sedation

82491 Chromatography, quantitative, column (eg, gas liquid or HPLC); single analyte not elsewhere specified, single stationary and mobile phase

82492 multiple analytes, single stationary and mobile phase

82495 Chromium

82507 Citrate

82520 Cocaine or metabolite

(Cocaine, qualitative analysis, see 80100-80103)

(Codeine, qualitative analysis, see 80100-80103)

(Codeine, quantitative analysis, see 82101)

(Complement, see 86160-86162)

82523 Collagen cross links, any method

82525 Copper

(Coproporphyrin, see 84119, 84120)

(Corticosteroids, use 83491)

82528 Corticosterone

82530 Cortisol; free

82533 total

(C-peptide, use 84681)

82540 Creatine

82541 Column chromatography/mass spectrometry (eg, GC/MS, or HPLC/MS), analyte not elsewhere specified; qualitative, single stationary and mobile phase

82542 quantitative, single stationary and mobile phase

82543 stable isotope dilution, single analyte, quantitative, single stationary and mobile phase

82544 stable isotope dilution, multiple analytes, quantitative, single stationary and mobile phase

| | Separate Procedure | | Unlisted Procedure | | CCI Comp. Code | | Non-specific Procedure | **1005** |

82550 Creatine kinase (CK), (CPK); total

82552   isoenzymes

82553   MB fraction only

82554   isoforms

82565 Creatinine; blood

82570   other source

82575   clearance

82585 Cryofibrinogen

82595 Cryoglobulin, qualitative or semi-quantitative (eg,cryocrit)

(For quantitative, cryoglobulin, see 82784, 82785)

(Crystals, pyrophosphate vs. urate, use 89060)

82600 Cyanide

82607 Cyanocobalamin (Vitamin B-12);

82608   unsaturated binding capacity

(Cyclic AMP, use 82030)

(Cyclic GMP, use 83008)

(Cyclosporine, use 80158)

82610 Cystatin C

82615 Cystine and homocystine, urine, qualitative

82626 Dehydroepiandrosterone (DHEA)

82627 Dehydroepiandrosterone-sulfate (DHEA-S)

(Delta-aminolevulinic acid (ALA), use 82135)

82633 Desoxycorticosterone, 11-

82634 Deoxycortisol, 11-

● New Code ▲ Revised Code + Add-On Code ⊘ Modifier -51 Exempt ⊙ Moderate Sedation

(Dexamethasone suppression test, use 80420)

(Diastase, urine, use 82150)

82638 Dibucaine number

(Dichloroethane, use 84600)

(Dichloromethane, use 84600)

(Diethylether, use 84600)

82646 Dihydrocodeinone

(For qualitative analysis, see 80100-80103)

82649 Dihydromorphinone

(For qualitative analysis, see 80100-80103)

82651 Dihydrotestosterone (DHT)

82652 This code is out of order. See page 1002

82654 Dimethadione

(For qualitative analysis, see 80100-80103)

(Diphenylhydantoin, use 80185)

(Dipropylacetic acid, use 80164)

(Dopamine, see 82382-82384)

(Duodenal contents, see individual enzymes; for intubation and collection, see 43756, 43757)

82656 Elastase, pancreatic (EL-1), fecal, qualitative or semi-quantitative

82657 Enzyme activity in blood cells, cultured cells, or tissue, not elsewhere specified; nonradioactive substrate, each specimen

82658   radioactive substrate, each specimen

82664 Electrophoretic technique, not elsewhere specified

(Endocrine receptor assays, see 84233-84235)`

82666 Epiandrosterone

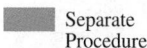 Separate Procedure

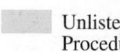 Unlisted Procedure

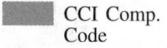 CCI Comp. Code

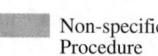 Non-specific Procedure

1007

(Epinephrine, see 82382-82384)

82668 Erythropoietin

82670 Estradiol

82671 Estrogens; fractionated

82672 total

(Estrogen receptor assay, use 84233)

82677 Estriol

82679 Estrone

(Ethanol, see 82055 and 82075)

82690 Ethchlorvynol

(Ethyl alcohol, see 82055 and 82075)

82693 Ethylene glycol

82696 Etiocholanolone

(For fractionation of ketosteroids, use 83593)

82705 Fat or lipids, feces; qualitative

82710   quantitative

82715 Fat differential, feces, quantitative

82725 Fatty acids, nonesterified

82726 Very long chain fatty acids

(For long-chain (C20-22) omega-3 fatty acids in red blood cell (RBC) membranes, use Category III code 0111T)

82728 Ferritin

(Fetal hemoglobin, see hemoglobin 83030, 83033, and 85460)

(Fetoprotein, alpha-1, see 82105, 82106)

82731 Fetal fibronectin, cervicovaginal secretions, semi-quantitative

---

1008 ● New Code ▲ Revised Code + Add-On Code ⊘ Modifier -51 Exempt ⊙ Moderate Sedation

82735 Fluoride

82742 Flurazepam

(For qualitative analysis, see 80100-80103)

(Foam stability test, use 83662)

82746 Folic acid; serum

82747 RBC

(Follicle stimulating hormone (FSH), use 83001)

82757 Fructose, semen

(Fructosamine, use 82985)

(Fructose, TLC screen, use 84375)

82759 Galactokinase, RBC

82760 Galactose

82775 Galactose-1-phosphate uridyl transferase; quantitative

82776 screen

● **82777** Galectin-3

82784 Gammaglobulin (immunoglobulin); IgA, IgD, IgG, IgM, each

82785 IgE

(For allergen specific IgE, see 86003, 86005)

82787 immunoglobulin subclasses (eg, IgG1, 2, 3, or 4), each

(Gamma-glutamyltransferase (GGT), use 82977)

82800 Gases, blood, pH only

82803 Gases, blood, any combination of pH, pCO_2, pO_2, CO_2, HCO_3 (including calculated O_2 saturation);

(Use 82803 for two or more of the above listed analytes)

82805 with O_2 saturation, by direct measurement, except pulse oximetry

	Separate Procedure		Unlisted Procedure		CCI Comp. Code		Non-specific Procedure

1009

82810	Gases, blood, O_2 saturation only, by direct measurement, except pulse oximetry

(For pulse oximetry, use 94760)

82820 Hemoglobin-oxygen affinity (pO2 for 50% hemoglobin saturation with oxygen)

(82926 deleted 2010 [2011 edition])

(82928 deleted 2010 [2011 edition])

(For gastric acid analysis, use 82930)

82930 Gastric acid analysis, includes pH if performed, each specimen

82938 Gastrin after secretin stimulation

82941 Gastrin

(Gentamicin, use 80170)

(GGT, use 82977)

(GLC, gas liquid chromatography, use 82486)

82943 Glucagon

82945 Glucose, body fluid, other than blood

82946 Glucagon tolerance test

82947 Glucose; quantitative, blood, (except reagent strip)

82948 blood, reagent strip

82950 post glucose dose (includes glucose)

82951 tolerance test (GTT), 3 specimens (includes glucose)

+ **82952** tolerance test, each additional beyond 3 specimens (List separately in addition to code for primary procedure)

(Use 82952 in conjunction with 82951)

82953 tolbutamide tolerance test

(For insulin tolerance test, see 80434, 80435)

● New Code　▲ Revised Code　+ Add-On Code　⊘ Modifier -51 Exempt　⊙ Moderate Sedation

(For leucine tolerance test, use 80428)

(For semiquantitative urine glucose, see 81000, 81002, 81005, 81099)

82955   Glucose-6-phosphate dehydrogenase (G6PD); quantitative

82960   screen

(For glucose tolerance test with medication, use 96374 in addition)

82962   Glucose, blood by glucose monitoring device(s) cleared by the FDA specifically for home use

82963   Glucosidase, beta

82965   Glutamate dehydrogenase

82975   Glutamine (glutamic acid amide)

82977   Glutamyltransferase, gamma (GGT)

82978   Glutathione

82979   Glutathione reductase, RBC

82980   Glutethimide

(Glycohemoglobin, use 83036)

82985   Glycated protein

(Gonadotropin, chorionic, see 84702, 84703)

83001   Gonadotropin; follicle stimulating hormone (FSH)

83002   luteinizing hormone (LH)

(For luteinizing releasing factor (LRH), use 83727)

83003   Growth hormone, human (HGH) (somatotropin)

(For antibody to human growth hormone, use 86277)

83008   Guanosine monophosphate (GMP), cyclic

1011

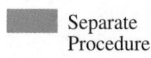 Separate Procedure   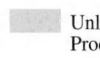 Unlisted Procedure   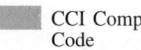 CCI Comp. Code   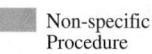 Non-specific Procedure

83009 Helicobacter pylori, blood test analysis for urease activity, non-radioactive isotope (eg, C-13)

(For H. pylori, breath test analysis for urease activity, see 83013, 83014)

83010 Haptoglobin; quantitative

83012 phenotypes

83013 Helicobacter pylori; breath test analysis for urease activity, non-radioactive isotope (eg, C-13)

83014 drug administration

(For H. pylori, stool, use 87338. For H. pylori, liquid scintillation counter, see 78267, 78268. For H. pylori, enzyme immunoassay, use 87339)

(For H. pylori, blood test analysis for urease activity, use 83009)

83015 Heavy metal (eg, arsenic, barium, beryllium, bismuth, antimony, mercury); screen

83018 quantitative, each

83020 Hemoglobin fractionation and quantitation; electrophoresis (eg, A2, S, C, and/or F)

83021 chromotography (eg, A2, S, C,and/or F)

(For glycosylated [A1c] hemoglobin analysis, by chromatography, in the absence of an identified hemoglobin variant, use 83036)

83026 Hemoglobin; by copper sulfate method, non-automated

83030 F (fetal), chemical

83033 F (fetal), qualitative

83036 glycosylated (A1C)

(For glycosylated [A1c] hemoglobin analysis, by chromatography, in the setting of an identified hemoglobin variant, use 83021)

(For fecal hemoglobin detection by immunoassay, use 82274)

1012 ● New Code   ▲ Revised Code   + Add-On Code   ⊘ Modifier -51 Exempt   ⊙ Moderate Sedation

83037   glycosylated (A1C) by device cleared by FDA for home use

83045   methemoglobin, qualitative

83050   methemoglobin, quantitative

(For transcutaneous quantitative methemoglobin determination, use 88741)

83051   plasma

83055   sulfhemoglobin, qualitative

83060   sulfhemoglobin, quantitative

83065   thermolabile

83068   unstable, screen

83069   urine

83070   Hemosiderin; qualitative

83071   quantitative

(Heroin, see 80100-80103)

(HIAA, use 83497)

(High performance liquid chromatography (HPLC), use 82486)

83080   b-Hexosaminidase, each assay

83088   Histamine

(Hollander test, see 43754, 43755)

83090   Homocystine

83150   Homovanillic acid (HVA)

(Hormones, see individual alphabetic listings in Chemistry section)

(Hydrogen breath test, use 91065)

83491   Hydroxycorticosteroids, 17- (17-OHCS)

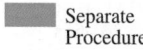 Separate Procedure   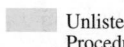 Unlisted Procedure   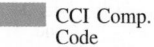 CCI Comp. Code   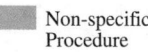 Non-specific Procedure   **1013**

(For cortisol, see 82530, 82533. For deoxycortisol, use 82634)

83497   Hydroxyindolacetic acid, 5-(HIAA)

(For urine qualitative test, use 81005)

(5-Hydroxytryptamine, use 84260)

83498   Hydroxyprogesterone, 17-d

83499   Hydroxyprogesterone, 20-

83500   Hydroxyproline; free

83505   total

83516   Immunoassay for analyte other than infectious agent antibody or infectious agent antigen; qualitative or semiquantitative, multiple step method

83518   qualitative or semiquantitative, single step method (eg, reagent strip)

83519   quantitative, by radioimmunoassay (eg, RIA)

83520   quantitative, not otherwise specified

(For immunoassays for antibodies to infectious agent antigens, see analyte and method specific codes in the Immunology section)

(For immunoassay of tumor antigen not elsewhere specified, use 86316)

(Immunoglobulins, see 82784, 82785)

83525   Insulin; total

(For proinsulin, use 84206)

83527   free

83528   Intrinsic factor

(For intrinsic factor antibodies, use 86340)

83540   Iron

83550   Iron binding capacity

● New Code   ▲ Revised Code   ✚ Add-On Code   ⊘ Modifier -51 Exempt   ⊙ Moderate Sedation

83570   Isocitric dehydrogenase (IDH)

(Isonicotinic acid hydrazide, INH, see code for specific method)

(Isopropyl alcohol, use 84600)

83582   Ketogenic steroids, fractionation

(Ketone bodies, for serum, see 82009, 82010; for urine, see 81000-81003)

83586   Ketosteroids, 17- (17-KS); total

83593   fractionation

83605   Lactate (lactic acid)

83615   Lactate dehydrogenase (LD), (LDH);

83625   isoenzymes, separation and quantitation

83630   Lactoferrin, fecal; qualitative

83631   quantitative

83632   Lactogen, human placental (HPL) human chorionic somatomammotropin

83633   Lactose, urine; qualitative

83634   quantitative

(For tolerance, see 82951, 82952)

(For breath hydrogen test for lactase deficiency, use 91065)

83655   Lead

83661   Fetal lung maturity assessment; lecithin-sphingomyelin ratio (L/S ratio)

83662   foam stability test

83663   fluorescence polarization

83664   lamellar body density

(For phosphatidylglycerol, use 84081)

| | Separate Procedure | | Unlisted Procedure | | CCI Comp. Code | | Non-specific Procedure |

83670 Leucine aminopeptidase (LAP)

83690 Lipase

83695 Lipoprotein (a)

83698 Lipoprotein-associated phospholipase A_2, (Lp-PLA_2)

83700 Lipoprotein, blood; electrophoretic separation and quantitation

83701 high resolution fractionation and quantitation of lipoproteins including lipoprotein subclasses when performed (eg, electrophoresis, ultracentrifugation)

83704 quantitation of lipoprotein particle numbers and lipoprotein particle subclasses (eg, by nuclear magnetic resonance spectroscopy)

83718 Lipoprotein, direct measurement; high density cholesterol (HDL cholesterol)

83719 VLDL cholesterol

83721 LDL cholesterol

(For fractionation by high resolution electrophoresis or ultracentrifugation, use 83701)

(For lipoprotein particle numbers and subclasses analysis by nuclear magnetic resonance spectroscopy, use 83695)

83727 Luteinizing releasing factor (LRH)

(Luteinizing hormone (LH), use 83002)

(For qualitative analysis, see 80100-80103)

(Macroglobulins, alpha-2, use 86329)

83735 Magnesium

83775 Malate dehydrogenase

(Maltose tolerance, see 82951, 82952)

(Mammotropin, use 84146)

83785 Manganese

● New Code   ▲ Revised Code   + Add-On Code   ⊘ Modifier -51 Exempt   ⊙ Moderate Sedation

(Marijuana, see 80100-80103)

83788 Mass spectrometry and tandem mass spectrometry (MS, MS/MS), analyte not elsewhere specified; qualitative, each specimen

83789   quantitative, each specimen

83805 Meprobamate

(For qualitative analysis, see 80100-80103)

83825 Mercury, quantitative

(Mercury screen, use 83015)

83835 Metanephrines

(For catecholamines, see 82382-82384)

83840 Methadone

(For methadone qualitative analysis, see 80100-80103)

(Methamphetamine, see 80100-80103, 82145)

(Methanol, use 84600)

83857 Methemalbumin

(Methemoglobin, see hemoglobin 83045, 83050)

83858 Methsuximide

(Methyl alcohol, use 84600)

(Microalbumin, see 82043 for quantitative, see 82044 for semiquantitative)

83861 Microfluidic analysis utilizing an integrated collection and analysis device, tear osmolarity

(Microglobulin, beta-2, use 82232)

(For microfluidic tear osmolarity of both eyes, report 83861 twice)

83864 Mucopolysaccharides, acid; quantitative

83866   screen

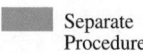 Separate Procedure   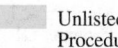 Unlisted Procedure   CCI Comp. Code   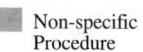 Non-specific Procedure   **1017**

83872   Mucin, synovial fluid (Ropes test)

83873   Myelin basic protein, cerebrospinal fluid
(For oligoclonal bands, use 83916)

83874   Myoglobin
(Nalorphine, use 83925)

83876   Myeloperoxidase (MPO)

83880   Natriuretic peptide

83883   Nephelometry, each analyte not elsewhere specified

83885   Nickel

83887   Nicotine

(83890   deleted 2012 [2013 edition]. To report, see 81200-81479)

(83891   deleted 2012 [2013 edition]. To report, see 81200-81479)

(83892   deleted 2012 [2013 edition]. To report, see 81200-81479)

(83893   deleted 2012 [2013 edition]. To report, see 81200-81479)

(83894   deleted 2012 [2013 edition]. To report, see 81200-81479)

(83896   deleted 2012 [2013 edition]. To report, see 81200-81479)

(83897   deleted 2012 [2013 edition]. To report, see 81200-81479)

(83898   deleted 2012 [2013 edition]. To report, see 81200-81479)

(83900   deleted 2012 [2013 edition]. To report, see 81200-81479)

(83901   deleted 2012 [2013 edition]. To report, see 81200-81479)

(83902   deleted 2012 [2013 edition]. To report, see 81200-81479)

(83903   deleted 2012 [2013 edition]. To report, see 81200-81479)

(83904   deleted 2012 [2013 edition]. To report, see 81200-81479)

(83905   deleted 2012 [2013 edition]. To report, see 81200-81479)

(83906   deleted 2012 [2013 edition]. To report, see 81200-81479)

(83907   deleted 2012 [2013 edition]. To report, see 81200-81479)

(83908   deleted 2012 [2013 edition]. To report, see 81200-81479)

(83909   deleted 2012 [2013 edition]. To report, see 81200-81479)

(83912   deleted 2012 [2013 edition]. To report, see 81200-81479)

(83913   deleted 2012 [2013 edition]. To report, see 81200-81479)

(83914   deleted 2012 [2013 edition]. To report, see 81200-81479)

83915   Nucleotidase 5-

83916   Oligoclonal immune (oligoclonal bands)

83918   Organic acids; total, quantitative, each specimen

83919   qualitative, each specimen

83921   Organic acid, single; quantitative

83925   Opiate(s), drug and metabolites, each procedure

83930   Osmolality; blood

83935   urine

     (For tear osmolarity using microfluidic analysis, use 83861)

83937   Osteocalcin (bone gla protein)

83945   Oxalate

83950   Oncoprotein; HER-2/neu

     (For tissue, see 88342, 88365)

83951   des-gamma-carboxy-prothrombin (DCP)

83970   Parathormone (parathyroid hormone)

1019

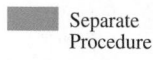 Separate Procedure   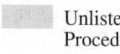 Unlisted Procedure   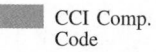 CCI Comp. Code   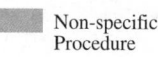 Non-specific Procedure

(Pesticide, quantitative, see code for specific method. For screen for chlorinated hydrocarbons, use 82441)

83986 pH; body fluid, not otherwise specified

83987 exhaled breath condensate

(For blood pH, see 82800, 82803)

83992 Phencyclidine (PCP)

(For qualitative analysis, see 80100-80103)

(Phenobarbital, use 80184)

83993 Calprotectin, fecal

84022 Phenothiazine

(For qualitative analysis, see 80100, 80101)

84030 Phenylalanine (PKU), blood

(Phenylalanine-tyrosine ratio, see 84030, 84510)

84035 Phenylketones, qualitative

84060 Phosphatase, acid; total

84061 forensic examination

84066 prostatic

84075 Phosphatase, alkaline;

84078 heat stable (total not included)

84080 isoenzymes

84081 Phosphatidylglycerol

(Phosphates inorganic, use 84100)

(Phosphates, organic, see code for specific method. For cholinesterase, see 82480, 82482)

84085 Phosphogluconate, 6-, dehydrogenase, RBC

● New Code   ▲ Revised Code   ✚ Add-On Code   ⊘ Modifier -51 Exempt   ⊙ Moderate Sedation

84087   Phosphohexose isomerase

84100   Phosphorus inorganic (phosphate);

84105   urine

(Pituitary gonadotropins, see 83001-83002)

(PKU, see 84030, 84035)

84106   Porphobilinogen, urine; qualitative

84110   quantitative

84112   Placental alpha microglobulin-1 (PAMG-1), cervicovaginal secretion, qualitative

84119   Porphyrins, urine; qualitative

84120   quantitation and fractionation

84126   Porphyrins, feces; quantitative

84127   qualitative

(Porphyrin precursors, see 82135, 84106, 84110)

(For protoporphyrin, RBC, see 84202, 84203)

84132   Potassium; serum, plasma or whole blood

84133   urine

84134   Prealbumin

(For microalbumin, see 82043, 82044)

84135   Pregnanediol

84138   Pregnanetriol

84140   Pregnenolone

84143   17-hydroxypregnenolone

84144   Progesterone

(Progesterone receptor assay, use 84234)

| Separate Procedure | Unlisted Procedure | CCI Comp. Code | Non-specific Procedure |

(For proinsulin, use 84206)

84145 Procalcitonin (PCT)

84146 Prolactin

84150 Prostaglandin, each

84152 Prostate specific antigen (PSA); complexed (direct measurement)

84153   total

84154   free

84155 Protein, total, except by refractometry; serum, plasma or whole blood

84156   urine

84157   other source (eg, synovial fluid, cerebrospinal fluid)

84160 Protein, total, by refractometry, any source

(For urine total protein by dipstick method, use 81000-81003)

84163 Pregnancy-associated plasma protein-A (PAPP-A)

84165 Protein; electrophoretic fractionation and quantitation, serum

84166 electrophoretic fractionation and quantitation, other fluids with concentration (eg, urine, CSF)

84181 Western Blot, with interpretation and report, blood or other body fluid

84182 Western Blot, with interpretation and report, blood or other body fluid, immunological probe for band identification, each

(For Western Blot tissue analysis, use 88371)

84202 Protoporphyrin, RBC; quantitative

84203   screen

84206 Proinsulin

● New Code   ▲ Revised Code   ✚ Add-On Code   ⊘ Modifier -51 Exempt   ⊙ Moderate Sedation

(Pseudocholinesterase, use 82480)

84207 Pyridoxal phosphate (Vitamin B-6)

84210 Pyruvate

84220 Pyruvate kinase

84228 Quinine

84233 Receptor assay; estrogen

84234 progesterone

84235 endocrine, other than estrogen or progesterone (specify hormone)

84238 non-endocrine (specify receptor)

84244 Renin

84252 Riboflavin (Vitamin B-2)

(Salicylates, use 80196)

(Secretin test, see 99070, 43756, 43757 and appropriate analyses)

84255 Selenium

84260 Serotonin

(For urine metabolites (HIAA), use 83497)

84270 Sex hormone binding globulin (SHBG)

84275 Sialic acid

(Sickle hemoglobin, use 85660)

84285 Silica

84295 Sodium; serum, plasma or whole blood

84300 urine

84302 other source

1023

 Separate Procedure   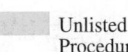 Unlisted Procedure   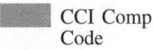 CCI Comp. Code   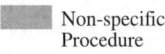 Non-specific Procedure

(Somatomammotropin, use 83632)

(Somatotropin, use 83003)

84305 Somatomedin

84307 Somatostatin

84311 Spectrophotometry, analyte not elsewhere specified

84315 Specific gravity (except urine)

(For specific gravity, urine, see 81000-81003)

(Stone analysis, see 82355-82370)

84375 Sugars, chromatographic, TLC or paper chromatography

84376 Sugars (mono, di, and oligosaccharides); single qualitative, each specimen

84377   multiple qualitative, each specimen

84378   single quantitative, each specimen

84379   multiple quantitative, each specimen

84392 Sulfate, urine

(Sulfhemoglobin, see hemoglobin, 83055, 83060)

(T-3, see 84479-84481)

(T-4, see 84436-84439)

84402 Testosterone; free

84403   total

84425 Thiamine (Vitamin B-1)

84430 Thiocyanate

84431 Thromboxane metabolite(s), including thromboxane if performed, urine

(For concurrent urine creatinine determination, use 84431 in conjunction with 82470)

● New Code ▲ Revised Code + Add-On Code ⊘ Modifier -51 Exempt ⊙ Moderate Sedation

84432 Thyroglobulin

(Thyroglobulin, antibody, use 86800)

(Thyrotropin releasing hormone (TRH) test, see 80438, 80439)

84436 Thyroxine; total

84437 requiring elution (eg, neonatal)

84439 free

84442 Thyroxine binding globulin (TBG)

84443 Thyroid stimulating hormone (TSH)

84445 Thyroid stimulating immune globulins (TSI)

(Tobramycin, use 80200)

84446 Tocopherol alpha (Vitamin E)

(Tolbutamide tolerance, use 82953)

84449 Transcortin (cortisol binding globulin)

84450 Transferase; aspartate amino (AST) (SGOT)

84460 alanine amino (ALT) (SGPT)

84466 Transferrin

(Iron binding capacity, use 83550)

84478 Triglycerides

84479 Thyroid hormone (T3 or T4) uptake or thyroid hormone binding ratio (THBR)

84480 Triiodothyronine T3; total (TT-3)

84481 free

84482 reverse

84484 Troponin, quantitative

(For Troponin, qualitative assay, use 84512)

	Separate Procedure		Unlisted Procedure		CCI Comp. Code		Non-specific Procedure

1025

84485   Trypsin; duodenal fluid

84488   feces, qualitative

84490   feces, quantitative, 24-hour collection

84510   Tyrosine

(Urate crystal identification, use 89060)

84512   Troponin, qualitative

(For Troponin, quantitative assay, use 84484)

84520   Urea nitrogen; quantitative

84525   semiquantitative (eg, reagent strip test)

84540   Urea nitrogen, urine

84545   Urea nitrogen, clearance

84550   Uric acid; blood

84560   other source

84577   Urobilinogen, feces, quantitative

84578   Urobilinogen, urine; qualitative

84580   quantitative, timed specimen

84583   semiquantitative

(Uroporphyrins, use 84120)

(Valproic acid (dipropylacetic acid), ues 80164)

84585   Vanillylmandelic acid (VMA), urine

84586   Vasoactive intestinal peptide (VIP)

84588   Vasopressin (antidiuretic hormone, ADH)

84590   Vitamin A

(Vitamin B-1, use 84425)

● New Code ▲ Revised Code ＋ Add-On Code ⊘ Modifier -51 Exempt ⊙ Moderate Sedation

(Vitamin B-2, use 84252)

(Vitamin B-6, use 84207)

(Vitamin B-12, use 82607)

(Vitamin B-12, absorption (Schilling), see 78270, 78271)

(Vitamin C, use 82180)

(Vitamin D, see 82306, 82652)

(Vitamin E, use 84446)

84591 Vitamin, not otherwise specified

84597 Vitamin K

(VMA, use 84585)

84600 Volatiles (eg, acetic anhydride, carbon tetrachloride, dichloroethane, dichloromethane, diethylether, isopropyl alcohol, methanol)

(For acetaldehyde, use 82000)

(Volume, blood, RISA or Cr-51, see 78110, 78111)

84620 Xylose absorption test, blood and/or urine

(For administration, use 99070)

84630 Zinc

84681 C-peptide

84702 Gonadotropin, chorionic (hCG); quantitative

84703 qualitative

(For urine pregnancy test by visual color comparison, use 81025)

84704 free beta chain

84830 Ovulation tests, by visual color comparison methods for human luteinizing hormone

84999 Unlisted chemistry procedure

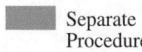 Separate Procedure

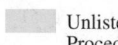 Unlisted Procedure

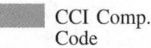 CCI Comp. Code

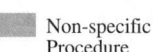 Non-specific Procedure

HEMATOLOGY AND COAGULATION

(For blood banking procedures, see Transfusion Medicine)

(Agglutinins, see Immunology)

(Antiplasmin, use 85410)

(Antithrombin III, see 85300, 85301)

85002 Bleeding time

85004 Blood count; automated differential WBC count

85007 blood smear, microscopic examination with manual differential WBC count

85008 blood smear, microscopic examination without manual differential WBC count

(For other fluids (eg, CSF), see 89050, 89051)

85009 manual differential WBC count, buffy coat

(Eosinophils, nasal smear, use 89190)

85013 spun microhematocrit

85014 hematocrit (Hct)

85018 hemoglobin (Hgb)

(For other hemoglobin determination, see 83020-83069)

(For immunoassay, hemoglobin, fecal, use 82274)

(For transcutaneous hemoglobin measurement, use 88738)

85025 complete (CBC), automated (Hgb, Hct, RBC, WBC and platelet count) and automated differential WBC count

85027 complete (CBC), automated (Hgb, Hct, RBC, WBC and platelet count)

85032 manual cell count (erythrocyte, leukocyte, or platelet) each

85041 red blood cell (RBC), automated

● New Code ▲ Revised Code + Add-On Code ⊘ Modifier -51 Exempt ⊙ Moderate Sedation

(Do not report code 85041 in conjunction with 85025 or 85027)

85044   reticulocyte, manual

85045   reticulocyte, automated

85046   reticulocytes, automated, including 1 or more cellular parameters (eg, reticulocyte hemoglobin content [CHr], immature reticulocyte fraction [IRF], reticulocyte volume [mrv], RNA content), direct measurement

85048   leukocyte (WBC), automated

85049   platelet, automated

85055   Reticulated platelet assay

85060   Blood smear, peripheral, interpretation by physician with written report

85097   Bone marrow, smear interpretation

(For special stains, see 85540, 88312, 88313)

(For bone biopsy, see 20220, 20225, 20240, 20245, 20250, 20251)

85130   Chromogenic substrate assay

(Circulating anti-coagulant screen (mixing studies), see 85611, 85732)

85170   Clot retraction

85175   Clot lysis time, whole blood dilution

(Clotting factor I (fibrinogen), see 85384, 85385)

85210   Clotting; factor II, prothrombin, specific

(See also 85610-85613)

85220   factor V (AcG or proaccelerin), labile factor

85230   factor VII (proconvertin, stable factor)

85240   factor VIII (AHG), 1 stage

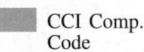

				1029
Separate Procedure	Unlisted Procedure	CCI Comp. Code	Non-specific Procedure	

85244	factor VIII related antigen
85245	factor VIII, VW factor, ristocetin cofactor
85246	factor VIII, VW factor antigen
85247	factor VIII, von Willebrands factor, multimetric analysis
85250	factor IX (PTC or Christmas)
85260	factor X (Stuart-Prower)
85270	factor XI (PTA)
85280	factor XII (Hageman)
85290	factor XIII (fibrin stabilizing)
85291	factor XIII (fibrin stabilizing), screen solubility
85292	prekallikrein assay (Fletcher factor assay)
85293	high molecular weight kininogen assay (Fitzgerald factor assay)
85300	Clotting inhibitors or anticoagulants; antithrombin III, activity
85301	antithrombin III, antigen assay
85302	protein C, antigen
85303	protein C, activity
85305	protein S, total
85306	protein S, free
85307	Activated Protein C (APC) resistance assay
85335	Factor inhibitor test
85337	Thrombomodulin

(For mixing studies for inhibitors, use 85732)

● New Code   ▲ Revised Code   + Add-On Code   ⊘ Modifier -51 Exempt   ⊙ Moderate Sedation

85345	Coagulation time; Lee and White

85347   activated

85348   other methods

(Differential count, see 85007 et seq)

(Duke bleeding time, use 85002)

(Eosinophils, nasal smear, use 89190)

85360 Euglobulin lysis

(Fetal hemoglobin, see 83030, 83033, 85460)

85362 Fibrin(ogen) degradation (split) products (FDP)(FSP); agglutination slide, semiquantitative

(Immunoelectrophoresis, use 86320)

85366   paracoagulation

85370   quantitative

85378 Fibrin degradation products, D-dimer; qualitative or semiquantitative

85379   quantitative

(For ultrasensitive and standard sensitivity quantitative D-dimer, use 85379)

85380   ultrasensitive (eg., for evaluation for venous thromboembolism), qualitative or semiquantitative

85384 Fibrinogen; activity

85385   antigen

85390 Fibrinolysins or coagulopathy screen, interpretation and report

85396 Coagulation/fibrinolysis assay, whole blood (eg, viscoelastic clot assessment), including use of any pharmacologic additive(s), as indicated, including interpretation and written report, per day

85397 Coagulation and fibrinolysis, functional activity, not otherwise specified (eg, adamts-13), each analyte

1031

	Separate Procedure		Unlisted Procedure		CCI Comp. Code		Non-specific Procedure

85400	Fibrinolytic factors and inhibitors; plasmin
85410	alpha-2 antiplasmin
85415	plasminogen activator
85420	plasminogen, except antigenic assay
85421	plasminogen, antigenic assay

(Fragility, red blood cell, see 85547, 85555-85557)

85441	Heinz bodies; direct
85445	induced, acetyl phenylhydrazine

(Hematocrit (PCV), see 85014)

(Hemoglobin, see 83020-83068, 85018-85027)

85460	Hemoglobin or RBCs, fetal, for fetomaternal hemorrhage; differential lysis (Kleihauer-Betke)

(See also 83030, 83033)

(Hemolysins, see 86940, 86941)

85461	rosette
85475	Hemolysin, acid

(See also 86940, 86941)

85520	Heparin assay
85525	Heparin neutralization
85530	Heparin-protamine tolerance test
85536	Iron stain, peripheral blood

(For iron stains on bone marrow or other tissues with physician evaluation, use 88313)

85540	Leukocyte alkaline phosphatase with count
85547	Mechanical fragility, RBC

● New Code   ▲ Revised Code   + Add-On Code   ⊘ Modifier -51 Exempt   ⊙ Moderate Sedation

85549 Muramidase

(Nitroblue tetrazolium dye test, use 86384)

85555 Osmotic fragility, RBC; unincubated

85557   incubated

(Packed cell volume, use 85013)

(Partial thromboplastin time, see 85730, 85732)

(Parasites, blood (eg, malaria smears), use 87207)

(Plasmin, use 85400)

(Plasminogen, use 85420)

(Plasminogen activator, use 85415)

85576 Platelet; aggregation (in vitro), each agent

(For thromboxane metabolite[s], including thromboxane, if performed, measurement[s] in urine, use 84431)

85597 Phospholipid neutralization; platelet

85598   hexagonal phospholipid

85610 Prothrombin time;

85611   substitution, plasma fractions, each

85612 Russell viper venom time (includes venom); undiluted

85613   diluted

(Red blood cell count, see 85025, 85027, 85041)

85635 Reptilase test

(Reticulocyte count, see 85044, 85045)

85651 Sedimentation rate, erythrocyte; non-automated

85652   automated

85660 Sickling of RBC, reduction

1033

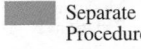 Separate Procedure    Unlisted Procedure   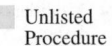 CCI Comp. Code   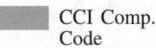 Non-specific Procedure

(Hemoglobin electrophoresis, use 83020)

(Smears (eg, for parasites, malaria), use 87207)

85670 Thrombin time; plasma

85675 titer

85705 Thromboplastin inhibition, tissue

(For individual clotting factors, see 85245-85247)

85730 Thromboplastin time, partial (PTT); plasma or whole blood

85732 substitution, plasma fractions, each

85810 Viscosity

(von Willebrand factor assay, see 85245-85247)

(WBC count, see 85025-85031, 85048, 89050)

85999 Unlisted hematology and coagulation procedure

IMMUNOLOGY

(Acetylcholine receptor antibody, see 83519, 86255, 86256)

(Actinomyces, antibodies to, use 86602)

(Adrenal cortex antibodies, see 86255, 86256)

86000 Agglutinins, febrile (eg, Brucella, Francisella, Murine typhus, Q fever, Rocky Mountain spotted fever, scrub typhus), each antigen

(For antibodies to infectious agents, see 86602-86804)

86001 Allergen specific IgG quantitative or semiquantitative, each allergen

(Agglutinins and autohemolysins, see 86940, 86941)

86003 Allergen specific IgE; quantitative or semiquantitative, each allergen

(For total quantitative IgE, use 82785)

86005 qualitative, multiallergen screen (dipstick, paddle or disk)

1034 ● New Code   ▲ Revised Code   + Add-On Code   ⊘ Modifier -51 Exempt   ⊙ Moderate Sedation

(For total qualitative IgE, use 83518)

(Alpha-1 antitrypsin, see 82103, 82104)

(Alpha-1 feto-protein, see 82105, 82106)

(Anti-AChR (acetylcholine receptor) antibody titer, see 86255, 86256)

(Anticardiolipin antibody, use 86147)

(Anti-DNA, use 86225)

(Anti-deoxyribonuclease titer, use 86215)

86021 Antibody identification; leukocyte antibodies

86022 platelet antibodies

86023 platelet associated immunoglobulin assay

86038 Antinuclear antibodies (ANA);

86039 titer

(Antistreptococcal antibody, ie, anti-DNAse, use 86215)

(Antistreptokinase titer, use 86590)

86060 Antistreptolysin 0; titer

(For antibodies to infectious agents, see 86602-86804)

86063 screen

(For antibodies to infectious agents, see 86602-86804)

(Blastomyces, antibodies to, use 86612)

86077 Blood bank physician services; difficult cross match and/or evaluation of irregular antibody(s), interpretation and written report

86078 investigation of transfusion reaction including suspicion of transmissible disease, interpretation and written report

86079 authorization for deviation from standard blood banking procedures (eg, use of outdated blood, transfusion of Rh incompatible units), with written report

(Brucella, antibodies to, use 86622)

1035

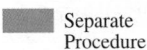 Separate Procedure   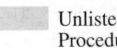 Unlisted Procedure   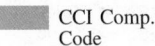 CCI Comp. Code   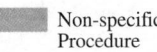 Non-specific Procedure

(Candida, antibodies to, use 86628. For skin testing, use 86485)

86140   C-reactive protein;

(Candidiasis, use 86628)

86141   high sensitivity (hsCRP)

86146   Beta 2 Glycoprotein 1 antibody, each

86147   Cardiolipin (phospholipid) antibody, each Ig class

● **86152**   Cell enumeration using immunologic selection and identification in fluid specimen (eg, circulating tumor cells in blood);

(For physician interpretation and report, use 86153. For cell enumeration with interpretation and report, use 86152 and 86153)

● **86153**   physician interpretation and report, when required

(For cell enumeration, use 86152. For cell enumeration with interpretation and report, use 86152 and 86153)

(For flow cytometric immunophenotyping, see 88184-88189)

(For flow cytometric quantitation, see 86355, 86356, 86357, 86359, 86360, 86361, 86367)

86148   Anti-phosphatidylserine (phospholipid) antibody

(To report antiprothrombin (phospholipid cofactor) antibody, use 86849)

(For cell enumeration using immunologic selection and identification in fluid specimen [eg, circulating tumor cells in blood], see 0279T, 0280T)

86152   Code out of order. See page 1036

86153   Code out of order. See page 1036

86155   Chemotaxis assay, specify method

(Clostridium difficile toxin, use 87230)

(Coccidioides, antibodies, to, see 86635. For skin testing, use 86490)

86156   Cold agglutinin; screen

| ● New Code | ▲ Revised Code | + Add-On Code | ⊘ Modifier -51 Exempt | ⊙ Moderate Sedation |

86157   titer

86160 Complement; antigen, each component

86161   functional activity, each component

86162   total hemolytic (CH50)

86171 Complement fixation tests, each antigen

(Coombs test, see 86880-86886)

86185 Counterimmunoelectrophoresis, each antigen

(Cryptococcus, antibodies to, use 86641)

86200 Cyclic citrullinated peptide (CCP), antibody

86215 Deoxyribonuclease, antibody

86225 Deoxyribonucleic acid (DNA) antibody; native or double stranded

(Echinococcus, antibodies to, see code for specific method)

(For HIV antibody tests, see 86701-86703)

86226   single stranded

(Anti D.S., DNA, IFA, eg, using C.Lucilae, see 86255 and 86256)

86235 Extractable nuclear antigen, antibody to, any method (eg, nRNP, SS-A, SS-B, Sm, RNP, Sc170, J01), each antibody

86243 Fc receptor

(Filaria, antibodies to, see code for specific method)

86255 Fluorescent noninfectious agent antibody; screen, each antibody

86256   titer, each antibody

(Fluorescent technique for antigen identification in tissue, use 88346; for indirect fluorescence, use 88347)

(FTA, use 86780)

(Gel (agar) diffusion tests, use 86331)

| | Separate Procedure | | Unlisted Procedure | | CCI Comp. Code | | Non-specific Procedure | **1037** |

86277   Growth hormone, human (HGH), antibody

86280   Hemagglutination inhibition test (HAI)

(For rubella, use 86762)

(For antibodies to infectious agents, see 86602-86804)

86294   Immunoassay for tumor antigen, qualitative or semiquantitative (eg, bladder tumor antigen)

(for qualitative NMP22 protein, use 86386)

86300   Immunoassay for tumor antigen, quantitative; CA 15-3 (27.29)

86301   CA 19-9

86304   CA 125

(For measurement of serum HER-2/neu oncoprotein, see 83950)

(For hepatitis delta agent, antibody, use 86692)

86305   Human epididymis protein 4 (HE4)

86308   Heterophile antibodies; screening

(For antibodies to infectious agents, see 86602-86804)

86309   titer

(For antibodies to infectious agents, see 86602-86804)

86310   titers after absorption with beef cells and guinea pig kidney

(Histoplasma, antibodies to, use 86698. For skin testing, use 86510)

(For antibodies to infectious agents, see 86602-86804)

(Human growth hormone antibody, use 86277)

86316   Immunoassay for tumor antigen, other antigen, quantitative (eg, CA 50, 72-4, 549), each

86317   Immunoassay for infectious agent antibody, quantitative, not otherwise specified

(For immunoassay techniques for antigens, see 83516, 83518, 83519, 83520, 87301-87450, 87810-87899)

1038   ● New Code   ▲ Revised Code   + Add-On Code   ⦸ Modifier -51 Exempt   ⊙ Moderate Sedation

(For particle agglutination procedures, use 86403)

86318 Immunoassay for infectious agent antibody, qualitative or semiquantitative, single step method (eg, reagent strip)

86320 Immunoelectrophoresis; serum

86325 other fluids (eg, urine, cerebrospinal fluid) with concentration

86327 crossed (2-dimensional assay)

86329 Immunodiffusion; not elsewhere specified

86331 gel diffusion, qualitative (Ouchterlony), each antigen or antibody

86332 Immune complex assay

86334 Immunofixation electrophoresis; serum

86335 other fluids with concentration (eg, urine, CSF)

86336 Inhibin A

86337 Insulin antibodies

86340 Intrinsic factor antibodies

(Leptospira, antibodies to, use 86720)

(Leukoagglutinins, use 86021)

86341 Islet cell antibody

86343 Leukocyte histamine release test (LHR)

86344 Leukocyte phagocytosis

86352 Cellular function assay involving stimulation (eg, mitogen or antigen) and detection of biomarker (eg, ATP)

86353 Lymphocyte transformation, mitogen (phytomitogen) or antigen induced blastogenesis

(Malaria antibodies, use 86750)

1039

| | Separate Procedure | | Unlisted Procedure | | CCI Comp. Code | | Non-specific Procedure |

(For cellular function assay involving stimulation and detection of biomarker, use 86352)

86355 B cells, total count

86356 Mononuclear cell antigen, quantitive (eg, flow cytometry), not otherwise specified, each antigen

(Do not report 88187-88189 for interpretation of 86355, 86356, 86357, 86359, 86360, 86361, 86367)

86357 Natural killer (NK) cells, total count

86359 T cells; total count

86360 absolute CD4 and CD8 count, including ratio

86361 absolute CD4 count

86367 Stem cells (ie, CD34), total count

(For flow cytometric immunophenotyping for the assessment of potential hematolymphoid neoplasia, see 88184-88189)

86376 Microsomal antibodies (eg, thyroid or liver-kidney), each

86378 Migration inhibitory factor test (MIF)

(Mitochondrial antibody, liver, see 86255, 86256)

(Mononucleosis, see 86308-86310)

86382 Neutralization test, viral

86384 Nitroblue tetrazolium dye test (NTD)

86386 Nuclear Matrix Protein 22 (NMP22), qualitative

(Ouchterlony diffusion, use 86331)

(Platelet antibodies, see 86022, 86023)

86403 Particle agglutination; screen, each antibody

86406 titer, each antibody

(Pregnancy test, see 84702, 84703)

(Rapid plasma reagin test (RPR), see 86592, 86593)

86430 Rheumatoid factor; qualitative

86431   quantitative

(Serologic test for syphilis, see 86592, 86593)

86480 Tuberculosis test, cell mediated immunity antigen response measurement; gamma interferon

86481   enumeration of gamma interferon-producing T-cells in cell suspension

86485 Skin test; candida

(For antibody, candida, use 86628)

86486   unlisted antigen, each

86490   coccidioidomycosis

86510   histoplasmosis

(For histoplasma, antibody, use 86698)

86580   tuberculosis, intradermal

(For tuberculosis test, cell mediated immunity measurement of gamma interferon antigen response, use 86480)

(For skin tests for allergy, see 95012-95199)

(Smooth muscle antibody, see 86255, 86256)

(Sporothrix, antibodies to, see code for specific method)

(For skin testing, unlisted antigen, use 86486. For flow cytometry, quantitative, not otherwise specified, use 86356)

86590 Streptokinase, antibody

(For antibodies to infectious agents, see 86602-86804)

(Streptolysin O antibody, see antistreptolysin O, 86060, 86063)

86592 Syphilis test, non-treponemal antibody; qualitative (eg, VDRL, RPR, ART)

(For antibodies to infectious agents, see 86602-86804)

86593   quantitative

| | Separate Procedure | | Unlisted Procedure | | CCI Comp. Code | | Non-specific Procedure | **1041** |

(For antibodies to infectious agents, see 86602-86804)

(Tetanus antibody, use 86774)

(Thyroglobulin antibody, use 86800)

(Thyroglobulin, use 84432)

(Thyroid microsomal antibody, use 86376)

(For toxoplasma antibody, see 86777-86778)

The following codes (86602-86804) are qualitative or semiquantitative immunoassays performed by multiple-step methods for the detection of antibodies to infectious agents. For immunoassays by single-step method (eg., reagent strips), use code 86318. Procedures for the identification of antibodies should be coded as precisely as possible. For example, an antibody to a virus could be coded with increasing specificity for virus, family, genus, species or type. In some cases, further precision may be added to codes by specifying the class of immunoglobulin being detected. When multiple tests are done to detect antibodies to organisms classified more precisely than the specificity allowed by available codes, it is appropriate to code each as a separate service. For example, a test for antibody to an enterovirus is coded as 86658. Coxsackie viruses are enteroviruses, but there are no codes for the individual species of enterovirus. If assays are performed for antibodies to coxsackie A and B species, each assay should be separately coded. Similarly, if multiple assays are performed for antibodies of different immunoglobulin classes, each assay should be coded separately. When a coding option exists for reporting IgM specific antibodies (eg., 86632), the corresponding nonspecific code (eg., 86631) may be reported for performance of either an antibody analysis not specific for a particular immunoglobulin class or for an IgG analysis.

(For the detection of antibodies other than those to infectious agents, see specific antibody [eg, 86021, 86022, 86023, 86376, 86800, 86850-86870] or specific method [eg, 83516, 86255, 86256])

(For infectious agent/antigen detection, see 87260-87899)

86602   Antibody; actinomyces

86603   adenovirus

86606   Aspergillus

86609   bacterium, not elsewhere specified

86611   Bartonella

86612	Blastomyces
86615	Bordetella
86617	Borrelia burgdorferi (Lyme disease) confirmatory test (eg, Western blot or immunoblot)
86618	Borrelia burgdorferi (Lyme disease)
86619	Borrelia (relapsing fever)
86622	Brucella
86625	Campylobacter
86628	Candida

(For skin test, candida, use 86485)

86631	Chlamydia
86632	Chlamydia, IgM

(For chlamydia antigen, see 87270, 87320. For fluorescent antibody technique, see 86255, 86256)

86635	Coccidioides
86638	Coxiella Brunetii (Q fever)
86641	Cryptococcus
86644	cytomegalovirus (CMV)
86645	cytomegalovirus (CMV), IgM
86648	Diphtheria
86651	encephalitis, California (La Crosse)
86652	encephalitis, Eastern equine
86653	encephalitis, St. Louis
86654	encephalitis, Western equine

1043

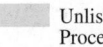 Separate Procedure   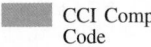 Unlisted Procedure   CCI Comp. Code   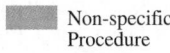 Non-specific Procedure

86658   enterovirus (eg, coxsackie, echo, polio)

(Trichinella, antibodies to, use 86784)

(Trypanosoma, antibodies to, see code for specific method)

(Tuberculosis, use 86580 for skin testing)

(Viral antibodies, see code for specific method)

86663   Epstein-Barr (EB) virus, early antigen (EA)

86664   Epstein-Barr (EB) virus, nuclear antigen (EBNA)

86665   Epstein-Barr (EB) virus, viral capsid (VCA)

86666   Ehrlichia

86668   Francisella Tularensis

86671   fungus, not elsewhere specified

86674   Giardia Lamblia

86677   Helicobacter Pylori

86682   helminth, not elsewhere specified

86684   Hemophilus influenza

86687   HTLV-I

86688   HTLV-II

86689   HTLV or HIV antibody, confirmatory test (eg, Western Blot)

86692   hepatitis, delta agent

(For hepatitis delta agent, antigen, use 87380)

86694   herpes simplex, non-specific type test

86695   herpes simplex, type 1

86696   herpes simplex, type 2

1044 ● New Code   ▲ Revised Code   + Add-On Code   ⊘ Modifier -51 Exempt   ⊙ Moderate Sedation

86698   histoplasma

86701   HIV-1

86702   HIV-2

86703   HIV-1 and HIV-2, single result

(For HIV-1 antigen(s) with HIV-1 and HIV-2 antibodies, single result, use 87389)

(When HIV immunoassay [HIV testing 86701-86703 or 87389] is performed using a kit or transportable instrument that wholly or in part consists of a single use, disposable analytical chamber, the service may be identified by adding modifier 92 to the usual code)

(For HIV-1 antigen, use 87390)

(For HIV-2 antigen, use 87391)

(For confirmatory test for HIV antibody (eg, Western Blot), use 86689)

86704   Hepatitis B core antibody (HBcAb); total

86705   IgM antibody

86706   Hepatitis B surface antibody (HBsAb)

86707   Hepatitis Be antibody (HBeAb)

86708   Hepatitis A antibody (HAAb); total

86709   IgM antibody

86710   Antibody; influenza virus

● **86711**   JC (John Cunningham) virus

86713   Legionella

86717   Leishmania

86720   Leptospira

86723   Listeria monocytogenes

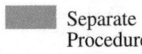 Separate Procedure    Unlisted Procedure   CCI Comp. Code   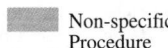 Non-specific Procedure

86727	lymphocytic choriomeningitis
86729	Lymphogranuloma Venereum
86732	mucormycosis
86735	mumps
86738	Mycoplasma
86741	Neisseria meningitidis
86744	Nocardia
86747	parvovirus
86750	Plasmodium (malaria)
86753	protozoa, not elsewhere specified
86756	respiratory syncytial virus
86757	Rickettsia
86759	rotavirus
86762	rubella
86765	rubeola
86768	Salmonella
86771	Shigella
86774	tetanus
86777	Toxoplasma
86778	Toxoplasma, IgM
86780	Treponema pallidum

(86781   Deleted 2009 [2010 edition])

(For syphilis testing by non-treponemal antibody analysis, see 86592-86593)

● New Code   ▲ Revised Code   + Add-On Code   ⃠ Modifier -51 Exempt   ☉ Moderate Sedation

86784	Trichinella
86787	varicella-zoster
86788	West Nile virus, IgM
86789	West Nile virus
86790	virus, not elsewhere specified
86793	Yersinia
86800	Thyroglobulin antibody

(For thyroglobulin, use 84432)

86803	Hepatitis C antibody;
86804	confirmatory test (eg, immunoblot)

TISSUE TYPING

86805	Lymphocytotoxicity assay, visual crossmatch; with titration
86806	without titration
86807	Serum screening for cytotoxic percent reactive antibody (PRA); standard method
86808	quick method
86812	HLA typing; A, B, or C (eg, A10, B7, B27), single antigen
86813	A, B, or C, multiple antigens
86816	DR/DQ, single antigen
86817	DR/DQ, multiple antigens
86821	lymphocyte culture, mixed (MLC)
86822	lymphocyte culture, primed (PLC)

(For HLA typing by molecular pathology techniques, see 81370-81383)

1047

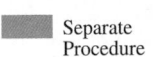 Separate Procedure   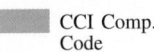 Unlisted Procedure   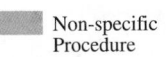 CCI Comp. Code   Non-specific Procedure

86825   Human leukocyte antigen (HLA) crossmatch, non cytotoxic (eg, using flow cytometry); first serum sample or dilution

+ 86826   each additional serum sample or sample dilution (List separately in addition to primary procedure)

     (Use 86826 in conjunction with 86825)

     (Do not report 86825, 86826 in conjunction with 86355, 86359, 88184-88189 for antibody surface markers integral to crossmatch testing)

     (For autologous HLA crossmatch, see 86825, 86826)

     (For lymphocytotoxicity visual crossmatch, see 86805, 86806)

● 86828   Antibody to human leukocyte antigens (HLA), solid phase assays (eg, microspheres or beads, ELISA, flow cytometry); qualitative assessment of the presence of absence of antibody(ies) to HLA Class I and Class II HLA antigens

● 86829   qualitative assessment of the presence or absence of antibody(ies) to HLA Class I or Class II HLA antigens

     (If solid phase testing is performed to assess presence or absence of antibody to both HLA classes, use 86828)

● 86830   antibody identification by qualitative panel using complete HLA phenotypes, HLA Class I

● 86831   antibody identification by qualitative panel using complete HLA phenotypes, HLA Class II

● 86832   high definition qualitative panel for identification of antibody sepcificities (eg, individual antigen per bead methodology), HLA Class I

● 86833   high definition qualitative panel for identification of antibody specificities (eg, individual antigen per bead methodology), HLA Class II

     (If solid phase testing is performed to test for HLA Class I or II antibody after treatment [eg, to remove IgM antibodies or other interfering substances], report 86828-86833 once for each panel with the untreated serum and once for each panel with the treated serum)

● 86834   semi-quantitative panel (eg, titer), HLA Class I

● 86835   semi-quantiative panel (eg, titer), HLA Class II

86849   Unlisted immunology procedure

● New Code   ▲ Revised Code   + Add-On Code   ⊘ Modifier -51 Exempt   ⊙ Moderate Sedation

TRANSFUSION MEDICINE

(For apheresis, see 36511-36512)

(For therapeutic phlebotomy, use 99195)

86850 Antibody screen, RBC, each serum technique

86860 Antibody elution (RBC), each elution

86870 Antibody identification, RBC antibodies, each panel for each serum technique

86880 Antihuman globulin test (Coombs test); direct, each antiserum

86885 indirect, qualitative, each reagent red cell

86886 indirect, each antibody titer

(For indirect antihuman globulin [Coombs] test for RBC antibody screening, use 86850)

(For indirect antihuman globulin [Coombs] test for RBC antibody identification using reagent red cell panels, use 86870)

86890 Autologous blood or component, collection processing and storage; predeposited

86891 intra-or postoperative salvage

86900 Blood typing; ABO

86901 Rh (D)

86902 antigen testing of donor blood using reagent serum, each antigen test

(If multiple blood units are tested for the same antigen, 86902 should be reported once for each antigen for each unit tested.)

(86903 deleted 2010 [2011 edition]. To report, use 86902.)

86904 antigen screening for compatible unit using patient serum, per unit screened

86905 RBC antigens, other than ABO or Rh (D), each

1049

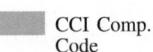

| Separate Procedure | Unlisted Procedure | CCI Comp. Code | Non-specific Procedure |

86906   Rh phenotyping, complete

86910   Blood typing, for paternity testing, per individual; ABO, Rh and MN

86911   each additional antigen system

86920   Compatibility test each unit; immediate spin technique

86921   incubation technique

86922   antiglobulin technique

86923   electronic

            (Do not use 86923 in conjunction with 86920-86922 for same unit crossmatch)

86927   Fresh frozen plasma, thawing, each unit

86930   Frozen blood, each unit; freezing (includes preparation)

86931   thawing

86932   freezing (includes preparation) and thawing

86940   Hemolysins and agglutinins; auto, screen, each

86941   incubated

86945   Irradiation of blood product, each unit

86950   Leukocyte transfusion

            (For leukapheresis, see 36511-36512)

86960   Volume reduction of blood or blood product (eg, red blood cells or platelets), each unit

86965   Pooling of platelets or other blood products

            (For injection(s) of platelet rich plasma, use 0232T)

86970   Pretreatment of RBCs for use in RBC antibody detection, identification, and/or compatibility testing; incubation with chemical agents or drugs, each

---

1050   ● New Code   ▲ Revised Code   ＋ Add-On Code   ⊘ Modifier -51 Exempt   ⊙ Moderate Sedation

86971   incubation with enzymes, each

86972   by density gradient separation

86975   Pretreatment of serum for use in RBC antibody identification; incubation with drugs, each

86976   by dilution

86977   incubation with inhibitors, each

86978   by differential red cell absorption using patient RBCs or RBCs of known phenotype, each absorption

86985   Splitting of blood or blood products, each unit

86999   Unlisted transfusion medicine procedure

MICROBIOLOGY

Includes bacteriology, mycology, parasitology, and virology.

Presumptive identification of microorganisms is defined as identification by colony morphology, growth on selective media, Gram stains, or up to three tests (eg., catalase, oxidase, indole, urease). Definitive identification of microorganisms is defined as an identification to the genus or species level that requires additional tests (eg., biochemical panels, slide cultures). If additional studies involve molecular probes, nucleic acid sequencing, chromatography, or immunologic techniques, these should be separately coded using 87140-87158, in addition to definitive identification codes. The molecular diagnostic codes (eg., 81200-81408) are not to be used in combination with or instead of the procedures represented by 87140-87158. For multiple specimens/sites, used modifier 59. For repeat laboratory tests performed on the same day, use modifier 91.

87001   Animal inoculation, small animal; with observation

87003   with observation and dissection

87015   Concentration (any type), for infectious agents

(Do not report 87015 in conjunction with 87177)

87040   Culture, bacterial; blood, aerobic, with isolation and presumptive identification of isolates (includes anaerobic culture, if appropriate)

1051

 Separate Procedure   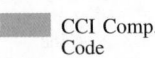 Unlisted Procedure   CCI Comp. Code   Non-specific Procedure

87045 stool, aerobic, with isolation and preliminary examination (eg, KIA, LIA), Salmonella and Shigella species

87046 stool, aerobic, additional pathogens, isolation and presumptive identification of isolates, each plate

87070 any other source except urine, blood or stool, aerobic, with isolation and presumptive identification of isolates

(For urine, use 87088)

87071 quantitative, aerobic with isolation and presumptive identification of isolates, any source except urine, blood or stool

(For urine, use 87088)

87073 quantitative, anaerobic with isolation and presumptive identification of isolates, any source except urine, blood or stool

(For definitive identification of isolates, use 87076 or 87077. for typing of isolates see 87140-87158)

87075 any source, except blood, anaerobic with isolation and presumptive identification of isolates

87076 anaerobic isolate, additional methods required for definitive identification, each isolate

87077 aerobic isolate, additional methods required for definitive identification, each isolate

87081 Culture, presumptive, pathogenic organisms, screening only;

87084 with colony estimation from density chart

87086 Culture, bacterial; quantitative colony count, urine

87088 with isolation and presumptive identification of each isolate, urine

87101 Culture, fungi (mold or yeast) isolation, with presumptive identification of isolates; skin, hair, or nail

87102 other source (except blood)

87103 blood

● New Code   ▲ Revised Code   + Add-On Code   ⊘ Modifier -51 Exempt   ⊙ Moderate Sedation

87106 Culture, fungi, definitive identification, each organism; yeast

87107 mold

87109 Culture, mycoplasma, any source

87110 Culture, chlamydia, any source

(For immunofluorescence staining of shell vials, use 87140)

87116 Culture, tubercle or other acid-fast bacilli (eg, TB, AFB, mycobacteria) any source, with isolation and presumptive identification of isolates

(For concentration, use 87015)

87118 Culture, mycobacterial, definitive identification, each isolate

87140 Culture, typing; immunofluorescent method, each antiserum

87143 gas liquid chromatography (GLC) or high pressure liquid chromotography (HPLC) method

87147 immunologic method, other than immunofluorescence (eg, agglutination grouping), per antiserum

87149 identification by nucleic acid (DNA or RNA) probe, direct probe technique, per culture or isolate, each organism probed

(Do not report 87149 in conjunction with 81200-81408)

87150 identification by nucleic acid (DNA or RNA) probe, amplified probe technique, per culture or isolate, each organism probed

(Do not report 87150 in conjunction with 81200-81408)

87152 identification by pulse field gel typing

(Do not report 87152 in conjunction with 81200-81408)

87153 identification by nucleic acid sequencing method, each isolate (eg, sequencing of the 16S rRNA gene)

87158 other methods

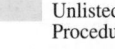 Separate Procedure   Unlisted Procedure   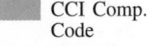 CCI Comp. Code   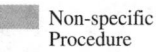 Non-specific Procedure   **1053**

87164 Dark field examination, any source (eg, penile, vaginal, oral, skin); includes specimen collection

87166 without collection

87168 Macroscopic examination; arthropod

87169 parasite

87172 Pinworm exam (eg, cellophane tape prep)

87176 Homogenization, tissue, for culture

87177 Ova and parasites, direct smears, concentration and identification

(Do not report 87177 in conjunction with 87015)

(For direct smears from a primary source, use 87207)

(For coccidia or microsporidia exam, use 87207)

(For complex special stain (trichrome, iron hematoxylin), use 87209)

(For nucleic acid probes in cytologic material, use 88365)

87181 Susceptibility studies, antimicrobial agent; agar diffusion method, per agent (eg, antibiotic gradient strip)

87184 disk method, per plate (12 or fewer disks)

87185 enzyme detection (eg, beta lactamase), per enzyme

87186 microdilution or agar dilution (minimum inhibitory concentration [MIC] or breakpoint), each multi-antimicrobial, per plate

+ 87187 microdilution or agar dilution, minimum lethal concentration (MLC), each plate ((List separately in addition to code for primary procedure)

(Use 87187 in conjunction with 87186 or 87188)

87188 macrobroth dilution method, each agent

87190 mycobacteria, proportion method, each agent

● New Code ▲ Revised Code + Add-On Code ⊘ Modifier -51 Exempt ⊙ Moderate Sedation

(For other mycobacterial susceptibility studies, see 87181, 87184, 87186, or 87188)

87197   Serum bactericidal titer (Schlicter test)

87205   Smear, primary source with interpretation; Gram or Giemsa stain for bacteria, fungi, or cell types

87206   fluorescent and/or acid fast stain for bacteria, fungi, or cell types

87207   special stain for inclusion bodies or parasites (eg, malaria, coccidia, microsporidia, trypanosomes, herpes viruses)

(For direct smears with concentration and identification, use 87177)

(For thick smear preparation, use 87015)

(For fat, meat, fibers, nasal eosinophils, and starch, see miscellaneous section)

87209   complex special stain (eg, trichrome, iron hemotoxylin) for ova and parasites

87210   wet mount for infectious agents (eg, saline, India ink, KOH preps)

(For KOH examination of skin, hair or nails, see 87220)

87220   Tissue examination by KOH slide of samples from skin, hair, or nails for fungi or ectoparasite ova or mites (eg, scabies)

87230   Toxin or antitoxin assay, tissue culture (eg, Clostridium difficile toxin)

87250   Virus isolation; inoculation of embryonated eggs, or small animal, includes observation and dissection

87252   tissue culture inoculation, observation, and presumptive identification by cytopathic effect

87253   tissue culture, additional studies or definitive identification (eg, hemabsorption, neutralization, immunofluorescence stain) each isolate

(Electron microscopy, use 88348)

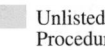 Separate Procedure   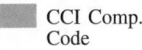 Unlisted Procedure   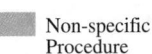 CCI Comp. Code   Non-specific Procedure

(Inclusion bodies in tissue sections, see 88304-88309; in smears, see 87207-87210; in fluids, use 88106)

87254   centrifuge enhanced (shell vial) technique, includes identification with immunofluorescence stain, each virus

(Report 87254 in addition to 87252 as appropriate)

87255   including identification by non-immunologic method, other than by cytopathic effect (eg., virus specific enzymatic activity)

These codes are intended for primary source only. For similar studies on culture material, refer to codes 87140-87158. Infectious agents by antigen detection, immunofluorescence microscopy, or nucleic acid probe techniques should be reported as precisely as possible. The molecular pathology procedure codes (eg., 81200-81408) are not to be used in combination with or instead of the procedures represented by 87470-87801. The most specific code possible should be reported. If there is no specific agent code, the general methodology code (eg., 87299, 87449, 87450, 87797, 87798, 87799, 87899) should be used. For identification of antibodies to many of the listed infectious agents, see 86602-86804. When separate results are reported for different species or strain of organisms, each result should be coded separately. Use modifier 59 when separate results are reported for different species or strains that are described by the same code.

87260   Infectious agent antigen detection by immunofluorescent technique; adenovirus

87265   Bordetella pertussis/parapertussis

87267   Enterovirus, direct fluorescent antibody (DFA)

87269   giardia

87270   Chlamydia trachomatis

87271   Cytomegalovirus, direct fluorescent antibody (DFA)

87272   cryptosporidium

87273   Herpes simplex virus type 2

87274   Herpes simplex virus 1

87275   Influenza B virus

87276   influenza A virus

● New Code   ▲ Revised Code   + Add-On Code   ⊘ Modifier -51 Exempt   ⊙ Moderate Sedation

87277 Legionella micdadei

87278 Legionella pneumophila

87279 Parainfluenza virus, each type

87280 respiratory syncytial virus

87281 Pneumocystis carinii

87283 Rubeola

87285 Treponema pallidum

87290 Varicella zoster virus

87299 not otherwise specified, each organism

87300 Infectious agent antigen detection by immunofluorescent technique, polyvalent for multiple organisms, each polyvalent antiserum

(For physican evaluation of infectious disease agents by immunofluorescence, use 88346)

87301 Infectious agent antigen detection by enzyme immunoassay technique, qualitative or semiquantitative, multiple step method; adenovirus enteric types 40/41

87305 Aspergillus

87320 Chlamydia trachomatis

87324 Clostridium difficile toxin(s)

87327 Cryptococcus neoformans

(For Cryptococcus latex agglutination, use 86403)

87328 cryptosporidium

87329 giardia

87332 cytomegalovirus

87335 Escherichia coli 0157

| | Separate Procedure | | Unlisted Procedure | | CCI Comp. Code | | Non-specific Procedure | **1057** |

(For giardia antigen, use 87329)

87336   Entamoeba histolytica dispar group

87337   Entamoeba histolytica group

87338   Helicobacter pylori, stool

87339   Helicobacter pylori

(For H. pylori, stool, use 87338. For H. pylori, breath and blood by mass spectrometry, see 83013, 83014. For H. pylori, liquid scintillation counter, see 78267, 78268)

87340   hepatitis B surface antigen (HBsAg)

87341   hepatitis B surface antigen (HBsAg) neutralization

87350   hepatitis Be antigen (HBeAg)

87380   hepatitis, delta agent

87385   Histoplasma capsulatum

87389   HIV-1 antigen(s), with HIV-1 and HIV-2 antibodies, single result

87390   HIV-1

87391   HIV-2

87400   Influenza, A or B, each

87420   respiratory syncytial virus

87425   rotavirus

87427   Shiga-like toxin

87430   Streptococcus, group A

87449   Infectious agent antigen detection by enzyme immunoassay technique qualitative or semiquantitative; multiple step method, not otherwise specified, each organism

87450   single step method, not otherwise specified, each organism

1058   ● New Code   ▲ Revised Code   ✚ Add-On Code   ⊘ Modifier -51 Exempt   ⊙ Moderate Sedation

87451   multiple step method, polyvalent for multiple organisms, each polyvalent antiserum

87470   Infectious agent detection by nucleic acid (DNA or RNA); Bartonella henselae and Bartonella quintana, direct probe technique

87471   Bartonella henselae and Bartonella quintana, amplified probe technique

87472   Bartonella henselae and Bartonella quintana, quantification

87475   Borrelia burgdorferi, direct probe technique

87476   Borrelia burgdorferi, amplified probe technique

87477   Borrelia burgdorferi, quantification

87480   Candida species, direct probe technique

87481   Candida species, amplified probe technique

87482   Candida species, quantification

87485   Chlamydia pneumoniae, direct probe technique

87486   Chlamydia pneumoniae, amplified probe technique

87487   Chlamydia pneumoniae, quantification

87490   Chlamydia trachomatis, direct probe technique

87491   Chlamydia trachomatis, amplified probe technique

87492   Chlamydia trachomatis, quantification

87493   Clostridium difficile, toxin gene(s), amplified probe technique

87495   cytomegalovirus, direct probe technique

87496   cytomegalovirus, amplified probe technique

87497   cytomegalovirus, quantification

1059

	Separate Procedure		Unlisted Procedure		CCI Comp. Code		Non-specific Procedure

▲ 87498   enterovirus, reverse transcription and amplified probe technique

87500   vancomycin resistance (eg, enterococcus species van A, van B), amplified probe technique

87501   influenza virus, reverse transcription and amplified probe technique, each type or subtype

87502   influenza virus, for multiple types or sub-types, multiplex reverse transcription and amplified probe technique, first 2 types or sub-types

+ 87503   influenza virus, for multiple types or sub-types, multiplex reverse transcription and amplified probe technique, each additional influenza virus type or sub-type beyond 2 (List separately in addition to code for primary procedure)

(Use 87503 in conjunction with 87502)

87510   Gardnerella vaginalis, direct probe technique

87511   Gardnerella vaginalis, amplified probe technique

87512   Gardnerella vaginalis, quantification

87515   hepatitis B virus, direct probe technique

87516   hepatitis B virus, amplified probe technique

87517   hepatitis B virus, quantification

87520   hepatitis C, direct probe technique

▲ 87521   hepatitis C, reverse transcription and amplified probe technique

▲ 87522   hepatitis C, reverse transcription and quantification

87525   hepatitis G, direct probe technique

87526   hepatitis G, amplified probe technique

87527   hepatitis G, quantification

87528   Herpes simplex virus, direct probe technique

● New Code   ▲ Revised Code   + Add-On Code   ⊘ Modifier -51 Exempt   ⊙ Moderate Sedation

87529	Herpes simplex virus, amplified probe technique
87530	Herpes simplex virus, quantification
87531	Herpes virus-6, direct probe technique
87532	Herpes virus-6, amplified probe technique
87533	Herpes virus-6, quantification
87534	HIV-1, direct probe technique
▲ 87535	HIV-1, reverse transcription and amplified probe technique
▲ 87536	HIV-1, reverse transcription and quantification
87537	HIV-2, direct probe technique
▲ 87538	HIV-2, reverse transcription and amplified probe technique
▲ 87539	HIV-2, reverse transcription and quantification
87540	Legionella pneumophila, direct probe technique
87541	Legionella pneumophila, amplified probe technique
87542	Legionella pneumophila, quantification
87550	Mycobacteria species, direct probe technique
87551	Mycobacteria species, amplified probe technique
87552	Mycobacteria species, quantification
87555	Mycobacteria tuberculosis, direct probe technique
87556	Mycobacteria tuberculosis, amplified probe technique
87557	Mycobacteria tuberculosis, quantification
87560	Mycobacteria avium-intracellulare, direct probe technique
87561	Mycobacteria avium-intracellulare, amplified probe technique

	Separate Procedure		Unlisted Procedure		CCI Comp. Code		Non-specific Procedure

1061

| 87562 | Mycobacteria avium-intracellulare, quantification |

| 87580 | Mycoplasma pneumoniae, direct probe technique |

| 87581 | Mycoplasma pneumoniae, amplified probe technique |

| 87582 | Mycoplasma pneumoniae, quantification |

| 87590 | Neisseria gonorrhoeae, direct probe technique |

| 87591 | Neisseria gonorrhoeae, amplified probe technique |

| 87592 | Neisseria gonorrhoeae, quantification |

| 87620 | papillomavirus, human, direct probe technique |

| 87621 | papillomavirus, human, amplified probe technique |

| 87622 | papillomavirus, human, quantification |

● **87631**   respiratory virus (eg, adenovirus, invluenza virus, coronavirus, metapneumovirus, parainfluenza virus, respiratory syncytial virus, rhinovirus), multiplex reverse transcription and amplified probe technique, multiple types or subtypes, 3-5 targets

● **87632**   respiratory virus (eg, adenovirus, influenza virus, coronavirus metapneumovirus, parainfluenza virus, respiratory syncytial virus, rhinovirus), multiplex reverse transcription and amplified probe technique, multiple types or subtypes, 6-11 targets

● **87633**   respiratory virus (eg, adenovirus, influenza virus, coronavirus, metapneumovirus, parainfluenza virus, respiratory syncytial virus, rhinovirus), multiplex reverse transcription and amplified probe technique, multiple types or subtypes, 12-25 targets

(Use 87631-87633 for nucleic acid assays which detect multiple respiratory viruses in a multiplex reaction [ie, single procedure with multiple results])

(For assays that are used to type or subtype influenza viruses only, see 87501-87503)

(For assays that include influenza viruses with additional respiratory viruses, see 87631-87633)

● New Code   ▲ Revised Code   + Add-On Code   ⊘ Modifier -51 Exempt   ⊙ Moderate Sedation

(For detection of multiple infectious agents not otherwise specified which report a single result, see 87800, 87801)

87640   Staphylococcus aureus, amplified probe technique

87641   Staphylococcus aureus, methicillin resistant, amplified probe technique

(For assays that detect methicillin resistance and identify Staphylococcus aureus using a single nucleic acid sequenc, use 87641)

87650   Streptococcus, group A, direct probe technique

87651   Streptococcus, group A, amplified probe technique

87652   Streptococcus, group A, quantification

87653   Streptococcus, group B, amplified probe technique

87660   Trichomonas vaginalis, direct probe technique

87797   Infectious agent detection by nucleic acid (DNA or RNA), not otherwise specified; direct probe technique, each organism

87798   amplified probe technique, each organism

87799   quantification, each organism

87800   Infectious agent detection by nucleic acid (DNA or RNA), multiple organisms; direct probe(s) technique

87801   amplified probe(s) technique

(For each specific organism nucleic acid detection from a primary source, see 87470-87660. For detection of specific infectious agents not otherwise specified, see 87797, 87798 or 87799 one time for each agent)

(For detection of multiple infectious agents not otherwise specified which report a single result, see 87800, 87801)

(Do not use 87801 for nucleic acid assays that detect multiple respiratory viruses in a multiplex reaction [ie, single procedure with multiple results], see 87631-87633)

87802   Infectious agent antigen detection by immunoassay with direct optical observation; Streptococcus, group B

1063

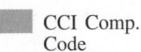

Separate Procedure   Unlisted Procedure   CCI Comp. Code   Non-specific Procedure

87803	Clostridium difficile toxin A
87804	Influenza
87807	respiratory syncytial virus
87808	Trichomonas vaginalis
87809	adenovirus
87810	Chlamydia trachomatis
87850	Neisseria gonorrhoeae
87880	Streptococcus, group A
87899	not otherwise specified

87900 Infectious agent drug susceptibility phenotype prediction using regularly updated genotypic bioinformatics

● **87910** Infectious agent genotype analysis by nucleic acid (DNA or RNA); cytomegalovirus

▲ **87901** HIV-1, reverse transciptase and protease regions

87906 HIV-1, other region (eg, integrase, fusion)

(For infectious agent drug susceptibility phenotype prediction for HIV-1, use 87900)

● **87912** Hepatitis B virus

87902 Hepatitis C virus

87903 Infectious agent phenotype analysis by nucleic acid (DNA or RNA) with drug resistance tissue culture analysis, HIV 1; first through 10 drugs tested

+ **87904** each additional drug tested (List separately in addition to code for primary procedure)

(Use 87904 in conjunction with code 87903)

87905 Infectious agent enzymatic activity other than virus (eg, sialidase activity in vaginal fluid)

(For virus isolation including identification by non-immunologic method, other than by cytopathic effect, use 87255)

87906   This code is out of order. See page 1064

87910   This code is out of order. See page 1064

87912   This code is out of order. See page 1064

87999   Unlisted microbiology procedure

ANATOMIC PATHOLOGY

POSTMORTEM EXAMINATION

Procedures 88000 through 88099 represent physician services only. Use modifier 90 for outside laboratory services.

88000   Necropsy (autopsy), gross examination only; without CNS

88005   with brain

88007   with brain and spinal cord

88012   infant with brain

88014   stillborn or newborn with brain

88016   macerated stillborn

88020   Necropsy (autopsy), gross and microscopic; without CNS

88025   with brain

88027   with brain and spinal cord

88028   infant with brain

88029   stillborn or newborn with brain

88036   Necropsy (autopsy), limited, gross and/or microscopic; regional

88037   single organ

88040   Necropsy (autopsy); forensic examination

1065

	Separate Procedure		Unlisted Procedure		CCI Comp. Code		Non-specific Procedure

88045   coroner's call

88099   Unlisted necropsy (autopsy) procedure

CYTOPATHOLOGY

When cytopathology codes are reported, the appropriate CPT code to bill is that which describes, to the highest level of specificity, what services were rendered. Accordingly, for a given specimen, only one code from a group of related codes describing a group of services that could be performed on a specimen with the same end result (e.g. 88104-88112, 88142- 88143, 88150-88154, 88164-88167, etc.) is to be reported.

If multiple services (i.e., separate specimens from different anatomic sites) are reported, modifier -59 should be used to indicate that different levels of service were provided for different specimens from different anatomic sites. This should be reflected in the cytopathologic reports. A cytopathology preparation from a fluid, washing, or brushing is to be reported using one code from the range of CPT codes 88104-88112. It is inappropriate to additionally use CPT codes 88160-88162 because the smears are included in the codes referable to fluids (or washings or brushings) and 88160-88162 references any other source which would exclude fluids, washings, or brushings.

88104   Cytopathology, fluids, washings or brushings, except cervical or vaginal; smears with interpretation

88106   simple filter method with interpretation

(Do not report 88106 in conjunction with 88104)

(88107   deleted 2011 [2012 edition]. To report smears and simple filter preparation, see 88104, 88106)

(For nongynecological selective cellular enhancement including filter transfer techniques, use 88112)

88108   Cytopathology, concentration technique, smears and interpretation (eg, Saccomanno technique)

(For cervical or vaginal smears, see 88150-88155)

(For gastric intubation with lavage, see 43754, 43755)

(For x-ray localization, use 74340)

88112   Cytopathology, selective cellular enhancement technique with interpretation (eg, liquid based slide preparation method), except cervical or vaginal

● New Code	▲ Revised Code	+ Add-On Code	⊘ Modifier -51 Exempt	⊙ Moderate Sedation

(Do not report 88112 with 88108)

88120 Cytopathology, in situ hybridization (eg, fish), urinary tract specimen with morphometric analysis, 3-5 molecular probes, each specimen; manual

88121 using computer-assisted technology

(For morphometric in situ hybridization on cytologic specimens other than urinary tract, see 88367, 88368)

(For more than 5 probes, use 88399)

88125 Cytopathology, forensic (eg, sperm)

88130 Sex chromatin identification; Barr bodies

88140 peripheral blood smear, polymorphonuclear drumsticks

(For Guard stain, use 88313)

Codes 88141-88155, 88164-88167, 88174-88175 are used to report cervical or vaginal screening by various methods and to report physician interpretation services. Use codes 88150-88154 to report conventional Pap smears that are examined using non-Bethesda reporting. Use codes 88164-88167 to report conventional Pap smears that are examined using the Bethesda System of reporting. Use codes 88142-88143 to report liquid-based specimens processed as thin-layer preparations that are examined using any system of reporting (Bethesda or non-Bethesda). Use codes 88174-88175 to report automated screening of liquid-based specimens that are examined using any system of reporting (Bethesda or non-Bethesda). Within each of these three code families choose the one code that describes the screening method(s) used. Codes 88141 and 88155 should be reported in addition to the screening code chosen when the additional services are provided. Manual rescreening requires a complete visual reassessment of the entire slide initially screened by either an automated or manual process. Manual review represents an assessment of selected cells or regions of a slide identified by initial automated review.

88141 Cytopathology, cervical or vaginal (any reporting system), requiring interpretation by physician

(Use 88141 in conjunction with 88142-88154, 88164-88167, 88174-88175)

88142 Cytopathology, cervical or vaginal (any reporting system), collected in preservative fluid, automated thin layer preparation; manual screening under physician supervision

| Separate Procedure | Unlisted Procedure | CCI Comp. Code | Non-specific Procedure |

88143   with manual screening and rescreening under physician supervision

(For automated screening of automated thin layer preparation, see 88174, 88175)

88147 Cytopathology smears, cervical or vaginal; screening by automated system under physician supervision

88148   screening by automated system with manual rescreening under physician supervision

88150 Cytopathology, slides, cervical or vaginal; manual screening under physician supervision

88152   with manual screening and computer-assisted rescreening under physician supervision

88153   with manual screening and rescreening under physician supervision

88154   with manual screening and computer-assisted rescreening using cell selection and review under physician supervision

+ 88155 Cytopathology, slides, cervical or vaginal, definitive hormonal evaluation (eg, maturation index, karyopyknotic index, estrogenic index) (List separately in addition to code[s] for other technical and interpretation services)

(Use 88155 in conjunction with 88142-88154, 88164-88167, 88174-88175)

88160 Cytopathology, smears, any other source; screening and interpretation

88161   preparation, screening and interpretation

88162   extended study involving over 5 slides and/or multiple stains

(For aerosol collection of sputum, use 89350)

(For special stains, see 88312-88314)

88164 Cytopathology, slides, cervical or vaginal (the Bethesda System); manual screening under physician supervision

88165   with manual screening and rescreening under physician supervision

88166   with manual screening and computer-assisted rescreening under physician supervision

88167   with manual screening and computer-assisted rescreening using cell selection and review under physician supervision

(To report collection of specimen via fine needle aspiration, see 10021, 10022)

88172   Cytopathology, evaluation of fine needle aspirate; immediate cytohistologic study to determine adequacy for diagnosis, first evaluation episode, each site

(The evaluation episode represents a complete set of cytologic material submitted for evaluation and is independent of the number of needle passes or slides prepared. A separate evaluation episode occurs if the proceduralist provider obtains additional material from the same site, based on the prior immediate adequacy assessment, or a separate lesion is aspirated.)

88173   interpretation and report

(Report one unit of 88173 for the interpretation and report from each anatomic site, regardless of the number of passes or evaluation episodes performed during the aspiration procedure)

(For fine needle aspirate, see 10021, 10022)

(Do not report 88172, 88173 in conjunction with 88333 and 88334 for the same specimen)

+ 88177   immediate cytohistologic study to determine adequacy for diagnosis, each separate additional evaluation episode, same site (List separately in addition to code for primary procedure)

(When repeat immediate evaluation episode(s) is required on subsequent cytologic material from the same site, eg, following determination the prior sampling that was not adequate for diagnosis, use 1 unit of 88177 for each additional evaluation episode)

(Use 88177 in conjunction with 88172)

1069

▉ Separate Procedure	▉ Unlisted Procedure	▉ CCI Comp. Code	▉ Non-specific Procedure

88174 Cytopathology, cervical or vaginal (any reporting system), collected in preservative fluid, automated thin layer preparation; screening by automated system, under physician supervision

88175 with screening by automated system and manual rescreening or review, under physician supervision

(For manual screening, see 88142, 88143)

88177 This code is out of order. See page 1069

88182 Flow cytometry; cell cycle or DNA analysis

(For DNA ploidy analysis by morphometric techniques, use 88358)

88184 Flow cytometry, cell surface, cytoplasmic, or nuclear marker, technical component only; first marker

+ **88185** each additional marker (List separately in addition to code for first marker)

(Report 88185 in conjunction with 88184)

88187 Flow cytometry, interpretation; 2 to 8 markers

88188 9 to 15 markers

88189 16 or more markers

(Do not report 88187-88189 for interpretation of 86355, 86356, 86357, 86359, 86360, 86361, 86367)

(For assessment of circulating antibodies by flow cytometric techniques, see analyte and method-specific codes in the Chemistry section [83516-83520] or Immunology section [86000-86849])

(For cell enumeration using immunologic selection and identification in fluid specimen [eg, circulating tumor cells in blood], see 0279T, 0280T)

88199 Unlisted cytopathology procedure

(For electron microscopy, see 88348, 88349)

● New Code ▲ Revised Code + Add-On Code ⊘ Modifier -51 Exempt ⊙ Moderate Sedation

CYTOGENETIC STUDIES

Molecular pathology procedures should be reported using either the appropriate Tier 1 (81200-81383), Tier 2 (81400-81408), or the unlisted molecular pathology procedure code, 81479.

(For acetylcholinesterase, use 82013)

(For alpha-fetoprotein, serum or amniotic fluid, see 82105, 82106)

(For laser microdissection of cells from tissue sample, see 88380)

88230 Tissue culture for non-neoplastic disorders; lymphocyte

88233 skin or other solid tissue biopsy

88235 amniotic fluid or chorionic villus cells

88237 Tissue culture for neoplastic disorders; bone marrow, blood cells

88239 solid tumor

88240 Cryopreservation, freezing and storage of cells, each cell line

(For therapeutic cryopreservation and storage, use 38207)

88241 Thawing and expansion of frozen cells, each aliquot

(For therapeutic thawing of previous harvest, use 38208)

88245 Chromosome analysis for breakage syndromes; baseline Sister Chromatid Exchange (SCE), 20-25 cells

88248 baseline breakage, score 50-100 cells, count 20 cells, 2 karyotypes (eg, for ataxia telangiectasia, Fanconi anemia, fragile X)

88249 score 100 cells, clastogen stress (eg, diepoxybutane, mitomycin C, ionizing radiation, UV radiation)

88261 Chromosome analysis; count 5 cells, 1 karyotype, with banding

88262 count 15-20 cells, 2 karyotypes, with banding

88263 count 45 cells for mosaicism, 2 karyotypes, with banding

1071

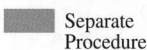 Separate Procedure	Unlisted Procedure	CCI Comp. Code	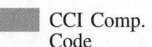 Non-specific Procedure	

| 88264 | analyze 20-25 cells |

| 88267 | Chromosome analysis, amniotic fluid or chorionic villus, count 15 cells, 1 karyotype, with banding |

| 88269 | Chromosome analysis, in situ for amniotic fluid cells, count cells from 6-12 colonies, 1 karyotype, with banding |

| 88271 | Molecular cytogenetics; DNA probe, each (eg, FISH) |

| 88272 | chromosomal in situ hybridization, analyze 3-5 cells (eg, for derivatives and markers) |

| 88273 | chromosomal in situ hybridization, analyze 10-30 cells (eg, for microdeletions) |

| 88274 | interphase in situ hybridization, analyze 25-99 cells |

| 88275 | interphase in situ hybridization, analyze 100-300 cells |

| 88280 | Chromosome analysis; additional karyotypes, each study |

| 88283 | additional specialized banding technique (eg, NOR, C-banding) |

| 88285 | additional cells counted, each study |

| 88289 | additional high resolution study |

| 88291 | Cytogenetics and molecular cytogenetics, interpretation and report |

| 88299 | Unlisted cytogenetic study |

SURGICAL PATHOLOGY

The CPT codes 88321-88325 are to be used to review slides, tissues, or other material obtained and prepared at a different location and referred to a pathologist for a second opinion. (These codes should not be reported by pathologists reporting a second opinion on slides, tissue, or material also examined and reported by another pathologist in the same provider group. Medicare generally does not pay twice for an interpretation of a given technical service (e.g., EKGs, radiographs, etc.).

CPT codes 88321- 88325 are reported with one unit of service regardless of the number of specimens, paraffin blocks, stained slides, etc. When reporting CPT

● New Code ▲ Revised Code + Add-On Code ⊘ Modifier -51 Exempt ⊙ Moderate Sedation

codes 88321-88325, providers should not report other pathology CPT codes such as 88312, 88313, 88342, 88187, 88188, 88189, etc., for interpretation of stains, slides or material previously interpreted by another pathologist. CPT codes 88312, 88313 and 88342 may be reported with CPT code 88323 if provider performs and interprets these stains de novo.

CPT codes 88321-88325 are not to be used for a face-to-face evaluation of a patient. In the event that a physician provides an evaluation and management service to a patient and, in the course of this service, specimens obtained elsewhere are reviewed as well, this is part of the evaluation and management service and is not to be reported separately. Only the evaluation and management service would be reported.

Medicare does not pay for duplicate testing. CPT codes 88342 (immuno-cytochemistry, each antibody) and 88184, 88187, 88188, 88189 (flow cytometry) should not in general be reported for the same or similar specimens. The diagnosis should be established using one of these methods. The provider may report both CPT codes if both methods are required because the initial method is nondiagnostic or does not explain all the light microscopic findings. The provider can report both methods utilizing modifier -59 and document the need for both methods in the medical record.

If the abnormal cells in two or more specimens are morphologically similar and testing on one specimen by one method (88342 or 88184, 88187, 88188, 88189) establishes the diagnosis, the same or other method should not be reported on the same or similar specimen. Similar specimens would include, but are not limited to: (1) blood and bone marrow; (2) bone marrow aspiration and bone marrow biopsy; (3) two separate lymph nodes; or (4) lymph node and other tissue with lymphoid infiltrate.

Services 88300 through 88309 include accession, examination, and reporting. They do not include the services designated in codes 88311 through 88365 and 88399, which are coded in addition when provided.

The unit of service for codes 88300 through 88309 is the specimen.

A specimen is defined as tissue or tissues that is (are) submitted for individual and separate attention, requiring individual examination and pathologic diagnosis. Two or more such specimens from the same patient (eg., separately identified endoscopic biopsies, skin lesions), are each appropriately assigned an individual code reflective of its proper level of service.

Service code 88300 is used for any specimen that in the opinion of the examining pathologist can be accurately diagnosed without microscopic examination. Service code 88302 is used when gross and microscopic examination is performed on a specimen to confirm identification and the absence of disease. Service codes 88304 through 88309 describe all other specimens requiring gross and microscopic

1073

	Separate Procedure		Unlisted Procedure		CCI Comp. Code		Non-specific Procedure

examination, and represent additional ascending levels of physician work. Levels 88302 through 88309 are specifically defined by the assigned specimens.

Any unlisted specimen should be assigned to the code which most closely reflects the physician work involved when compared to other specimens assigned to that code.

(Do not report 88302-88309 on the same specimen as part of Mohs surgery)

88300   Level I - Surgical pathology, gross examination only

88302   Level II - Surgical pathology, gross and microscopic examination

Appendix, Incidental
Fallopian Tube, Sterilization
Fingers/Toes, Amputation, Traumatic
Foreskin, Newborn
Hernia Sac, Any Location
Hydrocele Sac
Nerve
Skin, Plastic Repair
Sympathetic Ganglion
Testis, Castration
Vaginal Mucosa, Incidental
Vas Deferens, Sterilization

88304   Level III - Surgical pathology, gross and microscopic examination

Abortion, Induced
Abscess
Aneurysm - Arterial/Ventricular
Anus, Tag
Appendix, Other than Incidental
Artery, Atheromatous Plaque
Bartholin's Gland Cyst
Bone Fragment(s), Other than Pathologic Fracture
Bursa/Synovial Cyst
Carpal Tunnel Tissue
Cartilage, Shavings
Cholesteatoma
Colon, Colostomy Stoma
Conjunctiva - Biopsy/Pterygium
Cornea
Diverticulum - Esophagus/Small Intestine
Dupuytren's Contracture Tissue
Femoral Head, Other than Fracture
Fissue/Fistula

● New Code   ▲ Revised Code   + Add-On Code   ⊘ Modifier -51 Exempt   ⊙ Moderate Sedation

Foreskin, Other than Newborn
Gallbladder
Ganglion Cyst
Hematoma
Hemorrhoids
Hydatid of Morgagni
Intervertebral Disc
Joint, Loose Body
Meniscus
Mucocele, Salivary
Neuroma - Morton's/Traumatic
Pilonidal Cyst/Sinus
Polyps, Inflammatory - Nasal/Sinusoidal
Skin - Cyst/Tag/Debridement
Soft Tissue, Debridement
Soft Tissue, Lipoma
Spermatocele
Tendon/Tendon Sheath
Testicular Appendage
Thrombus or Embolus
Tonsil and/or Adenoids
Varicocele
Vas Deferens, Other than Sterilizaton
Vein, Varicosity

88305 Level IV - Surgical pathology, gross and microscopic examination

Abortion - Spontaneous/Missed
Artery, Biopsy
Bone Marrow, Biopsy
Bone Exostosis
Brain/Meninges, Other than for Tumor Resection
Breast Biopsy, Not Requiring Microscopic Evaluation of
    Surgical Margins
Breast, Reduction Mammoplasty
Bronchus, Biopsy
Cell Block, Any Source
Cervix, Biopsy
Colon, Biopsy
Duodenum, Biopsy
Endocervix, Curettings/Biopsy
Endometrium, Currettings/Biopsy
Esophagus, Biopsy
Extremity, Amputation, Traumatic
Fallopian Tube, Biopsy
Fallopian Tube, Ectopic Pregnancy
Femoral Head, Fracture
Fingers/Toes, Amputation, Non-Traumatic
Gingiva/Oral Mucosa, Biopsy

1075

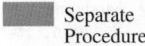 Separate Procedure   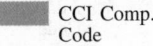 Unlisted Procedure   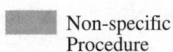 CCI Comp. Code   Non-specific Procedure

Heart Valve
Joint, Resection
Kidney, Biopsy
Larynx, Biopsy
Leiomyoma(s), Uterine Myomectomy - without Uterus
Lip, Biopsy/Wedge Resection
Lung, Transbronchial Biopsy
Lymph Node, Biopsy
Muscle, Biopsy
Nasal Mucosa, Biopsy
Nasopharynx/Oropharynx, Biopsy
Nerve, Biopsy
Odontogenic/Dental Cyst
Omentum, Biopsy
Ovary with or without Tube, Non-neoplastic
Ovary, Biopsy/Wedge Resection
Parathyroid Gland
Peritoneum, Biopsy
Pituitary Tumor
Placenta, Other than Third Trimester
Pleura/Pericardium - Biopsy/Tissue
Polyp, Cervical/Endometrial
Polyp, Colorectal
Polyp, Stomach/Small Intestine
Prostate, Needle Biopsy
Prostate, TUR
Salivary Gland, Biopsy
Sinus, Paranasal Biopsy
Skin, Other than Cyst/Tag/Debridement/Plastic Repair
Small Intestine, Biopsy
Soft Tissue, Other than Tumor/Mass/Lipoma/Debridement
Spleen
Stomach, Biopsy
Synovium
Testis, Other than Tumor/Biopsy/Castration
Thyroglossal Duct/Brachial Cleft Cyst
Tongue, Biopsy
Tonsil, Biopsy
Trachea, Biopsy
Ureter, Biopsy
Urethra, Biopsy
Urinary Bladder, Biopsy
Uterus, with or without Tubes and Ovaries, for Prolapse
Vagina, Biopsy
Vulva/Labia, Biopsy

88307 Level V - Surgical pathology, gross and microscopic examination

Adrenal, Resection

● New Code   ▲ Revised Code   + Add-On Code   ⊘ Modifier -51 Exempt   ⊙ Moderate Sedation

Bone - Biopsy/Curettings
Bone Fragment(s), Pathologic Fracture
Brain, Biopsy
Brain/Meninges, Tumor Resection
Breast, Excision of Lesion, Requiring Microscopic Evaluation
   of Surgical Margins
Breast, Mastectomy - Partial/Simple
Cervix, Conization
Colon, Segmental Resection, Other than for Tumor
Extremity, Amputation, Non-traumatic
Eye, Enucleation
Kidney, Partial/Total Nephrectomy
Larynx, Partial/Total Resection
Liver, Biopsy - Needle/Wedge
Lung, Wedge Biopsy
Lymph Nodes, Regional Resection
Mediastinum, Mass
Myocardium, Biopsy
Odontogenic Tumor
Ovary with or without Tube, Neoplastic
Pancreas, Biopsy
Placenta, Third Trimester
Prostate, Except Radical Resection
Salivary Gland
Sentinel Lymph Node
Small Intestine, Resection, Other Than for Tumor
Soft Tissue Mass (except Lipoma) - Biopsy/Simple Excision
Stomach - Subtotal/Total Resection, Other than for Tumor
Testis, Biopsy
Thymus, Biopsy
Thyroid, Total/Lobe
Ureter, Resection
Urinary Bladder, TUR
Uterus, with or without Tubes and Ovaries, Other than
   Neoplastic/Prolapse

88309 Level VI - Surgical pathology, gross and microscopic
examination

Bone Resection
Breast, Mastectomy - with Regional Lymph Nodes
Colon, Segmental Resection for Tumor
Colon, Total Resection
Esophagus, Partial/Total Resection
Extremity, Disarticulation
Fetus, with Dissection
Larynx, Partial/Total Resection - with Regional Lymph Nodes
Lung - Total/Lobe/Segment Resection
Pancreas, Total/Subtotal Resection
Prostate, Radical Resection

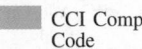

	Separate		Unlisted		CCI Comp.		Non-specific	**1077**
	Procedure		Procedure		Code		Procedure	

Small Intestine, Resection for Tumor
Soft Tissue Tumor, Extensive Resection
Stomach - Subtotal/Total Resection for Tumor
Testis, Tumor
Tongue/Tonsil - Resection for Tumor
Urinary Bladder, Partial/Total Resection
Uterus, with or without Tubes and Ovaries, Neoplastic
Vulva, Total/Subtotal Resection

(For fine needle aspiration, see 10021, 10022)

(For evaluation of fine needle aspirate, see 88172-88173)

(Do not report 88302-88309 on the same specimen as part of Mohs surgery)

+ **88311**   Decalcification procedure (List separately in addition to code for surgical pathology examination)

88312   Special stain including interpretation and report; Group I for microorganisms (eg, acid fast, methenamine silver)

(Report one unit of 88312 for each special stain, on each surgical pathology block, cytologic specimen, or hematologic smear)

88313   Group II, all other, (eg, iron, trichrome), except stain for microorganisms, stains for enzyme constituents, or immunocytochemistry and immunohistochemistry

(Report one unit of 88313 for each special stain, on each surgical pathology block, cytologic specimen, or hematologic smear)

(For immunocytochemistry and immunohistochemistry, use 88342)

+ **88314**   histochemical stain on frozen tissue block (List separately in addition to code for primary procedure)

(Use 88314 in conjunction with 17311-17315, 88302-88309, 88331, 88332)

(Do not report 88314 with 17311-17315 for routine frozen section stain [eg., hematoxylin and eosin, toluidine blue], performed during Mohs surgery. When a nonroutine histochemical stain on frozen tissue during Mohs surgery is utilized, report 88314 with modifier 59)

(Report one unit of 88314 for each special stain on each frozen surgical pathology block)

● New Code   ▲ Revised Code   + Add-On Code   ⊘ Modifier -51 Exempt   ⊙ Moderate Sedation

(For a special stain performed on frozen tissue section material to identify enzyme constituents, use 88319)

(88318   deleted 2011 [2012 edition])

(For determinative histochemistry to identify chemical components, use 88313)

88319   Group III, for enzyme constituents

(For each stain on each surgical pathology block, cytologic specimen, or hematologic smear, use one unit of 88319)

(For detection of enzyme constituents by immunohistochemical or immunocytochemical technique, use 88342)

88321   Consultation and report on referred slides prepared elsewhere

88323   Consultation and report on referred material requiring preparation of slides

88325   Consultation, comprehensive, with review of records and specimens, with report on referred material

88329   Pathology consultation during surgery;

88331   first tissue block, with frozen section(s), single specimen

+ **88332**   each additional tissue block with frozen section(s) (List separately in addition to code for primary procedure)

(Use 88332 in conjunction with 88331)

88333   cytologic examination (eg, touch prep, squash prep), initial site

+ **88334**   cytologic examination (eg, touch prep, squash prep), each additional site (List separately in addition to code for primary procedure)

(Use 88334 in conjunction with 88331, 88333)

(For intraoperative consultation on a specimen requiring both frozen section and cytologic evaluation, use 88331 and 88334)

(For percutaneous needle biopsy requiring intraprocedural cytologic examination, use 88333)

(Do not report 88333 and 88334 for non-intraoperative cytologic examination, see 88160-88162)

1079

	Separate Procedure		Unlisted Procedure		CCI Comp. Code		Non-specific Procedure

(Do not report 88333 and 88334 for intraprocedural cytologic evaluation of fine needle aspirate, see 88172).

88342 Immunohistochemistry (including tissue immunoperoxidase), each antibody

(Do not report 88342 in conjunction with 88360 or 88361 for the same antibody)

(For quantitative or semiquantitative immunohistochemistry, see 88360, 88361)

88346 Immunofluorescent study, each antibody; direct method

88347 indirect method

88348 Electron microscopy; diagnostic

88349 scanning

88355 Morphometric analysis; skeletal muscle

88356 nerve

88358 tumor (eg, DNA ploidy)

(Do not report 88358 with 88313 unless each procedure is for a different special stain)

88360 Morphometric analysis, tumor immunohistochemistry (eg, Her-2/neu, estrogen receptor/progesterone receptor), quantitative or semiquantitative, each antibody; manual

88361 using computer-assisted technology

(Do not report 88360, 88361 with 88342 unless each procedure is for a different antibody)

(For morphometric analysis, in situ hybridization, see 88367, 88368)

(When semi-thin plastic-embedded sections are performed in conjunction with morphometric analysis, only the morphometric analysis should be coded; if performed as an independent procedure, see codes 88300-88309 for surgical pathology)

88362 Nerve teasing preparations

88363   Examination and selection of retrieved archival (ie, previously diagnosed) tissue(s) for molecular analysis (eg, Kras mutational analysis)

88365   In situ hybridization (eg, FISH), each probe

(Do not report 88365 in conjunction with 88367, 88368 for the same probe)

88367   Morphometric analysis, in situ hybridization, (quantitative or semi-quantitative) each probe; using computer-assisted technology

88368   manual

(For morphometric in situ hybridization evaluation of urinary tract cytologic specimens, see 88120, 88121)

88371   Protein analysis of tissue by Western Blot, with interpretation and report;

88372   immunological probe for band identification, each

● **88375**   Optical endomicroscopic image(s), interpretation and report, real-time or referred, each endoscopic session

(Do not report 88375 in conjunction with 43206 or 43252)

88380   Microdissection (ie, sample preparation of microscopically identified target); laser capture

88381   manual

(Do not report 88380 in conjunction with 88381)

(88384   deleted 2012 [2013 edition]. To report, see 81200-81479)

(88385   deleted 2012 [2013 edition]. To report, see 81200-81479)

(88386   deleted 2012 [2013 edition]. To report, see 81200-81479)

88387   Macroscopic examination, dissection, and preparation of tissue for non microscopic analytical studies (eg, nucleic acid based molecular studies); each tissue preparation (eg, a single lymph node)

(Do not report 88387 for tissue preparation for microbiologic cultures or flow cytometric studies)

Separate Procedure	Unlisted Procedure	CCI Comp. Code	Non-specific Procedure

1081

(Do not report 88387 in conjunction with 88388, 88329-88334)

+ **88388** in conjunction with a touch imprint, intraoperative consultation, or frozen section, each tissue preparation (eg, a single lymph node) (List separately in addition to code for primary procedure)

(Use 88388 in conjunction with 88329-88334)

(Do not report 88387 or 88388 for tissue preparation for microbiologic cultures or flow cytometric studies)

88399 Unlisted surgical pathology procedure

(88400 deleted 2009 edition; see 88720)

IN VIVO (eg, TRANSCUTANEOUS) LABORATORY PROCEDURES

(For all in vivo measurements not specifically listed, use 88749)

(For wavelength fluorescent spectroscopy of advanced glycation end products [skin], use 0233T)

(For transcutaneous oxyhemoglobin measurement in a lower extremity wound by near infrared spectroscopy, use 0286T)

88720 Bilirubin, total, transcutaneous

(For transdermal oxygen saturation, see 94760-94762)

88738 Hemoglobin (Hgb), quantitative, transcutaneous

(For in vitro hemoglobin measurement, use 85018)

88740 Hemoglobin, quantitative, transcutaneous, per day; carboxyhemoglobin

(For in vitro carboxyhemoglobin measurement, use 82375)

88741 methemoglobin

(For in vitro quantitative methemoglobin determination, use 83050)

88749 Unlisted in vivo (eg, transcutaneous) laboratory service

OTHER PROCEDURES

89049 Caffeine halothane contracture test (CHCT) for malignant hyperthermia susceptibility, including interpretation and report

89050 Cell count, miscellaneous body fluids (eg, cerebrospinal fluid, joint fluid), except blood;

89051   with differential count

89055 Leukocyte assessment, fecal, qualitative or semiquantitative

89060 Crystal identification by light microscopy with or without polarizing lens analysis, tissue or any body fluid (except urine)

(Do not report 89060 for crystal identification on paraffin-embedded tissue)

(89100   deleted 2010 [2011 edition]. To report, see 43756, 43757)

(89105   deleted 2010 [2011 edition]. To report, see 43756, 43757)

89125 Fat stain, feces, urine, or respiratory secretions

(89130   deleted 2010 [2011 edition]. To report, see 43754, 43755)

(89132   deleted 2010 [2011 edition]. To report, see 43754, 43755)

(89135   deleted 2010 [2011 edition]. To report, see 43754, 43755)

(89136   deleted 2010 [2011 edition]. To report, see 43754, 43755)

(89140   deleted 2010 [2011 edition]. To report, see 43754, 43755)

(89141   deleted 2010 [2011 edition]. To report, see 43754, 43755)

89160 Meat fibers, feces

89190 Nasal smear for eosinophils

(Occult blood, feces, use 82270)

(Paternity tests, use 86910)

89220 Sputum, obtaining specimen, aerosol induced technique (separate procedure)

1083

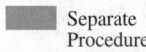 Separate Procedure   Unlisted Procedure   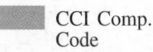 CCI Comp. Code   Non-specific Procedure

(89225   deleted 2010 [2011 edition])

89230   Sweat collection by iontophoresis

(89235   deleted 2010 [2011 edition])

89240   Unlisted miscellaneous pathology test

REPRODUCTIVE MEDICINE PROCEDURES

89250   Culture of oocyte(s)/embryo(s), less than 4 days;

89251   with co-culture of oocyte(s)/embryo(s)

(For extended culture of oocyte(s)/embryo(s), see 89272)

89253   Assisted embryo hatching, microtechniques (any method)

89254   Oocyte identification from follicular fluid

89255   Preparation of embryo for transfer (any method)

89257   Sperm identification from aspiration (other than seminal fluid)

(For semen analysis, see 89300-89320)

(For sperm identification from testis tissue, use 89264)

89258   Cryopreservation; embryo(s)

89259   sperm

(For cryopreservation of reproductive tissue, testicular, use 89335)

89260   Sperm isolation; simple prep (eg, sperm wash and swim-up) for insemination or diagnosis with semen analysis

89261   complex prep (eg, Percoll gradient, albumin gradient) for insemination or diagnosis with semen analysis

(For semen analysis without sperm wash or swim-up, use 89320)

89264   Sperm identification from testis tissue, fresh or cryopreserved

(For biopsy of testis, see 54500, 54505)

● New Code   ▲ Revised Code   + Add-On Code   ⊘ Modifier -51 Exempt   ⊙ Moderate Sedation

(For sperm identification from aspiration, use 89257)

(For semen analysis, see 89300-89320)

89268 Insemination of oocytes

89272 Extended culture of oocyte(s)/embryo(s), 4-7 days

89280 Assisted oocyte fertiliation, microtechnique; less than or equal to 10 oocytes

89281 greater than 10 oocytes

89290 Biopsy, oocyte polar body or embryo blastomere, microtechnique (for pre-implantation genetic diagnosis); less than or equal to 5 embryos

89291 greater than 5 embryos

89300 Semen analysis; presence and/or motility of sperm including Huhner test (post coital)

89310 motility and count (not including Huhner test)

89320 volume, count, motility, and differential

(Skin tests, see 86485-86580 and 95012-95199)

89321 sperm presence and motility of sperm, if performed

(To report Hyaluronan binding assay [HBA], use 89398)

89322 volume, count, motility, and differential using strict morphologic criteria (eg, Kruger)

89325 Sperm antibodies

(For medicolegal identification of sperm, use 88125)

89329 Sperm evaluation; hamster penetration test

89330 cervical mucus penetration test, with or without spinnbarkeit test

89331 Sperm evaluation, for retrograde ejaculation, urine (sperm concentration, motility, and morphology, as indicated)

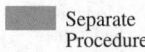 Separate Procedure   Unlisted Procedure   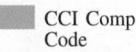 CCI Comp. Code   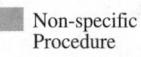 Non-specific Procedure

(For semen analysis on concurrent semen specimen, see 89300-89322 in conjunction with 89331)

(For detection of sperm in urine, use 81015)

89335 Cryopreservation, reproductive tissue, testicular

(For cryopreservation of embryo(s), use 89258. For cryopreservation of sperm, use 89259)

(For cryopreservation, ovarian reproductive tissue, oocytes, use 89240)

89342 Storage, (per year); embryo(s)

89343   sperm/semen

89344   reproductive tissue, testicular/ovarian

89346   oocyte(s)

89352 Thawing of cryopreserved; embryo(s)

89353   sperm/semen, each aliquot

89354   reproductive tissue, testicular/ovarian

89356   oocytes, each aliquot

89398 Unlisted reproductive medicine laboratory procedure

MEDICINE

MEDICINE SECTION OVERVIEW

The sixth section of the CPT coding system is the medicine section, which includes codes for immunizations, therapeutic or diagnostic injections, psychiatric services, dialysis, ophthalmology services, specialty specific diagnostic services, chemotherapy administration, physical medicine and rehabilitation services, osteopathic and chiropractic services. Within each subsection, the CPT codes are arranged by the type of service provided.

MEDICINE SUBSECTIONS

The MEDICINE section of CPT is divided into the following subsections:

Immune Globulins	90281-90399
Immunization Administration for Vaccines/Toxoids	90460-90474
Vaccines, Toxoids	90476-90749
Psychiatry	90801-90899
Biofeedback	90901-90911
Dialysis	90935-90999
Gastroenterology	91010-91299
Ophthalmology	92002-92499
Special Otorhinolaryngologic Services	92502-92700
Cardiovascular	92920-93779
Noninvasive Vascular Diagnostic Studies	93880-93998
Pulmonary	94002-94799
Allergy and Clinical Immunology	95004-95199
Endocrinology	95250-95251
Neurology and Neuromuscular Procedures	95782-96020
Medical Genetics and Genetic Counseling	96040
Central Nervous System Assessments/Tests	96101-96125
Health and Behavior Assessment/Intervention	96150-96155
Hydration, Therapeutic, Prophylactic, Diagnostic Injections and Infusions and Chemotherapy	96360-96549
Photodynamic Therapy	96567-96571
Special Dermatological Procedures	96900-96999
Physical Medicine and Rehabilitation	97001-97799
Medical Nutrition Therapy	97802-97804
Acupuncture	97810-97814
Osteopathic Manipulative Treatment	98925-98929
Chiropractic Manipulative Tretment	98940-98943
Education/Training for Patient Self-Management	98960-98962

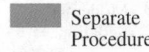 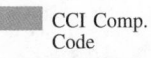

continued

1087

Separate Procedure   Unlisted Procedure   CCI Comp. Code   Non-specific Procedure

Non-Face-to-Face Physician Services	98966-98969
Special Services, Procedures and Reports	99000-99091
Qualifying Circumstances for Anesthesia	99100-99140
Moderate (Conscious) Sedation	99143-99150
Other Services and Procedures	99170-99199
Home Health Procedures/Services	99500-99602
Medication Therapy Management	99605-99607

Most of the subsections have special needs or instructions unique to that section which should be reviewed carefully before reporting.

MEDICINE SERVICES MODIFIERS

MEDICINE services and procedures may be modified under certain circumstances. When applicable, the modifying circumstance is identified by the addition of the appropriate modifier code. The following modifiers are frequently used with MEDICINE services.

-22 Unusual services

-26 Professional component

-51 Multiple procedures

This modifier may be used to report multiple medical procedures performed at the same session, as well as a combination of medical and surgical procedures.

-52 Reduced services

-76 Repeat procedure by same physician

-77 Repeat procedure by another physician

-90 Reference (outside) laboratory

-99 Multiple modifiers

● New Code   ▲ Revised Code   + Add-On Code   ⊘ Modifier -51 Exempt   ⊙ Moderate Sedation

MEDICINE CODES

IMMUNE GLOBULINS, SERUM OR RECOMBINANT PRODUCTS

Codes 90281-90399 identify the serum globulins, extracted from human blood; or recombinant immune globulin products created in a laboratory through genetic modification of human and/or animal proteins. Both are reported in addition to the administration codes 96365-96368, 96372, 96374, 96375 as appropriate. Modifier 51 should not be reported with this section of products codes when performed with another procedure. The serum or recombinant globulin products listed here include broad-spectrum anti-infective immune globulins, antitoxins, various isoantibodies, and monoclonal antibodies.

90281 Immune globulin (Ig), human, for intramuscular use

90283 Immune globulin (IgIV), human, for intravenous use

90284 Immune globulin (SCIg), human, for use in subcutaneous infusions, 100 mg, each

90287 Botulinum antitoxin, equine, any route

90288 Botulism immune globulin, human, for intravenous use

90291 Cytomegalovirus immune globulin (CMV-IgIV), human, for intravenous use

90296 Diphtheria antitoxin, equine, any route

90371 Hepatitis B immune globulin (HBIg), human, for intramuscular use

90375 Rabies immune globulin (RIg), human, for intramuscular and/or subcutaneous use

90376 Rabies immune globulin, heat-treated (RIg-HT), human, for intramuscular and/or subcutaneous use

90378 Respiratory syncytial virus monoclonal antibody, recombinant, for intramuscular use, 50 mg, each

(**90379** Deleted 2009 [2010 edition])

1089

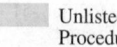 Separate Procedure	Unlisted Procedure	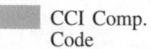 CCI Comp. Code	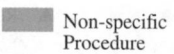 Non-specific Procedure

90384   Rho(D) immune globulin (RhIg), human, full-dose, for intramuscular use

90385   Rho(D) immune globulin (RhIg), human, mini-dose, for intramuscular use

90386   Rho(D) immune globulin (RhIgIV), human, for intravenous use

90389   Tetanus immune globulin (TIg), human, for intramuscular use

90393   Vaccinia immune globulin, human, for intramuscular use

90396   Varicella-zoster immune globulin, human, for intramuscular use

90399   Unlisted immune globulin

IMMUNIZATION ADMINISTRATION FOR VACCINES/TOXOIDS

Immunization is the administration of a vaccine or toxoid to stimulate the immune system to provide protection against disease. Immunizations are usually given in conjunction with an evaluation and management service. When an immunization is the only service performed, a minimal evaluation and management service code may be listed in addition to the injection code.

Coding Rules

1.   *When an immunization is the only service provided, evaluation and management service code 99211, Minimal service, may be reported in addition to the immunization.*

2.   *Immunization administration CPT codes must be reported in addition to the vaccine and toxoid CPT codes.*

3.   *Supplies or equipment used to inject the vaccine or toxoid are not reported separately.*

Report vaccine immunization administration codes 90460, 90461, 90471-90474 in addition to the vaccine and toxoid code(s) 90476-90749.

Report codes 90460 and 90461 only when the physician or qualified health care professional provides face-to-face counseling of the patient/family during the administration of a vaccine. For immunization administration of any vaccine that is not accompanied by face-to-face physician or qualified health care professional counseling to the patient/family, or for administration of vaccines to patients over 18 years of age, report codes 90471-90474.

  ● New Code   ▲ Revised Code   + Add-On Code   ⊘ Modifier -51 Exempt   ⊙ Moderate Sedation

If a significant separately identifiable Evaluation and Management service (eg., new or established patient office or other outpatient services [99201-99215], office or other outpatient consultations [99241-99245], emergency department services [99281-99285], preventive medicine services[99381-99429]) is performed, the appropriate E/M service code should be reported in addition to the vaccine and toxoid administration codes.

A component refers to all antigen in a vaccine that prevent disease(s) caused by one organism (90460 and 90461). Multi-valent antigens or multiple serotypes of antigens against a single organism are considered a single component of vaccines. Combination vaccines are those vaccines that contain multiple vaccine components. Conjugates or adjuvants contained in vaccines are not considered to be component parts of the vaccine as defined above.

IMMUNIZATION ADMINISTRATION

> (For allergy testing, see 95004 et seq)
>
> (For skin testing of bacterial, viral, fungal extracts, see 86485-86580)
>
> (For therapeutic or diagnostic injections, see 96372-96379)

90460   Immunization administration through 18 years of age via any route of administration, with counseling by physician or other qualified health care professional; first or only component of each vaccine or toxoid administered

+ 90461   each additional vaccine or toxoid component administered (List separately in addition to code for primary procedure)

> (Use 90460 for each vaccine administered. For vaccines with multiple components [combination vaccines], report 90460 in conjunction with 90461 for each additional component in a given vaccine)

(90465   deleted 2010 [2011 edition]. To report, see 90460, 90461, 90471-90474.)

(90466   deleted 2010 [2011 edition]. To report, see 90460, 90461, 90471-90474.)

(90467   deleted 2010 [2011 edition]. To report, see 90460, 90461, 90471-90474.)

(90468   deleted 2010 [2011 edition]. To report, see 90460, 90461, 90471-90474.)

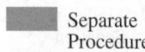 Separate Procedure   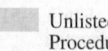 Unlisted Procedure   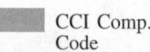 CCI Comp. Code   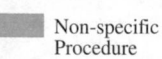 Non-specific Procedure   **1091**

(90470   deleted 2011 [2012 edition]

90471   Immunization administration (includes percutaneous, intradermal, subcutaneous, or intramuscular injections); 1 vaccine (single or combination vaccine/toxoid)

(Do not report 90471 in conjunction with 90473)

+ **90472**   each additional vaccine (single or combination vaccine/toxoid) (List separately in addition to code for primary procedure)

(Use 90472 in conjunction with 90460, 90471, 90473)

(For administration of immune globulins, see 90281-90399, 96360, 96361, 96365-96368, 96374)

(For intravesical administration of BCG vaccine, use 51720, and see 90586)

90473   Immunization administration by intranasal or oral route; 1 vaccine (single or combination vaccine/toxoid)

(Do not report 90473 in conjunction with 90471)

+ **90474**   each additional vaccine (single or combination vaccine/toxoid) (List separately in addition to code for primary procedure)

(Use 90474 in conjunction with 90460, 90471, 90473)

VACCINES, TOXOIDS

Vaccines and toxoids are administered to provide protection from hepatitis, influenza, typhoid, measles, mumps, polio, and other diseases. Vaccine and toxoid CPT codes 90476-90749 identify the vaccine or toxoid only and must be reported in addition to immunization administration CPT codes.

Codes 90476-90748 identify the vaccine product **only**. To report the administration of a vaccine/toxoid, the vaccine/toxoid product codes 90476-90749 must be used in addition to an immunization administration code(s) 90460-90474. Modifier -51 should not be reported for the vaccines, toxoids when performed with administration procedures.

If a significant separately identifiable E/M service (eg., office or other outpatient services, preventive medicine services) is performed, the appropriate E/M service code should be reported in addition to the vaccine and toxoid administration codes.

To meet the reporting requirements of immunization registries, vaccine distribution programs, and reporting systems (eg., Vaccine Adverse Event Reporting System) the exact vaccine product administered needs to be reported. Multiple codes for a particular vaccine are provided in the CPT codebook when the schedule (number of doses or timing) differs for two or more products of the same vaccine type (eg., hepatitis A, Hib) or the vaccine product is available in more than one chemical formulation, dosage, or route of administration.

The "when administered to" age descriptions included in CPT vaccine codes are not intended to identify a product's licensed age indication. The term "preservative free" includes use for vaccines that contain no preservative and vaccines that contain trace amounts of preservative agents that are not present in a sufficient concentration for the purpose of preserving the final vaccine formulation. The absence of a designation regarding a preservative does not necessarily indicate the presence or absence of preservative in the vaccine. Refer to the product's prescribing information (PI) for the licensed age indication before administering vaccine to a patient.

Separate codes are available for combination vaccines (eg., DTP-Hib, DtaP-Hib, HepB-Hib). It is inappropriate to code each component of a combination vaccine separately. If a specific vaccine code is not available, the unlisted procedure code should be reported, until a new code becomes available.

(For immune globulins, see codes 90281-90399, 96365-96368, 96372-96375 for administration of immune globulins)

90476 Adenovirus vaccine, type 4, live, for oral use

90477 Adenovirus vaccine, type 7, live, for oral use

90581 Anthrax vaccine, for subcutaneous or intramuscular use

90585 Bacillus Calmette-Guerin vaccine (BCG) for tuberculosis, live, for percutaneous use

90586 Bacillus Calmette-Guerin vaccine (BCG) for bladder cancer, live, for intravesical use

90632 Hepatitis A vaccine, adult dosage, for intramuscular use

90633 Hepatitis A vaccine, pediatric/adolescent dosage-2 dose schedule, for intramuscular use

90634 Hepatitis A vaccine, pediatric/adolescent dosage-3 dose schedule, for intramuscular use

90636 Hepatitis A and hepatitis B vaccine (HepA-HepB), adult dosage, for intramuscular use

90644 Meningococcal conjugate vaccine, serogroups C & Y and Hemophilus influenza B vaccine (Hib-MenCY), 4 dose schedule, when administered to children 2-15 months of age, for intramuscular use

90645 Hemophilus influenza B vaccine (Hib), HbOC conjugate (4 dose schedule), for intramuscular use

90646 Hemophilus influenza B vaccine (Hib), PRP-D conjugate, for booster use only, intramuscular use

90647 Hemophilus influenza B vaccine (Hib), PRP-OMP conjugate (3 dose schedule), for intramuscular use

90648 Hemophilus influenza B vaccine (Hib), PRP-T conjugate (4 dose schedule), for intramuscular use

90649 Human papilloma virus (HPV) vaccine, types 6, 11, 16, 18 (quadrivalent), 3 dose schedule, for intramuscular use

90650 Human papilloma virus (HPV) vaccine, types 16, 18, bivalent, 3 dose schedule, for intramuscular use

● **90653** Influenza vaccine, inactivated, subunit, adjuvanted, for intramuscular use

(FDA approval pending)

90654 Influenza virus vaccine, split virus, preservative-free, for intradermal use

▲ **90655** Influenza virus vaccine, trivalent, split virus, preservative free, when administered to children 6-35 months of age, for intramuscular use

▲ **90656** Influenza virus vaccine, trivalent, split virus, preservative free, when administered to individuals 3 years of age and older, for intramuscular use

▲ **90657** Influenza virus vaccine, trivalent, split virus, when administered to children 6-35 months of age, for intramuscular use

▲ **90658** Influenza virus vaccine, trivalent, split virus, when administered to individuals 3 years of age and older, for intramuscular use

● New Code   ▲ Revised Code   + Add-On Code   ⊘ Modifier -51 Exempt   ⊙ Moderate Sedation

▲ **90660**   Influenza virus vaccine, trivalent, live, for intranasal use

● **90672**   Influenza virus vaccine, quadrivalent, live, for intranasal

90661   Influenza virus vaccine, derived from cell cultures, subunit, preservative and antibiotic free, for intramuscular use

(FDA approval pending)

90662   Influenza virus vaccine, split virus, preservative free, enhanced immunogenicity via increased antigen content, for intramuscular use

(90663   deleted 2011 [2012 edition]

90664   Influenza virus vaccine, pandemic formulation, live, for intranasal use

(90665   deleted 2012 [2013 edition])

90666   Influenza virus vaccine, pandemic formulation, split virus, preservative free, for intramuscular use

(FDA approval pending)

90667   Influenza virus vaccine, pandemic formulation, split virus, adjuvanted, for intramuscular use

(FDA approval pending)

90668   Influenza virus vaccine, pandemic formulation, split virus, for intramuscular use

(FDA approval pending)

90669   Pneumococcal conjugate vaccine, 7 valent, for intramuscular use

90670   Pneumococcal conjugate vaccine, 13 valent, for intramuscular use

90672   This code is out of order. See page 1095

90675   Rabies vaccine, for intramuscular use

90676   Rabies vaccine, for intradermal use

90680   Rotavirus vaccine, pentavalent, 3 dose schedule, live, for oral use

1095

| | Separate Procedure | | Unlisted Procedure | | CCI Comp. Code | | Non-specific Procedure |

90681 Rotavirus vaccine, human, attenuated, 2 dose schedule, live, for oral use

90690 Typhoid vaccine, live, oral

90691 Typhoid vaccine, Vi capsular polysaccharide (ViCPs), for intramuscular use

90692 Typhoid vaccine, heat- and phenol-inactivated (H-P), for subcutaneous or intradermal use

90693 Typhoid vaccine, acetone-killed, dried (AKD), for subcutaneous use (U.S. military)

90696 Diphtheria, tetanus toxoids, acellular pertussis vaccine and poliovirus vaccine, inactivated (DTAP-IPV), when administered to children 4 through 6 years of age, for intramuscular use

90698 Diphtheria, tetanus toxoids, acellular pertussis vaccine, haemophilus influenza Type B, and poliovirus vaccine, inactivated (DTaP-Hib-IPV), for intramuscular use

90700 Diphtheria, tetanus toxoids, and acellular pertussis vaccine (DTaP), when administered to individuals younger than 7 years, for intramuscular use

(90701 deleted 2012 [2013 edition])

90702 Diphtheria and tetanus toxoids (DT) adsorbed, when administered to individuals younger than 7 years, for intramuscular use

90703 Tetanus toxoid adsorbed, for intramuscular use

90704 Mumps virus vaccine, live, for subcutaneous use

90705 Measles virus vaccine, live, for subcutaneous use

90706 Rubella virus vaccine, live, for subcutaneous use

90707 Measles, mumps and rubella virus vaccine (MMR), live, for subcutaneous use

90708 Measles and rubella virus vaccine, live, for subcutaneous use

● New Code   ▲ Revised Code   + Add-On Code   ⊘ Modifier -51 Exempt   ⊙ Moderate Sedation

90710 Measles, mumps, rubella, and varicella vaccine (MMRV), live, for subcutaneous use

90712 Poliovirus vaccine, (any type(s)) (OPV), live, for oral use

90713 Poliovirus vaccine, inactivated, (IPV), for subcutaneous or intramuscular use

90714 Tetanus and diphtheria toxoids (Td) adsorbed, preservative free, when administered to individuals 7 years or older, for intramuscular use

90715 Tetanus, diphtheria toxoids and acellular pertussis vaccine (Tdap), when administered to individuals 7 years or older, for intramuscular use

90716 Varicella virus vaccine, live, for subcutaneous use

90717 Yellow fever vaccine, live, for subcutaneous use

(**90718** deleted 2012 [2013 edition])

90719 Diphtheria toxoid, for intramuscular use

90720 Diphtheria, tetanus toxoids, and whole cell pertussis vaccine and Hemophilus influenza B vaccine (DTP-Hib), for intramuscular use

90721 Diphtheria, tetanus toxoids, and acellular pertussis vaccine and Hemophilus influenza B vaccine (DtaP-Hib), for intramuscular use

90723 Diphtheria, tetanus toxoids, acellular pertussis vaccine, Hepatitis B, and poliovirus vaccine, inactivated (DtaP-HepB-IPV), for intramuscular use

90725 Cholera vaccine for injectable use

90727 Plague vaccine, for intramuscular use

90732 Pneumococcal polysaccharide vaccine, 23-valent, adult or immunosuppressed patient dosage, when administered to individuals 2 years or older, for subcutaneous or intramuscular use

90733 Meningococcal polysaccharide vaccine (any group(s)), for subcutaneous use

| | Separate Procedure | | Unlisted Procedure | | CCI Comp. Code | | Non-specific Procedure | **1097** |

90734 Meningococcal conjugate vaccine, serogroups A, C, Y and W-135 (tetravalent), for intramuscular use

90735 Japanese encephalitis virus vaccine, for subcutaneous use

90736 Zoster (shingles) vaccine, live, for subcutaneous injection

90738 Japanese encephalitis virus vaccine, inactivated, for intramuscular use

● **90739** Hepatitis B vaccine, adult dosage (2 dose schedule), for intramuscular use

(FDA approval pending)

90740 Hepatitis B vaccine, dialysis or immunosuppressed patient dosage (3 dose schedule), for intramuscular use

90743 Hepatitis B vaccine, adolescent (2 dose schedule), for intramuscular use

90744 Hepatitis B vaccine, pediatric/adolescent dosage (3 dose schedule), for intramuscular use

▲ **90746** Hepatitis B vaccine, adult dosage (3 dose schedule), for intramuscular use

90747 Hepatitis B vaccine, dialysis or immunosuppressed patient dosage (4 dose schedule), for intramuscular use

90748 Hepatitis B and Hemophilus influenza B vaccine (HepB-Hib), for intramuscular use

90749 Unlisted vaccine/toxoid

PSYCHIATRY

Psychiatry is the study, treatment and prevention of mental disorders. Psychiatric services include diagnostic services, psychotherapy, and other services to an individual, family or group. Services are provided in all settings of care, and may be provided by a physician or other qualified health care professional. Psychiatric service CPT codes are used to report general psychiatry, clinical psychiatry, and psychiatric therapeutic services and procedures. Key coding issues include the type of psychotherapy, the place of service, the face-to-face time spent with the patient during psychotherapy, and whether evaluation and management services are furnished on the same date of service as psychotherapy.

● New Code ▲ Revised Code + Add-On Code ⊘ Modifier -51 Exempt ⊙ Moderate Sedation

Patient condition, characteristics, or situational factors may require services described as being with interactive complexity. Services may be provided to a patient in crisis. Services are provided in all settings of care and psychiatry services codes are reported without regard to setting. Services may be provided by a physician or other qualified health care professional. Some psychiatry services may be reported with E/M services (99201-99255, 99281-99285, 99304-99337, 99341-99350) or other services when performed. Evaluation and Management Services (99201-99285, 99304-99337, 99341-99350) may be reported for treatment of psychiatric conditions rather than using Psychiatry Services codes, when appropriate.

Hospital care in treating a psychiatric inpatient or partial hospitalization may be initial or subsequent in nature (see 99221-99233).

Some patients receive hospital evaluation and management services only and others receive evaluation and management services and other procedures. If other procedures such as electroconvulsive therapy or psychotherapy are rendered in addition to hospital evaluation and management services, these should be listed separately (ie., hospital care services [99221-99223, 99231-99233] plus electroconvulsive therapy [90870] or when psychotherapy is done, with appropriate code(s) defining psychotherapy services.

Consultation for psychiatric evaluation of a patient includes examination of a patient and exchange of information with the primary physician and other informants, such as nurses or family members, and preparation of a report. These services may be reported usin consultation codes.

INTERACTIVE COMPLEXITY

Code 90785 is an add-on code for interactive complexity to be reported in conjunction with codes for diagnostic psychiatric evaluation (90791, 90792), psychotherapy (90832, 90834, 90837), psychotherapy when performed with an E/M service (90833, 90836, 90838, 99201-99255, 99304-99337, 99341-99350), and group psychotherapy (90853).

Interactive complexity refers to specific communication factors that complicate the delivery of a psychiatric procedure. Common factors include more difficult communication with discordant or emotional family members and engagement of young and verbally undeveloped or impaired patients. Typical patients are those who have third parties, such as parents, guardians, other family members, interpreters, language translators, agencies, court officers, or schools involved in their psychaitric care.

Psychiatric procedures may be reported "with interactive complexity" when at least one of the following is present:

	Separate Procedure		Unlisted Procedure		CCI Comp. Code		Non-specific Procedure

1. The need to manage maladaptive communication (related to, eg, high anxiety, high reactivity, repeated questions, or disagreement) among participants that complicates delivery of care.

2. Caregiver emotions or behavior that interferes with the caregiver's understanding and ability to assist in the implementation of the treatment plan.

3. Evidence or disclosure of a sentinel event and mandated report to third party (eg, abuse or neglect with report to state agency) with initiation of discussion of the sentinel event and/or report with patient and other visit participants.

4. Use of play equipment, other physical devices, interpreter or translator to communicate with the patient to overcome barriers to therapeutic or diagnostic interaction between the physician or other qualified health care professional and a patient who:

> * is not fluent in the same language as the physician or other qualified health care professional, or

> * has not developed or has lost either the expressive language communication skills to explain his/her symptoms and response to treatment, or the receptive communication skills to understand the physician or other qualified health care professional if he/she were to use typical language for communication.

When provided in conjunction with the psychotherapy services (90832-90838), the amount of time spent by a physician or other qualified health care professional providing interactive complexity services should be reflected in the timed service code for psychotherapy (90832, 90834, 90837) or the psychotherapy add-on code performed with an evaluation and management service (90833, 90836, 90838) and must relate to the psychotherapy service only. Interactive complexity is not a factor for E/M services selection (99201-99255, 99281-99285, 99304-99337, 99341-99350), except as it directly affects key components as defined in the E/M services guidelines (ie, history, examination, and medical decision making).

●+**90785**   Interactive complexity (List separately in addition to the code for primary procedure)

> (Use 90785 in conjunction with codes for diagnostic psychiatric evaluation [90791, 90792], psychotherapy [90832, 90834, 90837], psychotherapy when performed with an evaluation and management service [90833, 90836, 90838, 99201-99255, 99304-99337, 99341-99350], and group psychotherapy [90853])

> (Do not report 90785 in conjunction with 90839, 90840, or in conjunction with E/M services when no psychotherapy service is also reported.)

PSYCHIATRIC DIAGNOSTIC PROCEDURES

Psychiatric diagnostic evaluation is an integrated biopsychosocial assessment, including history, mental status and recommendations. The evaluation may include communication with family or other sources and review and ordering of diagnostic services.

Psychiatric diagnostic evaluation with medical services is an integrated biopsychosocial and medical assessment, including history, mental status, other physical examination elements as indicated, and recommendations. The evaluation may include communication with family or other sources, prescription of medications, and review and ordering of laboratory or other diagnostic studies.

In certain circumstances one or more other informants (family members, guardians, or significant others) may be seen in lieu of the patient. Codes 90791, 90792 may be reported more than once for the patient when separate diagnostic evaluations are conducted with the patient and other informants. Report services as being provided to the patient and not the informant or other party in such circumstances. Codes 90791, 90792 may be reported once per day and not on the same day as an evaluation and management service performed by the same individual for the same patient.

The psychiatric diagnostic evaluation may include interactive complexity services when factors exist that complicate the delivery of the psychiatric procedure. These services should be reported with add-on code 90785 used in conjunction with the diagnostic psychiatric evaluation codes 90791, 90792.

Codes 90791, 90792 are used for the diagnostic assessment(s) or reassessment(s) if required, and do not include psychotherapeutic services. Psychotherapy services, including for crisis, may not be reported on the same day.

- **90791** Psychiatric diagnostic evaluation

- **90792** Psychiatric diagnostic evaluation with medical services

   (Do not report 90791 or 90792 in conjunction with 99201-99337, 99341-99350, 99366-99368, 99401-99444)

   (Use 90785 in conjunction with 90791, 90792 when the diagnostic evaluation includes interactive complxity services)

(90801 deleted 2012 [2013 edition]. To report diagnostic evaluations, see 90791, 90792)

(90802 deleted 2012 [2013 edition]. To report diagnostic evaluations, see 90791, 90792)

Separate Procedure | Unlisted Procedure | CCI Comp. Code | Non-specific Procedure

(90804   deleted 2012 [2013 edition]. To report, see psychotherapy codes 90832, 90834, 90837 or psychotherapy add-on codes when performed with an evaluation and management service [90833, 90836, 90838, 99201-99255, 99304-99337, 99341-99350])

(90805   deleted 2012 [2013 edition]. To report, see psychotherapy codes 90832, 90834, 90837 or psychotherapy add-on codes when performed with an evaluation and management service [90833, 90836, 90838, 99201-99255, 99304-99337, 99341-99350])

(90806   deleted 2012 [2013 edition]. To report, see psychotherapy codes 90832, 90834, 90837 or psychotherapy add-on codes when performed with an evaluation and management service [90833, 90836, 90838, 99201-99255, 99304-99337, 99341-99350])

(90807   deleted 2012 [2013 edition]. To report, see psychotherapy codes 90832, 90834, 90837 or psychotherapy add-on codes when performed with an evaluation and management service [90833, 90836, 90838, 99201-99255, 99304-99337, 99341-99350])

(90808   deleted 2012 [2013 edition]. To report, see psychotherapy codes 90832, 90834, 90837 or psychotherapy add-on codes when performed with an evaluation and management service [90833, 90836, 90838, 99201-99255, 99304-99337, 99341-99350])

(90809   deleted 2012 [2013 edition]. To report, see psychotherapy codes 90832, 90834, 90837 or psychotherapy add-on codes when performed with an evaluation and management service [90833, 90836, 90838, 99201-99255, 99304-99337, 99341-99350])

(90810   deleted 2012 [2013 edition]. To report interactive psychotherapy, report 90785 in conjunction with psychotherapy codes 90832, 90834, 90837 or psychotherapy add-on codes when performed with an evaluation and management service [90833, 90836, 90838, 99201-99255, 99304-99337, 99341-99350])

(90811   deleted 2012 [2013 edition]. To report interactive psychotherapy, report 90785 in conjunction with psychotherapy codes 90832, 90834, 90837 or psychotherapy add-on codes when performed with an evaluation and management service [90833, 90836, 90838, 99201-99255, 99304-99337, 99341-99350])

(90812   deleted 2012 [2013 edition]. To report interactive psychotherapy, report 90785 in conjunction with psychotherapy codes 90832, 90834, 90837 or psychotherapy add-on codes when performed with an evaluation and management service [90833, 90836, 90838, 99201-99255, 99304-99337, 99341-99350])

(90813   deleted 2012 [2013 edition]. To report interactive psychotherapy, report 90785 in conjunction with psychotherapy codes 90832, 90834, 90837 or psychotherapy add-on codes when performed with an evaluation and management service [90833, 90836, 90838, 99201-99255, 99304-99337, 99341-99350])

(90814   deleted 2012 [2013 edition]. To report interactive psychotherapy, report 90785 in conjunction with psychotherapy codes 90832, 90834, 90837 or psychotherapy add-on codes when performed with an evaluation and management service [90833, 90836, 90838, 99201-99255, 99304-99337, 99341-99350])

(90815   deleted 2012 [2013 edition]. To report interactive psychotherapy, report 90785 in conjunction with psychotherapy codes 90832, 90834, 90837 or psychotherapy add-on codes when performed with an evaluation and management service [90833, 90836, 90838, 99201-99255, 99304-99337, 99341-99350])

(90816   deleted 2012 [2013 edition]. To report, see psychotherapy codes 90832, 90834, 90837 or psychotherapy add-on codes when performed with an evaluation and management service [90833, 90836, 90838, 99201-99255, 99304-99337, 99341-99350])

(90817   deleted 2012 [2013 edition]. To report, see psychotherapy codes 90832, 90834, 90837 or psychotherapy add-on codes when performed with an evaluation and management service [90833, 90836, 90838, 99201-99255, 99304-99337, 99341-99350])

(90818   deleted 2012 [2013 edition]. To report, see psychotherapy codes 90832, 90834, 90837 or psychotherapy add-on codes when performed with an evaluation and management service [90833, 90836, 90838, 99201-99255, 99304-99337, 99341-99350])

(90819   deleted 2012 [2013 edition]. To report, see psychotherapy codes 90832, 90834, 90837 or psychotherapy add-on codes when performed with an evaluation and management service [90833, 90836, 90838, 99201-99255, 99304-99337, 99341-99350])

(90821   deleted 2012 [2013 edition]. To report, see psychotherapy codes 90832, 90834, 90837 or psychotherapy add-on codes when performed with an evaluation and management service [90833, 90836, 90838, 99201-99255, 99304-99337, 99341-99350])

(90822   deleted 2012 [2013 edition]. To report, see psychotherapy codes 90832, 90834, 90837 or psychotherapy add-on codes when performed with an evaluation and management service [90833, 90836, 90838, 99201-99255, 99304-99337, 99341-99350])

■ Separate Procedure   ■ Unlisted Procedure   ■ CCI Comp. Code   ■ Non-specific Procedure   **1103**

(90823 deleted 2012 [2013 edition]. To report interactive psychotherapy, report 90785 in conjunction with psychotherapy codes 90832, 90834, 90837 or psychotherapy add-on codes wehn performed with an evaluation and management service [90833, 90836, 90838, 99201-99255, 99304-99337, 99341-99350])

(90824 deleted 2012 [2013 edition]. To report interactive psychotherapy, report 90785 in conjunction with psychotherapy codes 90832, 90834, 90837 or psychotherapy add-on codes wehn performed with an evaluation and management service [90833, 90836, 90838, 99201-99255, 99304-99337, 99341-99350])

(90826 deleted 2012 [2013 edition]. To report interactive psychotherapy, report 90785 in conjunction with psychotherapy codes 90832, 90834, 90837 or psychotherapy add-on codes wehn performed with an evaluation and management service [90833, 90836, 90838, 99201-99255, 99304-99337, 99341-99350])

(90827 deleted 2012 [2013 edition]. To report interactive psychotherapy, report 90785 in conjunction with psychotherapy codes 90832, 90834, 90837 or psychotherapy add-on codes wehn performed with an evaluation and management service [90833, 90836, 90838, 99201-99255, 99304-99337, 99341-99350])

(90828 deleted 2012 [2013 edition]. To report interactive psychotherapy, report 90785 in conjunction with psychotherapy codes 90832, 90834, 90837 or psychotherapy add-on codes wehn performed with an evaluation and management service [90833, 90836, 90838, 99201-99255, 99304-99337, 99341-99350])

(90829 deleted 2012 [2013 edition]. To report interactive psychotherapy, report 90785 in conjunction with psychotherapy codes 90832, 90834, 90837 or psychotherapy add-on codes wehn performed with an evaluation and management service [90833, 90836, 90838, 99201-99255, 99304-99337, 99341-99350])

PSYCHOTHERAPY

Psychotherapy is the treatment of menal illness and behavioral disturbances in which the physician or other qualified health care professional, through definitive therapeutic communication, attempts to alleviate the emotional disturbances, reverse or change maladaptive patterns of behavior, and encourage personality growth and development.

The psychotherapy service codes 90832-90838 include ongoing assessment and adjustment of psychotherapeutic interventions, and may include involvement of family member(s) or others in the treatment process.

● New Code   ▲ Revised Code   + Add-On Code   ⊘ Modifier -51 Exempt   ⊙ Moderate Sedation

Psychotherapy times are for face-to-face services with patient and/or family member. the patient must be present for all or some of the service. For family psychotherapy without the patient present, use 90846. In reporting, choose the code closest to the actual time (ie, 16-37 minutes for 90832 and 90833, 38-52 minutes for 90834 and 90836, and 53 minutes or more for 90837 and 90838). Do not report psychotherapy of less than 16 minutes duration.

Psychotherapy provided to a patient in crisis state is reported with codes 90839 and 90840 and cannot be reported in addition to the psychotherapy codes 90832-90838. For psychotherapy for crisis, see "Other Psychotherapy."

Code 90785 is an add-on code to report interactive complexity services when provided in conjunction with the psychotherapy codes 90832-90838. The amount of time spent by a physician or other qualified health care professional providing interactive complexity services should be reflected in the timed service code for psychotherapy (90832, 90834, 90837) or the psychotherapy add-on code performed with an evaluation and management service (90833, 90836, 90838).

Some psychiatric patients receive a medical evaluation and management (E/M) service on the same day as the psychotherapy service by the same physician or other qualified health care professional. To report both E/M and psychotherapy, the two services must be significant and separately identifiable. These services are reported by using codes specific for psychotherapy when performed with evaluation and managment services (90833, 90836, 90838) as add-on codes to the evaluation and management service.

Medical symptoms and disorders inform treatment choices of psychotherapeutic interventions, and data from therapeutic communications are used to evaluate the presence, type, and severity of medical symptoms and disorders. For the purposes of reporting, the medical and psychotherapeutic components of the service may be separately identified as follows:

1. The type and level of E/M service is selected first based upon the key components of history, examination and medical decision making

2. Time associated with activities used to meet criteria for the E/M service is not included in the time used for reporting the psychotherapy service (ie, time spent on history, examination and medical decision making **when used for the E/M service** is not psychotherapy time). Time may not be used as the basis of E/M code selection and Prolonged Services may not be reported when psychotherapy with E/M (90833, 90836, 90838) are reported.

3. A separate diagnosis is not required for the reportin of E/M and psychotherapy on the same date of service.

● **90832** Psychotherapy, 30 minutes with patient and/or family member

| | Separate Procedure | | Unlisted Procedure | | CCI Comp. Code | | Non-specific Procedure |

●+**90833**   Psychotherapy, 30 minutes with patient and/or family member when performed with an evaluation and management service (List separately in addition to the code for primary procedure)

(Use 90833 in conjunction with 99201-99255, 99304-99337, 99341-99350)

● **90834**   Psychotherapy, 45 minutes with patient and/or family member

●+**90836**   Psychotherapy, 45 minutes with patient and/or family member when performed with an evaluation and management service (List separately in addition to the code for primary procedure)

(Use 90836 in conjunction with 99201-99255, 99304-99337, 99341-99350)

● **90837**   Psychotherapy, 60 minutes with patient and/or family member

●+**90838**   Psychotherapy, 60 minutes with patient and/or family member when performed with an evaluation and management service (List separately in addition to the code for primary procedure)

(Use 90838 in conjunction with 99201-99255, 99304-99337, 99341-99350)

(Use the appropriate prolonged services code [99354-99357] for psychotherapy services 68 minutes or longer)

(Use 90785 in conjunction with 90832, 90833, 90834, 90836, 90837, 90838 when psychotherapy includes interactive complexity services)

OTHER PSYCHOTHERAPY

Psychotherapy For Crisis

Psychotherapy for crisis is an urgent assessment and history of a crisis state, a mental status exam, and a disposition. The treatment includes psychotherapy, mobilization of resources to defuse the crisis and restore safety, and implementation of psychotherapeutic interventions to minimize the potential for psychological trauma. The presenting problem is typically life threatening or complex and requires immediate attention to a patient in high distress.

Codes 90839, 90840 are used to report the total duration of time face-to-face with the patient and/or family spent by the physician or other qualified health care professional providing psychotherapy for crisis, even if the time spent on that date is not continuous. For any given period of time spent providing psychotherapy for crisis state, the physician or other qualified health care professional must devote his or her full attention to the patient and, therefore, cannot provide services to any

● New Code   ▲ Revised Code   + Add-On Code   ⊘ Modifier -51 Exempt   ⊙ Moderate Sedation

other patients during the same time period. The patient must be present for all or some of the service. Do not report with 90791 or 90792.

Code 90839 is used to report the first 30-74 minutes of psychotherapy for crisis on a given date. It should be used only once per date if the time spent by the physician or other qualified health care professional is not continuous on that date. Psychotherapy for crisis of less than 30 minutes total duration on a given date should be reported with 90832 or 90833 (when provided with evaluation and management services). Code 90840 is used to report additional block(s) of time, up to 30 minutes each beyond the first 74 minutes.

● **90839**   Psychotherapy for crisis; first 60 minutes

●+**90840**   each additional 30 minutes (List separately in addition to code for primary service)

(Use 90840 in conjunction with 90839)

(Do not report 90839, 90840 in conjunction with 90791, 90792, psychotherapy codes 90832-90838 or other psychiatric services, or 90785-90899)

90845 Psychoanalysis

90846 Family psychotherapy (without the patient present)

90847 Family psychotherapy (conjoint psychotherapy) (with patient present)

90849 Multiple-family group psychotherapy

90853 Group psychotherapy (other than of a multiple-family group)

(Use 90853 in conjunction with 90785 for the specified patient when group psychotherapy includes interactive complexity)

(90857   deleted 2012 [2013 edition]. To report, use 90785 in conjunction with 90853)

OTHER PSYCHIATRIC SERVICES OR PROCEDURES

(For analysis / programming of neurostimulators used for vagus nerve stimulation therapy, see 95970, 95974, 95975)

(90862   deleted 2012 [2013 edition]. To report, see 90863 or evaluation and management services codes 99201-99255, 99281-99285, 99304-99337, 99341-99350)

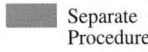 Separate Procedure   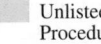 Unlisted Procedure   CCI Comp. Code   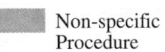 Non-specific Procedure

●+**90863**   Pharmacologic management, including prescription and review of medication, when performed with psythotherapy services (List separately in addition to the code for primary procedure)

(Use 90863 in conjunction with 90832, 90834, 90837)

(For pharmacologic management with psychotherapy services performed by a physician or other qualified health care professional who may report evaluation adn management codes, use the appropriate evaluation and management codes 99201-99255, 99281-99285, 99304-99337, 99341-99350 and the appropriate psychotherapy with evaluation and management service 90833, 90836, 90838)

(Do not count time spent on providing pharmacologic management services in the time used for selection of the psychotherapy service)

90865   Narcosynthesis for psychiatric diagnostic and therapeutic purposes (eg, sodium amobarbital (Amytal) interview)

90867   Therapeutic repetitive transcranial magnetic stimulation (TMS) treatment; initial, including cortical mapping, motor threshold determination, delivery and management

(Report only once per course of treatment)

(Do not report 90867 in conjunction with 90868, 90869, 95860-95870, 95928, 95929, 95939)

90868   subsequent delivery and management, per session

90869   subsequent motor threshold re-determination with delivery and management

(Do not report 90869 in conjunction with 90867, 90868, 95860-95870, 95928, 95929, 95939)

(If a significant, separately identifiableevaluation and management, medication management, or psychotherapy service is performed, the appropriate E/M or psychotherapy code may be reported in addition to 90867-90869. Evaluation and management activities directly related to cortical mapping, motor threshold determination, delivery and management of TMS are not separately reported)

(For transcranial magnetic stimulation motor function mapping for therapeutic planning other than for repetitive transcranial magnetic stimulation, use 0310T)

(Do not count time spent on providing pharmacologic management services in the time used for selection of the psychotherapy service)

90870 Electroconvulsive therapy (includes necessary monitoring)

▲ **90875** Individual psychophysiological therapy incorporating biofeedback training by any modality (face-to-face with the patient), with psychotherapy (eg, insight oriented, behavior modifying or supportive psychotherapy); 30 minutes

▲ **90876** 45 minutes

90880 Hypnotherapy

90882 Environmental intervention for medical management purposes on a psychiatric patients behalf with agencies, employers, or institutions

90885 Psychiatric evaluation of hospital records, other psychiatric reports, psychometric and/or projective tests, and other accumulated data for medical diagnostic purposes

90887 Interpretation or explanation of results of psychiatric, other medical examinations and procedures, or other accumulated data to family or other responsible persons, or advising them how to assist patient

▲ **90889** Preparation of report of patient's psychiatric status, history, treatment, or progress (other than for legal or consultative purposes) for other individuals, agencies, or insurance carriers

90899 Unlisted psychiatric service or procedure

BIOFEEDBACK

Biofeedback is the process of detecting information about a patient's biological functions, eg. heart rate, breathing rate, skin temperature, and amount of muscle tension, picked up by surface electrodes (sensors) and electronically amplified to provide feedback, usually in the form of an audio-tone and/or visual read-out to the patient. Biofeedback training uses the information that has been monitored from the sensors attached to a muscle on the skin's surface, or to the skin only for thermal or other readings. With the help of a trained clinician, the patient can learn how to make voluntary changes in those biological functions and bring them under control.

				1109
Separate Procedure	Unlisted Procedure	CCI Comp. Code	Non-specific Procedure	

Biofeedback services involve the use of electromyographic techniques to detect and record muscle activity. The CPT codes 95860- 95872 (EMG) should not be reported with biofeedback services based on the use of electromyography during a biofeedback session. If an EMG is performed as a separate medically necessary service for diagnosis or follow-up of organic muscle dysfunction, the appropriate EMG codes (e.g. CPT codes 95860-95872) may be reported.

Modifier -59 should be added to indicate that the service performed was a separately identifiable diagnostic service. Reporting only an objective electromyographic response to biofeedback is not sufficient to bill the codes referable to diagnostic EMG.

(For psychophysiological therapy incorporating biofeedback training, see 90875, 90876)

90901 Biofeedback training by any modality

90911 Biofeedback training, perineal muscles, anorectal or urethral sphincter, including EMG and/or manometry

(For testing of rectal sensation, tone and compliance, use 91120)

(For incontinence treatment by pulsed magnetic neuromodulation, use 53899)

DIALYSIS

(90918 deleted 2009 edition. To report ESRD-related services for patients younger than 2 years of age, see 90951-90953, 90963, 90967)

(90919 deleted 2009 edition. To report ESRD-related services for patients between 2 and 11 years of age, see 90954-90956, 90964, 90968)

(90920 deleted 2009 edition. To report ESRD-related services for patients between 12 and 19 years of age, see 90957-90959, 90965, 90969)

(90921 deleted 2009 edition. To report ESRD-related services for patients 20 years of age and older, see 90960-90962, 90966, 90970)

(90922 deleted 2009 edition. To report ESRD-related services for patients younger than 2 years of age, see 90951-90953, 90963, 90967)

● New Code ▲ Revised Code + Add-On Code ⊘ Modifier -51 Exempt ⊙ Moderate Sedation

(90923   deleted 2009 edition. To report ESRD-related services for patients between 2 and 11 years of age, see 90954-90956, 90964, 90968)

(90924   deleted 2009 edition. To report ESRD-related services for patients between 12 and 19 years of age, see 90957-90959, 90965, 90969)

(90925   deleted 2009 edition. To report ESRD-related services for patients 20 years of age and older, see 90960-90962, 90966, 90970)

HEMODIALYSIS

Codes 90935, 90937 are reported to describe the hemodialysis procedure with all evaluation and management services related to the patient's renal disease on the day of the hemodialysis procedure. These codes are used for inpatient ESRD and non-ESRD procedures or for outpatient non-ESRD dialysis services. Code 90935 is reported if only one evaluation of the patient is required related to that hemodialysis procedure. Code 90937 is reported when patient re-evaluation(s) is required during a hemodialysis procedure. Use modifier 25 with E/M codes, including new or established patient office or other outpatient services (99201-99215), office or other outpatient consultations (99241-99245), observation care (99217-99220, 99224-99226), observation or inpatient care including admission and discharge (99234-99236), initial hospital care (99221-99226, 99231-99239), new or established patient emergency department services (99281-99285), critical care services (99291, 99292), inpatient neonatal intensive care services and pediatric and neonatal critical care services (99466-99480), nursing facility services (99304-99318), domiciliary, rest home services, or custodial care (99324-99337), and home services (99341-99350), for separately identifiable services unrelated to the dialysis procedure or renal failure which cannot be rendered during the dialysis session.

(For home visit hemodialysis services performed by a non-physician health care professional, use 99512)

(For cannula declotting, see 36831, 36833, 36860, 36861)

(For declotting of implanted vascular access device or catheter by thrombolytic agent, use 36593)

(For collection of blood specimen from a partially or completely implantable venous access device, use 36591)

(For prolonged attendance by a physician or other qualified health care professional, see 99354-99360)

▲ **90935**   Hemodialysis procedure with single evaluation by a physician or other qualified health care professional

---

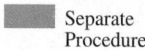 Separate Procedure   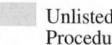 Unlisted Procedure   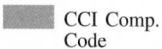 CCI Comp. Code   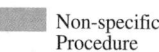 Non-specific Procedure   **1111**

90937 Hemodialysis procedure requiring repeated evaluation(s) with or without substantial revision of dialysis prescription

90940 Hemodialysis access flow study to determine blood flow in grafts and arteriovenous fistulae by an indicator method

(For duplex scan of hemodialysis access, use 93990)

MISCELLANEOUS DIALYSIS PROCEDURES

Codes 90945, 90947 describe dialysis procedures other than hemodialysis (eg., peritoneal dialysis, hemofiltration or continuous renal replacement therapies), and all evaluation and management services related to the patient's renal disease on the day of the procedure. Code 90945 is reported if only one evaluation of the patient is required related to that procedure. Code 90947 is reported when patient re-evaluation(s) is required during a procedure. Use modifier 25 with E/M codes, including new or established patient office or other outpatient services (99201-99215), office or other outpatient consultations (99241-99245), observation care (99217-99220, 99224-99226), observation or inpatient care including admission and discharge (99234-99239), hospital care (99221-99226, 99231-99239), new or established patient emergency department services (99281-99285), critical care services (99291, 99292), inpatient neonatal intensive care services and pediatric and neonatal critical care services (99466-99480), nursing facility services (99304-99318), domiciliary, rest home or custodial care (99324-99337), and home services (99341-99350) for separately identifiable services unrelated to the procedure or the renal failure which cannot be rendered during the dialysis session.

(For percutaneous insertion of intraperitoneal tunneled catheter, use 49418. For open insertion of tunneled intraperitoneal catheter, use 49421.)

(For prolonged attendance by a physician or other qualified heatlh care professional, see 99354-99360)

▲ **90945** Dialysis procedure other than hemodialysis (eg, peritoneal dialysis, hemofiltration or other continuous renal replacement therapies), with single evaluation by a physician or other qualified health care professional

(For home infusion of peritoneal dialysis, use 99559)

▲ **90947** Dialysis procedure other than hemodialysis (eg, peritoneal dialysis, hemofiltration, or other continuous renal replacement therapies) requiring repeated evaluation by a physician or other qualified health care professional, with or without substantial revision of dialysis prescription

---

1112 ● New Code ▲ Revised Code ＋ Add-On Code ⊘ Modifier -51 Exempt ⊙ Moderate Sedation

END-STAGE RENAL DISEASE SERVICES

Codes 90951-90962 are reported **once** per month to distinguish age-specific services related to the patient's end-stage renal disease (ESRD) performed in an outpatient setting with three levels of service based on the number of face-to-face visits. ESRD-related services by a physician or other qualified health care professional include establishment of a dialyzing cycle, outpatient evaluation and management of the dialysis visits, telephone calls, and patient management during the dialysis provided during a full month. In circumstances in which the patient has had a complete assessment visit during the month and services are provided over a period of less than a month, 90951-90962 may be used according to the number of visits performed.

Codes 90963-90966 are reported once per month for a full month of service to distinguish age-specific services for end-stage renal disease (ESRD) services for home dialysis patients.

For ESRD and non-ESRD dialysis services performed in an inpatient setting, and for non-ESRD dialysis services performed in an outpatient setting, see 90935-90937 and 90945-90947.

Evaluation and Management services unrelated to ESRD services that cannot be performed during the dialysis session may be reported separately.

Codes 90967-90970 are reported to distinguish age-specific services for end-stage renal disease (ESRD) services for less than a full month of service, per day, for services provided under the following circumstances: home dialysis patients less than a full month, transient patients, partial month where there was one or more face-to-face visits without the complete assessment, the patient was hospitalized before a complete assessment was furnished, dialysis was stopped due to recovery or death, or the patient received a kidney transplant. For reporting purposes, each month is considered 30 days.

>(Do not report 90951-90970 during the same month in conjunction with 99487-99489)

>(Do not report 90951-90970 during the service time of 99495-99496)

▲ **90951** End-stage renal disease (ESRD) related services monthly, for patients younger than 2 years of age to include monitoring for the adequacy of nutrition, assessment of growth and development, and counseling of parents; with 4 or more face-to-face visits by a physician or other qualified health care professional, per month

▲ **90952** with 2-3 face-to-face visits by a physician or other qualified health care professional, per month

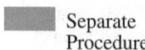 Separate Procedure   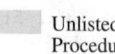 Unlisted Procedure   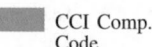 CCI Comp. Code   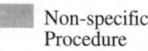 Non-specific Procedure

▲ **90953** with 1 face-to-face visit by a physician or other qualified health care professional per month

▲ **90954** End-stage renal disease (ESRD) related services monthly, for patients 2-11 years of age to include monitoring for the adequacy of nutrition, assessment of growth and development, and counseling of parents; with 4 or more face-to-face visits by a physician or other qualified health care professional per month

▲ **90955** with 2-3 face-to-face visits by a physician or other qualified health care professional per month

▲ **90956** with 1 face-to-face visits by a physician or other qualified health care professional per month

▲ **90957** End-stage renal disease (ESRD) related services monthly, for patients 12-19 years of age to include monitoring for the adequacy of nutrition, assessment of growth and development, and counseling of parents; with 4 or more face-to-face visits by a physician or other qualified health care professional per month

▲ **90958** with 2-3 face-to-face visits by a physician or other qualified health care professional per month

▲ **90959** with 1 face-to-face visit by a physician or other qualified health care professional per month

▲ **90960** End-stage renal disease (ESRD) related services monthly, for patients 20 years of age and older; with 4 or more face-to-face visits by a physician or other qualified health care professional per month

▲ **90961** with 2-3 face-to-face visits by a physician or other qualified health care professional per month

▲ **90962** with 1 face-to-face visit by a physician or other qualified health care professional per month

90963 End-stage renal disease (ESRD) related services for home dialysis per full month, for patients younger than 2 years of age to include monitoring for the adequacy of nutrition, assessment of growth and development, and counseling of parents

90964 End-stage renal disease (ESRD) related services for home dialysis per full month, for patients 2-11 years of age to include

● New Code   ▲ Revised Code   + Add-On Code   ⊘ Modifier -51 Exempt   ⊙ Moderate Sedation

monitoring for the adequacy of nutrition, assessment of growth and development, and counseling of parents

90965 End-stage renal disease (ESRD) related services for home dialysis per full month, for patients 12-19 years of age to include monitoring for the adequacy of nutrition, assessment of growth and development, and counseling of parents

90966 End-stage renal disease (ESRD) related services for home dialysis per full month, for patients 20 years of age and older

90967 End-stage renal disease (ESRD) related services for dialysis less than a full month of service, per day; for patients younger than 2 years of age

90968 for patients 2-11 years of age

90969 for patients 12-19 years of age

90970 for patients 20 years of age and older

OTHER DIALYSIS PROCEDURES

90989 Dialysis training, patient, including helper where applicable, any mode, completed course

90993 Dialysis training, patient, including helper where applicable, any mode, course not completed, per training session

90997 Hemoperfusion (eg, with activated charcoal or resin)

90999 Unlisted dialysis procedure, inpatient or outpatient

GASTROENTEROLOGY

Gastroenterology is the study and treatment of diseases of the stomach and digestive system. CPT codes listed in this subsection are used to report diagnostic services of the esophagus and/or stomach contents, and therapeutic services such as gastric intubation and lavage. Gastroenterology services are usually performed in conjunction with an evaluation and management service, such as a consultation or visit, and should be reported separately in addition to the evaluation and management service.

Gastroenterological tests included in CPT codes 91000-91299 are frequently complementary to endoscopic procedures. Esophageal and gastric washings for cytology are described as part of upper endoscopy (e.g. CPT code 43235);

	Separate Procedure		Unlisted Procedure		CCI Comp. Code		Non-specific Procedure	**1115**

therefore, CPT codes 91000 (esophageal intubation) and 91055 (gastric intubation) are not separately reported when performed as part of an upper endoscopy.

Provocative testing (CPT code 91052) can be expedited during GI endoscopy (procurement of gastric specimens). When performed at the same time as GI endoscopy, CPT code 91052 is reported with modifier -52 indicating that a reduced level of service was performed.

(For duodenal intubation and aspiration, see 43756, 43757)

(For gastrointestinal radiologic procedures, see 74210-74363)

(For esophagoscopy procedures, see 43200-43228; upper GI endoscopy 43235-43259; endoscopy, small intestine and stomal 44360-44393; proctosigmoidoscopy 45300-45321; sigmoidoscopy 45330-45339; colonscopy 45355-45385; anoscopy 46600-46615)

(91000   deleted 2010 [2011 edition])

91010   Esophageal motility (manometric study of the esophagus and/or gastroesophageal junction) study with interpretation and report;

(91011   deleted 2010 [2011 edition]. To report esophageal motility studies with stimulant or perfusion, use 91013 in conjunction with 91010)

(91012   deleted 2010 [2011 edition]. To report esophageal motility studies with stimulant or perfusion, use 91013 in conjunction with 91010)

+ **91013**   with stimulation or perfusion (eg, stimulant, acid or alkali perfusion) (List separately in addition to code for primary procedure)

(Use 91013 in conjunction with 91010)

(Do not report 91013 more than once per session)

(To report esophageal motility studies with high resolution esophageal pressure topography, use 0240T adn with stimulant or perfusion, use 0241T)

91020   Gastric motility (manometric) studies

91022   Duodenal motility (manometric) study

(If gastrointestinal endoscopy is performed, use 43235)

1116   ● New   ▲ Revised   + Add-On   ⊘ Modifier -51   ⊙ Moderate
             Code   Code   Code   Exempt   Sedation

(If fluoroscopy is performed, use 76000)

(If gastric motility study is performed, use 91020)

(Do not report 91020, 91022 in conjunction with 91112)

91030 Esophagus, acid perfusion (Bernstein) test for esophagitis

91034 Esophagus, gastroesophageal reflux test; with nasal catheter pH electrode(s) placement, recording, analysis and interpretation

91035 with mucosal attached telemetry pH electrode placement, recording, analysis and interpretation

91037 Esophageal function test, gastroesophageal reflux test with nasal catheter intraluminal impedance electrode(s) placement, recording, analysis and interpretation;

91038 prolonged (greater than 1 hour, up to 24 hours)

91040 Esophageal balloon distension provocation study

(For balloon dilatation with endoscopy, see 43220, 43249, 43456, or 43458)

(91052 deleted 2010 [2011 edition]. To report, see 43754, 43755)

(91055 deleted 2010 [2011 edition]. To report, see 43754, 43755)

91065 Breath hydrogen test (eg, for detection of lactase deficiency), fructose intolerance, bacterial overgrowth, or oro-cecal gastrointestinal transit)

(For H. pylori breath test analysis, use 83013 for non-radioactive (C-13) isotope or 78268 for radioactive (C-14) isotope)

(91100 deleted 2009 edition)

(To report placement of an esophageal tamponade tube for management of variceal bleeding, use 43460. To report placement of a long intestinal Miller-Abbott tube, use 44500)

(91105 deleted 2010 [2011 edition]. To report, use 43753)

(For cholangiography, see 47500, 74320)

(For abdominal paracentesis, see 49082, 49083, 49084; with instillation of medication, see 96440, 96446)

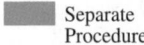 Separate Procedure   Unlisted Procedure   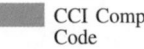 CCI Comp. Code   Non-specific Procedure   **1117**

(For peritoneoscopy, use 49320; with biopsy, use 49321)

(For peritoneoscopy and guided transhepatic cholangiography, use 47560; with biopsy, use 47561)

(For splenoportography, see 38200, 75810)

▲ **91110** Gastrointestinal tract imaging, intraluminal (eg, capsule endoscopy), esophagus through ileum, with interpretation and report

(Visualization of the colon is not reported separately)

(Append modifier -52 if the ileum is not visualized)

▲ **91111** Gastrointestinal tract imaging, intraluminal (eg, capsule endoscopy), esophagus with interpretation and report

(Do not report 91111 in conjunction with 91110)

(For measurement of gastrointestinal tract transit times or pressure using wireless capsule, use 91112)

● **91112** Gastrointestinal transit and pressure measurement, stomach through colon, wireless capsule, with interpretation and report

(Do not report 91112 in conjunction with 83986, 91020, 91022, 91117)

91117 Colon motility (manometric) study, minimum 6 hours continuous recording (including provocation tests, eg, meal, intracolonic balloon distension, pharmacologic agents, if performed), with interpretation and report

(For wireless capsule pressure measurements, use 91112)

(Do not report 91117 in conjunction with 91120, 91122)

91120 Rectal sensation, tone, and compliance test (ie, response to graded balloon distention)

(For biofeedback training, use 90911)

(For anorectal manometry, use 91122)

91122 Anorectal manometry

(Do not report 91120, 91122 in conjunction with 91117)

(91123 deleted 2010 [2011 edition])

● New Code   ▲ Revised Code   ✚ Add-On Code   ⊘ Modifier -51 Exempt   ⊙ Moderate Sedation

GASTRIC PHYSIOLOGY

91132 Electrogastrography, diagnostic, transcutaneous;

91133 with provocative testing

OTHER PROCEDURES

91299 Unlisted diagnostic gastroenterology procedure

OPHTHALMOLOGY

(For surgical procedures, see Surgery, Eye and Ocular Adnexa, 65091 et seq)

Ophthalmology is the study and treatment of diseases of the eye. Ophthalmological diagnostic and treatment services are reported using CPT Medicine codes 92002-92499.

Coding Rules

1. *Minimal, brief and limited office services, and hospital, home, extended care, emergency department and consultations are reported using appropriate evaluation and management service codes.*

2. *Surgical procedures on the eye(s) are reported using CPT codes from the Eye and Ocular Adnexa subsection of the SURGERY section of CPT.*

3. *To report intermediate ophthalmological services, the following must be performed and documented: a) evaluation of new or existing condition, b) complications of new diagnostic or management problems (not necessarily related to the primary diagnosis), c) history, d) general medical observation e) external ocular and adnexal examination, f) other diagnostic procedures as indicated, and g) may include the use of mydriasis. Intermediate ophthalmological services do not usually include determination of refractive state but may in an established patient under continuing active treatment.*

4. *To report comprehensive ophthalmological services the following must be performed and documented: a) reported as a single service but may be performed at more than one session, b) history, c) general medical observation, d) external and ophthalmoscopic examination, e) gross visual fields, f) basic sensorimotor examination, g. may include, as indicated; biomicroscopy, examination with cycloplegia or mydriasis and tonometry, h) always includes initiation of diagnostic and treatment programs.*

5. *For both intermediate and comprehensive ophthalmological services, service components, such as slip lamp examination, keratomy,*

Separate
Procedure

Unlisted
Procedure

CCI Comp.
Code

Non-specific
Procedure

ophthalmoscopy, retinoscopy, tonometry and motor evaluation are not reported separately.

For procedures requiring intravenous injection of dye or other diagnostic agent, insertion of an intravenous catheter and dye injection are necessary to accomplish the procedure and are included in the procedure. Accordingly, HCPCS/CPT codes 36000 (introduction of a needle or catheter), 36410 (venipuncture), G0345-G0350 (90760-90768 in 2006)(IV infusion), and G0353-G0354 (90774-90775 in 2006)(IV injection)as well as selective vascular catheterization codes are not to be separately reported with services requiring intravenous injection (e.g. CPT codes 92230, 92235, 92240, 92287, for angioscopy and angiography).

Fundus photography (CPT code 92250) and scanning ophthalmic computerized diagnostic imaging (CPT code 92135) are generally mutually exclusive of one another in that a provider would use one technique or the other to evaluate fundal disease. However, there are a limited number of clinical conditions where both techniques are medically reasonable and necessary on the ipsilateral eye. In these situations, both CPT codes may be reported appending modifier -59 to CPT code 92250.

GENERAL OPHTHALMOLOGICAL SERVICES

General ophthalmological services (e.g. CPT codes 92002-92014) describe components of the ophthalmologic examination. When evaluation and management codes are reported, these general ophthalmological service codes (e.g. CPT codes 92002-92014) are not to be reported; the same services would be represented by both series of codes.

NEW PATIENT

(For distinguishing between new and established patients, see E/M guidelines)

92002 Ophthalmological services: medical examination and evaluation with initiation of diagnostic and treatment program; intermediate, new patient

92004 comprehensive, new patient, 1 or more visits

ESTABLISHED PATIENT

(For distinguishing between new and established patients, see E/M guidelines)

92012 Ophthalmological services: medical examination and evaluation, with initiation or continuation of diagnostic and treatment program; intermediate, established patient

● New Code ▲ Revised Code + Add-On Code ⊘ Modifier -51 Exempt ⊙ Moderate Sedation

92014 comprehensive, established patient, 1 or more visits

(For surgical procedures, see Surgery, Eye and Ocular Adnexa, 65091 et seq)

SPECIAL OPHTHALMOLOGICAL SERVICES

Special ophthalmological services are defined as a level of service in which a special evaluation of part of the visual system is made which goes beyond the services usually included under general ophthalmological services, or in which special treatment is given. Fluorescein angioscopy, quantitative visual field examination, or extended color vision examination should be specifically reported as special ophthalmological services.

Special ophthalmologic services represent specific services not described as part of a general or routine ophthalmological examination. Special ophthalmological services are recognized as significant, separately identifiable services.

92015 Determination of refractive state

(For intrumen based ocular screening, use 99174)

92018 Ophthalmological examination and evaluation, under general anesthesia, with or without manipulation of globe for passive range of motion or other manipulation to facilitate diagnostic examination; complete

92019 limited

92020 Gonioscopy (separate procedure)

(For gonioscopy under general anesthesia, use 92018)

92025 Computerized corneal topography, unilateral or bilateral, with interpretation and report

(Do not report 92025 in conjunction with 65710-65771)

(92025 is not used for manual keratoscopy, which is part of a single system of E/M or ophthalmological service)

92060 Sensorimotor examination with multiple measurements of ocular deviation (eg, restrictive or paretic muscle with diplopia) with interpretation and report (separate procedure)

92065 Orthoptic and/or pleoptic training, with continuing medical direction and evaluation

(92070 deleted 2011 [2012 edition]. To report, see 92071, 92072)

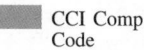

	Separate Procedure		Unlisted Procedure		CCI Comp. Code		Non-specific Procedure

1121

92071 Fitting of contact lens for treatment of ocular surface disease

(Do not report 92071 in conjunction with 92072)

(Report supply of lens separately with 99070 or appropriate supply codes)

92072 Fitting of contact lens for management of keratoconus, initial fitting

(For subsequent fittings, report using E/M services or General Ophthalmological services)

(Do not report 92072 in conjunction with 92071)

(Report supply of lens separately with 99070 or appropriate supply code)

92081 Visual field examination, unilateral or bilateral, with interpretation and report; limited examination (eg, tangent screen, Autoplot, arc perimeter, or single stimulus level automated test, such as Octopus 3 or 7 equivalent)

92082 intermediate examination (eg, at least 2 isopters on Goldmann perimeter, or semiquantitative, automated suprathreshold screening program, Humphrey suprathreshold automatic diagnostic test, Octopus program 33)

92083 extended examination (eg, Goldmann visual fields with at least 3 isopters plotted and static determination within the central 30 degrees, or quantitative, automated threshold perimetry, Octopus programs G-1, 32 or 42, Humphrey visual field analyzer full threshold programs 30-2, 24-2, or 30/60-2)

(Gross visual field testing (eg, confrontation testing) is a part of general ophthalmological services and is not reported separately)

92100 Serial tonometry (separate procedure) with multiple measurements of intraocular pressure over an extended time period with interpretation and report, same day (eg, diurnal curve or medical treatment of acute elevation of intraocular pressure)

(92120 deleted 2011 [2012 edition])

(92130 deleted 2011 [2012 edition])

● New Code ▲ Revised Code + Add-On Code ⊘ Modifier -51 Exempt ⊙ Moderate Sedation

(Ocular blood flow measurements are reported with 0198T. Single-episode tonomemtry is a component of general ophthalmological service or E/M service)

92132   Scanning computerized ophthalmic diagnostic imaging, anterior segment, with interpretation and report, unilateral or bilateral

(For spectral microscopy and endothelial cell analysis, use 92286)

92133   Scanning computerized ophthalmic diagnostic imaging, posterior segment, with interpretation and report, unilateral or bilateral; optic nerve

92134   retina

(Do not report 92133 and 92134 at the same patient encounter)

(92135   deleted 2010 [2011 edition])

(For scanning computerized ophthalmic diagnostic imaging of the optic nerve and retina, see 92133, 92134)

92136   Ophthalmic biometry by partial coherence interferometry with intraocular lens power calculation

92140   Provocative tests for glaucoma, with interpretation and report, without tonography

OPHTHALMOSCOPY

Routine ophthalmoscopy is part of general and special ophthalmologic services whenever indicated. It is a non-itemized service and is not reported separately.

92225   Ophthalmoscopy, extended, with retinal drawing (eg, for retinal detachment, melanoma), with interpretation and report; initial

92226   subsequent

92227   Remote imaging for detection of retinal disease (eg, retinopathy in a patient with diabetes) with analysis and report under physician supervision, unilateral or bilateral

(Do not report 92227 in conjunction with 92002-92014, 92133, 92134, 92250, 92228 or with the evaluation and management of the single organ system, the eye, 99201-99350)

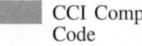 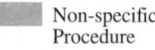

| Separate Procedure | Unlisted Procedure | CCI Comp. Code | Non-specific Procedure |

92228 Remote imaging for monitoring and management of active retinal disease (eg, diabetic retinopathy) with physician review, interpretation and report, unilateral or bilateral

(Do not report 92228 in conjunction with 92002-92014, 92133, 92134, 92250, 92227 or with the evaluation and management of the single organ system, the eye, 99201-99350)

92230 Fluorescein angioscopy with interpretation and report

92235 Fluorescein angiography (includes multiframe imaging) with interpretation and report

92240 Indocyanine-green angiography (includes multiframe imaging) with interpretation and report

92250 Fundus photography with interpretation and report

92260 Ophthalmodynamometry

(For opthalmoscopy under general anesthesia, use 92018)

OTHER SPECIALIZED SERVICES

For prescription, fitting, and/or medical supervision of ocular prosthetic (artificial eye) adaptation by a physician, see E/M services including Office or Other Outpatient services (99201-99215), Office or Other Outpatient Consultations (99241-99245) or General Ophthalmological service codes (92002-92014)

92265 Needle oculoelectromyography, 1 or more extraocular muscles, one or both eyes, with interpretation and report

92270 Electro-oculography with interpretation and report

92275 Electroretinography with interpretation and report

(For electronystagmography for vestibular function studies, see 92541 et seq)

(For ophthalmic echography (diagnostic ultrasound), see 76511-76529)

92283 Color vision examination, extended, eg, anomaloscope or equivalent

(Color vision testing with pseudoisochromatic plates (such as HRR or Ishihara) is not reported separately. It is included in the appropriate general or ophthalmological service, or 99172)

● New Code   ▲ Revised Code   + Add-On Code   ⊘ Modifier -51 Exempt   ⊙ Moderate Sedation

92284 Dark adaptation examination with interpretation and report

92285 External ocular photography with interpretation and report for documentation of medical progress (eg, close-up photography, slit lamp photography, goniophotography, stereo-photography)

▲ **92286** Anterior segment imaging with interpretation and report; with specular microscopy and endothelial cell analysis

▲ **92287** with fluorescein angiography

CONTACT LENS SERVICES

Follow-up of successfully fitted extended wear lenses is reported as part of a general ophthalmological service (92012 et seq).

The supply of contact lenses may be reported as part of the service of fitting. It may also be reported separately by using the appropriate supply codes.

(For therapeutic or surgical use of contact lens, see 68340, 92071, 92072)

92310 Prescription of optical and physical characteristics of and fitting of contact lens, with medical supervision of adaptation; corneal lens, both eyes, except for aphakia

(For prescription and fitting of one eye, add modifier -52)

92311 corneal lens for aphakia, 1 eye

92312 corneal lens for aphakia, both eyes

92313 corneoscleral lens

92314 Prescription of optical and physical characteristics of contact lens, with medical supervision of adaptation and direction of fitting by independent technician; corneal lens, both eyes except for aphakia

(For prescription and fitting of one eye, add modifier -52)

92315 corneal lens for aphakia, 1 eye

92316 corneal lens for aphakia, both eyes

92317 corneoscleral lens

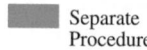 Separate Procedure 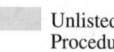 Unlisted Procedure 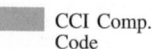 CCI Comp. Code 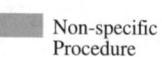 Non-specific Procedure **1125**

92325 Modification of contact lens (separate procedure), with medical supervision of adaptation

92326 Replacement of contact lens

(For prescription, fitting, and/or medical supervision of ocular prosthetic adaptation by a physician, see Evaluation and Management services or General Ophthalmological service codes 92002-92014)

SPECTACLE SERVICES (INCLUDING PROSTHESIS FOR APHAKIA)

Prescription of lenses, when required, is included in 92015, Determination of refractive state. It includes specification of lens type (monofocal, bifocal, other), lens power, axis, prism, absorptive factor, impact resistance, and other factors.

When provided, fitting of spectacles is a separate service and is reported as indicated by 92340-92371.

Fitting includes measurement of anatomical facial characteristics, the writing of laboratory specifications, and the final adjustment of the spectacles to the visual axes and anatomical topography. Presence of the physician or other qualified health care professional is not required.

Supply of materials is a separate service component; it is not part of the service of fitting spectacles.

92340 Fitting of spectacles, except for aphakia; monofocal

92341 bifocal

92342 multifocal, other than bifocal

92352 Fitting of spectacle prosthesis for aphakia; monofocal

92353 multifocal

92354 Fitting of spectacle mounted low vision aid; single element system

92355 telescopic or other compound lens system

92358 Prosthesis service for aphakia, temporary (disposable or loan, including materials)

92370 Repair and refitting spectacles; except for aphakia

● New Code	▲ Revised Code	+ Add-On Code	⊘ Modifier -51 Exempt	☉ Moderate Sedation

92371   spectacle prosthesis for aphakia

OTHER PROCEDURES

92499   Unlisted ophthalmological service or procedure

SPECIAL OTORHINOLARYNGOLOGIC SERVICES

Otorhinolaryngology is the study and treatment of diseases of the head and neck, including the ears, nose and throat.

Code 92506 is used to report evaluation of speech production, receptive language, and expressive language abilities. Tests may examine speech sound production, articulatory movements of oral musculature, the patient's ability to understand the meaning and intent of written and verbal expressions, and the appropriate formulation and utterance of expressive thought. In contrast, 92626 and 92627 are reported for an evaluation of auditory rehabilitation status determining the patient's ability to use residual hearing in order to identify the acoustic characteristics of sounds associated with speech communication.

CPT coding for otorhinolaryngologic services involves a number of tests that can be performed qualitatively by confrontation during physical examination or quantitatively with electrical recording equipment. The CPT definition specifies which is the case for each code. CPT codes 92552-92557, and 92561- 92588 can be performed qualitatively or quantitatively but according to CPT definition these can be reported only if calibrated electronic equipment is used. Confrontational estimation of these tests by the physician is part of the evaluation and management service.

Speech language pathologists may perform services coded as CPT codes 92507, 92508, or 92526. They do not perform services coded as CPT codes 97110, 97112, 97150, 97530, or 97532 which are generally performed by physical or occupational therapists. Speech language pathologists should not report CPT codes 97110, 97112, 97150, 97530, or 97532 as unbundled services included in the services coded as 92507, 92508, or 92526.

Coding Rules

1.   *Component procedures, such as otoscopy, rhinoscopy, tuning fork test, which may be provided as part of a comprehensive service are not reported separately.*

2.   *Special otorhinolaryngologic diagnostic or treatment services not usually included in a comprehensive otorhinolaryngologic evaluation or office visit are reported separately.*

1127

| Separate Procedure | Unlisted Procedure | CCI Comp. Code | Non-specific Procedure |

3. *All otorhinolaryngologic services include medical diagnostic evaluation. Technical procedures, which may or may not be performed by the physician personally, are often part of the service, but should not be mistaken to constitute the service itself.*

Diagnostic or treatment procedures that are reported as evaluation and management services (eg., otoscopy, anterior rhinoscopy, tuning fork test, removal of non-impacted cerumen) are not reported separately.

Special otorhinolaryngologic services are those diagnostic and treatment services not included in an Evaluation and Management service, including office or other outpatient services (99201-99215), or office or other outpatient consultations (99241-99245).

Code 92506 is used to report evaluation of speech production, receptive language, and expressive language abilities. Tests may examine speech sound production, articulatory movements of oral musculature, the patient's ability to understand the meaning and intent of written and verbal expressions, and the appropriate formulations and utterance of expressive thought. In contrast, 92626 and 92627 are reported for an evaluation of auditory rehabilitation status determining the patient's ability to use residual hearing in order to identify the acoustic characteristics of sounds associated with speech communications.

(For laryngoscopy with stroboscopy, use 31579)

92502 Otolaryngologic examination under general anesthesia

92504 Binocular microscopy (separate diagnostic procedure)

92506 Evaluation of speech, language, voice, communication, and/or auditory processing

92507 Treatment of speech, language, voice, communication, and/or auditory processing disorder; individual

92508 group, two or more individuals

(For auditory rehabilitation, prelingual hearing loss, use 92630)

(For auditory rehabilitation, postlingual hearing loss, use 92633)

(For cochlear implant programming, see 92601-92604)

92511 Nasopharyngoscopy with endoscope (separate procedure)

92512 Nasal function studies (eg, rhinomanometry)

92516 Facial nerve function studies (eg, electroneuronography)

● New Code ▲ Revised Code + Add-On Code ⊘ Modifier -51 Exempt ⊙ Moderate Sedation

92520 Laryngeal function studies (ie, aerodynamic testing and acoustic testing)

(For performance of a single test, use modifier 52)

(To report flexible fiberoptic laryngeal evaluation of swallowing and laryngeal sensory testing, see 92611-92617)

(To report other testing of laryngeal function (eg, electroglottography), use 92700)

92526 Treatment of swallowing dysfunction and/or oral function for feeding

VESTIBULAR FUNCTION TESTS, WITHOUT ELECTRICAL RECORDING

92531 Spontaneous nystagmus, including gaze

92532 Positional nystagmus test

(Do not report 92531, 92532 with evaluation and management services including office or other outpatient services [99201-99215], observation care [99218-99220, 99224-99226], observation of inpatient care including admission and discharge [99234-99236], hospital care [99221-99223, 99231-99233], office or other outpatient consultations [99241-99245], nursing facility services [99304-99318], and domiciliary, rest home or custodial care services [99324-99337])

92533 Caloric vestibular test, each irrigation (binaural, bithermal stimulation constitutes 4 tests)

92534 Optokinetic nystagmus test

VESTIBULAR FUNCTION TESTS, WITH RECORDING (eg, ENG)

92540 Basic vestibular evaluation, includes spontaneous nystagmus test with eccentric gaze fixation nystagmus, with recording, positional nystagmus test, minimum of 4 positions, with recording, optokinetic nystagmus test, bidirectional foveal and peripheral stimulation, with recording, and oscillating tracking test, with recording

(Do not report 92540 in conjunction with 92541, 92542, 92544, 92545)

▨ Separate Procedure	▨ Unlisted Procedure	▨ CCI Comp. Code	▨ Non-specific Procedure	**1129**

92541 Spontaneous nystagmus test, including gaze and fixation nystagmus, with recording

(Do not report 92541 in conjunction with 92540 or the set of 92542, 92544, and 92545)

92542 Positional nystagmus test, minimum of 4 positions, with recording

(Do not report 92542 in conjunction with 92540 or the set of 92541, 92544, and 92545)

92543 Caloric vestibular test, each irrigation (binaural, bithermal stimulation constitutes 4 tests), with recording

92544 Optokinetic nystagmus test, bidirectional, foveal or peripheral stimulation, with recording

(Do not report 92544 in conjunction with 92540 or the set of 92541, 92542, and 92545)

92545 Oscillating tracking test, with recording

(Do not report 92545 in conjunction with 92540 or the set of 92541, 92542, and 92544)

92546 Sinusoidal vertical axis rotational testing

+ 92547 Use of vertical electrodes (List separately in addition to code for primary procedure)

(Use 92547 in conjunction with codes 92540-92546)

(For unlisted vestibular tests, use 92700)

92548 Computerized dynamic posturography

AUDIOLOGIC FUNCTION TESTS

The audiometric tests listed below require the use of calibrated electronic equipment, recording of results and a report with interpretation. Hearing tests (such as whispered voice, tuning fork) that are otorhinolaryngologic E/M services are not reported separately. All services include testing of both ears. Use modifier 52 if a test is applied to one ear instead of two ears. All codes (except 92559) apply to testing of individuals. For testing of groups, use 92559 and specify test(s) used.

(For evaluation of speech, language and/or hearing problems through observation and assessment of performance, use 92506)

● New Code ▲ Revised Code + Add-On Code ⊘ Modifier -51 Exempt ⊙ Moderate Sedation

92550 Tympanometry and reflex threshold measurements

(Do not report 92550 in conjunction with 92567, 92568)

92551 Screening test, pure tone, air only

92552 Pure tone audiometry (threshold); air only

92553 air and bone

92555 Speech audiometry threshold;

92556 with speech recognition

92557 Comprehensive audiometry threshold evaluation and speech recognition (92553 and 92556 combined)

(For hearing aid evaluation and selection, see 92590-92595)

(For automated audiometry, see 0208T-0212T)

92558 Code out of order. See page 1132

92559 Audiometric testing of groups

92560 Bekesy audiometry; screening

92561 diagnostic

92562 Loudness balance test, alternate binaural or monaural

92563 Tone decay test

92564 Short increment sensitivity index (SISI)

92565 Stenger test, pure tone

92567 Tympanometry (impedance testing)

92568 Acoustic reflex testing; threshold

(**92569** Deleted 2009 [2010 edition]. For acoustic reflex decay testing performed in conjunction with tympanometry, use 92570)

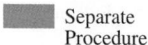 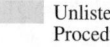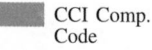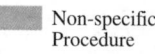

92570 Acoustic immittance testing, includes tympanometry (impedance testing), acoustic reflex threshold testing, and acoustic reflex decay testing

(Do not report 92570 in conjunction with 92567, 92568)

92571 Filtered speech test

92572 Staggered spondaic word test

92575 Sensorineural acuity level test

92576 Synthetic sentence identification test

92577 Stenger test, speech

92579 Visual reinforcement audiometry (VRA)

92582 Conditioning play audiometry

92583 Select picture audiometry

92584 Electrocochleography

92585 Auditory evoked potentials for evoked response audiometry and/or testing of the central nervous system; comprehensive

92586 limited

92558 Evoked otoacoustic emissions, screening (qualitative measurement of distortion product or transient evoked otoacoustic emissions), automated analysis

92587 Distortion product evoked otoacoustic emissions; limited evaluation (to confirm the presence or absence of hearing disorder, 3-6 frequencies) or transient evoked otoacoustic emissions, with interpretation and report

92588 comprehensive diagnostic evaluation (quantitative analysis of outer hair cell function by cochlear mapping, minimum of 12 frequencies), with interpretation and report

(For central auditory function evaluation, see 92620, 92621)

92590 Hearing aid examination and selection; monaural

92591 binaural

● New Code   ▲ Revised Code   + Add-On Code   ⊘ Modifier -51 Exempt   ⊙ Moderate Sedation

92592   Hearing aid check; monaural

92593   binaural

92594   Electroacoustic evaluation for hearing aid; monaural

92595   binaural

92596   Ear protector attenuation measurements

92597   Evaluation for use and/or fitting of voice prosthetic device to supplement oral speech

(To report augmentative and alternative communication device services, see 92605, 92607, 92608)

EVALUATIVE AND THERAPEUTIC SERVICES

Codes 92601 and 92603 describe post-operative analysis and fitting of previously placed external devices, connection to the cochlear implant, and programming of the stimulator. Codes 92602 and 92604 describe subsequent sessions for measurements and adjustments of the external transmitter and re-programming of the internal stimulator.

(For placement of cochlear implant, use 69930)

92601   Diagnostic analysis of cochlear implant, patient under 7 years of age; with programming

92602   subsequent reprogramming

(Do not report 92602 in addition to 92601)

(For aural rehabilitation services following cochlear implant, including evaluation of rehabilitation status, see 92626-92627, 92630-92633)

92603   Diagnostic analysis of cochlear implant, age 7 years or older; with programming

92604   subsequent reprogramming

(Do not report 92604 in addition to 92603)

92605   Evaluation for prescription of non-speech-generating augmentative and alternative communication device, face-to-face with the patient; first hour

1133

	Separate Procedure		Unlisted Procedure		CCI Comp. Code		Non-specific Procedure

+ 92618   each additional 30 minutes (List separately in addition to code for primary procedure)

(Use 92618 in conjunction with 92605)

92606   Therapeutic service(s) for the use of non-speech-generating device, including programming and modification

92607   Evaluation for prescription for speech-generating augmentative and alternative communication device, face-to-face with the patient; first hour

(For evaluation for prescription of a non-speech-generating device, use 92605)

+ 92608   each additional 30 minutes (List separately in addition to code for primary procedure)

(Use 92608 in conjunction with 92607)

92609   Therapeutic services for the use of speech-generating device, including programming and modification

(For therapeutic service(s) for the use of a non-speech-generating device, use 92606)

92610   Evaluation of oral and pharyngeal swallowing function

(For motion fluoroscopic evaluation of swallowing function, use 92611)

(For flexible endoscopic examination, use 92612-92617)

92611   Motion fluoroscopic evaluation of swallowing function by cine or video recording

(For radiological supervision and interpretation, use 74230)

(For evaluation of oral and pharyngeal swallowing function, use 92610)

(For flexible fiberoptic diagnostic laryngoscopy, use 31575. Do not report 31575 in conjunction with 92612-92617)

92612   Flexible fiberoptic endoscopic evaluation of swallowing by cine or video recording;

(If flexible fiberoptic or endoscopic evaluation of swallowing is performed without cine or video recording, use 92700)

▲ 92613   interpretation and report only

1134

● New Code	▲ Revised Code	+ Add-On Code	⊘ Modifier -51 Exempt	⊙ Moderate Sedation

(To report an evaluation of oral and pharyngeal swallowing function, use 92610)

(To report motion fluoroscopic evaluation of swallowing function, use 92611)

92614 Flexible fiberoptic endoscopic evaluation, laryngeal sensory testing by cine or video recording;

(If flexible fiberoptic or endoscopic evaluation of swallowing is performed without cine or video recording, use 92700)

▲ **92615** interpretation and report only

92616 Flexible fiberoptic endoscopic evaluation of swallowing and laryngeal sensory testing by cine or video recording;

(If flexible fiberoptic or endoscopic evaluation of swallowing is performed without cine or video recording, use 92700)

▲ **92617** interpretation and report only

92618 Code out of order. See page 1134

92620 Evaluation of central auditory function, with report; initial 60 minutes

+ **92621** each additional 15 minutes (List separately in addition to code for primary procedure)

(Use 92621 in conjunction with 92620)

(Do not report 92620, 92621 in conjunction with 92506)

92625 Assessment of tinnitus (includes pitch, loudness matching, and masking)

(Do not report 92625 in conjunction with 92562)

(For unilateral assessment, use modifier 52)

92626 Evaluation of auditory rehabilitation status; first hour

+ **92627** each additional 15 minutes (List separately in addition to code for primary procedure)

(Use 92627 in conjunction with 92626)

(When reporting 92626, 92627, use the face-to-face time with the patient or family)

1135

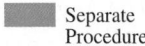 Separate Procedure

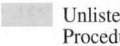 Unlisted Procedure

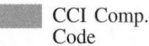 CCI Comp. Code

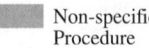 Non-specific Procedure

92630   Auditory rehabilitation; pre-lingual hearing loss

92633   post-lingual hearing loss

SPECIAL DIAGNOSTIC PROCEDURES

92640   Diagnostic analysis with programming of auditory brainstem implant, per hour

(Report nonprogramming services separately [eg., cardiac monitoring])

OTHER PROCEDURES

92700   Unlisted otorhinolaryngological service or procedure

CARDIOVASCULAR

Cardiovascular services refers to the study and treatment of diseases of the heart and vascular (arteries and veins) system. Cardiovascular services CPT codes are used to report therapeutic services such as cardiopulmonary resuscitation (CPR), cardioversion and percutaneous transluminal coronary angioplasty (PTCA) and diagnostic procedures such as electrocardiography, echocardiography and cardiac catheterization.

Cardiovascular medicine services include non-invasive and invasive diagnostic testing (including intracardiac testing) as well as therapeutic services (e.g. electrophysiological procedures).

When cardiopulmonary resuscitation is performed without other evaluation and management services (e.g. a physician responds to a "code blue" and directs cardiopulmonary resuscitation with the patient's attending physician then resuming the care of the patient after the patient has been revived), only the CPT code 92950 for CPR should be reported. Levels of critical care services and prolonged management services are determined by time; when CPT code 92950 is reported, the time required to perform CPR is not included in critical care or other timed evaluation and management services.

In keeping with the policies outlined previously, procedures routinely performed as part of a comprehensive service are included in the comprehensive service and not separately reported. A number of therapeutic and diagnostic cardiovascular procedures (e.g. CPT codes 92950-92998, 93501-93545, 93600-93624, 93640-93652) routinely utilize intravenous or intra-arterial vascular access, routinely require electrocardiographic monitoring, and frequently require agents administered by injection or infusion techniques; accordingly, separate codes for routine access, monitoring, injection or infusion services are not to be reported.

● New Code   ▲ Revised Code   + Add-On Code   ⊘ Modifier -51 Exempt   ⊙ Moderate Sedation

Fluoroscopic guidance procedures are integral to invasive intravascular procedures and are included in those services. In unique circumstances, where these services are performed, not as an integral part of the procedure, the appropriate code can be separately reported with modifier -59. When supervision and interpretation codes are identified in the CPT code book for a given procedure, these can be separately reported.

Cardiac output measurement (e.g. CPT codes 93561-93562) is routinely performed during cardiac catheterization procedures per CPT definition and, therefore, CPT codes 93561-93562 are not to be reported with cardiac catheterization codes.

THERAPEUTIC SERVICES AND PROCEDURES

92920   This code is out of order. See page 1142

92921   This code is out of order. See page 1142

92924   This code is out of order. See page 1142

92925   This code is out of order. See page 1142

92928   This code is out of order. See page 1143

92929   This code is out of order. See page 1143

92933   This code is out of order. See page 1143

92934   This code is out of order. See page 1143

92937   This code is out of order. See page 1143

92938   This code is out of order. See page 1143

92941   This code is out of order. See page 1143

92943   This code is out of order. See page 1143

92944   This code is out of order. See page 1143

OTHER THERAPEUTIC SERVICES AND PROCEDURES

(For nonsurgical septal reduction therapy [eg, alcohol ablation], use 93799)

92950   Cardiopulmonary resuscitation (eg, in cardiac arrest)

1137

| | Separate Procedure | | Unlisted Procedure | | CCI Comp. Code | | Non-specific Procedure |

(See also critical care services, 99291, 99292)

⊙ **92953** Temporary transcutaneous pacing

(For direction of ambulance or rescue personnel outside the hospital by a physician or other qualified health care professional, use 99288)

⊙ **92960** Cardioversion, elective, electrical conversion of arrhythmia; external

⊙ **92961** internal (separate procedure)

(Do not report 92961 in conjunction with 93282-93284, 93287, 93289, 93295, 93296, 93618-93624, 93631, 93640-93642, 93650, 93653-93657, 93662)

92970 Cardioassist-method of circulatory assist; internal

92971 external

(For balloon atrial-septostomy, use 92992)

(For placement of catheters for use in circulatory assist devices such as intra-aortic balloon pump, use 33970)

92973 This code is out of order. See page 1144

92974 This code is out of order. See page 1144

92975 This code is out of order. See page 1144

92977 This code is out of order. See page 1144

92978 This code is out of order. See page 1144

92979 This code is out of order. See page 1144

(92980 deleted 2012 [2013 edition]. To report, see 92920-92944)

(92981 deleted 2012 [2013 edition]. To report, see 92920-92944)

(92982 deleted 2012 [2013 edition]. To report, see 92920-92944)

(92984 deleted 2012 [2013 edition]. To report, see 92920-92944)

⊙ **92986** Percutaneous balloon valvuloplasty; aortic valve

● New Code ▲ Revised Code + Add-On Code ⊘ Modifier -51 Exempt ⊙ Moderate Sedation

⊙ **92987**   mitral valve

92990   pulmonary valve

92992   Atrial septectomy or septostomy; transvenous method, balloon (eg, Rashkind type) (includes cardiac catheterization)

92993   blade method (Park septostomy) (includes cardiac catheterization)

(92995   deleted 2012 [2013 edition]. To report, see 92924, 92925, 92933-92944)

(92996   deleted 2012 [2013 edition]. To report, see 92924, 92925, 92933-92944)

92997   Percutaneous transluminal pulmonary artery balloon angioplasty; single vessel

+ **92998**   each additional vessel (List separately in addition to code for primary procedure)

(Use 92998 in conjunction with code 92997)

CORONARY THERAPEUTIC SERVICES AND PROCEDURES

Codes 92920-92944 describe percutaneous revascularization services performed for occlusive disease of the coronary vessels (major coronary arteries, coronary artery branches, or coronary artery bypass grafts). These percutaneous coronary intervention (PCI) codes are built on progressive hierarchies with more intensive services inclusive of lesser intensive services. These PCI codes all include the work of accessing and selectively catheterizing the vessel, traversing the lesion, radiological supervision and interpretation directly related to the intervention(s) performed, closure of the arteriotomy when performed through the access sheath, and imaging performed to document completion of the intervention in addition to the intervention(s) performed. These codes include angioplasty (eg, balloon, cutting balloon, wired balloons, cryoplasty), atherectomy (eg, directional, rotational, laser), and stenting (eg, balloon expandable, self-expanding, bare metal, drug eluting, covered). Each code in this family includes balloon angioplasty, when performed. Diagnostic coronary angiography may be reported separately under specific circumstances.

Diagnostic coronary angiography codes (93454-93461) and injection procedure codes (93563-93564) should not be used with percutaneous coronary revascularization services (92920-92944) to report:

1. Contrast injections, angiography, roadmapping, and/or fluoroscopic guidance for the coronary intervention,

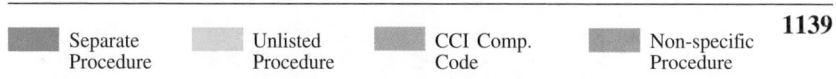

1139

Separate Procedure | Unlisted Procedure | CCI Comp. Code | Non-specific Procedure

2.Vessel measurement for the coronary intervention, or

3. Post-coronary angioplasty/stent/atherectomy angiography, as this work is captured in the percutaneous coronary revascularization services codes (92920-92944).

Diagnostic angiography performed at the time of a coronary interventional procedure may be separately reportable if:

1. No prior catheter-based coronary angiography study is available, and a full diagnostic study is performed, and a decision to intervene is based on the diagnostic angiography, OR

2. A prior study is available, but as documented in the medical record:

a. The patient's condition with respect to the clinical indication has changed since the prior study, OR

b. There is inadequate visualization of the anatomy and/or pathology, OR

c. There is a clinical change during the procedure that requires a new evaluation outside the target area of intervention.

Diagnostic coronary angiography performed at a separate session from an interventional procedure is separately reportable.

Major coronary arteries: The major coronary arteries are the left main, left anterior descending, left circumflex, right, and ramus intermediate arteries. All PCI procedures performed in all segments (proximal, mid, distal) of a single major coronary artery through the native coronary circulation are reported with one code. When one segment of a major coronary artery is treated through the native circulation and treatment of another segment of the same artery requires access through a coronary artery bypass graft, the intervention through the bypass graft is reported separately.

Coronary artery branches: Up to two coronary artery branches of the left anterior descending (diagonals), left circumflex (marginals), and right (posterior descending, posterolaterals) coronary arteries are recognized. The left main and ramus intermedius coronary arteries do not have recognized branches for reporting purposes. All PCI(s) performed in any segment (proximal, mid, distal) of a coronary of artery branch is reported with one code. PCI is reported for up to two branches of a major coronary artery. Additional PCI in a third branch of the same major coronary artery is not separately reportable.

Coronary artery bypass grafts: Each coronary artery bypass graft represents a coronary vessel. A sequential bypass graft with more than one distal anastomosis represents only one graft. A branching bypass graft (eg, Y graft) represents a coronary vessel for the main graft, and each branch off the main graft constitutes an additional coronary vessel. PCI performed on major coronary arteries or coronary artery branches by access through a bypass graft is reported using the bypass graft PCI codes. All bypass graft PCI codes include the use of coronary artery embolic protection devices when performed.

Only one base code from this family may be reported for revascularization of a major coronary artery and its recognized branches. Only one base code should be reported for revascularization of a coronary artery bypass graft, its subtended coronary artery, and recognized branches of the subtended coronary artery. If one segment of a major coronary artery and its recognized branches is treated through the native circulation, and treatment of another segment of the same vessel requires access through a coronary artery bypass graft, an additional base code is reported to describe the intervention performed through the bypass graft. The PCI base codes are 92920, 92924, 92928, 92933, 92937, 92941, and 92943. The PCI base code that includes the most intensive service provided for the target vessel should be reported. The hierarchy of these services is built on an intensity of service ranked from highest to lowest as 92943 = 92941 = 92933 > 92924 > 92937 = 92928 > 92920.

PCI performed during the same session in additional recognized branches of the target vessel should be reported using the applicable add-on code(s). The add-on codes are 92921, 92925, 92929, 92934, 92938, and 92944 and follow the same principle in regard to reporting the most intensive service provided. The intensity of service is ranked from highest to lowest as 92944 = 92938 > 92934 > 92925 > 92929 > 92921.

PCI performed during the same session in additional major coronary or in additional coronary artery bypass grafts should be reported using the applicable additional base code(s). PCI performed during the same session in additional coronary artery branches should be reported using the applicable additional add-on code(s).

If a single lesion extends from one target vessel (major coronary artery, coronary artery bypass graft, or coronary artery branch) into another target vessel, but can be revascularized with a single intervention bridging the two vessels, this PCI should be reported with a single code despite treating more than one vessel. For example, if a left main coronary lesion extends into the proximal left circumflex coronary artery and a single stent is placed to treat the entire lesion, this PCI should be reported as a single vessel stent (92928). In this example, a code for additional vessel treatment (92929) would not be additionally reported.

When bifurcation lesions are treated, PCI is reported for both vessels treated. For example, when a bifurcation lesion involving the left anterior descending artery and the first diagonal artery is treated by stenting both vessels, 92928 and 92929 are both reported.

Target vessel PCI for acute myocardial infarction is inclusive of all balloon angioplasty, atherectomy, stenting, manual aspiration thrombectomy, distal

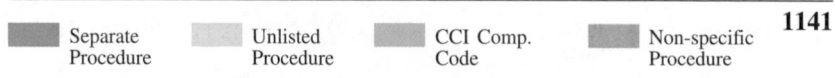

Separate Procedure Unlisted Procedure CCI Comp. Code Non-specific Procedure

protection, and intracoronary rheolytic agent administration performed. Mechanical thrombectomy is reported separately.

Chronic total occlusion of a coronary vessel is present when there is no antegrade flow through the true lumen, accompanied by suggestive angiographic and clinical criteria (eg, antegrade "bridging" collaterals present, calcification at the occlusion site, no current presentation with ST elevation or Q wave acute myocardial infarction attributable to the occluded target lesion). Current presentation with ST elevation or Q wave acute myocardial infarction attributable to the occluded target lesion, subtotal occlusion, and occlusion with dye staining at the site consistent with fresh thrombus are not considered chronic total occlusion.

Codes 92973 (percutaneous transluminal coronary thrombectomy, mechanical), 92974 (coronary brachytherapy), 92978 and 92979 (intravascular ultrasound), and 93571 and 93572 (intravascular Doppler velocity and/or pressure [fractional flow reserve (FFR) or coronary flow reserve (CFR)]) are add-on codes for reporting procedures performed in addition to coronary and bypass graft diagnostic and interventional services unless included in the base code. Non-mechanical, aspiration thrombectomy is not reported with 92973, and is included in the PCI code for acute myocardial infarction (92941), when performed.

> (To report transcatheter placement of radiation delivery device for coronary intravascular brachytherapy, use 92974)
>
> (For intravascular radioelement application, see 77785-77787)
>
> (For nonsurgical septal reduction therapy [eg, alcohol ablation], use 93799)

●⊙**92920**   Percutaneous transluminal coronary angioplasty; single major coronary artery or branch

●⊙+**92921**   each additional branch of a major coronary artery (List separately in addition to code for primary procedure)

> (Use 92921 in conjunction with 92920, 92924, 92928, 92933, 92937, 92941, 92943)

●⊙**92924**   Percutaneous transluminal coronary atherectomy, with coronary angioplasty when performed; single major coronary artery or branch

●⊙+**92925**   each additional branch of a major coronary artery (List separately in addition to code for primary procedure)

> (Use 92925 in conjunction with 92924, 92928, 92933, 92937, 92941, 92943)

● New Code   ▲ Revised Code   + Add-On Code   ⊘ Modifier -51 Exempt   ⊙ Moderate Sedation

●⊙**92928** Percutaneous transcatheter placement of intracoronary stent(s), with coronary angioplasty when performed; single majore coronary artery or branch

●⊙**+92929**   each additional branch of a major coronary artery (List separately in addition to code for primary procedure)

    (Use 92929 in conjunction with 92928, 92933, 92937, 92941, 92943)

●⊙**92933** Percutaneous transluminal coronary atherectomy, with intracoronary stent, with coronary angioplasty when performed; single major coronary artery or branch

●⊙**+92934**   each additional branch of a major coronary artery (List separately in addition to code for primary procedure)

    (Use 92934 in conjunction with 92933, 92937, 92941, 92943)

●⊙**92937** Percutaneous transluminal revascularization of or through coronary artery bypass graft (internal mammary, free arterial, venous), any combination of intracoronary stent, atherectomy and angioplasty, including distal protection when performed; single vessel

●⊙**+92938**   each additional branch subtended by the bypass graft (List separately in addition to code for primary procedure)

    (Use 92938 in conjunction with 92937)

●⊙**92941** Percutaneous transluminal revascularization of acute total/subtotal occlusion during acute myocardial infarction, coronary artery or coronary artery bypass graft, any combination of intracoronary stent, atherectomy and angioplasty, including aspiration thrombectomy when performed; single vessel

    (For additional vessels treated, see 92920-92938, 92943, 92944)

●⊙**92943** Percutaneous transluminal revascularization of chronic total occlusion, coronary artery, coronary artery branch, or coronary artery bypass graft, any combination of intracoronary stent, atherectomy and angioplasty; single vessel

●⊙**+92944**   each additional coronary artery, coronary artery branch, or bypass graft (List separately in addition to code for primary procedure)

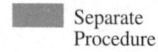 Separate Procedure   Unlisted Procedure   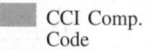 CCI Comp. Code   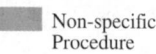 Non-specific Procedure   **1143**

(Use 92944 in conjunction with 92924, 92928, 92933, 92937, 92941, 92943)

(To report transcatheter placement of radiation delivery device for coronary intravascular brachytherapy, use 92974)

(For intravascular radioelement application, see 77785-77787)

▲⊙+**92973** Percutaneous transluminal coronary thrombectomy, mechanical (List separately in addition to code for primary procedure)

(Use 92973 in conjunction with codes 92920, 92924, 92928, 92933, 92937, 92941, 92943, 92975, 93454-93461, 93563, 93564)

(Do not report 92973 for aspiration thrombectomy)

⊙+**92974** Transcatheter placement of radiation delivery device for subsequent coronary intravascular brachytherapy (List separately in addition to code for primary procedure)

(Use 92974 in conjunction with 92920, 92924, 92928, 92933, 92937, 92941, 92943, 93454-93461)

(For intravascular radioelement application, see 77785-77787)

⊙ **92975** Thrombolysis, coronary; by intracoronary infusion, including selective coronary angiography

92977   by intravenous infusion

(For thrombolysis of vessels other than coronary, see 37211-37214)

(For cerebral thrombolysis, use 37195)

⊙+**92978** Intravascular ultrasound (coronary vessel or graft) during diagnostic evaluation and/or therapeutic intervention including imaging supervision, interpretation and report; initial vessel (List separately in addition to code for primary procedure)

(Use 92978 in conjunction with 92975, 92920, 92924, 92928, 92933, 92937, 92941, 92943, 93454-93461, 93563, 93564)

⊙+**92979**   each additional vessel (List separately in addition to code for primary procedure)

(Use 92979 in conjunction with code 92978)

(Intravascular ultrasound services include all transducer manipulations and repositioning within the specific vessel being

1144 ● New   ▲ Revised   + Add-On   ⊘ Modifier -51   ⊙ Moderate
              Code   Code   Code   Exempt   Sedation

examined, both before and after therapeutic intervention (eg, stent placement)

(For intravascular spectroscopy, use 0205T)

(For intravascular optical coherence tomography, see 0291T, 0292T)

CARDIOGRAPHY

Routine monitoring of EKG rhythm and review of daily hemodynamics, including cardiac outputs, is a part of critical care evaluation and management. Separate billing for review of EKG rhythm strips and cardiac output measurements (e.g. CPT codes 93040-93042, 93561, 93562) and critical care services is inappropriate.

An exception to this may include a sudden change in patient status associated with a change in cardiac rhythm requiring a return to the ICU or telephonic transmission to review a rhythm strip. If reported separately, time included for this service is not included in the critical care time calculated for the critical care service.

Codes 93040-93042 are appropriate when an order for the test is triggered by an event, the rhythm strip is used to help diagnose the presence or absence of an arrhythmia, and a report is generated.

(For echocardiography, see 93303-93350)

(For electrocardiogram, 64 leads or greater, with graphic presentation and analysis, see 0178T-0180T)

(For acoustic cardiography services, see 0223T-0225T)

93000 Electrocardiogram, routine ECG with at least 12 leads; with interpretation and report

93005 tracing only, without interpretation and report

93010 interpretation and report only

(For ECG monitoring, see 99354-99360)

(93012 deleted 2010 [2011 edition]. To report telephonic transmission of post-symptom electrocardiogram rhythm strips, see 93268-93272.)

(93014 deleted 2010 [2011 edition]. To report telephonic transmission of post-symptom electrocardiogram rhythm strips, see 93268-93272.)

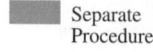 Separate Procedure   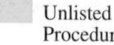 Unlisted Procedure   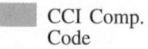 CCI Comp. Code   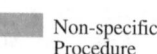 Non-specific Procedure   **1145**

▲ **93015** Cardiovascular stress test using maximal or submaximal treadmill or bicycle exercise, continuous electrocardiographic monitoring, and/or pharmacological stress; with supervision, with interpretation and report

▲ **93016** supervision only, without interpretation and report

93017 tracing only, without interpretation and report

93018 interpretation and report only

93024 Ergonovine provocation test

93025 Microvolt T-wave alternans for assessment of ventricular arrhythmias

93040 Rhythm ECG, 1 to 3 leads; with interpretation and report

93041 tracing only without interpretation and report

93042 interpretation and report only

CARDIOVASCULAR MONITORING SERVICES

Cardiovascular monitoring services are diagnostic medical procedures using in-person and remote technology to assess cardiovascular rhythm (ECG) data. Holter monitors (93224-93227) include up to 48 hours of continuous recording. Mobile cardiac telemetry monitors (93228, 93229) have the capability of transmitting a tracing at any time, always have internal ECG analysis algorithms designed to detect major arrhythmias, and transmit to an attended surveillance center. Event monitors (93268-93272) record segments of ECGs with recording initiation triggered either by patient activation or by an internal automatic, pre-programmed detection algorithm (or both) and transmit the recorded electrocardiographic data when requested (but cannot transmit immediately based upon the patient or algorighmic activation rhythm) and require attended surveillance.

▲ **93224** External electrocardiographic recording up to 48 hours by continuous rhythm recording and storage; includes recording, scanning analysis with report, review and interpretation

93225 recording (includes connection, recording, and disconnection)

93226 scanning analysis with report

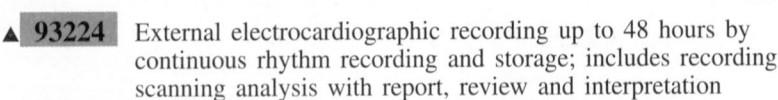

● New Code   ▲ Revised Code   + Add-On Code   ⊘ Modifier -51 Exempt   ⊙ Moderate Sedation

▲ **93227**   review and interpretation by a physician or other qualified health care professional

(For less than 12 hours of continuous recording, use modifier 52)

(For greater than 48 hours of monitoring, see 0295T-0298T0

▲ **93228** External mobile cardiovascular telemetry with electrocardiographic recording, concurrent computerized real time data analysis and greater than 24 hours of accessible ECG data storage (retrievable with query) with ECG triggered and patient selected events transmitted to a remote attended surveillance center for up to 30 days; review and interpretation with report by a physician or other qualified health care professional

(Report 93228 only once per 30 days)

(Do not report 93228 in conjunction with 93224, 93227)

▲ **93229**   technical support for connection and patient instructions for use, attended surveillance, analysis and transmission of daily and emergent data reports as prescribed by a physician or other qualified health care professional

(Report 93229 only once per 30 days)

(Do not report 93229 in conjunction with 93224, 93226)

(For external cardiovascular monitors that do not perform automatic ECG triggered transmissions to an attended surveillance center, see 93224-93227, 932268-93272)

(93230   deleted 2010 [2011 edition]. To report external electrocardiographic rhythm derived monitoring for up to 48 hours, see 93224-93227)

(93231   deleted 2010 [2011 edition]. To report external electrocardiographic rhythm derived monitoring for up to 48 hours, see 93224-93227)

(93232   deleted 2010 [2011 edition]. To report external electrocardiographic rhythm derived monitoring for up to 48 hours, see 93224-93227)

(93233   deleted 2010 [2011 edition]. To report external electrocardiographic rhythm derived monitoring for up to 48 hours, see 93224-93227)

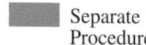 Separate Procedure   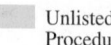 Unlisted Procedure   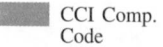 CCI Comp. Code   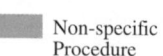 Non-specific Procedure

(93235   deleted 2010 [2011 edition]. To report external electrocardiographic rhythm derived monitoring for up to 48 hours, see 93224-93227)

(93236   deleted 2010 [2011 edition]. To report external electrocardiographic rhythm derived monitoring for up to 48 hours, see 93224-93227)

(93237   deleted 2010 [2011 edition]. To report external electrocardiographic rhythm derived monitoring for up to 48 hours, see 93224-93227)

▲ **93268**   External patient and, when performed, auto activated electrocardiographic rhythm derived event recording with symptom-related memory loop with remote download capability up to 30 days, 24-hour attended monitoring; includes transmission, review and interpretation by a physician or other qualified health care professional

93270   recording (includes connection, recording, and disconnection)

93271   transmission download and analysis

▲ **93272**   review and interpretation by a physician or other qualified health care professional

(For implanted patient activated cardiac event recording, see 33282, 93285, 93291, 93298)

93278   Signal-averaged electrocardiography (SAECG), with or without ECG

(For interpretation and report only, use 93278 with modifier -26)

(For unlisted cardiographic procedure, use 93799)

IMPLANTABLE AND WEARABLE CARDIAC DEVICE EVALUATIONS

Cardiovascular monitoring services are diagnostic medical procedures using face-to-face and remote monitoring technology to record cardiovascular data and assess the effectiveness of treatment.

Codes 93279-93299 describe this technology and technical/professional and service center practice. Codes 93279-93292 are reported per procedure. Codes 93293-93296 are reported no more than **once** every 90 days. Do not report

93293-93296 if the monitoring period is less than 30 days. Codes 93297, 93298 are reported no more than once up to every 30 days. Do not report 93297-93299 if the monitoring period is less than 10 days.

Cardiovascular devices defined by codes from this section include:

> *Implantable Cardiovascular Monitor (ICM)*
> *Implantable Cardioverter-Defibrillator (ICD)*
> *Implantable Loop Recorder (ILR)*
> *Pacemaker*

Monitoring services reported using codes from this section include:

> *Electrocardiographic rhythm derived*
> *Interrogation device evaluation*
> *Peri-procedural device evaluation and programming*
> *Physiologic cardiovascular data elements*
> *Programming device evaluation*
> *Transtelephonic rhythm strip pacemaker evaluation*

Consider the following coding notes when selecting codes from this section:

Codes 93279-93292 are reported per procedure.

Codes 93293-93296 are reported no more than once every 90 days.

Do not report 93293-93296 if the monitoring period is less than 30 days.

Codes 93297, 93298 are reported no more than once up to every 30 days.

Do no report 93297-93299 if the monitoring period is less than 10 days.

For monitoring by wearable devices, see 93224-93272.

For other services related to wearable defibrillator, use 93745.

Do not report 93012, 93014 when performing 93279-93289, 93291-93296 or 93298-93299.

Do no report 93040-93042 when performing 93279-93289, 93291-93296, or 93298-93299.

A service center may report 93296 or 93299 during a period in which a physician or other qualified health care professional performs an in-person interrogation device evaluation. The same individual may not report an in-person and remote interrogation of the same device during the same period. Report only remote services when an in-person interrogation device evaluation is performed during a period of remote interrogation device evaluation. A period is established by the initiation of the remote monitoring or the 91st day of a pacemaker or implantable

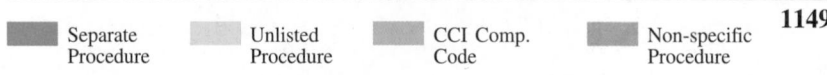

| | Separate Procedure | | Unlisted Procedure | | CCI Comp. Code | | Non-specific Procedure |

cardioverter-defibrillator (ICD) monitoring or the 31st day of an implantable loop recorder (ILR) or implantable cardiovascular monitor (ICM) monitoring and extends for the subsequent 90 or 30 days, respectively, for which remote monitoring is occurring. Programming device evaluations and in-person interrogation device evaluations may not be reported on the same date by the same individual. Programming device evaluations and remote interrogation device evaluations may both be reported during the remote interrogation device evaluation period.

For monitoring by wearable devices, see 93224-93272.

ECG rhythm derived elements are distinct from physiologic data, even when the same device is capable of producing both. ICM device services are always separately reported from ICD services. When ILR data is derived from an ICD or pacemaker, do not report ILR services with pacemaker or ICD services.

Do not report 93268-93272 when performing 93279-93289, 93291-93296 or 93298-93299. Do not report 93040-93042 when performing 93279-93289, 93291-93296, or 93298-93299.

The pacemaker and ICD interrogation device evaluations, peri-procedural device evaluations and programming, and programming device evaluations may not be reported in conjunction with pacemaker or ICD device and/or lead insertion or revision services by the same individual.

The following definitions and instructions apply to codes 93279-93299:

Attended surveillance: the immediate availability of a remote technician to respond to rhythm or device alert transmissions from a patient, either from an implanted or wearable monitoring or therapy device, as they are generated and transmitted to the remote surveillance location or center.

Device, single lead: a pacemaker or implantable cardioverter-defibrillator with pacing and sensing function in only one chamber of the heart.

Device, dual lead: a pacemaker or implantable cardioverter-defibrillator with pacing and sensing function in only two chambers of the heart.

Device, multiple lead: a pacemaker or implantable cardioverter-defibrillator with pacing and sensing function in three or more chambers of the heart.

Electrocardiographic rhythm derived elements: elements derived from recordings of the electrical activation of the heart including, but not limited to heart rhythm, rate, ST analysis, heart rate variability, T-wave alternans.

Implantable cardiovascular monitor (ICM): an implantable cardiovascular device used to assist the physician in the management of non-rhythm related cardiac conditions such as heart failure. The device collects longitudinal

● New Code	▲ Revised Code	+ Add-On Code	⊘ Modifier -51 Exempt	⊙ Moderate Sedation

physiologic cardiovascular data elements from one or more internal sensors (such as right ventricular pressure, left atrial pressure or an index of lung water) and/or external sensors (such as blood pressure or body weight) for patient assessment and management. The data are stored and transmitted by either local telemetry or remotely to an Internet based file server or surveillance technician. The function of the ICM may be an additional function of an implantable cardiac device (eg., implantable cardioverter-defibrillator) or a function of a stand-alone device. When ICM functionality is included in an ICD device or pacemaker, the ICM data and the ICD or pacemaker, heart rhythm data such as sensing, pacing and tachycardia detection therapy are distinct and therefore, the monitoring processes are distinct.

Implantable cardioverter-defibrillator (ICD): an implantable device that provides high-energy and low-energy stimulation to one or more chambers of the heart to terminate rapid heart rhythms called tachycardia or fibrillation. ICDs also have pacemaker functions to treat slow heart rhythms called bradycardia. In addition to the tachycardia and bradycardia functions, the ICD may or may not include the functionality of an implantable cardiovascular monitor or an implantable loop recorder.

Implantable loop recorder (ILR): an implantable device that continuously records the electrocardiographic rhythm triggered automatically by rapid and slow heart rates or by the patient during a symptomatic episode. The ILR function may be the only function of the device or it may be part of a pacemaker or implantable cardioverter-defibrillator device. The data are stored and transmitted either local telemetry or remotely to an Internet based file server or surveillance technician. Extraction of data and compilation or report for physician or qualified health care profesional interpretation is usually performed in the office setting.

Interrogation device evaluation: an evaluation of an implantable device such as a cardiac pacemaker, implantable cardioverter-defibrillator, implantable cardiovascular monitor, or implantable loop recorder. Using an office, hospital, or emergency room instrument or via a remote interrogation system, stored and measured information about the lead(s) when present, sensor(s) when present, battery and the implanted device function, as well as data collected about the patient's heart rhythm and heart rate is retrieved. The retrieved information is evaluated to determine the current programming of the device and to evaluate certain aspects of the device function such as battery voltage, lead impedance, tachycardia detection settings, and rhythm treatment settings.

The components that must be evaluated for the various types of implantable cardiac devices are listed below. (The required components for both remote and in-person interrogations are the same.)

Pacemaker: Programmed parameters, lead(s), battery, capture and sensing function and heart rhythm.

Separate Procedure Unlisted Procedure CCI Comp. Code Non-specific Procedure

Implantable cardioverter-defibrillator: Programmed parameters, lead(s), battery, capture and sensing function, presence or absence of therapy for ventricular tachyarrhythmias and underlying heart rhythms.

Implantable cardiovascular monitor: Programmed parameters and analysis of at least one recorded physiologic cardiovascular data element from either internal or external sensors.

Implantable loop recorder: Programmed parameters and the heart rate and rhythm during recorded episodes from both patient initiated and device algorithm detected events, when present.

Interrogation device evaluation (remote): a procedure performed for patients with pacemakers, implantable cardioverter-defibrillators or implantable loop recorders using data obtained remotely. All device functions, including the programmed parameters, lead(s), battery, capture and sensing function, presence or absence of therapy for ventricular tachyarrhythmias (for ICDs) and underlying heart rhythm are evaluated.

The components that must be evaluated for the various types of implantable cardiac devices are listed below. (The required components for both remote and in person interrogations are the same.)

Pacemaker: Programmed parameters, lead(s), battery, capture and sensing function and heart rhythm.

Implantable cardioverter-defibrillator: Programmed parameters, lead(s), battery, capture and sensing function, presence or absence of therapy for ventricular tachyarrhythmias and underlying heart rhythms.

Implantable cardiovascular monitor: Programmed parameters and analysis of at least one recorded physiologic cardiovascular data element from either internal or external sensors.

Implantable loop recorder: Programmed parameters and the heart rate and rhythm during recorded episodes from both patient initiated and device algorithm detected events, when present.

Pacemaker: an implantable device that provides low energy localized stimulation to one or more chambers of the heart to initiate contraction in that chamber.

Peri-procedural device evaluation and programming: an evaluation of an implantable device system (either a pacemaker or implantable cardioverter defibrillator) to adjust the device to settings appropriate for the patient prior to a surgery, procedure, or test. The device system data are interrogated to evaluate the lead(s), sensor(s), and battery in addition to review of stored information including patient and system measurements. The device is programmed to settings appropriate for the surgery, procedure, or test, as required. A second evaluation and programming are performed after the surgery, procedure, or test to provide settings

● New Code	▲ Revised Code	+ Add-On Code	⊘ Modifier -51 Exempt	⊙ Moderate Sedation

appropriate to the post procedural situation, as required. If one performs both the pre- and post-evaluation and programming service, the appropriate code, either 93286 or 93287, would be reported two times. If one performs the pre-surgical service and a separate provider performs the post-surgical service, each reports either 93286 or 93287 only one time.

Physiologic cardiovascular data elements: data elements from one or more internal sensors (such as right ventricular pressure, left atrial pressure, or an index of lung water) and/or external sensors (such as blood pressure or body weight) for patient assessment and management. It does not include ECG rhythm derived data elements.

Programming device evaluations (in person): a procedure performed for patients with a pacemaker, implantable cardioverter-defibrillator, or implantable loop recorder. All device functions, including the battery, programmable settings and lead(s), when present, are evaluated. To assess capture thresholds, iterative adjustments (eg., progressive changes in pacing output of a pacing lead) of the programmable parameters are conducted. The iterative adjustments provide information that permits the operator to assess and select the most appropriate final program parameters to provide for consistent delivery of the appropriate therapy and to verify the function of the device. The final program parameters may or may not change after evaluation.

The programming device evaluation includes all of the components of the interrogation device evaluation (remote) or the interrogation device evaluation (in person), and it includes the selection of patient specific programmed parameters depending on the type of device.

The components that must be evaluated for the various types of programming device evaluations are listed below. (See also required interrogation device evaluation [remote and in person] components above.)

Pacemaker: Programmed parameters, lead(s), battery, capture and sensing function and heart rhythm. Often, but not always, the sensor rate response, lower and upper heart rates, AV intervals, pacing voltage and pulse duration, sensing value, and diagnostics will be adjusted during a programming evaluation.

Implantable cardioverter-defibrillator: Programmed parameters, lead(s), battery, capture and sensing function, presence or absence of therapy for ventricular tachyarrhythmias and underlying heart rhythms. Often, but not always, the sensor rate response, lower and upper heart rates, AV intervals, pacing voltage and pulse duration, sensing value, and diagnostics will be adjusted during a programming evaluation. In addition, ventricular tachycardia detection and therapies are sometimes altered depending on the interrogated data, patient's rhythm, symptoms, and condition.

| Separate Procedure | Unlisted Procedure | CCI Comp. Code | Non-specific Procedure |

Implantable loop recorder: Programmed parameters and the heart rhythm during recorded episodes from both patient initiated and device algorithm detected events. Often, but not always, the tachycardia and bradycardia detection criteria will be adjusted during a programming evaluation.

Transtelephonic rhythm strip pacemaker evaluation: service of transmission of an electrocardiographic rhythm strip over the telephone by the patient using a transmitter and recorded by a receiving location using a receiver/recorder (also commonly known as transtelephonic pacemaker monitoring). The electrocardiographic rhythm strip is recorded both with and without a magnet applied over the pacemaker. The rhythm strip is evaluated for heart rate and rhythm, atrial and ventricular capture (if observed) and atrial and ventricular sensing (if observed). In addition, the battery status of the pacemaker is determined by measurement of the paced rate on the electrocardiographic rhythm strip recorded with the magnet applied.

▲ **93279**   Programming device evaluation (in person) with iterative adjustment of the implantable device to test the function of the device and select optimal permanent programmed values with analysis, review and report by a physician or other qualified health care professional; single lead pacemaker system

(Do not report 93279 in conjunction with 93286, 93288)

▲ **93280**   dual lead pacemaker system

(Do not report 93280 in conjunction with 93286, 93288)

▲ **93281**   multiple lead pacemaker system

(Do not report 93281 in conjunction with 93286, 93288)

▲ **93282**   single lead implantable cardioverter-defibrillator system

(Do not report 93282 in conjunction with 93287, 93289, 93745)

▲ **93283**   dual lead implantable cardioverter-defibrillator system

(Do not report 93283 in conjunction with 93287, 93289)

▲ **93284**   multiple lead implantable cardioverter-defibrillator system

(Do not report 93284 in conjunction with 93287, 93289)

▲ **93285**   implantable loop recorder system

(Do not report 93285 in conjunction with 33282, 93279-93284, 93291)

▲ 93286 Peri-procedural device evaluation (in person) and programming of device system parameters before or after a surgery, procedure, or test with analysis, review and report by a physician or other qualified health care professional; single, dual, or multiple lead pacemaker system

(Report 93286 once before and once after surgery, procedure, or test, when device evaluation and programming is performed before and after surgery, procedure, or test)

(Do not report 93286 in conjunction with 93279-93281, 93288)

▲ 93287 single, dual, or multiple lead implantable cardioverter-defibrillator system

(Report 93287 once before and once after surgery, procedure, or test, when device evaluation and programming is performed before and after surgery, procedure, or test)

(Do not report 93287 in conjunction with 93282-93284, 93289)

▲ 93288 Interrogation device evaluation (in person) with analysis, review and report by a physician or other qualified health care professional, includes connection, recording and disconnection per patient encounter; single, dual, or multiple lead pacemaker system

(Do not report 93288 in conjunction with 93279-93281, 93286, 93294, 93296)

▲ 93289 single, dual, or multiple lead implantable cardioverter-defibrillator system, including analysis of heart rhythm derived data elements

(For monitoring physiologic cardiovascular data elements derived froman ICD, use 93290)

(Do not report 93289 in conjunction with 93282-93284, 93287, 93295, 93296)

▲ 93290 implantable cardiovascular monitor system, including analysis of 1 or more recorded physiologic cardiovascular data elements from all internal and external sensors

(For heart rhythm derived data elements, use 93289)

(Do not report 93290 in conjunction with 93297, 93299)

▲ 93291 implantable loop recorder system, including heart rhythm derived data analysis

1155

 Separate Procedure   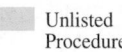 Unlisted Procedure   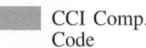 CCI Comp. Code   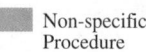 Non-specific Procedure

(Do not report 93291 in conjunction with 93282, 93288-93290, 93298, 93299)

▲ 93292   wearable defibrillator system

(Do not report 93292 in conjunction with 93745)

▲ 93293   Transtelephonic rhythm strip pacemaker evaluation(s) single, dual, or multiple lead pacemaker system, includes recording with and without magnet application with analysis, review and report(s) by a physician or other qualified health care professional, up to 90 days

(Do not report 93293 in conjunction with 93294)

(For in person evaluation, see 93040, 93041, 93042)

(Report 93293 only once per 90 days)

▲ 93294   Interrogation device evaluation(s) (remote), up to 90 days; single, dual, or multiple lead pacemaker system with interim analysis, review(s) and report(s) by a physician or other qualified health care professional

(Do not report 93294 in conjunction with 93288, 93293)

(Report 93294 only once per 90 days)

▲ 93295   single, dual, or multiple lead implantable cardioverter-defibrillator system with interim analysis, review(s) and report(s) by a physician or other qualified health care professional

(For remote monitoring of physiologic cardiovascular data elements derived from an ICD, use 93297)

(Do not report 93295 in conjunction with 93289)

(Report 93295 only once per 90 days)

93296   single, dual, or multiple lead pacemaker system or implantable cardioverter-defibrillator system, remote data acquisition(s), receipt of transmissions and technician review, technical support and distribution of results

(Do not report 93296 in conjunction with 93288, 93289, 93299)

(Report 93296 only once per 90 days)

▲ 93297   Interrogation device evaluation(s), (remote) up to 30 days; implantable cardiovascular monitor system, including analysis of

● New Code   ▲ Revised Code   + Add-On Code   ⊘ Modifier -51 Exempt   ⊙ Moderate Sedation

1 or more recorded physiologic cardiovascular data elements from all internal and external sensors, analysis, review(s) and report(s) by a physician or other qualified health care professional

(For heart rhythm derived data elements, use 93295)

(Do not report 93297 in conjunction with 93290, 93298)

(Report 93297 only once per 30 days)

▲ **93298**   implantable loop recorder system, including analysis of recorded heart rhythm data, analysis, review(s) and report(s) by a physician or other qualified health care professional

(Do not report 93298 in conjunction with 33282, 93291, 93297)

(Report 93298 only once per 30 days)

93299   implantable cardiovascular monitor system or implantable loop recorder system, remote data acquisition(s), receipt of transmissions and technician review, technical support and distribution of results

(Do not report 93299 in conjunction with 93290, 93291, 93296)

(Report 93299 only once per 30 days)

ECHOCARDIOGRAPHY

An echocardiogram is an ultrasound of the heart. Using standard ultrasound techniques, two-dimensional slices of the heart can be imaged. The latest ultrasound systems employ 3D real-time imaging. The standard echocardiogram is also known as a transthoracic echocardiogram, or TTE. In this case, the echocardiography transducer (or probe) is placed on the chest wall (or thorax) of the subject, and images are taken through the chest wall. This is a non-invasive, highly accurate and quick assessment of the overall health of the heart.

Another method to perform an echocardiogram is to insert a specialized scope containing an echocardiography transducer (TOE probe) into the patient's esophagus and record pictures from there. This is known as a transesophageal echocardiogram, or TEE. The advantages of TEE over TTE are clearer images, since the transducer is closer to the heart. Some structures are better imaged with the TEE. These structures include the aorta, the pulmonary artery, the valves of the heart, and the left and right atria. While TTE can be performed easily and without pain for the patient, TEE may require light sedation and a local anesthetic lubricant for the esophagus. Unlike the TTE, the TEE is considered an invasive procedure.

 Separate Procedure   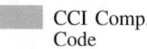 Unlisted Procedure   CCI Comp. Code   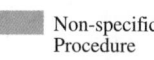 Non-specific Procedure   **1157**

In addition to creating two-dimensional pictures of the cardiovascular system, the echocardiogram can also produce accurate assessment of the direction of blood flow and the velocity of blood and cardiac tissue at any arbitrary point using Doppler ultrasound. This allows assessment of cardiac valve areas and function, any abnormal communications between the left and right side of the heart, any leaking of blood through the valves (valvular regurgitation), and calculation of the cardiac output as well as the ejection fraction.

Echocardiography includes obtaining ultrasonic signals from the heart and great vessels, with real time image and/or Doppler ultrasonic signal documentation, with interpretation and report. When interpretation is performed separately, use modifier 26.

A complete transthoracic echocardiogram without spectral or color flow Doppler (93307) is a comprehensive procedure that includes 2-dimensional and, when performed, selected M-mode examination of: the left and right atria; left and right ventricles; the aortic, mitral, and tricuspid valves; the pericardium; and adjacent portions of the aorta. Multiple views are required to obtain a complete functional and anatomic evaluation, and appropriate measurements are obtained and recorded. Despite significant effort, identification and measurement of some structures may not always be possible. In such instances, the reason that an element could not be visualized must be documented. Additional structures that may be visualized (eg., pulmonary veins, pulmonary artery, pulmonic valve, inferior vena cava) would be included as part of the service.

A complete transthoracic echocardiogram with spectral and color flow Doppler (93306) is a comprehensive procedure that includes spectral Doppler and color flow Doppler in addition to the 2-dimensional and selected M-mode examinations, when performed. Spectral Doppler (93320, 93321) and color flow Doppler (93325) provide information regarding intracardiac blood flow and hemodynamics.

A follow-up or limited echocardiographic study (93308) is an examination that does not evaluate or document the attempt to evaluate all the structures that comprise the complete echocardiographic exam. This is typically limited to, or performed in follow-up of a focused clinical concern.

When a stress echocardiogram is performed with a complete cardiovascular stress test (continuous electrocardiographic monitoring, supervision, interpretation and report by a physician or other qualified health care professional), use 93351. When only the professional components of a complete stress test and a stress echocardiogram are provided (eg, in a facility setting) by the same physician, use 93351 with modifier 26. When all professional services of a stress test are not performed by the same physician performing the stress echocardiogram, use 93350 in conjunction with the appropriate codes (93016-93018) for the components of the cardiovascular stress test that are provided.

When left ventricular endocardial borders cannot be adequately identified by standard echocardiographic imaging, echocardiographic contrast may be infused

● New Code	▲ Revised Code	＋ Add-On Code	⊘ Modifier -51 Exempt	⊙ Moderate Sedation

intravenously both at rest and with stress to achieve that purpose. Code 93352 is used to report the administration of echocardiographic contrast agent in conjunction with the stress echocardiography codes (93350 or 93351). Supply of contrast agent and/or drugs used for pharmacological stress is reported separately in addition to the procedure code.

Report of an echocardiographic study, whether complete or limited, includes an interpretation of all obtained information, documentation of all clinically relevant findings including quantitative measurements obtained, plus a description of any recognized abnormalities. Pertinent images, videotape, and/or digital data are archived for permanent storage and are available for subsequent review. Use of echocardiography not meeting these criteria is not separately reportable.

Use of ultrasound, without thorough evaluation of organ(s) or anatomic region, image documentation and final, written report, is not separately reportable.

(For fetal echocardiography, see 76825-76828)

93303 Transthoracic echocardiography for congenital cardiac anomalies; complete

93304 follow-up or limited study

93306 Echocardiography, transthoracic, real-time with image documentation (2D), includes M-mode recording, when performed, complete, with spectral doppler echocardiography, and with color flow doppler echocardiography

(For transthoracic echocardiography without spectral and color Doppler, use 93307)

93307 Echocardiography, transthoracic, real-time with image documentation (2D) includes M-mode recording, when performed, complete, without spectral or color Doppler echocardiography

(Do not report 93307 in conjunction with 93320, 93321, 93325)

93308 Echocardiography, transthoracic, real-time with image documentation (2D), includes M-mode recording, when performed, follow-up or limited study

⊙ **93312** Echocardiography, transesophageal, real-time with image documentation (2D) (with or without M-mode recording); including probe placement, image acquisition, interpretation and report

⊙ **93313** placement of transesophageal probe only

| Separate Procedure | Unlisted Procedure | CCI Comp. Code | Non-specific Procedure | **1159** |

⊙ **93314**   image acquisition, interpretation and report only

⊙ **93315**   Transesophageal echocardiography for congenital cardiac anomalies; including probe placement, image acquisition, interpretation and report

⊙ **93316**   placement of transesophageal probe only

⊙ **93317**   image acquisition, interpretation and report only

⊙ **93318**   Echocardiography, transesophageal (TEE) for monitoring purposes, including probe placement, real time 2-dimensional image acquisition and interpretation leading to ongoing (continuous) assessment of (dynamically changing) cardiac pumping function and to therapeutic measures on an immediate time basis

\+ **93320**   Doppler echocardiography, pulsed wave and/or continuous wave with spectral display (List separately in addition to codes for echocardiographic imaging); complete

(Use 93320 in conjunction with 93303, 93304, 93312, 93314, 93315, 93317, 93350, 93351)

\+ **93321**   follow-up or limited study (List separately in addition to codes for echocardiographic imaging)

(Use 93321 in conjunction with 93303, 93304, 93308, 93312, 93314, 93315, 93317, 93350, 93351)

\+ **93325**   Doppler echocardiography color flow velocity mapping (List separately in addition to codes for echocardiography)

(Use 93325 in conjunction with 76825, 76826, 76827, 76828, 93303, 93304, 93308, 93312, 93314, 93315, 93317, 93350, 93351)

93350   Echocardiography, transthoracic, real-time with image documentation (2D), includes M-mode recording, when performed, during rest and cardiovascular stress test using treadmill, bicycle exercise and/or pharmacologically induced stress, with interpretation and report

(Stress testing codes 93016-93018 should be reported, when appropriate, in conjunction with 93350 to capture the cardiovascular stress portion of the study)

(Do not report 93350 in conjunction with 93015)

▲ 93351   including performance of continuous electrocardiographic monitoring, with supervision by a physician or other qualified health care professional

(Do not report 93351 in conjunction with 93015-93018, 93350. Do not report 93351-26 in conjunction with 93016, 93018, 93350-26))

+ 93352   Use of echocardiographic contrast agent during stress echocardiography (list separately in addition to code for primary procedure)

(Do not report 93352 more than once per stress echocardiogram)

(Use 93352 in conjunction with 93350, 93351)

CARDIAC CATHETERIZATION

A coronary catheterization is a minimally invasive procedure to access the coronary circulation and blood filled chambers of the heart using a catheter. It is performed for both diagnostic and interventional (treatment) purposes.

Specifically, coronary catheterization is a visually interpreted test performed to recognize occlusion, stenosis, restenosis, thrombosis or aneurysmal enlargement of the coronary artery lumens, heart chamber size, heart muscle contraction performance and some aspects of heart valve function. Important internal heart and lung blood pressures, not measurable from outside the body, can be accurately measured during the test. The relevant problems that the test deals with most commonly occur as a result of advanced atherosclerosis, atheroma activity within the wall of the coronary arteries. Less frequently, other issues, valvular, heart muscle or arrhythmia issues are the primary focus of the test.

Coronary artery luminal narrowing reduces the flow reserve for oxygenated blood to the heart, typically producing intermittent angina if very advanced; luminal occlusion usually produces a heart attack. However, it has been increasingly recognized, since the late 1980s, that coronary catheterization does not allow the recognition of the presence or absence of coronary atherosclerosis itself, only significant luminal changes which have occurred as a result of end stage complications of the atherosclerotic process. See IVUS and atheroma for a better understanding of this issue.

Coronary catheterization is performed in a cardiac catheterization lab, usually located within a hospital.

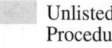 Separate Procedure   Unlisted Procedure   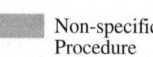 CCI Comp. Code   Non-specific Procedure

Catheterization to treat luminal disease

By changing the diagnostic catheter to a guiding catheter, physicians can also pass a variety of instruments through the catheter and into the artery to a lesion site. The most commonly used are guide wires and the balloon dilation catheters.

By injecting radiocontrast agent through a tiny passage extending down the balloon catheter and into the balloon, the balloon is progressively expanded. The hydraulic pressures are chosen and applied by the physician, according to how the balloon within the stenosis responds. The radiocontrast filled balloon is watched under fluoroscopy (it typically assumes a "dog bone" shape imposed on the outside of the balloon by the stenosis as the balloon is expanded), as it opens. As much hydraulic brute force is applied as judged needed and visualized to be effective to make the stenosis of the artery lumen visibly enlarge.

Additionally, several other devices can be advanced into the artery via a guiding catheter. These include laser catheters, stent catheters, IVUS catheters, Doppler catheter, pressure or temperature measurement catheter and various clot and grinding or removal devices. Most of these devices have turned out to be niche devices, only useful in a small percentage of situations or for research.

Stents, specially manufactured expandable stainless steel mesh tubes, mounted on a balloon catheter, are the most commonly used device beyond the balloon catheter. When the stent/balloon device is positioned within the stenosis, the balloon is inflated which, in turn, expands the stent and the artery. The balloon is removed and the stent remains in place, supporting the inner artery walls in the more open, dilated position.

There are two code families for cardiac catheterization: one for congenital heart disease, and one for all other conditions. Anomalous coronary arteries, patent foramen ovale, mitral valve prolapse, and bicuspid aortic valve are to be reported with 93451-93464, 93566-93568.

Right heart catheterization includes catheter placement in one or more right-sided cardiac chamber(s) or structures (ie, the right atrium, right ventricle, pulmonary artery, pulmonary wedge), obtaining blood samples for measurement of blood gases, and cardiac output measurements (Fick or other method), when performed. Left heart catheterization involves catheter placement in a left-sided (systemic) cardiac chamber(s) (left ventricle or left atrium) and includes left ventricular injection(s) when performed. Do not report code 93503 in conjunction with other diagnostic cardiac catheterization codes. When right heart catheterization is performed in conjunction with other cardiac catheterization services, report 93453, 93456, 93457, 93460 or 93461. For placement of a flow directed catheter (eg, Swan-Ganz) performed for hemodynamic monitoring purposes not in conjunction with other catheterization services, use 93503. Right heart catheterization does not include right ventricular or right atrial angiography (93566). When left heart catheterization if performed using either transapical puncture of the left ventricle or transeptal puncture of an intact septum, report 93462 in conjunction with 93452,

● New Code   ▲ Revised Code   + Add-On Code   ⊘ Modifier -51 Exempt   ⊙ Moderate Sedation

93453, 93458-93461, 93653, 93654. Catheter placement(s) in coronary artery(ies) involves selective engagement of the origins of the native coronary artery(ies) for the purpose of coronary angiography. Catheter placement(s) in bypass graft(s) (venous, internal mammary, free arterial graft[s]) involve selective engagement of the origins of the graft(s) for the purpose of bypass angiography. It is typically performed only in conjunction with coronary angiography of native vessels.

The cardiac catheterization codes (93452-93462), other than those for congenital heart disease, include contrast injection(s), imaging supervision, interpretation, and report for imaging typically performed. Codes for left heart catheterization (93452, 93453, 93458-93461) other than those for congenital heart disease, include intraprocedural injection(s) for left ventricular/left atrial angiography, imaging supervision, and interpretation, when performed. Codes for coronary catheter placement(s) (93454-93461), other than those for congenital heart disease, include intraprocedural injection(s) for coronary angiography, imaging supervision, and interpretation. Codes for catheter placement(s) in bypass graft(s) (93455, 93457, 93459, 93461) other than those for congenital heart disease, include intraprocedural injection(s) for bypass graft angiography, imaging supervision, and interpretation. Do not report 93563-93565 in conjunction with 93452-93461.

For cardiac catheterization for congenital cardiac anomalies, see 93530-93533. When contrast injection(s) are performed in conjunction with cardiac catheterization for congenital anomalies, see 93563-93568.

Cardiac catheterization (93451-93461) includes all roadmapping angiography in order to place the catheters, including any injections and imaging supervision, interpretation, and report. It does not include contrast injection(s) and imaging supervision, interpretation, and report for imaging that is separately identified by specific procedure code(s). For right ventricular or right atrial angiography performed in conjunction with cardiac catheterization for congenital or noncongenital heart disease (93451-93461, 93530-93533), use 93566. For aortography, use 93567. For pulmonary angiography, use 93568. For angiography of noncoronary arteries and veins, performed as a distinct service, use appropriate codes from the Radiology section and the Vascular Injection Procedures section.

When cardiac catheterization is combined with pharmacologic agent administration with the specific purpose of repeating hemodynamic measurements to evaluate hemodynamic response, use 93463 in conjunction with 93451-93453 and 93456-93461. Do not report 93463 for intracoronary administration of pharmacologic agents during percutaneous coronary interventional procedures, during intracoronary assessment of coronary pressure, flow or resistance, or during intracoronary imaging procedures. Do not report 93463 in conjunction with 92920-92944, 92975, 92977.

When cardiac catheterization is combined with exercise (eg, walking or arm or leg ergometry protocol) with the specific purpose of repeating hemodynamic measurements to evaluate hemodynamic response, report 93464 in conjunction with 93451-93453, 93456-93461, and 93530-93533.

| Separate Procedure | Unlisted Procedure | CCI Comp. Code | Non-specific Procedure |

Contrast injection to image the access site(s) for the specific purpose of placing a closure device is inherent to the catheterization procedure and not separately reportable. Closure device placement at the vascular access site is inherent to the catheterization procedure and not separately reportable.

Modifier 51 should not be appended to 93451, 93456, 93503.

Please see the cardiac catheterization table, located following 93572.

⊘⊙**93451**   Right heart catheterization including measurement(s) of oxygen saturation and cardiac output, when performed

(Do not report 93451 in conjunction with 93453, 93456, 93457, 93460, 93461)

⊙ **93452**   Left heart catheterization including intraprocedural injection(s) for left ventriculography, imaging supervision and interpretation, when performed

(Do not report 93452 in conjunction with 93453, 93458-93461)

⊙ **93453**   Combined right and left heart catheterization including intraprocedural injection(s) for left ventriculography, imaging supervision and interpretation, when performed

(Do not report 93453 in conjunction with 93451, 93452, 93456-93461)

⊙ **93454**   Catheter placement in coronary artery(s) for coronary angiography, including intraprocedural injection(s) for coronary angiography, imaging supervision and interpretation

⊙ **93455**   with catheter placement(s) in bypass graft(s) (internal mammary, free arterial venous grafts) including intraprocedural injection(s) for bypass graft angiography

⊘⊙**93456**   with right heart catheterization

⊙ **93457**   with catheter placement(s) in bypass graft(s) (internal mammary, free arterial, venous grafts) including intraprocedural injection(s) for bypass graft angiography and right heart catheterization

⊙ **93458**   with left heart catheterization including intraprocedural injection(s) for left ventriculography, when performed

⊙ **93459**   with left heart catheterization including intraprocedural injection(s) for left ventriculography, when performed, catheter placement(s) in bypass graft(s) (internal mammary, free arterial, venous grafts) with bypass graft angiography

⊙ **93460** with right and left heart catheterization including intraprocedural injection(s) for left ventriculography, when performed

⊙ **93461** with right and left heart catheterization including intraprocedural injection(s) for left ventriculography, when performed, catheter placement(s) in bypass graft(s) (internal mammary, free arterial, venous grafts) with bypass graft angiography

⊙+**93462** Left heart catheterization by transseptal puncture through intact septum or by transapical puncture (List separately in addition to code for primary procedure)

(Use 93462 in conjunction with 93452, 93453, 93458-93461, 93653, 93654)

(Do not report 93462 in conjunction with 93656)

⊙+**93463** Pharmacologic agent administration (eg, inhaled nitric oxide, intravenous infusion of nitroprusside, dobutamine, milrinone, or other agent) including assessing hemodynamic measurements before, during, after and repeat pharmacologic agent administration, when performed (List separately in addition to code for primary procedure)

(Use 93463 in conjunction with 93451-93453, 93456-93461, 93563, 93564, 93580, 93581)

(Report 93463 only once per catheterization procedure)

(Do not report 93463 for pharmacologic agent administration in conjunction with coronary interventional procedure codes 92920-92944, 92975, 92977)

⊙+**93464** Physiologic exercise study (eg, bicycle or arm ergometry) including assessing hemodynamic measurements before and after (List separately in addition to code for primary procedure)

(Use 93464 in conjunction with 93451-93453, 93456-93461, 93530-93533)

(Report 93464 only once per catheterization procedure)

(For pharmacologic agent administration, use 93463)

(For bundle of His recording, use 93600)

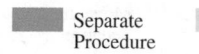 Separate Procedure 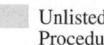 Unlisted Procedure 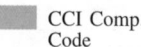 CCI Comp. Code 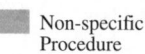 Non-specific Procedure

(93501   deleted 2010 [2011 edition]. To report, see 93451-93461.)

⊘ **93503**   Insertion and placement of flow directed catheter (eg, Swan-Ganz) for monitoring purposes

(For subsequent monitoring, see 99356-99357)

⊙ **93505**   Endomyocardial biopsy

(To report transcatheter placement of radiation delivery device for coronary intravascular brachytherapy, use 92974)

(For intravascular radioelement application, see 77785-77787)

(93508   deleted 2010 [2011 edition]. To report, see 93451-93461.)

(93510   deleted 2010 [2011 edition]. To report, see 93451-93461.)

(93511   deleted 2010 [2011 edition]. To report, see 93451-93461.)

(93514   deleted 2010 [2011 edition]. To report, see 93451-93461.)

(93524   deleted 2010 [2011 edition]. To report, see 93451-93461.)

(93526   deleted 2010 [2011 edition]. To report, see 93451-93461.)

(93527   deleted 2010 [2011 edition]. To report, see 93451-93461.)

(93528   deleted 2010 [2011 edition]. To report, see 93451-93461.)

(93529   deleted 2010 [2011 edition]. To report, see 93451-93461.)

⊙ **93530**   Right heart catheterization, for congenital cardiac anomalies

93531   Combined right heart catheterization and retrograde left heart catheterization, for congenital cardiac anomalies

93532   Combined right heart catheterization and transseptal left heart catheterization through intact septum with or without retrograde left heart catheterization, for congenital cardiac anomalies

93533   Combined right heart catheterization and transseptal left heart catheterization through existing septal opening, with or without retrograde left heart catheterization, for congenital cardiac anomalies

● New Code   ▲ Revised Code   + Add-On Code   ⊘ Modifier -51 Exempt   ⊙ Moderate Sedation

INJECTION PROCEDURES

All injection codes include radiological supervision, interpretation, and report. Cardiac catheterization codes (93452-93461), other than those for congenital heart disease, include contrast injection(s) for imaging typically performed during these procedures (see Cardiac Catheterization above.) Do not report 93563-93565 in conjunction with 93452-93461. When injection procedures for right ventricular, right atrial, aortic, or pulmonary angiography are performed in conjunction with cardiac catheterization, these services are reported separately (93566-93568). When right ventricular or right atrial angiography is performed at the time of heart catheterization, use 93566 with the appropriate catheterization code ((93451, 93453, 93456, 93457, 93460, or 93461). Use 93567 when supravalvular ascending aortography is performed at the t ime of heart catheterization. Use 93568 with the appropriate right heart catheterization code when pulmonary angiography is preformed. Separately reported injection procedures do not include introduction of catheters but do include repositioning of catheters when necessary and use of automatic power injectors, when performed.

When contrast injection(s) are performed in conjunction with cardiac catheterization for congenital cardiac anomalies (93530-93533), see 93563-93568. Injection procedure codes 93563-93568 include imaging supervision, interpretation, and report.

Injection procedures 93563-93568 represent separate identifiable services and may be coded in conjunction with one another when appropriate. The technical details of angiography, supervision of filming and processing, interpretation, and report are included.

(93539   deleted 2010 [2011 edition]. To report, see 93451-93461, 93563-93568.)

(93540   deleted 2010 [2011 edition]. To report, see 93451-93461, 93563-93568.)

(93541   deleted 2010 [2011 edition]. To report, see 93451-93461, 93563-93568.)

(93542   deleted 2010 [2011 edition]. To report, see 93451-93461, 93563-93568.)

(93543   deleted 2010 [2011 edition]. To report, see 93451-93461, 93563-93568.)

(93544   deleted 2010 [2011 edition]. To report, see 93451-93461, 93563-93568.)

(93545   deleted 2010 [2011 edition]. To report, see 93451-93461, 93563-93568.)

1167

| Separate Procedure | Unlisted Procedure | CCI Comp. Code | Non-specific Procedure |

(93555   deleted 2010 [2011 edition]. See introductory guidelines for Cardiac Catheterization and Injection Procedures.)

93556   deleted 2010 [2011 edition]. See introductory guidelines for Cardiac Catheterization and Injection Procedures.)

⊙ **93561**   Indicator dilution studies such as dye or thermodilution, including arterial and/or venous catheterization; with cardiac output measurement (separate procedure)

⊙ **93562**   subsequent measurement of cardiac output

(Do not report 93561, 93562 in conjunction with 93451-93462)

(For radioisotope method of cardiac output, see 78472, 78473 or 78481)

⊙+**93563**   Injection procedure during cardiac catheterization including imaging supervision, interpretation, and report; for selective coronary angiography during congenital heart catheterization (List separately in addition to code for primary procedure)

⊙+**93564**   for selective opacification of aortocoronary venous or arterial bypass graft(s) (eg, aortocoronary saphenous vein, free radial artery, or free mammary artery graft) to one or more coronary arteries and in situ arterial conduits (eg, internal mammary), whether native or used for bypass to one or more coronary arteries during congenital heart catheterization, when performed (List separately in addition to code for primary procedure)

⊙+**93565**   for selective left ventricular or left atrial angiography (List separately in addition to code for primary procedure)

(Do not report 93563-93565 in conjunction with 93452-93461)

(Use 93563-93565 in conjunction with 93530-93533)

⊙+**93566**   for selective right ventricular or right atrial angiography (List separately in addition to code for primary procedure)

(Use 93566 in conjunction with 93451, 93453, 93456, 93457, 93460, 93461, 93530-93533)

⊙+**93567**   for supravalvular aortography (List separately in addition to code for primary procedure)

(Use 93567 in conjunction with 93451-93461, 93530-93533)

  ● New Code   ▲ Revised Code   + Add-On Code   ⊘ Modifier -51 Exempt   ⊙ Moderate Sedation

Table of Catheterization Codes

CPT Code	Catheter Placement Type				Add-On Procedures (Can be reported separately)					
	RHC	LHC	Coronary Artery Placement	Bypass Graft(s)	With Transseptal or Transapical Puncture	With Pharmacological Study	With Exercise Study	Injection Procedure for Selective Rt Ventricular or Rt Atrial Angiography	Injection Procedure for Supravalvular Aortography	Injection Procedure for Pulmonary Angiography
					93462	93463	93464	93566	93567	93568
93451	•					•	•	•		•
93452		•			•	•	•		•	
93453	•	•			•	•	•	•	•	•
93454			•						•	
93455			•	•					•	
93456	•		•		•	•	•	•	•	•
93457	•		•	•	•	•	•	•	•	•
93458		•	•		•	•	•		•	
93459		•	•	•	•	•	•		•	
93460	•	•	•		•	•	•	•	•	•
93461	•	•	•	•	•	•	•	•	•	•

(For non-supravalvular thoracic aortography or abdominal aortography performed at the time of cardiac catheterization, use the appropriate radiological supervision and interpretation codes [36221, 75600-75630])

⊙+**93568**   for pulmonary angiography (List separately in addition to code for primary procedure)

(Use 93568 in conjunction with 93451, 93453, 93456, 93457, 93460, 93461, 93530-93533)

⊙+**93571**   Intravascular Doppler velocity and/or pressure derived coronary flow reserve measurement (coronary vessel or graft) during coronary angiography including pharmacologically induced stress; initial vessel (List separately in addition to code for primary procedure)

(Use 93571 in conjunction with 92920, 92924, 92928, 92933, 92937, 92941, 92943, 92975, 93454-93461, 93563, 93564)

⊙+**93572**   each additional vessel (List separately in addition to code for primary procedure)

(Use 93572 in conjunction with 93571)

	Separate Procedure		Unlisted Procedure		CCI Comp. Code		Non-specific Procedure

1169

(Intravascular distal coronary blood flow velocity measurements include all Doppler transducer manipulations and repositioning within the specific vessel being examined, during coronary angiography or therapeutic intervention (eg, angioplasty))

(For unlisted cardiac catheterization procedure, use 93799)

REPAIR OF SEPTAL DEFECT

93580 Percutaneous transcatheter closure of congenital interatrial communication (i.e., fontan fenestration, atrial septal defect) with implant

(Percutaneous transcatheter closure of atrial septal defect includes a right heart catheterization procedure. Code 93580 includes injection of contrast for atrial and ventricular angiograms. Codes 93451-93453, 93455-93461, 93530-93533, 93564-93566 should not be reported separately in addition to code 93580)

93581 Percutaneous transcatheter closure of a congenital ventricular septal defect with implant

(Percutaneous transcatheter closure of ventricular septal defect includes a right heart catheterization procedure. Code 93581 includes injection of contrast for atrial and ventricular angiograms. Codes 93451-93453, 93455-93461, 93530-93533, 93564-93566 should not be reported separately in addition to 93581)

(For echocardiographic services performed in addition to 93580, 93581, see 93303-93317 as appropriate)

INTRACARDIAC ELECTROPHYSIOLOGICAL PROCEDURES/STUDIES

Intracardiac electrophysiology study (EPS) involves placing wire electrodes within the heart to determine the characteristics of heart arrhythmias. Before performing EPS, which is invasive, the cardiologist will try to identify a suspected arrhythmia using other, less invasive tests like ambulatory cardiac monitoring. If the abnormal rhythm is not detected by these other methods and symptoms suggest an arrhythmia, EPS may be recommended. Additional reasons that EPS may be considered include:

- *To find the location of a known arrhythmia and determine the best therapy*

- *To assess the severity of the arrhythmia and determine if the patient is at risk for future cardiac events, especially sudden cardiac death*

| ● New Code | ▲ Revised Code | + Add-On Code | ⊘ Modifier -51 Exempt | ⊙ Moderate Sedation |

- *To evaluate the effectiveness of medication in controlling an arrhythmia*

- *To determine if the focus (the place where the arrhythmia is coming from) should be ablated*

- *To evaluate the need for a permanent pacemaker or an implantable cardioverter-defibrillator (ICD)*

During EPS, the cardiologist inserts a catheter through a small incision in a groin vein after cleansing the site and numbing it with a local anesthetic. This catheter is equipped with an electrode connected to electrocardiographic monitors. The catheter is then carefully threaded into the heart using an x-ray imaging technique called fluoroscopy to guide the insertion. Electrodes are placed in the heart to measure electrical activity along the heart's conduction system and within heart muscle cells themselves.

Normal electrical activity is signaled from the heart's natural pacemaker known as the sinoatrial (SA) node. It then travels through the atria, the atrioventricular (AV) node, and the ventricles. Abnormal electrical activity can occur anywhere along this conduction system, including in the muscle cells of either the atria or ventricles. The electrodes inserted during EPS will map the type of arrhythmia the patient has and where the problem arises in the heart.

If ablation is thought to be the appropriate therapy, it is performed at the time of EPS.

Definitions

Arrhythmia Induction: In most electrophysiologic studies, an attempt is made to induce arrhythmia(s) from single or multiple sites within the heart. Arrhythmia induction may be achieved by multiple techniques, eg. by performing pacing at different rates or programmed stimulation (introduction of critically timed electrical impulses). Because arrhythmia induction occurs via the same catheter(s) inserted for the electrophysiologic study(ies), catheter insertion and temporary pacemaker codes are not additionally reported. Codes 93600-93603, 93610-93612 and 93618 are used to describe unusual situations where there may be recording, pacing or an attempt at arrhythmia induction from only one site in the heart. Code 93619 describes only evaluation of the sinus node, atrioventricular node, and His-Purkinje conduction system, without arrhythmia induction. Codes 93620-93624, 93640-93642, 93653, 93654 and 93656 all include recording, pacing and attempted arrhythmia induction from one or more site(s) in the heart.

Mapping: When a tachycardia is induced, the site of tachycardia origination or its electrical path through the heart is often defined by mapping. Mapping is a distinct procedure performed in addition to a diagnostic electrophysiologic study or ablation procedure and may be separately reported using 93609 or 93613. Do not report standard mapping (93609) in addition to 3-dimensional mapping (93613).

	Separate Procedure		Unlisted Procedure		CCI Comp. Code		Non-specific Procedure

Ablation: Once the part of the heart involved in the tachycardia is localized, the tachycardia may be treated by ablation (the delivery of a radiofrequency or cryo-energy to the area to selectively destroy cardiac tissue). Ablation procedures (93653-93657) are performed at the same session as electrophysiology studies and therefore represent a combined code description. When reporting ablation therapy codes (93653-93657), the single site electrophysiology studies (93600-93603, 93610, 93612, 93618) and the comprehensive electrophysiology studies (93619, 93620) may not be reported separately. Codes 93622 and 93623 may be reported separately with 93656 for treatment of atrial fibrillation. However, 93621 for left atrial pacing and recording from coronary sinus or left atrium should not be reported in conjunction with 93656 as this is a component of 93656.

The differences in the techniques involved for ablation of supraventricular arrhythmias, ventricular arrhythmias, and atrial fibrillation are reflected within the descriptions for 93653-93657. Code 93653 is a primary code for catheter ablation for treatment of supraventricular tachycardia caused by dual atrioventricular nodal pathways, accessory atrioventricular connections, or other atrial foci. Code 93654 describes catheter ablation for treatment of ventricular tachycardia or focus of ventricular ectopy. Code 93656 is a primary code for reporting treatment of atrial fibrillation by ablation to achieve complete pulmonary vein electrical isolation. Codes 93653, 93654 and 93656 are distinct primary procedure codes and may not be reported together.

Codes 93655 and 93657 are add-on codes listed in addition to the primary ablation code to report ablation of sites distinct from the primary ablation site. After ablation of the primary target site, post-ablation electrophysiologic evaluation is performed as part of those ablation services (93653, 93654, 93656) and additional mechanisms of tachycardia may be identified. For example, if the primary tachycardia ablated was atrioventricular nodal reentrant tachycardia and during post-ablation testing an atrial tachycardia, atrial flutter, or accessory pathway with orthodromic reentry tachycardia was identified, this would be considered a separate mechanism of tachycardia. Pacing maneuvers are performed to define the mechanism(s) of the new tachycardia(s). Catheter ablation of this distinct mechanism of tachycardia is then performed at the newly discovered atrial or ventricular origin. Appropriate post-ablation attempts at re-induction and observation are again performed. Code 93655 is listed in conjunction with 93653 when repeat ablation is for treatment of an additional supraventricular tachycardia mechanism and with 93654 when the repeat ablation is for treatment of an additional ventricular tachycardia mechanism. Code 93655 may be reported with 93656 when an additional non-atrial fibrillation tachycardia is separately diagnosed after pulmonary vein isolation. Code 93657 is reported in conjunction with 93656 when successful pulmonary vein isolation is achieved, attempts at re-induction of atrial fibrillation identify an additional left or right atrial focus for atrial fibrillation, and further ablation of this new focus is performed.

In certain circumstances, depending on the chamber of origin, a catheter or catheters may be maneuvered into the left ventricle to facilitate arrhythmia diagnosis. This may be accomplished via a retrograde aortic approach by means of the arterial access or through a transseptal puncutre. For ablation treatment of supraventricular tachycardia (93653) and ventricular tachycardia (93654), the left heart catheterization by transseptal puncture through intact septum (93462) may be reported separately as an add-on code. However, for ablation treatment of atrial fibrillation (93656), the transseptal puncture (93462) is a standard component of the procedure and may not be reported separately. Do not report 93462 in conjunction with 93656.

Modifier 51 should not be appended to 93600-93603, 93610, 93612, 93615-93618, 93631.

⊘ **93600** Bundle of His recording

⊘ **93602** Intra-atrial recording

⊘ **93603** Right ventricular recording

⊙+**93609** Intraventricular and/or intra-atrial mapping of tachycardia site(s) with catheter manipulation to record from multiple sites to identify origin of tachycardia (List separately in addition to code for primary procedure)

(Use 93609 in conjunction with 93620, 93653)

(Do not report 93609 in conjunction with 93613, 93654)

⊘ **93610** Intra-atrial pacing

⊘ **93612** Intraventricular pacing

(Do not report 93612 in conjunction with 93620-93622)

⊙+**93613** Intracardiac electrophysiologic 3-dimensional mapping (List separately in addition to code for primary procedure)

(Use 93613 in conjunction with 93620, 93653)

(Do not report 93613 in addition to 93609, 93654)

⊘⊙**93615** Esophageal recording of atrial electrogram with or without ventricular electrogram(s);

⊘⊙**93616** with pacing

⊘⊙**93618** Induction of arrhythmia by electrical pacing

(For intracardiac phonocardiogram, use 93799)

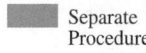 Separate Procedure   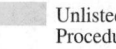 Unlisted Procedure   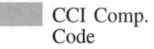 CCI Comp. Code   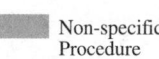 Non-specific Procedure   **1173**

⊙ **93619** Comprehensive electrophysiologic evaluation with right atrial pacing and recording, right ventricular pacing and recording, His bundle recording, including insertion and repositioning of multiple electrode catheters without induction or attempted induction of arrhythmia

(Do not report 93619 in conjunction with 93600, 93602, 93610, 93612, 93618 or 93620-93622)

⊙ **93620** Comprehensive electrophysiologic evaluation including insertion and repositioning of multiple electrode catheters with induction or attempted induction of arrhythmia; with right atrial pacing and recording, right ventricular pacing and recording, His bundle recording

(Do not report 93620 in conjunction with 93600, 93602, 93610, 93612, 93618 or 93619)

⊙**+93621** with left atrial pacing and recording from coronary sinus or left atrium (List separately in addition to code for primary procedure)

(Use 93621 in conjunction with 93620)

(Do not report 93621 in conjunction with 93656)

⊙**+93622** with left ventricular pacing and recording (List separately in addition to code for primary procedure)

(Use 93622 in conjunction with 93620)

+ 93623 Programmed stimulation and pacing after intravenous drug infusion (List separately in addition to code for primary procedure)

(Use 93623 in conjunction with 93619, 93620)

⊙ **93624** Electrophysiologic follow-up study with pacing and recording to test effectiveness of therapy, including induction or attempted induction of arrhythmia

⊘ **93631** Intra-operative epicardial and endocardial pacing and mapping to localize the site of tachycardia or zone of slow conduction for surgical correction

(For operative ablation of an arrhythmogenic focus or pathway by a separate individual, see 33250-33261)

⊙ **93640** Electrophysiologic evaluation of single or dual chamber pacing cardioverter-defibrillator leads including defibrillation threshold

---

1174 ● New Code   ▲ Revised Code   + Add-On Code   ⊘ Modifier -51 Exempt   ⊙ Moderate Sedation

evaluation (induction of arrhythmia, evaluation of sensing and pacing for arrhythmia termination) at time of initial implantation or replacement;

⊙ **93641** with testing of single or dual chamber pacing cardioverter-defibrillator pulse generator

(For subsequent or periodic electronic analysis and/or reprogramming of single or dual chamber pacing cardioverter-defibrillators, see 93282, 93283, 93289, 93292, 93295, 93642)

⊙ **93642** Electrophysiologic evaluation of single or dual chamber pacing cardioverter-defibrillator (includes defibrillation threshold evaluation, induction of arrhythmia, evaluation of sensing and pacing for arrhythmia termination, and programming or reprogramming of sensing or therapeutic parameters)

⊙ **93650** Intracardiac catheter ablation of atrioventricular node function, atrioventricular conduction for creation of complete heart block, with or without temporary pacemaker placement

(93651 deleted 2012 [2013 edition]. To report, see 93653-93657)

(93652 deleted 2012 [2013 edition]. To report, see 93653-93657)

●⊙**93653** Comprehensive electrophysiologic evaluation including insertion and repositioning of multiple electrode catheters with induction or attempted induction of an arrhythmia with right atrial pacing and recording, right ventricular pacing and recording, His recording with intracardiac catheter ablation of arrhythmogenic focus; with treatment of supraventricular tachycardia by ablation of fast or slow atrioventricular pathway, accessory atrioventricular connection, cavo-tricuspid isthmus or other single atrial focus or source of atrial re-entry.

(Do not report 93653 in conjunction with 93600-93603, 93610, 93612, 93618-93620, 93642, 93654)

●⊙**93654** with treatment of ventricular tachycardia or focus of ventricular ectopy including intracardiac electrophysiologic 3D mapping, when performed, and left ventricular pacing and recording, when performed

(Do not report 93654 in conjunction with 93279-93284, 93286-93289, 93600-93603, 93609, 93610, 93612, 93613, 93618-93620, 93622, 93642, 93653)

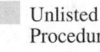 Separate Procedure   Unlisted Procedure   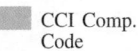 CCI Comp. Code   Non-specific Procedure

●⊙+**93655**   Intracardiac catheter ablation of a discrete mechanism of arrhythmia which is distinct from the primary ablated mechanism, including repeat diagnostic maneuvers, to treat a spontaneous or induced arrhythmia (List separately in addition to code for primary procedure)

(Use 93655 in conjunction with 93653, 93654, 93656)

●⊙**93656**   Comprehensive electrophysiologic evaluation including transseptal catheterizations, insertion and repositioning of multiple electrode catheters with induction or attempted induction of an arrhythmia with atrial recording and pacing, when possible, right ventricular pacing and recording, His bundle recording with intracardiac catheter ablation of arrhythmogenic focus, with treatment of atrial fibrillation by ablation by pulmonary vein isolation

(Do not report 93656 in conjunction with 93279-93284, 93286-93289, 93462, 93600, 93602, 93603, 93610, 93612, 93618, 93619, 93620, 93621, 93653, 93654)

●⊙+**93657**   Additional linear or focal intracardiac catheter ablation of the left or right atrium for treatment of atrial fibrillation remaining after completion of pulmonary vein isolation (List separately in addition to code for primary procedure)

(Use 93657 in conjunction with 93656)

93660   Evaluation of cardiovascular function with tilt table evaluation, with continuous ECG monitoring and intermittent blood pressure monitoring, with or without pharmacological intervention

(For testing of autonomic nervous system function, see 95921, 95924, 95943)

+ **93662**   Intracardiac echocardiography during therapeutic/diagnostic intervention, including imaging supervision and interpretation (List separately in addition to code for primary procedure)

(Use 93662 in conjunction with 92987, 93453, 93460-93462, 93532, 93580, 93581, 93621, 93622, 93653, 93654, 93656 as appropriate)

(Do not report 92961 in addition to 93662)

● New Code   ▲ Revised Code   + Add-On Code   ⊘ Modifier -51 Exempt   ⊙ Moderate Sedation

PERIPHERAL ARTERIAL DISEASE REHABILITATION

Peripheral Arterial Disease (PAD) rehabilitation is an outpatient service for patients diagnosed with peripheral artery disease—a disorder of the vessels of the legs or arms resulting in pain. PAD rehabilitation requires a physician's referral. The referring physician receives progress notes about his or her patient's progress in the program.

ehabilitation consists of a series of sessions involving physical exercise, using a motorized treadmill and various other pieces of exercise equipment to permit each patient to achieve symptom-limited claudication. Claudication is taken from the Latin word 'to limp' and refers to the pain that occurs in PAD patients when they exercise. A medically supervised walking program can improve the symptoms of claudication and lead to an enhanced quality of life. Each rehabilitation session lasts about 45 to 60 minutes and is supervised by an exercise physiologist or nurse. A patient's claudication threshold and other cardiovascular limitations are monitored and adjustments are made to the workload during the exercises.

During this supervised rehabilitation program, the development of new arrhythmias, symptoms that might suggest angina or the continued inability of the patient to progress to an adequate level of exercise may require review and examination of the patient by a physician or other qualified health care professional. These services would be separately reported with an appropriate E/M service code including office or other outpatient services (99201-99215), initial hospital care (99221-99223), subsequent hospital care (99231-99233), or crirical care services (99291-99292).

93668   Peripheral arterial disease (PAD) rehabilitation, per session

NONINVASIVE PHYSIOLOGIC STUDIES AND PROCEDURES

(For arterial cannulization and recording of direct arterial pressure, use 36620)

(For radiographic injection procedures, see 36000-36299)

(For vascular cannulization for hemodialysis, see 36800-36821)

(For chemotherapy for malignant disease, see 96409-96549)

(For penile plethysmography, use 54240)

93701   Bioimpedance-derived physiologic cardiovascular analysis

(For left ventricular filling pressure indirect measurement by computerized calibration of the arterial waveform response to Valsalva, use 93799)

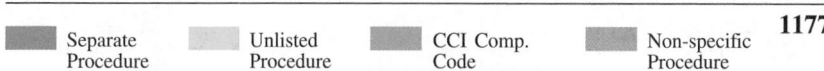

1177

| ■ Separate Procedure | ▨ Unlisted Procedure | ■ CCI Comp. Code | ■ Non-specific Procedure |

(93720   deleted 2011 [2012 edition])

(93721   deleted 2011 [2012 edition])

(93722   deleted 2011 [2012 edition])

93724   Electronic analysis of antitachycardia pacemaker system (includes electrocardiographic recording, programming of device, induction and termination of tachycardia via implanted pacemaker, and interpretation of recordings)

(93727   deleted 2009 edition. For programming of implantable loop recorder, use 93285. For interrogation of implantable loop recorder, see 93291, 93298)

(93731   deleted 2009 edition. For interrogation of dual lead pacemaker, see 93288, 93294. For programming of dual chamber pacemaker, use 93280)

(93732   deleted 2009 edition. For interrogation of dual lead pacemaker, see 93288, 93294. For programming of dual chamber pacemaker, use 93280)

(93733   deleted 2009 edition. For transtelephonic rhythm strip pacemaker, single and dual, or multiple lead pacemaker evaluatino, use 93293)

(93734   deleted 2009 edition. For interrogation of single lead pacemaker, see 93288, 93294. For programming of single lead pacemaker, use 93279)

(93735   deleted 2009 edition. For interrogation of single lead pacemaker, see 93288, 93294. For programming of single lead pacemaker, use 93279)

(93736   deleted 2009 edition. For transtelephonic rhythm strip pacemaker, single and dual, or multiple lead pacemaker evaluation, use 93293))

93740   Temperature gradient studies

(93741   deleted 2009 edition. For interrogation of single implantable cardioverter-defibrillator [ICD], see 93289, 93295. For programming of single ICD, use 93282. For interrogation of wearable cardioverter-defibrillator, use 93292)

● New Code   ▲ Revised Code   + Add-On Code   ⊘ Modifier -51 Exempt   ⊙ Moderate Sedation

(93742   deleted 2009 edition. For interrogation of single implantable cardioverter-defibrillator [ICD], see 93289, 93295. For programming of single ICD, use 93282. For interrogation of wearable cardioverter-defibrillator, use 93292)

(93743   deleted 2009 edition. For interrogation of dual implantable cardioverter-defibrillator [ICD], see 93289, 93295. For programming of dual ICD, use 93283.)

(93744   deleted 2009 edition. For interrogation of dual implantable cardioverter-defibrillator [ICD], see 93289, 93295. For programming of dual ICD, use 93283.)

▲ **93745**   Initial set-up and programming by a physician or other qualified health care professional of wearable cardioverter-defibrillator includes initial programming of system, establishing baseline electronic ECG, transmission of data to data repository, patient instruction in wearing system and patient reporting of problems or events

    (Do not report 93745 in conjunction with 93282, 93292)

▲ **93750**   Interrogation of ventricular assist device (VAD), in person, with physician or other qualified health care professional analysis of device parameters (eg, drivelines, alarms, power surges), review of device function (eg, flow and volume status, septum status, recovery), with programming, if performed, and report

    (Do not report 93750 in conjunction with 33975, 33976, 33979, 33981-33983)

(93760   deleted 2009 edition)

(93762   deleted 2009 edition)

93770   Determination of venous pressure

    (For central venous cannulization see 36555-36556, 36500)

93784   Ambulatory blood pressure monitoring, utilizing a system such as magnetic tape and/or computer disk, for 24 hours or longer; including recording, scanning analysis, interpretation and report

93786   recording only

93788   scanning analysis with report

▲ **93790**   review with interpretation and report

▨ Separate Procedure	▨ Unlisted Procedure	▨ CCI Comp. Code	▨ Non-specific Procedure	**1179**

OTHER PROCEDURES

▲ **93797**   Physician or other qualified health care professional services for outpatient cardiac rehabilitation; without continuous ECG monitoring (per session)

▲ **93798**   with continuous ECG monitoring (per session)

93799   Unlisted cardiovascular service or procedure

NON-INVASIVE VASCULAR DIAGNOSTIC STUDIES

Vascular studies refers to diagnostic procedures performed to determine blood flow and/or the condition of arteries and/or veins. Vascular studies include patient care required to perform the studies, supervision of the studies and interpretation of the study results with copies for patient records of hard copy output with analysis of all data, including bi-directional vascular flow or imaging when provided.

The use of a simple hand-held or other Doppler device that does not produce hard copy output, or that produces a record that does not permit analysis of bi-directional vascular flow, is considered to be part of the physical examination of the vascular system and is not reported separately. To report unilateral non-invasive diagnostic studies, add modifier -52 to the basic code.

Coding Rules

1.   *Non-invasive vascular studies are usually performed in addition to evaluation and management service, such as a consultation or visit, and should be reported separately in addition to the evaluation and management service.*

2.   *All of the non-invasive vascular services fall under the Medicare Purchased Diagnostic Services guidelines; therefore, reporting should be as instructed by your local Medicare carrier.*

The use of a simple hand-held or other Doppler device that does not produce hard copy output, or that produces a record that does not permit analysis of bidirectional vascular flow, is considered to be part of the physical examination of the vascular system and is not separately reported. The Ankle-Brachial Index (or ABI) is reportable with 93922 or 93923 as logn as simultaneous Doppler recording and analysis of bidirectional blood flow, volume plethysmography, or transcutaneous oxygen tension measurements are also performed.

Duplex scan (eg., 93880, 93882) describes an ultrasonic scanning procedure for characterizing the pattern and direction of blood flow in arteries or veins with the

---

1180   ● New Code   ▲ Revised Code   ＋ Add-On Code   ⊘ Modifier -51 Exempt   ⊙ Moderate Sedation

production of real-time images integrating B-mode two-dimensional vascular structure, Doppler spectral analysis and color flow Doppler imaging.

Physiologic studies: Noninvasive physiologic studies are performed using equipment separate and distinct from the duplex ultrasound imager. Codes 93922, 93923, 93924 and 93965 describe the evaluation of non-imaging physiologic recordings of pressures with Doppler analysis of bi-directional blood flow, plethysmography, and/or oxygen tension measurements appropriate for the anatomic area studied.

CEREBROVASCULAR ARTERIAL STUDIES

A complete transcranial Doppler (TCD) study (93886) includes ultrasound evaluation of the right and left anterior circulation territories and the posterior circulation territory (to include vertebral arteries and basilar artery). In a limited TCD study (93888) there is ultrasound evaluation of two or fewer of these territories. For TCD, ultrasound evaluation is a reasonable and concerted attempt to identify arterial signals through an acoustic window.

(93875   deleted 2011 [2012 edition])

93880 Duplex scan of extracranial arteries; complete bilateral study

93882   unilateral or limited study

          (To report common carotid intima-media thickness (IMT) study for evaluation of atherosclerotic burden or coronary heart disease risk factor assessment, use Category III code 0126T)

93886 Transcranial Doppler study of the intracranial arteries; complete study

93888   limited study

93890   vasoreactivity study

93892   emboli detection without intravenous microbubble injection

93893   emboli detection with intravenous microbubble injection

          (Do not report 93890-93893 in conjunction with 93888)

EXTREMITY ARTERIAL STUDIES (INCLUDING DIGITS)

93922 Limited bilateral non-invasive physiologic studies of upper or lower extremity arteries, (eg, for lower extremity: ankle/brachial

1181

Separate Procedure	Unlisted Procedure	CCI Comp. Code	Non-specific Procedure

indices at distal posterior tibial and anterior tibial/dorsalis pedis arteries plus bidirectional, Doppler waveform recording and analysis at 1-2 levels, or ankle/brachial indices at distal posterior tibial and anterior tibial/dorsalis pedis arteries plus volume plethysmography at 1-2 levels, or ankle/brachial indices at distal posterior tibial and anterior tibial/dorsalis pedis arteries with transcutaneous oxygen tension measurements at 1-2 levels)

(When only 1 arm or leg is available for study, report 93922 with modifier 52 for a unileal study when recording 1-2 levels. Report 93922 when recording 3 or more levels or performing provocative functional maneuvers.)

(Report 93922 only once in the upper extremity(s) and/or once in the lower extremity(s). When both the upper and lower extremities are evaluated in the same setting, 93922 may be reported twice by adding modifier 59 to the second procedure)

(For transcutaneous oxyhemoglobin measurement in a lower extremity wound by near infrared spectroscopy, use 0286T)

93923   Complete bilateral non-invasive physiologic studies of upper or lower extremity arteries, 3 or more levels (eg, for lower extremity: ankle/brachial indices at distal posterior tibial and anterior tibial/dorsalis pedis arteries plus segmental blood pressure measurements with bidirectional Doppler waveform recording and analysis, at 3 or more levels, or ankle/brachial indices at distal posterior tibial and anterior tibial/dorsalis pedis arteries plus segmental volume plethysmography at 3 or more levels, or ankle/brachial indices at distal posterior tibial and anterior tibial/dorsalis pedis arteries plus segmental transcutaneous oxygen tension measurements at 3 or more levels), or single level study—with provocative functional maneuvers (eg, measurements with postural provocative tests or measurements with reactive hyperemia)

(When only 1 arm or leg is available for study, report 93922 for a unilateral study when recording 3 or more levels or when performing provocative functional maneuvers.)

(Report 93923 only once in the upper extremity(s) and/or once in the lower extremity(s). When both the upper and lower extremities are evaluated in the same setting, 93923 may be reported twice by adding modifier 59 to the second procedure.)

(For transcutaneous oxyhemoglobin measurement in a lower extremity wound by near infrared spectroscopy, use 0286T)

93924   Non-invasive physiologic studies of lower extremity arteries, at rest and following treadmill stress testing, (ie, bidirectional Doppler waveform or volume plethysmography recording and

● New Code   ▲ Revised Code   + Add-On Code   ⊘ Modifier -51 Exempt   ⊙ Moderate Sedation

analysis at rest with ankle/brachial indices immediately after and at timed intervals following performance of a standardized protocol on a motorized treadmill plus recording of time of onset of claudication or other symptoms, maximal walking time, and time to recovery) complete bilateral study

(Do not report 93924 in conjunction with 93922, 93923)

93925 Duplex scan of lower extremity arteries or arterial bypass grafts; complete bilateral study

93926 unilateral or limited study

93930 Duplex scan of upper extremity arteries or arterial bypass grafts; complete bilateral study

93931 unilateral or limited study

EXTREMITY VENOUS STUDIES (INCLUDING DIGITS)

93965 Non-invasive physiologic studies of extremity veins, complete bilateral study (eg, Doppler waveform analysis with responses to compression and other maneuvers, phleborheography, impedance plethysmography)

93970 Duplex scan of extremity veins including responses to compression and other maneuvers; complete bilateral study

93971 unilateral or limited study

VISCERAL AND PENILE VASCULAR STUDIES

93975 Duplex scan of arterial inflow and venous outflow of abdominal, pelvic, scrotal contents and/or retroperitoneal organs; complete study

93976 limited study

93978 Duplex scan of aorta, inferior vena cava, iliac vasculature, or bypass grafts; complete study

93979 unilateral or limited study

93980 Duplex scan of arterial inflow and venous outflow of penile vessels; complete study

93981 follow-up or limited study

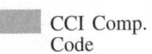

1183

Separate Procedure　Unlisted Procedure　CCI Comp. Code　Non-specific Procedure

93982 Noninvasive physiologic study of implanted wireless pressure sensor in aneurysmal sac following endovascular repair, complete study including recording, analysis of pressure and waveform tracings, interpretation and report

(Do not report 93982 in conjunction with 34806)

EXTREMITY ARTERIAL-VENOUS STUDIES

93990 Duplex scan of hemodialysis access (including arterial inflow, body of access and venous outflow)

(For measurement of hemodialysis access flow using indicator dilution methods, use 90940)

OTHER NONINVASIVE VASCULAR DIAGNOSTIC STUDIES

93998 Unlisted noninvasive vascular diagnostic study

PULMONARY

Pulmonary disease is concerned with diseases of the lungs and airways. The Pulmonologist diagnoses and treats pneumonia, cancer, pleurisy, asthma, occupational diseases, bronchitis, sleep disorders, emphysema, and other complex disorders of the lungs. Pulmonologists test lung functions in many ways, endoscope the bronchial airways and prescribe and monitor mechanical assistance to ventilation. Many pulmonary disease physicians are also expert in critical care.

Pulmonary services refer to diagnostic procedures performed to determine air flow, blood gases, and the condition of the lungs and respiratory system. Pulmonary services include the laboratory procedure(s), interpretation, and physician's services (except surgical and anesthesia services) unless otherwise stated. It is common for pulmonologists to provide interpretation services only, under contract to medical facilities.

CPT coding for pulmonary function tests includes both comprehensive and component codes to accommodate variation among pulmonary function laboratories. As a result of these code combinations, several issues are addressed in this policy section.

Alternate methods of reporting data obtained during a spirometry or other pulmonary function session cannot be separately reported. Specifically, the flow volume loop is an alternative method of calculating a standard spirometric parameter. The CPT code 94375 is included in standard spirometry (rest and exercise) studies.

● New Code   ▲ Revised Code   ＋ Add-On Code   ⊘ Modifier -51 Exempt   ⊙ Moderate Sedation

When a physician who is in attendance for a pulmonary function study, obtains a limited history, and performs a limited examination referable specifically to the pulmonary function testing, separately coding for an evaluation and management service is not appropriate. If a significant, separately identifiable service is performed unrelated to the technical performance of the pulmonary function test, an evaluation and management service may be reported.

When multiple spirometric determinations are necessary (e.g. CPT code 94070) to complete the service described in the CPT code, only one unit of service is reported.

Complex pulmonary stress testing (e.g. CPT code 94621) is a comprehensive stress test with a number of component tests separately defined in the CPT code book. It is inappropriate to separately code venous access, EKG monitoring, spirometric parameters performed before, during and after exercise, oximetry, O2 consumption, CO2 production, rebreathing cardiac output calculations, etc., when performed as part of a complex pulmonary stress test. It is also inappropriate to bill for a cardiac stress test and the component codes used to perform a simple pulmonary stress test (CPT code 94620), when a complex pulmonary stress test is performed. If using a standard exercise protocol, serial electrocardiograms are obtained, and a separate report describing a cardiac stress test (professional component) is included in the medical record, the professional components for both a cardiac and pulmonary stress test may be reported. Modifier -59 should be reported with the secondary procedure. Both tests must satisfy the requirement for medical necessity. (Since a complex pulmonary stress test includes electrocardiographic recordings, the technical components for both the cardiac stress test and the pulmonary stress test should not be reported separately.)

VENTILATOR MANAGEMENT

94002   Ventilation assist and management, initiation of pressure or volume preset ventilators for assisted or controlled breathing; hospital inpatient/observation, initial day

94003   hospital inpatient/observation, each subsequent day

94004   nursing facility, per day

(Do not report 94002-94004 in conjunction with E/M services 99201-99499)

94005   Home ventilator management care plan oversight of a patient (patient not present) in home, domiciliary or rest home (eg, assisted living) requiring review of status, review of laboratories and other studies and revision of orders and respiratory care plan (as appropriate),within a calendar month, 30 min. or more

1185

■ Separate Procedure	▨ Unlisted Procedure	■ CCI Comp. Code	■ Non-specific Procedure

(Do not report 94005 in conjunction with 99339-99340, 99374-99378)

(Ventilator management care plan oversight is reported separately from home or domiciliary, rest home [eg., assisted living] services. A physician or other qualified health care professional may report 94005, when performed, including when a different Individual reports 99339, 99340, 99374-99378 for the same 30 days)

PULMONARY DIAGNOSTIC TESTING AND THERAPIES

Codes 94010-94799 include laboratory procedure(s) and interpretation of test results. If a separate identifiable E/M service is performed, the appropriate E/M service code (including new or established patient office or other outpatient services [99201-99215], office or other outpatient consultations [99241-99245], emergency department services [99281-99285], nursing facility services [99304-99318], domiciliary, rest home or custodial care services [99324-99337] and home services [99341-99350]) may be reported in addition to 94010-94799.

Spirometry (94010) measures expiratory airflow and volumes and forms the basis of most pulmonary function testing. When spirometry is performed before and after administration of a bronchodilator, report 94060. Measurement of vital capacity (94150) is a component of spirometry and is only reported when performed alone. The flow-volume loop (94375) is used to identify patterns of inspiratory and/or expiratory obstruction in central or peripheral airways. Spirometry (94010, 94060) includes maximal breathing capacity (94200) and flow-volume loop (94375), when performed.

Measurement of lung volumes may be performed using plethysmography, helium dilution, or nitrogen washout. Plethysmyography (94726) is utilized to determine total lung capacity, residual volume, functional residual capacity, and airway resistance. Nitrogen washout or heliu dilution (94727) may be used to measure lung volumes, distribution of ventilation and closing volume. Impulse oscillometry (94728) assesses airway resistance and may be reported in addition to gas dilution techniques. Spirometry (94010, 94060) and bronchial provocation (94070) are not included in 94726 and 94727 and may be reported separately.

Diffusing capacity (94729) is most commonly performed in conjunction with lung volumes or spirometry and is an add-on code to 94726-94728, 94010, 94060, 94070, and 94375.

Pulmonary function tests (94011-94013) are reported for measurements in infants and young children though 2 years of age.

Pulmonary function testing measurements are reported as actual values and as a percent of predicted values by age, gender, height and race.

94010 Spirometry, including graphic record, total and timed vital capacity, expiratory flow rate measurement(s), with or without maximal voluntary ventilation

(Do not report 94010 in conjunction with 94150, 94200, 94375, 94728)

94011 Measurement of spirometric forced expiratory flows in an infant or child through 2 years of age

94012 Measurement of spirometric forced expiratory flows, before and after bronchodilator, in an infant or child through 2 years of age

94013 Measurement of lung volumes (ie, functional residual capacity [FRC], forced vital capacity [FVC], and expiratory reserve volume [ERV]) in an infant or child through 2 years of age

▲ **94014** Patient-initiated spirometric recording per 30-day period of time; includes reinforced education, transmission of spirometric tracing, data capture, analysis of transmitted data, periodic recalibration, and review and interpretation by a physician or other qualified health care professional

94015 recording (includes hook-up, reinforced education, data transmission, data capture, trend analysis, and periodic recalibration)

▲ **94016** review and interpretation only by a physician or other qualified health care professional

94060 Bronchodilation responsiveness, spirometry as in 94010, pre- and post-bronchodilator administration

(Do not report 94060 in conjunction with 94150, 94200, 94375, 94728)

(Report bronchodilator supply separately with 99070 or appropriate supply code)

(For prolonged exercise test for bronchospasm with pre- and post-spirometry, use 94620)

94070 Bronchospasm provocation evaluation, multiple spirometric determinations as in 94010, with administered agents (eg, antigen(s), cold air, methacholine)

(Report antigen(s) administration separately with 99070 or appropriate supply code)

1187

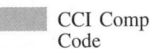 Separate Procedure   Unlisted Procedure   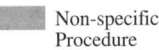 CCI Comp. Code   Non-specific Procedure

94150   Vital capacity, total (separate procedure)

(Do not report 94150 in conjunction with 94010, 94060, 94728. To report thoracic gas volumes, see 94726, 94727)

94200   Maximum breathing capacity, maximal voluntary ventilation

(Do not report 94200 in conjunction with 94010, 94060)

(94240   deleted 2011 [2012 edition]. To report thoracic gas volumes, see 94726, 94727)

94250   Expired gas collection, quantitative, single procedure (separate procedure)

(94260   deleted 2011 [2012 edition]. To report thoracic gas volumes, see 94726, 94727)

(94350   deleted 2011 [2012 edition]. To report, use 94727)

(94360   deleted 2011 [2012 edition]. To report, see 94726, 94728)

(94370   deleted 2011 [2012 edition]. To report, see 94726, 94727)

94375   Respiratory flow volume loop

(Do not report 94375 in conjunction with 94010, 94060)

94400   Breathing response to CO2 (CO2 response curve)

94450   Breathing response to hypoxia (hypoxia response curve)

(For high altitude simulation test (HAST), see 94452, 94453)

▲ **94452**   High altitude simulation test (HAST), with interpretation and report by a physician or other qualified health care professional;

(For obtaining arterial blood gases, use 36600)

(Do not report 94452 in conjunction with 94453, 94760, 94761)

▲ **94453**   with supplemental oxygen titration

(For obtaining arterial blood gases, use 36600)

(Do not report 94453 in conjunction with 94452, 94760, 94761)

⊘▲**94610**   Intrapulmonary surfactant administration by a physician or other qualified health care professional through endotracheal tube

1188 ● New Code   ▲ Revised Code   + Add-On Code   ⊘ Modifier -51 Exempt   ⊙ Moderate Sedation

(Do not report 94610 in conjunction with 99468-99472)

(For endotracheal intubation, use 31500)

(Report 94610 once per dosing episode)

94620 Pulmonary stress testing; simple (eg, 6-minute walk, prolonged exercise test for bronchospasm with pre- and post-spirometry and oximetry)

94621 complex (including measurements of CO2 production, O2 uptake, and electrocardiographic recordings)

94640 Pressurized or nonpressurized inhalation treatment for acute airway obstruction or for sputum induction for diagnostic purposes (eg., with an aerosol generator, nebulizer, metered dose inhaler or intermittent positive pressure breathing (IPPB) device)

(For more than one inhalation treatment performed on the same date, append modifier -76)

(For continuous inhalation treatment of 1 hour or more, see 94644, 94645)

94642 Aerosol inhalation of pentamidine for pneumocystis carinii pneumonia treatment or prophylaxis

94644 Continuous inhalation treatment with aerosol medication for acute airway obstruction; first hour

(For services of less than 1 hour, use 94640)

+ 94645 each additional hour (List separately in addition to code for primary procedure)

(Use 94645 in conjunction with 94644)

94660 Continuous positive airway pressure ventilation (CPAP), initiation and management

94662 Continuous negative pressure ventilation (CNP), initiation and management

94664 Demonstration and/or evaluation of patient utilization of an aerosol generator, nebulizer, metered dose inhaler or IPPB device

(94664 can be reported one time only per day of service)

1189

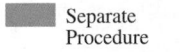 Separate Procedure   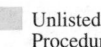 Unlisted Procedure   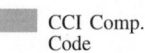 CCI Comp. Code   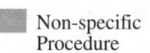 Non-specific Procedure

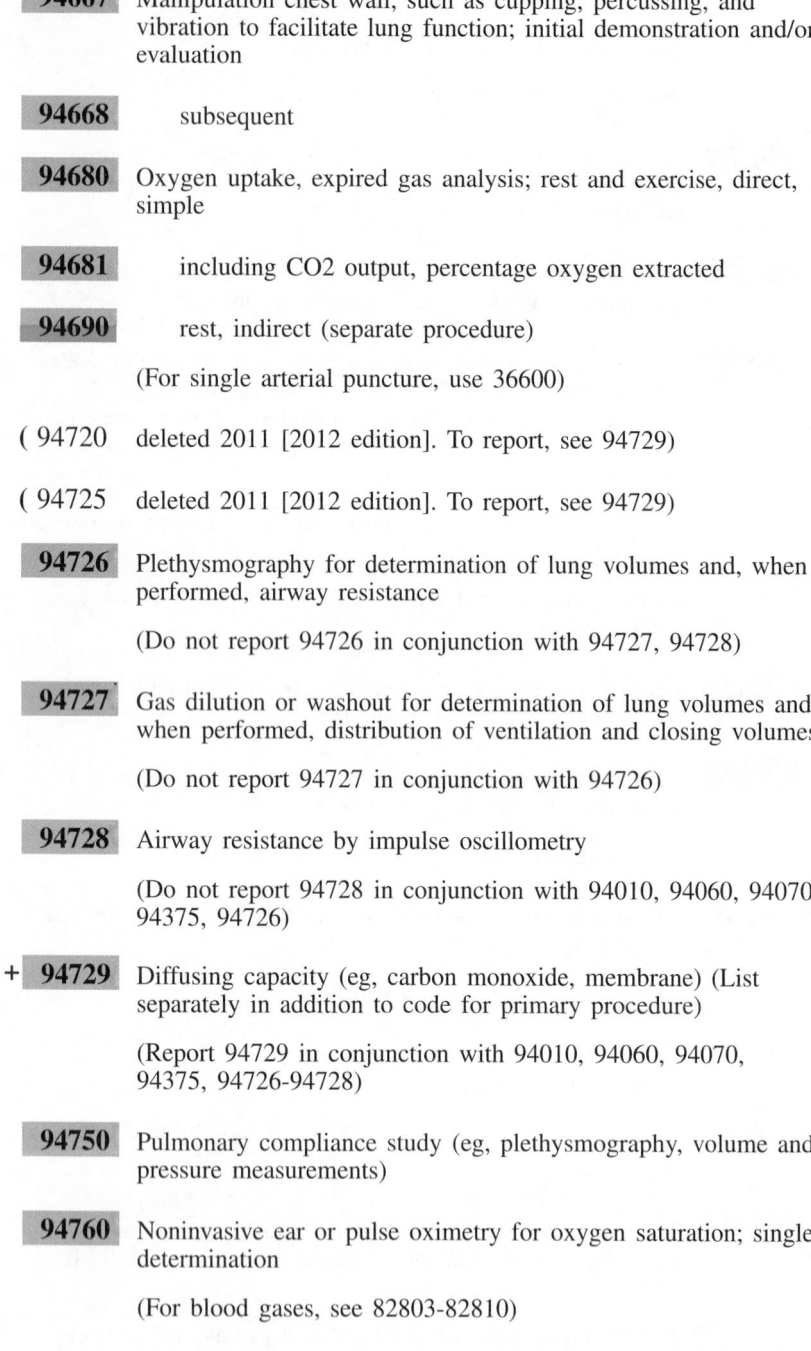

94667   Manipulation chest wall, such as cupping, percussing, and vibration to facilitate lung function; initial demonstration and/or evaluation

94668   subsequent

94680   Oxygen uptake, expired gas analysis; rest and exercise, direct, simple

94681   including CO2 output, percentage oxygen extracted

94690   rest, indirect (separate procedure)

(For single arterial puncture, use 36600)

(94720   deleted 2011 [2012 edition]. To report, see 94729)

(94725   deleted 2011 [2012 edition]. To report, see 94729)

94726   Plethysmography for determination of lung volumes and, when performed, airway resistance

(Do not report 94726 in conjunction with 94727, 94728)

94727   Gas dilution or washout for determination of lung volumes and, when performed, distribution of ventilation and closing volumes

(Do not report 94727 in conjunction with 94726)

94728   Airway resistance by impulse oscillometry

(Do not report 94728 in conjunction with 94010, 94060, 94070, 94375, 94726)

+ **94729**   Diffusing capacity (eg, carbon monoxide, membrane) (List separately in addition to code for primary procedure)

(Report 94729 in conjunction with 94010, 94060, 94070, 94375, 94726-94728)

94750   Pulmonary compliance study (eg, plethysmography, volume and pressure measurements)

94760   Noninvasive ear or pulse oximetry for oxygen saturation; single determination

(For blood gases, see 82803-82810)

● New Code   ▲ Revised Code   ✛ Add-On Code   ⊘ Modifier -51 Exempt   ⊙ Moderate Sedation

94761   multiple determinations (eg, during exercise)

94762   by continuous overnight monitoring (separate procedure)

(For other in vivo laboratory procedures, see 88720-88741)

94770   Carbon dioxide, expired gas determination by infrared analyzer

(For bronchoscopy, see 31622-31646)

(For placement of flow directed catheter, use 93503)

(For venipuncture, use 36410)

(For central venous catheter placement, see 36555-36556)

(For arterial puncture, use 36600)

(For arterial catheterization, use 36620)

(For thoracentesis, use 32554, 32555)

(For phlebotomy, therapeutic, use 99195)

(For lung biopsy, needle, use 32405)

(For intubation, orotracheal or nasotracheal, use 31500)

94772   Circadian respiratory pattern recording (pediatric pneumogram), 12 to 24 hour continuous recording, infant

(Separate procedure codes for electromyograms, EEG, ECG, and recordings of respiration are excluded when 94772 is reported)

▲ **94774**   Pediatric home apnea monitoring event recording including respiratory rate, pattern and heart rate per 30-day period of time; includes monitor attachment, download of data, review, interpretation, and preparation of a report by a physician or other qualified health care professional

(Do not report 94774 in conjunction with 94775-94777 during the same reporting period)

94775   monitor attachment only (includes hook-up, initiation of recording and disconnection)

94776   monitoring, download of information, receipt of transmission(s) and analyses by computer only

▮ Separate Procedure	▮ Unlisted Procedure	▮ CCI Comp. Code	▮ Non-specific Procedure

▲ 94777   review, interpretation and preparation of report only by a physician or other qualified health care professional

(When oxygen saturation monitoring is used in addition to heart rate and respiratory monitoring, it is not reported separately)

(Do not report 94774-94777 in conjunction with 93224-93272)

(Do not report apnea recording device separately)

(For sleep study, see 95805-95811)

94780   Car seat/bed testin for airway integrity, neonate, with continual nursing observation and continuous recording of pulse oximetry, heart rate and respiratory rate, with interpretation and report; 60 minutes

(Do not report 94780 for less than 60 minutes)

(Do not report 94780 in conjunction with 93040-93042, 94760, 94761, 99468-99472, 99477-99480)

+ 94781   each additional full 30 minutes (List separately in addition to code for primary procedure)

(Use 94781 in conjunction with 94780)

94799   Unlisted pulmonary service or procedure

ALLERGY AND CLINICAL IMMUNOLOGY

Allergy and Immunology refers to diagnostic services performed to determine a patient's sensitivity to specific substances, the treatment of patients with allergens by the administration or allergenic extracts, and/or medical conference services.

The CPT coding system divides allergy and clinical immunology into testing and immunotherapy. Immunotherapy is divided into codes that include preparation of the antigen when it is administered at the same session and when it is prepared but delivered for immunotherapy by a different physician. Several specific issues are identified regarding allergy testing and immunotherapy.

If percutaneous or intracutaneous (intradermal)single test (CPT codes 95004 or 95024) and "sequential and incremental" tests (CPT codes 95010, 95015, or 95027) are performed on the same date of service, both the "sequential and incremental" test and single test codes may be reported if the tests are for different allergens or different dilutions of the same allergen. The unit of service to report is the number of separate tests. Do not report both a single test and a sequential and incremental test for the same dilution of an allergen. For example, if the single test for an antigen is positive and the provider proceeds to sequential and incremental

| ● New Code | ▲ Revised Code | + Add-On Code | ⊘ Modifier -51 Exempt | ⊙ Moderate Sedation |

tests with three additional different dilutions of the same antigen, the provider may report one unit of service for the single test code and three units of service for the sequential and incremental test code.

When photo patch tests (e.g. CPT code 95052) are performed (same antigen/same session) with patch or application tests, only the photo patch testing should be reported. Additionally, if photo testing is performed including application or patch testing, the code for photo patch testing (CPT code 95052) is to be reported, not CPT code 95044 (patch or application tests) and CPT code 95056 (photo tests).

Evaluation and management codes reported with allergy testing or allergy immunotherapy are appropriate only if a significant, separately identifiable service is administered. Obtaining informed consent, is included in the immunotherapy. If E & M services are reported, medical documentation of the separately identifiable service should be in the medical record.

Allergy testing is not performed on the same day as allergy immunotherapy in standard medical practice. These codes should, therefore, not be reported together. Additionally, the testing becomes an integral part to rapid desensitization kits (CPT code 95180) and would therefore not be reported separately.

Do not report Evaluation and Management (E/M) services for test interpretation and report.

If a significant separately identifiable E/M service is performed, the appropriate E/M service code should be reported using modifier -25.

ALLERGY TESTING

(For allergy laboratory tests, see 86000-86999)

(For administration of medications [eg, epinephrine, steroidal agents, antihistamines] for therapy for severe or intractable allergic reaction, use 96372)

▲ **95004** Percutaneous tests (scratch, puncture, prick) with allergenic extracts, immediate type reaction, including test interpretation and report, specify number of tests

(95010 deleted 2012 [2013 edition]. To report, see 95017 and 95018)

95012 Nitric oxide expired gas determination

(95015 deleted 2012 [2013 edition]. To report, see 95017 and 95018)

● **95017** Allergy testing, any combination of percutaneous (scratch, puncture, prick) and intracutaneous (intradermal), sequential and

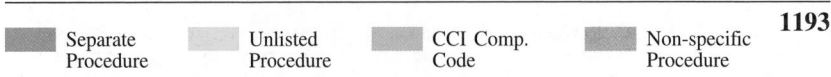

1193

	Separate Procedure		Unlisted Procedure		CCI Comp. Code		Non-specific Procedure

incremental, with venoms, immediate type reaction, including test interpretation and report, specify number of tests

● 95018　Allergy testing, any combination of percutaneous (scratch, puncture, prick) and intracutaneous (intradermal), sequential and incremental, with drugs or biologicals, immediate type reaction, including test interpretation and report, specify number of tests

▲ 95024　Intracutaneous (intradermal) tests with allergenic extracts, immediate type reaction, including test interpretation and report, specify number of tests

▲ 95027　Intracutaneous (intradermal) tests, sequential and incremental, with allergenic extracts for airborne allergens, immediate type reaction, including test interpretation and report, specify number of tests

95028　Intracutaneous (intradermal) tests with allergenic extracts, delayed type reaction, including reading, specify number of tests

95044　Patch or application test(s) (specify number of tests)

95052　Photo patch test(s) (specify number of tests)

95056　Photo tests

95060　Ophthalmic mucous membrane tests

95065　Direct nasal mucous membrane test

95070　Inhalation bronchial challenge testing (not including necessary pulmonary function tests); with histamine, methacholine, or similar compounds

95071　with antigens or gases, specify

(For pulmonary function tests, see 94060, 94070)

(95075　deleted 2012 [2013 edition]. For ingestion challenge testing, see 95076, 95079)

INGESTION CHALLENGE TESTING

Codes 95076 and 95079 re used to report ingestion challenge testing. Report 95076 for initial 120 minutes of testing time (ie, not physician face-to-face time). Report 95079 for each additional 60 minutes of testing time (ie, not physician

　● New Code　▲ Revised Code　+ Add-On Code　⊘ Modifier -51 Exempt　⊙ Moderate Sedation

face-to-face time). For total testing time less than 61 minutes (eg, positive challenge resulting in cessation of testing), report and evaluation and management service, if appropriate. Patient assessment/monitoring activities for allergic reactin (eg, blood pressure testing, peak flow meter testing) are not separately reported. Intervention therapy (eg, injection of steroid or epinephrine) may be reported separately as appropriate.

For purposes of reporting testing times, if an E/M service is required, then testing time ends.

- **95076**   Ingestion challenge test (sequential and incremental ingestion of test items, eg. food, drug or other substance); initial 120 minutes of testing

- **+95079**   each additional 60 minutes of testing (List separately in addition to code for primary procedure

    (Use 95079 in conjunction with 95076)

ALLERGEN IMMUNOTHERAPY

Allergen immunotherapy CPT codes include the professional services necessary for allergen immunotherapy. Evaluation and management service codes may be reported in addition to allergen immunotherapy if other identifiable services are provided at the same time.

Codes 95115-95199 include the professional services necessary for allergen immunotherapy. Office visit codes may be used in addition to allergen immunotherapy if other identifiable services are provided at that time.

95115   Professional services for allergen immunotherapy not including provision of allergenic extracts; single injection

95117   2 or more injections

▲ **95120**   Professional services for allergen immunotherapy in the office or institution of the prescribing physician or other qualified health care professional, including provision of allergenic extract; single injection

▲ **95125**   2 or more injections

▲ **95130**   single stinging insect venom

▲ **95131**   2 stinging insect venoms

▲ **95132**   3 stinging insect venoms

1195

	Separate Procedure		Unlisted Procedure		CCI Comp. Code		Non-specific Procedure

▲ **95133**   4 stinging insect venoms

▲ **95134**   5 stinging insect venoms

95144 Professional services for the supervision of preparation and provision of antigens for allergen immunotherapy; single dose vials(s) (specify number of vials)

(A single dose vial contains a single dose of antigen administered in one injection)

95145 Professional services for the supervision of preparation and provision of antigens for allergen immunotherapy (specify number of doses); single stinging insect venom

95146 2 single stinging insect venoms

95147 3 single stinging insect venoms

95148 4 single stinging insect venoms

95149 5 single stinging insect venoms

95165 Professional services for the supervision of preparation and provision of antigens for allergen immunotherapy; single or multiple antigens (specify number of doses)

95170 whole body extract of biting insect or other arthropod (specify number of doses)

(For allergy immunotherapy reporting, a dose is the amount of antigen(s) administered in a single injection from a multiple dose vial)

95180 Rapid desensitization procedure, each hour (eg, insulin, penicillin, equine serum)

95199 Unlisted allergy/clinical immunologic service or procedure

(For skin testing of bacterial, viral, fungal extracts, see 86485-86580, 95028)

(For special reports on allergy patients, use 99080)

(For testing procedures such as radioallergosorbent testing (RAST), rat mast cell technique (RMCT), mast cell degranulation test (MCDT), lymphocytic transformation test (LTT), leukocyte histamine release (LHR), migration inhibitory factor test (MIF), transfer factor test (TFT), nitroblue

1196 ● New Code   ▲ Revised Code   ✛ Add-On Code   ⊘ Modifier -51 Exempt   ⊙ Moderate Sedation

tetrazolium dye test (NTD), see Immunology section in
Pathology or use 95199)

ENDOCRINOLOGY

95250 Ambulatory continuous glucose monitoring of interstitial tissue
fluid via a subcutaneous sensor for a minimum of 72 hours;
sensor placement, hook-up, calibration of monitor, patient
training, removal of sensor, and printout of recording

(Do not report 95250 more than once per month)

(Do not report 95250 in conjunction with 99091)

95251 interpretation and report

(Do not report 95251 more than once per month)

(Do not report 95251 in conjunction with 99091)

NEUROLOGY AND NEUROMUSCULAR PROCEDURES

*Neurology refers to the study and treatment of the nervous system. Neurology
services are usually performed in conjunction with a medical consultation. The
consultation should be reported separately using the appropriate evaluation and
management consultation code.*

*Neurologic services are typically consultative, and any of the levels of consultation
(99241-99255) may be appropriate.*

*The EEG, autonomic function, evoked potential, reflex tests, EMG, NCV, and MEG
services (95812-95829 and 95860-95967) include recording, interpretation by a
physician, and report. For interpretation only, use modifier 26. For EMG guidance,
see 95873, 95874.*

*The CPT coding system defines codes for neuromuscular diagnostic or therapeutic
services not requiring surgical procedures. Sleep testing, nerve and muscle testing
and electroencephalographic procedures are included. The CPT code book
guidelines regarding sleep testing are very precise and should be reviewed
carefully before billing for these services.*

*Sleep testing differs from polysomnography in that the latter requires the presence
of sleep staging. Sleep staging includes a qualitative and quantitative assessment of
sleep as determined by standard sleep scoring techniques. Accordingly, at the same
session, a "sleep study" and "polysomnography" are not reported together.*

1197

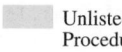 Separate Procedure 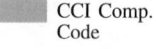 Unlisted Procedure 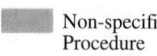 CCI Comp. Code Non-specific Procedure

Polysomnography requires at least one central and usually several other EEG electrodes. EEG procurement for polysomnography (sleep staging) differs greatly from that required for diagnostic EEG testing (i.e. speed of paper, number of channels, etc.). Accordingly, EEG testing is not to be reported with polysomnography unless performed separately; the EEG tests, if rendered with a separate report, are to be reported with modifier -59, indicating that this represents a different session from the sleep study.

Continuous electroencephalographic monitoring services (CPT codes 95950-95962) represent different services than those provided during sleep testing; accordingly these codes are only to be reported when a separately identifiable service is performed and documented. Additionally, billing standard EEG services would only be appropriate if a significant, separately identifiable service is provided. These codes are to be reported with modifier -59 to indicate that a different service is clearly documented.

When nerve testing (EMG, nerve conduction velocity, etc.) is performed to assess the level of paralysis during anesthesia or during mechanical ventilation, the series of CPT codes 95851-95937 are not to be separately reported; these codes reflect significant, separately identifiable diagnostic services requiring a formal report in the medical record. Additionally, electrical stimulation used to identify or locate nerves as part of a procedure involving treatment of a cranial or peripheral nerve (e.g. nerve block, nerve destruction, neuroplasty, transection, excision, repair, etc.) is part of the primary procedure.

Intraoperative neurophysiology testing (CPT code 95920) should not be reported by the physician performing an operative procedure since it is included in the global package. However, when performed by a different physician during the procedure, it is separately reportable by the second physician. The physician performing an operative procedure should not bill other 90000 neurophysiology testing codes for intraoperative neurophysiology testing since they are also included in the global package.

The NCCI edit with column one CPT code 95903 (Motor nerve conduction studies with F-wave study, each nerve) and column two CPT code 95900 (Motor nerve conduction studies without F-wave study, each nerve) is often bypassed by utilizing modifier -59. Use of modifier -59 with the column two CPT code 95900 of this NCCI edit is only appropriate if the two procedures are performed on different nerves or in separate patient encounters.

Neurologic services are typically consultative, and any of the levels of consultation (99241-99255) may be appropriate. In addition, services and skills outlined under Evaluation and Management levels of service appropriate to neurologic illnesses should be reported similarly.

The EEG, autonomic function, evoked potential, reflex tests, EMG, NCV, and MEG services (95812-95829 and 95860-95967) include recording, interpretation

---

1198   ● New Code   ▲ Revised Code   + Add-On Code   ⊘ Modifier -51 Exempt   ⊙ Moderate Sedation

and report by a physician or other qualified health care professional. For interpretation only, use modifier 26. For EMG guidelines, see 95873, 95874.

Codes 95812-95822, 95950-95953 and 95956 use recording time as a basis for code use. Recording time is when the recording is underway and data is being collected. Recording time excludes set up and take down time. Codes 95961-95962 use physician or other qualified health care professional attendance time as a basis for code use.

(Do not report codes 95860-95875 in addition to 96000-96004)

SLEEP MEDICINE TESTING

Polysomnography includes sleep staging that is refined to include a 1-4 lead electroencephalogram (EEG), an electro-oculogram (EOG), and a submental electromyogram (EMG). For a study to be reported as polysomnography, sleep must be recorded and staged. Additional parameters of sleep include:

> *Electrocardiogram (ECG)*

> *airflow*

> *ventilation and respiratory effort*

> *gas exchange by oximetry, transcutaneous monitoring, or end tidal gas analysis*

> *extremity muscle activity, motor activity-movement*

> *extended EEG monitoring*

> *penile tumescence*

> *gastroesophageal reflux*

> *continuous blood pressure monitoring*

> *snoring*

> *body positions, etc.*

For a study to be reported as a polysomnogram:

> *studies must be performed for 6 hours*

> *sleep must be recorded and staged*

> *an attendant must be present throughout the course of the study*

1199

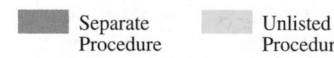 Separate Procedure

 Unlisted Procedure

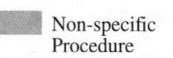 CCI Comp. Code

Non-specific Procedure

Diagnostic testing is covered when a patient has the symptoms or complaints of one of the following conditions:

Narcolepsy - Narcolepsy is a neurologic disorder of unknown etiology characterized predominantly by abnormalities of REM, some abnormalities of NREM sleep and the presence of excessive daytime sleepiness often with involuntary daytime sleep episodes (e.g., while driving, in the middle of a meal, amnesiac episodes).

Sleep Apnea - Sleep Apnea is defined as a cessation of airflow for at least 10 seconds. These cessations of breathing may be due to either an occlusion of the airway (obstructive sleep apnea), absence of respiratory effort (central sleep apnea), or a combination of these factors (mixed sleep apnea).

Parasomnias - Parasomnias are a group of behavioral disorders during sleep that are associated with brief or partial arousals but not with marked sleep disruption or impaired daytime alertness. The presenting complaint is usually related to the behavior itself.

All sleep services (95800-95811) include recording, interpretation and report. (Report with modifier 52 if less than 6 hours of recording for 95800, 95801 and 95806, 95807, 95810, 95811; if less than 7 hours of recording for 95782, 95783, or if less than 4 nap opportunities are recorded for 95805).

(Report with modifier 52 if less than 6 hours of recording or in other cases of reduced services as appropriate)

(For unattended sleep study, use 95806)

95782 This code is out of order. See page 1201

95783 This code is out of order. See page 1202

95800 This code is out of order. See page 1201

95801 This code is out of order. See page 1201

95803 Actigraphy testing, recording, analysis, interpretation, and report (minimum of 72 hours to 14 consecutive days of recording)

(Do not report 95803 more than once in any 14 day period)

(Do not report 95803 in conjunction with 95806-95811)

95805 Multiple sleep latency or maintenance of wakefulness testing, recording, analysis and interpretation of physiological measurements of sleep during multiple trials to assess sleepiness

● New Code ▲ Revised Code + Add-On Code ⊘ Modifier -51 Exempt ⊙ Moderate Sedation

95806 Sleep study, unattended, simultaneous recording of heart rate, oxygen saturation, respiratory airflow and respiratory effort (eg, thoracoabdominal movement)

(Do not report 95806 in conjunction with 93041-93227, 93228, 93229, 93268-93272, 95800, 95801)

(For unattended sleep study that measures heart rate, oxygen saturation, respiratory analysis, and sleep time, use 95800)

(For unattended sleep study that measures a minimum heart rate, oxygen saturation, and respiratory analysis, use 95801)

95800 Sleep study, unattended, simultaneous recording; heart rate, oxygen saturation, respiratory analysis (eg, by airflow or peripheral arterial tone), and sleep time

(Do not report 95800 in conjunction with 93041-93227, 93228, 93229, 93268-93272, 95803, 95806, 95801)

(For unattended sleep study that measures a minimum of heart rate, oxygen saturation, and respiratory analysis, use 95801)

95801 minimum of heart rate, oxygen saturation, and respiratory analysis (eg, by airflow or peripheral arterial tone)

(Do not report 95801 in conjunction with 93041-93227, 93228, 93229, 93268-93272, 95806, 95800)

(For unattended sleep study that measures heart rate, oxygen saturation, respiratory analysis, and sleep time, use 95800)

95807 Sleep study, simultaneous recording of ventilation, respiratory effort, ECG or heart rate, and oxygen saturation, attended by a technologist

▲ **95808** Polysomnography; any age, sleep staging with 1-3 additional parameters of sleep, attended by a technologist

▲ **95810** age 6 years or older, sleep staging with 4 or more additional parameters of sleep, attended by a technologist

▲ **95811** age 6 years or older, sleep staging with 4 or more additional parameters of sleep, with initiation of continuous positive airway pressure therapy or bilevel ventilation, attended by a technologist

● **95782** younger than 6 years, sleep staging with 4 or more additional parameters of sleep, attended by a technolgist

---

1201

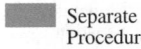 Separate Procedure 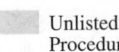 Unlisted Procedure 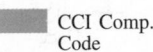 CCI Comp. Code 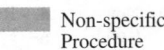 Non-specific Procedure

● **95783**   younger than 6 years, sleep staging with 4 or more additional parameters of sleep, with initiation of continuous positive airway pressure therapy or bi-level ventilation, attended by a technologist

ROUTINE ELECTROENCEPHALOGRAPHY (EEG)

EEG codes 95812-95822 include hyperventilation and/or photic stimulation when appropriate. Routine EEG codes 95816-95822 include 20 to 40 minutes of recording. Extended EEG codes 95812-95813 include reporting times longer than 40 minutes.

95812   Electroencephalogram (EEG) extended monitoring; 41-60 minutes

95813   greater than 1 hour

95816   Electroencephalogram (EEG) including recording awake and drowsy

95819   including recording awake and asleep

95822   recording in coma or sleep only

95824   cerebral death evaluation only

95827   all night recording

(For 24-hour EEG monitoring, see 95950-95953 or 95956)

(For EEG during nonintracranial surgery, use 95955)

(For Wada test, use 95958)

(For digital analysis of EEG, use 95957)

95829   Electrocorticogram at surgery (separate procedure)

▲ **95830**   Insertion by physician or other qualified health care professional of sphenoidal electrodes for electroencephalographic (EEG) recording

MUSCLE AND RANGE OF MOTION TESTING

95831   Muscle testing, manual (separate procedure) with report; extremity (excluding hand) or trunk

95832   hand, with or without comparison with normal side

● New Code   ▲ Revised Code   + Add-On Code   ⊘ Modifier -51 Exempt   ⊙ Moderate Sedation

95833   total evaluation of body, excluding hands

95834   total evaluation of body, including hands

95851   Range of motion measurements and report (separate procedure); each extremity (excluding hand) or each trunk section (spine)

95852   hand, with or without comparison with normal side

95857   Cholinesterase inhibitor challenge test for myasthenia gravis

ELECTROMYOGRAPHY

Needle electromyographic (EMG) procedures include the interpretation of electrical waveforms measured by equipment that produces both visible and audible components of electrical signals recorded from the muscle(s) studied by the needle electrode.

Use 95870 or 95885 when four or fewer muscles are tested in an extremity. Use 95860-95864 or 95886 when five or more muscles are tested in an extremity.

Use EMG codes (95860-95864 and 95867-95870) when no nerve conduction studies (95907-95913) are performed on that day. Use 95885, 95886 and 95887 for EMG services when nerve conduction studies (95907-95913) are performed in conjunction with EMG on the same day.

Report either 95885 or 95886 once per extremity. Codes 95885 and 95886 can be reported together up to a combined total of four units of service per patient when all four extremities are tested.

95860   Needle electromyography; 1 extremity with or without related paraspinal areas

95861   2 extremities with or without related paraspinal areas

(For dynamic electromyography performed during motion analysis studies, see 96002-96003)

95863   3 extremities with or without related paraspinal areas

95864   4 extremities with or without related paraspinal areas

95865   larynx

(Do not report modifier 50 in conjunction with 95865)

(For unilateral procedure, report modifier 52 in conjunction with 95865)

1203

Separate Procedure   Unlisted Procedure   CCI Comp. Code   Non-specific Procedure

95866   hemidiaphragm

95867   cranial nerve supplied muscle(s), unilateral

95868   cranial nerve supplied muscles, bilateral

95869   thoracic paraspinal muscles (excluding T1 or T12

95870   limited study of muscles in 1 extremity or non-limb (axial) muscles (unilateral or bilateral), other than thoracic paraspinal, cranial nerve supplied muscles, or sphincters

(To report a complete study of the extremities, see 95860-95864)

(For anal or urethral sphincter, detrusor, urethra, perineum musculature, see 51785-51792)

(For eye muscles, use 92265)

95872   Needle electromyography using single fiber electrode, with quantitative measurement of jitter, blocking and/or fiber density, any/all sites of each muscle studied

+ 95885   Needle electromyography, each extremity, with related paraspinal areas, when performed, done with nerve conduction, amplitude and latency/velocity study; limited (List separately in addition to code for primary procedure)

+ 95886   complete, five or muscles studied, innervated by three or more nerves or four or more spinal levels (List separately in addition to code for primary procedure)

(Use 95885, 95886 in conjunction with 95907-95913)

(Do not report 95885, 95886 in conjunction with 95860-95864, 95870, 95905)

+ 95887   Needle electromyography, non-extremity (cranial nerve supplied or axial) muscle(s) done with nerve conduction, amplitude and latency/velocity study (List separately in addition to code for primary procedure)

(Use 95887 in conjunction with 95907-95913)

(Do not report 95887 in conjunction with 95867-95870, 95905)

● New Code   ▲ Revised Code   + Add-On Code   ⊘ Modifier -51 Exempt   ⊙ Moderate Sedation

GUIDANCE FOR CHEMODENERVATION AND ISCHEMIC MUSCLE TESTING

+ 95873 Electrical stimulation for guidance in conjunction with chemodenervation (List separately in addition to code for primary procedure)

+ 95874 Needle electromyography for guidance in conjunction with chemodenervation (List separately in addition to code for primary procedure)

(Use 95873, 95874 in conjunction with 64612-64614)

(Do not report 95874 in conjunction with 95873)

(Do not report 95873, 95874 in conjunction with 95860-95870)

95875 Ischemic limb exercise test with serial specimen(s) acquisition for muscle(s) metabolite(s)

95885 Code out of order. See page 1204

95886 Code out of order. See page 1204

95887 Code out of order. See page 1204

NERVE CONDUCTION TESTS

Codes 95907-95913 describe nerve conduction tests when performed with individually placed stimulating, recording, and ground electrodes.

For the purposes of coding, a single conduction study is defined as a sensory conduction test, a motor conduction test with or without a F wave test, or an H-reflex test. Each type of study (sensory, motor with or without F wave, or H-reflex) for each nerve includes all orthodromic and antidromic impulses associated with that nerve and constitutes a distinct study when determining the number of studies in each grouping (eg. 1-2 or 3-4 nerve conduction studies). Each type of nerve conduction study is counted only once when multiple sites on the same nerve are stimulated or recorded. The numbers of these separate tests should be added to determine which code to use. Use 95885-95887 in conjunction with 95907-95913 when performing eletromyography with nerve conduction studies.

Code 95905 describes nerve conduction tests when performed with preconfigured electrodes customized to a specific anatomic site.

(95900 deleted 2012 [2013 edition]. For nerve conduction studies, see 95907-95913)

Separate Procedure	Unlisted Procedure	CCI Comp. Code	Non-specific Procedure

(95903   deleted 2012 [2013 edition]. For nerve conduction studies, see
          95907-95913)

(95904   deleted 2012 [2013 edition]. For nerve conduction studies, see
          95907-95913)

⊘ **95905**   Motor and/or sensory nerve conduction, using preconfigured
             electrode array(s), amplitude and latency/velocity study, each
             limb, includes F wave study when performed, with
             interpretation and report

             (Report 95905 only once per limb studied)

             (Do not report 95905 in conjunction with 95885, 95886,
             95907-95913)

● **95907**   Nerve conduction studies; 1-2 studies

● **95908**   3-4 studies

● **95909**   5-6 studies

● **95910**   7-8 studies

● **95911**   9-10 studies

● **95912**   11-12 studies

● **95913**   13 or more studies

INTRAOPERATIVE NEUROPHYSIOLOGY

Codes 95940, 95941 describe ongoing neurophysiologic monitoring, testing, and
data interpretation distinct from performance of specific type(s) of baseline
neurophysiologic study(s) performed during surgical procedures. When the service
is performed by a surgeon or anesthesiologist, the professional services are
included in the surgeon's or anesthesiologist's primary service code(s) for the
procedure and are not reported separately. Do not report these codes for automated
monitoring devices that do not require continuous attendance by a professional
qualified to interpret the testing and monitoring.

Recording and testing are performed either personally or by a technologist who is
physically present with the patient during the service. Supervision is performed
either in the operating room or by real time connection outside the operating room.
The monitoring professional must be solely dedicated to performing the
intraoperative neurophysiologic monitoring and must be available to intervene at
all times during the service as necessary, for the reported time period(s). For any
given period of time spent providing these services, the service takes full attention

● New Code   ▲ Revised Code   + Add-On Code   ⊘ Modifier -51 Exempt   ⊙ Moderate Sedation

and therefore other clinical activities beyond providing and interpreting of monitoring cannot be provided during the same period.

Throughout the monitoring, there must be provisions for continuous and immediate communication directly with the operating room team in the surgical suite. One or more simultaneous cases may be reported (95941). When monitoring more than one procedure, there must be the immediate ability to transfer patient monitoring to another monitoring professional during the surgical procedure should that individual's exclusive attention be required for another procedure. Report 95941 for all remote or non-one-on-one monitoring time connected to each case regardless of overlap with other cases.

Codes 95940, 95941 include only the ongoing neurophysiologic monitoring time distinct from performance of specific type(s) of baseline neurophysiologic study(s) or other services such as intraoperative functional cortical or subcortical mapping. Codes 95940 and 95941 are reported based upon the time spent monitoring only and not the number of baseline tests performed or parameters monitored. The time spent performing or interpreting the baseline neurophysiologic study(ies) should not be counted as intraoperative monitoring, but represents separately reportable procedures. When reporting 95940 and 95941, the same neurophysiologic study(ies) performed at baseline should be reported not more than once per operative session. Baseline study reporting is based on the total unique studies performed. For example, if during the course of baseline testing and one-on-one monitoring, two separate nerves have motor testing performed in conjunction with limited single extremity EMG, then 95885 and 95907 would be reported in addition to 95940. For procedures that last beyond midnight, report services using the day on which the monitoring began and using the total time monitored.

Code 95940 is reported per 15 minutes of service. Code 95940 requires reporting only the portion of time the monitoring professional was physically present in the operating room providing one-on-one patient monitoring, and no other cases may be monitored at the same time. Report continuous intraoperative neurophysiologic monitoring in the operating room (95940) in addition to the services related to monitoring from outside the operating room (95941).

Code 95941 should be used once per hour even if multiple methods of neurophysiologic monitoring are used during the time. Code 95941 requires the monitoring of neurophysiological data that is collected from the operating room continuously on-line in real time via a secure data link. When reporting 95941, real-time ability must be available through sufficient data bandwidth transfer rates to view and interrogate the neurophysiologic data contemporaneously.

Report 95941 for all cases in which there was no physical presence by the monitoring professional in the operating room during the monitoring time or when monitoring more than one case in an operating room. It is also used to report the time of monitoring physically performed outside of the operating room in those cases where monitoring occurred both within and outside the operating room. Do not report 95941 if monitoring lasts 30 minutes or less.

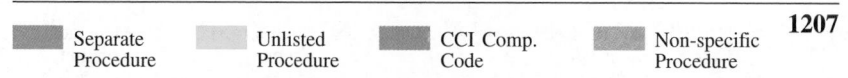

1207

| Separate Procedure | Unlisted Procedure | CCI Comp. Code | Non-specific Procedure |

Intraoperative neurophysiology monitoring codes 95940 and 95941 are each used to report the total duration of respective time spent providing each service, even if that time is not in a single continuous block.

(95920   deleted 2012 [2013 edition]. To report, see 95940, 95941)

●+95940   Continuous intraoperative neurophysiology monitoring in the operating room, one on one monitoring requiring personal attendance, each 15 minutes (List separately in addition to code for primary procedure)

(Use 95940 in conjunction with the study performed, 92585, 95822, 95860-95870, 95907-95913, 95925, 95926, 95927, 95928, 95929, 95930-95937, 95938, 95939)

●+95941   Continuous intraoperative neurophysiology monitoring, from outside the operating room (remote or nearby) or for monitoring of more than one case while in the operating room, per hour (List separately in addition to code for primary procedure)

(Use 95941 in conjunction with the study performed, 92585, 95822, 95860-95870, 95907-95913, 95925, 95926, 95927, 95928, 95929, 95930-95937, 95938, 95939)

(For time spent waiting on standby before monitoring, use 99360)

(For electrocorticography, use 95829)

(For intraoperative EEG during nonintracranial surgery, use 95955)

(For intraoperative functional cortical or subcortical mapping, see 95961-95962)

(For intraoperative neurostimulator programming and analysis, see 95970-95975)

AUTONOMIC FUNCTION TESTS

The purpose of autonomic nervous sytem function testing is to determine the presence of autonomic dysfunction, the site of autonomic dysfunction, and the various autonomic subsystems that may be disordered.

Code 95921 should be reported only when electrocardiographic monitoring of heart rate derived from the time elapsing between two consecutive R waves in the electrocardiogram, or the R-R interval, is displayed on a monitor and stored for subsequent analysis of waveforms. Testing is typically performed in the prone position. A tilt table may be used, but is not required equipment for testing of the parasympathetic function. At least two of the following components need to be included in testing:

1. Heart rate response to deep breathing derived from a visual quantitative analysis of recording with subject breathing at a rate of 5-6 breaths per minute

2. Valsalva ratio determined by dividing the maximum heart rate by the lowest heart rate. The initial heart rate responses to sustained oral pressure (blowing into a tube with an open glottis) consist of tachycardia followed by a bradycardia at 15-45 seconds after the Valsalva pressure has been released. A minimum of two Valsalva maneuvers are to be performed. The initial cardioacceleration is an exercise reflex while the subsequent tachycardia and bradycardia are baroreflex-mediated.

3. A 30:15 ratio (R-R interval at beat 30)/(R-R interval at beat 15) used as an index of cardiovascular function.

Code 95922 should be reported only when all of the following components are included in testing:

1. Continuous recording of beat-to-beat BP and heart rate. The heart rate needs to be derived from an electrocardiogram (ECG) unit such that an accurate quantitative graphical measurement of the R-R interval is obtained.

2. A period of supine rest of at least 20 minutes prior to testing.

3. The performance and recording of beat-to-beat blood pressure and heart rate during a minimum of two (2) Valsalva maneuvers.

4. The performance of passive head-up tilt with continuous recording of beat-to-beat blood pressure and heart rate for a minimum of five minutes, followed by passive tilt-back to the supine position. This must be performed using a tilt table.

Code 95924 should be reported only when both the parasympathetic function and the adrenergic function are tested together with the use of a tilt table.

> (To report autonomic function testing that does not include beat-to-beat recording or for testing without use of a tilt table, use 95943)

95921 Testing of autonomic nervous system function; cardiovagal innervation (parasympathetic function), including 2 or more of the following: heart rate response to deep breathing with recorded R-R interval, Valsalva ratio, and 30:15 ratio

95922 vasomotor adrenergic innervation (sympathetic adrenergic function), including beat-to-beat blood pressure and R-R

1209

	Separate Procedure		Unlisted Procedure		CCI Comp. Code		Non-specific Procedure

interval changes during Valsalva maneuver and at least 5 minutes of passive tilt

(Do not report 95922 in conjunction with 95921)

95923   sudomotor, including 1 or more of the following: quantitative sudomotor axon reflex test (QSART), silastic sweat imprint, thermoregulatory sweat test, and changes in sympathetic skin potential

● **95924**   combined parasympathetic and sympathetic adrenergic function testing with at least 5 minutes of passive tilt

(Do not report 95924 in conjunction with 95921 or 95922)

● **95943**   Simultaneous, independent, quantitative measures of both parasympathetic function and sympathetic function, based on time-frequency analysis of heart rate variability concurrent with time-frequency analysis of continuous respiratory activity, with mean heart rate and blood pressure measures, during rest, paced (deep) breathing, Valsalva maneuvers, and head-up postural change

(Do not report 95943 in conjunction with 93040, 95921, 95922, 95924)

EVOKED POTENTIALS AND REFLEX TESTS

95925   Short-latency somatosensory evoked potential study, stimulation of any/all peripheral nerves or skin sites, recording from the central nervous system; in upper limbs

(Do not report 95925 in conjunction with 95926)

95926   in lower limbs

(Do not report 95926 in conjunction with 95925)

95938   in upper and lower limbs

(Do not report 95938 in conjunction with 95925, 95926)

95927   in the trunk or head

(To report a unilateral study, use modifier -52)

(For auditory evoked potentials, use 92585)

95928   Central motor evoked potential study (transcranial motor stimulation); upper limbs

● New Code   ▲ Revised Code   + Add-On Code   ⊘ Modifier -51 Exempt   ⊙ Moderate Sedation

(Do not report 95928 in conjunction with 95929)

95929   lower limbs

(Do not report 95929 in conjunction with 95928)

95939   in upper and lower limbs

(Do not report 95939 in conjunction with 95928, 95929)

95930   Visual evoked potential (VEP) testing central nervous system, checkerboard or flash

95933   Orbicularis oculi (blink) reflex, by electrodiagnostic testing

(95934   deleted 2012 [2013 edition]. To report H-reflex testing, see 95907-95913)

(95936   deleted 2012 [2013 edition]. To report H-reflex testing, see 95907-95913)

95937   Neuromuscular junction testing (repetitive stimulation, paired stimuli), each nerve, any 1 method

95938   Code out of order, See page 1210

95939   Code out of order. See page 1211

95940   Code out of order. See page 1208

95941   Code out of order. See page 1208

95943   Code out of order. See page 1210

SPECIAL EEG TESTS

Codes 95950-95953 and 95956 are used per 24 hours of recording. For recording more than 12 hours, do not use modifier 52. For recording 12 hours or less, use modifier 52. Codes 95951 and 95956 are used for recording in which interpretations can be made throughout the recording time, with interventions to alter or end the recording or to alter the patient care during the recordings as needed.

Codes 95961 and 95962 use physician or other qualified health care professional time as a basis for unit of service. Report 95961 for the first hour of attendance. Use modifier 52 with 95961 for 30 minutes or less. Report 95962 for each additional hour of attendance.

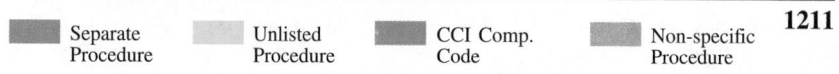

| | Separate Procedure | | Unlisted Procedure | | CCI Comp. Code | | Non-specific Procedure | **1211** |

95950 Monitoring for identification and lateralization of cerebral seizure focus, electroencephalographic (eg, 8 channel EEG) recording and interpretation, each 24 hours

95951 Monitoring for localization of cerebral seizure focus by cable or radio, 16 or more channel telemetry, combined electroencephalographic (EEG) and video recording and interpretation (eg, for presurgical localization), each 24 hours

95953 Monitoring for localization of cerebral seizure focus by computerized portable 16 or more channel EEG, electroencephalographic (EEG) recording and interpretation, each 24 hours, unattended

▲ **95954** Pharmacological or physical activation requiring physician or other qualified health care professional attendance during EEG recording of activation phase (eg, thiopental activation test)

95955 Electroencephalogram (EEG) during nonintracranial surgery (eg, carotid surgery)

95956 Monitoring for localization of cerebral seizure focus by cable or radio,16 or more channel telemetry, electroencephalographic (EEG) recording and interpretation, each 24 hours, attended by a technologist or nurse

95957 Digital analysis of electroencephalogram (EEG) (eg, for epileptic spike analysis)

95958 Wada activation test for hemispheric function, including electroencephalographic (EEG) monitoring

▲ **95961** Functional cortical and subcortical mapping by stimulation and/or recording of electrodes on brain surface, or of depth electrodes, to provoke seizures or identify vital brain structures; initial hour of attendance by a physician or other qualified health care professional

▲**+95962** each additional hour of attendance by a physician or other qualified health care professional (List separately in addition to code for primary procedure)

(Use 95962 in conjunction with code 95961)

95965 Magnetoencephalography (MEG), recording and analysis; for spontaneous brain magnetic activity (eg, epileptic cerebral cortex localization)

1212 ● New Code   ▲ Revised Code   + Add-On Code   ⊘ Modifier -51 Exempt   ⊙ Moderate Sedation

95966   for evoked magnetic fields, single modality (eg, sensory, motor, language, or visual cortex localization)

+ 95967   for evoked magnetic fields, each additional modality (eg, sensory, motor, language, or visual cortex localization) (List separately in addition to code for primary procedure)

(Use 95967 in conjunction with code 95966)

(For electroencephalography performed in addition to magnetoencephalography, see 95812-95827)

(For somatosensory evoked potentials, auditory evoked potentials, and visual evoked potentials performed in addition to magnetic evoked field responses, see 92585, 95925, 95926, and/or 95930)

(For computerized tomography performed in addition to magnetoencephalography, see 70450-70470, 70496)

(For magnetic resonance imaging performed in addition to magnetoencephalography, see 70551-70553)

NEUROSTIMULATORS, ANALYSIS-PROGRAMMING

Simple intraoperative or subsequent programming of the neurostimulator pulse generator/transmitter (95971) includes changes to three or fewer of the following parameters: rate, pulse amplitude, pulse duration, pulse frequency, eight or more electrode contacts, cycling, stimulation train duration, train spacing, number of programs, number of channels, alternating electrode polarities, dose time (stimulation parameters changing in time periods of minutes including dose lockout times), more than one clinical feature (eg., rigidity, dyskinesia, tremor). Complex intraoperative or subsequent programming (95972-95979) includes changes to more than three of the above.

Code 95970 describes subsequent electronic analysis of a previously-implanted simple or complex brain, spinal cord, or peripheral neurostimulator pulse generator system, without reprogramming. Code 95971 describes intraoperative or subsequent electronic analysis of an implanted simple spinal cord, or peripheral (ie., peripheral nerve, autonomic nerve, neuromuscular) neurostimulator pulse generator system, with programming. Codes 95972 and 95973 describe intraoperative (at initial insertion/revision) or subsequent electronic analysis of an implanted complex spinal cord or peripheral (except cranial nerve) neurostimulator pulse generator system, with programming. Codes 95974 and 95975 describe intraoperative (at initial insertion/revision) or subsequent electronic analysis of an implanted complex cranial nerve neurostimulator pulse generator system, with programming. Codes 95978 and 95979 describe initial or subsequent electronic analysis of an implanted brain neurostimulator pulse generator system, with programming.

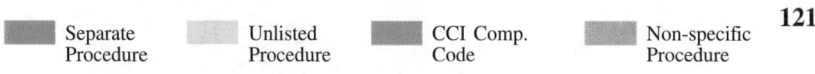

1213

| | Separate Procedure | | Unlisted Procedure | | CCI Comp. Code | | Non-specific Procedure |

Code 95980 describes intraoperative electronic analysis of an implanted gastric neurostimulator pulse generator system, with programming. Code 95981 describes subsequent analysis of the device; code 95982 describes subsequent analysis and re-programming. For electronic analysis and reprogramming of gastric neurostimulator, lesser curvature, see 95980-95982.

For 95972, 95974 and 95978, use modifier 52 if less than 31 minutes in duration.

(For electronic analysis and reprogramming of a peripheral subcutaneous field stimulation pulse generator, use 0285T)

(For insertion of neurostimulator pulse generator, see 61885, 63685, 64590)

(For revision or removal of neurostimulator pulse generator or receiver, see 61888, 63688, 64595)

(For implantation of neurostimulator electrodes, see 43647, 43881, 61850-61875, 63650-63655, 64553-64580. For revision or removal of neurostimulator electrodes, see 43648, 43882, 61880, 63661-63664, 64585)

95970 Electronic analysis of implanted neurostimulator pulse generator system (eg, rate, pulse amplitude, pulse duration, configuration of wave form, battery status, electrode selectability, output modulation, cycling, impedance and patient compliance measurements); simple or complex brain, spinal cord, or peripheral (ie, cranial nerve, peripheral nerve, sacral nerve, neuromuscular) neurostimulator pulse generator/transmitter, without reprogramming

95971 simple spinal cord, or peripheral (ie, peripheral nerve, sacral nerve, neuromuscular) neurostimulator pulse generator/transmitter, with intraoperative or subsequent programming

95972 complex spinal cord, or peripheral (ie, peripheral nerve, sacral nerve, neuromuscular) (except cranial nerve) neurostimulator pulse generator/transmitter, with intraoperative or subsequent programming, first hour

+ **95973** complex spinal cord, or peripheral (ie, peripheral nerve, sacral nerve, neuromuscular) (except cranial nerve) neurostimulator pulse generator/transmitter, with intraoperative or subsequent programming, each additional 30 minutes after first hour (List separately in addition to code for primary procedure)

(Use 95973 in conjunction with code 95972)

● New Code ▲ Revised Code + Add-On Code ⊘ Modifier -51 Exempt ⊙ Moderate Sedation

95974 complex cranial nerve neurostimulator pulse generator/transmitter, with intraoperative or subsequent programming, with or without nerve interface testing, first hour

+ 95975 complex cranial nerve neurostimulator pulse generator/transmitter, with intraoperative or subsequent programming, each additional 30 minutes after first hour (List separately in addition to code for primary procedure)

(Use 95975 in conjunction with code 95974)

(For electronic analysis, programming, and reprogramming of gastric neurostimulator pulse generator, lesser curvature [morbid obesity], use Category III code 0162T)

95978 Electronic analysis of implanted neurostimulator pulse generator system (eg, rate, pulse amplitude and duration, battery status, electrode selectability and polarity, impedance and patient compliance measurements), complex deep brain neurostimulator pulse generator/transmitter, with initial or subsequent programming; first hour

+ 95979 each additional 30 minutes after first hour (List separately in addition to code for primary procedure)

(Use 95979 in conjunction with 95978)

95980 Electronic analysis of implanted neurostimulator pulse generator system (eg, rate, pulse amplitude and duration, configuration of wave form, battery status, electrode selectability, output modulation, cycling, impedance and patient measurement(s) gastric neurostimulator pulse generator/transmitter; intraoperative, with programming

95981 subsequent, without reprogramming

95982 subsequent, with reprogramming

(For intraoperative or subsequent analysis, with programming, when performed, of vagus nerve trunk stimulator used for blocking therapy [morbid obesity], see 0312T, 0317T)

OTHER PROCEDURES

95990 Refilling and maintenance of implantable pump or reservoir for drug delivery, spinal (intrathecal, epidural) or brain (intraventricular), includes electronic analysis of pump, when performed;

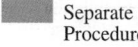 Separate Procedure   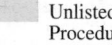 Unlisted Procedure   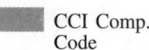 CCI Comp. Code   Non-specific Procedure

1215

▲ **95991**   requiring skill of a physician or other qualified health care professional

(Do not report 95990, 95991 in conjunction with 62367-62370. For analysis and/or reprogramming of implantable infusion pump, see 62367-62370)

(For refill and maintenance of implanted infusion pump or reservoir for systemic drug therapy [eg, chemotherapy] use 96522)

⊘ **95992**   Canalith repositioning procedure(s) (eg, Epley maneuver, Semont maneuver), per day

(Do not report 95992 in conjunction with 92531, 92532)

95999   Unlisted neurological or neuromuscular diagnostic procedure

MOTION ANALYSIS

Codes 96000-96004 describe services performed as part of a major therapeutic or diagnostic decision making process. Motion analysis is performed in a dedicated motion analysis laboratory (ie., facility capable of performing videotaping from the front, back and both sides, computerized 3D kinematics, 3D kinetics, and dynamic electromyography). Code 96000 may include 3D kinetics and stride characteristics. Codes 96002-96003 describe dynamic electromyography.

Code 96004 should only be reported once regardless of the number of studies reviewed/interpreted.

(For performance of needle electromyography procedures, see 95860-95870, 95872, 95885-95887)

(For gait training, use 97116)

96000   Comprehensive computer-based motion analysis by video-taping and 3-D kinematics;

96001   with dynamic plantar pressure measurements during walking

96002   Dynamic surface electromyography, during walking or other functional activities, 1-12 muscles

96003   Dynamic fine wire electromyography, during walking or other functional activities, 1 muscle

(Do not report 96002, 96003 in conjunction with 95860-95866, 95869-95872, 95885-95887)

▲ **96004** Review and interpretation by physician or other qualified health care professional of comprehensive computer-based motion analysis, dynamic plantar pressure measurements, dynamic surface electromyography during walking or other functional activities, and dynamic fine wire electromyography, with written report

FUNCTIONAL BRAIN MAPPING

Code 96020 includes selection and administration of testing of language, memory, cognition, movement, sensation, and other neurological functions when conducted in association with functional neuroimaging, monitoring of performance of this testing, and determination of validity of neurofunctional testing relative to separately interpreted functional magnetic resonance images.

▲ **96020** Neurofunctional testing selection and administration during noninvasive imaging functional brain mapping, with test administered entirely by a physician or other qualified health care professional (ie, psychologist), with review of test results and report

(For functional magnetic resonance imaging [fMRI], brain, use 70555)

(Do not report 96020 in conjunction with 96101-96103, 96116-96120)

(Do not report 96020 in conjunction with 70554)

(Evaluation and Management services codes should not be reported on the same day as 96020)

MEDICAL GENETICS AND GENETIC COUNSELING SERVICES

These sevices are provided by trained genetic counselors and may include obtaining a structured family genetic history, pedigree construction, analysis for genetic risk assessment, and counseling of the patient and family. These activities may be provided during one or more sessions and may include review of medical data and family information, face-to-face interviews, and counseling services.

Code 96040 is reported for each 30-minute increment of face-to-face time. Do not report 96040 for 15 minutes or less of face-to-face time. Report 96040 once for 16 to 30 minutes of face-to-face time.

96040 Medical genetics and genetic counseling services, each 30 minutes face-to-face with patient/family

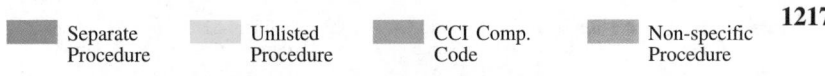

1217

	Separate Procedure		Unlisted Procedure		CCI Comp. Code		Non-specific Procedure

(For genetic counseling and education provided to an individual by a physician or other qualified health care professional who may report E/M services, see the appropriate E/M codes)

(For genetic counseling and education provided to a group by a physician or other qualified health care professional, use 99078)

(For education regarding genetic risks by a nonphysician to a group, see 98961, 98962)

(For genetic counseling and/or risk factor reduction intervention provided to patient(s) without symptoms or established disease, by a physician or other qualified health care professional who may report evaluation and management services, see 99401-99412)

CENTRAL NERVOUS SYSTEM ASSESSMENTS/TESTS (eg, NEURO-COGNITIVE, MENTAL STATUS, SPEECH TESTING)

The following codes are used to report the services provided during testing of the cognitive function of the central nervous system. The testing of cognitive processes, visual motor responses, and abstractive abilities is accomplished by the combination of several types of testing procedures. It is expected that the administration of these tests will generate material that will be formulated into a report. A minimum of 31 minutes must be provided to report any per hour code. Services 96101, 96116, 96118, and 96125 report time as face-to-face time with the patient and the time spent interpreting and preparing the report.

(For development of cognitive skills, see 97532, 97533)

(For mini-mental status examination performed by a physician, see E/M services codes)

96101 Psychological testing (includes psychodiagnostic assessment of emotionality, intellectual abilities, personality and psychopathology, eg, MMPI, Rorshach, WAIS), per hour of the psychologist's or physician's time, both face-to-face time administering tests to the patient and time interpreting test results and preparing the report

(96101 is also used in those circumstances when additional time is necessary to integrate other sources of clinical data, including previously completed and reported technician- and computer-administered tests)

(Do not report 96101 for the interpretation and report of 96102, 96103)

● New Code ▲ Revised Code + Add-On Code ⊘ Modifier -51 Exempt ⊙ Moderate Sedation

96102 Psychological testing (includes psychodiagnostic assessment of emotionality, intellectual abilities, personality and psychopathology, eg, MMPI and WAIS), with qualified health care professional interpretation and report, administered by technician, per hour of technician time, face-to-face

96103 Psychological testing (includes psychodiagnostic assessment of emotionality, intellectual abilities, personality and psychopathology, eg, MMPI), administered by a computer, with qualified health care professional interpretation and report

96105 Assessment of aphasia (includes assessment of expressive and receptive speech and language function, language comprehension, speech production ability, reading, spelling, writing, eg, by Boston Diagnostic Aphasia Examination) with interpretation and report, per hour

96110 Developmental screening, with interpretation and report, per standardized instrument form

96111 Developmental testing, (includes assessment of motor, language, social, adaptive and/or cognitive functioning by standardized developmental instruments) with interpretation and report

96116 Neurobehavioral status exam (clinical assessment of thinking, reasoning and judgment, eg, acquired knowledge, attention, language, memory, planning and problem solving, and visual spatial abilities), per hour of the psychologist's or physician's time, both face-to-face time with the patient and time interpreting test results and preparing the report

96118 Neuropsychological testing (eg, Halstead-Reitan Neuropsychological Battery, Wechsler Memory Scales and Wisconsin Card Sorting Test), per hour of the psychologist's or physician's time, both face-to-face time administering tests to the patient and time interpreting these test results and preparing the report

(96118 is also used in those circumstances when additional time is necessary to integrate other sources of clinical data, including previously completed and reported technician- and computer-administered tests)

(Do not report 96118 for the interpretation and report of 96119 or 96120)

96119 Neuropsychological testing (eg, Halstead-Reitan Neuropsychological Battery, Wechsler Memory Scales and Wisconsin Card Sorting Test), with qualified health care

	Separate Procedure		Unlisted Procedure		CCI Comp. Code		Non-specific Procedure

1219

professional interpretation and report, administered by technician, per hour of technician time, face-to-face

96120 Neuropsychological testing (eg, Wisconsin Card Sorting Test), administered by a computer, with qualified health care professional interpretation and report

96125 Standardized cognitive performance testing (eg, Ross Information Processing Assessment) per hour of a qualified health care professional's time, both face-to-face time administering tests to the patient and time interpreting these test results and preparing the report

(For psychological and neuropsychological testing by a physician or psychologist, see 96101-96103, 96118-96120)

HEALTH AND BEHAVIOR ASSESSMENT/ INTERVENTION

Codes 96150-96155 describe services offered to patients who present with primary physical illnesses, diagnoses, or symptoms and may benefit from assessments and interventions that focus on the biopsychosocial factors related to the patient's health status. These services do not represent preventive medicine counseling and risk factor reduction interventions.

For patients that require psychiatric services (90801-90899) as well as health and behavior assessment/intervention (96150-96155), report the predominant service performed. Do not report 96150-96155 in conjunction with 90801-90899 on the same date.

Evaluation and Management services codes (including Counseling Risk Factor Reduction and Behavior Change Intervention [99401-99412]), should not be reported on the same day.

(For health and behavior assessment and/or intervention performed by a physician or other qualified health care professional who may report evaluation and management services, see Evaluation and Management or Preventive Medicine services codes)

96150 Health and behavior assessment (eg, health-focused clinical interview, behavioral observations, psychophysicological monitoring, health-oriented questionnaires), each 15 minutes face-to-face with the patient; intial assessment

96151 re-assessment

● New Code ▲ Revised Code ✚ Add-On Code ⊘ Modifier -51 Exempt ⊙ Moderate Sedation

| 96152 | Health and behavior intervention, each 15 minutes, face-to-face; individual |

96153   group (2 or more patients)

96154   family (with the patient present)

96155   family (without the patient present)

HYDRATION, THERAPEUTIC, PROPHYLACTIC, DIAGNOSTIC INJECTIONS AND INFUSIONS, AND CHEMOTHERAPY AND OTHER HIGHLY COMPLEX DRUG OR HIGHLY COMPLEX BIOLOGIC ADMINISTRATION

Coding Rules

1. If a significant E/M service is performed, report the E/M service code with modifier -25 in addition to the infusion/injection codes.

2. Local anesthesia, IV start, access to indwelling IV, subcutaneous catheter or port, fFlush at the conclusion of infusion and standard tubing, syringes and supplies are included and not reported separately if performed to facilitate the infusion/injection.

3. When multiple drugs are administered, the service(s) and specific drugs or materials for each are reported.

4. When administering multiple infusions, injections or combinations, report only one "initial" service code unless two IV sites must be used.

5. When reported by the physician, report the "initial" code that best describes the primary reason for the encounter regardless of the order in which the infusions or injections are administered.

6. When reported by the facility, the "initial" code should reported in the order of chemotherapy services, followed by therapeutic/prophylactic/diagnostic services, followed by hydrationi services, followed by infusions, followed by pushes, and finally injections.

Physician or other qualified health care professional work related to hydration, injection, and infusion services predominantly involves affirmation of treatment plan and direct supervision of staff.

Codes 96360-96379, 96401, 96402, 96409-96425, 96521-96523 are not intended to be reported by the physician in the facility setting. If a significant, separately

| Separate Procedure | Unlisted Procedure | CCI Comp. Code | Non-specific Procedure |

identifiable office or other outpatient E/M service is performed, the appropriate E/M service (99201-99215, 99241-99245, 99354-99355) should be reported using modifier 25 in addition to 96360-96549. For same day E/M service, a different diagnosis is not required.

If performed to facilitate the infusion or injection, the following services are included and are not reported separately:

a. Use of local anesthesia

b. IV start

c. Access to indwelling IV, subcutaneous catheter or port

d. Flush at conclusion of infusion

e. Standard tubing, syringes, and supplies

> (For declotting a catheter or port, use 36593)

When multiple drugs are administered, report the service(s) and the specific materials or drugs for each.

When administering multiple infusions, injections or combinations, only one "initial" service code should be reported for a given date, unless protocol requires that two separate IV sites must be used. Do not report a second initial service on the same date due to an intravenous line requiring a re-start, an IV rate not being able to be reached without two lines, or for accessing a port of a nulti-lumen catheter. If an injection or infusion is of a subsequent or concurrent nature, even if it is the first such service within that group of services, then a subsequent or concurrent code from the appropriate section should be reported (eg., the first IV push given subsequent to an initial one-hour infusion is reported using a subsequent IV push code).

In order to determine which service should be reported as the initial service when there is more than one type of service, hierarchies have been created. These vary by whether they physician or other qualified health care professional or a facility is reporting. The order of selection for reporting is based upon the physician's or other qualified health care professional's knowledge of the clinical condition(s) and treatment(s). The hierarchy that facilities are to use is based upon a structural algorithm. When these codes are reported by the physician or other qualified health care professional, the "initial" code that best describes the key or primary reason for the encounter should always be reported irrespective of the order in which the infusions or injections occur.

When these codes are reported *by the facility,* the following instructions apply: The initial code should be selected using a hierarchy whereby chemotherapy services are primary to therapeutic, prophylactic, and diagnostic services which are primary to hydration services. Infusions are primary to pushes, which are primary to

● New Code	▲ Revised Code	+ Add-On Code	⊘ Modifier -51 Exempt	⊙ Moderate Sedation

injections. This hierarchy is to be followed by facilities and supersedes parenthetical instructions for add-on codes that suggest an add-on of a higher hierarchical position may be reported in conjunction with a base code of a lower position. (For example, the hierarchy would not permit reporting 96376 with 96360, as 96376 is a higher order code. IV push is primary to hydration.)

When reporting multiple infusions of the same drug/substance on the same date of service, the initial code should be selected. The second and subsequent infusion(s) should be reported based on the individual time(s) of each additional infusion(s) of the same drug/substances using the appropriate add-on code.

When reporting codes for which infusion time is a factor, use the actual time over which the infusion is administered. Intravenous or intra-arterial push is defined as: (a) an injection in which the health care professional who administers the drug/substance is continuously present to administer the injection and observe the patient; or (b) an infusion of 15 minutes or less. If intravenous hydration (96360, 96361) is given from 11 p.m. to 2 a.m., 96360 would be reported once and 96361 twice. For continuous services that last beyond midnight, use the date in which the service began and report the total units of time provided continuously. However, if instead of a continuous infusion, a medication was given by intravenous push at 10 pm and 2 am, as the service was not continuous, the two administrations would be reported as an initial service (96374) and sequential (96376) as: (1) no other infusion services were performed; and (2) the push of the same drug was performed more than 30 minutes beyond the initial administration. A "keep open" infusion of any type is not separately reported.

HYDRATION

Codes 96360-96361 are intended to report a hydration IV infusion to consist of a pre-packaged fluid and electrolytes (eg., normal saline, D5-1/2 normal saline + 30mEq KCl/liter), but are not used to report infusion of drugs or other substances. Hydration IV infusions typically require direct supervision for purposes of consent, safety oversight, or intraservice supervision of staff. Typically, such infusions require little special handling to prepare or dispose of, and staff that administer these do not typically require advanced practice training. After initial set-up, infusion typically entails little patient risk and thus little monitoring. These codes are not intended to be reported by the physician or other qualified health care profesional in the facility setting.

Some chemotherapeutic agents and other therapeutic agents require pre- and/or post-hydration to be given in order to avoid specific toxicities. A minimum time duration of 31 minutes of hydration infusion is required to report the service. However, the hydration codes 96360 or 96361 are not used when the purpose of the intravenous fluid is to "keep open" and IV line prior or subsequent to a therapeutic infusion, or as a free-flowing IV during chemotherapy or other therapeutic infusion.

Separate Procedure | Unlisted Procedure | CCI Comp. Code | Non-specific Procedure

96360   Intravenous infusion, hydration; initial, 31 minutes to 1 hour

(Do not report 96360 if performed as a concurrent infusion service)

(Do not report intravenous infusion for hydration of 30 minutes or less)

+ 96361   each additional hour (list separately in addition to code for primary procedure)

(Use 96361 in conjunction with 96360)

(Report 96361 for hydration infusion intervals of greater than 30 minutes beyond 1 hour increments)

(Report 96361 to identify hydration if provided as a secondary or subsequent service after a different initial service [96360, 96365, 96374, 96409, 96413] is administered through the same IV access)

THERAPEUTIC, PROPHYLACTIC, AND DIAGNOSTIC INJECTIONS AND INFUSIONS (EXCLUDES CHEMOTHERAPY AND OTHER HIGHLY COMPLEX DRUG OR HIGHLY COMPLEX BIOLOGIC AGENT ADMINISTRATION)

A therapeutic, prophylactic or diagnostic IV infusion or injection (other than hydration) is for the administration of substances/drugs. When fluids are used to administer the drug(s), the administration of the fluid is considered incidental hydration and is not separately reportable. These services typically require direct supervision for any or all purposes of patient assessment, provision of consent, safety oversight, and intra-service supervision of staff. Typically, such infusions require special consideration to prepare, dose or dispose of, require practice training and competency for staff who administer the infusions, and require periodic patient assessment with vital sign monitoring during the infusion. These codes are not intended to be reported by the physician or other qualified health care professional in the facility setting.

See codes 96401-96549 for the administration of chemotherapy or other highly complex drug or highly complex biologic agent services. These highly complex services require advanced practice training and competency for staff who provide these services; special considerations for preparation, dosage or disposal; and commonly, these services entail significant patient risk and frequent monitoring. Examples are frequent changes in the infusion rate, prolonged presence of nurse administering the solution for patient monitoring and infusion adjustments, and frequent conferring with the physician or other qualified health care profesisonal about these issues.

(Do not report 96365-96379 with codes for which IV push or infusion is an inherent part of the procedure [eg, administration of contrast material for a diagnostic imaging study])

96365 Intravenous infusion, for therapy, prophylaxis, or diagnosis (specify substance or drug); initial, up to 1 hour

+ **96366** each additional hour (list separately in addition to code for primary procedure)

(Report 96366 in conjunction with 96365, 96367)

(Report 96366 for additional hour[s] of sequential infusion)

(Report 96366 for infusion intervals of greater than 30 minutes beyond 1 hour increments)

(Report 96366 in conjunction with 96365 to identify each second and subsequent infusions of the same drug/substance)

+ **96367** additional sequential infusion of a new drug/substance, up to 1 hour (list separately in addition to code for primary procedure)

(Report 96367 in conjunction with 96365, 96374, 96409, 96413 to identify the infusion of a new drug/substance provided as a secondary or subsequent service after a different initial service is administered through the same IV access. Report 96367 only once per sequential infusion of same infusate mix)

+ **96368** concurrent infusion (list separately in addition to code for primary procedure)

(Report 96368 only once per date of service)

(Report 96368 in conjunction with 96365, 96366, 96413, 96415, 96416)

96369 Subcutaneous infusion for therapy or prophylaxis (specify substance or drug); initial, up to 1 hour, including pump set-up and establishment of subcutaneous infusion site(s)

(For infusions of 15 minutes or less, use 96372)

+ **96370** each additional hour (list separately in addition to code for primary procedure)

(Use 96370 in conjunction with 96369)

(Use 96370 for infusion intervals of greater than 30 minutes beyond 1 hour increments)

				1225
Separate Procedure	Unlisted Procedure	CCI Comp. Code	Non-specific Procedure	

+ **96371**   additional pump set-up with establishment of new subcutaneous infusion site(s) (list separately in addition to code for primary procedure)

(Use 96371 in conjunction with 96369)

(Use 96369, 96371 only once per encounter)

96372   Therapeutic, prophylactic, or diagnostic injection (specify substance or drug); subcutaneous or intramuscular

(For administration of vaccines/toxoids, see 90465, 90466, 90471, 90472)

(Report 96372 for non-antineoplastic hormonal therapy injections)

(Report 96401 for antineoplastic nonhormonal injection therapy)

(Report 96402 for antineoplastic hormonal injection therapy)

(Do not report 96372 for injections given without direct physician or other qualified health care professional supervision. To report, use 99211. Hospitals may report 96372 when the physician or other qualified health care professional is not present)

(96372 does not include injections for allergen immunotherapy. For allergen immunotherapy injections, see 95115-95117)

96373   intra-arterial

96374   intravenous push, single or initial substance/drug

+ **96375**   each additional sequential intravenous push of a new substance/drug (list separately in addition to code for primary procedure)

(Use 96375 in conjunction with 96365, 96374, 96409, 96413)

(Report 96375 to identify intravenous push of a new substance/drug if provided as a secondary or subsequent service after a different initial sevice is administered through the same IV access)

+ **96376**   each additional sequential intravenous push of the same substance/drug provided in a facility (list separately in addition to code for primary procedure)

(Do not report 96376 for a push performed within 30 minutes of a reported push of the same substance or drug)

1226   ● New Code   ▲ Revised Code   + Add-On Code   ⊘ Modifier -51 Exempt   ⊙ Moderate Sedation

(96376 may be reported by facilities only)

(Report 96376 in conjunction with 96365, 96374, 96409, 96413)

96379   Unlisted therapeutic, prophylactic, or diagnostic intravenous or intra-arterial injection or infusion

(For allergy immunology, see 95004 et seq)

CHEMOTHERAPY AND OTHER HIGHLY COMPLEX DRUG OR HIGHLY COMPLEX BIOLOGIC AGENT ADMINISTRATION

Chemotherapy administration codes 96401-96549 apply to parenteral administration of non-radionuclide anti-neoplastic drugs; and also to anti-neoplastic agents provided for treatment of noncancer diagnoses (eg, cyclophosphamide for auto-immune conditions) or to substances such as certain monoclonal antibody agents, and other biologic response modifiers. The highly complex infusion of chemotherapy or other drug or biologic agents requires physician or other qualified health care professional work and/or clinical staff monitoring well beyond that of therapeutic drug agents (96360-96379) because the incidence of severe adverse patient reactions are typically greater. These services can be provided by any physician or other qualified health care professional. Chemotherapy services are typically highly complex and require direct supervision for any or all purposes of patient assessment, provision of consent, safety oversight, and intra-service supervision of staff. Typically, such chemotherapy services require advanced practice training and competency for staff who provide these services; special considerations for preparation, dosage, or disposal; and commonly, these services entail significant patient risk and frequent monitoring. Examples are frequent changes in the infusion rate, prolonged presence of the nurse administering the solution for patient monitoring and infusion adjustments, and frequent conferring with the physician or other qualified health care professional about these issues. When performed to facilitate the infusion of injection, preparation of chemotherapy agent(s), highly complex agent(s), or other highly complex drug is included and is not reported separately. To report infusions that do not require this level of complexity, see 96360-96379. Codes 96401-96402, 96409-96425, 96521-96523 are not intended to be reported by the physician or other qualified health care professional in the facility setting.

The term "chemotherapy" in 96401-96549 includes other highly complex drugs or highly complex biologic agents.

Report separate codes for each parenteral method of administration employed when chemotherapy is administered by different techniques. The administration of medications (eg., antibiotics, steroidal agents, antiemetics, narcotics, analgesics) administered independently or sequentially as supportive management of

1227

| | Separate Procedure | | Unlisted Procedure | | CCI Comp. Code | | Non-specific Procedure |

chemotherapy administration, should be separately reported using 96360, 96361, 96365, 96379 as appropriate.

Report both the specific service as well as code(s) for the specific substance(s) or drug(s) provided. The fluid used to administer the drug(s) is considered incidental hydration and is not separately reportable.

Regional (isolation) chemotherapy perfusion should be reported using the codes for arterial infusion (96420-96425). Placement of the intra-arterial catheter should be reported using the appropriate code from the Cardiovascular Surgery section. Placement of arterial and venous cannula(s) for extracorporeal circulation via a membrane oxygenator perfusion pump should be reported using 36823. Code 36823 includes dose calculation and administration of the chemotherapy agent by injection into the perfusate. Do not report 96409-96425 in conjunction with 36823.

(For home infusion services, see 99601-99602)

INJECTION AND INTRAVENOUS INFUSION CHEMOTHERAPY AND OTHER HIGHLY COMPLEX DRUG OR HIGHLY COMPLEX BIOLOGIC AGENT ADMINISTRATION

Intravenous or intra-arterial push is defined as: (a) an injection in which the healthcare professional who administers the substance/drug is continuously present to administer the injection and observe the patient, or (b) an infusion of 15 minutes or less.

96401 Chemotherapy administration, subcutaneous or intramuscular; non-hormonal anti-neoplastic

96402 hormonal anti-neoplastic

96405 Chemotherapy administration; intralesional, up to and including 7 lesions

96406 intralesional, more than 7 lesions

96409 intravenous, push technique, single or initial substance/drug

+ **96411** intravenous, push technique, each additional substance/drug (List separately in addition to code for primary procedure)

(Use 96411 in conjunction with 96409, 96413)

96413 Chemotherapy administration, intravenous infusion technique; up to 1 hour, single or initial substance/drug

(Report 96361 to identify hydration if administered as a secondary or subsequent service in association with 96413 through the same IV access)

● New Code   ▲ Revised Code   + Add-On Code   ⊘ Modifier -51 Exempt   ⊙ Moderate Sedation

(Report 96366, 96367, 96375 to identify therapeutic, prophylactic, or diagnostic drug infusion or injection, if administered as a secondary or subsequent service in association with 96413 through the same IV access)

+ 96415   each additional hour (List separately in addition to code for primary procedure)

(Use 96415 in conjunction with 96413)

(Report 96415 for infusion intervals of greater than 30 minutes beyond 1-hour increments)

96416   initiation of prolonged chemotherapy infusion (more than 8 hours), requiring use of a portable or implantable pump

(For refilling and maintenance of a portable pump or an implantable infusion pump or reservoir for drug delivery, see 96521-96523)

+ 96417   each additional sequential infusion (different substance/drug), up to 1 hour (List separately in addition to code for primary procedure)

(Use 96417 in conjunction with 96413)

(Report only once per sequential infusion. Report 96415 for additional hour(s) of sequential infusion)

INTRA-ARTERIAL CHEMOTHERAPY AND OTHER HIGHLY COMPLEX DRUG OR HIGHLY COMPLEX BIOLOGIC AGENT ADMINISTRATION

96420   Chemotherapy administration, intra-arterial; push technique

96422   infusion technique, up to 1 hour

+ 96423   infusion technique, each additional hour (List separately in addition to code for primary procedure)

(Use 96423 in conjunction with code 96422)

(Report 96423 for infusion intervals of greater than 30 minutes beyond 1-hour increments)

(For regional chemotherapy perfusion via membrane oxygenator perfusion pump to an extremity, use 36823)

96425   infusion technique, initiation of prolonged infusion (more than 8 hours), requiring the use of a portable or implantable pump

1229

▓	Separate Procedure	░	Unlisted Procedure	▓	CCI Comp. Code	▓	Non-specific Procedure

(For refilling and maintenance of a portable pump or an implantable infusion pump or reservoir for drug delivery, see 96521-96523)

OTHER INJECTION AND INFUSION SERVICES

Code 96523 does not require direct supervision. Codes 96521-96523 may be reported when these devices are used for therapeutic drugs other than chemotherapy.

(For collection of blood specimen from a completely implantable venous access device, use 36591)

96440 Chemotherapy administration into pleural cavity, requiring and including thoracentesis

(96445 deleted 2010 [2011 edition]. To report intraperitoneal chemotherapy administration, use 96446)

96446 Chemotherapy administration into the peritoneal cavity via indwelling port or catheter

96450 Chemotherapy administration, into CNS (eg, intrathecal), requiring and including spinal puncture

(For intravesical (bladder) chemotherapy administration, use 51720)

(For insertion of subarachnoid catheter and reservoir for infusion of drug, see 62350, 62351, 62360, 62361, 62362; for insertion of intraventricular catherter and reservoir, see 61210, 61215)

96521 Refilling and maintenance of portable pump

96522 Refilling and maintenance of implantable pump or reservoir for drug delivery, systemic (eg, intravenous, intra-arterial)

(For refilling and maintenance of an implantable infusion pump for spinal or brain drug infusion, use 95990-95991)

96523 Irrigation of implanted venous access device for drug delivery systems

(Do not report 96523 in conjunction with other services. To report collection of blood specimen, use 36591)

96542 Chemotherapy injection, subarachnoid or intraventricular via subcutaneous reservoir, single or multiple agents

| ● New Code | ▲ Revised Code | + Add-On Code | ⊘ Modifier -51 Exempt | ⊙ Moderate Sedation |

(For radioactive isotope therapy, use 79005)

96549 Unlisted chemotherapy procedure

PHOTODYNAMIC THERAPY

Photodynamic therapy (PDT) is a two-part treatment for esophageal cancer, gastric cancer, and lung cancer using a photosensitizing drug activated by red, non-thermal laser light.

(To report ocular photodynamic therapy, use 67221)

96567 Photodynamic therapy by external application of light to destroy premalignant and/or malignant lesions of the skin and adjacent mucosa (eg, lip) by activation of photosensitive drug(s), each phototherapy exposure session

+ 96570 Photodynamic therapy by endoscopic application of light to ablate abnormal tissue via activation of photosensitive drug(s); first 30 minutes (List separately in addition to code for endoscopy or bronchoscopy procedures of lung and gastrointestinal tract)

(Report 96570 with modifier 52 for service of less than 23 minutes with report)

+ 96571 each additional 15 minutes (List separately in addition to code for endoscopy or bronchoscopy procedures of lung and gastrointestinal tract)

(For 23-27 minutes of service, use 96570. For 38-52 minutes of service, use 96570 in conjunction with 96571)

(96570, 96571 are to be used in addition to bronchoscopy, endoscopy codes)

(Use 96570, 96571 in conjunction with codes 31641, 43228 as appropriate)

SPECIAL DERMATOLOGICAL PROCEDURES

See the **Evaluation and Management coding guidelines** for further instructions on reporting that is appropriate for management of dermatologic illnesses.

(For intralesional injections, see 11900, 11901)

(For Tzanck smear, see 88160-88161)

96900 Actinotherapy (ultraviolet light)

| Separate Procedure | Unlisted Procedure | CCI Comp. Code | Non-specific Procedure | **1231** |

(For rhinophototherapy, intranasal application of ultraviolet and visible light, use 30999)

96902 Microscopic examination of hairs plucked or clipped by the examiner (excluding hair collected by the patient) to determine telogen and anagen counts, or structural hair shaft abnormality

96904 Whole body integumentary photography, for monitoring of high risk patients with dysplastic nevus syndrome or a history of dysplastic nevi, or patients with a personal or familial history of melanoma

96910 Photochemotherapy; tar and ultraviolet B (Goeckerman treatment) or petrolatum and ultraviolet B

96912 psoralens and ultraviolet A (PUVA)

96913 Photochemotherapy (Goeckerman and/or PUVA) for severe photoresponsive dermatoses requiring at least 4 to 8 hours of care under direct supervision of the physician (includes application of medication and dressings)

96920 Laser treatment for inflammatory skin disease (psoriasis); total area less than 250 sq cm

96921 250 sq cm to 500 sq cm

96922 over 500 sq cm

(For laser destruction of premalignant lesions, see 17000-17004)

(For laser destruction of cutaneous vascular proliferative lesions, see 17106-17108)

(For laser destruction of benign lesions, see 17110-17111)

(For laser destruction of malignant lesions, see 17260-17286)

96999 Unlisted special dermatological service or procedure

PHYSICAL MEDICINE AND REHABILITATION

Physical medicine is the diagnosis, treatment, and prevention of disease with the aid of physical agents such as light, heat, cold, water, electricity or with mechanical devices. Physical medicine services may be provided by physicians or physical therapists. Physical medicine and rehabilitation CPT codes are divided into three sections: Modalities, Procedures and Tests and Measurements. Other services performed by medical professionals specializing in physical medicine

● New Code   ▲ Revised Code   + Add-On Code   ⊘ Modifier -51 Exempt   ⊙ Moderate Sedation

and/or physical therapy include: muscle testing, range of joint motion, electromyography, biofeedback training by EMG, and transcutaneous nerve stimulation (TNS).

With one exception providers should not report more than one physical medicine and rehabilitation therapy service for the same fifteen minute time period. The only exception involves a supervised modality defined by CPT codes 97010-97028 which may be reported for the same fifteen minute time period as other therapy services. Some CPT codes for physical medicine and rehabilitation services include an amount of time in their code descriptors.

Coding Rules

1. *The physician or therapist is required to be in constant attendance when reporting CPT codes for modalities and procedures.*

2. *The physical medicine procedure CPT codes specify treatment to one area, initial 30 minutes, and provide CPT codes to report each additional 15 minutes of treatment.*

SPECIAL PHYSICAL MEDICINE CODING ISSUES

Many worker's compensation and casualty insurance companies use pre-CPT coding systems, such as CRVS, and do not use any form of diagnostic coding, relying instead on special reports to justify the procedures performed and services provided. As the majority of physical medicine services are performed for accidents and injuries, many work related, the medical professional performing these services must be informed of the specific reporting requirements in the area that they practice.

Codes 97001-97755 should be used to report each distinct procedure performed. Do not append modifier 51 to 97001-97755.

The work of the physician or other qualified health care professional consists of face-to-face time with the patient (and caregiver, if applicable) delivering skilled services. For the purpose of determining the total time of a service, incremental intervals of treatment at the same visit may be accumulated.

> (For muscle testing, range of joint motion, electromyography, see 95831 et seq)

> (For biofeedback training by EMG, use 90901)

> (For transcutaneous nerve stimulation (TNS), use 64550)

97001 Physical therapy evaluation

97002 Physical therapy re-evaluation

 Separate Procedure   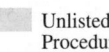 Unlisted Procedure   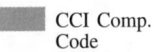 CCI Comp. Code   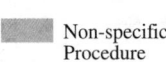 Non-specific Procedure

97003 Occupational therapy evaluation

97004 Occupational therapy re-evaluation

97005 Athletic training evaluation

97006 Athletic training re-evaluation

MODALITIES

SUPERVISED

The application of a modality that does not require direct (one-on-one) patient contact.

97010 Application of a modality to 1 or more areas; hot or cold packs

97012 traction, mechanical

97014 electrical stimulation (unattended)

(For acupuncture with electrical stimulation, see 97813, 97814)

97016 vasopneumatic devices

97018 paraffin bath

97022 whirlpool

97024 diathermy (eg, microwave)

97026 infrared

97028 ultraviolet

CONSTANT ATTENDANCE

The application of a modality that requires direct (one-on-one) patient contact.

97032 Application of a modality to 1 or more areas; electrical stimulation (manual), each 15 minutes

(For transcutaneous electrical modulation pain reprocessing (TEMPR/scrambler therapy], use 0278T)

97033 iontophoresis, each 15 minutes

1234 ● New Code   ▲ Revised Code   ✛ Add-On Code   ⊘ Modifier -51 Exempt   ⊙ Moderate Sedation

97034   contrast baths, each 15 minutes

97035   ultrasound, each 15 minutes

97036   Hubbard tank, each 15 minutes

97039   Unlisted modality (specify type and time if constant attendance)

THERAPEUTIC PROCEDURES

A manner of effecting change through the application of clinical skills and/or services that attempt to improve function. Physician or other qualified health care professional (ie, therapist) required to have direct (one-on-one) patient contact.

97110   Therapeutic procedure, 1 or more areas, each 15 minutes; therapeutic exercises to develop strength and endurance, range of motion and flexibility

97112   neuromuscular reeducation of movement, balance, coordination, kinesthetic sense, posture, and/or proprioception for sitting and/or standing activities

97113   aquatic therapy with therapeutic exercises

97116   gait training (includes stair climbing)

(Use 96000-96003 to report comprehensive gait and motion analysis procedures)

97124   massage, including effleurage, petrissage and/or tapotement (stroking, compression, percussion)

(For myofascial release, use 97140)

97139   Unlisted therapeutic procedure (specify)

97140   Manual therapy techniques (eg, mobilization/ manipulation, manual lymphatic drainage, manual traction), 1 or more regions, each 15 minutes

(Do not report 97140 in conjunction with 29581-29584)

97150   Therapeutic procedure(s), group (2 or more individuals)

(Report 97150 for each member of group)

(Group therapy procedures involve constant attendance of the physician or other qualified health care professional [ie,

---

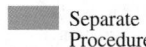 Separate Procedure   Unlisted Procedure   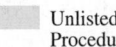 CCI Comp. Code   Non-specific Procedure   **1235**

therapist], but by definition do not require one-on-one patient contact by the same physician or other qualified health care professional)

(For manipulation under general anesthesia, see appropriate anatomic section in Musculoskeletal System)

(For osteopathic manipulative treatment (OMT), see 98925-98929)

▲ 97530 Therapeutic activities, direct (one-on-one) patient contact (use of dynamic activities to improve functional performance), each 15 minutes

▲ 97532 Development of cognitive skills to improve attention, memory, problem solving, (includes compensatory training), direct (one-on-one) patient contact, each 15 minutes

▲ 97533 Sensory integrative techniques to enhance sensory processing and promote adaptive responses to environmental demands, direct (one-on-one) patient contact, each 15 minutes

▲ 97535 Self-care/home management training (eg, activities of daily living (ADL) and compensatory training, meal preparation, safety procedures, and instructions in use of assistive technology devices/adaptive equipment) direct one-on-one contact, each 15 minutes

▲ 97537 Community/work reintegration training (eg, shopping, transportation, money management, avocational activities and/or work environment/modification analysis, work task analysis, use of assistive technology device/adaptive equipment), direct one-on-one contact, each 15 minutes

(For wheelchair management/propulsion training, use 97542)

97542 Wheelchair management (eg, assessment, fitting, training), each 15 minutes

97545 Work hardening/conditioning; initial 2 hours

+ 97546 each additional hour (List separately in addition to code for primary procedure)

(Use 97546 in conjunction with code 97545)

ACTIVE WOUND CARE MANAGEMENT

Active wound care procedures are performed to remove devitalized and/or necrotic tissue and promote healing. Services require direct (one-on-one) patient contact.

> (Do not report 97597-97602 in conjunction with 11042-11047 for the same wound)
>
> (For debridement of burn wounds, see 16020-16030)

97597 Debridement (eg, high pressure waterjet with/without suction, sharp selective debridement with scissors, scalpel and forceps), open wound, (eg, fibrin, devitalized epidermis and/or dermis, exudate, debris, biofilm) including topical application(s), wound assessment, use of a whirlpool, when performed, and instruction(s) for ongoing care, per session, total wound(s) surface area; first 20 square centimeters or less

+ 97598 each additional 20 square centimeters or part thereof (List separately in addition to code for primary procedure)

> (Use 97598 in conjunction with 97597)

97602 Removal of devitalized tissue from wound(s), non-selective debridement, without anesthesia (eg, wet-to-moist dressings, enzymatic, abrasion), including topical application(s), wound assessment, and instruction(s) for ongoing care, per session

97605 Negative pressure wound therapy (eg, vacuum assisted drainage collection), including topical application(s), wound assessment, and instruction(s) for ongoing care, per session; total wound(s) surface area less than or equal to 50 square centimeters

97606 total wound(s) surface area greater than 50 square centimeters

TESTS AND MEASUREMENTS

> (For muscle testing, manual or electrical, joint range of motion, electromyography or nerve velocity determination, see 95831-95857, 95860-95872, 95885-95887, 95907-95913)

97750 Physical performance test or measurement (eg, musculo-skeletal, functional capacity), with written report, each 15 minutes

▲ **97755** Assistive technology assessment (eg, to restore, augment or compensate for existing function, optimize functional tasks and/or maximize environmental accessibility), direct one-on-one contact, with written report, each 15 minutes

1237

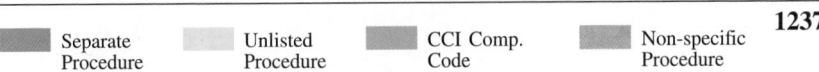

| Separate Procedure | Unlisted Procedure | CCI Comp. Code | Non-specific Procedure |

(To report augmentative and alternative communication devices, use 92605 or 92607)

ORTHOTIC MANAGEMENT AND PROSTHETIC MANAGEMENT

97760   Orthotic(s) management and training (including assessment and fitting when not otherwise reported), upper extremity(s), lower extremity(s) and/or trunk, each 15 minutes

(Code 97760 should not be reported with 97116 for the same extremity)

97761   Prosthetic training, upper and/or lower extremity(s), each 15 minutes

97762   Checkout for orthotic/prosthetic use, established patient, each 15 minutes

OTHER PROCEDURES

(For extracorporeal shock wave musculoskeletal therapy, see Category III codes 0019T, 0101T, 0102T)

97799   Unlisted physical medicine/rehabilitation service or procedure

MEDICAL NUTRITION THERAPY

Medical nutrition therapy (MNT) is the assessment of nutritional status followed by nutritional therapy. The nutrition assessment includes review and analysis of 1) medical, nutrition and medication histories, 2) physical examination, 3) anthropometric measurements, and 4) laboratory test values. Nutrition therapy may include 1) diet modification, 2) counseling and education, 3) disease self-management skills training, and 4) administration of specialized therapies such as medical foods, intravenous or tube feedings.

97802   Medical nutrition therapy; initial assessment and intervention, individual, face-to-face with the patient, each 15 minutes

97803   re-assessment and intervention, individual, face-to-face with the patient, each 15 minutes

97804   group (2 or more individual(s)), each 30 minutes

(Physicians and other qualified health care professional who may report evaluation and management services should use the appropriate E/M codes)

● New Code   ▲ Revised Code   + Add-On Code   ⊘ Modifier -51 Exempt   ⊙ Moderate Sedation

ACUPUNCTURE

Acupuncture refers to the insertion of thin needles through the skin at specific points on the body to control pain and other symptoms. It is a type of complementary and alternative medicine. The acupuncture needle is a stainless steel needle that is slightly thicker than a human hair. The specific spot on the body where a acupuncture needle may be inserted is call an acupuncture point or acupoint.

Acupuncture is reported based on 15-minute increments of personal (face-to-face) contact with the patient, not the duration of acupuncture needle(s) placement.

If no electrical stimulation is used during a 15-minute increment, use 97810, 97811. If electrical stimulation of any needle is used during a 15-minute increment, use 97813, 97814.

Only one code may be reported for each 15-minute increment. Use either 97810 or 97813 for the initial 15-minute increment. Only one initial code is reported per day.

Evaluation and Management services may be reported in addition to acupuncture procedures when performed by physicians or other qualified health care professionals who may report E/M services, including new or established patient office or other outpatient services (99201-99215), hospital observation care (99217-99220, 99224-99226), hospital care (99221-99223, 99231-99233), office or other outpatient consultations (99241-99245), inpatient consultations (99251-99255), critical care services (99291, 99292), inpatient neonatal intensive care services and pediatric and neonatal critical care services (99466-99480), emergency department service (99281-99285), nursing facility services (99304-99318), domiciliary, rest home, or custodial care services (99324-99337), and home services (99341-99350) may be reported separately, using modifier -25, if the patient's condition requires a significant separately identifiable E/M service above and beyond the usual preservice and postservice work associated with the acupuncture services. The time of the E/M service is not included in the time of the acupuncture service.

97810   Acupuncture, one or more needles; without electrical stimulation, initial 15 minutes of personal one-on-one contact with the patient

(Do not report 97810 in conjunction with 97813)

+ 97811   without electrical stimulation, each additional 15 minutes of personal one-on-one contact with the patient, with re-insertion of needle(s) (List separately in addition to code for primary procedure)

(Use 97811 in conjunction with 97810, 97813)

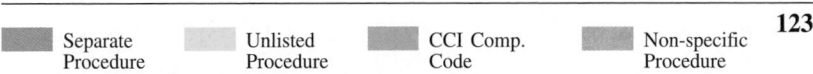

1239

Separate Procedure   Unlisted Procedure   CCI Comp. Code   Non-specific Procedure

97813   with electrical stimulation, initial 15 minutes of personal one-on-one contact with the patient

(Do not report 97813 in conjunction with 97810)

+ 97814   with electrical stimulation, each additional 15 minutes of personal one-on-one contact with the patient, with re-insertion of needle(s) (List separately in addition to code for primary procedure)

(Use 97814 in conjunction with 97810, 97813)

OSTEOPATHIC MANIPULATIVE TREATMENT

Osteopathic medicine is a system of therapy based on the theory that the body is capable of making its own remedies against disease and other toxic conditions when it is in normal structural relationship and has favorable environmental conditions and adequate nutrition. Osteopathic manipulative treatment (OMT) is a form of manual treatment applied by a physician to eliminate or alleviate somatic dysfunction and related disorders. This treatment may be accomplished by a variety of techniques.

Osteopathic Manipulative Treatment (OMT) is subject to Global Surgery Rules. Per Medicare Anesthesia Rules a provider performing OMT cannot separately report anesthesia services such as nerve blocks or epidural injections for OMT. In addition, per Medicare Global Surgery Rules, postoperative pain management after OMT (e.g., nerve block, epidural injection) is not separately reportable. Epidural or nerve block injections performed on the same date of service as OMT and unrelated to the MT may be reported with OMT using modifier -59.

Coding Rules

1.   *Evaluation and management services may be reported separately, if, and only if the patient's condition requires a significant separately identifiable evaluation and management service, above and beyond the usual pre-service and post service work associated with the osteopathic manipulation.*

2.   *CPT codes in this section are used to report OMT services provided in any location.*

Evaluation and Management services including new or established patient office or other outpatient services (99201-99215), hospital observation care (99217-99220, 99224-99226), hospital care (99221-99223, 99231-99233), office or other outpatient consultations (99241-99245), observation or inpatient care services (99234-99236), critical care services (99291, 99292), emergency department service (99281-99285), nursing facility services (99304-99318), domiciliary, rest home, or custodial care services (99324-99337), and home services (99341-99350)

1240   ● New Code   ▲ Revised Code   ➕ Add-On Code   ⊘ Modifier -51 Exempt   ⊙ Moderate Sedation

may be reported separately using modifier 25 if the patient's condition requires a significant separately identifiable E/M service, above and beyond the usual pre-service and post service work associated with the procedure. The E/M service may be caused or prompted by the same symptoms or condition for which the OMT service was provided. As such, different diagnoses are not required for the reporting of the OMT and E/M service on the same date.

98925   Osteopathic manipulative treatment (OMT); 1-2 body regions involved

98926   3-4 body regions involved

98927   5-6 body regions involved

98928   7-8 body regions involved

98929   9-10 body regions involved

CHIROPRACTIC MANIPULATIVE TREATMENT

Chiropractic medicine is a system of diagnosis and treatment based on the theory that irritation of the nervous system by mechanical, chemical or psychic factors is the cause of disease. Chiropractic services may include office visits, diagnostic tests, physical therapy, and/or chiropractic manipulation. Chiropractic manipulation treatment (CMT) is a form of manual treatment applied by a chiropractic physician to eliminate or alleviate somatic dysfunction and related disorders.

Coding Rules

1.   *Chiropractic manipulation treatment includes a pre-manipulation patient assessment.*

2.   *Evaluation and management services provided in conjunction with CMT may be reported separately with the addition of CPT modifier -25, along with any diagnostic tests or other therapy provided.*

REPORTING CHIROPRACTIC MANIPULATION TO MEDICARE

Medicare restricts the number of times the CMT code may be reported, provides a maximum reimbursement amount per year, and requires extensive supporting documentation as described below:

Documentation of Treatment Phase

Proper documentation of the treatment phase is extremely important when submitting claims for chiropractic services to Medicare. The treatment phase

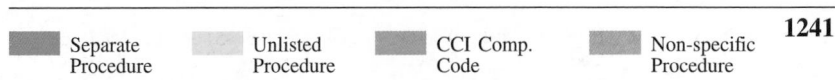

	Separate Procedure		Unlisted Procedure		CCI Comp. Code		Non-specific Procedure

consists of the date the course of treatment was initiated and the number of treatments rendered to date. Proper documentation enables Medicare to process your claims quickly and accurately. For payment of chiropractic claims, the following information must be on the CMS1500 claim form:

1. *The service must be manual manipulation of the spine. This service is reported by CPT codes 98940-98943.*

2. *The primary diagnosis must be subluxation of the spine, either so stated or identified by a term descriptive of the subluxation. The following diagnoses are acceptable because they would always involve a subluxation:*

Intervertebral disc disorders	*722.0-722.9*
Curvatures of the spine	*737.0-737.9*
Spondylolisthesis	*738.4,756.12*
Nonallopathic lesions	*739.1-739.4*
Spondylolysis	*756.11*

3. *The level of subluxation must be stated.*

4. *The symptoms related to the level of subluxation must be given.*

5. *The date of the confirming x-ray must be on the claim. Note that the x-ray must have been taken within 12 months prior to or 3 months after the course of treatment was initiated.*

6. *The date this course of treatment was initiated and the number of treatments rendered since the start of this course must be on the claim.*

Special Situations

If a patient returns with a new condition or injury, this represents a new treatment phase. The treatment phase information should reflect when you first saw the patient for this condition. Do not use the date you first saw the patient for an earlier course of treatment. Note on your CMS1500 claim form that this is a new condition. Remember that a new documenting x-ray may be required.

In the case of chronic conditions, an x-ray older than 12 months may be acceptable. For coverage of chronic conditions such as scoliosis, spondylolysis, and spondylolisthesis, there must be a reasonable expectation that there is a restorative potential. Remember that maintenance care is not covered by Medicare.

Chiropractic Manipulative Treatment Medicare covers chiropractic manipulative treatment (CMT) of five spinal regions. Physical therapy services described by CPT codes 97112, 97124 and 97140 are not separately reportable when performed in a spinal region undergoing CMT. If these physical therapy services are performed in a different region than CMT and the provider is eligible to report physical therapy codes under the Medicare program, the provider may report CMT and the above physical therapy codes using modifier -59.

The chiropractic manipulative treatment codes include a pre-manipulative patient assessment. Additional E/M services including office or other outpatient services (99201-99215), subsequent observation care (99224-99226), subsequent hospital care (99231-99233), office or other outpatient consultations (99241-99245), subsequent nursing facility services (99307-99310), domiciliary, rest home, or custodial care services (99324-99337), and home services (99341-99350) may be reported separately using modifier 25 if the patient's condition requires a significant separately identifiable E/M service, above and beyond the usual pre-service and postservice work associated with the procedure. The E/M service may be caused or prompted by the same symptoms or condition for which the CMT service was provided. As such, different diagnoses are not required for the reporting of the CMT and E/M service on the same date.

For purposes of CMT, the five spinal regions referred to are: cervical region (includes atlanto-occipital joint); thoracic region (includes costovertebral and costotransverse joints); lumbar region; sacral region; and pelvic (sacro-iliac joint) region. The five extraspinal regions referred to are: head (including temporomandibular joint, excluding atlanto-occipital) region; lower extremities; upper extremities; rib cage (excluding costotransverse and costovertebral joints) and abdomen.

98940 Chiropractic manipulative treatment (CMT); spinal, 1-2 regions

98941 spinal, 3-4 regions

98942 spinal, 5 regions

98943 extraspinal, 1 or more regions

EDUCATION AND TRAINING FOR PATIENT SELF-MANAGEMENT

The following codes are used to report educational and training services prescribed by a physician or other qualified health care professional and provided by a qualified, nonphysician health care professional using a standardized curriculum to an individual or group of patients for the treatment of established illness/disease(s) or to delay comorbidity(s). Education and training for patient self-management may be reported with these codes only when using a standardized curriculum as described below. This curriculum may be modified as necessary for the clinical needs, cultural norms and health literacy of the patient(s).

(For counseling and education provided by a physician to an individual, see the appropriate E/M codes, including office or other outpatient services [99201-99215], hospital observation care [99217-99220, 99224-99226], hospital care [99221-99223, 99231-99233], office or other outpatient consultations [99241-99245], inpatient consultations [99251-99255],

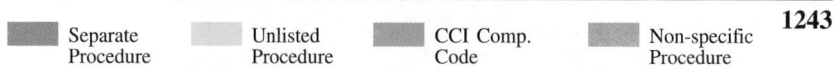

1243

| Separate Procedure | Unlisted Procedure | CCI Comp. Code | Non-specific Procedure |

emergency department services [99281-99285], nursing facility services [99304-99318], domiciliary, rest home, or custodial care services [99324-99337], home services [99341-99350], and counseling risk factor reduction and behavior change intervention [99401-99429].)

(For counseling and education provided by a physician to a group, use 99078)

(For counseling and/or risk factor reduction intervention provided by a physician to patient(s) without symptoms or established disease, see 99401-99412)

(For medical nutrition therapy, see 97802-97804)

(For health and behavior assessment/intervention that is not part of a standardized curriculum, see 96150-96155)

(For education provided as genetic counseling services, use 96040. For education to a group regarding genetic risks, see 98961, 98962)

98960   Education and training for patient self-management by a qualified, nonphysician health care professional using a standardized curriculum, face-to-face with the patient (could include caregiver/family) each 30 minutes; individual patient

98961   2-4 patients

98962   5-8 patients

NON-FACE-TO-FACE NONPHYSICIAN SERVICES

TELEPHONE SERVICES

Telephone services are non-face-to-face assessment and management services provided by a qualified health care professional to a patient via telephone. If the telephone call results in a decision to see the patient within 24 hours, the telephone call is not reported.

These codes are used to report episodes of care by the qualified health care professional initiated by an established patient or guardian of an established patient. If the telephone service ends with a decision to see the patient within 24 hours or the next available urgent visit appointment, the code is not reported; rather the encounter is considered part of the preservice work of the subsequent assessment and management service, procedure and visit. Likewise, if the telephone call refers to a service performed and reported by the qualified health care professional within the previous seven days (either qualified health care

● New Code   ▲ Revised Code   ✚ Add-On Code   ⊘ Modifier -51 Exempt   ⊙ Moderate Sedation

professional requested or unsolicited patient follow-up) or within the postoperative period of the previously completed procedure, then the service(s) are considered part of that previous service or procedure. (Do not report 98966-98969 if reporting 98966-98969 performed in the previous seven days.)

> (For telephone services provided by a physician, see 99441-99443)

98966 Telephone assessment and management service provided by a qualified nonphysician health care professional to an established patient, parent, or guardian not originating from a related assessment and management service provided within the previous 7 days nor leading to an assessment and management service or procedure within the next 24 hours or soonest available appointment; 5-10 minutes of medical discussion

98967 11-20 minutes of medical discussion

98968 21-30 minutes of medical discussion

> (Do not report 98966-98968 during the same month with 99487-99489)

> (Do not report 98966-98968 when performed during the service time of codes 99495, 99496)

ONLINE MEDICAL EVALUATION

An on-line electronic medical evaluation consists of non-face-to-face assessment and management services provided by a qualified health care professional to a patient via the internet in response to an on-line inquiry. To qualify for reporting, the service must include:

- *Timely response to the patient's inquiry by the health care professional*

- *Permanent storage of the on-line encounter (electronic or print copy is acceptable)*

- *The service may be reported only once per seven-day period for the same episode of care*

- *The reported service incorporates all related telephone calls, prescriptions, laboratory orders, etc. related to the on-line encounter.*

Reportable services involve the qualified health care professional's personal timely response to the patient's inquiry and must involve permanent storage (electronic or hard copy) of the encounter. This service is reported only once for the same episode of care during a seven-day period, although multiple qualified healthcare professionals could report their exchange with the same patient. If the on-line medical evaluation refers to an assessment and management service previously

Separate Procedure • Unlisted Procedure • CCI Comp. Code • Non-specific Procedure performed and reported by the qualified health care professional within the previous seven days (either qualified health care professional requested or unsolicited patient follow-up) or within the postoperative period of the previously completed procedure, then the service(s) are considered covered by the previous assessment and management office service or procedure. A reportable service encompasses the sum of communication (eg, related telephone calls, prescription provision, laboratory orders) pertaining to the on-line patient encounter.

(For an on-line medical evaluation provided by a physician, use 99444)

▲ **98969** Online assessment and management service provided by a qualified nonphysician health care profesional to an established patient or guardian, not originating from a related assessment and management service provided within the previous 7 days, using the internet or similar electronic communications network

(Do not report 98969 when using 99339-99340, 99374-99380 for the same communication[s])

(Do not report 98969 for anticoagulation management when reporting 99363, 99364)

(Do not report 98969 during the same month with 99487-99489)

(Do not report 98969 when performed during the service time of codes 99495, 99496)

SPECIAL SERVICES, PROCEDURES AND REPORTS

The MEDICINE section of CPT includes a subsection Special Services and Reports, with CPT codes 99000-99090 which provides the reporting physician with a means of identifying the completion of special reports and services that are an adjunct to the basic services rendered. The specific special services code reported indicates the special circumstances under which a basic procedure is performed.

The proper use of Special Services CPT codes can result in a significant increase in reimbursement. Most codes in this section are "add on" codes which means that they are used in addition to whatever other CPT codes describe the procedures or services performed.

The procedures with code numbers 99000 through 99091 provide the reporting physician or other qualified health care professional with the means of identifying the completion of special reports and services that are an adjunct to the basic services rendered. The specific number assigned indicates the special circumstances under which a basic procedure is performed.

● New Code   ▲ Revised Code   + Add-On Code   ⊘ Modifier -51 Exempt   ⊙ Moderate Sedation

Code 99091 should be reported no more than once in a 30-day period to include the physician or other qualified health care professional time involved with data accession, review and interpretation, modification of care plan as necessary (including communication to patient and/or caregiver), and associated documentation.

If the services described by 99091 are provided on the same day the patient presents for an E/M service, these services should be considered part of the E/M service and not separately reported.

Do not report 99091 if it occurs within 30 days of care plan oversight services 99374-99380. Do not report 99091 if other more specific CPT codes exist (eg, 93227, 93272 for cardiographic services; 95250 for continuous glucose monitoring). Do not report 99091 for transfer and interpretation of data from hospital or clinical laboratory computers.

Codes 99050-99060 are reported in addition to an associated basic service. Do not append modifier 51 to 99050-99060. Typically, only a single adjunct code from among 99050-99060 would be reported per patient encounter. However, there may be circumstances in which reporting multiple adjunct codes per patient encounter may be appropriate.

MISCELLANEOUS SERVICES

▲ **99000**   Handling and/or conveyance of specimen for transfer from the office to a laboratory

▲ **99001**   Handling and/or conveyance of specimen for transfer from the patient in other than an office to a laboratory (distance may be indicated)

▲ **99002**   Handling, conveyance, and/or any other service in connection with the implementation of an order involving devices (eg, designing, fitting, packaging, handling, delivery or mailing) when devices such as orthotics, protectives, prosthetics are fabricated by an outside laboratory or shop but which items have been designed, and are to be fitted and adjusted by the attending physician or other qualified health care professional

(For routine collection of venous blood, use 36415)

99024   Postoperative follow-up visit, normally included in the surgical package, to indicate that an evaluation and management service was performed during a postoperative period for a reason(s) related to the origianl procedure

(As a component of a surgical "package," see Surgery guidelines)

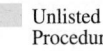 Separate Procedure   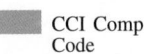 Unlisted Procedure   CCI Comp. Code   Non-specific Procedure

99026 Hospital mandated on call service; in-hospital, each hour

99027 out-of-hospital, each hour

(For standby services requiring prolonged attendance, use 99360, as appropriate. Time spent performing separately reportable procedure(s) or service(s) should not be included in the time reported as mandated on call service)

99050 Services provided in the office at times other than regularly scheduled office hours, or days when the office is normally closed (eg, holidays, Saturday or Sunday), in addition to basic service

99051 Service(s) provided in the office during regularly scheduled evening, weekend, or holiday office hours, in addition to basic service

99053 Service(s) provided between 10:00 PM and 8:00 AM at 24-hour facility, in addition to basic service

99056 Service(s) typically provided in the office, provided out of the office at request of patient, in addition to basic service

99058 Service(s) provided on an emergency basis in the office, which disrupts other scheduled office services, in addition to basic service

99060 Service(s) provided on an emergency basis, out of the office, which disrupts other scheduled office services, in addition to basic service

▲ **99070** Supplies and materials (except spectacles), provided by the physician or other qualified health care professional over and above those usually included with the office visit or other services rendered (list drugs, trays, supplies, or materials provided)

(For supply of spectacles, use the appropriate supply codes)

▲ **99071** Educational supplies, such as books, tapes, and pamphlets, for the patient's education at cost to physician or other qualified health care professional

99075 Medical testimony

▲ **99078** Physician or other qualified health care professional qualified by education, training, licensure/regulation (when applicable)

● New Code ▲ Revised Code ＋ Add-On Code ⃠ Modifier -51 Exempt ⊙ Moderate Sedation

educational services rendered to patients in a group setting (eg, prenatal, obesity, or diabetic instructions)

99080 Special reports such as insurance forms, more than the information conveyed in the usual medical communications or standard reporting form

(Do not report 99080 in conjunction with 99455, 99456 for the completion of Workmen's Compensation forms)

99082 Unusual travel (eg, transportation and escort of patient)

99090 Analysis of clinical data stored in computers (eg, ECGs, blood pressures, hematologic data)

(For physician or other qualified health care professional qualified by education, training, licensure/regulatin [when applicable] collection and interpretation of physiologic data stored/transmitted by patient/caregiver, see 99091)

(Do not report 99090 if other more specific CPT codes exist, eg, 93227, 93272, 0206T for cardiographic services; 95250 for continuous glucose monitoring; 97750 for musculoskeletal function testing)

▲ **99091** Collection and interpretation of physiologic data (eg, ECG, blood pressure, glucose monitoring) digitally stored and/or transmitted by the patient and/or caregiver to the physician or other qualified health care professional, qualified by education, training, licensure/regulation (when applicable) requiring a minimum of 30 minutes of time

QUALIFYING CIRCUMSTANCES FOR ANESTHESIA

(For explanation of these services, see Anesthesia guidelines)

+ 99100 Anesthesia for patient of extreme age, younger than 1 year and older than 70 (List separately in addition to code for primary anesthesia procedure)

(For procedure performed on infants less than 1 year of age at time of surgery, see 00326, 00561, 00834, 00836)

+ 99116 Anesthesia complicated by utilization of total body hypothermia (List separately in addition to code for primary anesthesia procedure)

1249

 Separate Procedure   Unlisted Procedure   ▨ CCI Comp. Code   ▨ Non-specific Procedure

+ 99135 Anesthesia complicated by utilization of controlled hypotension (List separately in addition to code for primary anesthesia procedure)

+ 99140 Anesthesia complicated by emergency conditions (specify) (List separately in addition to code for primary anesthesia procedure)

(An emergency is defined as existing when delay in treatment of the patient would lead to a significant increase in the threat to life or body part)

MODERATE (CONSCIOUS) SEDATION

Moderate sedation does not include minimal sedation (anxiolysis), deep sedation or monitored anesthesia care (00100-01999).

When providing moderate sedation, the following services are included and NOT reported separately:

* Assessment of the patient (not included in intraservice time);

* Establishment of IV access and fluids to maintain patency, when performed;

* Administration of agent(s);

* Maintenance of sedation;

* Monitoring of oxygen saturation, heart rate and blood pressure; and

* Recovery (not included in intraservice time).

Intraservice time starts with the administration of the sedation agent(s), requires continuous face-to-face attendance, and ends at the conclusion of personal contact by the physician providing the sedation.

Do not report 99143-99150 in conjunction with 94760-94762.

Do not report 99143-99145 in conjunction with codes listed in Appendix G. Do not report 99148-99150 in conjunction with codes listed in Appendix G when performed in the nonfacility setting.

When a second physician or other qualified health care professional other than the health care professional performing the diagnostic or therapeutic services provides moderate sedation in the facility setting (eg., hospital, outpatient hospital/ambulatory surgery center, skilled nursing facility) for the procedures listed in Appendix G, the second physician or other qualified health care professional reports 99148-99150. However, for the circumstances in which these services are performed by the second physician or other qualified health care

● New Code ▲ Revised Code + Add-On Code ⊘ Modifier -51 Exempt ⊙ Moderate Sedation

MEDICINE

professional in the nonfacility setting (eg., physician office, freestanding imaging center), codes 99148-99150 are not reported.

⊘▲**99143** Moderate sedation services (other than those services described by codes 00100-01999) provided by the same physician or other qualified health care professional performing the diagnostic or therapeutic service that the sedation supports, requiring the presence of an independent trained observer to assist in the monitoring of the patient's level of consciousness and physiological status; under 5 years of age, first 30 minutes intra-service time

⊘▲**99144** age 5 years or older, first 30 minutes intra-service time

▲**+99145** each additional 15 minutes intra-service time (List separately in addition to code for primary service)

(Use 99145 in conjunction with 99143, 99144)

▲ **99148** Moderate sedation services (other than those services described by codes 00100-01999), provided by a physician or other qualified health care professional other than the health care professional performing the diagnostic or therapeutic service that the sedation supports; younger than 5 years of age, first 30 minutes intra-service time

▲ **99149** age 5 years or older, first 30 minutes intra-service time

▲**+99150** each additional 15 minutes intra-service time (List separately in addition to code for primary service)

(Use 99150 in conjunction with 99148, 99149)

OTHER SERVICES AND PROCEDURES

99170 Anogenital examination with colposcopic magnification in childhood for suspected trauma

(For conscious sedation, use 99143-99150)

99172 Visual function screening, automated or semi-automated bilateral quantitative determination of visual acuity, ocular alignment, color vision by pseudoisochromatic plates, and field of vision (may include all or some screening of the determination(s) for contrast sensitivity, vision under glare)

(This service must employ graduated visual acuity stimuli that allow a quantitative determination of visual acuity (eg, Snellen

| ▨ Separate Procedure | ▨ Unlisted Procedure | ▨ CCI Comp. Code | ▨ Non-specific Procedure |

1251

chart). This service may not be used in addition to a gernal ophthalmological service or an E/M service)

(Do not report 99172 in conjunction with code 99173)

99173 Screening test of visual acuity, quantitative, bilateral

(The screening test used must employ graduated visual acuity stimuli that allow a quantitative estimate of visual acuity (eg, Snellen chart). Other identifiable services unrelated to this screening test provided at the same time may be reported separately (eg, preventive medicine services). When acuity is measured as part of a general ophthalmological service or of an E/M service of the eye, it is a diagnostic examination and not a screening test.)

(Do not report 99173 in conjunction with code 99172)

▲ **99174** Instrument-based ocular screening (ie, photoscreening, automated-refraction) bilateral

(Do not report 99174 in conjunction with 92002-92014, 99172, 99173)

99175 Ipecac or similar administration for individual emesis and continued observation until stomach adequately emptied of poison

(For diagnostic intubation, see 43754, 43755)

(For gastric lavage for diagnostic purposes, see 43754, 43755)

▲ **99183** Physician or other qualified health care professional attendance and supervision of hyperbaric oxygen therapy, per session

(Evaluation and Management services and/or procedures [eg, wound debridement] provided in a hyperbaric oxygen treatment facility in conjunction with a hyperbaric oxygen therapy session should be reported separately)

(99185 Deleted 2009 [2010 edition])

(99186 Deleted 2009 [2010 edition])

99190 Assembly and operation of pump with oxygenator or heat exchanger (with or without ECG and/or pressure monitoring); each hour

99191 45 minutes

● New Code   ▲ Revised Code   + Add-On Code   ⊘ Modifier -51 Exempt   ⊙ Moderate Sedation

99192   30 minutes

99195   Phlebotomy, therapeutic (separate procedure)

99199   Unlisted special service, procedure or report

HOME HEALTH PROCEDURES/SERVICES

Home health procedures/services codes are used by non-physician health care professionals to report services provided in the patient's residence.

Physicians should utilize the home visit codes 99341-99350 and utilize CPT codes other than 99500-99600 for any additional procedure/service provided to a patient living in a residence.

The following codes are used to report services provided in a patient's residence (including assisted living apartments, group homes, nontraditional private homes, custodial care facilities, or schools).

Health care professionals who are authorized to use Evaluation and Management (E/M) Home Visit codes (99341-99350) may report 99500-99600 in addition to 99341-99350 if both services are performed. E/M services may be reported separately, using modifier 25, if the patient's condition requires a significant separately identifiable E/M service, above and beyond the home health service(s)/procedure(s) codes 99500-99600.

99500   Home visit for prenatal monitoring and assessment to include fetal heart rate, non-stress test, uterine monitoring, and gestational diabetes monitoring

99501   Home visit for postnatal assessment and follow-up care

99502   Home visit for newborn care and assessment

99503   Home visit for respiratory therapy care (eg, bronchodilator, oxygen therapy, respiratory assessment, apnea evaluation)

99504   Home visit for mechanical ventilation care

99505   Home visit for stoma care and maintenance including colostomy and cystostomy

99506   Home visit for intramuscular injections

99507   Home visit for care and maintenance of catheter(s) (eg, urinary, drainage, and enteral)

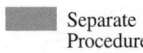 Separate Procedure   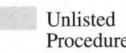 Unlisted Procedure   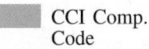 CCI Comp. Code   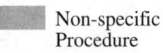 Non-specific Procedure

99509   Home visit for assistance with activities of daily living and personal care

(To report self-care/home management training, see 97535)

(To report home medical nutrition assessment and intervention services, see 97802-97804)

(To report home speech therapy services, see 92507-92508)

99510   Home visit for individual, family, or marriage counseling

99511   Home visit for fecal impaction management and enema administration

99512   Home visit for hemodialysis

(For home infusion of peritoneal dialysis, use 99601, 99602)

99600   Unlisted home visit service or procedure

HOME INFUSION PROCEDURES/SERVICES

Home infusion procedures codes are used to report per diem home visits for the purpose of administering infusions. With the exception of the infusion drug; all materials, equipments and supplies are included in the basic code. Drugs used for the infusion are coded separately.

99601   Home infusion/specialty drug administration, per visit (up to 2 hours)

+ 99602   each additional hour (List separately in addition to code for primary procedure)

(Use 99602 in conjunction with 99601)

MEDICATION THERAPY MANAGEMENT SERVICES

Medication Therapy Management Services or MTMS describes in-person patient assessment and intervention as appropriate by a pharmacist. The purpose of MTMS is to maximize medication response and/or managed medication interactions or complications. MTMS includes review of history, medication profile, and recommendations regarding outcomes and compliance. MTMS codes are not used to report product information at the point of dispensing or other routine activities related to dispensing.

● New Code   ▲ Revised Code   ✚ Add-On Code   ⊘ Modifier -51 Exempt   ⊙ Moderate Sedation

These codes are not to be used to describe the provision of product-specific information at the point of dispensing or any other routine dispensing-related activities.

99605 Medication therapy management service(s) provided by a pharmacist, individual, face-to-face with patient, with assessment and intervention if provided; initial 15 minutes, new patient

99606 initial 15 minutes, established patient

+ 99607 each additional 15 minutes (List separately in addition to code for primary service)

(Use 99607 in conjunction with 99605, 99606)

| Separate Procedure | Unlisted Procedure | CCI Comp. Code | Non-specific Procedure |

This page intentionally left blank.

● New
Code

▲ Revised
Code

✚ Add-On
Code

⊘ Modifier -51
Exempt

⊙ Moderate
Sedation

CATEGORY II CODES

This section of the CPT coding system is the Category II Performance Measurement section. The primary purpose of this section is to provide classification codes which will allow the collection of data for performance measurement.

The assignment of a Category II code to a given service or procedure does not mean that the particular service or procedure is endorsed, approved, safe or has applicability to clinical practice. The Category II code simply provides a mechanism to identify and review performance measurements.

The most current codes and their implementation dates can be found on the Web at http://www.ama-assn.org/go/cpt.

CPT Category II codes are arranged to the following categories:

Composite Measures	0001F-0015F
Patient Management	0500F-0575F
Patient History	1000F-1494F
Physical Examination	2060F
Diagnostic/Screening Pr	
Therapeutic, Preventi	
Follow-up or Other	
Patient Safety	
Structural Mea	

MOD

■ Not indicated (absence of organ/limb, already received/performed, other)

■ Contraindicated (patient allergic history, potential adverse drug interaction, other)

■ Other medical reason

2P Performance Measure Exclusion Modifier due to Patient Reason:

Reasons include:

■ Patient declined

■ Economic, social or religious reasons

■ Other patient reasons

3P Performance Measure Exclusion Modifier due to System Reason:

Reasons include:

■ Resources to perform the services not available

■ Insurance coverage/payor-related limitations

■ Other reasons attributable to health care delivery system

Modifier 8P is intended to be used as a "reporting modifier" to allow the reporting of circumstances when an action described in a measure's numerator is not performed and the reason is not otherwise specified.

8P Performance measure reporting modifier—action not performed, reason not otherwise specified

> (For blood pressure measured, use 2000F)

> (For tobacco use cessation intervention, pharmacologic therapy, use 4001F)

COMPOSITE CODES

Composite codes combine several measures grouped within a single code descriptor to facilitate reporting for a clinical condition when all components are met. If only some of the components are met, or if services are provided in addition to those included in the composite code, they may be reported individually using the corresponding CPT Category II codes for those services.

0001F Heart failure assessed (includes assessment of all the following components) (CAD)

Blood pressure measured (2000F)[1]

Level of activity assessed (1003F)[1]

Clinical symptoms of volume overload (excess) assessed (1004F)[1]

Weight, recorded (2001F)[1]

Clinical signs of volume overload (excess) assessed (2002F)[1]

(To report blood pressure measured, use 2000F)

0005F   Osteoarthritis assessed (OA)[1]

Includes assessment of all the following components:

Osteoarthritis symptoms and functional status assessed (1006F)[1]

Use of anti-inflammatory or over-the-counter (OTC) analgesic medications assessed (1007F)[1]

Initial examination of the involved joint(s) (includes visual inspection, palpation, range of motion) (2004F)[1]

(To report tobacco use cessation intervention, use 4001F)

0012F   Community-acquired bacterial pneumonia assessment (includes all of the following components) (CAP)[1]:

Co-morbid conditions assessed (1026F)[1]

Vital signs recorded (2010F)[1]

Footnotes

1-Physician Consortium for Performance Improvement (PCPI), www.physicianconsortium.org

2-National Committee on Quality Assurance (NCQA), Health Employer Data Information Set (HEDIS®), www.ncqa.org

3-Joint Commission on Accreditation of Healthcare Organizations (JCAHO), ORYX Initiative Performance Measures, www.jointcommission.org/performance_measurement.aspx

4-National Diabetes Quality Improvement Alliance (NDQIA), www.nationaldiabetesalliance.org

5-Joint measure from the Physician Consortium for Performance Improvement, www.physicianconsortium.org and National Committee on Quality Assurance (NCQA), www.ncqa.org

6-Society of Thoracic Surgeons, www.sts.org, and National Quality Forum, www.qualityforum.org

7-Ingenix, www.ingenix.com

8-American Academy of Neurology, www.aan.com/go/practic/quality/measurements or quality@aan.com

9-College of American Pathologists (CAP), www.cap.org/apps/docs/advocacy/pathology performance measurement.pdf

10-American Gastroenterological Assocation (AGA), www.gastro.org/quality

---

 Separate Procedure

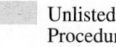 Unlisted Procedure

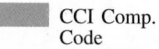 CCI Comp. Code

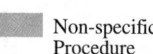 Non-specific Procedure

1259

Mental status assessed (2014F)[1]

Hydration status assessed (2018F)[1]

0014F   Comprehensive preoperative assessment performed for cataract surgery with intraocular lens (IOL) placement (includes assessment of all of the following components) (EC)[5]:

Dilated fundus evaluation performed within 12 months prior to cataract surgery (2020F)[5]

Pre-surgical (cataract) axial length, corneal power measurement and method of intraocular lens power calculation documented (must be performed within 12 months prior to surgery) (3073F)[5]

Preoperative assessment of functional or medical indication(s) for surgery prior to the cataract surgery with intraocular lens placement (must be performed within 12 months prior to cataract surgery) (3325F)[5]

0015F   Melanoma follow up completed (includes assessment of all of the following components) (ML)[5]:

History obtained regarding new or changing moles (1050F)[5]

Complete physical skin exam performed (2029F)[5]

Patient counseled to perform a monthly self skin examination (5005F)[5]

PATIENT MANAGEMENT

Patient management codes describe utilization measures or measures of patient care provided for specific clinical purposes (eg, prenatal care, pre- and post-surgical care).

0500F   Initial prenatal care visit (report at first prenatal encounter with health care professional providing obstetrical care. Report also date of visit and, in a separate field, the date of the last menstrual period [LMP]) (Prenatal)[2]

0501F   Prenatal flow sheet documented in medical record by first prenatal visit (documentation includes at minimum blood pressure, weight, urine protein, uterine size, fetal heart tones, and estimated date of delivery). Report also: date of visit and, in a separate field, the date of the last menstrual period [LMP] (Note: if reporting 0501F prenatal flow sheet, it is not necessary to report 0500F initial prenatal care visit) (Prenatal)[1]

● New Code   ▲ Revised Code   + Add-On Code   ⊘ Modifier -51 Exempt   ⊙ Moderate Sedation

0502F   Subsequent prenatal care visit (Prenatal)[2]

        [Excludes: patients who are seen for a condition unrelated to pregnancy or prenatal care (eg, an upper respiratory infection; patients seen for consultation only, not for continuing care)]

0503F   Postpartum care visit(Prenatal)[2]

0505F   Hemodialysis plan of care documented (ESRD, P_ESRD)[1]

0507F   Peritoneal dialysis plan of care documented (ESRD)[1]

0509F   Urinary incontinence plan of care documented (GER)[5]

0513F   Elevated blood pressure plan of care documented (CKD)[1]

0514F   Plan of care for elevated hemoglobin level documented for patient receiving Erythropoiesis-Stimulating Agent therapy (ESA) (CKD)[1]

0516F   Anemia plan of care documented (ESRD)[1]

0517F   Glaucoma plan of care documented (EC)[5]

0518F   Falls plan of care documented (GER)[5]

0519F   Planned chemotherapy regimen, including at a minimum: drug(s) prescribed, dose, and duration, documented prior to initiation of a new treatment regimen (ONC)[1]

Footnotes

1-Physician Consortium for Performance Improvement (PCPI), www.physicianconsortium.org

2-National Committee on Quality Assurance (NCQA), Health Employer Data Information Set (HEDIS®), www.ncqa.org

3-Joint Commission on Accreditation of Healthcare Organizations (JCAHO), ORYX Initiative Performance Measures, www.jointcommission.org/performance_measurement.aspx

4-National Diabetes Quality Improvement Alliance (NDQIA), www.nationaldiabetesalliance.org

5-Joint measure from the Physician Consortium for Performance Improvement, www.physicianconsortium.org and National Committee on Quality Assurance (NCQA), www.ncqa.org

6-Society of Thoracic Surgeons, www.sts.org, and National Quality Forum, www.qualityforum.org

7-Ingenix, www.ingenix.com

8-American Academy of Neurology, www.aan.com/go/practic/quality/measurements or quality@aan.com

9-College of American Pathologists (CAP), www.cap.org/apps/docs/advocacy/pathology performance measurement.pdf

10-American Gastroenterological Assocation (AGA), www.gastro.org/quality

---

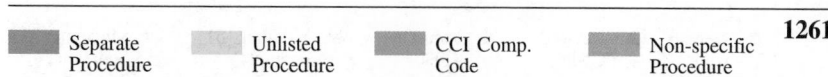

| | Separate Procedure | | Unlisted Procedure | | CCI Comp. Code | | Non-specific Procedure | **1261** |

0520F Radiation dose limits to normal tissues established prior to the initiation of a course of 3D conformal radiation for a minimum of 2 tissue/organ (ONC)[1]

0521F Plan of care to address pain documented (COA)[2] (ONC)[1]

0525F Initial visit for episode (BkP)[2]

0526F Subsequent visit for episode (BkP)[2]

0528F Recommended follow up interval for repeat colonoscopy of at least 10 years documented in colonoscopy report (End/Polyp)[5]

0529F Interval of 3 or more years since patient's last colonoscopy, documented (End/Polyp)[5]

0535F Dyspnea management plan of care, documented (Pall Cr)[5]

0540F Glucorticoid Management Plan Documented (RA)[5]

0545F Plan for follow-up care for major depressive disorder, documented (MDD ADOL)[1]

0550F Cytopathology report on routine nongynecologic specimen finalized within two working days of accession date (PATH)[9]

0551F Cytopathology report on nongynecologic specimen with documentation that the specimen was non-routine (PATH)[9]

0555F Symptom management plan of care documented (HF)[1]

0556F Plan of care to achieve lipid control documented (CAD)[1]

0557F Plan of care to manage anginal symptoms documented (CAD)[1]

0575F HIV RNA control plan of care, documented (HIV)[5]

PATIENT HISTORY

Patient history codes describe measures for select aspects of patient history or review of systems.

1000F Tobacco use assessed (CAD, CAP, COPD, PV)[1] (DM)[4]

1002F Anginal symptoms and level of activity, assessed(NMA- No Measure Associated)

● New Code	▲ Revised Code	+ Add-On Code	⊘ Modifier -51 Exempt	☉ Moderate Sedation

1003F Level of activity assessed (NMA-No Measure Associated)

1004F Clinical symptoms of volume overload (excess) assessed (NMA-No Measure Associated)

▲ **1005F** Asthma symptoms evaluated (includes documentation of numeric frequency of symptoms or patient completion of an asthma assessment tool/survey/questionnaire) (NMA-No Measure Associated)

1006F Osteoarthritis symptoms and functional status assessed (may include the use of a standardized scale or the completion of an assessment questionnaire, such as the SF-36, AAOS Hip & Knee Questionnaire) (OA)[1]

[Instructions: report when osteoarthritis is addressed during the patient encounter]

1007F Use of anti-inflammatory or analgesic over-the-counter (OTC) medications for symptom relief assessed (OA)[1]

1008F Gastrointestinal and renal risk factors assessed for patients on prescribed or OTC non-steroidal anti-inflammatory drug (NSAID) (OA)[1]

1010F Severity of angina assessed by level of activity (CAD)[1]

1011F Angina present (CAD)[1]

1012F Angina absent (CAD)[1]

Footnotes

1-Physician Consortium for Performance Improvement (PCPI), www.physicianconsortium.org

2-National Committee on Quality Assurance (NCQA), Health Employer Data Information Set (HEDIS®), www.ncqa.org

3-Joint Commission on Accreditation of Healthcare Organizations (JCAHO), ORYX Initiative Performance Measures, www.jointcommission.org/performance_measurement.aspx

4-National Diabetes Quality Improvement Alliance (NDQIA), www.nationaldiabetesalliance.org

5-Joint measure from the Physician Consortium for Performance Improvement, www.physicianconsortium.org and National Committee on Quality Assurance (NCQA), www.ncqa.org

6-Society of Thoracic Surgeons, www.sts.org, and National Quality Forum, www.qualityforum.org

7-Ingenix, www.ingenix.com

8-American Academy of Neurology, www.aan.com/go/practic/quality/measurements or quality@aan.com

9-College of American Pathologists (CAP), www.cap.org/apps/docs/advocacy/pathology performance measurement.pdf

10-American Gastroenterological Assocation (AGA), www.gastro.org/quality

---

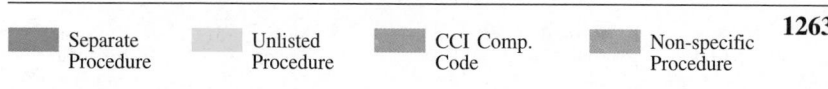

| Separate Procedure | Unlisted Procedure | CCI Comp. Code | Non-specific Procedure |

1263

1015F Chronic obstructive pulmonary disease (COPD) symptoms assessed (Includes assessment of at least one of the following: dyspnea, cough/sputum, wheezing), or respiratory symptom assessment tool completed (COPD)[1]

1018F Dyspnea assessed, not present (COPD)[1]

1019F Dyspnea assessed, present (COPD)[1]

1022F Pneumococcus immunization status assessed (CAP, COPD)[1]

1026F Co-morbid conditions assessed (eg, includes assessment for presence or absence of: malignancy, liver disease, congestive heart failure, cerebrovascular disease, renal disease, chronic obstructive pulmonary disease, asthma, diabetes, other co-morbid conditions) (CAP)[1]

1030F Influenza immunization status assessed (CAP)[1]

1031F Smoking status and exposure to second hand smoke in the home assessed (Asthma)[1]

1032F Current tobacco smoker OR currently exposed to secondhand smoke (Asthma)[1]

1033F Current tobacco non-smoker AND not currently exposed to secondhand smoke (Asthma)[1]

1034F Current tobacco smoker (CAD, CAP, COPD, PV)[1] (DM)[4]

1035F Current smokeless tobacco user (eg, chew, snuff) (PV)[1]

1036F Current tobacco non-user (CAD, CAP, COPD, PV)[1] (DM)[4]

1038F Persistent asthma (mild, moderate or severe) (Asthma)[1]

1039F Intermittent asthma (Asthma)[1]

1040F DSM-IV™ criteria for major depressive disorder documented at the initial evaluation (MDD, MDD ADOL)[1]

1050F History obtained regarding new or changing moles (ML)[5]

● **1052F** Type, anatomic location, and activity all assessed (IBD)[10]

1055F Visual functional status assessed (EC)[5]

● New Code	▲ Revised Code	+ Add-On Code	⊘ Modifier -51 Exempt	⊙ Moderate Sedation

1060F Documentation of permanent OR persistent OR paroxysmal atrial fibrillation (STR)[5]

1061F Documentation of absence of permanent AND persistent AND paroxysmal atrial fibrillation (STR)[5]

1065F Ischemic stroke symptom onset of less than 3 hours prior to arrival (STR)[5]

1066F Ischemic stroke symptom onset greater than or equal to 3 hours prior to arrival (STR)[5]

1070F Alarm symptoms (involuntary weight loss, dysphagia, or gastrointestinal bleeding) assessed; none present (GERD)[5]

1071F one or more present (GERD)[5]

(**1080F** deleted 2009 edition; to report surrogate decision maker or advance care plan documented in the medical record, report 1123F or 1124F)

1090F Presence or absence or urinary incontinence assessed (GER)[5]

1091F Urinary incontinence characterized (eg, frequency, volume, timing, type of symptoms, how bothersome) (GER)[5]

1100F Patient screened for future fall risk; documentation of two or more falls in the past year or any fall with injury in the past year (GER)[5]

Footnotes

1-Physician Consortium for Performance Improvement (PCPI), www.physicianconsortium.org

2-National Committee on Quality Assurance (NCQA), Health Employer Data Information Set (HEDIS®), www.ncqa.org

3-Joint Commission on Accreditation of Healthcare Organizations (JCAHO), ORYX Initiative Performance Measures, www.jointcommission.org/performance_measurement.aspx

4-National Diabetes Quality Improvement Alliance (NDQIA), www.nationaldiabetesalliance.org

5-Joint measure from the Physician Consortium for Performance Improvement, www.physicianconsortium.org and National Committee on Quality Assurance (NCQA), www.ncqa.org

6-Society of Thoracic Surgeons, www.sts.org, and National Quality Forum, www.qualityforum.org

7-Ingenix, www.ingenix.com

8-American Academy of Neurology, www.aan.com/go/practic/quality/measurements or quality@aan.com

9-College of American Pathologists (CAP), www.cap.org/apps/docs/advocacy/pathology performance measurement.pdf

10-American Gastroenterological Assocation (AGA), www.gastro.org/quality

---

1265

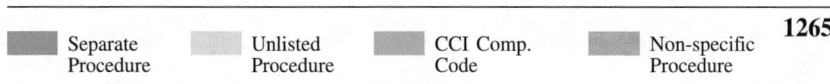

| Separate Procedure | Unlisted Procedure | CCI Comp. Code | Non-specific Procedure |

1101F documentation of no falls in the past year or only one fall without injury in the past year (GER)[5]

1110F Patient discharged from an inpatient facility (eg hospital, skilled nursing facility, or rehabilitation facility) within the last 60 days (GER)[5]

1111F Discharge medications reconciled with the current medication list in outpatient medical record (COA)[2] (GER)[5]

1116F Auricular or periauricular pain assessed (AOE)[1]

1118F Gerd symptoms assessed after 12 months of therapy (GERD)[5]

1119F Initial evaluation for condition (HEP C)[1] (EPI)[8]

1121F Subsequent evaluation for condition (HEP C)[1] (EPI)[8]

1123F Advance care planning discussed and documented advance care plan or surrogate decision maker documented in the medical record (DEM)[1] (GER, PallCr)[5]

1124F Advance care planning discussed and documented in the medical record patient did not wish or was not able to name a surrogate decision maker or provide an advance care plan (DEM)[1] (GER, PallCr)[5]

1125F Pain severity quantified; pain present (COA)[2] (ONC)[1]

1126F no pain present (COA)[2] (ONC)[1]

1127F New episode for condition (NMA-No Measure Associated)

1128F Subsequent episode for condition (NMA-No Measure Associated)

1130F Back pain and function assessed, including all of the following: Pain assessment AND functional status AND patient history, including notation of presence or absence of "red flags" (warning signs) AND assessment of prior treatment and response, AND employment status (BkP)[2]

1134F Episode of back pain lasting 6 weeks or less (BkP)[2]

1135F Episode of back pain lasting longer than 6 weeks (BkP)[2]

1136F Episode of back pain lasting 12 weeks or less (BkP)[2]

1266
● New Code	▲ Revised Code	+ Add-On Code	⊘ Modifier -51 Exempt	⊙ Moderate Sedation

1137F   Episode of back pain lasting longer than 12 weeks (BkP)[2]

1150F   Documentation that a patient has a substantial risk of death within 1 year (Pall Cr)[5]

1151F   Documentation that a patient does not have a substantial risk of death within one year (Pall Cr)[5]

1152F   Documentation of advanced disease diagnosis, goals of care prioritize comfort (Pall Cr)[5]

1153F   Documentation of advanced disease diagnosis, goals of care do not prioritize comfort (Pall Cr)[5]

1157F   Advance care plan or similar legal document present in the medical record (COA)[2]

1158F   Advance care planning discussion documented in the medical record (COA)[2]

1159F   Medication list documented in medical record (COA)[2]

1160F   Review of all medications by a prescribing practitioner or clinical pharmacist (such as, prescriptions, OTCs, herbal therapies and supplements) documented in the medical record (COA)[2]

1170F   Functional status assessed (COA)[2] (RA)[5]

Footnotes

1-Physician Consortium for Performance Improvement (PCPI), www.physicianconsortium.org

2-National Committee on Quality Assurance (NCQA), Health Employer Data Information Set (HEDIS®), www.ncqa.org

3-Joint Commission on Accreditation of Healthcare Organizations (JCAHO), ORYX Initiative Performance Measures, www.jointcommission.org/performance_measurement.aspx

4-National Diabetes Quality Improvement Alliance (NDQIA), www.nationaldiabetesalliance.org

5-Joint measure from the Physician Consortium for Performance Improvement, www.physicianconsortium.org and National Committee on Quality Assurance (NCQA), www.ncqa.org

6-Society of Thoracic Surgeons, www.sts.org, and National Quality Forum, www.qualityforum.org

7-Ingenix, www.ingenix.com

8-American Academy of Neurology, www.aan.com/go/practic/quality/measurements or quality@aan.com

9-College of American Pathologists (CAP), www.cap.org/apps/docs/advocacy/pathology performance measurement.pdf

10-American Gastroenterological Assocation (AGA), www.gastro.org/quality

---

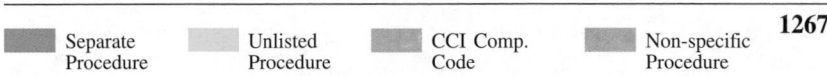

| | Separate Procedure | | Unlisted Procedure | | CCI Comp. Code | | Non-specific Procedure | **1267** |

1175F   Functional status for dementia assessed and results reviewed (DEM)[1]

1180F   All specified thromboembolic risk factors assessed (AFIB)[1]

1181F   Neuropsychiatric symptoms assessed and results reviewed (DEM)[1]

1182F   Neuropsychiatric symptoms, one or more present (DEM)[1]

1183F   Neuropsychiatric symptoms, absent (DEM)[1]

1200F   Seizure type(s) and current seizure frequency(ies) documented (EPI)[8]

1205F   Etiology of epilepsy or epilepsy syndrome(s) reviewed and documented (EPI)[8]

1220F   Patient screened for depression (SUD)[5]

1400F   Parkinson's disease diagnosis reviewed (PRKNS)[8]

1450F   Symptoms improved or remained consistent with treatment goals since last assessment (HF)[1]

1451F   Symptoms demonstrated clinically important deterioration since last assessment (HF)[1]

1460F   Qualifying cardiac event/diagnosis in previous 12 months (CAD)[1]

1461F   No qualifying cardiac event/diagnosis in previous 12 months (CAD)[1]

1490F   Dementia severity classified, mild (DEM)[1]

1491F   Dementia severity classified, moderate (DEM)[1]

1493F   Dementia severity classified, severe (DEM)[1]

1494F   Cognition assessed and reviewed (DEM)[1]

● New Code   ▲ Revised Code   + Add-On Code   ⊘ Modifier -51 Exempt   ⊙ Moderate Sedation

PHYSICAL EXAMINATION

Physical examination codes describe aspects of physical examination or clinical assessment.

2000F Blood pressure measured (CKD)[1] (DM)[2,4]

2001F Weight recorded(PAG)[1]

2002F Clinical signs of volume overload (excess) assessed (NMA-No Measure Associated)

2004F Initial examination of the involved joint(s) (includes visual inspection, palpation, range of motion) (OA)[1]

   [Instructions: report only for initial osteoarthritis visit or for visits for new joint involvement]

2010F Vital signs (temperature, pulse, respiratory rate, and blood pressure) documented and reviewed (CAP)[1](EM)[5]

2014F Mental status assessed (CAP)[1](EM)[5]

2015F Asthma impairment assessed (Asthma)[1]

2016F Asthma risk assessed (Asthma)[1]

2018F Hydration status assessed (normal/mildly dehydrated/severely dehydrated) (CAP)[1]

Footnotes

1-Physician Consortium for Performance Improvement (PCPI), www.physicianconsortium.org

2-National Committee on Quality Assurance (NCQA), Health Employer Data Information Set (HEDIS®), www.ncqa.org

3-Joint Commission on Accreditation of Healthcare Organizations (JCAHO), ORYX Initiative Performance Measures, www.jointcommission.org/performance_measurement.aspx

4-National Diabetes Quality Improvement Alliance (NDQIA), www.nationaldiabetesalliance.org

5-Joint measure from the Physician Consortium for Performance Improvement, www.physicianconsortium.org and National Committee on Quality Assurance (NCQA), www.ncqa.org

6-Society of Thoracic Surgeons, www.sts.org, and National Quality Forum, www.qualityforum.org

7-Ingenix, www.ingenix.com

8-American Academy of Neurology, www.aan.com/go/practic/quality/measurements or quality@aan.com

9-College of American Pathologists (CAP), www.cap.org/apps/docs/advocacy/pathology performance measurement.pdf

10-American Gastroenterological Assocation (AGA), www.gastro.org/quality

---

1269

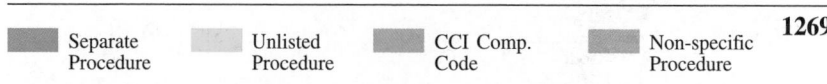

| Separate Procedure | Unlisted Procedure | CCI Comp. Code | Non-specific Procedure |

2019F   Dilated macular exam performed, including documentation of the presence or absence of macular thickening or hemorrhage AND the level of macular degeneration severity (EC)[5]

2020F   Dilated fundus evaluation performed within 12 months prior to cataract surgery (EC)[5]

2021F   Dilated macular or fundus exam performed, including documentation of the presence or absence of macular edema AND level of severity of retinopathy (EC)[5]

2022F   Dilated retinal eye exam with interpretation by an ophthalmologist or optometrist documented and reviewed (DM)[2,4]

2024F   7 standard field stereoscopic photos with interpretation by an ophthalmologist or optometrist documented and reviewed (DM)[2,4]

2026F   Eye imaging validated to match diagnosis from 7 standard field stereoscopic photos results documented and reviewed (DM)[2,4]

2027F   Optic nerve head evaluation performed (EC)[5]

2028F   Foot examination performed (includes examination through visual inspection, sensory exam with monofilament, and pulse exam — report when any of the 3 components are completed) (DM)[4]

2029F   Complete physical skin exam performed (ML)[5]

2030F   Hydration status documented, normally hydrated (PAG)[1]

2031F   Hydration status documented, dehydrated (PAG)[1]

2035F   Tympanic membrane mobility assessed with pneumatic otoscoopy or tympanometry (OME)[1]

2040F   Physical examination on the date of the initial visit for low back pain performed, in accordance with specifications (BkP)[2]

2044F   Documentation of mental health assessment prior to intervention (back surgery or epidural steroid injection) or for back pain episode lasting longer than 6 weeks (BkP)[2]

● New Code   ▲ Revised Code   ✚ Add-On Code   ⊘ Modifier -51 Exempt   ⊙ Moderate Sedation

2050F   Wound characteristics including size AND nature of wound base tissue AND amount of drainage prior to debridement documented (CWC)[5]

▲ **2060F**   Patient interviewed directly on or before date of diagnosis of major depressive disorder (MDD ADOL)[1]

DIAGNOSTIC/SCREENING PROCESSES OR RESULTS

Diagnostic/screening processes or results codes describe results of tests ordered (clinical laboratory tests, radiological or other procedural examinations and conclusions of medical decision making).

(To report blood pressure, use the corresponding systolic codes [3074F, 3075F, 3077F] and diastolic codes [3078F, 3079F, 3080F])

3006F   Chest X-ray results documented and reviewed (CAP)[1]

3008F   Body mass index (BMI), documented (PV)[1]

3011F   Lipid panel results documented and reviewed (must include total cholesterol, HDL-C, triglycerides and calculated LDL-C) (CAD)[1]

3014F   Screening mammography results documented and reviewed (PV)[1,2]

Footnotes

1-Physician Consortium for Performance Improvement (PCPI), www.physicianconsortium.org

2-National Committee on Quality Assurance (NCQA), Health Employer Data Information Set (HEDIS®), www.ncqa.org

3-Joint Commission on Accreditation of Healthcare Organizations (JCAHO), ORYX Initiative Performance Measures, www.jointcommission.org/performance_measurement.aspx

4-National Diabetes Quality Improvement Alliance (NDQIA), www.nationaldiabetesalliance.org

5-Joint measure from the Physician Consortium for Performance Improvement, www.physicianconsortium.org and National Committee on Quality Assurance (NCQA), www.ncqa.org

6-Society of Thoracic Surgeons, www.sts.org, and National Quality Forum, www.qualityforum.org

7-Ingenix, www.ingenix.com

8-American Academy of Neurology, www.aan.com/go/practic/quality/measurements or quality@aan.com

9-College of American Pathologists (CAP), www.cap.org/apps/docs/advocacy/pathology performance measurement.pdf

10-American Gastroenterological Assocation (AGA), www.gastro.org/quality

---

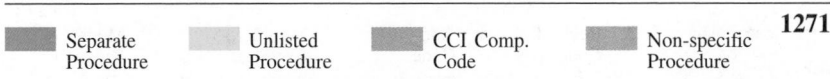

	Separate Procedure		Unlisted Procedure		CCI Comp. Code		Non-specific Procedure

1271

3015F   Cervical cancer screening results documented and reviewed (PV)[1]

3016F   Patient screened for unhealthy alcohol use using a systematic screening method (PV)[1]

3017F   Colorectal cancer screening results documented and reviewed (PV) [1,2]

3018F   Pre procedure risk assessment AND depth of insertion AND quality of the bowel prep AND complete description of polyp(s) found, including location of each polyp, size, number and gross morphology AND recommendations for follow up in final colonoscopy report documented (End/Polyp)[5]

3019F   Left ventricular ejection fracrtion (LVEF) assessment planned post discharge (HF)[1]

3020F   Left ventricular function (LVF) assessment (eg, echocardiography, nuclear test, or ventriculography) documented in the medical record (Includes quantitative or qualitative assessment results) (NMA-No Measure Associated)

3021F   Left ventricular ejection fraction (LVEF) 40% or documentation of moderately or severely depressed left ventricular systolic function (CAD, HF)[1]

3022F   Left ventricular ejection fraction (LVEF) 40% or documentation as normal or mildly depressed left ventricular systolic function (CAD, HF)[1]

3023F   Spirometry results documented and reviewed (COPD)[1]

3025F   Spirometry test results demonstrate FEV1/FVC70% with COPD symptoms (eg, dyspnea, cough/sputum, wheezing) (CAP, COPD)[1]

3027F   Spirometry test results demonstrate FEV1/FVC greater than or equal to 70% or patient does not have COPD symptoms (COPD)[1]

3028F   Oxygen saturation results documented and reviewed (Includes assessment through pulse oximetry or arterial blood gas measurement) (CAP, COPD)[1] (EM)[5]

3035F   Oxygen saturation less than or equal to 88 % or a Pa0$_2$ less than or equal to 55 mm Hg (COPD)[1]

● New Code   ▲ Revised Code   + Add-On Code   ⊘ Modifier -51 Exempt   ⊙ Moderate Sedation

3037F   Oxygen saturation greater than 88% or PaO_2 greater than 55 mmHg (COPD)[1]

3038F   Pulmonary function test performed within 12 months prior to surgery (Lung/Esop Cx)[6]

3040F   Functional expiratory volume (FEV_1) < 40% of predicted value (COPD)[1]

3042F   Functional expiratory volume (FEV_1) greater than or equal to 40% of predicted value (COPD)[1]

3044F   Most recent hemoglobin A1c (HbA1c) level < 7.0% (DM)[2,4]

3045F   Most recent hemoglobin A1c (HbA1c) level 7.0 - 9.0% (DM)[2,4]

3046F   Most recent hemoglobin A1c level greater than 9.0% (DM)[4]

   (To report most recent hemoglobin A1c level ≤ 9.0%, see codes 3044F-3045F)

3048F   Most recent LDL-C < 100 mg/dL (CAD)[1] (DM)[4]

3049F   Most recent LDL-C 100-129 mg/dL (CAD)[1] (DM)[4]

3050F   Most recent LDL-C≥ 130 mg/dL (CAD)[1] (DM)[4]

3055F   Left ventricular ejection fraction (LVEF) less than or equal to 35% (HF)[1]

Footnotes

1-Physician Consortium for Performance Improvement (PCPI), www.physicianconsortium.org

2-National Committee on Quality Assurance (NCQA), Health Employer Data Information Set (HEDIS®), www.ncqa.org

3-Joint Commission on Accreditation of Healthcare Organizations (JCAHO), ORYX Initiative Performance Measures, www.jointcommission.org/performance_measurement.aspx

4-National Diabetes Quality Improvement Alliance (NDQIA), www.nationaldiabetesalliance.org

5-Joint measure from the Physician Consortium for Performance Improvement, www.physicianconsortium.org and National Committee on Quality Assurance (NCQA), www.ncqa.org

6-Society of Thoracic Surgeons, www.sts.org, and National Quality Forum, www.qualityforum.org

7-Ingenix, www.ingenix.com

8-American Academy of Neurology, www.aan.com/go/practic/quality/measurements or quality@aan.com

9-College of American Pathologists (CAP), www.cap.org/apps/docs/advocacy/pathology performance measurement.pdf

10-American Gastroenterological Assocation (AGA), www.gastro.org/quality

---

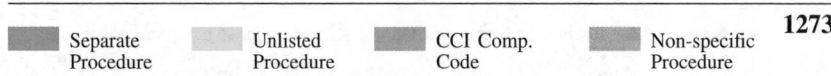

| ▮ Separate Procedure | ▮ Unlisted Procedure | ▮ CCI Comp. Code | ▮ Non-specific Procedure | **1273** |

3056F Left ventricular ejection fraction (LVEF) greater than 35% or no LVEF result available (HF)[1]

3060F Positive microalbuminuria test result documented and reviewed (DM)[2,4]

3061F Negative microalbuminuria test result documented and reviewed (DM)[2,4]

3062F Positive macroalbuminuria test result documented and reviewed (DM)[2,4]

3066F Documentation of treatment for nephropathy (eg, patient receiving dialysis, patient being treated for ESRD, CRF, ARF, or renal insufficiency, any visit to a nephrologist) (DM)[2,4]

3072F Low risk for retinopathy (no evidence of retinopathy in the prior year) (DM)[2,4]

3073F Pre-surgical (cataract) axial length, corneal power measurement and method of intraocular lens power calculation documented within 12 months prior to surgery (EC)[5]

3074F Most recent systolic blood pressure less than 130mm Hg (DM)[2,4](HTN,CKD, CAD)[1]

3075F Most recent systolic blood pressure 130-139 mm Hg (DM)[2,4](HTN,CKD, CAD)[1]

(To report most recent systolic blood pressure less than 140 mm Hg, see codes 3047F-3075F)

3077F Most recent systolic blood pressure greater than or equal to 140 mmHg (HTN,CKD, CAD)[1] (DM)[2,4]

3078F Most recent diastolic blood pressure less than 80 mm Hg (HTN,CKD, CAD)[1] (DM)[2,4]

3079F Most recent diastolic blood pressure 80-89 mm Hg (HTN,CKD, CAD)[1] (DM)[2,4]

3080F Most recent diastolic blood pressuregreater than or equal to 90 mmHg (HTN,CKD, CAD)[1] (DM)[2,4]

3082F Kt/V less than 1.2 (Clearance of urea [Kt]/volume [V]) (ESRD, P-ESRD)[1]

● New Code   ▲ Revised Code   + Add-On Code   ⊘ Modifier -51 Exempt   ⊙ Moderate Sedation

3083F   Kt/V equal to or greater than 1.2 and less than 1.7 (Clearance of urea [Kt]/volume [V]) (ESRD, P-ESRD)[1]

3084F   Kt/V greater than or equal to 1.7 (Clearance of urea [Kt]/volume [V]) (ESRD, P-ESRD)[1]

3085F   Suicide risk assessed (MDD, MDD ADOL)[1]

3088F   Major depressive disorder, mild (MDD)[1]

3089F   Major depressive disorder, moderate (MDD)[1]

3090F   Major depressive disorder, severe without psychotic features (MDD)[1]

3091F   Major depressive disorder, severe with psychotic features (MDD)[1]

3092F   Major depressive disorder, in remission (MDD)[1]

3093F   Documentation of new diagnosis of initial or recurrent episode of major depressive disorder (MDD)[1]

3095F   Central dual-energy x-ray absorptiometry (DXA) results documented (OP)[5]

3096F   Central dual-energy x-ray absorptiometry (DXA) ordered documented (OP)[5]

Footnotes

1-Physician Consortium for Performance Improvement (PCPI), www.physicianconsortium.org

2-National Committee on Quality Assurance (NCQA), Health Employer Data Information Set (HEDIS®), www.ncqa.org

3-Joint Commission on Accreditation of Healthcare Organizations (JCAHO), ORYX Initiative Performance Measures, www.jointcommission.org/performance_measurement.aspx

4-National Diabetes Quality Improvement Alliance (NDQIA), www.nationaldiabetesalliance.org

5-Joint measure from the Physician Consortium for Performance Improvement, www.physicianconsortium.org and National Committee on Quality Assurance (NCQA), www.ncqa.org

6-Society of Thoracic Surgeons, www.sts.org, and National Quality Forum, www.qualityforum.org

7-Ingenix, www.ingenix.com

8-American Academy of Neurology, www.aan.com/go/practic/quality/measurements or quality@aan.com

9-College of American Pathologists (CAP), www.cap.org/apps/docs/advocacy/pathology performance measurement.pdf

10-American Gastroenterological Assocation (AGA), www.gastro.org/quality

---

1275

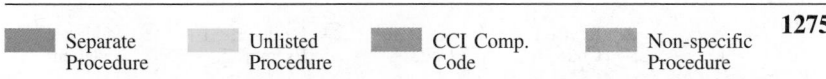

| | Separate Procedure | | Unlisted Procedure | | CCI Comp. Code | | Non-specific Procedure |

3100F Carotid imaging study report (includes direct or indirect reference to measurements of distal internal carotid diameter as the denominator for stenosis measurement) (STR, RAD)[5]

3110F Documentation in final CT or MRI report of presence or absence of hemorrhage and mass lesion and acute infarction (STR)[5]

3111F CT or MRI of the brain performed in the hospital within 24 hours of arrival OR performed in an outpatient imaging center, to confirm initial diagnosis of stroke, TIA, or intracranial hemorrhage (STR)[5]

3112F CT or MRI of the brain performed greater than 24 hours after arrival to the hospital OR performed in an outpatient imaging center for purpose other than confirmation of initial diagnosis of stroke, TIA, or intracranial hemorrhage (STR)[5]

3115F Quantitative results of an evaluation of current level of activity and clinical symptoms (HF)[1]

3117F Heart Failure disease specific structured assessment tool completed (HF)[1]

3118F New York Heart Association (NYHA) Class documented (HF)[1]

3119F No Evaluation of level of activity or clinical symptoms (HF)[1]

3120F 12-Lead ECG Performed (EM)[5]

3125F Esophageal biopsy report with statement about dysplasia (present, absent, or indefinite) (PATH)[9]

3130F Upper gastrointestinal endoscopy performed (GERD)[5]

3132F Documentation of referral for upper gastrointestinal endoscopy (GERD)[5]

3140F Upper gastrointestinal endoscopy report indicates suspicion of Barrett's esophagus (GERD)[5]

3141F Upper gastrointestinal endoscopy report indicates no suspicion of Barrett's esophagus (GERD)[5]

3142F Barium swallow test ordered (GERD)[1]

● New Code ▲ Revised Code + Add-On Code ⊘ Modifier -51 Exempt ⊙ Moderate Sedation

(To report documentation of barium swallow study, use code 3142F)

3150F Forceps esophageal biopsy performed (GERD)[5]

3155F Cytogenetic testing performed on bone marrow at time of diagnosis or prior to initiating treatment (HEM)[1]

3160F Documentation of iron stores prior to initiating erythropoietin therapy (HEM)[1]

3170F Flow cytometry studies performed at time of diagnosis or prior to initiating treatment (HEM)[1]

3200F Barium swallow test not ordered (GERD)[5]

3210F Group A Strep Test Performed (PHAR)[2]

3215F Patient has documented immunity to Hepatitis A (HEP-C)[1]

3216F Patient has documented immunity to Hepatitis B (HEP-C)[1]

(3217F deleted 2009 edtion)

3218F RNA testing for Hepatitis C documented as performed within 6 months prior to initiation of antiviral treatment for Hepatitis C (HEP-C)[1]

(3219F deleted 2009 edition)

Footnotes

1-Physician Consortium for Performance Improvement (PCPI), www.physicianconsortium.org

2-National Committee on Quality Assurance (NCQA), Health Employer Data Information Set (HEDIS®), www.ncqa.org

3-Joint Commission on Accreditation of Healthcare Organizations (JCAHO), ORYX Initiative Performance Measures, www.jointcommission.org/performance_measurement.aspx

4-National Diabetes Quality Improvement Alliance (NDQIA), www.nationaldiabetesalliance.org

5-Joint measure from the Physician Consortium for Performance Improvement, www.physicianconsortium.org and National Committee on Quality Assurance (NCQA), www.ncqa.org

6-Society of Thoracic Surgeons, www.sts.org, and National Quality Forum, www.qualityforum.org

7-Ingenix, www.ingenix.com

8-American Academy of Neurology, www.aan.com/go/practic/quality/measurements or quality@aan.com

9-College of American Pathologists (CAP), www.cap.org/apps/docs/advocacy/pathology performance measurement.pdf

10-American Gastroenterological Assocation (AGA), www.gastro.org/quality

---

1277

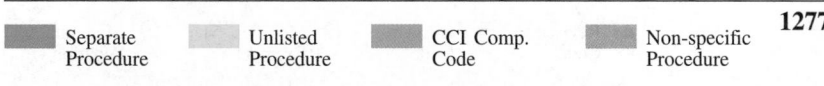

| | Separate Procedure | | Unlisted Procedure | | CCI Comp. Code | | Non-specific Procedure |

3220F   Hepatitis C quantitative RNA testing documented as performed at 12 weeks from initiation of antiviral treatment (HEP-C)[1]

3230F   Documentation that hearing test was performed within 6 months prior to tympanostomy tube insertion (OME)[1]

3250F   Specimen site other than anatomic location of primary tumor (PATH)[1]

3260F   pT category (primary tumor), pN category (regional lymph nodes), and histologic grade documented in pathology report (PATH)[1]

3265F   Ribonucleic acid (RNA) testing for Hepatitis C viremia ordered or results documented (HEP C)[1]

3266F   Hepatitis C genotype testing documented as performed prior to initiation of antiviral treatment for Hepatitis C (HEP C)[1]

3267F   Pathology report includes pT category, pN category, Gleason score, and statement about margin status (PATH)[9]

3268F   Prostate-specific antigen (PSA), AND primary tumor (T) stage, AND Gleason score documented prior to initiation of treatment (PRCA)[1]

3269F   Bone scan performed prior to initiation of treatment or at any time since diagnosis of prostate cancer (PRCA)[1]

3270F   Bone scan not performed prior to initiation of treatment nor at any time since diagnosis of prostate cancer (PRCA)[1]

3271F   Low risk of recurrence, prostate cancer (PRCA)[1]

3272F   Intermediate risk of recurrence, prostate cancer (PRCA)[1]

3273F   High risk of recurrence, prostate cancer (PRCA)[1]

3274F   Prostate cancer risk of recurrence not determined or neither low, intermediate nor high (PRCA)[1]

3278F   Serum levels of calcium, phosphorus, intact parathyroid hormone (PTH) and lipid profile ordered (CKD)[1]

3279F   Hemoglobin level greater than or equal to 13 g/dl (CKD, ESRD)[1]

● New Code   ▲ Revised Code   ✚ Add-On Code   ⊘ Modifier -51 Exempt   ⊙ Moderate Sedation

3280F Hemoglobin level 11 g/dl to 12.9 g/dl (CKD, ESRD)[1]

3281F Hemoglobin level less than 11 g/dl (CKD, ESRD)[1]

3284F Intraocular pressure (IOP) reduced by a value of greater than or equal to 15% from the pre-intervention level (EC)[5]

3285F Intraocular pressure (IOP) reduced by a value less than 15% from the pre-intervention level (EC)[5]

3288F Falls risk assessment documented (GER)[5]

3290F Patient is D (Rh) negative and unsensitized (Pre-Cr)[1]

3291F Patient is D (Rh) positive or sensitized (Pre-Cr)[1]

3292F HIV testing ordered or documented and reviewed during the first or second prenatal visit (Pre-Cr)[1]

3293F ABO and Rh blood typing documented as performed (Pre-Cr)[7]

3294F Group B streptococcus (GBS) screening documented as performed during week 35-37 gestation (Pre-Cr)[7]

3300F American Joint Committee on Cancer (AJCC) stage documented and reviewed (ONC)[1]

3301F Cancer stage documented in medical record as metastatic and reviewed (ONC)[1]

Footnotes

1-Physician Consortium for Performance Improvement (PCPI), www.physicianconsortium.org

2-National Committee on Quality Assurance (NCQA), Health Employer Data Information Set (HEDIS®), www.ncqa.org

3-Joint Commission on Accreditation of Healthcare Organizations (JCAHO), ORYX Initiative Performance Measures, www.jointcommission.org/performance_measurement.aspx

4-National Diabetes Quality Improvement Alliance (NDQIA), www.nationaldiabetesalliance.org

5-Joint measure from the Physician Consortium for Performance Improvement, www.physicianconsortium.org and National Committee on Quality Assurance (NCQA), www.ncqa.org

6-Society of Thoracic Surgeons, www.sts.org, and National Quality Forum, www.qualityforum.org

7-Ingenix, www.ingenix.com

8-American Academy of Neurology, www.aan.com/go/practic/quality/measurements or quality@aan.com

9-College of American Pathologists (CAP), www.cap.org/apps/docs/advocacy/pathology performance measurement.pdf

10-American Gastroenterological Assocation (AGA), www.gastro.org/quality

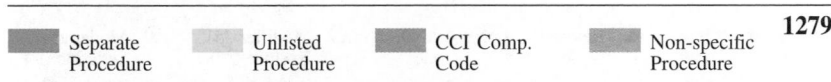

1279

Separate Procedure · Unlisted Procedure · CCI Comp. Code · Non-specific Procedure

(3302F Deleted 2009 [2010 edition]. To report measures for cancer staging, see 3321F-3390F)

(3303F Deleted 2009 [2010 edition]. To report measures for cancer staging, see 3321F-3390F)

(3304F Deleted 2009 [2010 edition]. To report measures for cancer staging, see 3321F-3390F)

(3305F Deleted 2009 [2010 edition]. To report measures for cancer staging, see 3321F-3390F)

(3306F Deleted 2009 [2010 edition]. To report measures for cancer staging, see 3321F-3390F)

(3307F Deleted 2009 [2010 edition]. To report measures for cancer staging, see 3321F-3390F)

(3308F Deleted 2009 [2010 edition]. To report measures for cancer staging, see 3321F-3390F)

(3309F Deleted 2009 [2010 edition]. To report measures for cancer staging, see 3321F-3390F)

(3310F Deleted 2009 [2010 edition]. To report measures for cancer staging, see 3321F-3390F)

(3311F Deleted 2009 [2010 edition]. To report measures for cancer staging, see 3321F-3390F)

(3312F Deleted 2009 [2010 edition]. To report measures for cancer staging, see 3321F-3390F)

(To report measures for cancer staging, see 3321F-3390F)

3315F Estrogen receptor (ER) or progesterone receptor (PR) positive breast cancer (ONC)[1]

3316F Estrogen receptor (ER) and progesterone receptor (PR) negative breast cancer (ONC)[1]

3317F Pathology report confirming malignancy documented in the medical record and reviewed prior to the initiation of chemotherapy (ONC)[1]

● New Code ▲ Revised Code ✛ Add-On Code ⊘ Modifier -51 Exempt ⊙ Moderate Sedation

3318F Pathology report confirming malignancy documented in the medical record and reviewed prior to the initiation of radiation therapy (ONC)[1]

3319F 1 of the following diagnostic imaging studies ordered: chest X-ray, CT, ultrasound, MRI, PET, or nuclear medicine scans (ML)[5]

3320F None of the following diagnostic imaging studies ordered: chest X-ray, CT, ultrasound, MRI, PET, or nuclear medicine scans (ML)[5]

3321F AJCC Cancer Stage 0 or IA Melanoma, documented (ML)[5]

3322F Melanoma greater than AJCC Stage 0 or IA (ML)[5]

3323F Clinical tumor, node and metastases (TNM) staging documented and reviewed prior to surgery (Lung/Esop Cx)[6]

3324F MRI or CT scan ordered, reviewed or requested (EPI)[8]

3325F Preoperative assessment of functional or medical indication(s) for surgery prior to the cataract surgery with intraocular lens placement (must be performed within twelve months prior to cataract surgery) (EC)[5]

3328F Performance status documented and reviewed within 2 weeks prior to surgery (Lung/Esop Cx)[6]

3330F Imaging study ordered (BkP)[2]

Footnotes

1-Physician Consortium for Performance Improvement (PCPI), www.physicianconsortium.org

2-National Committee on Quality Assurance (NCQA), Health Employer Data Information Set (HEDIS®), www.ncqa.org

3-Joint Commission on Accreditation of Healthcare Organizations (JCAHO), ORYX Initiative Performance Measures, www.jointcommission.org/performance_measurement.aspx

4-National Diabetes Quality Improvement Alliance (NDQIA), www.nationaldiabetesalliance.org

5-Joint measure from the Physician Consortium for Performance Improvement, www.physicianconsortium.org and National Committee on Quality Assurance (NCQA), www.ncqa.org

6-Society of Thoracic Surgeons, www.sts.org, and National Quality Forum, www.qualityforum.org

7-Ingenix, www.ingenix.com

8-American Academy of Neurology, www.aan.com/go/practic/quality/measurements or quality@aan.com

9-College of American Pathologists (CAP), www.cap.org/apps/docs/advocacy/pathology performance measurement.pdf

10-American Gastroenterological Assocation (AGA), www.gastro.org/quality

---

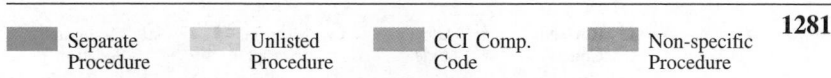

| Separate Procedure | Unlisted Procedure | CCI Comp. Code | Non-specific Procedure |

1281

3331F   Imaging study not ordered (BkP)[2]

3340F   Mammogram assessment category of "incomplete: need additional imaging evaluation", documented (RAD)[5]

3341F   Mammogram assessment category of "negative", documented (RAD)[5]

3342F   Mammogram assessment category of "benign", documented (RAD)[5]

3343F   Mammogram assessment category of "probably benign", documented (RAD)[5]

3344F   Mammogram assessment category of "suspicious", documented (RAD)[5]

3345F   Mammogram assessment category of "highly suggestive of malignancy", documented (RAD)[5]

3350F   Mammogram assessment category of "known biopsy proven malignancy", documented (RAD)[5]

3351F   Negative screen for depressive symptoms as categorized by using a standardized depression screening/assessment tool (MDD)[2]

3352F   No significant depressive symptoms as categorized by using a standardized depression assessment tool (MDD)[2]

3353F   Mild to moderate depressive symptoms as categorized by using a standardized depression screening/assessment tool (MDD)[2]

3354F   Clinically significant depressive symptoms as categorized by using a standardized depression screening/assessment tool (MDD)[2]

3370F   AJCC Breast Cancer Stage 0 documented (ONC)[1]

3372F   AJCC Breast Cancer Stage I: T1mic, T1a or T1b (tumor size <= 1 cm) documented (ONC)[1]

3374F   AJCC Breast Cancer Stage I: T1c (tumor size > 1 cm to 2 cm) documented (ONC)[1]

3376F   AJCC Breast Cancer Stage II documented (ONC)[1]

● New Code   ▲ Revised Code   + Add-On Code   ⊘ Modifier -51 Exempt   ⊙ Moderate Sedation

3378F AJCC Breast Cancer Stage III documented (ONC)[1]

3380F AJCC Breast Cancer Stage IV documented (ONC)[1]

3382F AJCC colon cancer, Stage 0 documented (ONC)[1]

3384F AJCC colon cancer, Stage I documented (ONC)[1]

3386F AJCC colon cancer, Stage II documented (ONC)[1]

3388F AJCC colon cancer, Stage III documented (ONC)[1]

3390F AJCC colon cancer, Stage IV documented (ONC)[1]

3394F Quantitative HER2 immunohistochemistry (IHC) evaluation of breast cancer consistent with the scoring system defined in the ASCO/CAP guidelines (PATH)[9]

3395F Quantitative non-HER2 immunohistochemistry (IHC) evaluation of breast cancer (eg, testing for estrogen or progesterone receptors [ER/PR]) performed (PATH)[9]

3450F Dyspnea screened, no dyspnea or mild dyspnea (Pall Cr)[5]

3451F Dyspnea screened, moderate or severe dyspnea (Pall Cr)[5]

3452F Dyspnea not screened (Pall Cr)[5]

Footnotes

1-Physician Consortium for Performance Improvement (PCPI), www.physicianconsortium.org

2-National Committee on Quality Assurance (NCQA), Health Employer Data Information Set (HEDIS®), www.ncqa.org

3-Joint Commission on Accreditation of Healthcare Organizations (JCAHO), ORYX Initiative Performance Measures, www.jointcommission.org/performance_measurement.aspx

4-National Diabetes Quality Improvement Alliance (NDQIA), www.nationaldiabetesalliance.org

5-Joint measure from the Physician Consortium for Performance Improvement, www.physicianconsortium.org and National Committee on Quality Assurance (NCQA), www.ncqa.org

6-Society of Thoracic Surgeons, www.sts.org, and National Quality Forum, www.qualityforum.org

7-Ingenix, www.ingenix.com

8-American Academy of Neurology, www.aan.com/go/practic/quality/measurements or quality@aan.com

9-College of American Pathologists (CAP), www.cap.org/apps/docs/advocacy/pathology performance measurement.pdf

10-American Gastroenterological Assocation (AGA), www.gastro.org/quality

---

1283

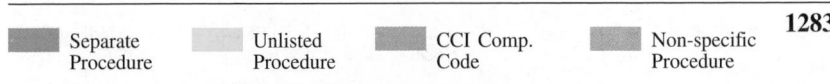

| | Separate Procedure | | Unlisted Procedure | | CCI Comp. Code | | Non-specific Procedure |

3455F   TB screening performed and results interpreted within six months prior to initiation of first time biologic disease modifying anti rheumatic drug therapy for RA (RA)[5]

3470F   Rheumatoid arthritis (RA) disease activity, low (RA)[5]

3471F   Rheumatoid arthritis (RA) disease activity, moderate (RA)[5]

3472F   Rheumatoid arthritis (RA) disease activity, high (RA)[5]

3475F   Disease prognosis for rheumatoid arthritis assessed, poor prognosis documented (RA)[5]

3476F   Disease prognosis for rheumatoid arthritis assessed, good prognosis documented (RA)[5]

3490F   History of AIDS defining condition (HIV)[5]

3491F   HIV indeterminate (infants of undetermined HIV status born of HIV infected mothers) (HIV)[5]

3492F   History of nadir CD4+ cell count <350 cells/mm (HIV)[5]

3493F   No history of nadir CD4+ cell count <350 cells/mm AND no history of AIDS defining condition (HIV)[5]

3494F   CD4+ cell count <200 cells/mm (HIV)[5]

3495F   CD4+ cell count 200 - 499 cells/mm (HIV)[5]

3496F   CD4+ cell count >=500 cells/mm (HIV)[5]

3497F   CD4+ cell percentage <15% (HIV)[5]

3498F   CD4+ cell percentage >=15% (HIV)[5]

3500F   CD4+ cell count or CD4+ cell percentage documented as performed (HIV)[5]

3502F   HIV RNA viral load below limits of quantification (HIV)[5]

3503F   HIV RNA viral load not below limits of quantification (HIV)[5]

3510F   Documentation that tuberculosis (TB) screening test performed and results interpreted (HIV)[5]

● New Code   ▲ Revised Code   + Add-On Code   ⊘ Modifier -51 Exempt   ⊙ Moderate Sedation

3511F Chlamydia and gonorrhea screenings documented as performed (HIV)[5]

3512F Syphilis screening documented as performed (HIV)[5]

3513F Hepatitis B screening documented as performed (HIV)[5]

3514F Hepatitis C screening documented as performed (HIV)[5]

3515F Patient has documented immunity to Hepatitis C (HIV)[5]

● **3517F** Hepatitis B Virus (HBV) status assessed and results interpreted within one year prior to receiving a first course of anti-TNF (tumor necrosis factor) therapy (IBD)[10]

● **3520F** Clostridium difficile testing performed (IBD)[10]

3550F Low risk for thromboembolism (AFIB)[1]

3551F Intermediate risk for thromboembolism (AFIB)[1]

3552F High risk for thromboembolism (AFIB)[1]

3555F Patient had International Normalized Ratio (INR) measurement performed (AFIB)[1]

3570F Final report for bone scintigraphy study includes correlation with existing relevant imaging studies (eg, x ray, MRI, CT) corresponding to the same anatomical region in question (NUC_MED)[1]

Footnotes

1-Physician Consortium for Performance Improvement (PCPI), www.physicianconsortium.org

2-National Committee on Quality Assurance (NCQA), Health Employer Data Information Set (HEDIS®), www.ncqa.org

3-Joint Commission on Accreditation of Healthcare Organizations (JCAHO), ORYX Initiative Performance Measures, www.jointcommission.org/performance_measurement.aspx

4-National Diabetes Quality Improvement Alliance (NDQIA), www.nationaldiabetesalliance.org

5-Joint measure from the Physician Consortium for Performance Improvement, www.physicianconsortium.org and National Committee on Quality Assurance (NCQA), www.ncqa.org

6-Society of Thoracic Surgeons, www.sts.org, and National Quality Forum, www.qualityforum.org

7-Ingenix, www.ingenix.com

8-American Academy of Neurology, www.aan.com/go/practic/quality/measurements or quality@aan.com

9-College of American Pathologists (CAP), www.cap.org/apps/docs/advocacy/pathology performance measurement.pdf

10-American Gastroenterological Assocation (AGA), www.gastro.org/quality

---

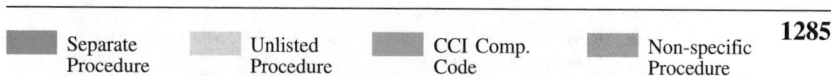

| Separate Procedure | Unlisted Procedure | CCI Comp. Code | Non-specific Procedure |

1285

3572F Patient considered to be potentially at risk for fracture in a weight bearing site (NUC_MED)[1]

3573F Patient not considered to be potentially at risk for fracture in a weight bearing site (NUC_MED)[1]

3650F Electroencephalogram (EEG) ordered, reviewed or requested (EPI)[8]

3700F Psychiatric disorders or disturbances assessed (Prkns)[8]

3702F Cognitive impairment or dysfunction assessed (Prkns)[8]

3725F Screening for depression performed (DEM)[1]

● **3750F** Patient not receiving dose of corticosteroids greater than or equal to 10 mg/day for 60 or greater consecutive days (IBD)[10]

THERAPEUTIC, PREVENTIVE OR OTHER INTERVENTIONS

Therapeutic, preventive or other interventions codes describe pharmacologic, procedural, or behavioral therapies, including preventive services such as patient education and counseling.

4000F Tobacco use cessation intervention, counseling (COPD, CAP, CAD, Asthma)[1](DM)[4](PV)[2]

4001F Tobacco use cessation intervention, pharmacologic therapy (COPD, CAD, CAP, PV, Asthma)[1] (DM)[4] (PV)[2]

(**4002F** deleted 2011 [2012 edition]. To report statin therapy, use 4013F)

4003F Patient education, written/oral, appropriate for patients with heart failure performed (NMA-No Measure Associated)

4004F Patient screened for tobacco use AND received tobacco cessation intervention (counseling, pharmacotherapy, or both), if identified as a tobacco user (PV, CAD)[1]

4005F Pharmacologic therapy (other than minerals/vitamins) for osteoporosis prescribed (OP)[5]

(**4006F** deleted 2011 [2012 edition]. To report beta blocker therapy, use 4008F)

● New Code   ▲ Revised Code   + Add-On Code   ⊘ Modifier -51 Exempt   ⊙ Moderate Sedation

(4007F   deleted 2009 edition. To report age related eye disease study (AREDS) formulation prescribed or recommended, use 4177F)

4008F   Beta-blocker therapy prescribed or currently being taken (CAD,HF)[1]

(4009F   deleted 2011 [2012 edition]. To report angiotensin converting enzyme [ACE] inhibitor or angiotensin receptor blocker [ARB] therapy, use 4010F)

4010F   Angiotensin converting enzyme (ACE) inhibitor or angiotensin receptor blocker (ARB) therapy prescribed or currently being taken (CAD, CKD, HF)[1] (DM)[2]

4011F   Oral antiplatelet therapy prescribed (CAD)[1]

4012F   Warfarin therapy prescribed (NMA-No Measure Associated)

4013F   Statin therapy prescrived or currently being taken (CAD)[1]

4014F   Written discharge instructions provided to heart failure patients discharged home. (Instructions include all of the following components: activity level, diet, discharge medications, follow-up appointment, weight monitoring, what to do if symptoms worsen) (NMA-No Measure Associated)

         [Excludes patients less than 18 years of age]

4015F   Persistent asthma, preferred long term control medication or an acceptable alternative treatment, prescribed (NMA-No Meausre Associated)

Footnotes

1-Physician Consortium for Performance Improvement (PCPI), www.physicianconsortium.org

2-National Committee on Quality Assurance (NCQA), Health Employer Data Information Set (HEDIS®), www.ncqa.org

3-Joint Commission on Accreditation of Healthcare Organizations (JCAHO), ORYX Initiative Performance Measures, www.jointcommission.org/performance_measurement.aspx

4-National Diabetes Quality Improvement Alliance (NDQIA), www.nationaldiabetesalliance.org

5-Joint measure from the Physician Consortium for Performance Improvement, www.physicianconsortium.org and National Committee on Quality Assurance (NCQA), www.ncqa.org

6-Society of Thoracic Surgeons, www.sts.org, and National Quality Forum, www.qualityforum.org

7-Ingenix, www.ingenix.com

8-American Academy of Neurology, www.aan.com/go/practic/quality/measurements or quality@aan.com

9-College of American Pathologists (CAP), www.cap.org/apps/docs/advocacy/pathology performance measurement.pdf

10-American Gastroenterological Assocation (AGA), www.gastro.org/quality

---

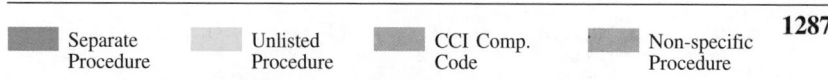

Separate Procedure	Unlisted Procedure	CCI Comp. Code	Non-specific Procedure

1287

[Note: There are no medical exclusion criteria]

(Do not report modifier 1P with 4015F)

(To report patient reasons for not prescribing, use modifier 2P)

4016F Anti-inflammatory/analgesic agent prescribed (OA)[1]

(Use for prescribed or continued medication(s), including over-the-counter medication[s])

4017F Gastrointestinal prophylaxis for NSAID use prescribed (OA)[1]

4018F Therapeutic exercise for the involved joint(s) instructed or physical or occupational therapy prescribed (OA)[1]

4019F Documentation of receipt of counseling on exercise AND either both calcium and vitamin D use or counseling regarding both calcium and vitamin D use (OP)[5]

4025F Inhaled bronchodilator prescribed (COPD)[1]

4030F Long term oxygen therapy prescribed (more than fifteen hours per day) (COPD)[1]

4033F Pulmonary rehabilitation exercise training recommended (COPD)[1]

(Report 4033F with 1019F)

4035F Influenza immunization recommended (COPD)[1]

4037F Influenza immunization ordered or administered (COPD, PV, CKD, ESRD)[1]

4040F Pneumococcal vaccine administered or previously received (COPD)[1], (PV)[1,2]

4041F Documentation of order for cefazolin OR cefurozime for antimicrobial prophylaxis (PERI 2)[5]

4042F Documentation that prophylactic antibiotics were neither given within 4 hours prior to surgical incision nor given intraoperatively (PERI 2)[5]

4043F Documentation that an order was given to discontinue prophylactic antibiotics within 48 hours of surgical end time, cardiac procedures (PERI 2)[5]

● New Code   ▲ Revised Code   + Add-On Code   ⊘ Modifier -51 Exempt   ⊙ Moderate Sedation

4044F Documentation that an order was given for venous thromboembolism (VTE) prophylaxis to be given within 24 hours prior to incision time or 24 hours after surgery end time (PERI 2)[5]

4045F Appropriate empiric antibiotic prescribed (CAP)[1] (EM)[5]

4046F Documentation that prophylactic antibiotics were given within 4 hours prior to surgical incision or given intraoperatively (PERI 2)[5]

4047F Documentation of order for prophylactic parenteral antibiotics to be given within 1 hour (if fluoroquinolone or vancomycin, 2 hours) prior to surgical incision (or start of procedure when no incision is required) (PERI 2)[5]

4048F Documentation that administration of prophylactic parenteral antibiotic was initiated within 1 hour (if fluoroquinolone or vancomycin, 2 hours) prior to surgical incision (or start of procedure when no incision is required), as ordered (PERI 2)[5]

4049F Documentation that order was given to discontinue prophylactic antibiotics within 24 hours of surgical end time, non-cardiac procedure (PERI 2)[5]

4050F Hypertension plan of care documented as appropriate (NMA-No Measure Associated)

4051F Referred for an arterio-venous (AV) fistula (ESRD, CKD)[1]

Footnotes

1-Physician Consortium for Performance Improvement (PCPI), www.physicianconsortium.org

2-National Committee on Quality Assurance (NCQA), Health Employer Data Information Set (HEDIS®), www.ncqa.org

3-Joint Commission on Accreditation of Healthcare Organizations (JCAHO), ORYX Initiative Performance Measures, www.jointcommission.org/performance_measurement.aspx

4-National Diabetes Quality Improvement Alliance (NDQIA), www.nationaldiabetesalliance.org

5-Joint measure from the Physician Consortium for Performance Improvement, www.physicianconsortium.org and National Committee on Quality Assurance (NCQA), www.ncqa.org

6-Society of Thoracic Surgeons, www.sts.org, and National Quality Forum, www.qualityforum.org

7-Ingenix, www.ingenix.com

8-American Academy of Neurology, www.aan.com/go/practic/quality/measurements or quality@aan.com

9-College of American Pathologists (CAP), www.cap.org/apps/docs/advocacy/pathology performance measurement.pdf

10-American Gastroenterological Assocation (AGA), www.gastro.org/quality

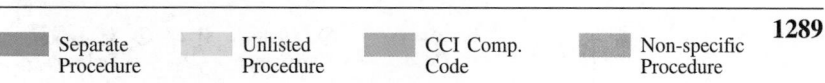

Separate Procedure Unlisted Procedure CCI Comp. Code Non-specific Procedure **1289**

4052F   Hemodialysis via functioning arteriovenous (AV) fistula (ESRD)[1]

4053F   Hemodialysis via functioning arteriovenous (AV) graft (ESRD)[1]

4054F   Hemodialysis via catheter (ESRD)[1]

4055F   Patient receiving peritoneal dialysis (ESRD)[1]

4056F   Appropriate oral rehydration solution recommended (PAG)[1]

4058F   Pediatric gastroenteritis education provided to caregiver (PAG)[1]

4060F   Psychotherapy services provided (MDD, MDD ADOL)[1]

4062F   Patient referral for psychotherapy documented (MDD, MDD ADOL)[1]

4063F   Antidepressant pharmacotherapy considered and not prescribed (MDD ADOL)[1]

4064F   Antidepressant pharmacotherapy prescribed (MDD, MDD ADOL)[1]

4065F   Antipsychotic pharmacotherapy prescribed (MDD)[1]

4066F   Electroconvulsive therapy (ECT) provided (MDD)[1]

4067F   Patient referral for electroconvulsive therapy (ECT) documented (MDD)[1]

● **4069F**   Venous thromboembolism (VTE) prophylaxis received (IBD)[10]

4070F   Deep vein thrombosis (DVT) prophylaxis received by end of hospital day 2 (STR)[5]

4073F   Oral antiplatelet therapy prescribed at discharge (STR)[5]

4075F   Anticoagulant therapy prescribed at discharge (STR)[5]

4077F   Documentation that tissue plasminogen activator (t-PA) administration was considered (STR)[5]

4079F   Documentation that rehabilitation services were considered (STR)[5]

● New Code   ▲ Revised Code   + Add-On Code   ⊘ Modifier -51 Exempt   ⊙ Moderate Sedation

4084F   Aspirin received within 24 hours before emergency department arrival or during emergency department stay (EM)[5]

4086F   Aspirin or clopidogrel prescribed or currently being taken (CAD)[1]

4090F   Patient receiving erythropoietin therapy (HEM)[1]

4095F   Patient not receiving erythropoietin therapy (HEM)[1]

4100F   Bisphosphonate therapy, intravenous, ordered or received (HEM)[1]

4110F   Internal mammary artery graft performed for primary, isolated coronary artery bypass graft procedure (CABG)[6]

4115F   Beta blocker administered within 24 hours prior to surgical incision (CABG)[6]

4120F   Antibiotic prescribed or dispensed (URI, PHAR)[2], (A-BRONCH)[2]

4124F   Antibiotic neither prescribed nor dispensed (URI, PHAR)[2], (A-BRONCH)[2]

4130F   Topical preparations (including OTC) prescribed for acute otitis externa (AOE)[1]

4131F   Systemic antimicrobial therapy prescribed (AOE)[1]

Footnotes

1-Physician Consortium for Performance Improvement (PCPI), www.physicianconsortium.org

2-National Committee on Quality Assurance (NCQA), Health Employer Data Information Set (HEDIS®), www.ncqa.org

3-Joint Commission on Accreditation of Healthcare Organizations (JCAHO), ORYX Initiative Performance Measures, www.jointcommission.org/performance_measurement.aspx

4-National Diabetes Quality Improvement Alliance (NDQIA), www.nationaldiabetesalliance.org

5-Joint measure from the Physician Consortium for Performance Improvement, www.physicianconsortium.org and National Committee on Quality Assurance (NCQA), www.ncqa.org

6-Society of Thoracic Surgeons, www.sts.org, and National Quality Forum, www.qualityforum.org

7-Ingenix, www.ingenix.com

8-American Academy of Neurology, www.aan.com/go/practic/quality/measurements or quality@aan.com

9-College of American Pathologists (CAP), www.cap.org/apps/docs/advocacy/pathology performance measurement.pdf

10-American Gastroenterological Assocation (AGA), www.gastro.org/quality

---

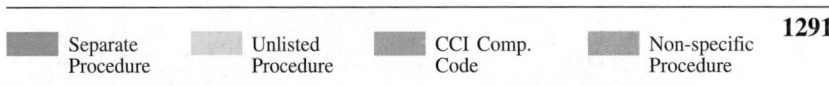

	Separate Procedure		Unlisted Procedure		CCI Comp. Code		Non-specific Procedure

4132F   Systemic antimicrobial therapy not prescribed (AOE)[1]

4133F   Antihistamines or decongestants prescribed or recommended (OME)[1]

4134F   Antihistamines or decongestants neither prescribed nor recommended (OME)[1]

4135F   Systemic corticosteroids prescribed (OME)[1]

4136F   Sysemic corticosteroids not prescribed (OME)[1]

4140F   Inhalded corticosteroids prescribed (Asthma)[1]

● **4142F**   Corticosteroid sparing therapy prescribed (IBD)[10]

4144F   Alternative long-term control medication prescribed (Asthma)[1]

4145F   Two or more anti-hypertensive agents prescribed or currently being taken (CAD, HTN)[1]

4148F   Hepatitis A vaccine injection administered or previously received (Hep-C)[1]

4149F   Hepatitis B vaccine injection administered or previously received (Hep-C, HIV)[1]

4150F   Patient receiving antiviral treatment for Hepatitis C (Hep-C)[1]

4151F   Patient not receiving antiviral treatment for Hepatitis C (Hep-C)[1]

(4152F   Deleted 2009 [2010 edition])

4153F   Combination peginterferon and ribavirin therapy prescribed (HEP-C)[1]

(4154F   Deleted 2009 [2010 edition])

4155F   Hepatitis A vaccine series previously received (Hep-C)[1]

(4156F   Deleted 2009 [2010 edition])

4157F   Hepatitis B vaccine series previously received (Hep-C)[1]

4158F   Patient counseled about risk of alcohol use (Hep-C)[1]

● New Code   ▲ Revised Code   + Add-On Code   ⊘ Modifier -51 Exempt   ⊙ Moderate Sedation

4159F   Counseling regarding contraception received prior to initiation of antiviral treatment (Hep-C)[1]

4163F   Patient counseling at a minimum on all of the following treatment options for clinically localized prostate cancer: active surveillance, AND interstitial prostate brachytherapy, AND external beam radiotherapy, AND radical prostatectomy, provided prior to initiation of treatment (PRCA)[1]

4164F   Adjuvant (ie, in combination with external beam radiotherapy to the prostate for prostate cancer) hormonal therapy (gonadotropin-releasing hormone [GNRH] agonist or antagonist) prescribed/administered (PRCA)[1]

4165F   Three-dimensional conformal radiotherapy (3D-CRT) or intensity modulated radiation therapy (IMRT) received (PRCA)[1]

4167F   Head of bed elevation (30-45 degrees) on first ventilator day ordered (CRIT)[1]

4168F   Patient receiving care in the intensive care unit (ICU) and receiving mechanical ventilation, 24 hours or less (CRIT)[1]

4169F   Patient either not receiving care in the intensive care unit (ICU) OR not receiving mechanical ventilation OR receiving mechanical ventilation greater than 24 hours (CRIT)[1]

4171F   patient receiving erythropoiesis-stimulating agents (ESA) therapy (CKD)[1]

Footnotes

1-Physician Consortium for Performance Improvement (PCPI), www.physicianconsortium.org

2-National Committee on Quality Assurance (NCQA), Health Employer Data Information Set (HEDIS®), www.ncqa.org

3-Joint Commission on Accreditation of Healthcare Organizations (JCAHO), ORYX Initiative Performance Measures, www.jointcommission.org/performance_measurement.aspx

4-National Diabetes Quality Improvement Alliance (NDQIA), www.nationaldiabetesalliance.org

5-Joint measure from the Physician Consortium for Performance Improvement, www.physicianconsortium.org and National Committee on Quality Assurance (NCQA), www.ncqa.org

6-Society of Thoracic Surgeons, www.sts.org, and National Quality Forum, www.qualityforum.org

7-Ingenix, www.ingenix.com

8-American Academy of Neurology, www.aan.com/go/practic/quality/measurements or quality@aan.com

9-College of American Pathologists (CAP), www.cap.org/apps/docs/advocacy/pathology performance measurement.pdf

10-American Gastroenterological Assocation (AGA), www.gastro.org/quality

---

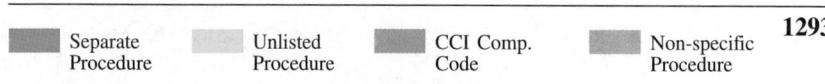

| Separate Procedure | Unlisted Procedure | CCI Comp. Code | Non-specific Procedure |

1293

4172F   Patient not receiving erythropoiesis-stimulating agents (ESA) therapy (CKD)[1]

4174F   Counseling about the potential impact of glaucoma on visual functioning and quality of life, and importance of treatment adherence provided to patient and/or caregiver(s) (EC)[5]

4175F   Best-corrected visual acuity of 20/40 or better (distance or near) achieved within the 90 days following cataract surgery (EC)[5]

4176F   Counseling about value of protection from UV light and lack of proven efficacy of nutritional supplements in prevention or progression of cataract development provided to patient and/or caregiver(s) (NMA-No Measure Associated)

4177F   Counseling about the benefits and/or risks of the age-related eye disease study (AREDS) formulation for preventing progression of age-related macular degeneration (AMD) provided to patient and/or caregiver(s) (EC)[5]

4178F   Anti-D immune globulin received between 26 and 30 weeks gestation (Pre-Cr)[1]

4179F   Tamoxifen or aromatase inhibitor (AI) prescribed (ONC)[1]

4180F   Adjuvant chemotherapy referred, prescribed or previously received for Stage III colon cancer (ONC)[1]

4181F   Conformal radiation therapy received (NMA-No Measure Assoc.)

4182F   Conformal radiation therapy not received (NMA-No Measure Assoc.)

4185F   Continuous (12-months) therapy with proton pump inhibitor (PPI) or histamine H2 receptor antagonist (H2RA) received (GERD)[5]

4186F   no continuous (12-months) therapy with either proton pump inhibitor (PPI) or histamine H2 receptor antagonist (H2RA) received (GERD)[5]

4187F   Disease modifying anti-rheumatic drug therapy prescribed or dispensed (RA)[2]

4188F   Appropriate angiotensin converting enzyme (ACE)/angiotensin receptor blockers (ARB) therapeutic monitoring test ordered or performed (AM)[2]

4189F   Appropriate digoxin therapeutic monitoring test ordered or performed (AM)[2]

4190F   Appropriate diuretic therapeutic monitoring test ordered or performed (AM)[2]

4191F   Appropriate anticonvulsant therapeutic monitoring test ordered or performed (AM)[2]

4192F   Patient not receiving glucocorticoid therapy (RA)[5]

4193F   Patient receiving <10 mg daily prednisone (or equivalent), or RA activity is worsening, or glucocorticoid use is for less than 6 months (RA)[5]

4194F   Patient receiving >=10 mg daily prednisone (or equivalent) for longer than 6 months, and improvement or no change in disease activity (RA)[5]

4195F   Patient receiving first time biologic disease modifying anti rheumatic drug therapy for rheumatoid arthritis (RA)[5]

4196F   Patient not receiving first time biologic disease modifying anti rheumatic drug therapy for rheumatoid arthritis (RA)[5]

Footnotes

1-Physician Consortium for Performance Improvement (PCPI), www.physicianconsortium.org

2-National Committee on Quality Assurance (NCQA), Health Employer Data Information Set (HEDIS®), www.ncqa.org

3-Joint Commission on Accreditation of Healthcare Organizations (JCAHO), ORYX Initiative Performance Measures, www.jointcommission.org/performance_measurement.aspx

4-National Diabetes Quality Improvement Alliance (NDQIA), www.nationaldiabetesalliance.org

5-Joint measure from the Physician Consortium for Performance Improvement, www.physicianconsortium.org and National Committee on Quality Assurance (NCQA), www.ncqa.org

6-Society of Thoracic Surgeons, www.sts.org, and National Quality Forum, www.qualityforum.org

7-Ingenix, www.ingenix.com

8-American Academy of Neurology, www.aan.com/go/practic/quality/measurements or quality@aan.com

9-College of American Pathologists (CAP), www.cap.org/apps/docs/advocacy/pathology performance measurement.pdf

10-American Gastroenterological Assocation (AGA), www.gastro.org/quality

---

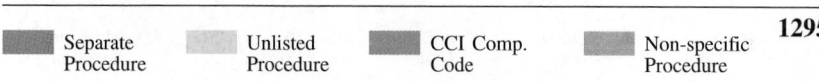

| Separate Procedure | Unlisted Procedure | CCI Comp. Code | Non-specific Procedure |

1295

4200F   External beam radiotherapy as primary therapy to prostate with or without nodal irradiation (PRCA)[1]

4201F   External beam radiotherapy with or without nodal irradiation as adjuvant or salvage therapy for prostate cancer patient (PRCA)[1]

4210F   Angiotensin converting enzyme (ACE) or angiotensin receptor blockers (ARB) medication therapy for 6 months or more (MM)[2]

4220F   Digoxin medication therapy for 6 months or more (MM)[2]

4221F   Diuretic medication therapy for 6 months or more (MM)[2]

4230F   Anticonvulsant medication therapy for 6 months or more (MM)[2]

▲ **4240F**   Instruction in therapeutic exercise with follow-up provided to patients during episode of back pain lasting longer than 12 weeks (BkP)[2]

4242F   Counseling for supervised exercise program provided to patients during episode of back pain lasting longer than 12 weeks (BkP)[2]

4245F   Patient counseled during the initial visit to maintain or resume normal activities (BkP)[2]

4248F   Patient counseled during the initial visit for an episode of back pain against bed rest lasting 4 days or longer (BkP)[2]

4250F   Active warming used intraoperatively for the purpose of maintaining normothermia, OR at least one body temperature equal to or greater than 36 degrees Centigrade (or 96.8 degrees Fahrenheit) recorded within the 30 minutes immediately before or the 15 minutes immediately after anesthesia end time (CRIT)[1]

4255F   Duration of general or neuraxial anesthesia 60 minutes or longer, as documented in the anesthesia record (CRIT)[5]

4256F   Duration of general or neuraxial anesthesia less than 60 minutes, as documented in the anesthesia record (CRIT)[5]

4260F   Wound surface culture technique used (CWC)[5]

● New Code   ▲ Revised Code   + Add-On Code   ⊘ Modifier -51 Exempt   ⊙ Moderate Sedation

4261F Technique other than surface culture of the wound exudate used (eg, Levine/deep swab technique, semi quantitative or quantitative swab technique) OR wound surface culture technique not used (CWC)[5]

4265F Use of wet to dry dressings prescribed or recommended (CWC)[5]

4266F Use of wet to dry dressings neither prescribed nor recommended (CWC)[5]

4267F Compression therapy prescribed (CWC)[5]

4268F Patient education regarding the need for long term compression therapy including interval replacement of compression stockings received (CWC)[5]

4269F Appropriate method of offloading (pressure relief) prescribed (CWC)[5]

4270F Patient receiving potent antiretroviral therapy for 6 months or longer (HIV)[5]

4271F Patient receiving potent antiretroviral therapy for less than 6 months or not receiving potent antiretroviral therapy (HIV)[5]

4274F Influenza immunization administered or previously received (HIV)[5] (P ESRD)[1]

(4275F deleted 2011 [2012 edition]. To report Hepatitis B vaccine injection administered or previously received, use 4149F)

Footnotes

1-Physician Consortium for Performance Improvement (PCPI), www.physicianconsortium.org

2-National Committee on Quality Assurance (NCQA), Health Employer Data Information Set (HEDIS®), www.ncqa.org

3-Joint Commission on Accreditation of Healthcare Organizations (JCAHO), ORYX Initiative Performance Measures, www.jointcommission.org/performance_measurement.aspx

4-National Diabetes Quality Improvement Alliance (NDQIA), www.nationaldiabetesalliance.org

5-Joint measure from the Physician Consortium for Performance Improvement, www.physicianconsortium.org and National Committee on Quality Assurance (NCQA), www.ncqa.org

6-Society of Thoracic Surgeons, www.sts.org, and National Quality Forum, www.qualityforum.org

7-Ingenix, www.ingenix.com

8-American Academy of Neurology, www.aan.com/go/practic/quality/measurements or quality@aan.com

9-College of American Pathologists (CAP), www.cap.org/apps/docs/advocacy/pathology performance measurement.pdf

10-American Gastroenterological Assocation (AGA), www.gastro.org/quality

1297

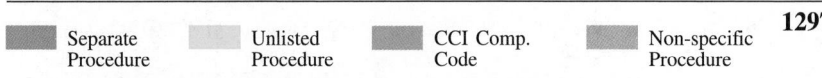

Separate Procedure   Unlisted Procedure   CCI Comp. Code   Non-specific Procedure

4276F   Potent antiretroviral therapy prescribed (HIV)[5]

4279F   Pneumocystis jiroveci pneumonia prophylaxis prescribed (HIV)[5]

4280F   Pneumocystis jiroveci pneumonia prophylaxis prescribed within 3 months of low CD4+ cell count or percentage (HIV)[5]

4290F   Patient screened for injection drug use (HIV)[5]

4293F   Patient screened for high risk sexual behavior (HIV)[5]

4300F   Patient receiving warfarin therapy for nonvalvular atrial fibrillation or atrial flutter (AFIB)[1]

4301F   Patient not receiving warfarin therapy for nonvalvular atrial fibrillation or atrial flutter (AFIB)[1]

4305F   Patient education regarding appropriate foot care AND daily inspection of the feet received (CWC)[5]

4306F   Patient counseled regarding psychosocial AND pharmacologic treatment options for opioid addiction (SUD)[1]

4320F   Patient counseled regarding psychosocial AND pharmacologic treatment options for alcohol dependence (SUD)[5]

4322F   Caregiver provided with education and referred to additional resources for support (DEM)[1]

4324F   Patient (or caregiver) queried about parkinson's disease medication related motor complications (Prkns)[8]

4325F   Medical and surgical treatment options reviewed with patient (or caregiver) (Prkns)[8]

4326F   Patient (or caregiver) queried about symptoms of autonomic dysfunction (Prkns)[8]

4328F   Patient (or caregiver) queried about sleep disturbances (Prkns)[8]

4330F   Counseling about epilepsy specific safety issues provided to patient (or caregiver(s)) (EPI)[8]

4340F   Counseling for women of childbearing potential with epilepsy (EPI)[8]

4350F   Counseling provided on symptom management, end of life decisions, and palliation (DEM)[1]

4400F   Rehabilitative therapy options discussed with patient (or caregiver) (Prkns)[8]

4450F   Self-care education provided to patient (HF)[1]

4470F   Implantable cardioverter-defibrillator (ICD) counseling provided (HF)[1]

4480F   Patient receiving ACE inhibitor/ARB therapy and beta-blocker therapy for 3 months or longer (HF)[1]

4481F   Patient receiving ACE inhibitor/ARB therapy and beta-blocker therapy for less than 3 months or patient not receiving ACE inhibitor/ARB therapy and beta blocker therapy (HF)[1]

4500F   Referred to an outpatient cardiac rehabilitation program (CAD)[1]

4510F   Previous cardiac rehabilitation for qualifying cardiac event completed (CAD)[1]

4525F   Neuropsychiatric intervention ordered (DEM)[1]

4526F   Neuropsychiatric intervention received (DEM)[1]

Footnotes

1-Physician Consortium for Performance Improvement (PCPI), www.physicianconsortium.org

2-National Committee on Quality Assurance (NCQA), Health Employer Data Information Set (HEDIS®), www.ncqa.org

3-Joint Commission on Accreditation of Healthcare Organizations (JCAHO), ORYX Initiative Performance Measures, www.jointcommission.org/performance_measurement.aspx

4-National Diabetes Quality Improvement Alliance (NDQIA), www.nationaldiabetesalliance.org

5-Joint measure from the Physician Consortium for Performance Improvement, www.physicianconsortium.org and National Committee on Quality Assurance (NCQA), www.ncqa.org

6-Society of Thoracic Surgeons, www.sts.org, and National Quality Forum, www.qualityforum.org

7-Ingenix, www.ingenix.com

8-American Academy of Neurology, www.aan.com/go/practic/quality/measurements or quality@aan.com

9-College of American Pathologists (CAP), www.cap.org/apps/docs/advocacy/pathology performance measurement.pdf

10-American Gastroenterological Assocation (AGA), www.gastro.org/quality

---

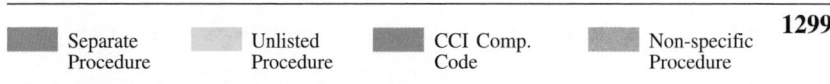

Separate Procedure   Unlisted Procedure   CCI Comp. Code   Non-specific Procedure

1299

FOLLOW-UP OR OTHER OUTCOMES

Follow-up or other outcomes codes describe review and communication of test results to patients, patient satisfaction or experience with care, patient functional status, and patient morbidity and mortality.

5005F Patient counseled on self-examination for new or changing moles (ML)[5]

▲ **5010F** Findings of dilated macular or fundus exam communicated to the physician or other qualified health care professional managing the diabetes care (EC)[5]

5015F Documentation of communication that a fracture occurred and that the patient was or should be tested or treated for osteoporosis (OP)[5]

▲ **5020F** Treatment summary report communicated to physician(s) or other qualified health care professional(s) managing continuing care and to the patient within 1 month of completing treatment (ONC)[1]

5050F Treatment plan communicated to provider(s) managing continuing care within 1 month of diagnosis (ML)[5]

5060F Findings from diagnostic mammogram communicated to practice managing patient's ongoing care within 3 business daysof exam interpretation(RAD)[5]

5062F Findings from diagnostic mammogram communicated to practic managingthe patient's on-going care within 5 business days of exam interpretation (RAD)[5]

▲ **5100F** Potential risk for fracture communicated to the referring physician or other qualified health care professional within 24 hours of completion of the imaging study (NUC_MED)[1]

5200F Consideration of referral for a neurological evaluation of appropriateness for surgical therapy for intractable epilepsy within the past 3 years (EPI)[8]

5250F Asthma discharge plan provided to patient (Asthma)[1]

● New Code ▲ Revised Code + Add-On Code ⊘ Modifier -51 Exempt ⊙ Moderate Sedation

PATIENT SAFETY

Patient safety codes that describe patient safety practices.

6005F   Rationale (eg, severity of illness and safety) for level of care (eg, home, hospital) documented (CAP)[1]

6010F   Dysphagia screening conducted prior to order for or receipt of any foods, fluids or medication by mouth (STR)[5]

6015F   Patient receiving or eligible to receive foods, fluids or medication by mouth (STR)[5]

6020F   NPO (nothing by mouth) ordered (STR)[5]

6030F   All elements of maximal sterile barrier technique followed including: cap AND mask AND sterile gown AND sterile gloves AND a large sterile sheet AND hand hygiene AND 2% chlorhexidine for cutaneous antisepsis (or acceptable alternative antiseptics, per current guideline) (CRIT)[1]

6040F   Use of appropriate radiation dose reduction devices or manual techniques for appropriate moderation of exposure, documented (RAD)[5]

6045F   Radiation exposure or exposure time in final report for procedure using fluoroscopy, documented (RAD)[5]

6070F   Patient queried and counseled about anti-epileptic drug (AED) side effects (EPI)[8]

Footnotes

1-Physician Consortium for Performance Improvement (PCPI), www.physicianconsortium.org

2-National Committee on Quality Assurance (NCQA), Health Employer Data Information Set (HEDIS®), www.ncqa.org

3-Joint Commission on Accreditation of Healthcare Organizations (JCAHO), ORYX Initiative Performance Measures, www.jointcommission.org/performance_measurement.aspx

4-National Diabetes Quality Improvement Alliance (NDQIA), www.nationaldiabetesalliance.org

5-Joint measure from the Physician Consortium for Performance Improvement, www.physicianconsortium.org and National Committee on Quality Assurance (NCQA), www.ncqa.org

6-Society of Thoracic Surgeons, www.sts.org, and National Quality Forum, www.qualityforum.org

7-Ingenix, www.ingenix.com

8-American Academy of Neurology, www.aan.com/go/practic/quality/measurements or quality@aan.com

9-College of American Pathologists (CAP), www.cap.org/apps/docs/advocacy/pathology performance measurement.pdf

10-American Gastroenterological Assocation (AGA), www.gastro.org/quality

---

1301

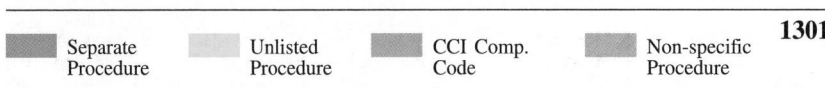

| ▨ Separate Procedure | ▨ Unlisted Procedure | ▨ CCI Comp. Code | ▨ Non-specific Procedure |

6080F patient (or caregiver) queried about falls (Prkns)[8]

6090F Patient (or caregiver) counseled about safety issues appropriate to patient's stage of disease (Prkns)[8]

6100F Timeout to verify correct patient, correct site, and correct procedure, documented (PATH)[8]

6101F Safety counseling for dementia provided (DEM)[1]

6102F Safety counseling for dementia ordered (DEM)[1]

6110F Counseling provided regarding risks of driving and the alternatives to driving (DEM)[1]

● **6150F** Patient not receiving a first course of anti-TNF (tumor necrosis factor) therapy (IBD)[10]

STRUCTURAL MEASURES

Structural measures codes are used to identify measures that address the setting or system of the delivered care. These codes also address aspects of the capabilities of the organization or health care professional providing the care.

7010F Patient information entered into a recall system that includes: target date for the next exam specified AND a process to follow up with patients regarding missed or unscheduled appointments (ML)[5]

7020F Mammogram assessment category [eg, Mammography Quality Standards Act (MQSA), Breast Imaging Reporting and Data System (BI-RADS®), or FDA approved equivalent categories] entered into an internal database to allow for analysis of abnormal interpretation (recall) rate (RAD)5

7025F Patient information entered into a reminder system with a target due date for the next mammogram (RAD)[5]

CATEGORY III CODES

CATEGORY III SECTION OVERVIEW

The eighth section of the CPT coding system is the Category III Emerging Technology section. The primary purpose of this section is to provide classification codes which will allow the collection of data on emerging technology services and procedures.

The assignment of a Category III code to a given service or procedure does not mean that the particular service or procedure is endorsed, approved, safe or has applicability to clinical practice. The Category III code simply provides a mechanism to identify and review emerging services and procedures.

Category III codes consist of four numbers followed by the letter "T." There is no particular organization to the codes listed in this section.

Services/procedures described in this section make use of alphanumeric characters. These codes have an alpha character as the 5th character in the string, preceded by four digits. The digits are not intended to reflect the placement of the code in the Category I section of CPT nomenclature. Codes in this section may or may not eventually receive a Category I CPT code. In either case, in general, a given Category III code will be archived five years from the date of initial publication or extension unless a modification of the archival date is specifically noted at the time of revision or change to a code (eg, addition of parenthetical instructions, reinstatement). Services/procedures described by Category III codes which have been archived after five years, without conversion, must be reported using the Category I unlisted code unless another specific cross reference is established at the time of archiving. New or revised codes in this section are released semi-annually via the AMA/CPT Internet site, to expedite dissemination for reporting. The full set of temporary codes for emerging technology, services and procedures are published annually in the CPT codebook. Go to www.ama-assn.org/go/cpt for the most current listing.

CATEGORY III CODES

(0016T   deleted 2010 [2011 edition])

(0017T   deleted 2010 [2011 edition])

> (For destruction of localized lesion of choroid by transpupillary thermotherapy, use 67299)

> (For destruction of macular drusen, photocoagulation, use 67299)

1303

	Separate Procedure		Unlisted Procedure		CCI Comp. Code		Non-specific Procedure

0019T Extracorporeal shock wave involving musculoskeletal system, not otherwise specified, low energy

(For application of high energy extracorporeal shock wave involving musculoskeletal system not otherwise specified, use 0101T)

(For application of high energy extracorporeal shock wave involving lateral humeral epicondyle, use 0102T)

(0024T deleted 2008 editio

(For non-surgical reduction therapy, use 93799)

(0026T deleted 2009 edition)

(For lipoprotein, direct measurement, intermediate density lipoproteins [IDL] [remnant lipoprotein], use 84999)

(0027T deleted 2009 edition)

(For endoscopic lysis of epidural adhesions with direct visualization using mechanical means or solution injection [eg, normal saline], use 64999)

(0028T deleted 2009 edition)

(For dual x-ray absorptiometry [DEXA] body composition study, use 76499)

(0029T deleted 2009 edition)

(For pulsed magnetic neuromodulation incontinence treatment, use 53899)

(0030T deleted 2013 editiion)

(To report antiprothrombin [phospholipid cofactor] antibody, use 86849)

(0031T deleted 2009 edition)

(0032T deleted 2009 edition)

(For speculoscopy, including sampling, use 58999)

(0041T deleted 2009 edition)

(For urinalysis infectious agent detection, semi-quantitative analysis of volatile compounds, use 81099)

● New Code   ▲ Revised Code   + Add-On Code   ⊘ Modifier -51 Exempt   ⊙ Moderate Sedation

0042T Cerebral perfusion analysis using computed tomography with contrast administration, including post-processing of parametric maps with determination of cerebral blood flow, cerebral blood volume, and mean transit time

(0043T deleted 2009 edition)

(For carbon monoxide, expired gas analysis [eg, ETC0/hemolysis greath test], use 84999)

(0046T deleted 2009 edition)

(0047T deleted 2009 edition)

(For mammary duct[s] catheter lavage, use 19499)

(0048T deleted 2013 edition. To report, use 33991)

(0049T deleted 2009 edition)

(0050T deleted 2013 edition. To report, see 33990-33993)

0051T Implantation of a total replacement heart system (artificial heart) with recipient cardiectomy

(For implantation of heart assist or ventricular assist device, see 33975, 33976)

0052T Replacement or repair of thoracic unit of a total replacement heart system (artificial heart)

(For replacement or repair of other implantable components in a total replacement heart system (artificial heart), use 0053T)

0053T Replacement or repair of implantable component or components of total replacement heart system (artificial heart), excluding thoracic unit

(For replacement or repair of a thoracic unit of a total replacement heart system (artificial heart), use 0052T)

+ **0054T** Computer-assisted musculoskeletal surgical navigational orthopedic procedure, with image-guidance based on fluoroscopic images (list separately in addition to code for primary procedure)

+ **0055T** Computer-assisted musculoskeletal surgical navigational orthopedic procedure, with image-guidance based on ct/mri

| Separate Procedure | Unlisted Procedure | CCI Comp. Code | Non-specific Procedure |

images (list separately in addition to code for primary procedure)

(When CT and MRI are both performed, report 0055T only once)

(0056T   deleted 2008 edition. To report, use 20985)

0058T   Cryopreservation; reproductive tissue, ovarian

0059T   oocyte(s)

(For cryopreservation of embryo(s), sperm, and testicular reproductive tissue, see 89258, 89259, 89335)

(0060T   deleted 2009 edition)

(For electrical impedance breast scan, use 76499)

(0061T   deleted 2009 edition)

(For destruction/reduction of malignant breast tumor, microwave phased array thermotherapy, use 19499)

(0062T   Deleted 2009 [2010 edition])

(0063T   Deleted 2009 [2010 edition])

(For percutaneous intradiscal annuloplasty, any method other than electrothermal, use 22899)

(For intradiscal electrothermal annuloplasty, see 22526-22527)

(0064T   Deleted 2009 [2010 edition]. To report, use 94799)

(0066T   Deleted 2009 [2010 edition])

(To report CT colon, screening, use 74263)

(0067T   Deleted 2009 [2010 edition])

(To report CT colon, diagnostic, use 74261-74262)

(0068T   Deleted 2009 [2010 edition])

(0069T   Deleted 2009 [2010 edition])

(0070T   Deleted 2009 [2010 edition])

(For acoustic heart sound recording and computer analysis, use 93799)

0071T Focused ultrasound ablation of uterine leiomyomata, including MR guidance; total leiomyomata volume less than 200 cc of tissue

0072T total leiomyomata volume greater or equal to 200 cc of tissue

(Do not report 0071T, 0072T in conjunction with 51702 or 77022)

0073T Compensator-based beam modulation treatment delivery of inverse planned treatment using 3 or more high resolution (milled or cast) compensator convergent beam modulated fields, per treatment session

(For treatment planning, use 77301)

(Do not report 0073T in conjunction with 77401-77416, 77418)

0075T Transcatheter placement of extracranial vertebral or intrathoracic carotid artery stent(s), including radiologic supervision and interpretation, percutaneous; initial vessel

+ 0076T each additional vessel (List separately in addition to code for primary procedure)

(Use 0076T in conjunction with 0075T)

(When the ipsilateral extracranial vertebral or intrathoracic carotid arteriogram (including imaging and selective catheterization) confirms the need for stenting, then 0075T and 0076T include all ipsilateral extracranial vertebral or intrathoracic selective carotid catheterization, all diagnostic imaging for ipsilateral extracranial vertebral or intrathoracic carotid artery stenting, and all related radiologic supervision and interpretation. If stenting is not indicated, then the appropriate codes for selective catheterization and imaging should be reported in lieu of code 0075T or 0076T.)

(0077T Deleted 2009 [2010 edition]. To report, see 61107, 61210)

(0078T-0081T should be reported in accordance with the Endovascular Abdominal Aneurysm Repair guidelines established for 34800-34826)

0078T Endovascular repair using prosthesis of abdominal aortic aneurysm, pseudoaneurysm or dissection, abdominal aorta

	Separate Procedure		Unlisted Procedure		CCI Comp. Code		Non-specific Procedure	**1307**

involving visceral branches (superior mesenteric, celiac and/or renal artery[s])

(Do not report 0078T in conjunction with 34800-34805, 35081, 35102, 35452, 35472)

(Report 0078T in conjunction with 37205-37208, 37220-37223, only when these procedures are performed outside the target zone of the endoprosthesis)

+ 0079T Placement of visceral extension prosthesis for endovascular repair of abdominal aortic aneurysm involving visceral vessels, each visceral branch (List separately in addition to code for primary procedure)

(Use 0079T in conjunction with 0078T)

0080T Endovascular repair using prosthesis of abdominal aortic aneurysm, pseudoaneurysm or dissection, abdominal aorta involving visceral vessels (superior mesenteric, celiac and/or renal artery[ies]), using fenestrated modular bifurcated prosthesis (2 docking limbs), radiological supervision and interpretation

(Do not report 0080T in conjunction with 34800-34805, 35081, 35102, 35452, 35472)

(Report 0080T in conjunction with 37205-37208, 37220-37223, only when these procedures are performed outside the target zone of the endoprosthesis)

+ 0081T Placement of visceral extension prosthesis for endovascular repair of abdominal aortic aneurysm involving visceral vessels, each visceral branch, radiological supervision and interpretation (List separately in addition to code for primary procedure)

(Use 0081T in conjunction with 0080T)

(0084T Deleted 2009 [2010 edition]. To report, use 53855)

0085T Breath test for heart transplant rejection

(0086T Deleted 2009 [2010 edition]. To report, use 93799)

(0087T Deleted 2009 [2010 edition]. To report, use 89398)

(0088T deleted 2009 edition. To report, use 41530)

(0089T deleted 2009 edition. For actigraphy testing, use 95803)

● New Code ▲ Revised Code + Add-On Code ⊘ Modifier -51 Exempt ⊙ Moderate Sedation

(0090T   deleted 2009 edition. To report total disc cervical arthroplasty, use 22856)

(To report total disc lumbar arthroplasty, use 22857)

+ **0092T**   Total disc arthroplasty (artificial disc), anterior approach, including discectomy with end plate preparation (includes osteophytectomy for nerve root or spinal cord decompression and microdissection), each additional interspace, cervical (List separately in addition to code for primary procedure)

(Use 0092T in conjunction with 22856)

(Do not report 0092T in conjunction with 22851 when performed at the same level)

(0093T   deleted 2009 edition. To report removal of total disc cervical arthroplasty, use 22864)

(To report removal of total disc lumbar arthroplasty, use 22865)

+ **0095T**   Removal of total disc arthroplasty (artificial disc), anterior approach, each additional interspace, cervical (List separately in addition to code for primary procedure)

(Use 0095T in conjunction with 22864)

(0096T   deleted 2009 edition; to report revision of total disc cervical arthroplasty, use 22861)

(To report revision of total disc lumbar arthroplasty, use 22862)

+ **0098T**   Revision including replacement of total disc arhtroplasty (artificial disc), anterior approach, each additional interspace, cervical (List separately in addition to code for primary procedure)

(Use 0098T in conjunction with 22861)

(Do not report 0098T in conjunction with 0095T)

(Do not report 0098T in conjunction with 22851 when performed at the same level)

(For decompression, see 63001-63048)

0099T   Implantation of intrastromal corneal ring segments

0100T   Placement of a subconjunctival retinal prosthesis receiver and pulse generator, and implantation of intra-ocular retinal electrode array, with vitrectomy

---

							1309
	Separate Procedure		Unlisted Procedure		CCI Comp. Code		Non-specific Procedure

0101T Extracorporeal shock wave involving musculoskeletal system, not otherwise specified, high energy

(For application of low energy musculoskeletal system extracorporeal shock wave, use 0019T)

(For extracorporeal shock wave therapy involving integumentary system not otherwise specified, se 0299T, 0300T)

(Do not report 0101T in conjunction with 0299T, 0300T when treating same area)

0102T Extracorporeal shock wave, high energy, performed by a physician, requiring anesthesia other than local, involving lateral humeral epicondyle

(For application of low energy musculoskeletal system extracorporeal shock wave, use 0019T)

0103T Holotranscobalamin, quantitative

(0104T deleted 2010 [2011 edition])

(0105T deleted 2010 [2011 edition])

(For inert gas rebreathing for cardiac output measurement during rest, use 93799)

(For intert gas rebreathing for cardiac output measurement during exercise, use 93799)

0106T Quantitative sensory testing (QST), testing and interpretation per extremity; using touch pressure stimuli to assess large diameter sensation

0107T using vibration stimuli to assess large diameter fiber sensation

0108T using cooling stimuli to assess small nerve fiber sensation and hyperalgesia

0109T using heat-pain stimuli to assess small nerve fiber sensation and hyperalgesia

0110T using other stimuli to assess sensation

0111T Long-chain (C20-22) omega-3 fatty acids in red blood cell (RBC) membranes

● New Code ▲ Revised Code + Add-On Code ⊘ Modifier -51 Exempt ⊙ Moderate Sedation

(For very long chain fatty acids, use 82726)

0123T Fistulization of sclera for glaucoma, through ciliary body

0124T Conjunctival incision with posterior extrascleral placement of pharmacological agent (does not include supply of medication)

(For suprachoroidal delivery of pharmacologic agent, use 0186T)

0126T Common carotid intima-media thickness (IMT) study for evaluation of atherosclerotic burden or coronary heart disease risk factor assessment

(0130T deleted 2010 [2011 edition])

(For validated, statistically reliable, randomized, controlled, single-patient clinical investigation of FDA approved chronic care drugs, provided by a pharmacist, interpretation and report to the prescribing health care professional, use 99199)

(0137T deleted 2009 edition. For transperineal stereotactic template guided saturation prostate biopsies, use 55706)

(0140T deleted 2010 [2011 edition])

(0141T deleted 2011 [2012 edition])

(0142T deleted 2011 [2012 edition])

(0143T deleted 2011 [2012 edition])

(To report pancreatic islet cell transplantation, use 48999)

(0144T Deleted 2009 [2010 edition]. To report, see 75571-75574.)

(0145T Deleted 2009 [2010 edition]. To report, see 75571-75574.)

(0146T Deleted 2009 [2010 edition]. To report, see 75571-75574.)

(0147T Deleted 2009 [2010 edition]. To report, see 75571-75574.)

(0148T Deleted 2009 [2010 edition]. To report, see 75571-75574.)

(0149T Deleted 2009 [2010 edition]. To report, see 75571-75574.)

(0150T Deleted 2009 [2010 edition]. To report, see 75571-75574.)

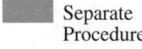 Separate Procedure   Unlisted Procedure   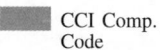 CCI Comp. Code   Non-specific Procedure

(0151T   Deleted 2009 [2010 edition]. To report, see 75571-75574.)

(0155T   deleted 2011 [2012 edition])

(0156T   deleted 2011 [2012 edition])

(For laparoscopic implantation, replacement, revision or removal of gastric stimulation electrodes, lesser curvature, use 43659)

(0157T   deleted 2011 [2012 edition])

(0158T   deleted 2011 [2012 edition])

(For open implantation, replacement, revision, or removal of gastric stimulation electrodes, lesser curvature, use 43999)

+ 0159T   Computer-aided detection, including computer algorithm analysis of MRI image data for lesion detection/characterization, pharmacokinetic analysis, with further physician review for interpretation, breast MRI (List separately in addition to code for primary procedure)

(Use 0159T in conjunction with 77058, 77059)

(Do not report 0159T in conjunction with 76376, 76377)

(0160T   deleted 2010 [2011 edition]. To report, see 90867, 90869)

(0161T   deleted 2010 [2011 edition]. To report, see 90867, 90869)

(0162T   deleted 2009 edition. To report, see 95980-95982)

+ 0163T   Total disc arthroplasty (artificial disc), anterior approach, including discectomy to prepare interspace (other than for decompression), each additional interspace, lumbar (List separately in addition to code for primary procedure)

(Use 0163T in conjunction with 22857)

+ 0164T   Removal of total disc arthroplasty, (artificial disc), anterior approach, each additional interspace, lumbar (List separately in addition to code for primary procedure)

(Use 0164T in conjunction with 22865)

+ 0165T   Revision including replacement of total disc arthroplasty, (artificial disc), anterior approach, each additional interspace, lumbar (List separately in addition to code for primary procedure)

1312   ● New Code   ▲ Revised Code   + Add-On Code   ⊘ Modifier -51 Exempt   ⊙ Moderate Sedation

(Use 0165T in conjunction with 22862)

(Do not report 0163T-0165T in conjunction with 22851, 49010, when performed at the same level)

(For decompression, see 63001-63048)

(0166T   deleted 2011 [2012 edition])

(0167T   deleted 2011 [2012 edition])

(For transmyocardial transcatheter closure of ventricular septal defect, with implant, including cadiopulmonary bypass if performed, use 33999)

(0168T   deleted 2011 [2012 edition])

(For rhinophototherapy, intranasal application of ultraviolet and visible light, use 30999)

0169T   Stereotactic placement of infusion catheter(s) in the brain for delivery of therapeutic agent(s), including computerized stereotactic planning and burr hole(s)

(Do not report code 0169T in conjunction with 20660, 61107, 61781, 61782, 61783)

(0170T   Deleted 2009 [2010 edition]. To report, use 46707)

0171T   Insertion of posterior spinous process distraction device (including necessary removal of bone or ligament for insertion and imaging guidance), lumbar; single level

+ 0172T   each additional level (List separately in addition to code for primary procedure)

(Use 0172T in conjunction with 0171T)

(0173T   deleted 2013 edition)

+ 0174T   Computer-aided detection (CAD) (computer algorithm analysis of digital image data for lesion detection) with further physician review for interpretation and report, with or without digitization of film radiographic images, chest radiograph(s), performed concurrent with primary interpretation (List separately in addition to code for primary procedure)

(Use 0174T in conjunction with 71010, 71020, 71021, 71022, 71030)

1313

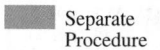 Separate Procedure   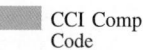 Unlisted Procedure   CCI Comp. Code   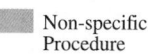 Non-specific Procedure

0175T Computer-aided detection (CAD) (computer algorithm analysis of digital image data for lesion detection) with further physician review for interpretation and report, with or without digitization of film radiographic images, chest radiograph(s), performed remote from primary interpretation

(Do not report 0175T in conjunction with 71010, 71020, 71021, 71022, 71030)

(0176T deleted 2010 [2011 edition]. To report, see 66174, 66175)

(0177T deleted 2010 [2011 edition]. To report, see 66174, 66175)

0178T Electrocardiogram, 64 leads or greater, with graphic presentation and analysis; with interpretation and report

0179T tracing and graphics only, without interpretation and report

0180T interpretation and report only

(For electrocardiogram, routine, with at least 12 leads separately performed, see 93000-93010)

0181T Corneal hysteresis determination, by air impulse stimulation, bilateral, with interpretation and report

0182T High dose rate electronic brachytherapy, per fraction

(Do not report 0182T in conjunction with 77761-77763, 77776-77778, 77785-77787, 77789)

0183T Low frequency, non-contact, non-thermal ultrasound, including topical application(s), when performed, wound assessment, and instruction(s) for ongoing care, per day

0184T Excision of rectal tumor, transanal endoscopic microsurgical approach (ie, TEMS), including muscularis propria (ie, full thickness)

(For non-endoscopic excision of rectal tumor, see 45160, 45171, 45172)

(Do not report 0184T in conjunction with 45300-45327, 69990)

0185T Multivariate analysis of patient-specific findings with quantifiable computer probability assessment, including report

(Do not report 0185T in conjunction with 99090)

● New Code ▲ Revised Code ✛ Add-On Code ⊘ Modifier -51 Exempt ⊙ Moderate Sedation

0186T   Suprachoroidal delivery of pharmacologic agent (does not include supply of medication)

(0187T   deleted 2010 [2011 edition]. To report, use 92132)

Remote Real-Time Interactive Videoconferenced Critical Care Service

In order to report remote real-time interactive video conferenced critical care, the physician(s) or other qualified health care professionals in the remote location must have real-time access to the patient's medical record including progress notes, nursing notes, current medications, vital signs, clinical laboratory test results, other diagnostic test results, and radiographic images. The remote physician or other qualified health care professional must have real-time capability to enter electronic orders; document the remote care services provided in the hospital medical record; videoconference with the on-site health care team in the patient room; assess patients in their individual rooms, using high fidelity audio and video capabilities, including clear observation of the patient, monitors, ventilators, and infusion pumps; and speak to patients and family members.

The review and/or interpretation of all diagnostic information is included in reporting remote real-time interactive video-conferenced critical care when performed during the critical period by the individual(s) providing remote real-time interactive video-conferenced critical care and should not be reported separately.

The remote real-time interactive video conferenced critical care codes 0188T and 0189T are used to report the total duration of time spent by the individual providing remote real-time interactive video conferenced critical care services to a critically ill or critically injured patient, even if the time spent by the physician on that date is not continuous. For any given period of time spent providing remote real-time interactive video-conferenced critical care services, the physician or other qualified health care professional must devote his or her full attention to the patient and, therefore, cannot provide services to any other patient during the same period of time.

Only one physician or other qualified health care professional may report either Critical Care Services (99291, 99292) or remote real-time interactive video-conferenced Critical Care for the same period of time. Do not report remote real-time interactive video-conferenced critical care if another individual reports Pediatric or Neonatal Critical Care or Intensive Care services (99468-99476).

Code 0188T is used to report the first 30 to 74 minutes of remote real-time interactive video-conferenced critical care on a given date. It should be used only once per date even if the time spent by the physician or other qualified health care professional is not continuous on that date. Remote real-time interactive video-conferenced critical care of less than 30 minutes total duration on a given date should not be reported.

Separate Procedure	Unlisted Procedure	CCI Comp. Code	Non-specific Procedure

Code 0189T is used to report additional block(s) of time, of up to 30 minutes each, beyond the first 74 minutes (see table below).

The following examples illustrate the correct reporting of remote critical care services:

Total Duration of Critical Care	Codes
less than 30 minutes (less than 1/2 hour)	Do not report
30-74 minutes (1/2 hr. - 1 hr. 14 min.)	0188T once
75-104 minutes (1 hr. 15 min. - 1 hr. 44 min.)	0188T once AND 0189T once
105-134 minutes (1 hr. 45 min. - 2 hr. 14 min.)	0188T once AND 0189T twice

0188T   Remote real-time interactive video-conferenced critical care, evaluation and management of the critically ill or critically injured patient; first 30- 74 minutes

+ 0189T   each additional 30 minutes (List separately in addition to code for primary service)

    (Use 0189T in conjunction with 0188T)

+ 0190T   Placement of intraocular radiation source applicator (list separately in addition to primary procedure)

    (Use 0190T in conjunction with 67036)

    (For application of the source by radiation oncologist, see Clinical Brachytherapy section)

0191T   Insertion of anterior segment aqueous drainage device, without extraocular resevoir; internal approach, into the trabecular meshwork

0253T   internal approach, into the suprachoroidal space

0192T   external approach

(0193T   deleted 2010 [2011 edition]. To report, use 53860)

(0194T   Deleted 2009 [2010 edition]. To report procalcitonin, use 84145)

▲ **0195T**   Arthrodesis, pre-sacral interbody technique, disc space preparation, discectomy, without instrumentation, with image guidance, includes bone graft when performed; L5-S1 interspace

1316 ● New Code   ▲ Revised Code   + Add-On Code   ⊘ Modifier -51 Exempt   ⊙ Moderate Sedation

▲ **+0196T**   L4-L5 interspace (List separately in addition to code for primary procedure)

(Use 0196T in conjunction with 0195T)

(Do not report 0195T, 0196T in conjunction with 20930-20938, 22558, 22840, 22845, 22848, 22851, 72275, 76000, 76380, 76496, 76497, 77002, 77003, 77011, 77012)

0197T   Intra fraction localization and tracking of target or patient motion during delivery of radiation therapy (eg, 3D positional tracking, gating, 3D surface tracking), each fraction of treatment

0198T   Measurement of ocular blood flow by repetitive intraocular pressure sampling, with interpretation and report

0199T   Physiologic recording of tremor using accelerometer(s) and/or gyroscope(s) (including frequency and amplitude), including interpretation and report

⊙ **0200T**   Percutaneous sacral augmentation (sacroplasty), unilateral injection(s), including the use of a balloon or mechanical device, when used, 1 or more needles

⊙ **0201T**   Percutaneous sacral augmentation (sacroplasty), bilateral injections, including the use of a balloon or mechanical device, when used, 2 or more needles

(For radiological supervision and interpretation, see 72291, 72292)

(If bone biopsy is performed, see 20220, 20225)

0202T   Posterior vertebral joint(s) arthroplasty (eg, facet joint[s] replacement), including facetectomy, laminectomy, foraminotomy, and vertebral column fixation, injection of bone cement, when performed, including fluoroscopy, single level, lumbar spine

(Do not report 0202T in conjunction with 22521, 22524, 22840, 22851, 63005, 63012, 63017, 63030, 63042, 63047, 63056 at the same level)

(0203T   deleted 2010 [2011 edition]. To report, use 95800)

(0204T   deleted 2010 [2011 edition]. To report, use 95801)

+ 0205T   Intravascular catheter based coronary vessel or graft spectroscopy (eg, infrared) during diagnostic evaluation and/or

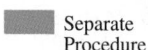 Separate Procedure   Unlisted Procedure   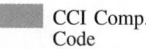 CCI Comp. Code   Non-specific Procedure

therapeutic intervention including imaging supervision, interpretation, and report, each vessel (List separately in addition to code for primary procedure)

(Use 0205T in conjunction with 92920, 92924, 92928, 92933, 92937, 92941, 92943, 92975, 93454-93461, 93563, 93564)

▲ **0206T** Computerized database analysis of multiple cycles of digitized cardiac electrical data from two or more ECG leads, including transmission to a remote center, application of multiple nonlinear mathematical transormations, with coronary artery obstruction severity assessment

(When a 12-lead ECG is performed, 93000-93010 may be reported, as appropriate)

0207T Evacuation of meibomian glands, automated, using heat and intermittent pressure, unilateral

0208T Pure tone audiometry (threshold), automated; air only

0209T air and bone

0210T Speech audiometry threshold, automated;

0211T with speech recognition

0212T Comprehensive audiometry threshold evaluation and speech recognition (0209T, 0211T combined), automated

(For audiometric testing using audiometers performed manually by a qualified health care professional, see 92551-92557)

0213T Injection(s), diagnostic or therapeutic agent, paravertebral facet (zygapophyseal) joint (or nerves innervating that joint) with ultrasound guidance, cervical or thoracic; single level

(To report bilateral procedure, use 0213T with modifier 50)

+ **0214T** second level (list separately in addition to code for primary procedure)

(To report bilateral procedure, use 0214T with modifier 50)

+ **0215T** third and any additional level(s) (list separately in addition to code for primary procedure)

(Do not report 0215T more than once per day)

(Use 0214T, 0215T in conjunction with 0213T)

● New Code ▲ Revised Code + Add-On Code ⊘ Modifier -51 Exempt ⊙ Moderate Sedation

(To report bilateral procedure, use 0215T with modifier 50)

0216T Injection(s), diagnostic or therapeutic agent, paravertebral facet (zygapophyseal) joint (or nerves innervating that joint) with ultrasound guidance, lumbar or sacral; single level

(To report bilateral procedure, use 0216T with modifier 50)

+ **0217T** second level (list separately in addition to code for primary procedure)

(To report bilateral procedure, use 0217T with modifier 50)

+ **0218T** third and any additional level(s) (list separately in addition to code for primary procedure)

(Do not report 0218T more than once per day)

(Use 0217T, 0218T in conjunction with 0216T)

(If injection(s) are performed using fluoroscopy or CT, see 64490-64495)

(To report bilateral procedure, use 0218T with modifier 50)

0219T Placement of a posterior intrafacet implant(s), unilateral or bilateral, including imaging and placement of bone graft(s) or synthetic device(s), single level; cervical

0220T thoracic

0221T lumbar

(Do not report 0219T-0221T in conjunction with any radiological service)

(Do not report 0219T-0221T in conjunction with 20930, 20931, 22600-22614, 22840, 22851 at the same level)

+ **0222T** each additional vertebral segment (list separately in addition to code for primary procedure)

(Use 0222T in conjunction with 0219T-0221T)

(For posterior or posterolateral arthrodesis technique, see 22600-22614)

Acoustic cardiography codes 0223T-0225T describe the evaluation and optimization of physiologic data including systolic and diastolic heart sounds and their temporal relationships to the electrocardiogram (ECG).

| Separate Procedure | Unlisted Procedure | CCI Comp. Code | Non-specific Procedure |

1319

Codes 0224T and 0225T also include interrogation and limited reprogramming of a cardiac pacing device to ensure hemodynamic optimization (heart rate parameter and/or automated timing modes, including explicit changes of AV/VV intervals) and facilitate device parameter optimization. Do not report 0224T or 0225T in conjunction with 93228 or 93289.

Acoustic cardiography services include a rhythm strip ECG. Do not report 93040-93042 in conjunction with 0223T-0225T.

For complete programming services as a separate procedure, see 93280, 93281, 93283, and 93284.

0223T   Acoustic cardiography, including automated analysis of combined acoustic and electrical intervals; single, with interpretation and report

0224T   multiple, including serial trended analysis and limited reprogramming of device parameter, AV or VV delays only, with interpretation and report

0225T   multiple, including serial trended analysis and limited reprogramming of device parameter, AV and VV delays, with interpretation and report

0226T   Anoscopy, high resolution (HRA) (with magnification and chemical agent enhancement); diagnostic, including collection of specimen(s) by brushing or washing when performed

0227T   with biopsy(ies)

0228T   Injection(s), anesthetic agent and/or steroid, transforaminal epidural, with ultrasound guidance, cervical or thoracic; single level

+ **0229T**   each additional level (list separately in addition to code for primary procedure)

(Use 0229T in conjunction with 0228T)

0230T   Injection(s), anesthetic agent and/or steroid, transforaminal epidural, with ultrasound guidance, lumbar or sacral; single level

+ **0231T**   each additional level (list separately in addition to code for primary procedure)

(Use 0231T in conjunction with 0230T)

   ● New Code   ▲ Revised Code   + Add-On Code   ⊘ Modifier -51 Exempt   ⊙ Moderate Sedation

(For transforaminal epidural injections performed under fluoroscopy or CT, see 64479-64484)

(Do not report 0228T-0231T in conjunction with 76942, 76998, 76999)

0232T Injection(s), platelet rich plasma, any site, including image guidance, harvesting and preparation when performed

(Do not report 0232T in conjunction with 20550, 20551, 20600-20610, 20926, 76942, 77002, 77012, 77021, 86965)

(Do not report 38220-38230 for bone marrow aspiration for platelet rich stem cell injection. For bone marrow aspiration for platelet rich stem cell injection, use 0232T)

0233T Skin advanced glycation endproducts (AGE) measurement by multi-wavelength fluorescent spectroscopy

Atherectomy (Open or Percutaneous) for Supra-Inguinal Arteries

Codes 0234T-0238T describe atherectomy performed by any method (eg, directional, rotational, laser) in arteries above the inguinal ligaments. These codes are structured differently than the codes describing atherectomy performed below the inguinal legaments (37225, 37227, 37229, 37231, 37233, 37235).

0234T Transluminal peripheral atherectomy, open or percutaneous, including radiological supervision and interpretation; renal artery

0235T visceral artery (except renal), each vessel

0236T abdominal aorta

0237T brachiocephalic trunk and branches, each vessel

0238T iliac artery, each vessel

0239T Bioimpedance spectroscopy (BIS), measuring 100 frequencies or greater, direct measurement of extracellular fluid differences between the limbs

0240T Esophageal motility (manometric study of the esophagus and/or gastroesophageal junction) study with interpretation and report; with high resolution esophageal pressure topography

(Do not report 0240T in conjunction with 91010 or 91013)

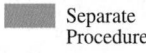 Separate Procedure   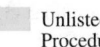 Unlisted Procedure   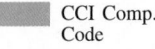 CCI Comp. Code   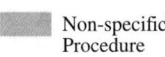 Non-specific Procedure

+ 0241T   with stimulation or perfusion during high resolution esophageal pressure topography study, (eg, stimulant, acid or alkali perfusion) (List separately in addition to code for primary procedure)

(Use 0241T in conjunction with 0240T)

(Do not report 0241T in conjunction with 91010 or 91013)

(Do not report 0241T more than once per session)

(To report esophageal motility studies without high-resolution esophageal pressure topography, use 91010 and with stimulant or perfusion, use 91013)

(0242T   deleted 2013 edition. To report, use 91112)

0243T   Intermittent measurement of wheeze rate for bronchodilator or bronchial-challenge diagnostic evaluation(s), with interpretation and report

(Use 0243T once per 24 hour period)

(Do not report 0243T in conjunction with 0244T for the same 24 hour period)

0244T   Continuous measurement of wheeze rate during treatment assessment or during sleep for documentation of nocturnal wheeze and cough for diagnostic evaluation 3 to 24 hours, with interpretation and report

0245T   Open treatment of rib fracture requiring internal fixation, unilateral; 1-2 ribs

0246T   3-4 ribs

0247T   5-6 ribs

0248T   7 or more ribs

0249T   Ligation, hemorrhoidal vascular bundle(s), including ultrasound guidance

(Do not report 0249T in conjunction with 46020, 46221, 46250-46262, 46600, 46945, 46946, 76872, 76942, 76998)

(0250T   deleted 2013 edition. For airway sizing and insertion and removal of bronchial valve[s], see 31647-31649)

● New Code   ▲ Revised Code   + Add-On Code   ⊘ Modifier -51 Exempt   ⊙ Moderate Sedation

(0251T   deleted 2013 edition. For airway sizing and insertion and removal of bronchial valve[s], see 31647-31649)

(0252T   deleted 2013 edition. For airway sizing and insertion and removal of bronchial valve[s], see 31647-31649)

0253T   This code is out of order. See page 1316

0254T   Endovascular repair of iliac artery bifurcation (eg, aneurysm, pseudoaneurysm, arteriovenous malformation, trauma) using bifurcated endoprosthesis from the common iliac artery into both the external and internal iliac artery, unilateral;

0255T   radiological supervision and interpretation

(0256T   deleted 2013 edition. To report, see 33361-33364)

(0257T   deleted 2013 edition. To report, see 33365, 0318T)

(0258T   deleted 2013 edition. To report, see 33365, 0318T)

(0259T   deleted 2013 edition. To report, see 33365-33369

0260T   Total body systemic hypothermia, per day, in the neonate 28 days of age or younger

0261T   Selective head hypothermia, per day, in the neonate 28 days of age or younger

0262T   Implantation of catheter-delivered prosthetic pulmonary valve, endovascular approach

(0262T includes all congenital cardiac catheterization(s), intraprocedural contrast injection[s], fluoroscopic radiological supervision and interpretation, and imaging guidance performed to complete the pulmonary valve procedure. Do not report 0262T in conjunction with 76000, 76001, 93530, 93563, 93566-93568)

0262T includes percutaneous balloon angioplasty/valvuloplasty of the pulmonary valve/conduit. Do not report 0262T in conjunction with 92990)

(0262T includes stent deployment within the pulmonary conduit. Do not report 37205, 37206, 75960 for stent placement within the pulmonary conduit. Report 37205, 37206, 92928-92944, 75960 separately when cardiovascular stent placement is performed at a site separate from the prosthetic

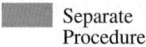 Separate Procedure   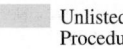 Unlisted Procedure   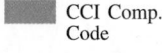 CCI Comp. Code   Non-specific Procedure   **1323**

valve delivery site. Report 92997, 92998 separately when pulmonary artery angioplasty is performed at a site separate from the prosthetic valve delivery site)

0263T Intramuscular autologous bone marrow cell therapy, with preparation of harvested cells, multiple injections, one leg, including ultrasound guidance, if performed; complete procedure including unilateral or bilateral bone marrow harvest

(Do not report 0263T in conjunction with 38204-38242, 76942, 93925, 93926)

0264T complete procedure excluding bone marrow harvest

(Do not report 0264T in conjunction with 38204-38242, 76942, 93925, 93926, 0265T)

0265T unilateral or bilateral bone marrow harvest only for intramuscular autologous bone marrow cell therapy

(Do not report 0265T in conjunction with 38204-38242, 0264T. For complete procedure, use 0263T)

0266T Implantation or replacement of carotid sinus baroreflex activation device; total system (includes generator placement, unilateral or bilateral lead placement, intra-operative interrogation, programming, and repositioning, when performed)

0267T lead only, unilateral (includes intra-operative interrogation, programming, and repositioning, when performed)

(For bilateral lead implantation or replacement, use 0267T with modifier 50)

0268T pulse generator only (includes intra-operative interrogation, programming, and repositioning, when performed)

(Do not report 0267T, 0268T in conjunction with 0266T, 0269T-0273T)

0269T Revision or removal of carotid sinus baroreflex activation device; total system (includes generator placement, unilateral or bilateral lead placement, intra-operative interrogation, programming, and repositioning, when performed)

(Do not report 0269T in conjunction with 0266T-0268T, 0270T-0273T)

0270T lead only, unilateral (includes intra-operative interrogation, programming, and repositioning, when performed)

1324

● New Code	▲ Revised Code	+ Add-On Code	⊘ Modifier -51 Exempt	⊙ Moderate Sedation

(Do not report 0270T in conjunction with 0266T-0269T, 0271T-0273T)

(For bilateral lead removal, use 0270T with modifier 50)

(For removal of total carotic sinus baroreflex activation device, use 0269T)

0271T   pulse generator only (includes intra-operative interrogation, programming, and repositioning, when performed)

(Do not report 0271T in conjunction with 0266T-0270T, 0272T, 0273T)

(For removal and replacement, see 0266T, 0267T, 0268T)

0272T   Interrogation device evaluation (in person), carotid sinus baroreflex activation system, including telemetric ineractive communication with the implantable device to monitor device diagnostics and programmed therapy values, with interpretation and report (eg, battery status, lead impedance, pulse amplitude, pulse width, therapy frequency, pathway mode, burst mode, therapy start/stop times each day);

(Do not report 0272T in conjunction with 0266T-0271T, 0273T)

0273T   with programming

(Do not report 0273T in conjunction with 0266T-0272T)

0274T   Percutaneous laminotomy/laminectomy (interlaminar approach) for decompression of neural elements, (with or without ligamentous resection, discectomy, facetectomy and/or foraminotomy), any method, under indirect image guidance (eg, fluoroscopic, CT), with or without the use of an endoscope, single or multiple levels, unilateral or bilateral; cervical or thoracic

0275T   lumbar

(For laminotomy/hemilaminectomy performed using an open and endoscopically-assisted approach, see 63020-63035)

(For percutaneous decompression of the nucleus pulposus of intervertebral disc utilizing needle based technique, use 62287)

(0276T   deleted 2013 edition. To report, see 31660, 31661)

(0277T   deleted 2013 edition. To report, see 31660, 31661)

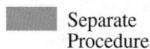

| | Separate Procedure | | Unlisted Procedure | | CCI Comp. Code | | Non-specific Procedure |

1325

0278T   Transcutaneous electrical modulation pain reprocessing (eg, scrambler therapy), each treatment session (includes placement of electrodes)

(0279T   deleted 2013 edition. To report, see 86152, 86153)

(0280T   deleted 2013 edition. To report, see 86152, 86153)

0281T   Percutaneous transcatheter closure of the left atrial appendage with implant, including fluoroscopy, transseptal puncture, catheter placement(s), left atrial angiography, left atrial appendage angiography, radiological supervision and interpretation.

(Do not report 0281T in conjunction with 93462 [left heart catheterization by transseptal puncture])

(Report cardiac catheterization procedures [93451-93461, 93530-93533] separately for indications distinct from the left atrial appendage closure procedure)

(For left ventriculography performed by transseptal approach for indications distinct from the left atrial appendage closure procedure, use 93565)

(Do not report 0281T in conjunction with 93452, 93453, 93458-93461, 93531-93533 unless catheterization of the left ventricle is performed by a non-transseptal approach for indications distinct from the left atrial appendage closure procedure)

(Do not report 0281T in conjunction with 93451, 93453, 93456, 93460, 93461, 93530-93533 unless complete right heart catheterization is performed for indications distinct from the left atrial appendage closure procedure)

⊙ **0282T**   Percutaneous or open implantation of neurostimulator electrode array(s), subcutaneous (peripheral subcutaneous field stimulation), including imaging guidance, when performed, cervical, thoracic or lumbar; for trial, including removal at the conclusion of trial period

⊙ **0283T**   permanent, with implantation of a pulse generator

⊙ **0284T**   Revision or removal of pulse generator or electrodes, including imaging guidance, when performed, including addition of new electrodes, when performed

● New Code   ▲ Revised Code   + Add-On Code   ⊘ Modifier -51 Exempt   ⊙ Moderate Sedation

0285T Electronic analysis of implanted peripheral subcutaneous field stimulation pulse generator, with reprogramming when performed

(Do not report 0282T-0285T in conjunction with 64550-64595, 77002, 77003, 95970-95973)

0286T Near-infrared spectroscopy studies of lower extremity wounds (eg, for oxyhemoglobin measurement)

0287T Near-infrared guidance for vascular access requiring real-time digital visualization of subcutaneous vasculature for evaluation of potential access sites and vessel patency

0288T Anoscopy, with delivery of thermal energy to the muscle of the anal canal (eg, for fecal incontinence)

(Do not report 0288T in conjunction with 46600-46615)

+ 0289T Corneal incisions in the donor cornea created using a laser, in preparation for penetrating or lamellar keratoplasty (List separately in addition to code for primary procedure)

(Use 0289T in conjunction with 65710, 65730, 65750, 65755)

+ 0290T Corneal incisions in the recipient cornea created using a laser, in preparation for penetrating or lamellar keratoplasty (List separately in addition to code for primary procedure)

(Use 0290T in conjunction with 65710, 65730, 65750, 65755)

●⊙+0291T Intravascular optical coherence tomography (coronary native vessel or graft) during diagnostic evaluation and/or therapeutic intervention, including imaging supervision, interpretation, and report; initial vessel (List separately in addition to primary procedure)

(Use 0291T in conjunction with cardiac catheterization codes 92920, 92924, 92928, 92933, 92937, 92941, 92943, 92975, 93454-93461, 93563, 93564)

(Intravascular optical coherence tomography services include all transducer manipulations and repositioning within the specific vessel being examined, both before and after therapeutic intervention [eg, stent placement])

●⊙+0292T each additional vessel (List separately in addition to primary procedure)

(Use 0292T in conjunction with 0291T)

| Separate Procedure | Unlisted Procedure | CCI Comp. Code | Non-specific Procedure | **1327** |

(For intravascular spectroscopy, use 0205T)

●⊙**0293T** Insertion of left atrial hemodynamic monitor; complete system, includes implanted communication module and pressure sensor lead in left atrium including transseptal access, radiological supervision and interpretation, and associated injection procedures, when performed

(Do not report 0293T in conjunction with 93462, 93662)

●⊙+**0294T** pressure sensor lead at time of insertion of pacing cardioverter-defibrillator pulse generator including radiological supervision and interpretation and associated injection procedures, when performed (List separately in addition to code for primary procedure)

(Use 0294T in conjunction with 33230, 33231, 33240, 33262-33264, 33249)

(Do not report 0294T in conjunction with 93462, 93662)

(Do not report 0293T or 0294T in conjunction with 33202-33249, 93451-93453 unless performed for separate and distinct clinical indication other than for placement or calibration of left atrial hemodynamic monitoring system)

● **0295T** External electrocardiographic recording for more than 48 hours up to 21 days by continuous rhythm recording and storage; includes recording, scanning analysis with report, review and interpretation

● **0296T** recording (includes connection and initial recording)

● **0297T** scanning analysis with report

● **0298T** review and interpretation

(Do not report 0295T-0298T in conjunction with 93224-93272 for same monitoring period)

● **0299T** Extracorporeal shock wave for integumentary wound healing, high energy, including topical application and dressing care; initial wound

●+**0300T** each additional wound (List separately in addition to code for primary procedure)

(Use 0300T in conjunction with 0299T)

(Do not report 0300T in conjunction with 28890, 0101T, 0102T when treating same area)

● New Code ▲ Revised Code + Add-On Code ⊘ Modifier -51 Exempt ⊙ Moderate Sedation

●⊙**0301T**   Destruction/reduction of malignant breast tumor with externally applied focused microwave, including interstitial placement of disposable catheter with combined temperature monitoring probe and microwave focusing sensocatheter under ultrasound thermotherapy guidance

(Do not report 0301T in conjunction with 76645, 76942, 76998, 77600-77615)

●⊙**0302T**   Insertion or removal and replacement of intracardiac ischemia monitoring system including imaging supervision and interpretation when performed and intra-operative interrogation and programming when performed; complete system (includes device and electrode)

●⊙**0303T**   electrode only

●⊙**0304T**   device only

(Do not report 0302T-0304T in conjunction with 93000-93010)

● **0305T**   Programming device evaluation (in person) of intracardiac ischemia monitoring system with iterative adjustment of programmed values, with analysis, review and report

(Do not report 0305T in conjunction with 93000-93010, 0302T-0304T, 0306T)

● **0306T**   Interrogation device evaluation (in person) of intracardiac ischemia monitoring system with analysis, review and report

(Do not report 0306T in conjunction with 93000-93010, 0302T-0304T)

●⊙**0307T**   Removal of intracardiac ischemia monitoring device

⊘⊙**0308T**   Insertion of ocular telescope prosthesis including removal of crystalline lens

(Do not report 0308T in conjunction with 65800-65815, 66020, 66030, 66600-66635, 66761, 66825, 66982-66986, 69990)

●+**0309T**   Arthrodesis, pre-sacral interbody technique, including disc space preparation, discectomy, with posterior instrumentation, with image guidance, includes bone graft, when performed, lumbar, L4-L5 interspace (List separately in addition to code for primary procedure)

(Use 0309T in conjunction with 22586)

| | Separate Procedure | | Unlisted Procedure | | CCI Comp. Code | | Non-specific Procedure | **1329** |

(Do not report 0309T in conjunction with 20930-20938, 22840, 22848, 72275, 77002, 77003, 77011, 77012)

● **0310T** Motor function mapping using non-invasive navigated transcranial magnetic stimulation (nTMS) for therapeutic treatment planning, upper and lower extremity

(Do not report 0310T in conjunction with 95860-95870, 95928, 95929, 95939)

● **0311T** Non-invasive calculation and analysis of central arterial pressure waveforms with interpretation and report

● **0312T** Vagus nerve blocking therapy (morbid obesity); laparoscopic implantation of neurostimulator electrode array, anterior and posterior vagal trunks adjacent to esophagogastric junction (EGJ), with implantation of pulse generator, includes programming

● **0313T** laparoscopic revision or replacement of vagal trunk neurostimulator electrode array, including connection to existing pulse generator

● **0314T** laparascopic removal of vagal trunk neurostimulator

● **0315T** removal of pulse generator

● **0316T** replacement of pulse generator

(Do not report 0315T in conjunction with 0316T)

● **0317T** neurostimulator pulse generator electronic analysis, includes reprogramming when performed

(For implantation, revision, replacement, and/or removal of vagus [cranial] nerve neurostimulator electrode array and/or pulse generator for vagus nerve stimulation performed other than at the ECJ [eg, epilepsy], see 64568-64570)

(For analsysis and/or [re]programming for vagus nerve stimulator, see 95970, 95974, 95975)

● **0318T** Implantation of catheter-delivered prosthetic aortic heart valve, open thoracic approach, (eg, transapical, other than transaortic)

(For percutaneous femoral artery, open femoral artery, open axillary artery, open iliac artery, or transaortic approach, see 33361-33365)

(To report cardiopulmonary bypass in conjunction with 0318T, see 33367, 33368, or 33369)

● New Code	▲ Revised Code	＋ Add-On Code	⊘ Modifier -51 Exempt	⊙ Moderate Sedation

ALPHABETICAL INDEX

The alphabetical index includes listings by procedure, CPT® headings and sub-headings and anatomic site. Procedures and services commonly known by their acronyms, eponyms, homonyms or other designations are also included. The alphabetical index of CPT® PLUS is unique in that both indexes to specific page numbers and indexes to CPT code numbers are included.

HOW TO USE THE ALPHABETICAL INDEX

When using the alphabetical index to locate CPT codes, use the following search sequence:

- Look for the CPT HEADING for the general category of surgical procedure(s) or medical service(s) or TOPIC for instructional and/or explanatory information.

- Look for the CPT Sub-heading for the organ system(s) involved or service(s) performed or the TOPIC sub-heading for the instructional or explanatory issue. Scan the index listings to determine if the specific procedure or service or topic is listed.

- For CPT codes, use the thumb-tab indexes to locate the appropriate CPT code section. If the specific procedure or service was listed in the index, locate the procedure or service in the CPT code section and verify the full description of the CPT code before using. If the specific procedure or service was not listed in the index, first locate the organ system and/or medical service sub-heading and then review the CPT code section until you locate the specific procedure and/or service.

- For instructional and/or explanatory topics, turn to the page number specified in the alphabetical index.

- Alternately, look for SYNONYMS, HOMONYMS, EPONYMS or ACRONYMS.

The alphabetic index is NOT a substitute for the main text of CPT. Even if codes are found in the index, the user must refer to the main text to ensure that the code selection is accurate.

This page intentionally left blank.

A

Abbe-Estlander procedure ~ 40527, 40761
Abdomen
  abdonminal aorta, angiography ~ 75635
  abdominal wall
    removal, mesh/prosthesis ~ 11008
    repair hernia ~ 49491-49496, 49501, 49507, 49521, 49590
    tumor, excision ~ 22900-22905
    unlisted services and procedures ~ 22999
  abscess
    incision and drainage ~ 49020, 49040
      open ~ 49040
      percutaneous ~ 49021
  angiography ~ 74174, 74175, 75635
  artery ligation ~ 37617
  biopsy ~ 49000
  bypass graft ~ 35907
  catheter removal ~ 49422
  celiotomy for staging ~ 49220
  CT scan ~ 74150-74178, 75635
  cyst destruction/excision ~ 49203-49205
  drainage fluid ~ 49082-49083
  ectopic pregnancy ~ 59130
  endometrioma destruction/excision ~ 49203-49205
  exploration ~ 49000-49002
    blood vessel ~ 35840
    staging ~ 58960
  incision ~ 49000
    staging ~ 58960
  incision and drainage pancreatitis ~ 48000
  infraumbilical panniculectomy ~ 15830
  injection
    air ~ 49400
    contrast material ~ 49400
  insertion
    catheter ~ 49324, 49418-49419, 49421
    venous shunt ~ 49425
  intraperitoneal
    catheter exit site ~ 49436
    catheter insertion ~ 49324, 49435
    catheter removal ~ 49422
    catheter revision ~ 49325
    shunt
      ligation ~ 49428
      removal ~ 49429
  laparotomy, staging ~ 49220
  magnetic resonance imaging (MRI) ~ 74181-74183
  needle biopsy, mass ~ 49180
  paracentesis ~ 49082-49083
  peritoneal lavage ~ 49084
  radical resection ~ 51597
  radiation therapy, guidance ~ 49411-49412

Abdomen ~ *continued*
  repair
    blood vessel ~ 35221
      with other graft ~ 35281
      with vein graft ~ 35251
    hernia ~ 49491-49525, 49560-49587
    suture ~ 49900
  revision venous shunt ~ 49426
  suture ~ 49900
  tumor destruction/excision ~ 49203-49205
  ultrasound ~ 76700-76705
  unlisted services and procedures ~ 49999
  wound exploration penetrating ~ 20102
  X-ray ~ 74000-74022
Abdominal aorta ~ *see* aorta, abdominal
Abdominal aortic aneurysm ~ 0078T-0081T, 34800-34805, 34825-34832, 35081-35103, 75952, 75953
Abdominal deliveries ~ *see* cesarean delivery
Abdominal hysterectomy ~ *see* hysterectomy, abdominal
Abdominal lymphangiogram ~ 75805, 75807
Abdominal paracentesis ~ *see* abdomen, drainage
Abdominal radiographies ~ 74000-74022
Abdominal wall
  debridement, infected ~ 11005-11006
  reconstruction ~ 49905
  removal
    mesh ~ 11008
    prosthesis ~ 11008
  surgery ~ 22999
  tumor excision ~ 22900-22905
Abdominohysterectomy ~ *see* hysterectomy, abdominal
Abdominopelvic amputation ~ 27290
Abdominoplasty
  excision ~ 15847
Ablation
  anal polyp or tumor ~ 46615
  bone tumor ~ 20982
  colon tumor ~ 44393, 45339
  cryosurgical
    fibroadenoma ~ 19105
    liver tumor ~ 47381
    renal mass ~ 50250
    renal tumor, percutaneous ~ 50593
  CT scan guidance ~ 77013
  endometrial ~ 58353, 58356, 58563
    with ultrasound guidance ~ 58356
  heart
    arrhythmogenic focus ~ 33250-33251, 33261, 93653, 93654, 93655
    atrioventricular ~ 93650, 93653, 93654
  liver tumor
    cryosurgical ~ 47381
    laparoscopic ~ 47370-47371
    open ~ 47380-47382
  lung tumor
    radiofrequency ~ 32998

Ablation ~ *continued*
parenchymal tissue
  CT scan guidance ~ 77013
  magnetic resonance guidance ~ 77022
  ultrasound guidance ~ 76940
prostate ~ 55873
pulmonry tumor ~ 32998
radiofrequency
  liver tumor ~ 47382
  lung tumor ~ 32998
  renal tumor ~ 50592
  tongue base ~ 41530
rectum, polyp or tumor ~ 45339
renal
  cyst ~ 50541
  mass ~ 50542
  tumor, percutaneous cryotherapy ~ 50593
tongue base, radiofrequency ~ 41530
turbinate mucosa ~ 30801-30802
uterine tumor, ultrasound, focused ~
  0071T-0072T
vein, endovenous ~ 36475-36479
Abortion
incomplete ~ 59812
induced by
  dilation and curettage ~ 59840
  dilation and evacuation ~ 59841
  saline ~ 59850-59851
  vaginal suppositories ~ 59855-59856
missed
  first trimester ~ 59820
  second trimester ~ 59821
septic ~ 59830
spontaneous ~ 59812
therapeutic
  by saline ~ 59850
    with dilation and curettage ~ 59851
    with hysterectomy ~ 59852
  with hysterectomy ~ 59100, 59852, 59857
Abrasion
skin
  chemical peel ~ 15788-15793
  dermabrasion ~ 15780-15783
  lesion ~ 15786-15787
  salabrasion ~ 15810-15811
Abscess
abdomen ~ 49040-49041
  incision and drainage
    open ~ 49040
    percutaneous ~ 49021
anal, incision and drainage ~ 46045-46050
ankle ~ 27603
appendix, incision and drainage ~ 44900
  open ~ 44900
  percutaneous ~ 44901
arm, lower ~ 25028
  excision ~ 25145
  incision and drainage ~ 25035
arm, upper, incision and drainage ~
  23930-23935
auditory canal, external ~ 69020

Abscess ~ *continued*
Bartholin's gland, incision and drainage ~
  56420
bladder, incision and drainage ~ 51080
brain
  drainage ~ 61150-61151
  excision ~ 61514, 61522
  incision and drainage ~ 61320-61321
breast, incision and drainage ~ 19020
carpals, incision, deep ~ 25035
clavicle sequestrectomy ~ 23170
drainage, with X-ray ~ 75989
ear, external
  complicated ~ 69005
  simple ~ 69000
elbow, incision and drainage ~ 23930-23935
epididymis, incision and drainage ~ 54700
excision
  olecranon process ~ 24138
  radius ~ 24136
  ulna ~ 24138
eyelid, incision and drainage ~ 67700
facial bones, excision ~ 21026
finger ~ 26010-26011
  incision and drainage ~ 26034
foot, incision ~ 28005
gums, incision and drainage ~ 41800
hand, incision and drainage ~ 26034
hematoma, incision and drainage ~ 27603
hip, incision and drainage ~ 26990-26992
humeral head ~ 23174
humerus
  excision ~ 24134
  incision and drainage ~ 23935
kidney incision and drainage ~ 50020
  open ~ 50020
  percutaneous ~ 50021
leg, lower,incision and drainage ~ 27603
liver ~ 47010
  drainage, open ~ 47010
  injection ~ 47015
  repair ~ 47300
localization, nuclear medicine ~ 78806-78807
lung, percutaneous drainage ~ 32200-32201
lymph node, incision and drainage ~
  38300-38305
lymphocele drainage ~ 49062
mandible, excision ~ 21025
mouth, incision and drainage ~ 40800-40801,
  41005-41009, 41015-41018
nasal septum, incision and drainage ~ 30020
neck, incision and drainage ~ 21501-21502
ovarian incision and drainage ~ 58820-58822
  abdominal approach ~ 58822
  vaginal approach ~ 58820
ovary, drainage, percutaneous ~ 58823
palate, incision and drainage ~ 42000
paraurethral gland, incision and drainage ~
  53060
parotid gland drainage ~ 42300-42305
pelvic, drainage, percutaneous ~ 58823

Abscess ~ *continued*
pelvis, incision and drainage ~ 26990-26992, 45000
pericolic, drainage, percutaneous ~ 58823
perineum, incision and drainage ~ 56405
perirenal or renal
drainage ~ 50020-50021
percutaneous ~ 50021
peritoneum
incision and drainage
open ~ 49020
percutaneous ~ 49021
prostate
incision and drainage ~ 55720-55725
transurethral drainage ~ 52700
radius, incision, deep ~ 25035
rectum, incision and drainage ~ 45005-45020, 46040, 46060
retroperitoneal ~ 49060-49061
drainage
open ~ 49060
percutaneous ~ 49061
salivary gland, drainage ~ 42300-42320
scapula, sequestrectomy ~ 23172
scrotum, incision & drainage ~ 54700, 55100
shoulder, drainage ~ 23030
Skene's gland, incision and drainage ~ 53060
skin
incision and drainage ~ 10060-10061
puncture aspiration ~ 10160
soft tissue, incision ~ 20005
subdiaphragmatic ~ 49040-49041
sublingual gland, drainage ~ 42310-42320
submaxillary gland, drainage ~ 42310-42320
subphrenic ~ 49040-49041
testis, incision and drainage ~ 54700
thoracostomy ~ 32551
thorax, incision and drainage ~ 21501-21502
throat, incision and drainage ~ 42700-42725
tongue, incision and drainage ~ 41000-41006
tonsil, incision and drainage ~ 42700
ulna, incision, deep ~ 25035
urethra, incision and drainage ~ 53040
uvula, incision and drainage ~ 42000
vagina, incision and drainage ~ 57010
vulva, incision and drainage ~ 56405
wrist
excision ~ 25145
incision and drainage ~ 25028, 25035
X-ray ~ 76080
Absorptiometry
dual energy ~ 3095F-3096F
bone
appendicular ~ 77081
axial skeleton ~ 77080
vertebral ~ 77082
dual photon, bone ~ 78351
single photon, bone ~ 78350
Absorption spectrophotometry, atomic ~ 82190
Accessory nerve, spinal ~ 63191
Accessory, toes ~ 28344

ACE (angiotensin converting enzyme) ~ 82164
Acetabuloplasty ~ 27120-27122
Acetabulum
fracture
closed treatment ~ 27220-27222
open treatment ~ 27226-27228
with manipulation ~ 27222
without manipulation ~ 27220
reconstruction ~ 27120
with resection, femoral head ~ 27122
tumor, excision ~ 27076
Acetaldehyde, blood ~ 82000
Acetaminophen, urine ~ 82003
Acetic anhydrides ~ 84600
Acetone, blood or urine ~ 82009-82010
Acetone body ~ 82009-82010
Acetylcholinesterase, blood or urine ~ 82013
AcG ~ 85220
Achilles tendon
incision ~ 27605-27606
lengthening ~ 27612
repair ~ 27650-27654
Achillotomy ~ 27605-27606
Acid(s)
adenylic ~ 82030
amino ~ 82127-82139
aminolevulinic ~ see aminolevulinic acid (ALA)
ascorbic ~ 82180
bile ~ 82239
deoxyribonucleic ~ 86225-86226
fatty ~ see fatty acid
folic ~ 82747
glycocholic ~ 82240
guanylic ~ 83008
lactic ~ 83605
n-acetylneuraminic ~ 84275
n-acetylneuraminic ~ 84275
phenylethylbarbituric ~ 82205
uric ~ see uric acid
Acidity/alkalinity ~ *see* pH
Acid diethylamide, lysergic ~ 80102-80103, 80299
Acid fast bacilli (AFB), culture ~ 87116
Acid fast stain ~ 88312
Acid perfusion test, esophagus ~ 91030
Acid phosphatase ~ 84060-84066
Acid probes, nucleic ~ *see* nucleic acid probes
Acid reflux test, esophagus ~ 91034-91038
Acne surgery
incision and drainage
abscess ~ 10060-10061
comedones ~ 10040
cyst ~ 10040
milia, multiple ~ 10040
pustules ~ 10040
Acne treatment
abrasion ~ 15786-15787
chemical peel ~ 15788-15793
cryotherapy ~ 17340
dermabrasion ~ 15780-15783

1335

Acne treatment ~ *continued*
exfoliation
chemical ~ 17360
salabrasion ~ 15810-15811
Acoustic evoked brain stem potential ~
92585-92586
Acoustic neuroma (*see also* brainstem, skull
base surgery) ~ 61510, 61518,
61520-61521, 61526-61530, 61545, 62164
Acoustic recording, heart sounds, with
computer analysis ~ 93799
Acromioclavicular joint, arthrocentesis ~
20605
arthrotomy ~ 23044
with biopsy ~ 23101
dislocation ~ 23540-23552
open treatment ~ 23550-23552
X-ray ~ 73050
Acromion,excision, shoulder ~ 23130
Acromionectomy, partial ~ 23130
Acromioplasty ~ 23415-23420
partial ~ 23130
ACTH releasing factor ~ 80412
Actigraphy, sleep study ~ 95803
Actinomyces, antibody ~ 86602
Actinomycosis ~ 86000
Actinomycotic infection ~ 86000
Actinotherapy ~ see dermatology ~ 96900
Activated factor X ~ 85260
Activated partial thromboplastin time ~
85730-85732
Activation, lymphocyte ~ 86353
Activities of daily living ~ *see* physical
medicine/therapy/occupational therapy
Activity, glomerular procoagulant ~ *see*
thromboplastin
Acupuncture
with electrical stimulation ~ 97813-97814
without electrical stimulation ~ 97810-97811
Acute poliomyelitis ~ *see* polio
Acylcarnitines ~ 82016-82017
Adamantinoma, pituitary ~ *see*
craniopharyngioma
Addam operation ~ 26040-26045
Adductor tenotomy of hip ~ 27000-27003
Adenoidectomy ~ 42820-42821, 42830-42836
Adenoids
excision ~ 42830-42836
with tonsils ~ 42820-42821
unlisted services and procedures ~ 42999
Adenoma
pancreas, excision ~ 48120
thyroid gland excision ~ 60200
Adenosine 3'5' monophosphate ~ 82030
Adenosine diphosphate, blood ~ 82030
Adenosine monophosphate (AMP), blood ~
82030
Adenovirus
antibody ~ 86603
antigen detection
enzyme immunoassay ~ 87301
immunofluorescense ~ 87260

Adenovirus vaccine ~ *see* vaccines
Adenylic acid ~ *see* adenosine monophosphate
(AMP)
ADH (antidiuretic hormone) ~ 84588
Adhesions
epidural ~ , 62263-62264
eye
corneovitreal ~ 65880
incision
anterior segment ~ 65860-65870
posterior segment ~ 65875
intermarginal, construction ~ 67880
transposition of tarsal plate ~ 67882
intestinal, enterolysis ~ 44005
laparoscopic ~ 44200
intracranial, lysis ~ 62161
intrauterine, lysis ~ 58559
labial, lysis ~ 56441
lungs, lysis ~ 32124
pelvic, lysis ~ 58660, 58662, 58740
penile, lysis, post-circumcision ~ 54162
preputial, lysis ~ 54450
urethral, lysis ~ 53500
Adipectomy ~ *see* lipectomy
ADL ~ *see* activities of daily living
Administration
immunization
each additional vaccine/toxoid ~ 90472,
90474
with counseling ~ 90461
one vaccine/toxoid ~ 90471, 90473
with counseling ~ 90460
occlusive substance ~ 31634
pharmacologic agent ~ 93463
ADP ~ *see* adenosine diphosphate
ADP phosphocreatine phosphotransferase ~
see CPK
Adrenal cortex hormone ~ *see* corticosteroids
Adrenal gland
biopsy ~ 60540-60545
excision
laparoscopy ~ 60650
retroperitoneal tumor ~ 60545
exploration ~ 60540-60545
nuclear medicine, imaging ~ 78075
Adrenal medulla ~ *see* medulla
Adrenalectomy ~ 60540
anesthesia ~ 00866
laparoscopic ~ 50545
Adrenalin ~ 80424, 82382-82384
blood ~ 82383
urine ~ 82384
Adrenaline-noradrenaline
testing ~ 82382-82384
Adrenocorticotropic hormone (ACTH) ~
80400-80406, 80412, 80418, 82024
blood or urine ~ 82024
stimulation panel ~ 80400-80406
Adrenogenital syndrome ~ 56805, 57335
Adult T cell leukemia lymphoma virus I ~
see HTLV I

Advanced life support ~ 99281-99288
  physician direction ~ 99288
Advancement
  genioglossus ~ 21199
  tendon foot ~ 28238
Advancement flap ~ 14000-14350
Aerosol inhalation ~ see pulmonology,
  therapeutic
  pentamidine ~ 94642
AFB ~ see acid fast bacilli
Afferent nerve ~ see sensory nerve
AFP ~ see alpha-fetoprotein
After hours medical services ~ 99050-99054
Agents, anticoagulant ~ 85300-85305, 85307
Agglutinin
  cold ~ 86156-86157
  febrile ~ 86000
Aggregation, platelet ~ 85576
AHG ~ 85210-85293
AICD (pacing cardioverter-defibrillator) ~ see
  defibrillator, heart; pacemaker, heart
Aid, hearing ~ see hearing aid
AIDS antibodies ~ 86689, 86701-86703
AIDS virus ~ see HIV-1
Akin operation ~ 28296-28299
ALA ~ see aminolevulinic acid
Alanine 2 oxoglutarate aminotransferase ~
  84460
Alanine amino (ALT) ~ 84460
Alanine transaminase ~ 84460
Albumin
  ischemia modified ~ 82045
  serum ~ 82040
  urine ~ 82042-82044
Alcohol
  breath ~ 82075
  ethyl
    blood ~ 82055
    urine ~ 82055
  ethylene glycol ~ 82693
  dehydrogenase ~ 84588
  isopropyl ~ 84600
  methyl ~ 84600
Aldolase, blood ~ 82085
Aldosterone
  blood ~ 82088
  suppression evaluation ~ 80408
  urine ~ 82088
Alimentary canal ~ see gastrointestinal tract
Alkaline phosphatase ~ 84075-84080
  leukocyte ~ 85540
  WBC ~ 85540
Alkaloids ~ see specific drug
  urine ~ 82101
Allergen bronchial provocation tests ~
  95070-95071
Allergen challenge, endobronchial ~
  95070-95071

Allergen immunotherapy
  allergen
    prescription/ supply/injection ~ 95120-95125
      with extract supply ~ 95144
    injection ~ 95115-95117
  antigens ~ 95144
  IgE ~ 86003-86005
  IgG ~ 86001
  insect venom
    prescription/supply ~ 95145-95149
    prescription/supply/injection ~ 95130-95134
  prescription/supply ~ 95165
    insect, whole body ~ 95170
  rapid desensitization ~ 95180
Allergy services/procedures ~ 95004-95199
  education and counseling ~ 99201-99215
  unlisted services and procedures ~ 95199
Allergy tests
  challenge test
    bronchial ~ 95070-95071
    ingestion ~ 95076, 95079
  eye allergy ~ 95060
  food allergy ~ 95076, 95079
  intradermal
    allergen extract ~ 95024-95028
    biologicals ~ 95018
    drugs ~ 95018
    incremental ~ 95027
    venoms ~ 95017
  nasal mucous membrane test ~ 95065
  nose allergy ~ 95065
  patch
    application tests ~ 95044
    photo patch ~ 95052
  photosensitivity ~ 95056
  skin tests
    allergen extract ~ 95004, 95024, 95027
    biologicals ~ 95018
    drugs ~ 95018
    venoms ~ 95017
Allogeneic donor, lymphocyte infusion ~
  38242
Allogeneic transplantation ~ see homograft
Allograft
  aortic valve ~ 33406, 33413
  bone, structural ~ 20931
  cartilage, knee ~ 27415
  lung transplant ~ 32850
  skin ~ 15350-15351
  skin substitute graft ~ 15271-15278
  spine surgery
    morselized ~ 20930
    structural ~ 20931
Allograft preparation
  heart ~ 33933, 33944
  intestines ~ 44715-44721
  kidney ~ 50323-50329
  liver ~ 47143-47147
  lung ~ 32855-32856, 33933
  pancrease ~ 48551-48552
  renal ~ 50323-50329

Allotransplantation
  intestines ~ 44135-44136
  renal ~ 50360-50365
  removal ~ 50370
Almen test ~ 82270
Alpha-1 antitrypsin ~ 82103-82104, 99565
Alpha-2 antiplasmin ~ 85410
Alpha-fetoprotein
  amniotic fluid ~ 82106
  serum ~ 82105, 82107
Alphatocopherol ~ 84446
ALT ~ 84460
Altemeier procedure ~ (see anus)
  45130-45135
Aluminum, blood ~ 82108
  Alveolafracture
  closed treatment ~ 21421
  open treatment ~ 21422-21423
Alveolar cleft
  ungrafted bilateral ~ 21147
  ungrafted unilateral ~ 21146
Alveolar nerve
  avulsion ~ 64738
  incision ~ 64738
  transection ~ 64738
Alveolar ridge fracture
  closed treatment ~ 21440
  open treatment ~ 21445
Alveolectomy ~ 41830
Alveoloplasty ~ 41874
Alveolus, excision ~ 41830
Amide, procaine ~ see procainamide
Amikacin, assay ~ 80150
Amine, vaginal fluid ~ 82120
Amino acids ~ 82127-82139
Aminolevulinic acid (ALA), blood or urine ~
  82135
Aminotransferase ~ see transaminase
Aminotransferase, alanine ~ 84460
Aminotransferase, aspartate ~ 84450
Amitriptyline, assay ~ 80152
Ammonia
  blood ~ 82140
  urine ~ 82140
Amniocenteses ~ 59000
  with amniotic fluid reduction ~ 59001
  induced abortion ~ 59850
    with dilation and curettage ~ 59851
    with dilation and evacuation ~ 59851
    with hysterectomy ~ 59852
Amnioinfusion, transabdominal ~ 59070
Amnion ~ 59001
  amniocentesis ~ 59000
    with amniotic fluid reduction ~ 59001
  amnioinfusion, transabdominal ~ 59070
Amniotic fluid
  alpha-fetoprotein ~ 82106
  scan ~ 82143
  testing ~ 83661, 83663-83664
Amniotic membrane ~ 59001
  ocular wound healing ~ 65778-65779
Amobarbital ~ 82205

AMP ~ 82030
AMP, cyclic ~ 82030
Amphetamine, blood or urine ~ 82145
Amputation ~ see radical resection; replantation
  ankle ~ 27888
  arm, lower ~ 25900-25905, 25915
    revision ~ 25907-25909
  arm, upper ~ 24900-24920
    and shoulder ~ 23900-23921
    revision ~ 24925-24930
    with implant ~ 24931-24935
  cervix, total ~ 57530
  ear
    partial ~ 69110
    total ~ 69120
  finger ~ 26910-26952
  foot ~ 28800-28805
  hand at metacarpal ~ 25927
    at wrist ~ 25920
      revision ~ 25922
    revision ~ 25924, 25929-25931
  interpelviabdominal ~ 27290
  interthoracoscapular ~ 23900
  leg, lower ~ 27598, 27880-27882
    revision ~ 27884-27886
  leg, upper ~ 27590-27592
    at hip ~ 27290-27295
    revision ~ 27594-27596
  metacarpal ~ 26910
  metatarsal ~ 28810
  nose ~ see resection, nose
  penis
    partial ~ 54120
    radical ~ 54130-54135
    total ~ 54125
  thumb ~ 26910-26952
  toe ~ 28810-28825
  tuft of distal phalanx ~ 11752
  upper extremity ~ 24940
    cineplasty ~ 24940
Amylase
  blood ~ 82150
  urine ~ 82150
ANA ~ 86038-86039
Anabolic steroid ~ see androstenedione
Anal abscess ~ see abscess, anal
Anal bleeding ~ see anus, hemorrhage
Anal fistula ~ see fistula, anal
Anal fistulectomy ~ 46288, 46706
Anal fistulotomy ~ 46270, 46280
Anal sphincter
  dilation ~ 45905
  incision ~ 46080
Anal ulceration ~ see anus, fissure
Analgesia ~ see anesthesia; sedation
  99141-99142
Analgesic cutaneous electrostimulation ~
  64550
Analysis
  computer data ~ 99090
    cardiovascular monitoring ~ 93290, 93297,
      93299

1338

Analysis ~ *continued*
  cardioverter-defibrillator ~ 93289,
    93295-93296
  loop recorder ~ 93291, 93298-93299
  multivariate probability assessment ~ 0185T
  pacemaker ~ 93288, 93293-93294
  electroencephalogram, digital ~ 95957
  electronic
    drug infusion pump ~ 62367-62368
    pacing cardioverter-defibrillator
      data analysis ~ 93289, 93295-93296
      evaluation of programming ~
        93282-93284, 93287, 93641-93642
      initial evaluation ~ 93640
      pulse generator ~ 95970-95971,
        95980-95982
  physiologic data, remote ~ 99091
  protein, tissue western blot ~ 88372
  semen ~ 89320-89322
    sperm isolation ~ 89260-89261
  spectrum ~ *see* spectrophotometry
Anaspadias ~ *see* epispadias
Anastomosis
  aorta-pulmonary artery ~ 33606
  arteriovenous fistula
    direct ~ 36821
    with bypass graft ~ 35686
    with graft ~ 36825-36830, 36832
  artery
    to aorta ~ 33606
    to artery, cranial ~ 61711
  bile duct
    to bile duct ~ 47800
    to intestines ~ 47760, 47780
  bile duct to gastrointestinal ~ 47785
  bladder, to intestine ~ 51960
  broncho-bronchial ~ 32486
  caval to mesenteric ~ 37160
  colorectal ~ 44620
  epididymis
    to vas deferens
      bilateral ~ 54901
      unilateral ~ 54900
  excision trachea ~ 31780-31781
  fallopian tube ~ 58750
  gallbladder to intestines ~ 47720-47740
  hepatic duct ~ see hepatic duct, anastomosis
  hepatic duct to intestines ~ 47765, 47802
  ileo-anal ~ 45113
  intestines
    colo-anal ~ 45119
    cystectomy ~ 51590
    enterocystoplasty ~ 51960
    resection, laparoscopic ~ 44202-44205
  intestine to intestine ~ 44130
  intrahepatic portosystemic ~ 37182-37183
  jejunum ~ 43825
  lacrimal sac to conjunctival sac ~ see
    conjunctivorhinostomy
  microvascular, free transfer, jejunum ~ 43496

Anastomosis ~ *continued*
  nerve
    facial to hypoglossal ~ 64868
    facial to phrenic ~ 64870
  oviduct ~ 58750
  pancreas ~ see pancreas, anastomosis
  pancreas to intestines ~ 48520-48540, 48548
  portocaval ~ 37140
  pulmonary ~ 33606
  renoportal ~ 37145
  splenorenal ~ 37180-37181
  stomach ~ 43825
    to duodenum ~ 43810, 43855
      revision ~ 43850
    to jejunum ~ 43820, 43860-43865
  tubotubal ~ 58750
  ureter
    to bladder ~ 50780-50785
    to colon ~ 50810-50815
      removal ~ 50830
    to intestine ~ 50800, 50820-50825
      removal ~ 50830
    to kidney ~ 50727-50750
    to ureter ~ 50727, 50760-50770
  vein, saphenopopliteal ~ 34530
  vein to vein ~ 37140-37160, 37182-37183
Anatomic pathology services ~ 88000-88099
Anderson tibial lengthening ~ see ankle
  27715
Androstanediol glucuronide ~ 82154
Androstanolone ~ 82651
Androstenedione, blood or urine ~ 82157
Androstenolone ~ 82626
Androsterone, blood or urine ~ 82160
Anesthesia ~ 00100-01999
  Abbe-Estlander procedure ~ 00102
  abdomen
    abdominal wall ~ 00700, 00730,
      00800-00802, 00820, 00836
      Halsted repair ~ 00750-00756
    blood vessels ~ 00770, 00880-00882
    endoscopy ~ 00740, 00810
    extraperitoneal ~ 00860-00862, 00866-00870
    hernia repair ~ 00830-00836
      Halsted repair ~ 00750-00756
    intraperitoneal ~ 00790-00797, 00840-00842
  abdominoperineal resection ~ 00844
  abortion, induced ~ 01964
  Achilles tendon repair ~ 01472
  acromioclavicular joint ~ 01620
  adrenalectomy ~ 00866
  amniocentesis ~ 00842
  aneurysm
    axillary-brachial ~ 01652
    knee ~ 01444
    popliteal artery ~ 01444
  angiography ~ 01920
  ankle ~ 00400, 01462-01522
  anorectal procedure ~ 00902
  anus ~ 00902

Anesthesia ~ continued
arm
lower ~ 00400, 01810-01820, 01830-01860
upper ~ 00400, 01710-01782
arrhythmias ~ 00410
arteriography ~ 01916
arteriovenous fistula ~ 01432, 01784
arthroplasty
hip ~ 01214-01215
knee ~ 01402
arthroscopic procedures
ankle ~ 01464
elbow ~ 01732-01740
foot ~ 01464
hip ~ 01202
knee ~ 01382, 01400
shoulder ~ 01622-01630
wrist ~ 01829-01830
auditory canal, external, removal foreign body
~ 69205
axilla ~ 00400, 01610-01682
back skin ~ 00300
Batch-Spittler-McFaddin operation ~ 01404
biopsy ~ 00100
liver ~ 00702
bladder ~ 00870, 00912
brain ~ 00210-00218, 00220-00222
breast ~ 00402-00406
bronchi ~ 00542
intrathoracic repair of trauma ~ 00548
reconstruction ~ 00539
bronchoscopy ~ 00520
burns
debridement and/or excision ~ 01951-01953
dressings and/or debridement ~ 16010-16015
burr hole ~ 00214
bypass graft
leg, lower ~ 01500
leg, upper ~ 01270
shoulder, axillary ~ 01654-01656
cardiac catheterization ~ 01920
cast, knee ~ 01420
cast application
forearm, wrist and hand ~ 01860
leg ~ 01490
pelvis ~ 01130
shoulder ~ 01680-01682
central venous circulation ~ 00532
cervical cerclage ~ 00948
cervix ~ 00948
cesarean delivery ~ 01961, 01963
chemonucleolysis ~ 00634
chest ~ 00400-00406, 00410, 00470-00474,
00522, 00530-00539, 00542, 00546-00550
chest skin ~ 00400
childbirth
cesarean delivery ~ 01961, 01963,
01968-01969
external cephalic version ~ 01958
vaginal delivery ~ 01960, 01967
clavicle ~ 00450-00454
cleft lip repair ~ 00102

Anesthesia ~ continued
cleft palate repair ~ 00172
colpectomy ~ 00942
colporrhaphy ~ 00942
colpotomy ~ 00942
corneal transplant ~ 00144
cranioplasty ~ 00215
culdoscopy ~ 00950
cystectomy ~ 00864
cystolithotomy ~ 00870
cystourethroscopy
local ~ 52265
spinal ~ 52260
decortication ~ 00542
defibrillator ~ 00534, 00560
diaphragm ~ 00540-00541
disarticulation
hip ~ 01212
knee ~ 01404
shoulder ~ 01634
diskography ~ 01935, 01936
dressing change ~ 15852
drug administration, epidural or subarachnoid
~ 01996
ear ~ 00120-00126
elbow ~ 00400, 01710-01782
electrocoagulation, intracranial nerve ~ 00222
electroconvulsive therapy ~ 00104
embolectomy
arm, upper ~ 01772
femoral ~ 01274
femoral artery ~ 01274
forearm, wrist and hand ~ 01842
leg, lower ~ 01502
endoscopy
arm, lower ~ 01830
gastrointestinal ~ 00740
intestines ~ 00810
uterus ~ 00952
vagina ~ 00950
esophagus ~ 00320, 00500
external cephalic version ~ 01958
external fixation system
adjustment/revision ~ 20693
removal ~ 20694
eye ~ 00140-00148
cornea ~ 00144
iridectomy ~ 00147
iris ~ 00147
eyelid ~ 00103
facial bones ~ 00190-00192
fallopian tube, ligation ~ 00851
femoral artery, ligation ~ 01272
femur ~ 01220-01234, 01340-01360
fibula ~ 01390-01392
foot ~ 00400, 01462-01522
forearm ~ 00400, 01810-01820, 01830-01860
Fowler-Stephens orchiopexy ~ 00930
gastrocnemius recession ~ 01474
gastrointestinal endoscopy ~ 00740

Anesthesia ~ *continued*
genitalia
  female ~ 00940-00952, 01958-01969
  male ~ 00920-00938
great vessels of chest ~ 00560-00563
hand ~ 00400, 01810-01820, 01830-01860
Harrington rod technique ~ 00670
head ~ 00222, 00300
  muscles ~ 00300
  nerves ~ 00300
heart ~ 00560-00567, 00580
  coronary artery bypass grafting ~
   00566-00567
  electrophysiology/ablation ~ 00537
  transplant ~ 00580
hepatectomy, partial ~ 00792
hernia repair, abdomen
  lower ~ 00830-00836
  upper ~ 00750-00752, 00756
hip ~ 01200-01215
humerus ~ 01620, 01730, 01742-01744, 01758
hysterectomy ~ 01962
  cesarean ~ 01963, 01969
  radical ~ 00846
  vaginal ~ 00944
hysterosalpingography ~ 00952
hysteroscopy ~ 00952
induced abortion ~ 01964
inferior vena cava ligation ~ 00882
injections, nerve ~ 01991-01992
integumentary system
  anterior trunk ~ 00400
  arm, upper ~ 00400
  axilla ~ 00400
  elbow ~ 00400
  extremity ~ 00400
  forearm ~ 00400
  hand ~ 00400
  head ~ 00300
  knee ~ 00400
  leg, lower ~ 00400
  leg, upper ~ 00400
  neck ~ 00300
  perineum ~ 00400
  popliteal area ~ 00400
  posterior pelvis ~ 00300
  posterior trunk ~ 00300
  shoulder ~ 00400
  wrist ~ 00400
intestines, endoscopy ~ 00810
intracranial procedures ~ 00210-00218,
  00220-00222
intraoral procedures ~ 00170-00176
intrathoracic procedures
  bronchi ~ 00539, 00548
  trachea ~ 00539, 00548
intrathoracic system ~ 00500, 00520-00529,
  00530-00539, 00540-00548, 00550,
  00560-00567, 00580
iridectomy ~ 00147
Keen operation ~ 00604
kidney ~ 00862, 00868, 00872-00873

Anesthesia ~ *continued*
knee ~ 00400, 01320-01444
knee skin ~ 00400
laminectomy ~ 00604
laparoscopy ~ 00790-00792, 00840
larynx ~ 00320, 00326
leg
  lower ~ 00400, 01462-01522
  upper ~ 01200-01274
lens ~ 00142
Leriche operation ~ 00622
life support for organ donor ~ 01990
ligation, fallopian tube ~ 00851
lithotripsy ~ 00872-00873
liver ~ 00702, 00796
  transplant ~ 00796
liver hemorrhage ~ 00792
lumbar puncture ~ 00635
lungs ~ 00522, 00539, 00540-00548
  transplant ~ 00580
lymphadenectomy ~ 00934-00936
lymphatic system ~ 00320
mammoplasty ~ 00402
marcellation operation ~ 00944
mediastinoscopy ~ 00528-00529
mediastinum ~ 00528-00529, 00540-00541
mouth ~ 00170-00172
myelography ~ 01935, 01936
myringotomy ~ 69421
neck ~ 00300, 00320-00322, 00350-00352
nephrectomy ~ 00862
neuraxial
  cesarean delivery ~ 01968-01969
  labor ~ 01967-01969
  vaginal delivery ~ 01967
neurectomy ~ 01180-01190
nose ~ 00160-00164
  removal, foreign body ~ 30310
omphalocele ~ 00754
ophthalmoscopy ~ 00148
orchiectomy ~ 00926-00928
orchiopexy ~ 00930
  Torek procedure ~ 00930
organ harvesting, brain dead patient ~ 01990
osteoplasty, tibia/fibula ~ 01484
osteotomy
  humerus ~ 01742
  tibia/fibula ~ 01484
other procedures ~ 01990, 01996-01999
otoscopy ~ 00124
pacemaker insertion ~ 00530
pacing cardioverter/defibrillator ~ 00534
pancreas ~ 00794
pancreatectomy ~ 00794
panniculectomy ~ 00802
patella ~ 01390-01392
pectus excavatum ~ 00474
pelvic exenteration ~ 00848
pelvis ~ 00400, 00865, 01112-01190
  amputation ~ 01140
  bone ~ 01120
  bone marrow ~ 01112

1341

Anesthesia ~ continued
examination ~ 57400
extraperitoneal ~ 00864
intraperitoneal ~ 00844-00848
repair ~ 01173
skin ~ 00300, 00400
penis ~ 00932-00938
pericardial sac ~ 00560-00563
perineum ~ 00904-00908
pharynx ~ 00174-00176
phleborrhaphy
arm, upper ~ 01782
forearm, wrist, and hand ~ 01852
pleura ~ 00540-00541
needle biopsy ~ 00522
pneumocentesis ~ 00524
popliteal area ~ 00400, 01320, 01430-01444
prognathism ~ 00192
prostate ~ 00865, 00908, 00914
prostatectomy
perineal ~ 00908
radical ~ 00865
Walsh modified radical ~ 00865
radiologic procedures ~ 01916-01936
arterial, therapeutic ~ 01924-01926
venous/lymphatic, therapeutic ~ 01930-01933
renal procedures ~ 00862
repair of skull ~ 00215
replacement
ankle ~ 01486
elbow ~ 01760
hip ~ 01212-01215
knee ~ 01402
shoulder ~ 01638
wrist ~ 01832
restriction, gastric
for obesity ~ 00797
retropharyngeal tumor excision ~ 00174
rib resection ~ 00470-00474
sacroiliac joint ~ 01160-01170, 27096
salivary glands ~ 00100
Scheie procedure ~ 00147
sedation, analgesia ~ 99141-99142
seminal vesicles ~ 00922
shoulder ~ 00400, 00450-00454, 01610-01682
dislocation, closed treatment ~ 23655
shunt, spinal fluid ~ 00220
sinuses, accessory ~ 00160-00164
skull ~ 00190
skull fracture, elevation ~ 00215
special circumstances
emergency ~ 99140
extreme age ~ 99100
hypotension ~ 99135
hypothermia ~ 99116
spinal instrumentation ~ 00670
spinal manipulation ~ 00640
spine and spinal cord ~ 00600-00604, 00620-00670
cervical ~ 00600-00604, 00640-00670

Anesthesia ~ continued
guided ~ 01935-01936
injection ~ 62310-62319
lumbar ~ 00630-00635, 00640, 00670
thoracic ~ 00620-00626, 00640, 00670
vascular ~ 00670
sternoclavicular joint ~ 01620
sternum ~ 00550
stomach, restriction, for obesity ~ 00797
Strayer procedure ~ 01474
subdural taps ~ 00212
suture removal ~ 15850-15851
sympathectomy
lumbar ~ 00632
thoracolumbar ~ 00622
symphysis pubis ~ 01160-01170
tenodesis ~ 01716
tenoplasty ~ 01714
tenotomy ~ 01712
testis ~ 00924-00930
thoracoplasty ~ 00472
thoracoscopy ~ 00528-00529, 00540-00541
thoracotomy ~ 00540-00541
thorax ~ 00400-00406, 00410, 00450-00454, 00470-00474
thromboendarterectomy ~ 01442
thyroid ~ 00320-00322
tibia ~ 01390-01392, 01484
trachea ~ 00320, 00326, 00542
reconstruction ~ 00539
transplantation
cornea ~ 00144
heart ~ 00580
kidney ~ 00868
liver ~ 00796, 01990
lungs ~ 00580
organ harvesting ~ 01990
transurethral procedures ~ 00910-00918
tubal ligation ~ 00851
tuffier vaginal hysterectomy ~ 00944
TURP ~ 00914
tympanostomy ~ 00120
tympanotomy ~ 00126
unlisted services and procedures ~ 01999
urethra ~ 00910, 00918-00920, 00942
urethrocystoscopy ~ 00910
urinary bladder ~ 00864, 00870, 00912
urinary tract ~ 00860
uterus ~ 00952
vagina ~ 00940-00942, 00950
dilation ~ 57400
removal, foreign body ~ 57415
vaginal delivery ~ 01960
vas deferens, excision ~ 00921
vascular access ~ 00532
vascular shunt ~ 01844
vascular surgery
abdomen, lower ~ 00880-00882
abdomen, upper ~ 00770
arm, lower ~ 01840-01852
arm, upper ~ 01770-01782

Anesthesia ~ *continued*
  brain ~ 00216
  elbow ~ 01770-01782
  hand ~ 01840-01852
  knee ~ 01430-01444
  leg, lower ~ 01500-01522
  leg, upper ~ 01260-01274
  neck ~ 00350-00352
  shoulder ~ 01650-01670
  wrist ~ 01840-01852
  vasectomy ~ 00921
  venography ~ 01916
  ventriculography ~ 00214, 01920
  vertebral process, fracture/dislocation, closed
    treatment ~ 22315
  vertebroplasty ~ 01935, 01936
  vitrectomy ~ 00145
  vitreoretinal surgery ~ 00145
  vitreous body ~ 00145
  vulva ~ 00906
  vulvectomy ~ 00906
  Wertheim operation ~ 00846
  wrist ~ 00400, 01810-01860
Aneurysm repair
  abdominal aorta ~ 0078T-0081T, 34800-34805,
    34825-34832, 35081-35103, 75952-75953
  axillary artery ~ 35011-35013
  basilar artery ~ 61698, 61702
  brachial artery ~ 35011-35013
  carotid artery ~ 35001-35002, 61613, 61697,
    61700, 61703
  celiac artery ~ 35121-35122
  femoral artery ~ 35141-35142
  hepatic artery ~ 35121-35122
  iliac artery ~ 34900, 35131-35132,
    75953-75954
  innominate artery ~ 35021-35022
  intracranial artery ~ 61705-61708
  mesenteric artery ~ 35121-35122
  popliteal artery ~ 35151-35152
  radial artery ~ 35045
  renal artery ~ 35121-35122
  splenic artery ~ 35111-35112
  subclavian artery ~ 35001-35002, 35021-35022
  thoracoabdominal aorta ~ 33877
  ulnar artery ~ 35045
  vascular malformation or carotid-cavernous
    fistula ~ 61710
  vertebral artery ~ 61698, 61702
Angel dust ~ 83992
Angina assessment ~ *see* performance measure
Angiocardiographies ~ *see* heart, angiography
Angiography
  abdomen ~ 74174, 74175, 74185, 75635,
    75726
  abdominal aorta ~ 0080T-0081T, 75635,
    75952-75953
  adrenal ~ 75731-75733
  aorta, injection ~ 93567
  arm artery ~ 73206, 75710-75716
  arteriovenous shunt ~ 75791

Angiography ~ *continued*
  atrial ~ 93565-93566
  brachial artery ~ 75658
  brain ~ 70496
  bypass graft ~ 93455, 93457, 93459-93461
  carotid artery ~ 36221-36228
  cervicocerebral arch ~ 36221-36226
  chest ~ 71275, 71555
  congenital heart ~ 93563-93564
  coronary artery ~ 93454-93461, 93563
    coronary calcium ~ 75571-75574
    flow velocity measurement during
      angiography ~ 93571-93572
  endovascular repair ~ 0080T-0081T,
    75952-75953
  extremity, lower ~ 73725
  extremity, upper ~ 73225
  fluorescein ~ 92235
  head ~ 70496, 70544-70546
    artery ~ 36221-36226
  heart vessels, injection ~ 93454-93461
  indocyanine-green ~ 92240
  left heart, injection ~ 93565
  leg artery ~ 73706, 75635, 75710-75716
  lung, injection ~ 93568
  mammary artery ~ 75756
  neck ~ 70498, 70547-70549
    artery ~ 36221-36226
  nuclear medicine ~ 78445
  other artery ~ 75774
  pelvic artery ~ 72198, 75736
  pelvis ~ 72191, 74174
  pulmonary ~ 75741-75746, 93568
  renal artery ~ 36251-36254
  right heart, injection ~ 93566
  spinal artery ~ 75705
  spinal canal ~ 72159
  thorax ~ 71275
  transcatheter therapy
    embolization ~ 75894, 75898
    infusion ~ 75894, 75898
  ventricular ~ 93565-93566
  vertebral ~ 36211, 36225-36226, 36228
Angioma ~ see lesion, skin
Angioplasties, coronary balloon ~ see
  percutaneous transluminal angioplasty
Angioplasty
  aorta
    intraoperative ~ 35452
    percutaneous ~ 35472
  axillary artery, intraoperative ~ 35458
  brachiocephalic artery
    intraoperative ~ 35458
    percutaneous ~ 35475
  coronary artery, percutaneous transluminal ~
    92982-92984
  femoral artery, intraoperative ~ 37224
  iliac artery, intraoperative ~ 37220, 37222
  intracranial, percutaneous ~ 61630
  percutaneous transluminal angioplasty ~
    92982-92984

1343

Angioplasty ~ continued
popliteal artery, intraoperative ~ 37224
pulmonary artery, percutaneous transluminal ~ 92997-92998
renal artery
  intraoperative ~ 35450
  percutaneous ~ 35471
subclavian artery, intraoperative ~ 35458
tibioperoneal artery, intraoperative ~ 37228
transluminal
  arterial ~ 75962-75968
  venous ~ 75978
venous
  intraoperative ~ 35460
  percutaneous ~ 35476
visceral artery
  intraoperative ~ 35450
  percutaneous ~ 35471
Angioscopy, non-coronary vessels ~ 35400
Angiotensin converting enzyme (ACE) ~ 82164
Angiotensin forming enzyme ~ 80408, 80416, 84244
Angiotensin I ~ 84244
riboflavin ~ 84252
Angiotensin II, blood or urine ~ 82163
Angle deformity, reconstruction toe ~ 28313
Anhydride, carbonic ~ 82374
Anhydrides, acetic ~ 84600
Animal inoculation ~ 87001-87003, 87250
Ankle
(see also fibula; leg, lower; tibia; tibiofibular joint)
abscess, incision and drainage ~ 27603
amputation ~ 27888
arthrocentesis ~ 20605
arthrodesis ~ 27870
arthrography ~ 73615
arthroplasty ~ 27700-27703
arthroscopy, surgical ~ 29891-29899
arthrotomy ~ 27610-27612, 27620-27626
biopsy ~ 27613-27614, 27620
bursa, incision and drainage ~ 27604
disarticulation ~ 27889
dislocation
  closed treatment ~ 27840-27842
  open treatment ~ 27846-27848
exploration ~ 27610, 27620
fracture
  bimalleolar ~ 27808-27814
  lateral ~ 27786-27814, 27792
  medial ~ 27760-27766, 27808-27814
  posterior ~ 27767-27769, 27808-27814
  trimalleolar ~ 27816-27823
fusion ~ 27870
hematoma, incision and drainage ~ 27603
incision ~ 27607
injection, radiologic ~ 27648
lesion excision ~ 27630
magnetic resonance imaging (MRI) ~ 73721-73723
manipulation ~ 27860

Ankle ~ continued
removal
  foreign body ~ 27610, 27620
  implant ~ 27704
  loose body ~ 27620
repair
  Achilles tendon ~ 27650-27654
  ligament ~ 27695-27698
  tendon ~ 27612, 27680-27687
  strapping ~ 29540
  synovium, excision ~ 27625-27626
  tenotomy ~ 27605-27606
  tumor, excision ~ 27615-27619, 27632, 27634
  unlisted services and procedures ~ 27899
X-ray ~ 73600-73610
  with contrast ~ 73615
Ankylosis (surgical) ~ see arthrodesis
Annuloplasty, percutaneous, intradiscal ~ 22526-22527
Anogenital region ~ see perineum
Anoplasty, stricture ~ 46700-46705
Anorectal myectomy ~ 45108
Anorectal procedure, biofeedback ~ 90911
Anorectovaginoplasty ~ 46744-46746
Anoscopy
ablation, polyp/tumor ~ 46615
biopsy ~ 46606
dilation ~ 46604
exploration ~ 46600
hemorrhage ~ 46614
removal
  foreign body ~ 46608
  polyp/tumor ~ 46610-46612
Antebrachium ~ 20805
Antecedent, plasma thromboplastin ~ 85270
Antepartum care
vaginal delivery ~ 59400, 59425-59426
with cesarean delivery ~ 59510
  previous ~ 59610, 59618
Anterior ramus of thoracic nerve ~ see intercostal nerve
Anthrax vaccine ~ 90476-90749
Anthrogon ~ 80418, 80426, 83001
Anti Australia antigens ~ see antibody, hepatitis B
Anti D immunoglobulin ~ 90384-90386
Anti-human globulin consumption test ~ 86880
Anti-phospholipid antibody ~ 86147
Antiactivator, plasmin ~ 85410
Antibiotic administration
injection ~ 96372
prescribed or dispensed ~ 4120F-4124F
Antibiotic sensitivity ~ 87181-87184, 87188
enzyme detection ~ 87185
minimum bactericidal concentration ~ 87187
minimum inhibitory concentration ~ 87186
Antibody detection
actinomyces ~ 86602
adenovirus ~ 86603
antinuclear ~ 86038-86039

Antibody ~ *continued*
antiphosphatidylserine (phospholipid) ~ 86148
antistreptolysin O ~ 86060-86063
aspergillus ~ 86606
bacterium ~ 86609
bartonella ~ 86611
beta 2 glycoprotein 1 ~ 86146
blastomyces ~ 86612
blood crossmatch ~ 86920-86923
bordetella ~ 86615
borrelia ~ 86618-86619
brucella ~ 86622
campylobacter ~ 86625
candida ~ 86628
cardiolipin ~ 86147
chlamydia ~ 86631-86632
coccidioides ~ 86635
coxiella burnetii ~ 86638
cryptococcus ~ 86641
cyclic citrullinated peptide (CCP)~ 86200
cytomegalovirus ~ 86644-86645
cytotoxic screen ~ 86807-86808
deoxyribonuclease ~ 86215
deoxyribonucleic acid (DNA) ~ 86225-86226
diphtheria ~ 86648
ehrlichia ~ 86666
encephalitis ~ 86651-86654
enterovirus ~ 86658
Epstein-Barr virus ~ 86663-86665
fluorescent ~ 86255-86256
francisella tularensis ~ 86668
fungus ~ 86671
giardia lamblia ~ 86674
growth hormone ~ 86277
helicobacter pylori ~ 86677
helminth ~ 86682
hemophilus influenza ~ 86684
hepatitis, delta agent ~ 86692
hepatitis A ~ 86708-86709
hepatitis B
  core ~ 86704
  IgM ~ 86705
  surface ~ 86706
hepatitis Be ~ 86707
hepatitis C ~ 86803-86804
herpes simplex ~ 86694-86696
heterophile ~ 86308-86310
histoplasma ~ 86698
HIV ~ 86689, 86701-86703
HIV 1 ~ 86701, 86703
HIV 2 ~ 86702-86703
HTLV I ~ 86687, 86689
HTLV II ~ 86688
influenza virus ~ 86710
insulin ~ 86337
intrinsic factor ~ 86340
islet cell ~ 86341
legionella ~ 86713
leishmania ~ 86717
leptospira ~ 86720

Antibody ~ *continued*
listeria monocytogenes ~ 86723
Lyme disease ~ 86617
lymphocytic choriomeningitis ~ 86727
lymphogranuloma venereum ~ 86729
microsomal ~ 86376
mucormycosis ~ 86732
mumps ~ 86735
mycoplasma ~ 86738
neisseria meningitidis ~ 86741
nocardia ~ 86744
nuclear antigen ~ 86235
other virus ~ 86790
parvovirus ~ 86747
phospholipid ~ 85597, 85598, 86147
plasmodium ~ 86750
platelet ~ 85597-85598, 86022-86023
protozoa ~ 86753
red blood cell ~ 86850-86870
respiratory syncytial virus (RSV) ~ 86756
rickettsia ~ 86757
rotavirus ~ 86759
rubella ~ 86762
rubeola ~ 86765
salmonella ~ 86768
shigella ~ 86771
sperm ~ 89325
streptokinase ~ 86590
tetanus ~ 86774
thyroglobulin ~ 86800
toxoplasma ~ 86777-86778
treponema pallidum ~ 86780
trichinella ~ 86784
varicella-zoster ~ 86787
West Nile virus ~ 86788-86789
white blood cell ~ 86021
yersinia ~ 86793
Antibody identification
leukocyte antibodies ~ 86021
platelet ~ 86022-86023
red blood cell, pretreatment ~ 86970-86972
serum, pretreatment ~ 86975-86978
Antibody neutralization test ~ 86382
Antibody receptor ~ 86243
Anticoagulant ~ 85300-85305, 85307
Antidiabetic hormone ~ 82943
Antidiuretic hormone measurement~ 84588
AntiDNA autoantibody ~ 86038-86039
Antigen(s)
allergen immunotherapy ~ 95144
Australia ~ 87340-87341
carcinoembryonic ~ 82378
CD4 ~ 86360
CD8 ~ 86360
CD142 ~ see thromboplastin
CD143 ~ 82164
E ~ 87350
hepatitis ~ see hepatitis antigen
hepatitis B ~ 87515-87517
prostate specific ~ 84152-84153

Antigen detection
direct fluorescence ~ 87265-87272, 87276,
87278, 87280, 87285-87290
bordetella ~ 87265
chlamydia trachomatis ~ 87270
cryptosporidium ~ 87272
cytomegalovirus ~ 87271
enterovirus ~ 87267
giardia ~ 87269
influenza A ~ 87276
legionella pneumophila ~ 87278
not otherwise specified ~ 87299
respiratory syncytial virus ~ 87280
treponema pallidum ~ 87285
varicella-zoster ~ 87290
enzyme immunoassay ~ 87301-87451
adenovirus ~ 87301
aspergillus ~ 87305
chlamydia trachomatis ~ 87320
clostridium difficile ~ 87324
cryptococcus neoformans ~ 87327
cryptosporidium ~ 87328
cytomegalovirus ~ 87332
entomoeba histolytica dispar group ~ 87336
entomoeba histolytica group ~ 87337
escherichia coli 0157 ~ 87335
giardia ~ 87329
helicobacter pylori ~ 87338-87339
hepatitis Be antigen (HBeAg) ~ 87350
hepatitis B surface antigen (HBsAg) ~ 87340
hepatitis B surface antigen (HBsAg)
neutralization ~ 87341
hepatitis delta agent ~ 87380
histoplasma capsulatum ~ 87385
HIV 1 ~ 87390
HIV 2 ~ 87391
influenza A ~ 87400
influenza B ~ 87400
multiple step method ~ 87301-87449
polyvalent ~ 87451
not otherwise specified ~ 87449, 87451
respiratory syncytial virus ~ 87420
rotavirus ~ 87425
shigella-like toxin ~ 87427
single step method ~ 87450
streptococcus, group A ~ 87430
immunofluorescence ~ 87260-87300
adenovirus ~ 87260
herpes simplex ~ 87273-87274
influenza B ~ 87275
legionella micdadei ~ 87277
not otherwise specified ~ 87299
parainfluenza virus ~ 87279
pneumocystis carinii ~ 87281
polyvalent ~ 87300
rubeola ~ 87283
Antihemophilic factor B ~ 85250
Antihemophilic factor C ~ 85270
Antihemophilic globulin (AHG) ~ 85240
Antihuman globulin ~ 86880-86886
Antimony ~ 83015
Antinuclear antibodies (ANA) ~ 86038-86039

Antiplasmin, alpha 2 ~ Antigen detection
Antiplatelet therapy ~ see performance
measures
Antiprotease, alpha 1 ~ 82103-82104, 99565
Antistreptococcal antibody ~ 86215
Antistreptokinase titer ~ 86590
Antistreptolysin O ~ 86060-86063
Antithrombin III ~ 85300-85301
Antithrombin VI (six) ~ 85362-85380
Antitoxin assay ~ 87230
Antiviral antibody ~ 86280
Antrostomy, sinus, maxillary ~ 31256-31267
Antrotomy, sinus
maxillary ~ 31020-31032
transmastoid ~ 69501
Antrum of highmore ~ see sinuses, maxillary
Antrum puncture
sinus
maxillary ~ 31000
sphenoid ~ 31002
Anus ~ see also hemorrhoids; rectum
ablation ~ 46615
abscess, incision and drainage ~ 46045-46050
biofeedback ~ 90911
biopsy, endoscopy ~ 46606
crypt, excision ~ 46999
dilation, endoscopy ~ 46604
endoscopy
biopsy ~ 46606
dilation ~ 46604
exploration ~ 46600
hemorrhage ~ 46614
removal
foreign body ~ 46608
polyp ~ 46610, 46612
tumor ~ 46610, 46612
excision, tag ~ 46220, 46230
exploration, endoscopy ~ 46600
fissure
destruction ~ 46940-46942
excision ~ 46200
fistula
excision ~ 46270-46285
repair ~ 46706
hemorrhage, endoscopic control ~ 46614
hemorrhoids
clot excision ~ 46320
destruction ~ 46930
excision ~ 46250-46262
injection ~ 46500
ligation ~ 46221, 46945-46946
stapling ~ 46947
suture ~ 46945-46946
imperforated, repair ~ 46715-46742
incision, septum ~ 46070
lesion
destruction ~ 46900-46917, 46924
excision ~ 45108, 46922
manometry ~ 91122
placement, seton ~ 46020

Anus ~ *continued*
reconstruction ~ 46742
  congenital absence ~ 46730-46740
  sphincter ~ 46750-46751, 46760-46762
  with graft ~ 46753
  with implant ~ 46762
removal
  foreign body ~ 46608
  seton ~ 46030
  suture ~ 46754
  wire ~ 46754
repair
  anovaginal fistula ~ 46715-46716
  cloacal anomaly ~ 46748
  fistula ~ 46706
  stricture ~ 46700-46705
sphincter
  electromyography ~ 51784-51785
  needle ~ 51785
unlisted services and procedures ~ 46999
Aorta
abdominal
  aneurysm ~ 0078T-0081T, 34800-34805,
    34825-34832, 35081-35103,
    75952-75953
  thromboendarterectomy ~ 35331
anastomosis, to pulmonary artery ~ 33606
angiogram, radiologic injection ~ 93567
angioplasty ~ 35452
aortography ~ 75600-75630
ascending, graft ~ 33864
balloon ~ 33967, 33970
catheterization
  catheter ~ 36200
  intracatheter/needle ~ 36160
circulation assist ~ 33967, 33970
conduit to heart ~ 33404
excision, coarctation ~ 33840-33851
insertion
  balloon device ~ 33967
  graft ~ 33330-33335, 33864
  intracatheter/needle ~ 36160
removal, balloon assist device ~ 33968, 33971
repair ~ 33320-33322, 33802-33803
  coarctation ~ 33840-33851
  graft ~ 33860-33877
    ascending ~ 33864
  hypoplastic or interrupted aortic arch
    with cardiopulmonary bypass ~ 33853
    without cardiopulmonary bypass ~ 33852
  sinus of Valsalva ~ 33702-33720
suspension ~ 33800
suture ~ 33320-33322
thoracic repair ~ 75956-75959
  endovascular ~ 33880-33891
translocation, aortic root ~ 33782-33783

Aorta ~ *continued*
valve
  implantation ~ 0318T, 33361-33365,
    33367-33369
  incision ~ 33415
  repair ~ 33400-33401, 33403
    left ventricle ~ 33414
    supravalvular stenosis ~ 33417
X-ray with contrast ~ 75600-75630
Aortic sinus ~ 33702-33720
Aortic stenosis
repair ~ 33415
supravalvular ~ 33417
Aortic valve ~ see heart, aortic valve
Aortic valve replacement ~ 33405-33413
Aortocoronary bypass ~ 33503-33505,
  33510-33516
Aortography ~ (see angiography)
  75600-75605, 75630, 93567
serial ~ 75625
with iliofemoral artery ~ 75630
Aortoiliac
embolectomy ~ 34151-34201
thrombectomy ~ 34151-34201
Aortopexy ~ 33800
Aortoplasty, supravalvular stenosis ~ 33417
AP ~ see voiding pressure studies
Apert-Gallais syndrome ~ see adrenogenital
  syndrome
Aphasia testing ~ (see neurology, diagnostic)
  96105
Apheresis, therapeutic ~ 36511-36516
Apical-aortic conduit ~ 33404
Apicectomy
with mastoidectomy ~ 69605
petrous ~ 69530
Apoaminotransferase, aspartate ~ see
  transaminase, glutamic oxaloacetic
Apolipoprotein, blood or urine ~ 82172
Appendectomy ~ 44950-44960
laparoscopic ~ 44970
Appendiceal abscess ~ see abscess, appendix
Appendico-vesicostomy, cutaneous ~ 50845
Appendix
abscess
  incision and drainage
    open ~ 44900
    percutaneous ~ 44901
  excision ~ 44950-44960
Application
allergy tests ~ 95044
bone fixation device
  multiplane ~ 20692
    stereotactic computer assisted ~
      20696-20697
  uniplane ~ 20690
caliper ~ 20660
cranial tongs ~ 20660
fixation device, shoulder ~ 23700

Application ~ *continued*
halo
  cranial ~ 20661
    thin skull osteology ~ 20664
  femoral ~ 20663
  maxillofacial fixation ~ 21100
  pelvic ~ 20662
interdental fixation device ~ 21110
intervertebral device ~ 22851
neurostimulation ~ 64550, 64566
radioelement ~ 77761-77778
  surface ~ 77789
  with ultrasound ~ 76965
stereotactic frame ~ 20660
  headframe ~ 61800
strapping, multi-layer compession system
  arm ~ 29583-29584
  leg ~ 29581-29582
Application of external fixation device ~ see
  fixation device, application, external
APPT ~ see thromboplastin, partial, time
Aquatic therapy ~ 97113
Aqueous shunt
to extraocular reservoir ~ 66180
revision ~ 66185
Arch, zygomatic ~ see zygomatic arch
Arm
see also radius; ulna; wrist
lower
  abscess ~ 25028
    excision ~ 25145
    incision and drainage, bone ~ 25035
  amputation ~ 24900-24920, 25900-25905, 25915
    cineplasty ~ 24940
    revision ~ 25907-25909
  angiography ~ 73206
  artery ligation ~ 37618
  biopsy ~ 25065-25066
  bursa, incision and drainage ~ 25031
  bypass graft ~ 35903
  cast ~ 29075
  CT scan ~ 73200-73206
  decompression ~ 25020-25025
  exploration, blood vessel ~ 35860
  fasciotomy ~ 24495, 25020-25025
  hematoma ~ 25028
  lesion, tendon sheath, excision ~ 25110
  magnetic resonance imaging (MRI) ~ 73218-73220, 73223
  reconstruction, ulna ~ 25337
  removal, foreign body ~ 25248
  repair
    blood vessel with other graft ~ 35266
    blood vessel with vein graft ~ 35236
    decompression ~ 24495
    muscle ~ 25260-25263, 25270
    secondary muscle or tendon ~ 25272-25274

Arm ~ *continued*
tendon ~ 25260-25263, 25270, 25280-25295, 25310-25316
  secondary ~ 25265
tendon sheath ~ 25275
replantation ~ 20805
splint ~ 29125-29126
tenotomy ~ 25290
tumor, excision ~ 25071-25078
unlisted services and procedures ~ 25999
X-ray ~ 73090
  with upper arm ~ 73092
removal, foreign body, forearm or wrist ~ 25248
repair
  muscle ~ 24341
  tendon ~ 24341
upper
  abscess, incision and drainage ~ see elbow; humerus ~ 23930
  amputation ~ 23900-23921, 24900-24920
    cineplasty ~ 24940
    revision ~ 24925-24930
    with implant ~ 24931-24935
  anesthesia ~ 00400, 01710-01782
  angiography ~ 73206
  artery, ligation ~ 37618
  biopsy ~ 24065-24066
  bypass graft ~ 35903
  cast ~ 29065
  CT scan ~ 73200-73206
  exploration, blood vessel ~ 35860
  hematoma, incision and drainage ~ 23930
  magnetic resonance imaging (MRI) ~ 73218-73220, 73223
  muscle revision ~ 24330-24331
  removal
    cast ~ 29705
    foreign body ~ 24200-24201
  repair
    blood vessel with other graft ~ 35266
    blood vessel with vein graft ~ 35236
    muscle transfer ~ 24301, 24320
    tendon ~ 24332
    tendon lengthening ~ 24305
    tendon revision ~ 24320
    tendon transfer ~ 24301
    tenotomy ~ 24310
  replantation ~ 20802
  splint ~ 29105
  tumor, excision ~ 24071-24079
  unlisted services and procedures ~ 24999
  wound exploration, penetrating ~ 20103
  X-ray, with lower arm, infant ~ 73092
Arnold-Chiari malformation repair ~ 61343
Arrest, epiphyseal ~ see epiphyseal arrest
Arrhythmogenic focus, heart
ablation ~ 33250-33251, 33261, 93653-93654, 93656
  catheter ~ 93655

Arsenic
blood or urine ~ 82175
detection ~ 83015
measurement ~ 82175, 83018
ART (syphilis test) ~ 86592, 86593
Arterial
catheterization ~ see cannulation, arterial
dilation, transluminal ~ see angioplasty,
transluminal
grafting for coronary artery bypass ~ see
bypass graft, coronary artery, arterial
pressure ~ see blood pressure
puncture ~ 36600
Arteriography, aorta ~ see aortography
Arteriosus, ductus ~ see ductus arteriosus
Arteriosus, truncus ~ see truncus arteriosus
Arteriotomy ~ see incision, artery; transection,
artery
Arteriovenous anastomosis ~ 36818-36820
Arteriovenous fistula
cannulization vein ~ 36815
hemodialysis via fistula ~ 4052F
referral ~ 4051F
repair
abdomen ~ 35182
acquired or traumatic ~ 35189
head ~ 35180
acquired or traumatic ~ 35188
lower extremity ~ 35184
acquired or traumatic ~ 35190
neck ~ 35180
acquired or traumatic ~ 35188
thorax ~ 35182
acquired or traumatic ~ 35189
upper extremity ~ 35184
acquired or traumatic ~ 35190
revision, hemodialysis graft or fistula
without thrombectomy ~ 36832
with thrombectomy ~ 36833
thrombectomy
dialysis graft, without revision ~ 36831
graft ~ 36870
Arteriovenous malformation
cranial, repair ~ 61680-61692, 61705-61708
spinal
excision ~ 63250-63252
injection ~ 62294
repair ~ 63250-63252
Arteriovenous shunt
angiography ~ 75791
catheterization ~ 36147-36148
Artery
abdomen
angiography ~ 75726
catheterization ~ 36245-36248
ligation ~ 37617
adrenal, angiography ~ 75731-75733
anastomosis, cranial ~ 61711
angioplasty ~ 75962-75968
aorta
angioplasty ~ 35452

Artery ~ *continued*
aortoiliac
embolectomy ~ 34151-34201
thrombectomy ~ 34151-34201
aortoiliofemoral ~ 35363
arm
angiography ~ 75710-75716
harvest of artery for coronary artery bypass
graft ~ 35600
axillary
aneurysm ~ 35011-35013
angioplasty ~ 35458
bypass graft ~ 35516-35522, 35533,
35616-35623, 35650, 35654
embolectomy ~ 34101
thrombectomy ~ 34101
thromboendarterectomy ~ 35321
basilar, aneurysm ~ 61698, 61702
biopsy, transcatheter ~ 75970
brachial
aneurysm ~ 35011-35013
angiography ~ 75658
bypass graft ~ 35510, 35512, 35522-35525
catheterization ~ 36120
embolectomy ~ 34101
exploration ~ 24495
exposure ~ 34834
thrombectomy ~ 34101
thromboendarterectomy ~ 35321
brachiocephalic
angioplasty ~ 35458
catheterization ~ 36215-36218
bypass graft, with composite graft ~
35681-35683
cannulization
for extra corporeal circulation ~ 36823
to vein ~ 36810-36815
carotid
aneurysm ~ 35001-35002, 61697-61705,
61708
vascular malformation or carotid-cavernous
fistula ~ 61710
bypass graft ~ 33891, 35501-35510,
35601-35606, 35642
catheterization ~ 36100, 36221-36224,
36227-36228
common, intima-media thickness (IMT)
study ~ 0126T
decompression ~ 61590-61591, 61595-61596
embolectomy ~ 34001
exploration ~ 35701
ligation ~ 37600-37606, 61611-61612
stenosis, imaging study measurement ~
3100F
thrombectomy ~ 34001
thromboendarterectomy ~ 35301, 35390
transection ~ 61611-61612
transposition ~ 33889
celiac
aneurysm ~ 35121-35122
bypass graft ~ 35531, 35631

1349

Artery ~ continued
  embolectomy ~ 34151
  thrombectomy ~ 34151
  thromboendarterectomy ~ 35341
  chest, ligation ~ 37616
  coronary
    atherectomy ~ 92995-92996
    bypass ~ 33517-33519
      arterial ~ 33533-33536
      bypass venous graft ~ 33510-33517, 35523
      internal mammary artery graft ~ 4110F
      graft ~ 33503-33505
      ligation ~ 33502
      repair ~ 33500-33507
      thrombectomy, percutaneous ~ 92973
  digital, sympathectomy ~ 64820
  ethmoidal, ligation ~ 30915
  extra corporeal circulation, for regional chemotherapy of extremity ~ 36823
  extremities, vascular studies ~ 93922-93923
  extremity
    bypass graft revision ~ 35879-35884
    catheterization ~ 36140
    ligation ~ 37618
  femoral
    aneurysm ~ 35141-35142
    angioplasty ~ 35456
    bypass graft ~ 35521, 35533, 35556-35558, 35566, 35621, 35646-35647, 35654-35661, 35666, 35700
    bypass graft revision ~ 35883-35884
    bypass in-situ ~ 35583-35585
    embolectomy ~ 34201
    exploration ~ 35721
    exposure ~ 34812-34813
    thrombectomy ~ 34201
    thromboendarterectomy ~ 35371-35372
  great vessel, repair ~ 33770-33781
  head, angiography ~ 36221-36226
  hepatic, aneurysm ~ 35121-35122
  iliac
    aneurysm ~ 35131-35132, 75954
    angioplasty ~ 37222
    bypass graft ~ 35563, 35632-35634, 35663
    embolectomy ~ 34151-34201
    endoprosthesis ~ 0254T-0255T
    exposure ~ 34820, 34833
    occlusion device ~ 34808
    revascularization ~ 37222
    thrombectomy ~ 34151-34201
    thromboendarterectomy ~ 35351, 35361-35363
    tube endoprosthesis ~ 34900, 75954
  iliofemoral
    bypass graft ~ 35565
    thromboendarterectomy ~ 35355, 35363
    X-ray with contrast ~ 75630
  innominate
    aneurysm ~ 35021-35022
    embolectomy ~ 34001-34101
    thrombectomy ~ 34001-34101
    thromboendarterectomy ~ 35311

Artery ~ continued
  leg
    angiography ~ 75710-75716
    catheterization ~ 36245-36248
  mammary, angiography ~ 75756
  maxillary, ligation ~ 30920
  mesenteric
    aneurysm ~ 35121-35122
    bypass graft ~ 35531, 35631
    embolectomy ~ 34151
    thrombectomy ~ 34151
    thromboendarterectomy ~ 35341
  middle cerebral artery, fetal, vascular studies ~ 76821
  neck
    angiography ~ 36221-36226
    ligation ~ 37615
  nose, incision ~ 30915-30920
  other angiography ~ 75774
  other artery, exploration ~ 35761
  pelvic
    angiography ~ 75736
    catheterization ~ 36245-36248
  peripheral arterial rehabilitation ~ 93668
  peroneal
    bypass graft ~ 35566-35571, 35666-35671
    bypass in-situ ~ 35585-35587
    embolectomy ~ 34203
    thrombectomy ~ 34203
    thromboendarterectomy ~ 35305-35306
  popliteal
    aneurysm ~ 35151-35152
    angioplasty ~ 37224
    atherectomy ~ 37225, 37227
    bypass graft ~ 35556, 35571, 35623, 35656, 35671, 35700
    bypass in-situ ~ 35583, 35587
    embolectomy ~ 34203
    exploration ~ 35741
    thrombectomy ~ 34203
    thromboendarterectomy ~ 35303
  pulmonary
    anastomosis ~ 33606
    angiography ~ 75741-75746
    banding ~ 33620
    repair ~ 33690, 33925-33926
  radial, aneurysm ~ 35045
    embolectomy ~ 34111
    sympathectomy ~ 64821
    thrombectomy ~ 34111
  rehabilitation ~ 93668
  reimplantation
    carotid ~ 35691, 35694-35695
    subclavian ~ 35693-35695
    vertebral ~ 35691-35693
    visceral ~ 35697
  renal
    aneurysm ~ 35121-35122
    angiography ~ 36251-36254
    angioplasty ~ 35450
    bypass graft ~ 35535-35536, 35560, 35631-35636

Artery ~ *continued*
  embolectomy ~ 34151
  thrombectomy ~ 34151
  thromboendarterectomy ~ 35341
  repair
    aneurysm ~ 61697-61708
    angioplasty ~ 75962-75968
  revision
    hemodialysis graft or fistula
      without thrombectomy ~ 36832
      with thrombectomy ~ 36833
  spine, angiography ~ 75705
  splenic
    aneurysm ~ 35111-35112
    bypass graft ~ 35536, 35636
  subclavian
    aneurysm ~ 35001-35002, 35021-35022
    angioplasty ~ 35458
    bypass graft ~ 35506, 35511-35516, 35526,
      35606-35616, 35626, 35645
    embolectomy ~ 34001-34101
    thrombectomy ~ 34001-34101
    thromboendarterectomy ~ 35301-35311
    unlisted services and procedures ~ 37799
  superficial palmar arch, sympathectomy ~
    64823
  temporal
    biopsy ~ 37609
    ligation ~ 37609
  thoracic, catheterization ~ 36215-36218
  thrombectomy
    hemodialysis graft or fistula ~ 36831
    other than hemodialysis graft or fistula ~
      35875, 36870
  tibial
    bypass graft ~ 35566-35571, 35623,
      35666-35671
    bypass in-situ ~ 35585-35587
    embolectomy ~ 34203
    revascularization ~ 37228-37235
    thrombectomy ~ 34203
    thromboendarterectomy ~ 35305-35306
  transcatheter therapy, with angiography ~
    75894-75898
  transposition
    carotid ~ 0037T, 35691, 35694-35695
    subclavian ~ 0037T, 35693-35695
    vertebral ~ 35691-35693
  ulnar
    aneurysm ~ 35045
    embolectomy ~ 34111
    sympathectomy ~ 64822
    thrombectomy ~ 34111
  unlisted services and procedures ~ 37799
  vertebral
    aneurysm ~ 35005, 61698, 61702
    angiography ~ 36211, 36225-36226, 36228
    bypass graft ~ 35508, 35515, 35642-35645
    catheterization ~ 36100
    decompression ~ 61597
    thromboendarterectomy ~ 35301

Artery ~ *continued*
  visceral
    angioplasty ~ 35450
    reimplantation ~ 35697
Artery catheterization, pulmonary ~ see
  catheterization, pulmonary artery
Arthrectomy, elbow ~ 24155
Arthrocentesis
  intermediate joint ~ 20605
  large joint ~ 20610
  small joint ~ 20600
Arthrodesis
  ankle ~ 27870
    tibiotalar and fibulotalar joints ~ 29899
  anterior interbody ~ 22551-22552
  carpometacarpal joint
    hand ~ 26843-26844
    thumb ~ 26841-26842
  cervical anterior, with discectomy ~ 22554
  elbow ~ 24800-24802
  finger joint ~ 26852
    interphalangeal ~ 26860-26863
    metacarpophalangeal ~ 26850
  foot joint ~ 28730-28735, 28740
    pantalar ~ 28705
    subtalar ~ 28725
    triple ~ 28715
    with advancement ~ 28737
    with lengthening ~ 28737
  hand joint ~ 26843-26844
  hip joint ~ 27284-27286
  intercarpal joint ~ 25820
    with autograft ~ 25825
  interphalangeal joint ~ 26860-26863
    great toe ~ 28755
    with tendon transfer ~ 28760
  knee ~ 27580
  metacarpophalangeal joint ~ 26850-26852
  metatarsophalangeal joint, great toe ~ 28750
  pubic symphysis ~ 27282
  radioulnar joint, with resection of ulna ~
    25830
  sacroiliac joint ~ 27280
  shoulder ~ see shoulder, arthrodesis
  shoulder joint ~ 23800
    with autogenous graft ~ 23802
  talus
    pantalar ~ 28705
    subtalar ~ 28725
    triple ~ 28715
  tarsal joint ~ 28730-28735, 28740
    with advancement ~ 28737
    with lengthening ~ 28737
  tarsometatarsal joint ~ 28730-28735, 28740
  thumb joint ~ 26841-26842
  tibiofibular joint ~ 27871
  vertebra
    additional interspace
      anterior/anterolateral approach ~ 22585
      lateral extracavitary ~ 22534
      posterior ~ 22632

1351

Arthrodesis ~ *continued*
  cervical
    anterior/anterolateral approach ~ 22548
    posterior/posterolateral and/or lateral
      traverse process ~ 22590-22600
  lumbar
    anterior/anterolateral approach ~ 22558
    lateral extracavitary ~ 22533
    pre-sacral interbody ~ 0195T, 0196T
    posterior/interbody ~ 22630
    posterior/posterolateral and/or lateral
      transverse process ~ 22612
  spinal deformity
    anterior approach ~ 22808-22812
    posterior approach ~ 22800-22804
  spinal fusion, exploration ~ 22830
  thoracic
    anterior/anterolateral approach ~ 22556
    lateral extracavitary ~ 22532
    posterior/posterolateral and/or lateral
      traverse process ~ 22610
  vertebrae, posterior ~ 22614
  wrist ~ 25800
    with graft ~ 25810
    with sliding graft ~ 25805
Arthrography
  ankle ~ 73615
    injection ~ 27648
  elbow ~ 73085
    injection ~ 24220
  hip ~ 73525
    injection ~ 27093-27095
  knee ~ 73580
    injection ~ 27370
  sacroiliac joint
    injection ~ 27096
  shoulder ~ 73040
    injection ~ 23350
  temporomandibular joint (TMJ) ~
    70328-70332
    injection ~ 21116
  wrist ~ 73115
    injection ~ 25426
Arthroplasties, knee replacement ~ 27438,
  27445
Arthroplasty
  ankle ~ 27700-27703
  elbow ~ 24360
    total replacement ~ 24363
    with implant ~ 24361-24362
  hip ~ 27132
    partial replacement ~ 27125
    revision ~ 27134-27138
    total replacement ~ 27130
  interphalangeal joint ~ 26535-26536
  intervertebral disc
    removal ~ 0164T, 22864-22865
    revision ~ 0165T, 22861-22862
    total replacement ~ 0163T, 22856-22857
    with osteophytectomy ~ 22856

Arthroplasty ~ *continued*
  knee ~ 27437-27443, 27446-27447
    revision ~ 27486-27487
    with prosthesis ~ 27438, 27445
  metacarpophalangeal joint ~ 26530-26531
  radius ~ 24365
    with implant ~ 24366
  reconstruction, prosthesis, hip ~ 27125
  shoulder joint with implant ~ 23470-23472
  temporomandibular joint ~ 21240-21243
  vertebral joint, lumbar spine ~ 0202T
  wrist ~ 25447
    carpal ~ 25443
    lunate ~ 25444
    navicular ~ 25443
    radius ~ 25441
    revision ~ 25449
    total replacement ~ 25446
    trapezium ~ 25445
    ulna ~ 25442
    with implant ~ 25441-25445
    wrist (pseudarthrosis type) ~ 25332
Arthropods, examination ~ 87168
Arthroscopy
  diagnostic
    elbow ~ 29830
    hip ~ 29860
    knee ~ 29870
    metacarpophalangeal joint ~ 29900
    shoulder ~ 29805
    temporomandibular joint ~ 29800
    wrist ~ 29840
  surgical
    ankle ~ 29891-29899
    elbow ~ 29834-29838
    hip ~ 29861-29863, 29914
    knee ~ 29871-29889
      cartilage allograft ~ 29867
      cartilage autograft ~ 29866
      meniscal transplantation ~ 29868
    metacarpophalangeal joint ~ 29901-29902
    shoulder ~ 29806-29828
      biceps tenodesis ~ 29828
    subtalar joint ~ 29904-29907, 29915-29916
      arthrodesis ~ 29907
      debridement ~ 29906
      with labral repair ~ 29916
      removal of loose or foreign body ~ 29904
      synovectomy ~ 29905
    temporomandibular joint ~ 29804
    wrist ~ 29843-29848
  unlisted services and procedures ~ 29999
Arthrotomy
  acromioclavicular joint ~ 23044
  ankle ~ 27610-27612, 27620
  ankle joint ~ 27625-27626
  carpometacarpal joint ~ 26070
    with biopsy, synovium
      with synovial biopsy ~ 26100

Arthrotomy ~ *continued*
 elbow ~ 24000
  capsular release ~ 24006
  with joint exploration ~ 24101
  with synovectomy ~ 24102
  with synovial biopsy ~ 24100
 finger joint ~ 26075
  interphalangeal
   with synovial biopsy ~ 26110
  metacarpophalangeal
   with biopsy, synovium ~ 26105
 glenohumeral joint ~ 23040
 hip ~ 27033
  for infection
   with drainage ~ 27030
  with synovectomy ~ 27054
 interphalangeal joint ~ 26080, 26110
  toe ~ 28024, 28054
 intertarsal joint ~ 28020, 28050
 knee ~ 27310, 27330-27335, 27403, 29868
 metacarpophalangeal joint ~ 26075, 26105
 metatarsophalangeal joint ~ 28022, 28052
 shoulder ~ 23044, 23105-23107
 shoulder joint ~ 23100-23101
  exploration and/or removal of loose or
   foreign body ~ 23107
 sternoclavicular joint ~ 23044
 tarsometatarsal joint ~ 28020, 28050
 temporomandibular joint ~ 21010
 with biopsy
  acromioclavicular joint ~ 23101
  glenohumeral joint ~ 23100
  hip joint ~ 27052
  knee joint ~ 27330
  sacroiliac joint
   hip joint ~ 27050
  sternoclavicular joint ~ 23101
 with synovectomy
  glenohumeral joint ~ 23105
  sternoclavicular joint ~ 23106
 wrist ~ 25040, 25100-25107
Articular ligament ~ see ligament
Artificial abortion ~ see abortion
Artificial cardiac pacemaker ~ see heart,
 pacemaker
Artificial eye ~ see prosthesis
Artificial genitourinary sphincter ~ see
 prosthesis, urethral sphincter
Artificial insemination ~ 58976
 intra-cervical ~ 58321
 intra-uterine ~ 58322
 sperm washing ~ 58323
Artificial knee joints ~ 27438, 27445
Artificial penis ~ see penile prosthesis
Artificial pneumothorax ~ 32960
Arytenoid, excision, endoscopic ~ 31560-31561
Arytenoid cartilage
 excision ~ 31400
 repair ~ 31400
Arytenoidectomy ~ 31400
 endoscopic ~ 31560
Arytenoidopexy ~ 31400

Ascorbic acid, blood ~ 82180
Aspartate aminotransferase ~ 84450
Aspergillus
 antibody ~ 86606
 antigen detection
  enzyme immunoassay ~ 87305
Aspiration ~ see puncture aspiration
 amniotic fluid
  diagnostic ~ 59000
  therapeutic ~ 59001
 bladder ~ 51100-51102
 bone marrow ~ 38220
 brain lesion, stereotactic ~ 61750-61751
 bronchi, endoscopy ~ 31645-31646
 bursa ~ 20600-20610
 catheter
  nasotracheal ~ 31720
  tracheobronchial ~ 31725
 chest ~ 32554-32555
 cyst
  bone ~ 20615
  kidney ~ 50390
  pelvis ~ 50390
  spinal cord ~ 62268
  thyroid ~ 60300
 disc ~ 62267
 duodenal ~ 43756-43757
 fetal fluid ~ 59074
 ganglion cyst ~ 20612
 gastric ~ 43753-43755
 hydrocele, tunica vaginalis ~ 55000
 joint ~ 20600-20610
 laryngoscopy
  direct ~ 31515
 lens material ~ 66840
 liver ~ 47015
 lung ~ 32405
 lung puncture ~ 32405
 nail ~ 11740
 nucleus of disk, lumbar ~ 62287
 orbital contents ~ 67415
 pelvis, endoscopy ~ 49322
 pericardium ~ 33010-33011
 pleural cavity ~ 32554-32555
 puncture, cyst, breast ~ 19000-19001
 spinal cord, stereotaxis ~ 63615
 spinal puncture ~ see spinal tap
 syrinx, spinal cord ~ 62268
 thyroid ~ 60300
 trachea
  nasotracheal ~ 31720
  puncture ~ 31612
 tunica vaginalis, hydrocele ~ 55000
 vitreous ~ 67015
Aspiration lipectomies ~ 15876-15879
Aspiration of bone marrow from donor for
 transplant ~ 38230
Assay, very long chain fatty acids ~ 82726
Assay tobramycin ~ 80200
Assisted circulation ~ see circulation assist
AST ~ 84450
Astragalectomy ~ 28130

1353

Astragalus ~ see talus
Asymmetry, face ~ 21247
Ataxia telangiectasia, chromosome analysis ~ 88248
Ataxy, telangiectasia ~ 88248
ATLV ~ see HTLV I
ATLV antibodies ~ 86688
Atomic absorption spectroscopy ~ 82190
ATP creatine phosphotranferase ~ 82550-82552
Atresia
  choanal ~ 30540-30545
  congenital, auditory canal, external, reconstruction ~ 69320
Atria
  ablation ~ 33254-33256, 33257-33259 33265-33266
  endoscopy, surgical ~ 33265-33266
  reconstruction ~ 33254-33256, 33265-33266
Atrial electrogram ~ see cardiology, diagnostic esophageal recording ~ 93615-93616
Atrial fibrillation ~ see fibrillation, atrial
Atrioseptopexy ~ see heart, repair, atrial septum
Atrioseptoplasty ~ see heart, repair, atrial septum
Attachment ~ see fixation
Atticotomy ~ 69631, 69635
Audiologic function tests ~ 92590-92595
  acoustic reflex ~ 92568
  acoustic reflex decay ~ 92570
  audiometry
    Bekesy ~ 92560-92561
    comprehensive ~ 92557
    conditioning play ~ 92582
    groups ~ 92559
    pure tone ~ 92552-92553
    select picture ~ 92583
    speech ~ 92555-92556
    visual reinforcement ~ 92579
  central auditory function ~ 92620-92621
  diagnostic analysis
    auditory brainstem implant ~ 92640
  electrocochleography ~ 92584
  evoked otoacoustic emission ~ 92587-92588
  filtered speech ~ 92571
  loudness balance ~ 92562
  screening ~ 92551
  sensorineural acuity ~ 92575
  short increment sensitivity index ~ 92564
  staggered spondaic word test ~ 92572
  Stenger test ~ 92565, 92577
  synthetic sentence test ~ 92576
  tinnitus assessment ~ 92625
  tone decay ~ 92563
  tympanometry ~ 92550, 92567, 92570
Audiometry
  Bekesy ~ 92560-92561
  brainstem evoked response ~ 92585-92586
  comprehensive ~ 0212T, 92557
  conditioning play ~ 92582
  groups ~ 92559

Audiometry ~ *continued*
  pure tone ~ 92552-92553
    automated 0208T-0209T
  select picture ~ 92583
  speech ~ 0210T-0211T, 92555-92556
  tympanometry ~ 92550, 92567, 92570
Auditory brain stem evoked response ~ 92585-92586
Auditory canal
  decompression ~ 61591
  external
    abscess, incision and drainage ~ 69020
    biopsy ~ 69105
    lesion, excision ~ 69140-69155
    reconstruction
      for congenital atresia ~ 69320
      for stenosis ~ 69310
    removal
      cerumen ~ 69210
      ear wax ~ 69210
      foreign body ~ 69200-69205
  internal, decompression ~ 69960
Auditory atresia, external ~ 69320
Auditory evoked otoacoustic emission ~ 92587-92588
Auditory evoked potentials ~ 92585-92586, 92590-92595
Auditory labyrinth ~ see ear, inner
Auditory meatus, X-ray ~ 70134
Auditory system surgical procedures ~ 69000-69990
Auditory tube ~ see eustachian tube
Augmentation
  chin ~ 21120, 21123
  malar ~ 21270
  mammoplasty ~ 19324-19325
  mandibular body
    with bone graft ~ 21127
    with prosthesis ~ 21125
  osteoplasty, facial bones ~ 21208
Aural rehabilitation ~ 92510
Auricle (heart) ~ see atria
Auricular fibrillation ~ fibrillation, atria
Auricular prosthesis ~ 21086
Australia antigen ~ 87340-87341
Autograft
  bone
    local ~ 20936
    morselized ~ 20937
    structural ~ 20938
  chondrocytes, knee ~ 27412
  for spine surgery
    local ~ 20936
    morselized ~ 20937
    structural ~ 20938
  osteochondral
    knee ~ 27416
    talus ~ 28446
  skin
    dermal ~ 15130-15136
    epidermal ~ 15110-15116, 15150-15157
    harvesting, for tissue culture ~ 15040

Autologous blood transfusion ~ 86890-86891
Autologous transplantation ~ see autograft
Autonomic nervous system function ~ see
  neurology, diagnostic; neurophysiologic
  testing
Autoprothrombin
  C ~ 85260
  I ~ 85230
  II ~ 85250
  III ~ 85260
Autopsy
  coroner's exam ~ 88045
  forensic exam ~ 88040
  gross and micro exam ~ 88020-88029
  gross exam ~ 88000-88016
  organ ~ 88037
  regional ~ 88036
  unlisted services and procedures ~ 88099
Autotransfusion, blood ~ 86890-86891
Autotransplant ~ see autograft
Autotransplantation, renal ~ 50380
Avulsion
  nails ~ 11730-11732
  nerve ~ 64732-64772
AV fistula ~ see arteriovenous fistula
AV shunt ~ see arteriovenous shunt
Axillary arteries ~ see artery, axillary
Axillary nerve, injection, anesthetic ~ 64417
Axis, dens ~ 22548

B

B antibodies, hepatitis ~ see antibody, hepatitis
  B
B antigens, hepatitis ~ 87515-87517
B complex vitamins, B12 absorption ~
  78270-78272
B-DNA ~ 86225-86226
B-hexosaminidase ~ 83080
B1 vitamin ~ see 84425
B6 vitamin ~ 84207
B12 vitamin ~ 82607-82608
Babcock operation ~ 37700-37735, 37780
Bacillus Calmette Guerin vaccine ~ see BCG
  vaccine
Back/ flank
  biopsy ~ 21920-21925
  repair, hernia ~ 49540
  strapping ~ 29799
  tumor
    excision ~ 21930-21936
    radical resection ~ 21935, 21936
  wound exploration
    penetrating ~ 20102
Backbone ~ see spine
Bacteria culture
  additional methods ~ 87077
  aerobic ~ 87040-87071

Bacteria culture ~ continued
  anaerobic ~ 87073-87076
  blood ~ 87040
  other source ~ 87070-87075
  screening ~ 87081
  stool ~ 87045-87046
  urine ~ 87086-87088
Bacterial endotoxins ~ 87176
Bacterial overgrowth breath test ~ 91065
Bactericidal titer, serum ~ 87197
Bacterium, antibody ~ 86609
Baer ~ 92585-92586
Baker's cyst ~ 27345
Baker tube, intestine decompression ~ 44021
Balanoplasty ~ see penis, repair
Baldy-Webster operation ~ 58400
Balkan grippe ~ 86000, 86638
Balloon
  angioplasties, coronary ~ see percutaneous
    transluminal angioplasty
  angioplasty ~ see angioplasty
  assisted device, aorta ~ 33967-33974
Band, pulmonary artery ~ 33690
Banding, artery
  fistula ~ 37607
  pulmonary ~ 33620, 33690
Bank, blood ~ see blood banking
Bankart procedure ~ 23450-23462
Barany caloric test ~ 92533
Barbiturates, blood or urine ~ 82205
Bardenheurer operation ~ 37616
Bariatric surgery ~ 43644-43645, 43842-43848
Barium ~ 83015
Barium enema ~ 74270-74280
Barker operation ~ 28120, 28130
Barr bodies ~ 88130
Barr procedure ~ 27690-27692
Bartholin's gland
  abscess, incision and drainage ~ 56420
  cyst, repair ~ 56440
  excision ~ 56740
  marsupialization ~ 56440
Bartonella
  antibody ~ 86611
  detection ~ 87470-87472
Basic life services ~ 99450
Basic proteins, myelin ~ 83873
Basilar arteries ~ 61698, 61702
Batch-Spittler-McFaddin operation ~ 27598
BCG vaccine ~ 90585, 90586
Be antigens, hepatitis ~ 87350
Bed sores ~ see debridement; skin graft and
  flap; 15920-15999
Bed testing ~ 94780, 94781
Bekesy audiometry ~ 92560-92561
Belsey IV procedure ~ see fundoplasty
Bender-Gestalt test ~ 96100
Benedict test for urea ~ 81005
Benign cystic mucinous tumour ~ see
  ganglion
Benign neoplasm of cranial nerves ~ see
  cranial nerve

Bennett fracture ~ see phalanx, finger; 26720-26727
Bennett procedure ~ see revision; 27385-27386, 27400, 27430
Benzidine test ~ 82270, 82272
Benzodiazepine, assay ~ 80154
Benzoyl cholinesterase ~ 82480-82482
Bernstein test ~ 91030
Beryllium ~ 83015
Beta-2 -microglobulin
blood ~ 82232
urine ~ 82232
Beta-hydroxydehydrogenase ~ 80406
Beta 2 glycoprotein 1 antibody ~ 86146
Beta blocker therapy ~ see performance measures
Beta glucosidase ~ 82963
Beta hypophamine ~ 84588
Beta lipoproteins ~ 83700-83704, 83721
Beta test ~ see psychiatric diagnosis ~ 96100
Bethesda system ~ 88164-88167
Bicarbonate ~ 82374
Biceps tendon, insertion ~ 24342
Bichloride, methylene ~ 84600
Bicuspid valve ~ see mitral valve
Bifrontal craniotomy ~ 61557
Bilaminate skin substitute/ neodermis ~ see tissue
repair ~ see tissue, culture; 15100-15101, 15120-15121
Bile acids ~ 82239
blood ~ 82240
Bile duct ~ see gallbladder
anastomosis
with intestines ~ 47760, 47780-47785
biopsy, endoscopy ~ 47553
catheterization ~ 75982
change catheter tube ~ 75984
cyst, excision ~ 47715
destruction, calculi (stone) ~ 43265
dilation, endoscopy ~ 43271, 47555-47556
drainage, transhepatic ~ 75980
endoscopy
biopsy ~ 47553
cannulation ~ 43273
destruction
calculi (stone) ~ 43265
tumor ~ 43272
dilation ~ 43271, 47555-47556
exploration ~ 47552
intraoperative ~ 47550
removal
calculi (stone) ~ 43264, 47554
foreign body ~ 43269
stent ~ 43269
specimen collection ~ 43260
sphincterotomy ~ 43262
sphincter pressure ~ 43263
tube placement ~ 43267-43268
exploration
atresia ~ 47700
endoscopy ~ 47552

Bile duct ~ *continued*
incision, sphincter ~ 43262, 47460
incision and drainage ~ 47420-47425
insertion
catheter ~ 47510, 47525, 75982
revision ~ 47530
stent ~ 47511, 47801
reconstruction, anastomosis ~ 47800
removal
calculi (stone) ~ 43264, 47420-47425
percutaneous ~ 47630
foreign body ~ 43269
stent ~ 43269
repair ~ 47701
gastrointestinal tract ~ 47785
with intestines ~ 47760, 47780
tube placement
nasobiliary ~ 43267
stent ~ 43268
tumor
destruction ~ 43271
excision ~ 47711-47712
unlisted services and procedures ~ 47999
X-ray
guide dilation ~ 74360
with contrast ~ 74300-74320
calculus removal ~ 74327
guide catheter ~ 74328, 74330
Bilirubin
blood ~ 82247-82248
feces ~ 82252
total
direct ~ 82247-82248
transcutaneous ~ 88720
Billroth I or II ~ 43631-43635, 43845
Bilobectomy ~ 32482
Bimone ~ 84402
Binding globulin, testosterone-estradiol ~ 84270
Binet-Simon test ~ 96100
Binet test ~ 96100
Binet-Simon test, binocular microscopy ~ 92504
Biofeedback ~ 90901-90911
anorectal ~ 90911
psychiatric treatment ~ 90875-90876
Biofeedback training ~ 90901-90911
Bioimpedance
thorax ~ 93701
Biometry, eye ~ 76516-76519, 92136
Biopsies, needle ~ see needle biopsy
Biopsy ~ see brush biopsy; needle biopsy
abdomen ~ 49000
adrenal gland ~ 60540-60545
anal, endoscopy ~ 46606
ankle ~ 27613-27614, 27620
arm, lower ~ 25065-25066
arm, upper ~ 24065-24066
artery, temporal ~ 37609
auditory canal, external ~ 69105
back/flank ~ 21920-21925

Biopsy ~ *continued*
bile duct, endoscopy ~ 47553
bladder ~ 52354
  cystourethroscope ~ 52204
  cystourethroscopy ~ 52224, 52250
blood vessel, transcatheter ~ 75970
bone ~ 20220-20245
bone marrow ~ 38221
brain ~ 61140
  stereotactic ~ 61750-61751
brainstem ~ 61575-61576
breast ~ 19100-19103
  stereotactic localization ~ 77031
bronchi
  catheterization ~ 31717
  endoscopic ~ 31625-31629, 31632-31633
brush
  bronchi ~ 31717
  renal pelvis ~ 52007
  ureter ~ 52007
  with cystourethroscopy ~ 52204
carpometacarpal joint, synovium ~ 26100
cervix ~ 57454-57455, 57460, 57500, 57520
chorionic villus ~ 59015
colon ~ 44025, 44100
  endoscopy ~ 44389, 45380, 45391, 45392
  multiple, with colostomy, cecostomy ~ 44322
colon-sigmoid, endoscopy ~ 45305, 45331
conjunctiva ~ 68100
cornea ~ 65410
duodenum ~ 44010
ear, external ~ 69100
elbow ~ 24065-24066, 24101
  synovium ~ 24100
embryo blastomere ~ 89290-89291
endometrium ~ 58100, 58558
epididymis ~ 54800-54865
esophagus, endoscopy ~ 43202
  forceps ~ 3150F
eye muscle ~ 67346
eyelid ~ 67810
forearm, soft tissue ~ 25065-25066
gallbladder, endoscopy ~ 43261
gastrointestinal, upper, endoscopy ~ 43239
hand joint, synovium ~ 26100
heart ~ 93505
hip ~ 27040-27041
  joint ~ 27052
hypopharynx ~ 42802
ileum, endoscopy ~ 44382
interphalangeal joint
  finger ~ 26110
  toe ~ 28054
intertarsal joint, toe ~ 28050
intestines, small ~ 44020, 44100
  endoscopy ~ 44361, 44377
kidney ~ 50200-50205
  endoscopic ~ 50555-50557, 50574-50576, 52354

Biopsy ~ *continued*
knee ~ 27323-27324
  synovium ~ 27330
knee joint, synovium ~ 27330
lacrimal gland ~ 68510
lacrimal sac ~ 68525
larynx, endoscopy ~ 31510, 31576
leg
  lower ~ 27613-27614
  upper ~ 27323-27324
lip ~ 40490
liver ~ 47000-47001, 47100
lung
  needle ~ 32405
  thoracoscopy ~ 32607-32608
  thoracotomy ~ 32096-32097
lymph nodes ~ 38500-38530
  injection procedure, for identification of sentinel node ~ 38792
  laparoscopic ~ 38570-38572
  needle ~ 38505
  open ~ 38500, 38510-38530
  superficial ~ 38500
mediastinum ~ 39400
  needle ~ 32405
metacarpophalangeal joint ~ 26105
metatarsophalangeal joint ~ 28052
mouth ~ 40808, 41108
muscle ~ 20200-20206
nail ~ 11755
nasopharynx ~ 42804-42806
neck ~ 21550
nerve ~ 64795
nose
  endoscopic ~ 31237
  intranasal ~ 30100
oocyte polar body ~ 89290-89291
orbit ~ 61332
  exploration ~ 67400, 67450
  fine needle aspiration ~ 67415
oropharynx ~ 42800
ovary ~ 58900
palate ~ 42100
pancreas ~ 48100
pelvis ~ 27040-27041
penis ~ 54100
  deep structures ~ 54105
percutaneous needle, spinal cord ~ 62269
perineum ~ 56605-56606
peritoneum, endoscopic ~ 47561
pharynx ~ 42800-42806
pleura
  needle ~ 32400
  thoracoscopy ~ 32609
  thoracotomy ~ 32098, 32400
prostate ~ 55700-55706
rectum ~ 45100
retroperitoneal area ~ 49010
sacroiliac joint ~ 27050
salivary gland ~ 42405

Biopsy ~ *continued*
shoulder
  deep ~ 23066
  soft tissue ~ 23065
shoulder joint ~ 23100-23101
sinus, sphenoid ~ 31050-31051
skin ~ see skin, biopsy
skin lesion ~ 11100-11101
spinal cord ~ 63275-63290
  percutaneous ~ 62269
  stereotaxis ~ 63615
stomach ~ 43605
tarsometatarsal joint, synovial ~ 28050
testis ~ 54500-54505
thorax ~ 21550
throat ~ 42800-42806
tongue ~ 41100-41105
transcatheter ~ 37200
ureter ~ 52354
  endoscopic ~ 50955-50957, 50974-50976
urethra ~ 52204, 52354, 53200
uterus
  endometrial ~ 58100
  endoscopic ~ 58558
uvula ~ 42100
vagina ~ 57100-57105, 57421
vein ~ 75970
vertebral body ~ 20250-20251
vulva ~ 56605-56606, 56821
with arthrotomy
  acromioclavicular joint ~ 23101
  glenohumeral joint ~ 23100
  sternoclavicular joint ~ 23101
with cystourethroscopy ~ 52354
wrist ~ 25065-25066, 25100-25101
Biostatistics ~ 76516-76519, 92136
Biosterol ~ 84590
Biotinidase ~ 82261
Birthing room, newborn care ~ 99465
Bischof procedure ~ 63170-63172
Bismuth ~ 83015
Bizzozero's corpuscle/cell ~ see blood, platelet
Bladder
abscess, incision and drainage ~ 51080
anastomosis ~ 51960
aspiration ~ 51100-51102
biopsy ~ 52204
catheterization ~ 51045, 51701-51703
change tube ~ 51705-51710
creation, stoma ~ 51980
cyst, urachal, excision ~ 51500
destruction, endoscopic ~ 52214-52224, 52354
dilation, ureter ~ 52260-52265, 52341-52342,
  52344-52345
diverticulum
  excision ~ 51525
  incision ~ 52305
  resection ~ 52305
endoscopy ~ 52000
  biopsy ~ 52204, 52354
  catheterization ~ 52005, 52010

Bladder ~ *continued*
destruction ~ 52214-52224, 52400
dilation ~ 52260-52265
diverticulum ~ 52305
evacuation, clot ~ 52001
excision, tumor ~ 52234-52240, 52355
exploration ~ 52351
injection ~ 52283
lithotripsy ~ 52353
radiotracer ~ 52250
removal
  calculus ~ 52310-52315, 52352
  foreign body ~ 52310-52315
sphincter surgery ~ 52277
tumor, excision ~ 52355
ureter surgery ~ 52290-52300
urethral syndrome ~ 52285
  with urethrotomy ~ 52270-52276
excision
  partial ~ 51550-51565
  total ~ 51570, 51580, 51590-51597
    with nodes ~ 51575, 51585, 51595
  transurethral ~ 52640
  tumor ~ 52234-52240
incision
  catheter ~ 51045
  with destruction ~ 51020-51030
  with radiotracer ~ 51020
incision and drainage ~ 51040
injection, radiologic ~ 51600-51610
insertion, stent ~ 51045, 52334
instillation, drugs ~ 51720
irrigation ~ 51700
lesion, destruction ~ 51030
neck, endoscopy, injection of implant material
  ~ 51715
excision ~ 51520
micro-remodeling ~ 53860
nuclear medicine, residual study ~ 78730
radiotracer ~ 52250
reconstruction, and urethra ~ 51800-51820
  with intestines ~ 51960
removal
  calculus ~ 51050, 52310-52315
  foreign body ~ 52310-52315
  urethral stent ~ 52310-52315
repair
  diverticulum ~ 52305
  exstrophy ~ 51940
  fistula ~ 44660-44661, 45800-45805,
    51880-51925
  neck ~ 51845
  wound ~ 51860-51865
resection ~ 52500
sphincter surgery ~ 52277
suspension ~ 51990
suture
  fistula ~ 44660-44661, 45800-45805,
    51880-51925
  wound ~ 51860-51865
tumor, excision ~ 51530

Bladder ~ *continued*
  unlisted services and procedures ~ 53899
  urethrocystography ~ 74450-74455
  urethrotomy ~ 52270-52276
  urinary incontinence procedures
    laparoscopy ~ 51990-51992
  plan of care documented ~ 0509F
  X-ray ~ 74430
    with contrast ~ 74450-74455
Bladder voiding pressure studies ~
  51728-51729
Blalock-Hanlon procedure ~ 33735-33737
Blalock-Taussig procedure ~ see shunt, great
  vessel
Blastocyst implantation ~ see implantation
Blastocyst transfer ~ see embryo transfer
Blastogenesis ~ 86353
Blastomyces, antibody ~ 86612
Blastomycosis, european ~ see cryptococcus
Blast cells ~ see stem cell
Blast transformation ~ 86353
Bleeding ~ see also hemorrhage
  anal ~ 46614
  disorder ~ 85390
  time ~ 85002
  tube, passage and placement ~ 43460
  uterine ~ 59160
  vaginal ~ 57180
Blepharoplasty ~ 15820-15823, 67950
  anesthesia ~ 00103
Blepharoptosis
  repair ~ 67901-67909
    frontalis muscle technique ~ 67901
      with fascial sling ~ 67902
    superior rectus technique with fascial sling ~
      67906
    tarso levator resection/advancement
      external approach ~ 67904
      internal approach ~ 67903
Blepharorrhaphy ~ 67875
Blepharospasm, chemodenervation ~ 64612
Blepharotomy ~ 67700
Blister ~ see bulla
Blom-Singer prosthesis ~ 31611
Blood ~ 85025-85027
  bleeding time ~ 85002
  collection, for autotransfusion
    intraoperative ~ 86891
    preoperative ~ 86890
  feces ~ 82270
    by hemoglobin immunoassay ~ 82274
  hemoglobin A1c (HbA1c) level ~ 3044F-3045F
  hemoglobin concentration ~ 85046
  nuclear medicine
    flow imaging ~ 78445
    plasma iron ~ 78160
    red cell ~ 78140
    red cell survival ~ 78130-78135
  osmolality ~ 83930

Blood ~ *continued*
  plasma, exchange ~ 36514-36516
  platelet
    aggregation ~ 85576
    automated count ~ 85049
    count ~ 85008
    manual count ~ 85032
  stem cell
    count ~ 86587
    donor search ~ 38204
    erythropoietin therapy ~ 3160F, 4090F-4095F
    harvesting ~ 38205-38206
    transplantation ~ 38240-38242
      cell concentration ~ 38215
      cryopreservation ~ 38207, 88240
      plasma depletion ~ 38214
      platelet depletion ~ 38213
      red blood cell depletion ~ 38212
      T-cell depletion ~ 38210
      thawing ~ 38208-38209, 88241
      tumor cell depletion ~ 38211
      washing ~ 38209
  transfusion ~ 36430
    exchange ~ 36455
      newborn ~ 36450
    fetal ~ 36460
    push, infant ~ 36440
  unlisted services and procedures ~ 85999
  urine ~ 83491
  viscosity ~ 85810
Blood, occult ~ 82270-82272
Blood banking
  frozen blood preparation ~ 86930-86932
  frozen plasma preparation ~ 86927
  physician services ~ 86077-86079
Blood cell
  CD4 and CD8, including ratio ~ 86360
  enzyme activity ~ 82657
  exchange ~ 36511-36513
  red ~ see red blood cell (RBC)
  sedimentation rate
    automated ~ 85652
    manual ~ 85651
  white ~ see leukocyte
Blood cell count
  automated ~ 85049
  B-cells ~ 86064
  blood smear ~ 85007-85008
  differential WBC count ~ 85004-85007, 85009
  hematocrit ~ 85014
  hemoglobin ~ 85018
  hemogram
    added indices ~ 85025-85027
    automated ~ 85025-85027
    manual ~ 85032
  microhematocrit ~ 85013
  natural killer (NK) cells ~ 86379
  red ~ 85032-85041
  red blood cells ~ 85032-85041
  reticulocyte ~ 85044-85046
  stem cells ~ 86587

Blood cell count ~ *continued*
T-cells ~ 86359-86361
white ~ 85032, 85048, 89055
white blood cells ~ 85032, 85048, 89055
Blood clot
assay ~ 85396
clotting factor ~ 85250-85293
clotting factor test ~ 85210-85244
clotting inhibitors ~ 85300-85302, 85305,
    85307
clot lysis time ~ 85175
clot retraction ~ 85170
coagulation time ~ 85345-85348
thrombolytic agent(s), tissue plasminogen
    activator (tPA) ~ 4077F
Blood coagulation
defect ~ 85390
disorders ~ 34401-34490, 35875-35876, 50230
factor ~ 85210-85293
factor I ~ 85384-85385
factor II ~ 85210
factor III ~ see thromboplastin
factor IV ~ see calcium
factor VII ~ 85230
factor VIII ~ 85210-85293
factor IX ~ 85250
factor X ~ 85260
factor X, activated ~ 85260
factor XI ~ 85270
factor XIII ~ 85290-85291
test ~ 85999
Blood component removal ~ 36511-36516
Blood count, complete ~ 85025-85027
Blood flow check, graft ~ 15860, 90939-90940
Blood gases
CO2 ~ 82803
HCO3 ~ 82803
O2 saturation ~ 82805-82810
pCO2 ~ 82803
pH ~ 82800-82803
pO2 ~ 82803
Blood letting ~ 99195
Blood lipoprotein ~ see lipoprotein
Blood pool imaging ~ 78472-78473,
    78481-78483, 78494-78496

Blood pressure ~ see performance measures
monitoring, 24 hour ~ 93784-93790
ocular ~ 0198T
systolic ~ 3074F-3075F
venous ~ 93770
Blood products
irradiation ~ 86945
pooling ~ 86965
splitting ~ 86985
Blood sample, fetal ~ 59030
Blood serum ~ see serum
Blood smear ~ 85060
Blood syndrome, chromosome analysis ~
    88245-88248

Blood tests
iron stores ~ 3160F
Kt/V ~ 3082F-3084F
nuclear medicine
    iron, chelatable ~ 78172
    iron absorption ~ 78162
    iron utilization ~ 78170
    plasma volume ~ 78110-78111
    platelet survival ~ 78190-78191
    red cell volume ~ 78120-78121
    whole blood volume ~ 78122
panels
    electrolyte ~ 80051
    general health panel ~ 80050
    hepatic function ~ 80076
    hepatitis, acute ~ 80074
    lipid panel ~ 80061
    metabolic
        basic, total calcium ~ 80048
        basic, ionized calcium ~ 80047
        comprehensive ~ 80053
    obstetric panel ~ 80055
    renal function ~ 80069
    volume determination ~ 78122
Blood transfusion, autologous ~ 86890-86891
Blood typing, ABO only ~ 86900
antigen screen ~ 86904
crossmatch ~ 86920-86922
other RBC antigens ~ 86905
paternity testing ~ 86910-86911
Rh (D) ~ 86901
Rh phenotype ~ 86906
Blood urea nitrogen ~ 84520-84525
Blood vessels ~ see also artery; vein
angioscopy, non-coronary ~ 35400
endoscopy, surgical ~ 37500
excision, arteriovenous malformation ~
    63250-63252
exploration
    abdomen ~ 35840
    chest ~ 35820
    extremity ~ 35860
    neck ~ 35800
great, suture ~ 33320-33322
harvest
    endoscopic ~ 33508
    lower extremity vein ~ 35572
    upper extremity artery ~ 35600
    upper extremity vein ~ 35500
kidney, repair ~ 50100
repair
    abdomen ~ see aneurysm repair; fistula,
        repair
        with composite graft ~ 35681-35683
        with other graft ~ 35281
        with vein graft ~ 35251
    aneurysm ~ 61705-61708
    arteriovenous malformation ~ 61680-61692,
        61705-61710, 63250-63252

Blood vessels ~ *continued*
  chest
    with composite graft ~ 35681-35683
    with other graft ~ 35271-35276
    with vein graft ~ 35241-35246
    direct ~ 35201-35226
    finger ~ 35207
    graft defect ~ 35870
    hand ~ 35207
    lower extremity ~ 35226
     with composite graft ~ 35681-35683
     with other graft ~ 35281
     with vein graft ~ 35251
    neck
     with composite graft ~ 35681-35683
     with other graft ~ 35261
     with vein graft ~ 35231
    upper extremity ~ 35206
     with composite graft ~ 35681-35683
     with other graft ~ 35266
     with vein graft ~ 35236
  shunt creation, direct ~ 36818, 36821
    thomas shunt ~ 36835
    with bypass graft ~ 35686
    with graft ~ 36825-36830
  shunt revision, with graft ~ 36832
Blood, occult ~ see occult blood
Bloom syndrome, chromosome analysis ~ 88245
Blotting, western ~ see western blot
Blot test, ink ~ 96100
Blow-out fracture, orbital floor ~ 21385-21395
Blue, dome cyst ~ 19000-19001
BMT ~ 38240-38242
Boarding home care ~ 99321-99333
Bodies
  acetone ~ 82009-82010
  Barr ~ 88130
  carotid ~ see carotid body
  ciliary ~ see ciliary body
  Heinz ~ 85441-85445
  inclusion ~ see inclusion bodies
  ketone ~ 82009-82010
Body cast
  halo ~ 29000
  removal ~ 29700, 29710-29715
  repair ~ 29720
  Risser jacket ~ 29010-29015
  turnbuckle jacket ~ 29020-29025
  upper body and head ~ 29040
  upper body and legs ~ 29046
  upper body and one leg ~ 29044
  upper body only ~ 29035
Body fluid, crystal identification ~ 89060
Body of vertebra ~ see vertebral, body
Body section
  X-ray ~ 76100
  motion ~ 76101-76102
Body system, neurologic ~ *78699*
Boil ~ 10060-10061
Boil, vulva ~ 56405

Bone ~ see also specific bone***
  ablation, tumor ~ 20982
  biopsy ~ 20220-20245
  carpal ~ see carpal bone
  cheek ~ see cheekbone
  CT scan, density study ~ 77078
  cyst
    drainage ~ 20615
    injection ~ 20615
  dual energy X-ray absorptiometry ~ 77080-77081
  excision
    epiphyseal bar ~ 20150
    facial bones ~ 21026
    mandible ~ 21025
  facial ~ see facial bone
  fixation
    caliper ~ 20660
    cranial tong ~ 20660
    halo ~ 20661-20663, 21100
    interdental ~ 21110
    multiplane ~ 20692
     stereotactic computer assisted ~ 20696-20697
    pin/wire ~ 20650
    skeletal, humeral epicondyle, percutaneous ~ 24566
    stereotactic frame ~ 20660
    uniplane ~ 20690
  fracture, osteoporosis screening ~ 5015F
  hyoid ~ 21495
  insertion
    needle ~ 36680
    osseointegrated implant, for external speech processor/cochlear stimulator ~ 69714-69718
  marrow, cytogenic testing ~ 3155F
  metatarsal ~ see metatarsal
  nasal ~ see nasal bone
  navicular ~ see navicular
  nuclear medicine
    density study ~ 78350-78351
    imaging ~ 78300-78320
    spect ~ 78320
    unlisted services and procedures ~ 78399
  osetoporosis, pharmacologic therapy ~ 4005F
  protein ~ 83937
  removal, fixation device ~ 20670-20680
  replacement, osseointegrated implant, for external speech processor/cochlear stimulator ~ 69717-69718
  scan ~ see bone, nuclear medicine; nuclear medicine
  semilunar ~ see lunate
  sesamoid ~ see sesamoid bone
  tarsal ~ see ankle
  temporal ~ see temporal bone
  X-ray
    age study ~ 77072
    dual energy absorptiometry ~ 77080-77081
    length study ~ 77073
    osseous survey ~ 77074-77077

1361

CPT PLUS! 2013

Bone 4-carboxyglutamic protein ~ 83937
Bone conduction hearing device,
  electromagnetic
  implantation/replacement ~ 69710
  removal/repair ~ 69711
Bone density study
  appendicular skeleton ~ 77081
  axial skeleton ~ 77078, 77080
  ultrasound ~ 76977
  vertebral fracture assessment ~ 77082
Bone graft
  augmentation mandibular body ~ 21127
  femur ~ 27170
  fracture orbit ~ 21408
  harvesting ~ 20900-20902
  malar area ~ 21210
  mandible ~ 21215
  mandibular ramus ~ 21194
  maxilla ~ 21210
  microvascular anastomosis
    fibula ~ 20955
    other ~ 20962
  nasal area ~ 21210
  nasomaxillary complex fracture ~ 21348
  open treatment, craniofacial separation ~
    21436
  osteocutaneous flap ~ 20969-20973
  reconstruction
    mandibular rami ~ 21194
    midface ~ 21145-21160
    skull ~ 61316
      excision ~ 62148
  spine surgery
    allograft
      morselized ~ 20930
      structural ~ 20931
    autograft
      local ~ 20936
      morselized ~ 20937
      structural ~ 20938
    vascular pedicle ~ 25430
Bone healing
  electrical stimulation
    invasive ~ 20975
    noninvasive ~ 20974
  ultrasound stimulation ~ 20979
Bone infection ~ 20005
Bone marrow
  aspiration ~ 38220
  cell therapy ~ 0263T-0265T
  harvesting
    allogenic ~ 38230
    autologous ~ 38232
  magnetic resonance imaging (MRI) ~ 77084
  needle biopsy ~ 38221
  nuclear medicine, imaging ~ 78102-78104
  smear ~ 85097
  T-cell transplantation ~ 38240-38242
  trocar biopsy ~ 38221
Bone plate, mandible ~ 21244
Bone scan ~ see bone, nuclear medicine;
  nuclear medicine

Bone spur ~ 69140
Bone wedge reversal, osteotomy ~ 21122
Bordetella
  antibody ~ 86615
  antigen detection, direct fluorescence ~ 87265
Borrelia, antibody ~ 86618-86619
Borrelia burgdorferi ab ~ 86617
Borreliosis, Lyme ~ 86617-86618
Borthen operation ~ 66165
Bost fusion ~ 25800
Bosworth operation ~ see arthrodesis,
  vertebrae; fasciotomy; 23540-23552
Bottle type procedure ~ 55060
Botulinum toxin ~ see chemodenervation
Boutonniere deformity ~ 26426-26428
Bowel ~ see intestine
Bowleg repair ~ 27455-27457
Boyce operation ~ 50040-50045
Boyd hip disarticulation ~ see radical
  resection; replantation; 27590-27592
Brace ~ see cast for leg cast ~ 29358
Brachial arteries ~ see artery, brachial
Brachial plexus
  decompression ~ 64713
  injection anesthetic ~ 64415-64416
  neuroplasty ~ 64713
  release ~ 64713
  repair/suture ~ 64861
Brachiocephalic artery ~ see artery,
  brachiocephalic
Brachycephaly ~ 21175
Brachytherapy ~ 57156, 77761-77778, 77789
  dose plan ~ 77326-77328
  high dose electronic ~ 0182T
  remote afterloading
    1 channel ~ 77785
    2-12 channels ~ 77786
    more than 1 channel 77786-77787
    more than 12 channels ~ 77787
  unlisted services and procedures ~ 77799
Bradykinin, blood or urine ~ 82286
Brain ~ see also brainstem; skull base surgery;
  61480
  abscess
    drainage ~ 61150-61151
    excision ~ 61514, 61522
    incision and drainage ~ 61320-61321
  adhesions, lysis ~ 62161
  anesthesia ~ 00210-00218, 00220-00222
  angiography ~ 70496
  biopsy ~ 61140
    stereotactic ~ 61750-61751
  catheter
    irrigation ~ 62194, 62225
    replacement ~ 62160, 62194, 62225
  cisternography ~ 70015
  cortex, magnetic stimulation ~ 90867-90868
  craniopharyngioma, excision ~ 61545
  CT scan ~ 0042T, 70450-70470, 70496
  cyst
    drainage ~ 61150-61151, 62161-62162
    excision ~ 61516, 61524, 62162

1362

Brain ~ *continued*
Doppler, transcranial ~ 93886-93893
epileptogenic focus, excision ~ 61534, 61536
excision
  amygdala ~ 61566
  choroid plexus ~ 61544
  hemisphere ~ 61542-61543
  hippocampus ~ 61566
  other lobe ~ 61323, 61539-61540
  temporal lobe ~ 61537-61538
exploration
  infratentorial ~ 61305
  supratentorial ~ 61304
hematoma
  drainage ~ 61154
  incision and drainage ~ 61312-61315
implantation
  chemotherapy agent ~ 61517
  electrode ~ 61850-61875
  pulse generator ~ 61885-61886
  receiver ~ 61885-61886
incision
  corpus callosum ~ 61541
  frontal lobe ~ 61490
  mesencephalic tract ~ 61480
  subpial ~ 61567
insertion, catheter ~ 61210
  electrode ~ 61531-61533, 61850-61875
  pulse generator ~ 61885-61886
  receiver ~ 61885-61886
  reservoir ~ 61210-61215
lesion
  aspiration stereotactic ~ 61750-61751
  excision ~ 61534, 61536, 61600-61608,
    61615-61616
magnetic resonance imaging (MRI) ~
  70551-77055
  intraoperative ~ 70557-70559
meningioma, excision ~ 61512, 61519
myelography ~ 70010
nuclear medicine
  blood flow ~ 78610
  cerebrospinal fluid ~ 78630-78650
  imaging ~ 78600-78607
  vascular flow ~ 78610
positron emission tomography ~ 78608-78609
removal
  electrode ~ 61535, 61880
  foreign body ~ 61570, 62163
  pulse generator ~ 61888
  receiver ~ 61888
  shunt ~ 62256-62258
repair
  dura ~ 61618
  wound ~ 61571
shunt
  creation ~ 62180-62192, 62200-62223
  removal ~ 62256-62258
  replacement ~ 62160, 62194, 62225-62230,
    62256-62258
  reprogramming ~ 62252

Brain ~ *continued*
skull
  transcochlear approach ~ 61596
  transcondylar approach ~ 61597
  transpetrosal approach ~ 61598
  transtemporal approach ~ 61595
skull base
  craniofacial approach ~ 61580-61585
  infratemporal approach ~ 61590-61591
  orbitocranial-zygomatic approach ~ 61592
stereotactic
  aspiration ~ 61750-61751
  biopsy ~ 61750-61751
  catheter placement ~ 0169T
  create lesion ~ 61720-61735, 61790-61791
  localization for placement of therapy fields ~
    61770
  radiation treatment ~ 77432
  radiosurgery ~ 61796-61800, 77371-77373,
    77435
  trigeminal tract ~ 61791
  transection, subpial ~ 61567
tumor, excision ~ 61510, 61518, 61520-61521,
  61526-61530, 61545, 62164
X-ray, with contrast ~ 70010-70015
Brainstem ~ see also brain
auditory evoked potential ~ 92585-92586
biopsy ~ 61575-61576
decompression ~ 61575-61576
evoked potentials ~ 92585-92586
lesion, excision ~ 61575-61576
Brain coverings ~ 61512, 61519
Brain death, determination ~ 95824
Brain surface electrode, stimulation ~
95961-95962
Brain tumor
acoustic neuroma ~ 61510, 61518,
  61520-61521, 61526-61530, 61545, 62164
craniopharyngioma ~ 61545
meningioma ~ 61512, 61519
Brain ventriculography ~ see ventriculography
Branchial cleft cyst excision ~ 42810-42815
Branchioma ~ 42810-42815
BRCA gene alaysis
BRCA1 ~ 81214, 81215
BRCA2 ~ 81216, 81217
BRCA1 and BRCA2 ~ 81211-81213
Breast
ablation
  cryosurgery ~ 19105
abscess
  incision and drainage ~ 19020
augmentation ~ 19324-19325
biopsy ~ 19100-19103
catheter placement, for interstitial radioelement
  application ~ 19296-19298
cyst, puncture aspiration ~ 19000-19001
excision
  biopsy ~ 19100-19103
  capsules ~ 19371
  chest wall tumor ~ 19260-19272

Breast ~ continued
cyst ~ 19120
lactiferous duct fistula ~ 19112
lesion ~ 19120-19126, 19301
by needle localization ~ 19125-19126
mastectomy ~ 19300-19307
nipple exploration ~ 19110
exploration ~ 19020
implants
insertion ~ 19340-19342
preparation of moulage ~ 19396
removal ~ 19328-19330
supply ~ 19396
incision, capsules ~ 19370
injection, radiologic ~ 19030
magnetic resonance imaging (MRI) ~ 77058-77059
mammoplasty
augmentation ~ 19324-19325
reduction ~ 19318
mastopexy ~ 19316
metallic localization clip placement ~ 19295
needle biopsy ~ 19100
needle wire placement ~ 19290-19291
periprosthetic capsulectomy ~ 19371
periprosthetic capsulotomy ~ 19370
reconstruction ~ 19357-19369
augmentation ~ 19324-19325
mammoplasty ~ 19318-19325
nipple ~ 19350-19355
areola ~ 19350
revision ~ 19380
with free flap ~ 19364
with latissimus dorsi flap ~ 19361
with other techniques ~ 19366
with tissue expander ~ 19357
with transverse rectus abdominis
myocutaneous flap ~ 19367-19369
reduction ~ 19318
removal
capsules ~ 19371
modified radical ~ 19307
partial ~ 19300-19302
radical ~ 19305-19306
simple, complete ~ 19303
subcutaneous ~ 19304
repair, suspension ~ 19316
stereotactic localization ~ 77031
ultrasound ~ 76645
unlisted services and procedures ~ 19499
X-ray ~ 77055-77057
localization nodule ~ 77032
with computer-aide detection ~ 77051-77052
Breath odor alcohol ~ 82075
Breath test
alcohol, ethyl ~ 82075
heart transplant rejection detection ~ 0085T
helicobacter pylori ~ 78267-78268, 83013-83014
hydrogen ~ 91065
Bricker procedure, intestines anastomosis ~ 50820

Bristow procedure ~ 23450-23462
Brock operation ~ 33470-33474
Broken, nose ~ see fracture, nasal bone
Bronchi
aspiration, endoscopic ~ 31645-31646
biopsy, endoscopic ~ 31625-31629, 31632-31633
catheterization
with bronchial brush biopsy ~ 31717
endoscopy
aspiration ~ 31645-31646
biopsy ~ 31625-31629, 31632-31633
destruction, tumor ~ 31641
dilation ~ 31630-31631, 31636-31638
excision, lesion ~ 31640
exploration ~ 31622
foreign body removal ~ 31635
fracture ~ 31630
injection ~ 31899
lesion ~ 31640-31641
stenosis ~ 31641
tumor ~ 31640-31641
ultrasound ~ 31620
exploration, endoscopic ~ 31622
fracture, endoscopy ~ 31630
injection, X-ray ~ 31899
needle biopsy ~ 31629, 31633
reconstruction ~ 31770
graft repair ~ 31770
stenosis ~ 31775
removal, foreign body ~ 31635
repair, fistula ~ 32815
stenosis, endoscopic treatment ~ 31641
stent
placement ~ 31636-31637
revision ~ 31638
tumor, excision ~ 31640
ultrasound ~ 31620
unlisted services and procedures ~ 31899
X-ray, with contrast ~ 76499
Bronchial
alveolar lavage ~ 31624
brushings/protected brushing ~ 31623
brush biopsy, with catheterization ~ 31717
challenge test ~ 95070-95071, 95076, 95079
with antigens, gases ~ 95070
with chemicals ~ 95071
lavage ~ 31624
Broncho-bronchial anastomosis ~ 32486
Bronchoalveolar lavage ~ 31624
Bronchography ~ 76499
injection, transtracheal ~ 31899
segmental, injection ~ 31899
Bronchoplasty ~ 32501
excision stenosis and anastomosis ~ 31775
graft repair ~ 31770
Bronchopneumonia, hiberno-vernal ~ 86000, 86638
Bronchopulmonary lavage ~ 31624

Bronchoscopy
alveolar lavage ~ 31624
aspiration ~ 31645-31646
biopsy ~ 31625-31629, 31632-31633
brushing/protected brushing ~ 31623
catheter placement, intracavitary radioelement
~ 31643
dilation ~ 31630-31631, 31636-31638
exploration ~ 31622
fracture ~ 31630
injection ~ 31899
needle biopsy ~ 31629, 31633
removal
foreign body ~ 31635
tumor ~ 31640-31641
stenosis ~ 31641
stent placement ~ 31631, 31636-31637
stent revision ~ 31638
ultrasound ~ 31620
X-ray contrast ~ 31899
Bronchospasm evaluation ~ 94010-94070
Bronkodyl ~ 80198
Brow ptosis, repair ~ 67900
Brucella ~ 86000
antibody ~ 86622
Bruise ~ see hematoma
Brunschwig operation ~ see hip ~ 45126,
58240
Brush biopsy ~ see biopsy; needle biopsy
bronchi ~ 31717
Brush border ab ~ 86308-86310
Bucca ~ see cheek
Buccal mucosa ~ 40818
Bulbourethral gland, excision ~ 53250
Bulla
incision and drainage
puncture aspiration ~ 10160
lung
excision-plication ~ 32141
endoscopic ~ 32655
Bun ~ see urea nitrogen ~ 84520-84525
Bunion repair ~ 28296-28299
Chevron procedure ~ 28296
concentric procedure ~ 28296
Joplin procedure ~ 28294
Keller procedure ~ 28292
Lapidus procedure ~ 28297
Mayo procedure ~ 28292
McBride procedure ~ 28292
Mitchell procedure ~ 28296
Silver procedure ~ 28290
with implant ~ 28293
Burgess amputation ~ 27889
Burhenne procedure ~ see gallbladder ~
43264, 47420-47425
Burkitt herpesvirus ~ 86663-86665
Burns
debridement ~ 01951-01953, 15002-15005,
16020-16030
dressings ~ 16020-16030
escharotomy ~ 16035-16036

Burns ~ *continued*
excision ~ 01951-01953
initial treatment ~ 16000
tissue cultured skin grafts ~ 15150-15157
Burrow's operation ~ 14000-14350
Burr hole
anesthesia ~ 00214
skull
biopsy brain ~ 61140
catheterization ~ 61210
drainage
abscess ~ 61150-61151
cyst ~ 61150-61151
hematoma ~ 61154-61156
exploration
infratentorial ~ 61253
supratentorial ~ 61250
for implant of neurostimulator array ~
61863-61868
injection, contrast media ~ 61120
insertion, catheter ~ 61210
reservoir ~ 61210
Bursa
ankle ~ 27604
arm, lower ~ 25031
elbow
excision ~ 24105
incision and drainage ~ 23931
femur, excision ~ 27062
foot, incision and drainage ~ 28001
hip, incision and drainage ~ 26991
injection ~ 20600-20610
ischial, excision ~ 27060
joint
aspiration ~ 20600-20610
drainage ~ 20600-20610
injection ~ 20600-20610
knee, excision ~ 27340
leg, lower ~ 27604
palm, incision and drainage ~ 26025-26030
pelvis, incision and drainage ~ 26991
shoulder, drainage ~ 23031
wrist ~ 25031
excision ~ 25115-25116
Bursectomy ~ see excision, bursa
Bursitis, radiohumeral ~ 24357-24359
Bursocentesis ~ 20600-20610
Button, nasal septal prosthesis, insertion ~
30220
Butyrylcholine esterase ~ 82480-82482
Bypass, cardiopulmonary ~ 33926
Bypass graft
aortobi-iliac ~ 35538, 35638
aortobifemoral ~ 35540
aortocarotid ~ 35526, 35626
aortofemoral ~ 35539
aortoiliac ~ 35537, 35637
aortosubclavian ~ 35526, 35626
axillary artery ~ 35516-35522, 35533,
35616-35623, 35650, 35654
brachial artery ~ 35510, 35512, 35522-35525

Bypass graft ~ *continued*
  carotid artery ~ 33891, 35501-35510,
    35601-35606, 35642
  celiac artery ~ 35531, 35631
  coronary artery
    arterial ~ 33533-33536
    venous graft ~ 33510-33516
  excision
    abdomen ~ 35907
    extremity ~ 35903
    neck ~ 35901
    thorax ~ 35905
  femoral artery ~ 35521, 35533, 35556-35558,
    35566, 35621, 35646-35647, 35654-35661,
    35666, 35700
  harvest
    endoscopic ~ 33508
    upper extremity vein ~ 35500
  hepatorenal venous graft ~ 35535
  iliac artery ~ 35563
  ilio-celiac artery ~ 35632
  iliofemoral artery ~ 35565, 35665
  ilio-mesenteric artery ~ 35633
  iliorenal artery ~ 35634
  mesenteric artery ~ 35531, 35631
  peroneal artery ~ 35566-35571, 35666-35671
  peroneal-tibial venous graft ~ 35570
  placement, vein patch ~ 35685
  popliteal artery ~ 35556-35558, 35571, 35623,
    35656, 35671, 35700
  renal artery ~ 35536, 35560, 35631-35636
  reoperation ~ 35700
  repair
    abdomen ~ 35907
    extremity ~ 35903
    lower extremity, with composite graft ~
      35681-35683
    neck ~ 35901
    thorax ~ 35905
  revascularization
    extremity ~ 35903
    neck ~ 35901
    thorax ~ 35905
  revision
    lower extremity
      femoral artery ~ 35883-35884
      with angioplasty ~ 35879
      with vein interposition ~ 35881
  secondary repair ~ 35870
  splenic artery ~ 35536, 35636
  subclavian artery ~ 35506, 35511-35516,
    35606-35616, 35645
  thrombectomy ~ 37184-37186
    other than hemodialysis graft or fistula ~
      35875-35876
  tibial artery ~ 35566-35571, 35623,
    35666-35671
  tibial-tibial venous graft ~ 35570
  vertebral artery ~ 35508, 35515, 35642-35645
  with composite graft ~ 35681

Bypass in-situ
  femoral artery ~ 35583-35585
  peroneal artery ~ 35585-35587
  popliteal artery ~ 35583, 35587
  tibial artery ~ 35585-35587
  ventricular restoration ~ 33548

C

C vitamin ~ 82180
C-13
  urea breath test ~ 83013-83014
  urease activity ~ 83013-83014
C-14
  urea breath test ~ 78267-78268
  urease activity ~ 83013-83014
C-peptide ~ 80432, 84681
C-reactive protein ~ 86140-86141
C-section ~ see cesarean delivery
CABG ~ see coronary artery bypass graft
    (CABG) ~ 33503-33505, 33510-33516
Cadmium, urine ~ 82300
Calcaneal spur ~ 28119
Calcaneus
  craterization ~ 28120
  cyst, excision ~ 28100-28103
  diaphysectomy ~ 28120
  excision ~ 28118-28120
  fracture
    open treatment ~ 28415-28420
    percutaneous fixation ~ 28406
    without manipulation ~ 28400
    with manipulation ~ 28405-28406
  repair, osteotomy ~ 28300
  saucerization ~ 28120
  tumor, excision ~ 27647, 28100-28103
  X-ray ~ 73650
Calcareous deposits, subdeltoid, removal ~
    23000
Calcifediol, blood or urine ~ 82306
Calciferol, blood or urine ~ 82306
Calcification ~ see calcium, deposits
Calciol ~ 82306
Calcitonin
  blood or urine ~ 82308
  stimulation panel ~ 80410
Calcium, blood, infusion test ~ 82331
  deposits ~ see removal, calculi (stone) ~
    65205-65265
  ionized ~ 82330
  total ~ 82310
  urine ~ 82340
**Calcium-binding protein, vitamin
    K-dependent ~** 83937
Calcium-pentagastrin stimulation ~ 80410

Calculus
analysis ~ 82355-82370
destruction
bile duct ~ 43265
pancreatic duct ~ 43265
removal
bile duct ~ 43264, 47554, 74327
bladder ~ 51050, 52310-52318, 52352
kidney ~ 50060-50081, 50130, 50561,
50580, 52352
pancreatic duct ~ 43264
ureter ~ 50610-50630, 50961, 50980,
51060-51065, 52320-52325, 52352
urethra ~ 52310-52315, 52352
Calculus of kidney ~ 50060-50081, 50130,
50561, 50580, 52352
Caldwell-Luc procedure ~ 21385
sinusotomy ~ 31030-31032
Caliper, application/removal ~ 20660
Callander knee disarticulation ~ 27598
Callosum, corpus ~ 61541
Calmette Guerin Bacillus vaccine ~ see BCG
vaccine
Caloric vestibular test ~ 92533
Calprotectin, fecal ~ 83993
Calycoplasty ~ 50405
Camey enterocystoplasty ~ 50825
CAMP ~ 82030
Campbell procedure ~ 27422
Campylobacter, antibody ~ 86625
Campylobacter pylori ~ see helicobacter pylori
Canal, ear ~ see auditory canal
Canal, semicircular ~ 69820, 69840
Canalith repositioning ~ 95992
Canaloplasty ~ 69631, 69635
Candida
antibody ~ 86628
skin test ~ 86485
Cannulation ~ 36821
arterial ~ 36620-36625
sinus
maxillary ~ 31000
sphenoid ~ 31002
thoracic duct ~ 38794
Cannulation, renoportal ~ 37145
Cannulization ~ see catheterization
arteriovenous ~ 36147-36148, 36810-36815
declotting ~ 36593, 36860-36861
ecmo ~ 36822
external, declotting ~ 36860-36861
vas deferens ~ 55200
vein to vein ~ 36800
Canthocystostomy ~ 68745, 68750
Canthopexy
lateral ~ 21282
medial ~ 21280
Canthoplasty ~ 67950
Canthorrhaphy ~ 67880-67882
Canthotomy ~ 67715
Canthus, reconstruction ~ 67950
Cap, cervical ~ 57170

Capsule ~ 26516-26518
elbow
arthrotomy ~ 24006
excision ~ 24006
foot ~ 28264
interphalangeal joint
excision ~ 26525
incision ~ 26525
knee ~ 27435
metacarpophalangeal joint
excision ~ 26520
incision ~ 26520
metatarsophalangeal joint, release ~ 28289
shoulder, incision ~ 23020
wrist, excision ~ 25320
Capsulectomy, breast, periprosthetic ~ 19371
Capsulodesis, metacarpophalangeal joint ~
26516-26518
Capsulorrhaphy
anterior ~ 23450-23462
multi-directional instability ~ 23466
posterior ~ 23465
wrist ~ 25320
Capsulotomy, breast, periprosthetic ~ 19370
foot ~ 28260-28262
hip, with release, flexor muscles ~ 27036
interphalangeal joint ~ 28272
knee ~ 27435
metacarpophalangeal joint ~ 26520
metatarsophalangeal joint ~ 28270
toe ~ 28270-28272
wrist ~ 25085
Captopril ~ 80416-80417
Car seat testing ~ 94780, 94781
Carbamazepine, assay ~ 80156-80157
Carbazepin ~ 80156-80157
Carbinol ~ 84600
Carbohydrate deficient transferrin ~ 82373
Carbon dioxide, blood or urine ~ 82374
Carbon monoxide, blood ~ 82375-82376
Carbon tetrachloride ~ 84600
Carboxycathepsin ~ 82164
Carboxyhemoglobin ~ 82375-82376, 88740
Carbuncle, incision and drainage ~
10060-10061
Carcinoembryonal antigen ~ 82378
Carcinoembryonic antigen ~ 82378
Cardiac ~ see coronary
Cardiac anomoly, reconstruction ~ 33622
Cardiac arrhythmia, tachycardia ~ 93609
Cardiac atria ~ see atria
Cardiac catheterization
combined left and right heart ~ 93460-93461
with left ventriculography ~ 93453,
93460-93461
combined right and retrograde left congenital
cardiac anomalies ~ 93531
combined right and transseptal left congenital
cardiac anomalies ~ 93532-93533
congenital cardiac anomalies ~ 0262T,
93530-93533

Cardiac catheterization ~ continued
for angiography
bypass graft(s) ~ 93455, 93457, 93459,
93461
congenital heart ~ 93563, 93564
coronary ~ 93454-93461, 93563, 93571
left atrial ~ 93565
left ventricular ~ 93565
pulmonary ~ 93568
right atrial ~ 93566
right ventricular ~ 93566
for biopsy ~ 93505
for congenital prosthetic valve implantation ~
0262T
for dilution studies ~ 93561-93562
for flow measurement ~ 93571-93572
imaging ~ 93452-93461, 93563-93568
injection ~ 93454-93461, 93563-93568
left heart ~ 93452, 93458-93459, 93462,
93565
pacemaker ~ 33210
right, congenital cardiac anomalies ~ 93530
right heart ~ 93451, 93456, 93503
Cardiac electroversion ~ 92960-92961
Cardiac event recorder
implantation ~ 33282
removal ~ 33284
Cardiac magnetic resonance imaging (CMRI)
~ 75557-75563, 75565
Cardiac massage, thoracotomy ~ 32160
Cardiac muscle ~ see myocardium
Cardiac neoplasm ~ 33120-33130
Cardiac output, indicator dilution ~
93561-93562
Cardiac pacemaker ~ see heart, pacemaker
Cardiac rehabilitation ~ 93797-93798
Cardiac septal defect ~ 33813-33814
Cardiac transplantation ~ 33935, 33945
Cardiectomy, donor ~ 33930, 33940
Cardioassist ~ 92970-92971
Cardiolipin antibody ~ 86147
Cardiology
diagnostic
acoustic cardiography ~ 0223T-0225T
arrhythmia induction ~ 93618-93624, 93640,
93641, 93653-93656
atrial electrogram ~ 93615-93616
esophageal recording ~ 93615-93616
bioimpedence derived analysis ~ 93701
echocardiography
Doppler ~ 76827-76828, 93306-93308,
93320-93350
intracardiac ~ 93662
transesophageal ~ 93318
transthoracic ~ 93303-93317
congenital cardiac anomoly
fetal ~ 76825-76826
doppler, fetal ~ 76827-76828
transesophageal ~ 93315-93317
transthoracic ~ 93303-93304

Cardiology ~ continued
ergonovine provocation test ~ 93024
intracardiac pacing and mapping
3-D mapping ~ 93613, 93654
follow-up study ~ 93624
localization ~ 93631
stimulation and pacing ~ 93623
intracardiac pacing and recording
arrhythmia induction ~ 93618-93624,
93653-93654, 93656
bundle of His ~ 93600, 93619-93620,
93653-93654, 93656
comprehensive ~ 93619-93622
intra-atrial ~ 93602, 93610, 93616, 93656
left ventricular ~ 93654
right ventricle ~ 93603, 93653, 93656
tachycardia sites ~ 93609
ventricular ~ 93612
intravascular ultrasound ~ 92978-92979
perfusion imaging ~ see nuclear medicine ~
78460-78461
stress tests
cardiovascular ~ 93015-93018
drug induced ~ 93024
multiple gated acquisition (MUGA) ~
78473
temperature gradient studies ~ 93740
tilt table evaluation ~ 93660
venous pressure determination ~ 93784,
93786, 93788, 93790
therapeutic
ablation ~ 93650, 93653-93656
cardioassist ~ 92970-92971
cardioversion ~ 92960-92961
intravascular ultrasound ~ 92978-92979
pacing, transcutaneous, temporary ~ 92953
rehabilitation ~ 93668, 93797-93798
thrombolysis ~ 92975-92977
thrombolysis, coronary ~ 92977
valvuloplasty, percutaneous ~ 92986-92990
Cardiomyotomy ~ 32665, 43330-43331
Cardioplasty ~ 43320
Cardiopulmonary bypass ~ 32852, 32854,
32851-32854, 33935
Cardiopulmonary resuscitation ~ 92950
Cardiotomy ~ 33310-33315
Cardiovascular stress test ~ 93015-93018
Cardiovascular system
medical services ~ 92950-93799
surgical procedures ~ 33000-39599
Cardioversion ~ 92960-92961
Cardioverter-Defibrillator
implantable system
data analysis ~ 93289, 93295-93296
electrode
insertion ~ 33216-33217, 33224-33225
removal ~ 33243-33244
repair ~ 33218-33220
repositioning ~ 33215
peri-procedural device evaluation ~ 93287

Cardioverter-Defibrillator ~ *continued*
programming device evaluation ~
93282-93284
revise chest pocket ~ 33223
pulse generator
insertion ~ 33230-33231, 33240
removal ~ 33241
repacement ~ 33262-33264
replacement ~ 33249
repositioning, electrodes ~ 33215, 33226
wearable device ~ 93745
data analysis ~ 93292
Care, custodial ~ see nursing facility services
Care, neonatal intensive ~ see intensive care,
neonatal
Care, self ~ see self care
Care plan oversight services ~ 99339-99340,
99374-99380
Carneous mole ~ see abortion
Carnitine ~ 82379
Carotene ~ 82380
Caroticum, glomus ~ 60605, 60600
Carotid artery
aneurysm repair
vascular malformation or carotid-cavernous
fistula ~ 61710
excision ~ 60605
ligation ~ 37600-37606
stenosis imaging ~ 3100F
stent, transcatheter placement ~ 0075T-0076T
transection, with skull base surgery ~ 61609
Carotid body
lesion
carotid artery ~ 60605
excision ~ 60600
Carpals, incision and drainage ~ 25035
Carpal bone ~ see wrist
arthroplasty, with implant ~ 25443
cyst, excision ~ 25130-25136
dislocation
closed treatment ~ 25690
open treatment ~ 25695
excision ~ 25210-25215
partial ~ 25145
fracture
closed treatment ~ 25622, 25630
open treatment ~ 25628, 25645
without manipulation ~ 25630
with manipulation ~ 25624, 25635
incision and drainage ~ 26034
insertion, vascular pedicle ~ 25430
osteoplasty ~ 25394
repair ~ 25431-25440
sequestrectomy ~ 25145
tumor, excision ~ 25130-25136
Carpal tunnel, injection, therapeutic ~ 20526
Carpal tunnel syndrome, decompression ~
64721
Carpectomy ~ 25210-25215

Carpometacarpal joint
arthrodesis
hand ~ 26843-26844
thumb ~ 26841-26842
arthrotomy ~ 26070
biopsy, synovium ~ 26100
dislocation
closed treatment ~ 26670
with manipulation ~ 26675-26676
open treatment ~ 26685-26686
exploration ~ 26070
fusion
hand ~ 26843-26844
thumb ~ 26841-26842
removal, foreign body ~ 26070
repair ~ 25447
synovectomy ~ 26130
Cartilage, arytenoid ~ 31560-31561
Cartilage, ear ~ 21235
Cartilage graft
ear to face ~ 21235
harvesting ~ 20910-20912
rib to face ~ 21230
Cartilaginous exostoses ~ 69140
Case management services
anticoagulant management ~ 99363-99364
team conferences ~ 99366-99368
telephone calls ~ 98966-98968
Cast ~ see also splint ~ 29358
body, Risser jacket ~ 29010-29015
body cast
halo ~ 29000
turnbuckle jacket ~ 29020-29025
upper body and head ~ 29040
upper body and legs ~ 29046
upper body and one leg ~ 29044
upper body only ~ 29035
clubfoot ~ 29450
cylinder ~ 29365
finger ~ 29086
hand ~ 29085
hip ~ 29305-29325
leg, rigid total contact ~ 29445
long arm ~ 29065
long leg ~ 29345-29355, 29365, 29450
long leg brace ~ 29358
patellar tendon bearing (PTB) ~ 29435
removal ~ 29700-29715
repair ~ 29720
short arm ~ 29075
short leg ~ 29405-29435, 29450
shoulder ~ 29049-29058
walking ~ 29355, 29425
revision ~ 29440
wedging ~ 29740-29750
windowing ~ 29730
wrist ~ 29085
Casting, unlisted services and procedures ~
29799
Castration ~ see orchiectomy

Castration, female ~ 58262-58263, 58291-58292, 58552, 58554, 58661, 58940-58943
Cat scan ~ see CT scan
Cataract
  excision ~ 66830
  dilated fundus evaluation ~ 2021F
  incision ~ 66820-66821
  laser ~ 66821
  stab incision ~ 66820
  removal/extraction
  extracapsular ~ 66982, 66984
  intracapsular ~ 66983
  presurgical measurement/calculation ~ 3073F
Catecholamines ~ 80424, 82382-82384
  blood ~ 82383
  urine ~ 82382
Cathepsin-D ~ 82387
Catheter ~ see also cannulization; venipuncture
  aspiration
  nasotracheal ~ 31720
  tracheobronchial ~ 31725
  bladder ~ 51701-51703
  irrigation ~ 51700
  declotting ~ 36593
  exchange
  arterial ~ 37211-37214
  peritoneal ~ 49423
  intracatheter, irrigation ~ 99507
  obstruction clearance ~ 36596
  intraperitoneal ~ 49418-49419
  pericatheter obstruction
  clearance ~ 36595
  placement
  breast
  for intracavitary radioelement application ~ 19296-19298
  bronchus
  for intracavitary radioelement application ~ 31643
  stent ~ 33621
  removal
  central venous ~ 36589
  peritoneum ~ 49422
  spinal cord ~ 62355
  repair, central venous ~ 36575
  replacement, central venous ~ 36580-36581, 36584
  repositioning ~ 36597
  tunneled intraperitoneal ~ 49418-49419
  transthoracic insertion for stent placement ~ 33621
Catheterization ~ see also catheter
  abdomen ~ 49421
  abdominal artery ~ 36245-36248
  aorta ~ 36160, 36200
  arterial system ~ 36215, 36245-36248
  cutdown ~ 36625
  intracatheter/needle ~ 36100-36140
  percutaneous ~ 36620
  arteriovenous shunt ~ 36147-36148

Catheterization ~ *continued*
  bile duct ~ 47530
  change ~ 47525
  percutaneous ~ 47510
  bladder ~ 51102, 51045, 51702-51703
  brachiocephalic artery ~ 36215-36218
  brain ~ 61210
  replacement ~ 62160, 62194, 62225
  stereotactic ~ 0169T
  breast ~ 19296-19298, 20555, 41019
  bronchus ~ 31643, 31710
  cardiac ~ see cardiac catheteriztaion
  carotid artery ~ 36100, 36221-36224, 36227-36228
  cerebral artery ~ 36215
  cholecystostomy ~ 47490
  coronary artery ~ 93455
  cystourethroscopy, ejaculatory duct ~ 52010
  ureteral ~ 52005
  dialysis ~ 49418-49419, 49421
  ear, middle ~ 69405
  electrode array ~ 63650
  eustachian tube ~ 69400, 69405
  extremity, artery ~ 36140
  fallopian tube ~ 58345, 74742
  gastrointestinal ~ 43241
  hepatic vein ~ 37182-37183
  innominate artery ~ 36222-36223, 36225
  intracardiac, ablation ~ 93650, 93653-93657
  intraperitoneal, tunneled ~ 49324, 49421
  jejunum, for enteral ~ 44015
  kidney
  drainage ~ 50392
  with ureter ~ 50393
  legs ~ 36245-36248
  nasotracheal ~ 31720
  newborn, umbilical vein ~ 36510
  pelvic artery ~ 36245-36248
  peripheral ~ 36568-36571
  pleural cavity ~ 32550-32552
  portal vein ~ 36481, 37182-37183
  pulmonary artery ~ 36013-36015
  radioelement application ~ 519296-19297, 20555, 31643, 41019, 55875, 55920
  removal
  fractured catheter ~ 37197
  obstructive material
  intracatheter ~ 36596
  pericatheter ~ 36595
  renal artery ~ 36251-36254
  rental pelvis ~ 50392-50393
  retrograde brachial artery ~ 36120
  salivary duct ~ 42660
  skull ~ 61107
  spinal cord ~ 62350-62351
  subclavian artery ~ 36225
  thoracic artery ~ 36215-36218
  tracheobronchi ~ 31725
  umbilical artery ~ 36660
  umbilical vein ~ 36510

ALPHABETICAL INDEX

Catheterization ~ *continued*
ureter
  endoscopic ~ 50553, 50572, 50953, 50972,
    52005
  injection ~ 50394, 50684
  manometric studies ~ 50396, 50686
uterus, radiology ~ 58340
vena cava ~ 36010
venous
  central line ~ see Central venous catheter
  first order ~ 36011
  intracatheter/needle ~ 36000
  organ blood ~ 36500
  second order ~ 36012
  umbilical vein ~ 36510
  vertebral artery ~ 36100, 36221, 36225-36226,
    36228
  ventricular ~ 61020-61026, 61210-61215,
    62160-62162, 62164, 62225
Cauda equina ~ see spinal cord
decompression ~ 63005-63011, 63017,
  63047-63048, 63055-63057, 63087-63091
exploration ~ 63005-63011, 63017
Cauterization
anal fissure ~ 46940-46942
cervix ~ 57522
  cryocautery ~ 57511
  electro or thermal ~ 57510
  laser ablation ~ 57513
chemical, granulation tissue ~ 17250
everted punctum ~ 68705
lower esophageal sphincter, thermal, via
  endoscopy ~ 0057T
nasopharyngeal hemorrhage ~ 42970
nose, hemorrhage ~ 30901-30906
skin lesion ~ 11055-11057, 17000-17004
skin tags ~ 11200-11201
turbinate mucosa ~ 30801-30802
Cavernitides, fibrous ~ see Peyronie disease
Cavernosography, corpora ~ 54230
Cavernosometry ~ 54231
Cavities, pleural ~ see pleural cavity
Cavus foot correction ~ 28309
CBC ~ see blood cell count ~ 85025-85027
CCL4 ~ 84600
CCU visit ~ see Critical Care Services
CD142 antigens ~ see thromboplastin
CD143 antigens ~ 82164
CD4 ~ 86360
CD8 ~ 86360
CEA ~ 82378
Cecil repair ~ 46744-46746
Cecostomy ~ 44300
contrast ~ 49465
insertion of tube ~ 49442
laparoscopic ~ 44188
obstructive material removal ~ 49460
radiological evaluation of tube ~ 49465
tube replacement ~ 49450

Celiac plexus
destruction ~ 64680
injection
  anesthetic ~ 64530
  neurolytic ~ 64680
Celiac trunk artery ~ see artery, celiac
Celioscopy ~ see endoscopy, peritoneum
Celiotomy ~ 49000
abdomen, for staging ~ 49220
Cell count, body fluid ~ 89050-89051
Cell, blood ~ see blood cell
Cell, islet ~ 86341
Cell, mother ~ see stem cell
Cell-stimulating hormone, interstitial ~ 80418,
  80426, 83002
Cellobiase ~ 82963
Cellular function assay ~ 86352
Cellular inclusion ~ see inclusion bodies
Central shunt ~ 33764
Central nervous system assessments or tests ~
  96101-96120
Central venous catheter placement
insertion
  central ~ 36555-36558
  peripheral ~ 36568-36569
repair ~ 36575
replacement ~ 36580-36585
repositioning ~ 36597
Central venous catheter removal ~ 36589
Cephalic version, of fetus, external ~ 59412
Cephalocele ~ 62120-62121
Cephalogram, orthodontic ~ 70350
Cerclage, cervix ~ 57700
abdominal ~ 59325
removal under anesthesia ~ 59871
vaginal ~ 59320
Cerebellopontine angle tumor ~ see brainstem;
  skull base surgery ~ 61480, 61510, 61518,
  61520-61521, 61526-61530, 61545, 62164
Cerebral cortex decortication ~ see
  decortication
Cerebral death ~ 95824
Cerebral hernia ~ 62120-62121
Cerebral perfusion analysis ~ 0042T
Cerebral ventriculographies ~ see
  ventriculography
Cerebral vessels, occlusion ~ 61623
Cerebrose ~ 82760
Cerebrospinal fluid ~ 86325
nuclear imaging ~ 78630-78650
Cerebrospinal fluid leak ~ 63744
brain, repair ~ 61618-61619, 62100
nasal/sinus endoscopy, repair ~ 31290-31291
spinal cord, repair ~ 63707-63709
Cerebrospinal fluid shunt ~ 63740, 63746
creation ~ 62180-62192, 62200-62223
irrigation ~ 62194
removal ~ 62256-62258
replacement ~ 62160, 62194, 62225-62230
reprogramming ~ 62252
Ceruloplasmin ~ 82390
Cerumen, removal ~ 69210

1371

Cervical cap ~ 57170
Cervical lymphadenectomy ~ 38720-38724
Cervical mucus penetration test ~ 89330
Cervical plexus, injection, anesthetic ~ 64413
Cervical pregnancy ~ 59140
Cervical puncture ~ 61050-61055
Cervical smears ~ 88141, 88155, 88164-88167, 88174-88175
Cervical spine ~ see vertebra, cervical
Cervical sympathectomy ~ 64802
Cervicectomy ~ 57530
Cervicography ~ 0003T
Cervicoplasty ~ 15819
Cervicothoracic ganglia ~ 64510
Cervix ~ see cytopathology
  amputation, total ~ 57530
  biopsy ~ 57500, 57520
    colposcopy ~ 57454-57455, 57460
  cauterization ~ 57522
    cryocautery ~ 57511
    electro or thermal ~ 57510
    laser ablation ~ 57513
  cerclage ~ 57700
    abdominal ~ 59325
    removal under anesthesia ~ 59871
    vaginal ~ 59320
  cervicography ~ 0003T
  colposcopy ~ 57452-57461
  conization ~ 57461, 57520-57522
  curettage, endocervical ~ 57454, 57456, 57505
  dilation
    canal ~ 57800
    stump ~ 57558
  dilation and curettage ~ 57558
  ectopic pregnancy ~ 59140
  excision
    radical ~ 57531
    stump
      abdominal approach ~ 57540-57545
      vaginal approach ~ 57550-57556
    total ~ 57530
  exploration, endoscopy ~ 57452
  insertion
    dilation ~ 59200
    laminaria ~ 59200
    prostaglandin ~ 59200
    sensor, fetal oximetry ~ 0021T
  repair, cerclage ~ 57700
    abdominal ~ 59325
    suture ~ 57720
    vaginal ~ 59320
  unlisted services and procedures ~ 58999
Cesarean delivery
  antepartum care ~ 59610, 59618
  delivery
    after attempted vaginal delivery ~ 59618
      delivery only ~ 59620
      postpartum care ~ 59622
      routine care ~ 59610, 59618
    delivery only ~ 59514
    postpartum care ~ 59515

Cesarean delivery ~ continued
  routine care ~ 59510
  tubal ligation at time of ~ 58611
  with hysterectomy ~ 59525
CGMP ~ 83008
Chalazion, excision ~ 67805
  multiple
    different lids ~ 67805
    same lid ~ 67801
  single ~ 67800
  under anesthesia ~ 67808
Challenge tests, bronchial/ingestion ~ 95070-95071, 95076-95079
Chambers procedure ~ 28300
Change
  catheter
    bile duct ~ 75984
  fetal position
    by manipulation ~ 59412
  tube or stent
    endoscopic
      bile or pancreatic duct ~ 43269
Change, gastrostomy tube ~ 43760
Change of, dressing ~ 15852
Cheek
  bone
    excision ~ 21030, 21034
    fracture
      closed treatment with manipulation ~ 21355
      open treatment ~ 21360-21366
    reconstruction ~ 21270
  fascia graft ~ 15840
  muscle graft ~ 15841-15845
  muscle transfer ~ 15845
Cheilectomy, metatarsophalangeal joint release ~ 28289
Cheiloplasty ~ 40650-40654
Cheiloschisis ~ 30460-30462, 40700-40761
Cheilotomy ~ 40806
Chemical cauterization, granulation tissue ~ 17250
Chemical exfoliation ~ 17360
Chemical peel ~ 15788-15793
Chemiluminescent assay ~ 82397
Chemistry tests ~ 82000-84999
Chemocauterization
  corneal epithelium ~ 65435
  with chelating agent ~ 65436
Chemodenervation
  anal sphincter ~ 46505
  bladder ~ 52287
  eccrine glands
    axillae ~ 64650
    other area ~ 64653
  extraocular muscle ~ 67345
  extremity muscle ~ 64614
  facial muscle ~ 64612, 64615
  guidance
    electrical stimulation ~ 95873
    needle electromyography ~ 95874

Chemodenervation ~ *continued*
    neck muscle ~ 64613, 64615
    salivary gland ~ 64611
    trunk muscle ~ 64614
Chemonucleolysis ~ 62292
Chemosurgery
    destruction of benign lesion ~ 17110-17111
    skin lesion ~ 17000-17004, 17110-17111,
        17270, 17280
Chemotaxis assay ~ 86155
Chemotherapy
    administration ~ 96401-96549
    arterial catheterization ~ 36640
    bladder instillation ~ 51720
    brain ~ 61517
    CNS ~ 61517, 96450
    extracorporeal circulation, extremity ~ 36823
    home infusion procedures ~ 99601-99602
    intra-arterial ~ 96420-96425
    intralesional ~ 96405-96406
    intramuscular ~ 96401-96402
    intravenous ~ 96409-96417
    kidney instillation ~ 50391
    peritoneal cavity ~ 96446
        catheterization ~ 49418
    pleural cavity ~ 96440
    pump services
        implantable ~ 96530
        maintenance ~ 95990-95991
        portable ~ 96520
    reservoir filling ~ 96542
    subcutaneous ~ 96400
    supply of agent ~ 96545
    unlisted services and procedures ~ 96549
    ureteral instillation ~ 50391
    venous cannulation ~ 36823
Chest ~ see mediastinum; thorax
    angiography ~ 71275
    artery, ligation ~ 37616
    CT scan ~ 71250-71275
    exploration, blood vessel ~ 35820
    magnetic resonance imaging (MRI) ~
        71550-71552
    repair, blood vessel ~ 35211-35216
        with other graft ~ 35271-35276
        with vein graft ~ 35241-35246
    ultrasound ~ 76604
    wound exploration, penetrating ~ 20101
    X-ray ~ 71010-71035
        complete (four views), with fluoroscopy ~
            71034
        partial (two views), with fluoroscopy ~
            71023
        stereo ~ 71015
        with computer-aided detection ~ 0174T-0175T
Chest, funnel ~ 21740, 21742-21743
Chest cavity, bypass graft ~ 35905
    endoscopy
        exploration ~ 32601-32606
        surgical ~ 32650-32665

Chest wall ~ 94667-94668
    manipulation ~ 94667-94668
    reconstruction ~ 49904
        trauma ~ 32820
    repair ~ 32905
        closure ~ 32810
        fistula ~ 32906
    tumor, excision ~ 19260-19272
    unlisted services and procedures ~ 32999
Chest wall fistula ~ 32906
Chevron procedure ~ 28296
Chiari osteotomy of the pelvis ~ 27158
Chicken pox vaccine ~ 90716
Child procedure ~ 48140-48146, 48150,
    48153-48154, 48160
Chin
    repair
        augmentation ~ 21120
        osteotomy ~ 21121-21123
Chinidin ~ 80194
Chiropractic manipulation (CMT) ~
    98940-98943
Chiropractic treatment
    spinal
        extraspinal ~ 98940-98943
Chlamydia
    antibody ~ 86631-86632
    antigen detection
        amplified nucleic acid probe ~ 87486, 87491
        direct nucleic acid probe ~ 87485, 87490
        direct optical ~ 87810
        enzyme immunoassay ~ 87320
        immunofluorescence ~ 87270
        nucleic acid quantification ~ 87487, 87492
    culture ~ 87110
Chloramphenicol ~ 82415
Chloride
    blood ~ 82435
    other source ~ 82438
    spinal fluid ~ 82438
    urine ~ 82436
Chloride, methylene ~ 84600
Chlorinated hydrocarbons ~ 82441
Chlorohydrocarbon ~ 82441
Chlorpromazine ~ 84022
Choanal atresia, repair ~ 30540-30545
Cholangiography
    injection ~ 47500-47505
    intraoperative ~ 74300-74301
    percutaneous ~ 74320
        with laparoscopy ~ 47560-47561
    postoperative ~ 74305
    repair
        with bile duct exploration ~ 47700
        with cholecystectomy ~ 47563, 47605,
            47620
Cholangiopancreatography ~ see bile duct;
    pancreatic duct ~ 43260
    repair ~ see bile duct; pancreatic duct
        with biopsy ~ 43261
        with surgery ~ 43262-43267, 43269
Cholangiostomy ~ 47400

1373

Cholangiotomy ~ 47400
Cholecalciferol ~ 82306
Cholecystectomy ~ 47562-47564, 47600-47620
  any method ~ 47562-47564
  with cholangiography ~ 47563, 47605,
    47620
  with exploration common duct ~ 47564,
    47610
Cholecystenterostomy ~ 47570, 47720-47741
Cholecystography ~ 74290-74291
Cholecystotomy ~ 47480, 48001
  percutaneous ~ 47490
Choledochoplasty ~ 47701
Choledochoscopy ~ 47550
Choledochostomy ~ 47420-47425
Choledochotomy ~ 47420-47425
Choledochus, cyst ~ see cyst, choledochal
Cholera vaccine, injectable ~ 90725
Cholesterol
  measurement ~ 83721
  serum ~ 82465
  testing ~ 83718-83719
Cholinesterase, blood ~ 82480-82482
Choline esterase I ~ 82013
Choline esterase II ~ 82480-82482
Cholylglycine, blood ~ 82240
Chondroitin sulfate ~ 82485
Chondromalacia patella, repair ~ 27418
Chondropathia patellae ~ 27418
Chondrosteoma ~ 69140
Chopart procedure ~ see radical resection;
  replantation ~ 28800-28805
Chordotomies ~ 63194-63199
Chorioangioma ~ see lesion, skin
Choriogonadotropin ~ 80414-80415,
  84702-84703
Choriomeningitides, lymphocytic ~ 86727
Chorionic gonadotropin ~ 80414, 84702-84704
  stimulation ~ 80414-80415
Chorionic growth hormone ~ 83632
Chorionic tumor ~ 59100, 59870
Chorionic villi ~ 59015
Chorionic villus, biopsy ~ 59015
Choroid, destruction, lesion ~ 67220-67225
Choroid plexus, excision ~ 61544
Christmas factor ~ 85250
Chromaffinoma, medullary ~ 80424
Chromatin, sex ~ 88130
Chromatography
  column/mass spectrometry ~ 82541-82544
  gas-liquid or HPLC ~ 82486, 82491-82492
  paper ~ 82487-82488
  thin-layer ~ 82489
Chromium ~ 82495
Chromogenic substrate assay ~ 85130
Chromosome analysis
  added study ~ 88280-88289
  amniotic fluid ~ 88267, 88269
    culture ~ 88235
  biopsy culture, tissue ~ 88233
  bone marrow culture ~ 88237

Chromosome analysis ~ *continued*
  chorionic villus ~ 88267
    5 cells ~ 88261
    15-20 cells ~ 88262
    20-25 cells ~ 88264
    45 cells ~ 88263
    culture ~ 88235
  for breakage syndromes ~ 88245-88249
  fragile-X ~ 88248
  lymphocyte culture ~ 88230
  pregnancy associated plasma protein-A ~
    84163
  skin culture, tissue ~ 88233
  tissue culture ~ 88239
  unlisted services and procedures ~ 88299
Chromotubation ~ 58350
  oviduct ~ 58350
Chronic erection ~ see priapism
Chronic interstitial cystitides ~ 52260-52265
Ciliary body
  cyst
    destruction
      cryotherapy ~ 66720
      cyclodialysis ~ 66740
      cyclophotocoagulation ~ 66710, 66711
      diathermy ~ 66700
      nonexcisional ~ 66770
    destruction ~ 66770
      cyclophotocoagulation ~ 66710, 66711
      endoscopic ~ 66711
    lesion, destruction ~ 66770
    repair ~ 66680
Cimino type procedure ~ 36821
Cinefluorographies ~ see cineradiography
Cineplasty, arm, lower or upper ~ 24940
Cineradiography
  esophagus ~ 74230
  pharynx ~ 70371, 74230
  speech evaluation ~ 70371
  swallowing evaluation ~ 74230
  unlisted services and procedures ~
    76120-76125
Circulation, extracorporeal ~ 33960-33961
Circulation assist
  aortic ~ 33967, 33970
  balloon ~ 33967, 33970
  external ~ 33960-33961
Circulatory assist ~ see circulation assist
Circumcision
  repair ~ 54163
  surgical excision ~ 54161
    newborn ~ 54160
  with clamp or other device ~ 54150
    newborn ~ 54150
Cisternal puncture ~ 61050-61055
Cisternography ~ 70015
  nuclear ~ 78630
Citrate, blood or urine ~ 82507
Clagett procedure ~ 32810

Clavicle
craterization ~ 23180
cyst
  excision ~ 23140
  with allograft ~ 23146
  with autograft ~ 23145
diaphysectomy ~ 23180
dislocation
  acromioclavicular joint
    closed treatment ~ 23540-23545
    open treatment ~ 23550-23552
  sternoclavicular joint
    closed treatment ~ 23520-23525
    open treatment ~ 23530-23532
    without manipulation ~ 23540
excision ~ 23170
  partial ~ 23120, 23180
  total ~ 23125
fracture
  closed treatment
    without manipulation ~ 23500
    with manipulation ~ 23505
  open treatment ~ 23515
pinning, wiring ~ 23490
prophylactic treatment ~ 23490
repair osteotomy ~ 23480-23485
saucerization ~ 23180
sequestrectomy ~ 23170
tumor, excision ~ 23140, 23146, 23200
  with autograft ~ 23145
  radical resection ~ 23200
X-ray ~ 73000
Clavicula ~ see clavicle
Claviculectomy
partial ~ 23120
total ~ 23125
Claw finger repair ~ 26499
Cleft, branchial ~ see branchial cleft
Cleft cyst, branchial ~ 42810-42815
Cleft foot, reconstruction ~ 28360
Cleft hand, repair ~ 26580
Cleft lip
repair ~ 40700-40761
rhinoplasty ~ 30460-30462
Cleft palate
repair ~ 42200-42225
rhinoplasty ~ 30460-30462
Clinical act of insertion ~ see insertion
Clinical chemistry test ~ 84999
Clinical pathology ~ 80500-80502
Clitoroplasty, intersex state ~ 56805
Closed [transurethral] biopsy of bladder ~ 52224, 52250
Clostridial tetanus ~ 86280
Clostridium botulinum toxin ~ see chemodenervation
Clostridium difficile
antigen detection
  enzyme immunoassay ~ 87324
by immunoassay
  with direct optical observation ~ 87803
Clostridium tetani AB ~ 86774

Closure
anal fistula ~ 46288
atrioventricular valve ~ 33600
cranial sutures, premature ~ see craniosynostosis
cystostomy ~ 51880
enterostomy ~ 44625-44626
esophagostomy ~ 43420-43425
fistula, vesicouterine ~ 51920-51925
gastrostomy ~ 43870
lacrimal fistula ~ 68770
lacrimal punctum
  plug ~ 68761
  thermocauterization, ligation or laser surgery ~ 68760
meningocele spinal ~ 63700-63702
rectovaginal fistula ~ 57300-57308
semilunar valve ~ 33602
septal defect ~ 33615
  ventricular ~ 33675-33677, 93581
sternotomy ~ 21750
vagina ~ 57120
ventricular tunnel ~ 33722
Clot ~ 34401-34490, 35875-35876, 50230
Clotting disorder ~ 85390
Clotting factor ~ 85210-85293
Clotting inhibitors ~ 85300-85305, 85307
Clotting operation ~ 11765
Clotting test
protein C ~ 85303, 85307
protein S ~ 85306
Clotting time ~ 85345-85348
Clot lysis time ~ 85175
Clot retraction ~ 85170
Clubfoot cast ~ 29450
wedging ~ 29750
CMG ~ 51725-51726
CMRI ~ see cardiac magnetic resonance imaging
CMV ~ see cytomegalovirus
CNPB (continuous negative pressure breathing) ~ 94662
Co-factor I , heparin ~ 85300-85301
CO2 ~ 82374
Coagulation
blood ~ see blood clot
defect ~ 85390
factor ~ 85210-85293
factor I (fibrinogen) ~ 85384, 85385
factor II (prothrombin) ~ 85210
factor III (thromboplastin) ~ 85730, 85732
factor IV (calcium) ~ 82310
factor V (AcG or proaccelerin) ~ 85220
factor VII (proconvertin) ~ 85230
factor VIII (AHG) ~ 85240-85247
factor IX (Christmas factor) ~ 85250
factor X (thrombokinase) (Stuart-Prower factor) ~ 85260
factor XI (plasma thromboplastin antecedent, PTA) ~ 85270
factor XII (Hageman factor) ~ 85280

Coagulation ~ continued
factor XIII (fibrin stabilizing factor) ~ 85290, 85291
light ~ see photocoagulation
time ~ 85345-85348
unlisted services and procedures ~ 85999
Coagulin ~ see thromboplastin
Coagulopathy ~ 85390
assay ~ 85130
Cocaine
blood or urine ~ 82520
screen ~ 82486
Coccidioides, antibody ~ 86635
Coccidioidin test ~ 86590
Coccidioidomycosis, skin test ~ 86490
Coccygeal spine fracture ~ 27200, 27202
Coccygectomy ~ 15920-15922, 27080
Coccyx
excision ~ 27080
fracture
closed treatment ~ 27200
open treatment ~ 27202
tumor, excision ~ 49215
X-ray ~ 72220
Cochlear device
insertion ~ 69930
programming ~ 92601-92604
Codeine, alkaloid screening ~ 82101
Codeine screen ~ 82486
Cofactor protein S ~ 85305, 85306
Coffey operation ~ 58400
Cognitive function tests ~ 96101-96125 (see also neurology, diagnostic)
Cognitive skills development ~ 97532
Cold agglutinin ~ 86156-86157
Cold pack treatment ~ 97010
Cold preservation ~ see cryopreservation
Cold therapies ~ see cryotherapy
Colectomy
partial ~ 44140
with anastomosis ~ 44140
laparoscopic ~ 44204, 44207-44208
with coloproctostomy ~ 44145-44146
with colostomy ~ 44141-44144
laparoscopic ~ 44206, 44208
with ileocolostomy, laparoscopic ~ 44205
with ileostomy ~ 44144
with ileum removal ~ 44160
with transcanal approach ~ 44147
total
laparoscopic ~ 44210-44212
with protectomy and ileostomy ~ 44210-44212
without protectomy ~ 44210
open
with complete proctectomy ~ 45121
with ileostomy ~ 44150-44151
with protectomy ~ 44155-44158
Collagen cross links ~ 82523
Collagen injection ~ 11950-11954
Collar bone ~ see clavicle

Collateral ligament
ankle repair ~ 27695-27698
interphalangeal joint ~ 26545
knee
joint repair ~ 27409
repair ~ 27405
metacarpophalangeal joint ~ 26540-26542
Collection and processing
allogeneic blood harvesting of stem cells ~ 38205
autologous blood
harvesting of stem cells ~ 38206
intraoperative ~ 86891
preoperative ~ 86890
specimen
capillary blood ~ 36416
venous blood ~ 36415, 36591
Colles fracture ~ 25600-25605
Colles fracture reversed ~ see Smith fracture
Collins syndrome, Treacher ~ 21150-21151
Collis procedure ~ 43283, 43842-43843
Colon ~ see also colon-sigmoid
biopsy ~ 44025, 44100, 44322
endoscopic ~ 44389, 45380, 45391, 45392
colostomy, revision ~ 44340-44346
colotomy ~ 44322
colostomy ~ 44320
CT scan
colonography ~ 74261-74263
destruction
lesion ~ 44393, 45383
tumor ~ 44393, 45383
endoscopy
biopsy ~ 44389, 45380, 45391, 45392
destruction
lesion ~ 44393
tumor ~ 44393, 45383
dilation ~ 45386
exploration ~ 44388, 45378, 45381, 45386
hemorrhage ~ 44391, 45382
injection, submucosal ~ 45381
placement, stent ~ 45387
removal
foreign body ~ 44390, 45379
polyp ~ 44392, 45384-45385
tumor ~ 45384-45385
specimen collection ~ 45380
ultrasound ~ 45391-45392
via colotomy ~ 45355
via stoma ~ 44388-44397
excision
partial ~ 44140-44147, 44160
laparoscopic ~ 44204-44208
total ~ 44150-44156
laparoscopic ~ 44210-44212
exploration ~ 44025
endoscopy ~ 44388, 45378, 45381, 45386
hemorrhage, endoscopic control ~ 44391, 45382
hernia ~ 44050

Colon ~ _continued_
incision
  creation, stoma ~ 44320-44322
  exploration ~ 44025
  revision, stoma ~ 44340-44346
lavage, intraoperative ~ 44701
lesion
  destruction ~ 45383
  excision ~ 44110-44111
lysis, adhesions ~ 44005
obstruction ~ 44025-44050
reconstruction, bladder from ~ 50810
removal
  foreign body ~ 44025, 44390, 45379
  polyp ~ 44392
repair
  diverticula ~ 44605
  fistula ~ 44650-44661
  hernia ~ 44050
  malrotation ~ 44055
  obstruction ~ 44050
  ulcer ~ 44605
  volvulus ~ 44050
  wound ~ 44605
stoma closure ~ 44620-44625
suture
  diverticula ~ 44605
  fistula ~ 44650-44661
  plication ~ 44680
  stoma ~ 44620-44625
  ulcer ~ 44605
  wound ~ 44605
tumor, destruction ~ 45383
ultrasound, endoscopic ~ 45391-45392
X-ray with contrast, barium enema ~
  74270-74280
Colon-sigmoid ~ see also colon
biopsy, endoscopy ~ 45331
dilation, endoscopy ~ 45340
endoscopy
  ablation
    polyp ~ 45339
    tumor ~ 45339
  biopsy ~ 45331
  dilation ~ 45340
  exploration ~ 45330, 45335
  hemorrhage ~ 45334
  needle biopsy ~ 45342
  placement, stent ~ 45327, 45345
  removal
    foreign body ~ 45332
    polyp ~ 45333, 45338
    tumor ~ 45333, 45338
  ultrasound ~ 45341-45342
  volvulus ~ 45337
exploration, endoscopy ~ 45330, 45335
hemorrhage, endoscopy ~ 45334
needle biopsy, endoscopy ~ 45342
removal, foreign body ~ 45332
repair, volvulus, endoscopy ~ 45337
ultrasound, endoscopy ~ 45341-45342
Colonna procedure ~ 27120

Colonography, CT scan
diagnostic ~ 74261-74262
screening ~ 74263
Colonoscopy
biopsy ~ 45380, 45392
collection specimen ~ 45380
  via colotomy ~ 45355
destruction, lesion or tumor ~ 45383
dilation ~ 45386
follow-up interval ~ 0528F-0529F
hemorrhage control ~ 45382
injection, submucosal ~ 45381
placement, stent ~ 45387
removal
  foreign body ~ 45379
  polyp ~ 45384-45385
  tumor ~ 45384-45385
surveillance intervals ~ 0528F-0529F
ultrasound ~ 45391-45392
via stoma ~ 44388-44390
  biopsy ~ 44389
  destruction
    of lesion ~ 44393
    of tumor ~ 44393
  exploration ~ 44388
  hemorrhage ~ 44391
  placement, stent ~ 44397
  removal
    foreign body ~ 44390
    polyp ~ 44392, 44394
    tumor ~ 44392, 44394
Colorrhaphy ~ 44604
Color vision examination ~ 92283
Colostomy ~ 44320, 45563
abdominal, establishment ~ 50810
home visit ~ 99505
intestine, large, with suture ~ 44605
perineal, establishment ~ 50810
revision ~ 44340
paracolostomy hernia ~ 44345-44346
Colotomy ~ 44025
Colpectomy
partial ~ 57106
total ~ 57110
with hysterectomy ~ 58275-58280
with repair of enterocele ~ 58280
Colpo-urethrocystopexy ~ 58152, 58267,
  58293
  Marshall-Marchetti-Krantz procedure ~ 58152,
    58267, 58293
  Pereyra procedure ~ 58267, 58293
Colpoceliocentesis ~ 57020
Colpocentesis ~ 57020
Colpocleisis ~ 57120
Colpohysterectomies ~ 58260, 58290-58294,
  58550, 58553
Colpoperineorrhaphy ~ 57210
Colpopexy
extra-peritoneal ~ 57282
intra-peritoneal ~ 57283
laparoscopic ~ 57425
open ~ 57280

1377

Colpoplasty ~ see repair, vagina
Colporrhaphy
  anterior ~ 57240, 57289
    with insertion of mesh ~ 57267
    with insertion of prosthesis ~ 57267
  anteroposterior ~ 57260-57265
    with enterocele repair ~ 57265
    with insertion of mesh ~ 57267
    with insertion of prosthesis ~ 57267
  nonobstetrical ~ 57200
  posterior ~ 57250
    with insertion of mesh ~ 57267
    with insertion of prosthesis ~ 57267
Colposcopy
  biopsy ~ 56821, 57421, 57454-57455, 57460
  cervix ~ 57421, 57452-57461
  exploration ~ 57452
  loop electrode excision ~ 57460
  loop electrode conization ~ 57461
  perineum ~ 99170
  vagina ~ 57420-57421
  vulva ~ 56820
    biopsy ~ 56821
Colpotomy
  drainage, abscess ~ 57010
  exploration ~ 57000
Colprosterone ~ 84144
Columna vertebralis ~ see spine
Column chromatography/mass spectrometry
  ~ 82541-82544
Combined heart-lung transplantation ~ 33935
Combined right and left heart cardiac
  catheterization ~ 93453
Comedones, removal ~ 10040
Commissurotomy, right ventricle ~
  33476-33478
Common sensory nerve, repair/suture ~
  64834
Common truncus ~ 33786
Communication device
  non-speech-generating ~ 92605-92606
  speech-generating ~ 92606-92609
Community/work reintegration training ~
  97537
Compatibility test, blood ~ 86920
Complement
  antigen ~ 86160
  fixation test ~ 86171
  functional activity ~ 86161
  hemolytic, total ~ 86162
  total ~ 86162
Complete blood count (CBC) ~ see also blood
  cell count ~ 85025-85027
Complete colectomy ~ see colectomy, total
Complete pneumonectomy ~ 32488
Complete transposition of great vessels ~
  33770-33781
Complex, factor IX ~ 85250
Complex, vitamin B ~ 78270-78272
Component removal, blood ~ 36511-36516
Composite graft ~ 15760-15770, 35681-35683
Compound B ~ 82528

Compound F ~ 80400-80406, 80418-80420,
  80436, 82530
Compression, nerve, median ~ 64721
Computed tomographic scintigraphy ~ 78607
Computed tomography (CT) ~ see CT scan;
  specific anatomic site
Computer assisted navigation, orthopedic
  surgery ~ 0054T-0055T, 20985
Computer analysis, acoustic recording, heart
  sounds ~ 93799
Computer data analysis ~ 99090
Computer-aided detection
  lesion, chest radiograph ~ 0174T-0175T
  mammography ~ 77051-77052
  MRI ~ 0159T
Computerized emission tomography ~ 78607
Concentration, hydrogen ion ~ see pH
Concentration, minimum inhibitory ~ 87186
Concentration of specimen ~ 87015
Concentric procedure ~ 28296
Conchae nasale ~ 30930
Concha Bullosa resection
  with nasal/sinus endoscopy ~ 31240
Conduction, nerve ~ see nerve conduction
Conduit, ileal ~ 50690
Condyle
  humerus
    fracture
      closed treatment ~ 24576-24577
      open treatment ~ 24579
      percutaneous ~ 24582
  mandibular ~ 21247, 21465
  metatarsal, excision ~ 28288
  phalanges, toe, excision ~ 28126
Condylectomy
  temporomandibular joint ~ 21050
  with skull base surgery ~ 61596-61597
Condyloma, destruction ~ 54050-54065
Conference, medical, with interdisciplinary
  team ~ 99366-99368
Confirmation, drug ~ 80102
Congenital arteriovenous malformation ~ see
  arteriovenous malformation
Congenital elevation of scapula ~ 23400
Congenital heart septum defect ~
  33813-33814
Congenital kidney abnormality
  nephrolithotomy ~ 50070
  pyeloplasty ~ 50405
  pyelotomy ~ 50135
Congenital laryngocele ~ 31300
Congenital vascular anomaly ~ see vascular
  malformation
Conisation ~ 57461, 57520-57522
Conization, cervix ~ 57461, 57520-57522
Conjoint psychotherapy ~ 90846-90849, 99510
Conjunctiva
  biopsy ~ 68100
  cyst, incision and drainage ~ 68020
  fistulize for drainage, with tube ~ 68750
    without tube ~ 68745

Conjunctiva ~ *continued*
graft ~ 65782
harvesting ~ 68371
harvesting ~ 68371
insertion stent ~ 68750
lesion
destruction ~ 68135
excision ~ 68110-68130
over 1 cm ~ 68115
with adjacent sclera ~ 68130
reconstruction ~ 68320-68335
symblepharon, with graft ~ 68335
with flap
bridge or partial ~ 68360
total ~ 68362
repair
symblepharon
division ~ 68340
with graft ~ 68335
without graft ~ 68330
wound
direct closure ~ 65270
mobilization and rearrangement ~ 65272-65273
unlisted services and procedures ~ 68399
Conjunctivo-tarso-Muller resection ~ 67908
Conjunctivocystorhinostomy ~ 68745-68750
Conjunctivodacryocystostomy ~ 68745-68750
Conjunctivoplasty ~ 68320-68330
reconstruction cul de sac, with extensive
rearrangement ~ 68326
with graft ~ 68326
buccal mucous membrane ~ 68328
with extensive rearrangement ~ 68320
with graft ~ 68320
buccal mucous membrane ~ 68325
Conjunctivorhinostomy
with tube ~ 68750
without tube ~ 68745
Conscious sedation ~ 99143-99150
Construction
finger, toe to hand transfer ~ 26551-26556
neobladder ~ 51596
vagina
with graft ~ 57292
without graft ~ 57291
Consultation(s) ~ 99241-99255
clinical pathology ~ 80500-80502
initial inpatient ~ 99251-99255
new or established patient ~ 99251-99255
office and/or other outpatient ~ 99241-99245
new or established patient ~ 99241-99245
psychiatric, with family ~ 90887
radiation therapy, radiation physics ~ 77336-77370
surgical pathology ~ 88321-88325
intraoperation ~ 88329-88332
X-ray ~ 76140
Consumption test, antiglobulin ~ 86880

Contact lens services
fittings and prescription ~ 92071-92072, 92310-92313
modification ~ 92325
prescription ~ 92314-92317
replacement ~ 92326
Continuous negative pressure breathing (CNPD) ~ 94662
Continuous positive airway pressure (CPAP) ~ 94660
Contouring
silicone injections ~ 11950-11954
tumor, facial bone ~ 21029
Contraception
cervical cap
fitting ~ 57170
diaphragm
fitting ~ 57170
intrauterine device (IUD)
insertion ~ 58300
removal ~ 58301
Contraceptive capsules, implantable
removal ~ 11976
Contraceptive device, intrauterine ~ 58300-58301
Contracture
elbow, release
with radical resection of capsule ~ 24149
palm, release ~ 26121-26125
thumb, release ~ 26508
Contracture of palmar fascia ~ 26040-26045
Contralateral ligament repair, knee ~ 27405
Contrast aortogram ~ 75600-75605, 75630, 93567
Contrast bath therapy ~ see also physical medicine/therapy/occupational therapy ~ 97034
Contrast material
injection via peritoneal catheter ~ 49424
Contrast phlebogram ~ see venography
Contusion ~ see hematoma
Converting enzyme, angiotensin ~ 82164
Coombs test ~ 86880
Copper ~ 82525
Coprobilinogen, feces ~ 84577
Coproporphyrin ~ 84120
Coracoacromial ligament release ~ 23415
Coracoid process transfer ~ 23462
Cord
spermatic ~ see spermatic cord
spinal ~ see spinal cord
vocal ~ see vocal cords
Cordectomy ~ 31300
Cordocentesis ~ 59012
Cordotomy ~ 63194-63199
Corectomy ~ see excision, iris
Coreoplasty ~ 66762
Cornea
biopsy ~ 65410
curettage ~ 65435-65436
with chelating agent ~ 65436

Cornea ~ *continued*
epithelium, excision ~ 65435-65436
  with chelating agent ~ 65436
hysteresis determination ~ 0181T
lesion
  destruction ~ 65450
  excision ~ 65400
    with graft ~ 65426
    without graft ~ 65420
pachymetry ~ 76514
prosthesis ~ 65770
pterygium, excision ~ 65420
puncture ~ 65600
relaxing incisions ~ 65772-65775
repair
  astigmatism ~ 65772-65775
  wedge resection ~ 65775
  with glue ~ 65286
  wound
    nonperforating ~ 65275
    perforating ~ 65280-65285
    tissue glue ~ 65286
reshape
  epikeratoplasty ~ 65765
  keratomileusis ~ 65760
  keratoprosthesis ~ 65767
scraping, smear ~ 65430
tattoo ~ 65600
thickness measurement ~ 76514
transplantation
  autograft or homograft
    allograft preparation ~ 65757
    endothelial ~ 65756
    lamellar ~ 65710
    penetrating ~ 65730-65755
    for aphakia ~ 65750
Coronary
atherectomy, percutaneous ~ 92995-92996
thrombectomy, percutaneous ~ 92973
Coronary angioplasty, transluminal balloon ~
  see percutaneous transluminal angioplasty
Coronary artery
CT scan ~ 75571-75573
insertion, stent ~ 92980-92981
ligation ~ 33502
placement, radiation delivery device ~ 92974
repair ~ 33500-33506
Coronary artery bypass graft (CABG) ~
  33503-33505, 33510-33516
arterial ~ 33533-33536
arterial-venous ~ 33517-33523
beta-blocker administration ~ 4115F
harvest, upper extremity artery ~ 35600
internal mammary artery graft ~ 4110F
reoperation ~ 33530
venous ~ 33510-33516
Coronary endarterectomy ~ 33572
Coroner's exam ~ 88045
Coronoidectomy, temporomandibular joint ~
  21070
Corpectomy ~ 63101-63103

Corpora cavernosa
corpus spongiosum shunt ~ 54430
glans penis fistulization ~ 54435
injection ~ 54235
irrigation, priapism ~ 54220
saphenous vein shunt ~ 54420
X-ray with contrast ~ 74445
Corpora cavernosa, plastic induration ~ see
  Peyronie disease
Corpora cavernosography ~ 74445
Corpus callosum, transection ~ 61541
Corpus vertebrae (vertebrale) ~ see vertebral
  body
Correction (of)
cleft palate ~ 42200-42225
lid retraction ~ 67911
malrotation of duodenum ~ 44055
syndactyly ~ 26560-26562
ureteropelvic junction ~ 50400-50405, 50544
Cortex decortication, cerebral ~ see
  decortication
Cortical mapping
transection, by electric stimulation ~
  95961-95962
Corticoids ~ 83491
Corticoliberin ~ 80412
Corticosteroids
blood ~ 83491
urine ~ 83491
Corticosteroid-binding globulin ~ 84449
Corticosteroid-binding protein ~ 84449
Corticosterone, blood or urine ~ 82528
Corticotropic releasing hormone (CRH) ~
  80412
Cortisol ~ 80400-80406, 80418-80420, 80436,
  82530
stimulation ~ 80412
total ~ 82533
Cortisol binding globulin ~ 84449
Costectomy ~ 19260-19272, 32900
Costen syndrome ~ see temporomandibular
  joint (TMJ)
Costotransversectomy ~ 21610
Cothromboplastin ~ 85230
Cotte operation ~ see revision ~ 58400-58410
Cotton procedure, Bohler procedure ~ 28405
Counseling and/or risk factor reduction
  intervention ~ 99401-99429
alcohol and/or substance abuse ~ 99408-99409
behavior change ~ 99406-99409
smoking and tobacco use ~ 99406-99407
Count
blood cell ~ see blood cell count
blood platelet ~ 85008
cell ~ 89050-89051
complete blood ~ 85025-85027
erythrocyte ~ 85032-85041
leukocyte ~ 85032, 85048, 89055
reticulocyte ~ 85044-85045
Counterimmunoelectrophoresis ~ 86185
Counters, cell ~ 89050-89051
Countershock, electric ~ 92960-92961

Coventry tibial wedge osteotomy ~
   27455-27457, 27705, 27709-27712
Cowper's gland, excision ~ 53250
Coxa ~ see hip
Coxiella burnetii, antibody ~ 86638
Coxsackie, antibody ~ 86658
CPAP ~ 94660
CPK, blood ~ 82550-82552
CPR (cardiopulmonary resuscitation) ~ 92950
Cranial bone
   halo, thin skull osteology ~ 20664
   reconstruction, extracranial ~ 21181-21184
   tumor, excision ~ 61563-61564
Cranial halo ~ 20661
Cranial nerve ~ see specific nerve
   avulsion ~ 64732-64760, 64771
   decompression ~ 61458, 61460, 64716
   implantation ~ 64568-64569
     electrode ~ 64553
   incision ~ 64568, 64732-64752, 64760, 65771
   injection
     anesthetic ~ 64400-64408, 64412
     neurolytic ~ 64600-64610
   insertion, electrode ~ 64553
   neuroplasty ~ 64716
   release ~ 64716
   removal, neurostimulator ~ 64570
   repair, suture, with or without graft ~
     64864-64865
   section ~ 61460
   transection ~ 64732-64760, 64771
   transposition ~ 64716
Cranial nerve II ~ see optic nerve
Cranial nerve V (five) ~ see trigeminal nerve
Cranial nerve VII (seven) ~ see facial nerve
Cranial nerve X (ten) ~ see vagus nerve
Cranial nerve XI ~ see accessory nerve
Cranial nerve XII (twelve) ~ 64868
Cranial tongs
   application/removal ~ 20660
   removal ~ 20665
Craniectomy ~ see also craniotomy ~ 61501
   decompression ~ 61322-61323, 61340-61343
   exploratory ~ 61304-61305
   extensive, for multiple suture craniosynostosis
     ~ 61558-61559
   for electrode ~ 61860-61875
   release stenosis ~ 61550-61552
   surgical ~ 61312-61315, 61320-61323,
     61440-61480, 61500-61516, 61518-61522
Craniofacial, unlisted procedures ~ 21299
Craniofacial separation
   closed treatment ~ 21431
   open treatment ~ 21432-21436
   wire fixation ~ 21431
Craniomegalic skull, reduction ~ 62115-62117
Craniopharyngioma, excision ~ 61545
Cranioplasty ~ 62120
   encephalocele repair ~ 62120
   for defect ~ 62140-62141, 62145
   with autograft ~ 62146-62147
   with bone graft ~ 61316, 62146-62147

Craniostenosis ~ see craniosynostosis
Craniosynostosis
   bifrontal craniotomy ~ 61557
   extensive craniectomy ~ 61558-61559
Craniotomy ~ see burr hole; drill hole;
    puncture ~ 61501
   bifrontal ~ 61557
   decompression ~ 61322-61323
   exploratory ~ 61304-61305
   for craniosynostosis ~ 61556-61557
   for encephalocele ~ 62121
   for implant of neurostimulators ~ 61850-61875
   frontal ~ 61556
   parietal ~ 61556
   surgery ~ 61312-61315, 61320-61323, 61440,
     61490, 61546, 61570-61571, 61582-61583,
     61590, 61592, 61760, 62120
   with bone flap ~ 61510-61516, 61526-61530,
     61533-61545, 61566-61567
Cranium ~ see skull
Craterization
   calcaneus ~ 28120
   clavicle ~ 23180
   femur ~ 27070-27071, 27360
   fibula ~ 27360, 27641
   hip ~ 27070
   humerus ~ 23184, 24140
   ileum ~ 27070
   metacarpal ~ 26230
   metatarsal ~ 28122
   olecranon process ~ 24147
   phalanges
     finger ~ 26235-26236
     toe ~ 28124
   pubis ~ 27070
   radius ~ 24145, 25151
   scapula ~ 23182
   talus ~ 28120
   tarsal ~ 28122
   tibia ~ 27360, 27640
   ulna ~ 24147, 25150
Creatine ~ 82553-82554
   blood or urine ~ 82540
Creatine kinase, total ~ 82550
Creatine phosphokinase
   blood ~ 82552
   total ~ 82550
Creatinine
   blood ~ 82565
   clearance ~ 82575
   other source ~ 82570
   urine ~ 82570-82575
Creation
   arteriovenous
     fistula/autogenous graft ~ 36825
   colonic reservoir ~ 45119
   complete heart block ~ 93650
   defect ~ 40720
   ileal reservoir ~ 44158, 45113
   lesion ~ 61790, 63600
   mucofistula ~ 44144
   pericardial window ~ 32659

Creation ~ *continued*
recipient site ~ 15002-15005
shunt
  cerebrospinal fluid ~ 62200
  subarachnoid, lumbar-peritoneal ~ 63740
  subarachnoid-subdural ~ 62190
  ventriculo ~ 62200
sigmoid bladder ~ 50810
speech prosthesis ~ 31611
stoma
  bladder ~ 51980
  kidney ~ 50395
  renal pelvis ~ 50395
  tympanic membrane ~ 69433-69436
  ureter ~ 50860
ventral hernia ~ 39503
CRF ~ 80412
CRH ~ see corticotropic releasing hormone
  (CRH)
Cricoid cartilage split, larynx ~ 31587
Cricothyroid membrane, incision ~ 31605
Cristobalite ~ 84285
Critical care services ~ 99291-99292
evaluation and management ~ 99291-99292
interfacility transport ~ 99466-99467
ipecac administration for poison ~ 99175
neonatal
  initial ~ 99468
  low birth weight infant ~ 99478-99479
  subsequent ~ 99469
pediatric
  initial ~ 99471, 99475
  interfacility transport ~ 99466-99467
  subsequent ~ 99472, 99476
Cross finger flap ~ 15574
Crossmatch ~ 86920-86922
Crossmatching, tissue ~ 86812-86817,
  86821-86822
Cruciate ligament
arthroscopic repair ~ 29888-29889
repair ~ 27407-27409
  knee, with collateral ligament ~ 27409
Cryoablation ~ 17000-17286, 47371, 47381
Cryofibrinogen ~ 82585
Cryofixation ~ see cryopreservation
Cryoglobulin ~ 82595
Cryopreservation
cells ~ 38207-38209, 88240-88241
embryo ~ 89258
for transplantation ~ 32850, 33930, 33940,
  44132, 47133, 47140, 48550,
  50300-50320, 50547
freezing and storage ~ 38207, 88240
sperm ~ 89259
testes ~ 89335
thawing
  embryo ~ 89352
  oocytes ~ 89353
  reproductive tissue ~ 89354
  sperm ~ 89356

Cryosurgery ~ see destruction ~ 17000-17286,
  47371, 47381
fibroadenoma, breast ~ 19105
labyrinthotomy ~ 69801
lesion
  mouth ~ 40820
  penis ~ 54056, 54065
  vagina ~ 57061-57065
  vulva ~ 56501-56515
Cryotherapy
ablation, renal tumor ~ 50593
acne ~ 17340
destruction, ciliary body ~ 66720
lesion
  cornea ~ 65450
  retina ~ 67208, 67227
retinal detachment
  prophylaxis ~ 67141
  repair ~ 67101
trichiasis, correction ~ 67825
Cryptectomy ~ 46999
Cryptococcus
antibody ~ 86641
antigen detection, enzyme immunoassay ~
  87327
Cryptococcus neoformans, antigen detection,
  enzyme immunoassay ~ 87327
Cryptorchism ~ 54550-54560
Cryptosporidium
antigen detection
  direct fluorescence ~ 87272
  enzyme immunoassay ~ 87328
Crystal identification, any body fluid ~ 89060
CSF ~ see cerebrospinal fluid leak
CT angiography ~ 75574
CT scan
3-D rendering ~ 76376-76377
abdomen ~ 74150-74178, 75635
arm ~ 73200-73206
bone, density study ~ 77078
brain ~ 3111F-3112F
drainage ~ 75989
follow-up study ~ 76380
guidance
  localization ~ 77011
  needle placement ~ 77012
  parenchymal tissue ablation ~ 77013
  radiation therapy ~ 77014
  vertebroplasty ~ 72292
  visceral tissue ablation ~ 77013
heart ~ 75571-75574
  hemorrhage documented ~ 3110F
  infarction documented ~ 3110F
  lesion documented ~ 3110F
unlisted services and procedures ~ 76497
with contrast ~ 70460
  abdomen ~ 74160, 74177
  arm ~ 73201
  brain ~ 0042T, 70460
  cerebral blood flow/volume ~ 0042T
  ear ~ 70481

CT scan ~ *continued*
  face ~ 70487
  head ~ 70460
  leg ~ 73701
  maxilla ~ 70487
  neck ~ 70491
  orbit ~ 70481
  pelvis ~ 72193, 74177
  sella tucica ~ 70481
  spine
    cervical ~ 72126
    lumbar ~ 72132
    thoracic ~ 72129
  thorax ~ 71260
  without and with contrast
    abdomen ~ 74170, 74174-74175, 74178,
      75635
    arm ~ 73202
    brain ~ 70470, 70496
    chest ~ 71275
    ear ~ 70482
    face ~ 70488
    head ~ 70470, 70496
    leg ~ 73702-73706, 75635
    maxilla ~ 70488
    neck ~ 70492, 70498
    orbit ~ 70482
    pelvis ~ 72194, 74174, 74178
    sella turcica ~ 70482
    spine, cervical ~ 72127
      lumbar ~ 72133
      thoracic ~ 72130
    thorax ~ 71270
  without contrast ~ 70450
    abdomen ~ 74150, 74176, 74178
    arm ~ 73200
    brain ~ 70450
    colonography ~ 74261-74263
    ear ~ 70480
    face ~ 70486
    head ~ 70450
    leg ~ 73700
    maxilla ~ 70486
    neck ~ 70490
    orbit ~ 70480
    pelvis ~ 72192, 74176, 74178
    sella turcica ~ 70480
    spine
      cervical ~ 72125
      lumbar ~ 72131
      thoracic ~ 72128
    thorax ~ 71250
CT scan, radionuclide ~ 78607
Cuff, rotator ~ 23410-23420
Culdocentesis ~ 57020
Culture
  acid fast bacilli ~ 87116
  amniotic fluid, chromosome analysis ~ 88235
  bacteria
    aerobic ~ 87040-87071, 87077
    anaerobic ~ 87073-87076

Culture ~ *continued*
  blood ~ 87040
    other ~ 87070-87075
    screening ~ 87081
    stool ~ 87045-87046
    urine ~ 87086-87088
  bone marrow, chromosome analysis ~ 88237
  chlamydia ~ 87110
  chorionic villus, chromosome analysis ~
    88235
  fertilized oocyte for in vitro fertilization ~
    89250
    co-culture of embryo ~ 89251
  fungus
    blood ~ 87103
    hair ~ 87101
    identification ~ 87106
    nail ~ 87101
    other ~ 87102
    skin ~ 87101
  lymphocyte
    chromosome analysis ~ 88230
    HLA typing ~ 86821-86822
  mold ~ 87107
  mycobacteria ~ 87118
  mycoplasma ~ 87109
  oocyte/embryo ~ 89250
    co-culture of oocyte/embryo ~ 89251
    extended culture ~ 89272
  pathogen ~ 87081-87084
  skin, chromosome analysis ~ 88233
  tissue
    homogenization ~ 87176
    infectious agent drug resistance ~
      87903-87904
    toxin/antitoxin ~ 87230
    virus ~ 87252-87253
  tubercle bacilli ~ 87116
  typing ~ 87140-87158
  unlisted services and procedures ~ 87999
  yeast ~ 87106
Curettage ~ 59840
  cervix, endocervical ~ 57454, 57456, 57505
  cornea ~ 65435-65436
    chelating agent ~ 65436
  hydatidiform mole ~ 59870
  postpartum ~ 59160
  uterus ~ 58356
Curettage and dilatation ~ 59840
Curettement, skin lesion ~ 11055-11057,
  17004, 17110, 17270, 17280
Curietherapy ~ 77761-77778, 77789
Custodial care ~ *see* domiciliary services;
  nursing facility services
Cutaneolipectomy ~ *see* lipectomy
Cutaneous-vesicostomy ~ 51980
Cutaneous electrostimulation, analgesic ~
  64550
Cutaneous tag ~ 11200-11201
Cutaneous tissue ~ see integumentary system
CVS ~ 59015
Cyanacobalamin ~ 82607-82608

Cyanide
blood ~ 82600
tissue ~ 82600
Cyanocobalamin ~ 82607-82608
Cyclic AMP ~ 82030
Cyclic GMP ~ 83008
Cyclic somatostatin ~ 84307
Cyclocryotherapy ~ 66720
Cyclodialysis, destruction ciliary body ~ 66740
Cyclophotocoagulation, destruction ciliary body ~ 66710
Cyclosporine, assay ~ 80158
Cyst
abdomen, destruction/excision ~ 49203-49205
ankle
capsule ~ 27630
tendon sheath ~ 27630
Bartholin's gland excision ~ 56740
repair ~ 56440
bile duct ~ 47715
bladder, excision ~ 51500
bone
drainage ~ 20615
injection ~ 20615
brain
drainage ~ 61150-61151, 61156, 62161-62162
excision ~ 61516, 61524, 62162
branchial cleft, excision ~ 42810-42815
breast
incision and drainage ~ 19020
puncture aspiration ~ 19000-19001
calcaneus ~ 28100-28103
carpal ~ 25130-25136
choledochal ~ 47715
ciliary body, destruction ~ 66770
clavicle, excision ~ 23140-23146
conjunctiva ~ 68020
dermoid, nose, excision ~ 30124-30125
drainage
contrast injection ~ 49424
with X-ray ~ 76080
excision
cheekbone ~ 21030
clavicle ~ 23140
with allograft ~ 23146
with autograft ~ 23145
femur ~ 27355-27358
ganglion ~ see ganglion
humerus
with allograft ~ 23156
with autograft ~ 23155
hydatid ~ 86171, 86280
lymphatic ~ 49062, 49323
maxilla ~ 21030
mediastinum ~ 32662
olecranon process
with allograft ~ 24126
with autograft ~ 24125
pericardial ~ 32661

Cyst ~ *continued*
pilonidal ~ 11770-11772
radius
with allograft ~ 24126
with autograft ~ 24125
scapula ~ 23140
with allograft ~ 23146
with autograft ~ 23145
ulna
with allograft ~ 24126
with autograft ~ 24125
zygoma ~ 21030
facial bones
excision ~ 21030
femur ~ 27065-27067
fibula ~ 27635-27638
ganglion, aspiration/injection ~ 20612
gums, incision and drainage ~ 41800
hip ~ 27065-27067
humerus
excision ~ 23150-23156, 24110
with allograft ~ 24116
with autograft ~ 24115
ileum ~ 27065-27067
incision and drainage ~ 10060-10061
pilonidal ~ 10080-10081
iris, destruction ~ 66770
kidney
ablation ~ 50541
aspiration ~ 50390
excision ~ 50280-50290
injection ~ 50390
X-ray ~ 74470
knee
Baker's ~ 27345
excision ~ 27347
leg, lower
capsule ~ 27630
tendon sheath ~ 27630
liver ~ 47010
drainage ~ 47010
open ~ 47010
repair ~ 47300
lung
incision and drainage ~ 32200
removal ~ 32140
lymph node
axillary/cervical
excision ~ 38550-38555
mandible, excision ~ 21040, 21046-21047
maxilla, excision ~ 21030, 21048-21049
mediastinal, excision ~ 39200
metacarpal ~ 26200-26205
metatarsal ~ 28104-28107
mouth ~ 41005-41009, 41015-41018
incision and drainage ~ 40800-40801
mullerian duct, excision ~ 55680
nose, excision ~ 30124-30125
olecranon ~ 24120
ovarian
excision ~ 58925
incision and drainage ~ 58800-58805

Cyst ~ *continued*
  pancreas ~ 48500
    anastomosis ~ 48520-48540
    excision ~ 48120
  pelvis
    aspiration ~ 50390
    injection ~ 50390
  pericardial, excision ~ 33050
  phalanges
    finger ~ 26210-26215
    toe ~ 28108
  pilonidal
    excision ~ 11770-11772
    incision and drainage ~ 10080-10081
  pubis ~ 27065-27067
  radius ~ 24120, 25120-25126
  Rathke's pouch ~ 61545
  removal, skin ~ 10040
  retroperitoneal, destruction/excision ~
    49203-49205, 58957, 58958
  salivary gland creation
    destruction/excision, fistula ~ 42325-42326
    drainage ~ 42409
    excision ~ 42408
  scapula, excision ~ 23140-23146
  seminal vesicle, excision ~ 55680
  skin, puncture aspiration ~ 10160
  spinal cord
    aspiration ~ 62268
    incision and drainage ~ 63172-63173
  sublingual gland drainage ~ 42409
    excision ~ 42408
  talus ~ 28100-28103
  tarsal ~ 28104-28107
  thyroglossal duct
    excision ~ 60280-60281
    incision and drainage ~ 60000
  thyroid gland aspiration ~ 60300
    excision ~ 60200
    injection ~ 60300
  tibia ~ 27635-27638
  tongue ~ 41000-41006, 41015
  ulna ~ 24120, 25120-25126
  urachal, bladder, excision ~ 51500
  vaginal, excision ~ 57135
  wrist ~ 25130-25136
    excision ~ 25111-25112
  zygoma
    excision ~ 21030
Cyst ovary ~ see ovary, cyst
Cystatin C ~ 82610
Cystatins, kininogen ~ 85293
Cystectomy
  complete ~ 51570
    with bilateral pelvic lymphadenectomy ~
      51575, 51585, 51595
    with continent diversion ~ 51596
    with ureteroileal conduit ~ 51590
    with ureterosigmoidostomy ~ 51580
  ovarian ~ 58925
    laparoscopic ~ 58661

Cystectomy ~ *continued*
  partial
    complicated ~ 51555
    reimplantation of ureters ~ 51565
    simple ~ 51550
Cystic hygroma ~ 38550-38555
Cystine, urine ~ 82615
Cystitis, interstitial ~ 52260-52265
Cystography ~ 74430
  injection ~ 52281
  radiologic ~ 51600
Cystolithotomy ~ 51050
Cystometrogram ~ 51725-51726
Cystoplasty ~ 51800
Cystorrhaphy ~ 51860-51865
Cystoscopy ~ 52000
Cystoscopy, with biopsy ~ 52224, 52250
Cystostomy
  change tube ~ 51705-51710
  closure ~ 51880
  home visit ~ 99505
  with fulguration ~ 51020
  with insertion radioactive material ~ 51020
  with urethrectomy
    female ~ 53210
    male ~ 53215
Cystotomy
  excision
    bladder diverticulum ~ 51525
    bladder tumor ~ 51530
    repair of ureterocele ~ 51535
    vesical neck ~ 51520
  repair of ureterocele ~ 51535
  with calculus basket extraction ~ 51065
  with destruction intravesical lesion ~ 51030
  with drainage ~ 51040
  with fulguration ~ 51020
  with insertion
    radioactive material ~ 51020
    ureteral catheter ~ 51045
  with removal calculus ~ 51050, 51065
Cystourethrogram, retrograde ~ 51610
Cystourethropexy ~ 51840-51841
Cystourethroplasty ~ 51800-51820
Cystourethroscopy ~ 52000, 52351, 52601,
  52647-52648, 53500
  biopsy ~ 52204, 52354
  brush ~ 52007
  calibration and/or dilation urethral stricture or
    stenosis ~ 52281
  catheterization
    ejaculatory duct ~ 52010
    ureteral ~ 52005
  destruction, lesion ~ 52400
  dilation
    bladder ~ 52260-52265
    intra-renal stricture ~ 52343, 52346
    ureter ~ 52341-52342, 52344-52345
    urethra ~ 52281
  evacuation, clot ~ 52001
  female urethral syndrome ~ 52285
  incision, ejaculatory duct ~ 52402

1385

Cystourethroscopy ~ *continued*
injection of implant material ~ 52327
insertion
  indwelling ureteral stent ~ 50947, 52332
    radioactive substance ~ 52250
    ureteral guide wire ~ 52334
    urethral stent ~ 52282
  lithotripsy ~ 52353
  manipulation of ureteral calculus ~ 52330
  meatotomy, ureteral ~ 52290-52305
  removal
    calculus ~ 52310-52315, 52320-52325,
      52352
    foreign body ~ 52310-52315
    urethral stent ~ 52310-52315
  resection
    ejaculatory duct ~ 52402
    external sphincter ~ 52277
    tumor ~ 52355
  urethral syndrome ~ 52285
  vasectomy, transurethral ~ 52402
  vasotomy
    transurethral ~ 52402
  with direct vision internal urethromtomy ~
    52276
  with ejaculatory duct catheterization ~ 52010
  with fulguration ~ 52214, 52354
    lesion ~ 52224
    tumor ~ 52234-52240
  with internal urethrotomy
    female ~ 52270
    male ~ 52275
  with steroid injection ~ 52283
  with ureteral catheterization ~ 52005
  with ureteral meatotomy ~ 52290-52305
Cytochrome reductase, lactic ~ 83615-83625
Cytogenetic studies
  bone marrow ~ 3155F
  molecular, DNA probe ~ 88271-88275, 88291,
    88365
  unlisted services and procedures ~ 88299
Cytomegalovirus
  antibody ~ 86644-86645
  antigen detection
    direct fluorescence ~ 87271
    enzyme immunoassay ~ 87332
    nucleic acid ~ 87495-87497
Cytometries, flow ~ 88184-88189
Cytopathology
  cervical or vaginal
    definitive hormone evaluationi ~ 88155
    Pap ~ 88164-88167
    requiring interpretation by physician ~
      88141
    thin layer prep ~ 88142-88143, 88174-88175
  evaluation ~ 88172, 88177
  fluids, washings, brushings ~ 88104, 88106
  forensic ~ 88125
  other source ~ 88160-88162
  sex chromatin identification ~ 88130, 88140

Cytopathology ~ *continued*
  selective cellular enhancement technique ~
    88112
  smears
    any other source ~ 88160-88162
    brushings ~ 88104
    cervical or vaginal
      automated screen ~ 88174
      hormone evaluation ~ 88155
      manual screen ~ 88150, 88153-88154,
        88164-88165
    washings ~ 88104
  unlisted services and procedures ~ 88199
  urinary tract specimen ~ 88120-88121
Cytoscopy ~ 52000
Cytosol aminopeptidase ~ 83670
Cytotoxic screen
  lymphocyte ~ 86805-86806
  percent reactive antibody (PRA) ~
    86807-86808
  serum antibodies ~ 86807-86808

D

D and C ~ 59840
D and E ~ 59841
D-xylose absorption test ~ 84620
Dacryoadenectomy
  partial ~ 68505
  total ~ 68500
Dacryocystectomy ~ 68520
Dacryocystogram ~ 68850, 70170
Dacryocystography ~ 68850, 70170
  nuclear imaging ~ 78660
Dacryocystorhinostomy ~ 68720
  total, with nasal/sinus endoscopy ~ 31239
Dacryocystostomies ~ 68420
Dacryocystotomy ~ 68420
Daily living activities ~ 97535, 99509
Damus-Kaye-Stansel procedure ~ 33606
Dana operation ~ 63185-63190
Dandy operation ~ 62180, 62200-62201
Dark adaptation examination ~ 92284
Dark field examination ~ 87164-87166
Darkroom test ~ 92140
Darrach procedure ~ 25150-25151, 25240
Day test ~ 82270, 82272
De Quervain's disease treatment ~ 25000
Death, brain ~ 95824
Debridement
  bone ~ 11044, 11047
  brain ~ 62010
  burns ~ 01951-01953, 16010-16030
  mastoid cavity
    complex ~ 69222
    simple ~ 69220
  metatarsophalangeal joint ~ 28289

Debridement ~ *continued*
muscle and/or fascia ~ 11043, 11046
  infected ~ 11004-11006
nails ~ 11720-11721
nose
  endoscopic ~ 31237
pancreatic tissue ~ 48105
skin
  eczematous ~ 11000-11001
  infected ~ 11000-11006
  with open fracture and/or dislocation ~
    11010-11012
  subcutaneous tissue ~ 11042, 11045
    infected ~ 11004-11006
sternum ~ 21627
wound
  non-selective ~ 97602
  selective ~ 97597-97598
Debulking procedure
ovary/pelvis ~ 58952-58954
Decompression ~ see section
arm, lower ~ 24495, 25020-25025
auditory canal, internal ~ 69960
brainstem ~ 61575-61576
cauda equina ~ 63011, 63017, 63047-63048,
  63056-63057, 63087-63091
cranial nerve ~ 61458
esophagogastric varices ~ 37181
facial nerve ~ 61590
  intratemporal
    lateral to geniculate ganglion ~ 69720,
      69740
    medial to geniculate ganglion ~ 69725,
      69745
  total ~ 69955
finger ~ 26035
gasserian ganglion
  sensory root ~ 61450
hand ~ 26035-26037
intestines
  small ~ 44021
jejunostomy
  laparoscopic ~ 44201
leg, fasciotomy ~ 27600-27602
nerve ~ 64702-64727
  root ~ 63020-63048, 63055-63103
nucleus of disk
lumbar ~ 62287
optic nerve ~ 67570
orbit ~ 61330
  removal of bone ~ 67414, 67445
skull ~ 61322-61323, 61340-61345
spinal cord ~ 63001-63017, 63045-63103,
  cauda equina ~ 63005
tarsal tunnel release ~ 28035
volvulus ~ 45321, 45337
with nasal/sinus endoscopy
  optic nerve ~ 31294
  orbit wall ~ 31292-31293
wrist ~ 25020-25025

Decortication
lung
  endoscopic ~ 32651-32652
  with parietal pleurectomy ~ 32320
  partial ~ 32225
  total ~ 32220
Decubiti ~ see pressure ulcer (decubitus)
Decubitus ulcers ~ see debridement; pressure
  ulcer (decubitus); skin graft and flap
Deetjeen's body ~ see blood, platelet
Defect, coagulation ~ 85390
Defect, heart septal ~ 33813-33814
Defect, septal closure, atrial ~ see heart, repair,
  atrial septum
Deferens, ductus ~ see vas deferens
Defibrillation ~ 92960-92961
Defibrillator, heart ~ see pacemaker, heart
  cardioverter-defibrillator, implantable
    data analysis ~ 93289, 93295-93296
    evaluation of programming ~ 93282-93284,
      93287, 93640-93642
  insertion single/dual chamber
    electrodes ~ 33216-33217, 33224-33225,
      33249
    pulse generator ~ 33240
  removal single/dual chamber
    electrodes ~ 33243-33244
    pulse generator ~ 33241
  repair ~ 33218-33220
  repositioning single/dual chamber
    electrodes ~ 33215, 33226
  revise pocket chest ~ 33223
  wearable device ~ 93745
Deformity, boutonniere ~ 26426-26428
Deformity, Sprengel's ~ 23400
Degenerative, articular cartilage, patella ~
  27418
Degradation products, fibrin ~ 85362-85380
Dehydroepiandrosterone ~ 82626
Dehydroepiandrosterone sulfate ~ 82627
Dehydrogenase, 6-phosphogluconate ~ 84085
Dehydrogenase, alcohol ~ 84588
Dehydrogenase, glucose-6-phosphate ~
  82955-82960
Dehydrogenase, glutamate ~ 82965
Dehydrogenase, isocitrate ~ 83570
Dehydrogenase, lactate ~ 83615-83625
Dehydrogenase, malate ~ 83775
Dehydroisoandrosterone sulfate ~ 82626
Delay of flap, skin graft ~ 15600-15630
Deligation, ureter ~ 50940
Deliveries, abdominal ~ see cesarean delivery
Delivery ~ see cesarean delivery; vaginal
  delivery
Delorme operation ~ see pericardiectomy
Denervation
hip
  femoral ~ 27035
  obturator ~ 27035
  sciatic ~ 27035
Denervation, sympathetic ~ 64802-64818

1387

Dens axis ~ 22548
Denver developmental screening test ~ 96100
Denver shuntpatency test ~ 78291
Denver Krupic procedure ~ 66180
Denver-Krupin procedure ~ 66180
Deoxycorticosterone ~ 82633
Deoxycortisol ~ 80436, 82634
Deoxyephedrine ~ 82145
Deoxyribonuclease antibody ~ 86215
Deoxyribonuclease I ~ 86215
Deoxyribonucleic acid antibody ~
  86225-86226
Depilation ~ see removal, hair
Depletion
  plasma ~ 38214
  platelet ~ 38213
  T-cell ~ 38210
  tumor cell ~ 38211
Deposit calcium ~ 82310, 82330, 82340
Depth electrode
  insertion ~ 61760
Derma-fat-fascia graft ~ 15770
Dermabrasion ~ 15780-15783
Dermatology medical procedures ~
  96900-96999
  actinotherapy ~ 96900
  examination of hair, microscopic ~ 96902
  ultraviolet A treatment ~ 96912
  ultraviolet B treatment ~ 96910-96913
  ultraviolet light treatment ~ 96900-96913
  unlisted services and procedures ~ 96999
Dermatoplasty, septal ~ 30620
Dermoid ~ 30124-30125
Derrick-Burnet disease ~ 86000, 86638
Descending abdominal aorta ~ see aorta,
  abdominal
Desipramine, assay ~ 80160
Desmotomy ~ 23415, 29848
Desoxycorticosterone ~ 82633
Desoxycortone ~ 82633
Desoxyephedrine ~ 82145
Desoxynorephedrin ~ 82145
Desoxyphenobarbital ~ 80188
Desquamation ~ 17360
Destruction
  acne ~ 17340-17360
    cryotherapy ~ 17340
  arrhythmogenic focus, heart ~ 33250-33251,
    33261
  bladder ~ 51020, 52214-52224, 52354
  calculus
    bile duct ~ 43265
    kidney ~ 50590
    pancreatic duct ~ 43265
  chemical cauterization, granulation tissue ~
    17250
  chemosurgery ~ 17110-17111
  ciliary body
    cryotherapy ~ 66720
    cyclodialysis ~ 66740
    cyclophotocoagulation ~ 66710-66711

Destruction ~ continued
  diathermy ~ 66700
  endoscopic ~ 66711
  cryosurgery ~ 17110-17111
  cyst
    abdomen ~ 49203-49205
    ciliary body ~ 66770
    iris ~ 66770
  endometrial ablation ~ 58356
  endometriomas
    abdomen ~ 49203-49205
  fissure, anal ~ 46940-46942
  hemorrhoids, thermal ~ 46930
  kidney ~ 52354
    endoscopic ~ 50557, 50576
  laser surgery ~ 17110-17111
  lesion
    anal ~ 46900-46917, 46924
    bladder ~ 51030
    choroid ~ 67220-67225
    ciliary body ~ 66770
    colon ~ 45383
    conjunctiva ~ 68135
    cornea ~ 65450
    eyelid ~ 67850
    facial ~ 17000-17004, 17280-17286
    gastrointestinal, upper ~ 43258
    gums ~ 41850
    intestines
      large ~ 44393
      small ~ 44369
    iris ~ 66770
    mouth ~ 40820
    nerve plantar ~ 64632
    nose, intranasal ~ 30117-30118
    palate ~ 42160
    penis
      cryosurgery ~ 54056
      electrodesiccation ~ 54055
      extensive ~ 54065
      laser surgery ~ 54057
      simple ~ 54050-54060
      surgical excision ~ 54060
    pharynx ~ 42808
    prostrate ~ 45320
      thermotherapy ~ 53850-53852
        microwave ~ 53850
        radio frequency ~ 53852
    rectum ~ 45320
    retina
      cryotherapy, diathermy ~ 67208, 67227
      photocoagulation ~ 67210, 67228-67229
      radiation by implantation of source ~ 67218
    skin
      benign ~ 17110-17111, 17106-17250
      malignant ~ 17260-17286, 96567
      premalignant ~ 17000-17004, 96567
    spinal cord ~ 62280-62282
    ureter ~ 52341-52342, 52344-52345
    urethra ~ 52400, 53265

Destruction ~ *continued*
uvula ~ 42160
vagina
  extensive ~ 57065
  simple ~ 57061
  vascular, cutaneous ~ 17106-17108
vulva
  extensive ~ 56515
  simple ~ 56501
molluscum contagiosum ~ 17110-17111
muscle endplate
  extraocular ~ 67345
  extremity ~ 64614
  facial ~ 64612
  neck ~ 64613
  trunk ~ 64614
nerve ~ 64600-64640, 64680-64681
  laryngeal, recurrent ~ 31595
polyp
  aural ~ 69540
  nose ~ 30110-30115
  urethra ~ 53260
prostate ~ 55873
prostate tissue, transurethral thermotherapy ~ 53850-53852
sinus, frontal ~ 31080-31085
Skene's gland ~ 53270
skin lesion
  benign ~ 17110-17111
  malignant ~ 17260-17286
    by photodynamic therapy ~ 96567
  premalignant ~ 17000-17004
    2-14 lesions ~ 17003
    15 or more lesions ~ 17004
    by photodynamic therapy ~ 96567
tonsil, lingual ~ 42870
tumor
  abdomen ~ 49203-49205
  bile duct ~ 43272
  colon ~ 45383
  intestines
    large ~ 44393
    small ~ 44369
  mesentery ~ 49203-49205
  pancreatic duct ~ 43272
  rectum ~ 45190, 46937-46938
  retroperitoneal ~ 49203-49205
  urethra ~ 53220
tumor or polyp, rectum ~ 45320
turbinate mucosa ~ 30801-30802
ureter ~ 52354
  endoscopic ~ 50957, 50976
urethra ~ 52214-52224, 52354
  prolapse ~ 53275
warts, flat ~ 17110-17111
with cystourethroscopy ~ 52354
Determination, blood pressure ~ see blood pressure
Developmental testing ~ 96110-96111

Device
iliac artery occlusion device insertion ~ 34808
venous access
  collection of blood specimen ~ 36591
  fluoroscopic guidance ~ 36598, 77001
  insertion
    central ~ 36560-36566
    peripheral ~ 36570-36571
  obstruction clearance ~ 36595-36596
    imaging ~ 75901-75902
  removal ~ 36590
  repair ~ 36576
  replacement ~ 36582-36583, 36585
    catheter ~ 36578
ventricular assist
  extracorporeal
    removal ~ 33990-33993
    replacement ~ 33981
  implantable
    removal ~ 33980
    replacement ~ 33982-33983
Device, intrauterine ~ 58300-58301
Device, orthotic ~ 97760, 97762
Device handling ~ 99002
Dexamethasone suppression test ~ 80420
DHA sulfate ~ 82627
Dhea ~ 82626
Dhea sulfate ~ 82627
DHT ~ 82651
Diagnosis, psychiatric ~ see psychiatric diagnosis
Diagnostic amniocentesis ~ 59000
Diagnostic aspiration of anterior chamber of eye ~ 65800
Diagnostic radiology ~ 70010-76499
Diagnostic skin and sensitization tests ~ see allergy tests
Diagnostic ultrasound ~ 76506-76999
Diagnostic ultrasound of heart ~ see echocardiography
Dialyses, peritoneal ~ 90945-90947
  plan of care documented ~ 0507F
Dialysis
arteriovenous fistula revision without thrombectomy ~ 36832
arteriovenous shunt ~ 36147-36148
  revision with thrombectomy ~ 36833
  thrombectomy ~ 36831
end stage renal disease ~ 90951-90970
hemodialysis ~ 90935-90937, 4051F-4054F
  blood flow study ~ 90940
  plan of care documented ~ 0505F
hemoperfusion ~ 90997
Kt/V level ~ 3082F-3084F
patient training
  completed course ~ 90989
  per session ~ 90993
peritoneal ~ 90945-90947, 4055F
  plan of care documented ~ 0507F
unlisted services and procedures ~ 90999
Dialysis, extracorporeal ~ 90935-90937

1389

Diaphragm
repair
for eventration ~ 39545
hernia ~ 39503-39541
laceration ~ 39501
resection ~ 39560-39561
unlisted procedures ~ 39599
vagina
fitting ~ 57170
Diaphragm contraception ~ 57170
Diaphysectomy
calcaneus ~ 28120
clavicle ~ 23180
femur ~ 27360
fibula ~ 27360, 27641
humerus ~ 23184, 24140
metacarpal ~ 26230
metatarsal ~ 28122
olecranon process ~ 24147
phalanges
finger ~ 26235-26236
toe ~ 28124
radius ~ 24145, 25151
scapula ~ 23182
talus ~ 28120
tarsal ~ 28122
tibia ~ 27360, 27640
ulna ~ 24147, 25150
Diastase ~ 82150
Diastasis ~ see separation
Diathermy ~ 97024
destruction ciliary body ~ 66700
lesion retina ~ 67208, 67227
retinal detachment
prophylaxis ~ 67141
repair ~ 67101
surgical ~ 17000-17286
Dibucaine number ~ 82638
Dichloride, methylene ~ 84600
Dichlorides, ethylene ~ 84600
Dichloroethane ~ 84600
Dichloromethane ~ 84600
Diethylamide, lysergic acid ~ 80102-80103, 80299
Diethylether ~ 84600
Differential count ~ 85032, 85048, 89055
Differentiation reversal factor ~ 85210
Diffusion test, gel ~ 86329-86331
Digestive system, surgical procedures ~ 40490-49999
Digestive tract ~ see gastrointestinal tract
Digit replantation ~ 20816-20822
Digital artery sympathectomy ~ 64820
Digital slit-beam radiograph ~ see scanogram
Digits pinch graft ~ 15050
Digoxin assay ~ 80162
Dihydrocodeinone ~ 82646
Dihydrocodeinone screen ~ 82486
Dihydroepitestosterone ~ 82651
Dihydrohydroxycodeinone ~ 80102-80103, 83925
Dihydromorphinone ~ 82486, 82649

Dihydrotestosterone ~ 82651
Dihydroxyethanes ~ 82693
Dihydroxyvitamin D ~ 82652
Dilatation, transluminal arterial ~ 75962-75968
Dilation ~ 59840
anal
endoscopy ~ 46604
sphincter ~ 45905
bile duct
endoscopy ~ 43271, 47555-47556
stricture ~ 74363
bladdercystourethroscopy ~ 52260-52265
bronchiendoscopy ~ 31630, 31636-31638
cervix
canal ~ 57800
stump ~ 57558
colon endoscopy ~ 45386
colon-sigmoid endoscopy ~ 45340
esophagus ~ 43450-43458
balloon ~ 43220, 43249
endoscopy ~ 43220, 43226, 43249
surgical ~ 43510
intestines, small endoscopy ~ 44370
kidney ~ 50395
intra-renal stricture ~ 52343, 52346
lacrimal punctum ~ 68801
larynx
endoscopy ~ 31528-31529
nasal/sinus endoscopy ~ 31295-31297
pancreatic duct
endoscopy ~ 43271
rectum
endoscopy ~ 45303
sphincter ~ 45910
salivary duct ~ 42650-42660
trachea
endoscopy ~ 31630-31631, 31636-31638
transluminal, aqueous outflow canal ~ 66174-66175
ureter ~ 50395, 52341-52342, 52344-52345
endoscopy ~ 50553, 50572, 50953, 50972
urethra ~ 52260-52265
general ~ 53665
suppository and/or instillation ~ 53660-53661
urethral
stenosis ~ 52281
stricture ~ 52281, 53600-53621
vagina ~ 57400
Dilation and curettage ~ 59840
cervix ~ 57558, 57800
corpus uteri ~ 58120
hysteroscopy ~ 58558
postpartum ~ 59160
with amniotic injections ~ 59851
with vaginal suppositories ~ 59856
Dilation and evacuation ~ 59841
with amniotic injections ~ 59851
Dimethadione ~ 82654
Dioxide, carbon ~ 82374
Dioxide, silicon ~ 84285
Dipeptidyl peptidase A ~ 82164

Diphenylhydantoin ~ 80185-80186
Diphosphate, adenosine ~ 82030
Diphtheria ~ 86648
Dipropylacetic acid assay ~ 80164
Direct pedicle flap formation ~ 15570-15576
Disability evaluation services
basic life and/or disability evaluation ~ 99450
work-related or medical disability evaluation ~ 99455-99456
Disarticulation
ankle ~ 27889
hip ~ 27295
knee ~ 27598
shoulder ~ 23920-23921
wrist ~ 25920, 25924
revision ~ 25922
Disc, intervertebral ~ see intervertebral disk
Discectomies ~ 63075-63078
percutaneous ~ 62287
Discharge, body substance ~ see drainage
Discharge services
hospital ~ 99238-99239
nursing facility ~ 99315-99316
observation care ~ 99234-99236
Discission
cataract
laser surgery ~ 66821
stab incision ~ 66820
vitreous strands ~ 67030
Discography ~ see diskography
Discolysis ~ 62292
Disease
Durand-Nicolas-Favre ~ 86729
Erb-Goldflam ~ 95857
Heine-Medin ~ see polio
hydatid ~ see echinococcosis
Lyme ~ see Lyme disease
Ormond ~ see retroperitoneal fibrosis
Peyronie ~ see Peyronie disease
Posada-Wernicke ~ 86490
Disease/organ panel ~ see organ or disease
oriented panel
Diskectomy ~ 63075-63078
additional segment ~ 22226
arthrodesis
additional interspace ~ 22534, 22585
cervical ~ 22554
lumbar ~ 22533, 22558, 22630
thoracic ~ 22532, 22556
cervical ~ 22220
lumbar ~ 22224, 22630
percutaneous ~ 62287
thoracic ~ 22222
Diskography
cervical disk ~ 72285
injection ~ 62290-62291
lumbar disk ~ 72295
thoracic ~ 72285
Disk chemolyses, intervertebral ~ 62292
Dislocated joint ~ see dislocation

Dislocation
acromioclavicular joint, open treatment ~
23550-23552
ankle
closed treatment ~ 27840-27842
open treatment ~ 27846-27848
carpal
closed treatment ~ 25690
open treatment ~ 25695
carpometacarpal joint ~ 26670
closed treatment
with manipulation ~ 26675-26676
open treatment ~ 26685-26686
percutaneous fixation ~ 26676
clavicle
closed treatment ~ 23540-23545
open treatment ~ 23550-23552
without manipulation ~ 23540
with manipulation ~ 23545
closed treatment
carpometacarpal joint ~ 26670-26675
metacarpophalangeal ~ 26700-26706
thumb ~ 26641
elbow
closed treatment ~ 24600-24605, 24640
open treatment ~ 24615
hip joint
closed treatment ~ 27250-27252,
27265-27266
congenital ~ 27256-27259
open treatment ~ 27253-27254, 27258-27259
without trauma ~ 27265-27266
interphalangeal joint
closed treatment ~ 26770-26775
open treatment ~ 26785
percutaneous fixation ~ 26776
toe
closed treatment ~ 28660-28665
open treatment ~ 28675
percutaneous fixation ~ 26770-26776,
28666
with manipulation ~ 26770
knee ~ 27560-27562
closed treatment ~ 27550-27552,
27560-27562
open treatment ~ 27556-27558, 27566,
27730
recurrent ~ 27420-27424
lunate
closed treatment ~ 25690
open treatment ~ 25695
with manipulation ~ 25690, 26670-26676,
26700-26706
metacarpophalangeal joint
closed treatment ~ 26700-26706
open treatment ~ 26715
metatarsophalangeal joint
closed treatment ~ 28630-28635
open treatment ~ 28645
percutaneous fixation ~ 28636
open treatment ~ 26685-26686

1391

Dislocation ~ *continued*
patella
  closed treatment ~ 27560-27562
  open treatment ~ 27566
  recurrent ~ 27420-27424
pelvic ring
  closed treatment ~ 27193-27194
  open treatment ~ 27217-27218
  percutaneous fixation ~ 27216
  without manipulation ~ 27193-27194
percutaneous fixation
  metacarpophalangeal ~ 26705
peroneal tendons ~ 27675-27676
radiocarpal joint ~ 25660
radio-ulnar joint ~ 25520-25526
radius
  closed treatment ~ 24640
  with fracture
    closed treatment ~ 24620
    open treatment ~ 24635
shoulder
  closed treatment with manipulation ~ 23650-23655
  open treatment ~ 23660
  with greater tuberosity fracture
    closed treatment ~ 23665
    open treatment ~ 23670
  with surgical or anatomical neck fracture
    closed treatment ~ 23675
    open treatment ~ 23680
skin debridement ~ 11010-11012
sternoclavicular joint
  closed treatment
    without manipulation ~ 23520
    with manipulation ~ 23525
  open treatment ~ 23530-23532
talotarsal joint
  closed treatment ~ 28570-28575
  open treatment ~ 28546
  percutaneous fixation ~ 28576
tarsal
  closed treatment ~ 28540-28545
  open treatment ~ 28555
  percutaneous fixation ~ 28546
tarsometatarsal joint
  closed treatment ~ 28600-28605
  open treatment ~ 28615
  percutaneous fixation ~ 28606
temporomandibular joint
  closed treatment ~ 21480-21485
  open treatment ~ 21490
thumb
  closed treatment ~ 26641-26645
  open treatment ~ 26665
  percutaneous fixation ~ 26650
  with fracture ~ 26645
    open treatment ~ 26665
    percutaneous fixation ~ 26650-26665
  with manipulation ~ 26641-26650
tibiofibular joint
  closed treatment ~ 27830-27831
  open treatment ~ 27832

Dislocation ~ *continued*
vertebra
  additional segment, open treatment ~ 22328
  cervical
    open treatment ~ 22326
    closed treatment ~ 22305
    without manipulation ~ 22310
    with manipulation, casting and/or bracing ~ 22315
  lumbar, open treatment ~ 22325
  thoracic, open treatment ~ 22327
wrist
  closed treatment ~ 25660, 25675, 25680
  intercarpal ~ 25660
    open treatment ~ 25670
  open treatment ~ 25670, 25685
  percutaneous fixation ~ 25671
  radiocarpal ~ 25660
    open treatment ~ 25670
  radioulnar
    closed treatment ~ 25675
    open treatment ~ 25676
    percutaneous fixation ~ 25671
  with fracture
    closed treatment ~ 25680
    open treatment ~ 25685
  with manipulation ~ 25660, 25675, 25680
Disorder
blood coagulation ~ 85390
penis ~ see penis
retinal ~ see retina
Displacement therapy
nose ~ 30210
Dissection
hygroma, cystic
  axillary/cervical ~ 38550-38555
lymph nodes ~ 38542
neck, radical ~ see radical neck dissection
Distention ~ see dilation
Diverticula, Meckel's ~ 44800
Diverticulectomy ~ 44800
esophagus ~ 43130-43135
Meckel's ~ 44800
Diverticulum
bladder ~ see bladder, diverticulum
Meckel's, excision ~ 44800
repair, urethra ~ 53400-53405
Division
isthmus, horseshoe kidney ~ 50540
muscle, foot ~ 28250
plantar fascia, foot ~ 28250
Division, scalenus anticus muscle ~ 21700-21705
Di-amphetamine ~ 82145
DMO ~ 82654
DNA antibody ~ 86225-86226
endonuclease ~ 86215
DNAse antibody ~ 86215
Domiciliary services ~ 99324-99340
discharge services ~ 99315-99316
established patient ~ 99331-99333
new patient ~ 99321-99323

1392

Donor procedures
conjunctival graft ~ 68371
heart/lung excision ~ 33930
heart excision ~ 33940
liver segment ~ 47140-47142
stem cells
donor search ~ 38204
Dopamine ~ 80424, 82382-82384
blood ~ 82383-82384
urine ~ 82382, 82384
Doppler echocardiography ~ 76827-76828,
93306-93308, 93320-93350
intracardiac ~ 93662
transesophageal ~ 93318
transthoracic ~ 93303-93317
Doppler scan
arterial studies
extremities ~ 93922-93924
fetal
middle cerebral artery ~ 76821
umbilical artery ~ 76820
extremities ~ 93965
intracranial arteries ~ 93886-93893
Dorsal vertebra ~ 22101, 22112
Dosimetry
radiation therapy ~ 77300, 77331
brachytherapy ~ 77326-77328
intensity modulation ~ 77301
teletherapy ~ 77305-77321
Double-stranded DNA ~ 86225-86226
Doxepin
assay ~ 80166
DPH ~ 80185-80186
Drainage ~ see also excision; incision; incision
and drainage
abdomen
abdomen fluid ~ 49082-49083
abscess
appendix ~ 44900-.44901
percutaneous ~ 44901
brain ~ 61150-61151
eyelid ~ 67700
liver ~ 47010-47011
ovary, percutaneous ~ 58823
pelvic, percutaneous ~ 58823
pericolic, percutaneous ~ 58823
perirenal or renal ~ 50020-50021
percutaneous ~ 50021
prostate ~ 52700
retroperitoneal ~ 49060-49061
percutaneous ~ 49061
subdiaphragmatic or subphrenic ~
49040-49041
percutaneous ~ 49040-49041
with X-ray ~ 75989
amniotic fluid
diagnostic aspiration ~ 59000
therapeutic aspiration ~ 59001
bile duct, transhepatic ~ 75980
brain fluid ~ 61070
bursa ~ 20600-20610

Drainage ~ continued
cerebrospinal fluid ~ 61000-61020, 61050,
61070, 62272
cervical fluid ~ 61050
cisternal fluid ~ 61050
cyst
bone ~ 20615
brain ~ 61150-61151, 62161-62162
breast ~ 19000-19001
ganglion ~ 20612
liver ~ 47010-47011
percutaneous ~ 47011
salivary gland ~ 42409
sublingual gland ~ 42409
with fistula ~ 42325-42326
extraperitoneal lymphocele
laparoscopic ~ 49323
open ~ 49062
eye
anterior chamber paracentesis
with diagnostic aspiration of aqueous ~
65800
with therapeutic release of aqueous ~
65800
removal blood ~ 65815
removal of vitreous and/or discission anterior
hyaloid membrane ~ 65810
fetal fluid ~ 59074
ganglion cyst ~ 20612
hematoma
brain ~ 61154-61156
vagina ~ 57022-57023
hematoma, subungual ~ 11740
joint ~ 20600-20610
liver
abscess or cyst ~ 47010-47011
percutaneous ~ 47011
lymphocele, endoscopic ~ 49323
onychia ~ 10060-10061
orbit ~ 67405, 67440
pancreas
pseudocyst ~ 48510-48511
percutaneous ~ 48511
paronychia ~ 10060-10061
pericardial sac ~ 32659
pericardium ~ 33010-33011
pseudocyst
gastrointestinal, upper
transmural endoscopic ~ 43240
pancreas ~ 48510
open ~ 48510
percutaneous ~ 48511
puncture
chest ~ 32554-32555
skin ~ 10040-10180
spinal cord
cerebrospinal fluid ~ 62272
subdural fluid ~ 61000-61001
urethra
extravasation ~ 53080-53085
ventricular fluid ~ 61020
Drainage implant, glaucoma ~ 66180, 66185

1393

Dressings
burns ~ 16010-16030
change
anesthesia ~ 15852
Drez procedure ~ see incision, spinal cord ~ 63200
Dril ~ 36838
Drill hole, skull
catheter ~ 61107
drain hematoma ~ 61108
exploration ~ 61105
implant electrode ~ 61850, 61863-61868
Drinking test for glaucoma ~ 92140
Drug ~ see drug assay; specific drug
analysis
tissue preparation ~ 80103
aspirin ~ 4084F
confirmation ~ 80102
infusion ~ 62360-62362
therapy
bisphosphonate ~ 4100F
Drugs, anticoagulant ~ 85300-85305, 85307
Drug assay
amikacin ~ 80150
amitriptyline ~ 80152
benzodiazepine ~ 80154
carbamazepine ~ 80156-80157
cyclosporine ~ 80158
desipramine ~ 80160
digoxin ~ 80162
dipropylacetic acid ~ 80164
doxepin ~ 80166
ethosuximide ~ 80168
gentamicin ~ 80170
gold ~ 80172
haloperidol ~ 80173
imipramine ~ 80174
lidocaine ~ 80176
lithium ~ 80178
nortriptyline ~ 80182
phenobarbital ~ 80184
phenytoin ~ 80185-80186
primidone ~ 80188
procainamide ~ 80190-80192
quantitative, other ~ 80299
quinidine ~ 80194
salicylate ~ 80196
tacrolimus ~ 80197
theophylline ~ 80198
Tobramycin ~ 80200
topiramate ~ 80201
vancomycin ~ 80202
Drug delivery implant
insertion ~ 11981
maintenance and refill
brain ~ 95990
epidural ~ 95990-95991
intra-arterial ~ 96530
intrathecal ~ 95990-95991
intravenous ~ 96530
intraventricular ~ 95990-95991

Drug delivery implant ~ *continued*
removal ~ 11982-11983
with reinsertion ~ 11983
Drug instillation ~ see instillation, drugs
Drug management
by pharmacist ~ 99605-99607
psychiatric ~ 90863
Drug screen ~ 80100-80101, 82486
Drug testing ~ 80100-80103
DST ~ 80420
DTaP-HepB-IPV immunization ~ 90723
DTaP immunization ~ 90721
DTP immunization ~ 90720
DT shots ~ 90702
Dual X-ray absorptiometry (DXA) ~ 3095F-3096F
appendicular ~ 77081
axial skeleton ~ 77080
vertebral fracture ~ 77082
Dual photon absorptiomety ~ 78351
Duct
bile ~ see bile duct
hepatic ~ see hepatic duct
nasolacrimal ~ see nasolacrimal duct
omphalomesenteric ~ 44800
pancreatic ~ see pancreatic duct
salivary ~ see salivary duct
Stensen's ~ see parotid duct
thoracic ~ see thoracic duct
Ductogram, mammary ~ galactogram
Ductus arteriosus repair ~ 33820-33824
Ductus deferens ~ see vas deferens
Duhamel procedure ~ 45110, 45112, 45119-45120
Dunn operation ~ 28730-28735, 28740
Duodenostomy
contrast ~ 49465
insertion ~ 49441
obstructive material removal ~ 49460
radiological evaluation ~ 49465
replacement ~ 49451
Duodenotomy ~ 44010
Duodenum
biopsy ~ 44010
exclusion ~ 48547
exploration ~ 44010
incision ~ 44010
intubation and aspiration ~ 43756-43757
removal, foreign body ~ 44010
X-ray ~ 74260
Duplex scan ~ see vascular studies
arterial studies
aorta ~ 93978-93979
extracranial ~ 93880-93882
lower extremity ~ 93925-93926
penile ~ 93980-93981
upper extremity ~ 93930-93931
visceral ~ 93975-93979
hemodialysis access ~ 93990
venous studies
extremity ~ 93970-93971
penile ~ 93980-93981

ALPHABETICAL INDEX

Dupuy-Dutemp operation ~ see reconstruction, eyelid; revision
Dupuytren's contracture
fasciotomy ~ 26040-26045
injection, enzyme ~ 20527
manipulation ~ 26341
Durand-Nicolas-Favre disease ~ 86729
Dust, Angel ~ 83992
Duvries operation ~ 01714
Dwyer procedure ~ 28300
DXA ~ see dual X-ray absorptiometry (DXA)
Dynamometry ~ 28300
venous studies ~ 28300
with ophthalmoscopy ~ 92260
D & C yellow no. 7 (seven) ~ see fluorescein
D 2, vitamin ~ 82306
D galactose ~ 82760
D glucose ~ 80422-80424, 80430-80435, 95250-95251
D vitamin ~ 82306, 82652

E

E1 ~ 82679
E2 ~ 82670
E3 ~ 82677
Ear
collection of blood ~ 36415-36416
drum ~ 69420-69421, 69433-69436, 69450, 69610-69620
external
abscess incision and drainage
complicated ~ 69005
simple ~ 69000
biopsy ~ 69100
excision
partial ~ 69110
total ~ 69120
hematoma, incision and drainage ~ 69000-69005
reconstruction ~ 69300
unlisted services and procedures ~ 69399
inner
CT scan ~ 70480-70482
excision labyrinth ~ 69905-69910
exploration endolymphatic sac ~ 69805-69806
incision ~ 69820
labyrinth ~ 69801
semicircular canal ~ 69840
insertion cochlear device ~ 69930
semicircular canal ~ 69820
unlisted services and procedures ~ 69949
middle
catheterization ~ 69405
CT scan ~ 70480-70482
exploration ~ 69440

Ear ~ *continued*
inflation
with catheterization ~ 69400
without catheterization ~ 69401
insertion
baffle ~ 69410
catheter ~ 69405
lesion excision ~ 69540
reconstruction
tympanoplasty with antrotomy or mastoidectomy ~ 69635-69637
tympanoplasty with mastoidectomy ~ 69641-69646
tympanoplasty without mastoidectomy ~ 69631-69633
removal ventilating tube ~ 69424
repair
oval window ~ 69666
round window ~ 69667
revision, stapes ~ 69662
tumor excision ~ 69550-69554
unlisted services and procedures ~ 69799
outer, CT scan ~ 70480-70482
Ear canal ~ see auditory canal
Ear cartilage graft to face ~ 21235
Ear lobes, pierce ~ 69090
Ear, nose, and throat ~ see also hearing aid
services ~ 92700
audiologic function tests
acoustic reflex ~ 92568
acoustic reflex decay ~ 92570
audiometry
Bekesy ~ 92560-92561
comprehensive ~ 92557
conditioning play ~ 92582
evoked response ~ 92585-92586
groups ~ 92559
pure tone ~ 92552-92553
select picture ~ 92583
speech ~ 92555-92556
brainstem evoked response ~ 92585-92586
central auditory function ~ 92620-92621
ear protector evaluation ~ 92596
electrocochleography ~ 92584
filtered speech ~ 92571
hearing aid evaluation ~ 92590-92595
Lombard test ~ 92700
loudness balance ~ 92562
screening test ~ 92551
sensorineural acuity ~ 92575
short increment sensitivity index (SISI) ~ 92564
staggered spondaic word test ~ 92572
Stenger test ~ 92565, 92577
synthetic sentence test ~ 92576
tone decay ~ 92563
tympanometry ~ 92567
audiometry
evoked otoacoustic emissions ~ 92587-92588
visual reinforcement ~ 92579
binocular microscopy ~ 92504

1395

Ear, nose, and throat ~ *continued*
facial nerve function study ~ 92516
hearing, language, and speech evaluation ~ 92506
laryngeal function study ~ 92520
nasal function study ~ 92512
nasopharyngoscopy ~ 92511
vestibular function tests
    additional electrodes ~ 92547
    basic ~ 92540
    caloric tests ~ 92533, 92543
    nystagmus
        optokinetic ~ 92534, 92544
        positional ~ 92532, 92542
        spontaneous ~ 92531, 92541
    posturography ~ 92548
    torsion swing test ~ 92546
    tracking tests ~ 92545
Ear protector attenuation ~ see also hearing aid services ~ 92596
Ear wax ~ 69210
Ebstein anomaly repair ~ 33468
ECG ~ see electrocardiography
Echinococcosis ~ 86171, 86280
Echocardiography
cardiac ~ 93320-93350
    intracardiac ~ 93662
    transesophageal ~ 93318
    transthoracic ~ 93303-93317
        with stress test ~ 93350-93352
    Doppler ~ 93303-93317, 93320-93321, 93662
fetal heart ~ 76825-76826
    Doppler
        complete ~ 76827
        follow-up or repeat study ~ 76828
for congenital anomalies
    transesophageal ~ 93315-93317
    transthoracic ~ 93303-93304
intracardiac ~ 93662
transesophageal ~ 93318
    for congenital anomalies ~ 93315-93317
transthoracic ~ 93303-93318, 93350
    for congenital anomalies ~ 93303-93304
    with stress test ~ 93350-93352
Echoencephalography ~ 76506
Echography
abdomen ~ 76700-76705
arm ~ 76881, 76882
breast ~ 76645
cardiac ~ 93303-93317, 93320-93321, 93350-93352, 93662
    guidance ~ 76932
chest ~ 76604
extracranial arteries ~ 93880-93882
eyes ~ 76510-76529
follow-up ~ 76970
head ~ 76536
heart imaging guidance ~ 76932
hip infant ~ 76885-76886
intracranial arteries ~ 93886-93893
intraoperative ~ 76998

Echography ~ *continued*
kidney transplant ~ 76776
leg ~ 76881, 76882
neck ~ 76536
pelvis ~ 76856-76857
placement therapy fields ~ 76950
pregnant uterus ~ 76801-76828
prostate ~ 76872-76873
retroperitoneal ~ 76770-76775
scrotum ~ 76870
spine ~ 76800
transvaginal ~ 76817, 76830
unlisted services and procedures ~ 76999
vagina ~ 76817, 76830
Echotomography ~ see echography
ECMO ~ see extracorporeal membrane oxygenation
ECS ~ see emission computerized tomography
ECSF (erythrocyte colony stimulating factor) ~ 82668
ECT ~ see emission computerized tomography
Ectasia ~ see dilation
Ectopic pregnancy ~ see obstetrical care
abdominal ~ 59130
cervix ~ 59140
interstitial
    partial resection uterus ~ 59136
    total hysterectomy ~ 59135
laparoscopy ~ 59150
    with salpingectomy and/or oophorectomy ~ 59151
tubal ~ 59121
    with salpingectomy and/or oophorectomy ~ 59120
Ectropion, repair
excision tarsal wedge ~ 67916
extensive ~ 67917
suture ~ 67914
thermocauterization ~ 67915
Education services
group ~ 98961-98962, 99078
individual
    pediatric gastroenteritis ~ 4058F
Education supplies ~ 99071
EEG ~ see electroencephalography (EEG)
Egg (ova) ~ 87177
Ehrlichia antibody ~ 86666
EKG ~ see electrocardiogram
Elastase ~ 82656
Elbow ~ see also humerus; radius; ulna
abscess, incision and drainage ~ 23930, 23935
anesthesia ~ 00400, 01710-01782
arthrectomy ~ 24155
arthrocentesis ~ 20605
arthrodesis ~ 24800-24802
arthroplasty ~ 24360
    with implant ~ 24361-24362
    total replacement ~ 24363
arthroscopy
    diagnostic ~ 29830
    surgical ~ 29834-29838

Elbow ~ *continued*
  arthrotomy ~ 24000
    capsular release ~ 24006
    with joint exploration ~ 24101
    with synovectomy ~ 24102
    with synovial biopsy ~ 24101
  biopsy ~ 24065-24066, 24101
  bursa, incision and drainage ~ 23931
  dislocation
    closed treatment ~ 24600-24605, 24640
    open treatment ~ 24615
    subluxate ~ 24640
  excision ~ 24155
    bursa ~ 24105
    synovium ~ 24102
  exploration ~ 24000, 24101
  fracture
    Monteggia ~ 24620-24635
      open treatment ~ 24586-24587
  hematoma, incision and drainage ~ 23930
  implant, removal ~ 24164
  incision and drainage ~ 24000
  injection, arthrography, radiologic ~ 24220
  magnetic resonance imaging (MRI) ~ 73221
  manipulation ~ 24300
  radical resection, capsule, soft tissue and bone
    with contracture release ~ 24149
  removal
    foreign body ~ 24000, 24101, 24200-24201
    implant ~ 24160
    loose body ~ 24101
  repair
    epicondylitis ~ 24357-24359
    flexorplasty ~ 24330
    hemiepiphyseal arrest ~ 24470
    ligament ~ 24343-24346
    muscle ~ 24341
    muscle transfer ~ 24301
    tendon ~ 24340-24342
      lengthening ~ 24305
      transfer ~ 24301
    tennis elbow ~ 24357-24359
  Steindler advancement ~ 24330
  strapping ~ 29260
  tumor excision ~ 24071-24079
  unlisted services and procedures ~ 24999
  X-ray ~ 73070-73080
    with contrast ~ 73085
Elbow, golfer ~ 24357-24359
Elbows, tennis ~ 24357-24359
Electrical stimulation
  bone healing
    invasive ~ 20975
    noninvasive ~ 20974
  brain surface ~ 95961-95962
  physical therapy
    attended, manual ~ 97032
    unattended ~ 97014
Electric countershock ~ 92960-92961
Electric stimulation, transcutaneous ~ 64550
Electro-hydraulic procedure ~ 52325

Electro-oculography ~ 92270
Electroanalgesia ~ 64550
Electrocardiography
  12-lead ~ 3120F
  24-hour monitoring ~ 93224-93229
  evaluation ~ 93000, 93010, 93660
  rhythm
    evaluation ~ 93042
    microvolt T-wave alternans ~ 93025
    tracing ~ 93041
    tracing and evaluation ~ 93040
  signal averaged ~ 93278
  wearable patient-activated recording
    transmission and evaluation ~ 93268, 93270
      interpretation ~ 93272
      monitoring ~ 93271
Electrocautery ~ see also destruction ~
  17000-17286
Electrochemistry ~ 17380
Electroconvulsive therapy ~ 90870-90871
Electrocortiogram, intraoperative ~ 95829
Electrode, depth ~ 61760
Electrodesiccation ~ 17000-17286
  lesion, penis ~ 54055
Electroejaculation ~ 55870
Electroencephalography (EEG) ~ 95816
  brain death ~ 95824
  coma ~ 95822
  digital analysis ~ 95957
  electrode placement ~ 95830
  intraoperative ~ 95955
  monitoring ~ 95812-95813, 95950-95953,
    95956
    with drug activation ~ 95954
    with physical activation ~ 95954
    with wada activation ~ 95958
  sleep ~ 95822, 95827
  standard ~ 95819
Electrogastrography ~ 91132-91133
Electrogram, atrial esophageal recording ~
  93615-93616
Electrolysis ~ 17380
Electromyography
  anorectal with biofeedback ~ 90911
  fine wire dynamic ~ 96004
  needle
    extremities ~ 95861-95864
    extremity ~ 95860
    face and neck muscles ~ 95867-95868
    ocular ~ 92265
    other than thoracic paraspinal ~ 95870
    single fiber electrode ~ 95872
    thoracic paraspinal muscles ~ 95869
  sphincter muscles
    anus ~ 51784-51785
      needle ~ 51785
    urethra ~ 51784-51785
      needle ~ 51785
  surface dynamic ~ 96002-96004
Electron microscopy ~ 88348-88349

Electronic analysis
  cardioverter-defibrillator, implantable
    data analysis ~ 93289, 93295-93296
    evaluation of programming ~ 93282-94284,
      93287, 93640, 93642
  drug infusion pump ~ 62367-62368
  loop recorder, implantable
    data analysis ~ 93291, 93298-93299
    evaluation of programming ~ 93285
  neurostimulator pulse generator ~
    95970-95982
Electrophoresis
  counterimmuno- ~ 86185
  immuno- ~ 86320-86327
  immunofixation ~ 86334-86335
  protein ~ 84165-84166
  unlisted services and procedures ~ 82664
Electrophysiology procedure ~ 93600-93660
Electroretinogram ~ 92275
Electroretinography ~ 92275
Electrostimulation, analgesic cutaneous ~
  64550
Electrosurgery, trichiasis correction ~ 67825
Electroversion, cardiac ~ 92960-92961
Elevation, scapula, congenital ~ 23400
Elliot operation ~ 66130
Eloesser procedure ~ 32035-32036
Eloesser thoracoplasty ~ 32905
Embolectomy
  aortoiliac artery ~ 34151-34201
  axillary artery ~ 34101
  brachial artery ~ 34101
  carotid artery ~ 34001
  celiac artery ~ 34151
  femoral ~ 34201
  iliac ~ 34151-34201
  innominate artery ~ 34001-34101
  mesentery artery ~ 34151
  peroneal artery ~ 34203
  popliteal artery ~ 34203
  pulmonary artery ~ 33910-33916
  radial artery ~ 34111
  renal artery ~ 34151
  subclavian artery ~ 34001-34101
  tibial artery ~ 34203
  ulnar artery ~ 34111
Embolization
  leiomyomata ~ 37210
Embryo
  biopsy ~ 89290-89291
  cryopreservation ~ 89258
  cryopreserved preparation thawing ~ 89352
  culture ~ 89250
    with co-culture oocyte ~ 89251
  hatching assisted microtechnique ~ 89253
  preparation for transfer ~ 89255
  storage ~ 89342
Embryonated eggs inoculation ~ 87250
Embryo/fetus monitoring ~ 59050-59051,
  99500

Embryo transfer
  in vitro fertilization ~ 58974-58976
  intrafallopian transfer ~ 58976
  intrauterine transfer ~ 58974
Emergency department services ~
  99281-99288
  anesthesia ~ 99140
  physician direction of advanced life support ~
    99288
Emesis induction ~ 99175
EMG ~ see electromyography, needle
Emission-computed tomography,
  single-photon ~ 78607
Emission computerized tomography ~ 78607
EMI scan ~ see CAT scan
Emmet operation ~ 59300
Empyema
  closure, chest wall ~ 32810
  lung ~ 21501-21502
  thoracostomy ~ 32035-32036, 32551
Empyemectomy ~ 32540
Encephalitis
  antibody ~ 86651-86654
Encephalitis virus vaccine ~ 90735
Encephalocele
  repair ~ 62120
    craniotomy ~ 62121
Encephalon ~ see brain
End stage renal disease services ~
  90951-90970
End-expiratory pressure, positive ~ 94660
Endarterectomy
  coronary artery ~ 33572
  pulmonary ~ 33916
Endemic flea-borne typhus ~ 86000
Endobronchial challenge tests ~ 95070-95071
Endocavitary fulguration ~ 17000-17286
Endocrine, pancreas ~ 86341
Endocrine system surgical procedures
  60000-60699
Endolymphatic sac
  exploration
    with shunt ~ 69806
    without shunt ~ 69805
Endometrial ablation ~ 0009T, 58353
  exploration via hysteroscopy ~ 58563
Endometrioma
  abdomen
    destruction/excision ~ 49203-49205, 58957,
      58958
  retroperitoneal
    destruction/excision ~ 49203-49205, 58957,
      58958
Endometriosis, adhesive ~ 58559
Endometrium
  ablation ~ 58356
  biopsy ~ 58100, 58558
Endonuclease, DNA ~ **86215**
Endoscopic retrograde cannulation of
  pancreatic duct (ERCP) ~ 43260
Endoscopies, pleural ~ see thoracoscopy

Endoscopy ~ see arthroscopy; thoracoscopy
  adrenal gland
    biopsy ~ 60650
    excision ~ 60650
  anus
    biopsy ~ 46606
    dilation ~ 46604
    exploration ~ 46600
    hemorrhage ~ 46614
    removal
      foreign body ~ 46608
      polyp ~ 46610, 46612
      tumor ~ 46610, 46612
  atria ~ 33265-33266
  bile duct ~ 43273
    biopsy ~ 47553
    destruction
      calculi (stone) ~ 43265
      tumor ~ 43272
    dilation ~ 43271, 47555-47556
    exploration ~ 47552
    intraoperative ~ 47550
    percutaneous ~ 47552-47555
    removal
      calculi (stone) ~ 43264, 47554
      foreign body ~ 43269
      stent ~ 43269
    specimen collection ~ 43260
    sphincter pressure ~ 43263
    sphincterotomy ~ 43262
    tube placement ~ 43267-43268
  bladder ~ 52000
    biopsy ~ 52204, 52354
    catheterization ~ 52005, 52010
    destruction ~ 52354
      lesion ~ 52400
    evacuation clot ~ 52001
    excision tumor ~ 52355
    exploration ~ 52351
    lithotripsy ~ 52353
    removal calculus ~ 52352
    urethral stent ~ 52282
  bladder neck
    injection of implant material ~ 51715
  brain shunt creation ~ 62201
  bronchi
    aspiration ~ 31645-31646
    biopsy ~ 31625-31629, 31632-31633
    destruction
      lesion ~ 31641
      tumor ~ 31641
    dilation ~ 31630-31631, 31636-31638
    exploration ~ 31622
    injection ~ 31899
    lesion destruction ~ 31641
    needle biopsy ~ 31629, 31633
    placement stent ~ 31631, 31636-31637
    revision stent ~ 31638
    specimen collection ~ 31623-61324
    stenosis ~ 31641
    tumor destruction ~ 31641
    ultrasound ~ 31620

Endoscopy ~ *continued*
  cervix
    biopsy ~ 57454-57455, 57460
    curettage ~ 57454, 57456
    exploration ~ 57452
    loop electrode biopsy ~ 57460
    loop electrode conization ~ 57461
  chest cavity
    exploration ~ 32601-32606
    surgical ~ 32650-32665
  colon
    biopsy ~ 44389, 45380, 45392
    destruction
      lesion ~ 44393, 45383
      tumor ~ 44393, 45383
    exploration ~ 45378
    hemorrhage ~ 44391, 45382
    injection ~ 45381
    placement stent ~ 45387
    removal
      foreign body ~ 44390, 45379
      polyp ~ 44392, 45384-45385
      tumor ~ 44392, 45384-45385
    specimen collection ~ 45380
    ultrasound ~ 45391-45392
    via colotomy ~ 45355
    via stoma ~ 44388-44393, 44397
  colon-sigmoid
    ablation
      polyp ~ 45339
      tumor ~ 45339
    biopsy ~ 45331
    dilation ~ 45340
    exploration ~ 45330, 45335
    hemorrhage ~ 45334
    needle biopsy ~ 45342
    placement stent ~ 45327, 45345
    removal
      foreign body ~ 45332
      polyp ~ 45333, 45338
      tumor ~ 45333, 45338
    specimen collection ~ 45331
    ultrasound ~ 45341-45342
    volvulus ~ 45337
  esophagus
    biopsy ~ 43202
    dilation ~ 43220-43226
    exploration ~ 43200
    hemorrhage ~ 43227
    injection ~ 43201, 43204
    insertion stent ~ 43219
    needle biopsy ~ 43232
    removal
      foreign body ~ 43215
      polyp ~ 43216-43217, 43228
      tumor ~ 43216, 43228
    ultrasound ~ 43231-43232
    vein ligation ~ 43205
  eye ~ 66990
  foot, plantar fasciotomy ~ 29893
  gastrointestinal, upper ~ 3130F-3132F,
    3140F-3141F

1399

Endoscopy ~ *continued*
biopsy ~ 43239
catheterization ~ 43241
destruction of lesion ~ 43258
dilation ~ 43245, 43248-43249
drainage of pseudocyst ~ 43240
exploration ~ -43235
foreign body ~ 43247
gastric bypass ~ 43644-43645
gastroenterostomy ~ 43644-43645
hemorrhage ~ 43255
inject varices ~ 43243
injection ~ 43236
needle biopsy ~ 43238, 43242
referral ~ 3132F
removal ~ 43247, 43250-43251
roux-en-y ~ 43644
stent placement ~ 43256
thermal radiation ~ 43257
tube placement ~ 43246
ultrasound ~ 43237-43242, 43259, 76975
vein ligation ~ 43244
ileum via stoma ~ 44383
intestines, small
biopsy ~ 44361, 44377
destruction
lesion ~ 44369
tumor ~ 44369
diagnostic ~ 44376
exploration ~ 44360
hemorrhage ~ 44366, 44378
insertion
stent ~ 44370, 44379
tube ~ 44379
pelvic pouch ~ 44385-44386
removal
foreign body ~ 44363
lesion ~ 44365
polyp ~ 44364-44365
tube placement ~ 44372
tube revision ~ 44373
via stoma ~ 44380-44383
tumor ~ 44364-44365
intracranial ~ 62160-62165
kidney
biopsy ~ 50555, 50574-50576, 52354
catheterization ~ 50553, 50572
destruction ~ 50557, 50576, 52354
dilation of ureter ~ 50553
excision tumor ~ 52355
exploration ~ 52351
lithotripsy ~ 52353
removal
calculus ~ 50561, 50580, 52352
foreign body ~ 50561, 50580
via incision ~ 50562-50580
via stoma ~ 50551-50561

Endoscopy ~ *continued*
larynx
biopsy ~ 31510, 31535-31536
direct ~ 31515-31571
exploration ~ 31505, 31520-31526, 31575
fiberoptic ~ 31575-31579
indirect ~ 31505-31513
operative ~ 31530-31561
removal
foreign body ~ 31530-31531
lesion ~ see endoscopic ~ 31511,
31545-31546
mediastinoscopy
biopsy ~ 39400
exploration ~ 39400
nose
diagnostic ~ 31231-31235
surgical ~ 31237-31297
unlisted services and procedures ~ 31299
pancreatic duct
cannulation ~ 43273
destruction
calculi (stone) ~ 43265
tumor ~ 43272
dilation ~ 43271
removal
calculi (stone) ~ 43264
foreign body ~ 43269
stent ~ 43269
specimen collection ~ 43260
sphincter pressure ~ 43263
sphincterotomy ~ 43262
tube placement ~ 43267-43268
pelvis
aspiration ~ 49322
destruction of lesion ~ 58662
lysis of adhesions ~ 58660
oviduct surgery ~ 58670-58671
removal of adnexal structures ~ 58661
peritoneum
biopsy ~ 47561
drainage lymphocele ~ 49323, 54690
radiologic ~ 47560
rectum
biopsy ~ 45305
destruction tumor ~ 45320
dilation ~ 45303
exploration ~ 45300
hemorrhage ~ 45317
removal
foreign body ~ 45307
polyp ~ 45308-45315
tumor ~ 45308-45315
volvulus ~ 45321
spleen, removal ~ 38120
testis, removal ~ 54690
trachea
dilation ~ 31630-31631, 31636-31638
via tracheostomy ~ 31615

Endoscopy ~ *continued*
ureter
  biopsy ~ 50955-50957, 50974-50976, 52354
  catheterize ~ 50953, 50972
  destruction ~ 50957, 50976, 52354
  excision tumor ~ 52355
  exploration ~ 52351
  injection of implant material ~ 52327
  lithotripsy ~ 52353
  manipulation of ureteral calculus ~ 52330
  placement stent ~ 50947
  removal
    calculus ~ 50961, 50980, 52352
    foreign body ~ 50961, 50980
  resection ~ 52355
  via incision ~ 50970-50980
  via stoma ~ 50951-50961
ureteral
  biopsy ~ 52007
  catheterization ~ 52005
urethra ~ 52000
  biopsy ~ 52204, 52354
  catheterization ~ 52010
  destruction ~ 52354
    lesion ~ 52400
  evacuation clot ~ 52001
  excision tumor ~ 52355
  exploration ~ 52351
  incision ejaculatory duct ~ 52402
  injection of implant material ~ 51715
  lithotripsy ~ 52353
  removal calculus ~ 52352
  resection ejaculatory duct ~ 52402
  vasectomy ~ 52402
  vasotomy ~ 52402
uterus
  anesthesia ~ 00952
  hysteroscopy
    diagnostic ~ 58555
    with division/resection intrauterine septum
      ~ 58560
    with lysis of intrauterine adhesions ~
      58559
    placement fallopian tube ~ 58565
    removal
      endometrial ~ 58563
      impacted foreign body ~ 58562
      leiomyomata ~ 58561
    surgical with biopsy ~ 58558
vagina
  anesthesia ~ 00950
  biopsy ~ 57454
  exploration ~ 57452
vascularsurgical ~ 33508, 37500-37501
Endosteal implant
reconstruction
  mandible ~ 21248-21249
  maxilla ~ 21248-21249
Endothelioma, dural ~ 61512, 61519
Endotracheal intubation ~ 31500
Endotracheal tube
intubation ~ 31500

Endovascular repair ~ 0033T-0040T,
  0078T-0081T, 34800-34805, 34812-34826,
  34833-34900
angiography ~ 75952-75954
imaging neck ~ 0037T
Endovascular revascularization ~ 37220-37235
Endovascular therapy
ablation, vein ~ 36475-36479
occlusion ~ 61623
Enema
home visit for fecal impaction ~ 99511
intussusception ~ 74283
therapeutic, for intussusception ~ 74283
Energies, electromagnetic ~ 86945
ENT ~ see ear nose and throat ~ 92700
Entamoeba histolytica
antigen detection
  enzyme immunoassay ~ 87336-87337
Enterectomy ~ 44120-44121, 44126-44128,
  44137, 44202
donor ~ 44132-44133
with enterostomy ~ 44125
Enterocele
repair ~ 57556
hysterectomy
  with colpectomy ~ 58280
Enterocystoplasty ~ 51960
Camey ~ 50825
Enteroenterostomy ~ see anastomosis,
  intestines
Enterolysis ~ 44005
laparoscopic ~ 44200
Enteropancreatostomy ~ see anastomosis,
  pancreas to intestines
Enterorrhaphy ~ 44602-44603, 44615
Enterostomy ~ 44300
closure ~ 44625-44626
with enterectomy
  intestine, small ~ 44125
Enterotomy ~ 44615
Enterovirus
antibody ~ 86658
Entropion
repair ~ 67921-67924
  excision tarsal wedge ~ 67923
  suture ~ 67921
  thermocauterization ~ 67922
Enucleation
eye
  with implant ~ 65103
    muscles attached ~ 65105
  without implant ~ 65101
pleural ~ 32540
Enucleation, cyst, ovarian ~ 58925
Environmental intervention
for psychiatric patients ~ 90882
Enzyme
angiotensin converting ~ 82164
angiotensin-forming ~ 80408, 80416, 84244
Enzyme activity ~ 82657
radioactive substrate ~ 82658
EOG ~ 92270

1401

Eosinocyte ~ 89190
Eosinophils
nasal smear ~ 89190
Epiandrosterone ~ 82666
Epicondylitides, lateral humeral ~
24357-24359
Epicondylitis, radiohumeral ~ 24357-24359
Epidemic parotitis ~ see mumps
Epididymectomy
bilateral ~ 54861
unilateral ~ 54860
Epididymis
abscess, incision and drainage ~ 54700
anastomosis
to vas deferens
bilateral ~ 54901
unilateral ~ 54900
biopsy ~ 54800, 54865
epididymography ~ 74440
excision
bilateral ~ 54861
unilateral ~ 54860
exploration biopsy ~ 54865
hematoma, incision and drainage ~ 54700
lesion
excision
local ~ 54830
spermatocele ~ 54840
needle biopsy ~ 54800
spermatocele excision ~ 54840
unlisted services and procedures ~ 55899
X-ray with contrast ~ 74440
Epididymograms ~ 55300
Epididymography ~ 74440
Epididymoplasty ~ 54900-54901
Epididymovasostomy
bilateral ~ 54901
unilateral ~ 54900
Epidural
electrode
insertion ~ 61531
removal ~ 61535
injection ~ 62281-62282 62310-62319,
64479-64484
lysis ~ , 62263-62264
Epidural anesthesia ~ see anesthesia; epidural
Epidurography ~ 72275
Epigastric hernia repair ~ 49572
Epiglottidectomy ~ 31420
Epiglottis excision ~ 31420
Epikeratoplasty ~ 65767
Epilation ~ 17380
Epinephrine ~ 80424, 82382-82384
blood ~ 82383-82384
urine ~ 82384
Epiphysis ~ see bone; specific bone
Epiphyseal arrest
femur ~ 20150, 27185, 27475, 27479-27485,
27742
fibula ~ 20150, 27477-27485, 27730-27742
radius ~ 20150, 25450-25455

Epiphyseal arrest ~ continued
tibia ~ 20150, 27477-27485, 27730,
27734-27742
ulna ~ 20150, 25450-25455
Epiphyseal separation
radius
closed treatment ~ 25600
open treatment ~ 25607-25609
Epiphysiodesis ~ see epiphyseal arrest
Epiploectomy ~ 49255
Episiotomy ~ 59300
Epispadias
penis reconstruction ~ 54385
repair ~ 54380-54390
with extrophy of bladder ~ 54390
with incontinence ~ 54380-54390
Epistaxis ~ 30901-30906
with nasal/sinus endoscopy ~ 31238
EPO ~ see erythropoietin
Epstein-Barr virus
antibody ~ 86663-86665
Equina, cauda ~ see cauda equina
ERCP ~ see bile duct; pancreatic duct ~ 43260
ERG ~ 92275
Ergocalciferol ~ 82306
Ergocalciferols ~ 82306
Ergonovine provocation test ~ 93024
Erythrocyte ~ see red blood cell (RBC)
Erythrocyte AB ~ see antibody, red blood cell
Erythrocyte count ~ 85032-85041
Erythropoietin ~ 82668
Escharotomy, burns ~ 16035-16036
Escherichia coli 0157
antigen detection, enzyme immunoassay ~
87335
ESD ~ see endoscopy, gastrointestinal, upper
Esophageal
acid infusion test ~ 91030
lengthening ~ 43283, 43338
polyp ~ 43228
tumor ~ 43228
varices
ligation ~ 43205, 43400
transection/repair ~ 43401
Esophagectomy
partial ~ 43116-43124
total ~ 43107-43113, 43124
Esophagoenterostomy with total gastrectomy
~ 43620
Esophagogastroduodenoscopies ~ see
endoscopy, gastrointestinal, upper
Esophagogastromyotomy ~ 32665,
43330-43331
Esophagogastrostomy ~ 43320
Esophagojejunostomy ~ 43340-43341
Esophagomyotomy ~ 32665, 43330-43331
with fundoplasty ~ 43279
Esophagorrhaphy ~ 43405
Esophagoscopies ~ see endoscopy, esophagus
Esophagostomy ~ 43350-43352
closure ~ 43420-43425
Esophagotomy ~ 43020, 43045

Ethmoidectomy ~ 31200-31205
  endoscopic ~ 31254-31255
  skull base surgery ~ 61580-61581
  with nasal/sinus endoscopy ~ 31254-31255
Ethosuccimid ~ 80168
Ethosuximide ~ 80168
  assay ~ 80168
Ethylene dichlorides ~ 84600
Ethyl alcohol ~ 82055, 82075
Ethylene glycol ~ 82693
Ethylmethylsuccimide ~ 80168
Etiocholanolone ~ 82696
Etiocholanolone measurement ~ 82696
ETOH ~ 82055
Euglobulin lysis ~ 85360
European blastomycosis ~ see cryptococcus
Eustachian tube
  catheterization ~ 69405
  inflation
    myringotomy ~ 69420
      anesthesia ~ 69421
    with catheterization ~ 69400
    without catheterization ~ 69401
  insertion, catheter ~ 69405
Eutelegenesis ~ 58976
Evacuation
  cervical pregnancy ~ 59140
  hematoma
    brain ~ 61312-61315
    subungual ~ 11740
  hydatidiform mole ~ 59870
Evaluation
  athletic training
    evaluation ~ 97005
    re-evaluation ~ 97006
Evaluation and management services
  assistive technology, assessment ~ 97755
  basic life and/or disability evaluation services
    ~ 99450
  care plan oversight services ~ 99339-99340,
    99374-99380
    home health agency care ~ 99374-99375
    home or rest home ~ 99339-99340
    hospice ~ 99377-99378
    nursing facility ~ 99379-99380
  case management services ~ 99366-99368
  consultation ~ 99241-99255
  critical care ~ 99291-99292
    interfacility pediatric transport ~
      99466-99467, 99485-99486
  domiciliary or rest home
    established patient ~ 99334-99337
    new patient ~ 99324-99328
  emergency department ~ 99281-99288
  health behavior
    assessment ~ 96150
    family intervention ~ 96154-96155
    group intervention ~ 96153
    individual intervention ~ 96152
    re-assessment ~ 96151
  home services ~ 99341-99350

Evaluation and management services ~
  continued
  hospital ~ 99221-99233
    discharge ~ 99238-99239
    observation care ~ 99217-99220,
      99224-99226, 99234-99236
  hyperbaric oxygen treatment facility ~ 99183
  insurance exam ~ 99455-99456
  internet communication ~ 98969, 99444
  low birthweight infant ~ 99478-99479
  medical team conferences ~ 99366-99368
  neonatal critical care ~ 99468-99469
  newborn care ~ 99460-99465
  nursing facility ~ see nursing facility services
    ~ 99304-99318
  occupation therapy evaluation ~ 97003
    re-evaluation ~ 97004
  office and other outpatient ~ 99201-99215
  online ~ 98969, 99444
  pediatric critical care ~ 99471-99476
  pediatric interfacility transport ~ 99466-99467,
    99485-99486
  physical therapy evaluation ~ 97001
    re-evaluation ~ 97002
  physician standby services ~ 99360
  post-discharge transitional care ~ 99495-99496
  preventive services ~ 99381-99429
  prolonged services ~ 99354-99360
  standby services ~ 99360
  team conferences ~ 99366-99368
  telephone services ~ 98966-98968,
    99441-99443
  unlisted services and procedures ~ 99499
  with psychotherapy ~ 90833, 90836, 90838
  work-related and/or medical disability
    evaluation ~ 99455
Evaluation studies, drug, pre-clinical ~
  80100-80101, 82486
Evisceration
  ocular contents
    with implant ~ 65093
    without implant ~ 65091
  pelvic ~ 45126, 58240
Evocative/suppression testing ~ 80400-80440
  stimulation panel ~ 80410
Evoked potential ~ see audiologic function
  tests
  auditory brainstem ~ 92585-92586
  central motor
    transcranial motor stimulation ~
      95928-95929
  somatosensory testing ~ 95925-95927
  visual, CNS ~ 95930
Ewart procedure ~ 42226-42227
Excavatum, pectus ~ 21740-21743
Exchange
  arterial catheter ~ 37211-37214
  drainage catheter
    under radiologic guidance ~ 49423
  intraocular lens ~ 66986
  transfusion ~ 36455

Excision ~ see debridement; destruction
  abscess
    brain ~ 61514, 61522
    olecranon process ~ 24138
    radius ~ 24136
    ulna ~ 24138
  acromion
    shoulder ~ 23130
  adenoids ~ 42830-42836
  adenoma thyroid gland ~ 60200
  adrenal gland ~ 60540
    with excision retroperitoneal tumor ~ 60545
    laparoscopic ~ 60650
  alveolus ~ 41830
  anal crypt ~ 46999
  anal fissure ~ 46200
  anal tag ~ 46220, 46230
  aorta coarctation ~ 33840-33851
  appendix ~ 44950-44960
  arteriovenous malformation
    spinal ~ 63250-63252
  arytenoid cartilage ~ 31400
    endoscopic ~ 31560-31561
  atrial septum ~ 33735-33737
  Bartholin's gland ~ 56740
  bladder
    diverticulum ~ 51525
    neck ~ 51520
    partial ~ 51550-51565
    total ~ 51570, 51580, 51590-51597
      with nodes ~ 51575, 51585, 51595
    transurethral ~ 52640
    tumor ~ 51530
  bladder neck contracture, postoperative ~ 52640
  bone
    facial ~ 21026
    mandible ~ 21025
    postoperative
      femur ~ 20150
      fibula ~ 20150
      radius ~ 20150
      tibia ~ 20150
      ulna ~ 20150
  bone abscess
    facial ~ 21026
    mandible ~ 21025
  brain
    amygdala ~ 61566
    epileptogenic focus ~ 61536
    hemisphere ~ 61542-61543
    hippocampus ~ 61566
    other lobe ~ 61323, 61539-61540
    temporal lobe ~ 61537-61538
  brain lobe ~ 61323, 61537-61540
  breast
    biopsy ~ 19100-19103
    chest wall tumor ~ 19260-19272
    cyst ~ 19120-19126
    lactiferous duct fistula ~ 19112

Excision ~ *continued*
    lesion ~ 19120-19126
      by needle localization ~ 19125-19126
    mastectomy ~ 19300-19307
    nipple exploration ~ 19110
  bulbourethral gland ~ 53250
  bullae
    lung ~ 32141
    endoscopic ~ 32655
  burns ~ 01951-01953, 15002-15005
  bursa
    elbow ~ 24105
    femur ~ 27062
    ischial ~ 27060
    knee ~ 27340
    wrist ~ 25115-25116
  bypass graft ~ 35901-35907
  calcaneus ~ 28118-28120
  calculi (stone)
    parotid gland ~ 42330, 42340
    salivary gland ~ 42330-42340
    sublingual gland ~ 42330
    submandibular gland ~ 42330-42335
  carotid artery ~ 60605
  carpal ~ 25145, 25210-25215
  cartilage
    knee joint ~ 27332-27333
    shoulder joint ~ 23101
    temporomandibular joint ~ 21060
    wrist ~ 25107
  caruncle
    urethra ~ 53265
  cataract
    secondary ~ 66830
  cervix
    radical ~ 57531
    stump
      abdominal approach ~ 57540-57545
      vaginal approach ~ 57550-57556
    total ~ 57530
  chalazion
    multiple
      different lids ~ 67805
      same lid ~ 67801
    single ~ 67800
    with anesthesia ~ 67808
  chest wall tumor ~ 19260-19272
  choroid plexus ~ 61544
  clavicle
    partial ~ 23120, 23180
    sequestrectomy ~ 23170
    total ~ 23125
    tumor
      radical resection ~ 23200
  coccyx ~ 27080
  colon
    excision
      partial ~ 44140-44147, 44160
        with anastomosis ~ 44140
      total ~ 44150-44158

Excision ~ *continued*
  laparoscopic
    with anastomosis ~ 44204, 44207-44208
    with colostomy ~ 44206, 44208
    with ileocolostomy ~ 44205
  condyle, temporomandibular joint ~ 21050
  constricting ring
    finger ~ 26596
  cornea
    epithelium ~ 65435
      with chelating agent ~ 65436
    scraping ~ 65430
  coronoidectomy ~ 21070
  Cowper's gland ~ 53250
  cranial bone tumor ~ 61563-61564
  cyst ~ see also ganglion cyst
    bile duct ~ 47715
    bladder ~ 51500
    brain ~ 61516, 61524, 62162
    branchial ~ 42810-42815
    calcaneus ~ 28100-28103
    carpal ~ 25130-25136
    cheekbone ~ 21030
    clavicle ~ 23140
      with allograft ~ 23146
      with autograft ~ 23145
    facial bone ~ 21030
    femur ~ 27065-27067, 27355-27358
    fibula ~ 27635-27638
    finger ~ 26160
    foot ~ 28090
    hand ~ 26160
    hip ~ 27065-27067
    humerus ~ 23150, 24110
      with allograft ~ 23156, 24116
      with autograft ~ 23155, 24115
    ileum ~ 27065-27067
    kidney ~ 50280-50290
    knee ~ 27345-27347
    lung ~ 32140
    mandible ~ 21040, 21046-21047
    maxilla ~ 21030, 21048-21049
    mediastinal ~ 39200
    mediastinum ~ 32662
    metacarpal ~ 26200-26205
    metatarsal ~ 28104-28107
    mullerian duct ~ 55680
    nose ~ 30124-30125
    olecranon ~ 24120
    olecranon process
      with allograft ~ 24126
      with autograft ~ 24125
    ovarian ~ 58925
    pericardial ~ 33050
      endoscopic ~ 32661
    phalanges ~ 26210-26215
      toe ~ 28108
    pilonidal ~ 11770-11772
    pubis ~ 27066-27067
    radius ~ 24120, 25120-25126
      with allograft ~ 24126

Excision ~ *continued*
      with autograft ~ 24125
    salivary gland ~ 42408
    scapula ~ 23140
      with allograft ~ 23146
      with autograft ~ 23145
    seminal vesicle ~ 55680
    sublingual gland ~ 42408
    talus ~ 28100-28103
    tarsal ~ 28104-28107
    thyroglossal duct ~ 60280-60281
    thyroid gland ~ 60200
    tibia ~ 27635-27638
    toe ~ 28092
    ulna ~ 24120, 25120-25126
      with allograft ~ 24126
      with autograft ~ 24125
    urachalbladder ~ 51500
    vaginal ~ 57135
  destruction of the vestibule of the mouth ~
    40808-40820
  diverticulum, Meckel's ~ 44800
  ear, external
    partial ~ 69110
    total ~ 69120
  elbow joint ~ 24155
  electrode ~ 57522
  embolectomy/thrombectomy
    aortoiliac artery ~ 34151-34201
    axillary artery ~ 34101
    brachial artery ~ 34101
    carotid artery ~ 34001
    celiac artery ~ 34151
    femoral artery ~ 34201
    heart ~ 33310-33315
    iliac artery ~ 34151-34201
    innominate artery ~ 34001-34101
    mesentery artery ~ 34151
    peroneal artery ~ 34203
    popliteal artery ~ 34203
    radial artery ~ 34111
    renal artery ~ 34151
    subclavian artery ~ 34001-34101
    tibial artery ~ 34203
    ulnar artery ~ 34111
  embolism, pulmonary artery ~ 33910-33916
  empyema
    lung ~ 32540
    pleural ~ 32540
  epididymis
    bilateral ~ 54861
    unilateral ~ 54860
  epiglottis ~ 31420
  esophagus
    diverticula ~ 43130-43135
    partial ~ 43116-43124
    total ~ 43107-43113, 43124
  eye ~ 65101, 65103, 65109
  fallopian tube
    salpingectomy ~ 58700
    salpingo-oophorectomy ~ 58720

Excision ~ *continued*
fascia ~ see fasciectomy
femur ~ 27360
  partial ~ 27070-27071
fibula ~ 27360, 27455-27457, 27641
fistula
  anal ~ 46270-46285
foot
  fasciectomy ~ 28060
    radical ~ 28060-28062
gallbladder ~ 47600-47620
  cholecystectomy ~ 47562-47564
    with cholangiography ~ 47563
    with exploration common duct ~ 47564
ganglion cyst
  knee ~ 27347
  wrist ~ 25111-25112
gingiva ~ 41820
gums ~ 41820
  alveolus ~ 41830
  operculum ~ 41821
heart
  donor ~ 33940
heart/lung
  donor ~ 33930
hemangioma ~ 11400-11446
hemorrhoids ~ 46221, 46250
  clot ~ 46320
  complex ~ 46260-46262
  with fissurectomy ~ 46257-46258
  simple ~ 46255
hip, partial ~ 27070-27071
hippocampus ~ 61566
humeral head
  resection ~ 23195
  sequestrectomy ~ 23174
humerus ~ 23184, 23220, 24134, 24140,
  24150
hydrocele
  spermatic cord ~ 55500
  tunica vaginalis ~ 55040-55041
    bilateral ~ 55041
    unilateral ~ 55040
hygroma, cystic, axillary/cervical ~
  38550-38555
hymenotomy ~ 56700
ileum
  ileoanal reservoir ~ 45136
  partial ~ 27070-27071
inner ear ~ 69905-69910
interphalangeal joint
  toe ~ 28160
intervertebral disk
  decompression ~ 63075-63078
  hemilaminectomy ~ 63040, 63043-63044
  herniated ~ 63020-63044, 63055-63066
intestine
  laparoscopic
    with anastomosis ~ 44202-44203
intestines
  donor ~ 44132-44133

Excision ~ *continued*
intestines, small ~ 44120-44128
  transplantation ~ 44137
iris
  iridectomy
    with corneoscleral or corneal section ~
      66600
    with cyclectomy ~ 66605
    optical ~ 66635
    peripheral ~ 66625
    sector ~ 66630
kidney
  donor ~ 50300-50320, 50547
  partial ~ 50240
  recipient ~ 50340
  transplantation ~ 50370
  with ureters ~ 50220-50236
kneecap ~ 27350
labyrinth
  with mastoidectomy ~ 69910
  transcanal ~ 69905
lacrimal gland
  partial ~ 68505
  total ~ 68500
lacrimal sac ~ 68520
larynx
  partial ~ 31367-31382
  with pharynx ~ 31390-31395
  total ~ 31360-31365
lesion
  anal ~ 45108, 46922
  ankle ~ 27630
    arthroscopic ~ 29891
  auditory canal, external
    exostosis ~ 69140
    radical with neck dissection ~ 69155
    radical without neck dissection ~ 69150
    soft tissue ~ 69145
  bladder ~ 52224
  brain ~ 61534, 61536-61540
  brainstem ~ 61575-61576
  carotid body ~ 60600-60605
  colon ~ 44110-44111
  conjunctiva ~ 68110-68130
    over 1cm ~ 68115
    with adjacent sclera ~ 68130
  cornea ~ 65400
    without graft ~ 65420
  ear, middle ~ 69540
  epididymis
    local ~ 54830
    spermatocele ~ 54840
  esophagus ~ 43100-43101
  eye ~ 65900
  eyelid
    multiple, different lids ~ 67805
    multiple, same lid ~ 67801
    single ~ 67800
    under anesthesia ~ 67808
    without closure ~ 67840

1407

Excision ~ *continued*
  femur ~ 27062
  finger ~ 26160
  foot ~ 28080, 28090
  gums ~ 41822-41828
  hand ~ 26160
  intestines ~ 44110
    small ~ 43250, 44111
  intraspinal ~ 63265-63273
  knee ~ 27347
  larynx, endoscopic ~ 31545-31546
  leg, lower ~ 27630
  meniscus ~ 27347
  mesentery ~ 44820
  mouth ~ 40810-40816, 41116
  nerve ~ 64774-64792
  neuroma ~ 64778
  nose, intranasal ~ 30117-30118
  orbit ~ 61333
    lateral approach ~ 67420
  palate ~ 42104-42120
  pancreas ~ 48120
  penis ~ 54060
    surgical excision penile plaque ~
      54110-54112
  pharynx ~ 42808
  rectum ~ 45108
  sclera ~ 66130
  skin
    benign ~ 11400-11471
    malignant ~ 11600-11646
  skull ~ 61500, 61615-61616
  spermatic cord ~ 55520
  spinal cord ~ 63300-63308
  stomach ~ 43611
  talus, arthroscopic ~ 29891
  testis ~ 54512
  tibia, arthroscopic ~ 29891
  toe ~ 28092
  tongue ~ 41110-41114
  urethra ~ 52224, 53265
  uterus ~ 59100
    leiomyomata ~ 58140, 58545-58546,
      58561
  uvula ~ 42104-42107
  wrist tendon ~ 25110
  lesion, arthroscopic
    ankle ~ 29891
    talus ~ 29891
    tibia ~ 29891
  lesion, tendon sheath
    arm, lower ~ 25110
  lip ~ 40500-40530
    frenum ~ 40819
  liver
    extensive ~ 47122
    lobectomy ~ 47125-47130
    partial ~ 47120, 47125-47130, 47140-47142
    total ~ 47133

Excision ~ *continued*
  lung
    bronchus resection ~ 32486
    bullae, completion ~ 32488
    lobe ~ 32480-32482
    pleurectomy ~ 32310, 32320
    pneumonectomy 32440-32445
    segment ~ 32484
    tumor, apical ~ 32503-32504
  lung/heart donor ~ 33930
  lymph nodes ~ 38500, 38510-38530
    abdominal ~ 38747
    inguinofemoral ~ 38760-38765
    limited, for staging
      para-aortic ~ 38562
      pelvic ~ 38562
      retroperitoneal ~ 38564
    pelvic ~ 38770
    radical
      axillary ~ 38740-38745
      cervical ~ 38720-38724
      suprahyoid ~ 38700
    retroperitoneal transabdominal ~ 38780
    thoracic ~ 38746
  mandibular exostosis ~ 21031
  mastoid
    complete ~ 69502
    radical ~ 69511
      modified ~ 69505
      petrous apicectomy ~ 69530
    simple ~ 69501
  maxilla exotosis ~ 21032
  maxillary torus palatinus ~ 21032
  meningioma, brain ~ 61512, 61519
  meniscectomy, temporomandibular joint ~
    21060
  metacarpal ~ 26230
  metatarsal ~ 28110-28114, 28122, 28140
    condyle ~ 28288
  mouth, frenum ~ 40819
  mucosa
    gums ~ 41828
    mouth ~ 40818
  nail fold ~ 11765
  nails ~ 11750-11752
  nerve
    foot ~ 28055
    leg, upper ~ 27325
    sympathetic ~ 64802-64818
  neurofibroma ~ 64788-64790
  neurolemmoma ~ 64788-64792
  neuroma ~ 64774-64786
  nose
    cyst ~ 30124-30125
    lesion ~ 30117-30118
    polyp ~ 30110-30115
    rhinectomy ~ 30150, 30160
    skin ~ 30120
    turbinate ~ 30130, 30140
  odontoid process ~ 22548
  olecranon process ~ 24147

Excision ~ *continued*
  omentum ~ 49255
  ovary ~ 58720
    cystectomy ~ 58925
    oophorectomy ~ 58940, 58943
    salpingo-oophorectomy ~ 58720
    wedge resection/bisection ~ 58920
  oviduct ~ 58700, 58720
  palate ~ 42120, 42145
    lesion ~ 42104, 42106-42107
  pancreas
    ampulla of Vater ~ 48148
    duct ~ 48148
    partial ~ 48140-48146, 48150, 48153-48154, 48160
    peripancreatic tissue ~ 48105
    total ~ 48155-48160
  parathyroid gland ~ 60500-60502
  parotid gland ~ 42340
    partial ~ 42410-42415
    total ~ 42420-42426
  patella ~ 27350, 27424
  penile adhesions, post-circumcision ~ 54162
  penis
    amputation ~ 54120, 54125, 54130, 54135
    circumcision ~ 54150, 54160-54161, 54163
    frenulum ~ 54164
    partial ~ 54120
    post circumcision adhesion ~ 54162
    prepuce ~ 54150-54161, 54163
    radical ~ 54130-54135
    total ~ 54125
  pericardium ~ 33030-33031
    endoscopic ~ 32659
  petrous temporal
    apex ~ 69530
  phalanges
    fingers ~ 26235-26236
    toe ~ 28124-28126, 28150-28160
  pharynx ~ 42145
    with larynx ~ 31390-31395
    partial ~ 42890
    resection ~ 42892-42894
  pituitary gland ~ 61546-61548
  pleura ~ 32310-32320
    endoscopic ~ 32656
  polyp
    nose
      endoscopic ~ 31237
      extensive ~ 30115
      simple ~ 30110
    urethra ~ 53260, 53265
  pressure ulcers ~ see also skin graft and flap ~ 15920-15999
  prostate
    abdominoperineal ~ 45119
    partial ~ 55801, 55821-55831
    perineal ~ 55801-55815
    radical ~ 55810-55815, 55840-55845
    regrowth ~ 52630
    residual obstructive tissue ~ 52630

Excision ~ *continued*
  retropubic ~ 55831-55845
  suprapubic ~ 55821
  transurethral ~ 52601, 52630
  pterygium, with graft ~ 65426
  pubis, partial ~ 27070-27071
  radical synovium wrist ~ 25115-25116
  radius ~ 24130, 24136, 24145, 24152, 25145
    styloid process ~ 25230
  rectum
    with colon ~ 45121
    partial ~ 45111, 45113-45116, 45123
    prolapse ~ 45130-45135
    stricture ~ 45150
    total ~ 45119-45120
  redundant skin of eyelid ~ 15820-15823
  ribs ~ 21600-21616, 32900
  scapula
    ostectomy ~ 23190
    partial ~ 23182
    sequestrectomy ~ 23172
    tumor/cyst ~ 23140, 23145, 23146
  sclera ~ 66150, 66155, 66160, 66165, 66170
  scrotum ~ 55150
  semilunar cartilage of knee ~ 27332-27333
  seminal vesicle ~ 55650
  sesamoid bone
    foot ~ 28315
  sinus
    ethmoid ~ 31200-31205
    maxillary ~ 31225-31230
  Skene's gland ~ 53270
  skin
    excess ~ 15830-15839, 15847
    lesion
      benign ~ 11400-11471
      malignant ~ 11600-11646
    nose ~ 30120
  skin graft, preparation of site ~ 15000
  skull ~ 61501
  spermatic veins ~ 55530-55540
    abdominal approach ~ 55535
    hernia repair ~ 55540
  spleen ~ 38100-38102
    laparoscopic ~ 38120
  stapes
    with footplate drill out ~ 69661
    without foreign material ~ 69660
  sternum ~ 21620, 21630-21632
  stomach
    partial ~ 43631-43639, 43845
    total ~ 43620-43622
  sublingual gland ~ 42450
  submandibular gland ~ 42440, 42508
  sweat glands
    axillary ~ 11450-11451
    inguinal ~ 11462-11463
    perianal ~ 11470-11471
    perineal ~ 11470-11471
    umbilical ~ 11470-11471

1409

Excision ~ _continued_
synovium
  ankle ~ 27625-27626
  carpometacarpal joint ~ 26130
  elbow ~ 24102
  hip joint ~ 27054
  interphalangeal joint ~ 26140
  intertarsal joint ~ 28070
  knee joint ~ 27334-27335
  metacarpophalangeal joint ~ 26135
  metatarsophalangeal joint ~ 28072
  shoulder ~ 23105-23106
  tarsometatarsal joint ~ 28070
  wrist ~ 25105, 25118-25119
talus ~ 28120, 28130
tarsal ~ 28116, 28122
temporal bone ~ 69535
temporal, petrous apex ~ 69530
tendon
  arm
    lower ~ 25109
  finger ~ 26180, 26390, 26415
  hand ~ 26390, 26415
  palm ~ 26170
tendon sheath
  finger ~ 26145
  foot ~ 28086-28088
  palm ~ 26145
  wrist ~ 25115-25116
testis
  laparoscopic ~ 54690
  partial ~ 54522
  radical ~ 54530-54535
  simple ~ 54520
  tumor ~ 54530-54535
thrombectomy
  axillary vein ~ 34490
  bypass graft ~ 35875-35876
  femoropopliteal vein ~ 34401-34451
  iliac vein ~ 34401-34451
  subclavian vein ~ 34471-34490
  vena cava ~ 34401-34451
thromboendarterectomy
  aorta, abdominal ~ 35331
  aortoiliofemoral ~ 35363
  axillary artery ~ 35321
  brachial artery ~ 35321
  carotid artery ~ 35301, 35390
  celiac artery ~ 35341
  femoral artery ~ 35371-35372
  iliac ~ 35361-35363
  iliac artery ~ 35351
  iliofemoral artery ~ 35355, 35363
  innominate artery ~ 35311
  mesenteric artery ~ 35341
  peroneal artery ~ 35305-35306
  popliteal artery ~ 35303
  renal artery ~ 35341
  subclavian artery ~ 35301-35311
  tibial artery ~ 35305-35306
  vertebral artery ~ 35301

Excision ~ _continued_
thymus gland ~ 60521
thyroid gland for malignancy
  partial ~ 60210-60225
  removal all thyroid tissue ~ 60260
  secondary ~ 60260
  total ~ 60240
    cervical approach ~ 60271
    sternal split/transthoracic approach ~ 60270
      limited neck dissection ~ 60252
      radical neck dissection ~ 60254
tibia ~ 27360, 27640
tongue
  complete ~ 41140-41155
  frenum ~ 41115
    with mouth resection ~ 41150-41153
  partial ~ 41120-41135
    with radical neck ~ 41135, 41145-41155
tonsils ~ 42825-42826
  lingual ~ 42870
  radical ~ 42842-42845
  tag ~ 42860
  with adenoids ~ 42820-42821
torus mandibularis ~ 21031
trachea stenosis ~ 31780-31781
transcervical approach ~ 60520
tricuspid valve ~ 33460
tumor
  abdominal wall ~ 22900-22905
  acetabulum ~ 27076
  ankle ~ 27615-27619, 27632, 27634
  arm, lower ~ 25071-25078
  arm, upper ~ 24071-24079
  back/flank ~ 21930
  bile duct ~ 47711-47712
  bladder ~ 51530, 52234-52240, 52355
  brain ~ 61510, 61518, 61520-61521, 61526-61530, 61545, 62164
  bronchi ~ 31640
  calcaneus ~ 27647, 28100-28103
  carpal ~ 25130-25136
  cheekbone ~ 21030, 21034, 21048-21049
  clavicle ~ 23140
    with allograft ~ 23146
    with autograft ~ 23145
  ear, middle
    extended ~ 69554
    transcanal ~ 69550
    transmastoid ~ 69552
  elbow ~ 24071-24079
  esophagus endoscopic ablation ~ 43228
  facial bones ~ 21029-21030, 21034-21040, 21046-21049
  facial tissue ~ 21011-21016
  femur ~ 27065-27067, 27355-27358, 27365
  fibula ~ 27635-27638, 27646
  finger ~ 26111-26118
  foot ~ 28039-28047
  gums ~ 41825-41827
  hand ~ 26111-26118

Excision ~ *continued*
  tumor ~ *continued*
    heart ~ 33120-33130
    hip ~ 27043-27045, 27049, 27059,
      27065-27067
      radical ~ 27075-27076
    humerus ~ 23150, 23220, 24110-24115
      with allograft ~ 23156, 24116
      with autograft ~ 23155, 24116
      radial head or neck ~ 24152
    ileum ~ 27065-27067
    innominate ~ 27077
    intestines, small ~ 43250
    ischial ~ 27078
    kidney ~ 52355
    knee ~ 27327-27328, 27337-27339, 27365
    lacrimal gland
      frontal approach ~ 68540
      involving osteotomy ~ 68550
    larynx ~ 31300
      endoscopic ~ 31540-31541, 31578
    leg, lower ~ 27615-27619, 27632, 27634
    leg, upper ~ 27327-27329, 27337-27339,
      27365
    mandible ~ 21040-21047
    maxilla ~ 21030, 21034, 21048-21049
    mediastinal ~ 39220
    mediastinum ~ 32662
    metacarpal ~ 26200-26205, 26250
    metatarsal ~ 28104-28107, 28173
    neck ~ 21552-21558
    olecranon process ~ 24120
      with allograft ~ 24126
      with autograft ~ 24125
    parotid gland ~ 42410-42426
    pelvis ~ 27043-27045, 27049, 27059
    pericardial ~ 33050
    pericardium ~ 32661
    phalanges ~ 26210-26215, 26260-26262
      toe ~ 26215, 28108, 28175
    pituitary gland ~ 61546-61548, 62165
    presacral ~ 49215
    pubis ~ 27065-27067
    radius ~ 24120-24125, 25120-25126, 25170
    rectum ~ 45160-45172
    sacrococcygeal ~ 49215
    scapula ~ 23140
      with allograft ~ 23146
      with autograft ~ 23145
    shoulder ~ 23071-23078
    skull ~ 61500
    spermatocele ~ 54840
    spinal cord ~ 63275-63290
    spleen, total ~ 38100
    sternum ~ 21630
    stomach ~ 43610
    talus ~ 27647, 28100-28103
    tarsal ~ 28104-28107, 28171
    thorax ~ 21552-21558
    thyroid ~ 60200
    tibia ~ 27635-27638, 27645-27646

Excision ~ *continued*
  tumor ~ *continued*
    trachea
      cervical ~ 31785
      thoracic ~ 31786
    ulna ~ 24120-24125, 25120-25126, 25170
    ureter ~ 52355
    urethra ~ 52234-52240, 52355, 53220
    uterus
      abdominal approach ~ 58140, 58146
      vaginal approach ~ 58145
    vagina ~ 57135
    vertebra, lumbar ~ 22102
    vertebra, thoracic ~ 22101
    wrist ~ 25071-25078
    zygoma ~ 21030, 21034
  turbinate ~ 30130-30140
  tympanic nerve ~ 69676
  ulcer
    stomach ~ 43610
  ulna ~ 24147, 25145
    complete ~ 25240
    partial ~ 25150-25151, 25240
  umbilicus ~ 49250
  ureter ~ 50650-50660
  ureterocele ~ 51535
  urethra
    diverticulum ~ 53230-53235
    prolapse ~ 53275
    total
      female ~ 53210
      male ~ 53215
  uterus
    laparoscopic ~ 58550
    leiomyomata ~ 58546
    partial ~ 58180
    radical ~ 58210, 58285
    removal tubes and/ or ovaries ~
      58262-58263, 58291, 58552, 58554
    total ~ 58150-58152, 58200
    vaginal ~ 58260, 58290-58294, 58550,
      58553
      with colpectomy ~ 58275-58280
      with colpo-urethrocystopexy ~ 58267,
        58293
      with repair of enterocele ~ 58270, 58292,
        58294
  uvula ~ 42140-42145
  vagina
    cyst ~ 57135
    lumen ~ 57120
    repair of enterocele ~ 58280
    septum ~ 57130
    total ~ 57110-57112
      with hysterectomy ~ 58275-58280
  varicocele
    spermatic cord ~ 55530-55540
      abdominal approach ~ 55535
      hernia repair ~ 55540
  vas deferens ~ 55250

Excision ~ *continued*
vascular malformation
finger ~ 26115
hand ~ 26115
vein, varicose ~ 37765-37766
vertebra
additional segment ~ 22103, 22116
cervical ~ 22110
for tumor ~ 22100, 22110
lumbar ~ 22102
for tumor ~ 22114
thoracic ~ 22112
for tumor ~ 22101
vertebral body
decompression ~ 63081-63103
lesion ~ 63300-63308
vitreous ~ 67039
with retinal surgery ~ 67041-67043
total
pars plana approach ~ 67036
with epiretinal membrane stripping ~
67041-67043
vulva
radical
complete ~ 56633-56640
partial ~ 56630-56632
simple
complete ~ 56625
partial ~ 56620
Exclusion
duodenum ~ 48547
small intestine ~ 44700
Exenteration
eye
removal orbital contents ~ 65110
therapeutic removal of bone ~ 65112
with muscle or myocutaneous flap ~ 65114
pelvis ~ 45126, 58240
Exercise stress tests ~ 93015-93018
Exercise test ~ see also electromyography,
needle
ischemic limb ~ 95875
Exercise therapy ~ 97110-97113
Exfoliation, chemical ~ 17360
Exocrine, pancreas ~ see pancreas
Exomphalos ~ 49600-49611
Exostectomy ~ 28288, 28290
Exostoses ~ 69140
Exostoses, cartilaginous ~ 69140
Exostosis excision ~ 69140
Expander, skin, inflatable ~ see tissue,
expander
Expired gas analysis ~ 94680-94690, 94770
nitric oxide ~ 95012
spectroscopic ~ 94799
Exploration
abdomen ~ 49000-49002
penetrating wound ~ 20102
staging ~ 58960
adrenal gland ~ 60540-60545
anal endoscopy ~ 46600

Exploration ~ *continued*
ankle ~ 27610, 27620
arm, lower ~ 25248
artery
brachial ~ 24495
carotid ~ 35701
femoral ~ 35721
other ~ 35761
popliteal ~ 35741
back, penetrating wound ~ 20102
bile duct
atresia ~ 47700
endoscopy ~ 47552-47553
blood vessel
abdomen ~ 35840
chest ~ 35820
extremity ~ 35860
neck ~ 35800
brain
via burr hole
infratentorial ~ 61253
supratentorial ~ 61250
infratentorial ~ 61305
supratentorial ~ 61304
breast ~ 19020
bronchi endoscopy ~ 31622
bronchoscopy ~ 31622
cauda equina ~ 63005-63011, 63017
chest penetrating wound ~ 20101
colon endoscopic ~ 44388, 45378
colon-sigmoid endoscopic ~ 45330, 45335
common bile duct with cholecystectomy ~
47610
duodenum ~ 44010
ear, inner
endolymphatic sac
with shunt ~ 69806
without shunt ~ 69805
ear, middle ~ 69440
elbow ~ 24000, 24101
epididymis ~ 54865
esophagus endoscopy ~ 43200
extremity penetrating wound ~ 20103
finger joint ~ 26075-26080
flank penetrating wound ~ 20102
gallbladder ~ 47480
gastrointestinal tract, upper endoscopy ~
43235-43236
hand joint ~ 26070
heart ~ 33310-33315
hepatic duct ~ 47400
hip ~ 27033
interphalangeal joint toe ~ 28024
intertarsal joint ~ 28020
intestines, small
endoscopy ~ 44360
enterotomy ~ 44020
kidney ~ 50010, 50045, 50120
knee ~ 27310, 27331
lacrimal duct ~ 68810
canaliculi ~ 68840
with anesthesia ~ 68811

Exploration ~ *continued*
with insertion tube or stent ~ 68815
larynx ~ 31320
endoscopy ~ 31505, 31520-31526, 31575
liver wound ~ 47361-47362
mediastinum ~ 39000-39010
metatarsophalangeal joint ~ 28022
nasolacrimal duct ~ 68810
with anesthesia ~ 68811
with insertion tube or stent ~ 68815
neck
lymph nodes ~ 38542
penetrating wound ~ 20100
nipple ~ 19110
nose endoscopy ~ 31231-31235
orbit ~ 61332-61334
with/without biopsy ~ 67450
without bone flap ~ 67400
parathyroid gland ~ 60500-60505
pelvis ~ 49320
prostate ~ 55860
with nodes ~ 55862-55865
rectum
endoscopic ~ 45300
injury ~ 45562-45563
retroperitoneal area ~ 49010
scrotum ~ 55110
shoulder joint ~ 23040-23044, 23107
sinus
frontal ~ 31070-31075
maxillary ~ 31020-31030
skull ~ 61105
spinal cord ~ 63001-63011, 63015-63017, 63040-63044
spine fusion ~ 22830
stomach ~ 43500
tarsometatarsal joint ~ 28020
testis, undescended ~ 54550-54560
toe joint ~ 28024
ureter ~ 50600
vagina ~ 57000
endocervical ~ 57452
wrist ~ 25101, 25248
joint ~ 25040
Exploration, larynx by incision ~ 31320
Exploratory laparotomy ~ 49000-49002
Expression lesion, conjunctiva ~ 68040
Exteriorization, small intestine ~ 44300
External auditory canal ~ see auditory canal
External cephalic version ~ 59412
External ear ~ see ear, external
External extoses ~ 69140
External fixation
adjustment/revision ~ 20693
application ~ 20690-20692
stereotactic computer assisted ~ 20696-20697
mandibular fracture
open treatment ~ 21454
percutaneous treatment ~ 21452
removal ~ 20694
Extirpation, lacrimal sac ~ 68520

Extracorporeal circulation ~ 33960-33961
for regional chemotherapy
extremity ~ 36823
Extracorporeal dialyses ~ 90935-90937
Extracorporeal membrane oxygenation cannulization ~ 36822
Extracorporeal photochemotherapies ~ 36522
Extracorporeal shock wave therapy ~ see lithotripsy
musculoskeletal ~ 0019T
plantar fascia ~ 0020T
Extracranial intracranial ~ 61623
Extraction lens
extracapsular ~ 66940
intracapsular ~ 66920
for dislocated lens ~ 66930
Extraction, cataract ~ 66830
Extradural injection ~ 62281-62282, 62310-62319, 64479-64484
Extraocular muscle ~ 67340
Extrauterine pregnancy ~ see ectopic pregnancy
Extravasation blood ~ see hemorrhage
Extremity
lower
harvest of vein for bypass graft ~ 35500
harvest of vein for vascular reconstruction ~ 35572
revision ~ 35879-35881
ultrasound ~ 76881-76882
upper
harvest of artery for coronary artery bypass graft ~ 35600
harvest of vein for bypass graft ~ 35500
repair blood vessel ~ 35206
wound exploration penetrating wound ~ 20103
Eye
age-related eye disease study (AREDS) ~ 4177F
biometry ~ 76516-76519, 92136
computerized corneal topography ~ 92025
dilation outflow canal ~ 66174-66175
discission of anterior hyaloid membrane ~ 65810
drainage, anterior chamber
with diagnostic aqueous aspiration ~ 65800
with removal of blood ~ 65815
with removal of vitreous ~ 65810
with therapeutic aqueous release ~ 65800
endoscopy ~ 66990
evaluation
dilated fundus ~ 2020F-2021F
dilated macular ~ 2019F
goniotomy ~ 65820
incision
adhesions
anterior synechiae ~ 65860, 65870
corneovitreal adhesions ~ 65880
goniosynechiae ~ 65865
posterior synechiae ~ 65875
anterior chamber ~ 65820
trabeculae ~ 65850

Eye ~ *continued*
  injection
    air ~ 66020
    medication ~ 66030
  insertion, implantation
    drug delivery system ~ 67027
    foreign material for reinforcement ~ 65155
    muscles attached ~ 65140
    muscles, not attached ~ 65135
    reinsertion ~ 65150
    scleral shell ~ 65130
  interferometry biometry ~ 92136
  lesion excision ~ 65900
  nerve
    destruction ~ 67345
    optic, head evaluation ~ 2027F
  paracentesis anterior chamber
    with diagnostic aspiration of aqueous ~ 65800
    removal of blood ~ 65815
    removal of vitreous and/or discission anterior
      hyaloid membrane ~ 65810
    with therapeutic release of aqueous ~
      65800
  radial keratotomy ~ 65771
  reconstruction
    graft
      conjunctiva ~ 65782
      stem cell ~ 65781
    transplantation
      amniotic membrane ~ 65780
  removal
    blood clot ~ 65930
    bone ~ 65112
    foreign body
      conjunctival embedded ~ 65210
      conjunctival superficial ~ 65205
      corneal with slit lamp ~ 65222
      corneal without slit lamp ~ 65220
      intraocular ~ 65235-65265
    implant ~ 65175
      anterior segment ~ 65920
      muscles, not attached ~ 65103
      posterior segment ~ 67120-67121
  repair
    amniotic membrane ~ 65778-65779
    conjunctiva
      by mobilization and rearrangement without
        hospitalization ~ 65272
      by mobilization and rearrangement with
        hospitalization ~ 65273
      direct closure ~ 65270
    cornea
      nonperforating ~ 65275
      perforating ~ 65280-65285
    muscles ~ 65290
    sclera
      anterior segment ~ 66250
      with graft ~ 66225
      without graft ~ 66220
      with tissue glue ~ 65286
    trabeculae ~ 65855

Eye ~ *continued*
  wound
    by mobilization and rearrangement ~
      65272-65273
    direct closure ~ 65270
  shunt, aqueous to extraocular reservoir ~
    66180
  transluminal dilation, aqueous outflow canal
    ~ 66174-66175
  ultrasound ~ 76510-76514
    biometry ~ 76516-76519
    foreign body ~ 76529
  unlisted services and procedures
    anterior segment ~ 66999
    posterior segment ~ 67299
  with muscle or myocutaneous flap ~ 65114
    muscles attached ~ 65105
  ocular contents
    without implant ~ 65091
    with implant ~ 65093
  orbital contents ~ 65110
    without implant ~ 65101
  X-ray ~ 70030
Eye and ocular adnexa, surgical procedures
  65091-68899
Eyebrow repair
  ptosis ~ 67900
Eyeglasses ~ 92340-92342
Eyelashes
  repair trichiasis
    epilation
      by forceps only ~ 67820
      by other than forceps ~ 67825
    incision of lid margin ~ 67830
      with free mucous membrane graft ~ 67835
Eyelid
  abscess, incision and drainage ~ 67700
  biopsy ~ 67810
  blepharoplasty ~ 15820-15823
  chalazion
    excision ~ 67805
      with anesthesia ~ 67808
      multiple ~ 67801-67805
      single ~ 67800
  closure by suture ~ 67875
  incision
    canthus ~ 67715
    sutures ~ 67710
  injection, subconjunctival ~ 68200
  lesion
    destruction ~ 67850
    excision
      with anesthesia ~ 67808
      without closure ~ 67840
      multiple ~ 67801-67805
      single ~ 67800
  reconstruction
    canthus ~ 67950
    total ~ 67973-67975
    total eyelid
      lower ~ 67973-67975
      second stage ~ 67975

Eyelid ~ *continued*
  upper ~ 67974
  transfer of tarsoconjunctival flap from
    opposing eyelid ~ 67971
  removal foreign body ~ 67938
  repair ~ 21280-21282
    blepharoptosis
      conjunctivo-tarso-muller's muscle-levator
        resection ~ 67908
      frontalis muscle technique ~ 67901-67094
      reduction overcorrection of ptosis ~ 67909
      superior rectus technique with fascial sling
        ~ 67906
    ectropion
      blepharoplasty ~ 67914
      suture ~ 67914
    entropion
      excision tarsal wedge ~ 67923
      extensive ~ 67924
      suture ~ 67921
      thermocauterization ~ 67922
    excisional ~ 67961
      over one-fourth of lid margin ~ 67966
    lagophthalmos ~ 67912
    lashes
      epilation, by forceps only ~ 67820
      epilation, by other than forceps ~ 67825
      lid margin ~ 67830-67835
    wound
      full thickness ~ 67935
      partial thickness ~ 67930
    repair with graft retraction ~ 67911
    skin graft
      full thickness ~ 67961
      split ~ 67961
    suture ~ 67880
      with transposition of tarsal plate ~ 67882
    tissue transfer, adjacent ~ 67961
    unlisted services and procedures ~ 67999
Eyelid ptoses ~ see blepharoptosis
Eye allergy test ~ 95060
Eye evisceration ~ 65091, 65093
Eye exam
  established patient ~ 92012-92014
  new patient ~ 92002-92004
  with anesthesia ~ 92018-92019
Eye exercises, training ~ 92065
Eye muscles
  biopsy ~ 67346
  repair
    strabismus
      adjustable sutures ~ 67335
      exploration and/or repair detached
        extraocular muscle ~ 67340
      one vertical muscle ~ 67314
      on patient with previous surgery ~ 67331
      posterior fixation suture ~ 67334
      recession or resection ~ 67311-67312
      release of scar tissue without detaching
        extraocular muscle ~ 67343
      two or more vertical muscles ~ 67316

Eye muscles ~ *continued*
    with scarring extraocular muscles ~ 67332
    with superior oblique muscle ~ 67318
  transposition ~ 67320
  unlisted services and procedures ~ 67399
Eye prosthesis ~ see prosthesis
Eye socket ~ see orbit ~ 21385-21395,
  21260-21263, 21267-21268, 67415
E antigens ~ 87350
E B virus ~ 86663-86665
E vitamin ~ 84446

F

Face
  CT scan ~ 70486-70488
  lesion
    destruction ~ 17000-17004, 17280-17286
  lift ~ 15824-15828
  magnetic resonance imaging (MRI) ~
    70540-70543
  tumor resection ~ 21015
Facial asymmetries ~ 21247
Facial bones ~ see also mandible; maxilla
  abscess excision ~ 21026
  reconstruction
    secondary ~ 21275
  repair ~ 21208-21209
  tumor
    excision ~ 21029-21034
    resection
      radical ~ 21015
  X-ray ~ 70140-70150
Facial nerve
  anastomosis
    to hypoglossal ~ 64868
    to phrenic nerve ~ 64870
    to spinal accessory ~ 64866
  avulsion ~ 64742
  chemodenervation, muscles ~ 64615
  decompression ~ 61590, 61596
    intratemporal
      lateral to geniculate ganglion ~ 69720,
        69740
      medial to geniculate ganglion ~ 69725,
        69745
    total ~ 69955
  function study ~ 92516
  incision ~ 64742
  injection, anesthetic ~ 64402
  mobilization ~ 61590
  repair
    lateral to geniculate ganglion ~ 69740
    medial to geniculate ganglion ~ 69745
  repair/suture
    with or without graft ~ 64864-64865

1415

Facial nerve ~ *continued*
suture
    lateral to geniculate ganglion ~ 69740
    medial to geniculate ganglion ~ 69745
    transection ~ 64742
Facial nerve paralysis
graft ~ 15840-15845
repair ~ 15840-15845
Facial prosthesis impression ~ 21088
Facial rhytidectomy ~ 15824-15828
Factor
ACTH-releasing ~ 80412
antinuclear ~ 86038-86039
blood coagulation ~ 85210-85293
Factor I ~ 85384-85385
Factor II ~ 85210
Factor III ~ see thromboplastin
Factor inhibitor test ~ 85335
Factor IV ~ see calcium
Factor IXix ~ 85250
Factor rheumatoid ~ 86430-86431
Factor VII ~ 85230
Factor VIII ~ 85210-85293
Factor X ~ 85260
Factor X, activated ~ 85260
Factor XA inhibitor ~ 85300-85301
Factor XI ~ 85270
Factor XII ~ 85280
Factor XIII ~ 85290-85291
Fitzgerald ~ 85293
Fletcher ~ 85293
hyperglycemic-glycogenolytic ~ 82943
intrinsic ~ 83528
sulfation ~ 84305
Fallopian tube
anastomosis ~ 58750
catheterization ~ 58345, 74742
destruction endoscopy ~ 58670
ectopic pregnancy ~ 59121
    with salpingectomy and/or oophorectomy ~ 59120
excision ~ 58700-58720
ligation ~ 58600-58611
lysis adhesions ~ 58740
occlusion ~ 58615
    endoscopy ~ 58671
    placement, implant for occlusion ~ 58568
pregnancy ~ 59121
repair ~ 58752
    anastomosis ~ 58750
    create stoma ~ 58770
tumor resection ~ 58950, 58952-58956
unlisted services and procedures ~ 58999
X-ray ~ 74742
Fallot, tetralogy of ~ 33692-33697, 33924
Family psychotherapy ~ 90846-90849, 99510
Fanconi anemia chromosome analysis ~ 88248
Farnsworth-Munsell color test ~ 92283
Farr test ~ 82784-82787
Fasanella-Servat procedure ~ 67908
Fascia graft ~ 15840

Fascia lata graft harvesting ~ 20920-20922
Fascial defect repair ~ 50728
Fascial graft
free microvascular anastomosis ~ 15758
open treatment, sternoclavicular dislocation ~ 23532
Fasciectomy
foot ~ 28060
    radical ~ 28060-28062
palm ~ 26121-26125
Fasciocutaneous flaps ~ 15732-15738
Fasciotomy
arm, lower ~ 24495, 25020-25025
buttock, decompression ~ 27027
    with debridement ~ 27057
foot ~ 28008
hand decompression ~ 26037
hip ~ 27025
knee ~ 27305, 27496-27499
leg, lower ~ 27600-27602, 27892-27894
leg, upper ~ 27305, 27496-27499, 27892-27894
palm ~ 26040-26045
pelvis, decompression ~ 27027
    with debridement ~ 27057
plantar endoscopic ~ 29893
thigh ~ 27025
toe ~ 28008
wrist ~ 25020-25023
FAST ~ see allergen immunotherapy
Fat
feces ~ 82705-82715
removal, lipectomy ~ 15876-15879
Fatty acid
blood ~ 82725
very long chain ~ 82726
Fat stain
feces ~ 89125
respiratory secretions ~ 89125
sputum ~ 89125
urine ~ 89125
Favre-durand disease ~ 86729
FC receptor ~ 86243
FDP ~ 85362-85380
Fe (iron) ~ 83540
Feedback, psychophysiologic (see biofeedback) ~ 90901-90911
Female castration ~ 58262-58263, 58291-58292, 58552, 58554, 58661, 58940-58943
Female genital system, surgical procedures ~ 56405-58999
Female gonad ~ see ovary
Femoral arteries ~ see artery, femoral
Femoral nerve
injection, anesthetic ~ 64447-64448
Femoral stem prosthesis ~ 27132
Femoral vein ~ 34501
Femur ~ see hip; knee; leg, upper
abscess, incision ~ 27303
bursa, excision ~ 27062
craterization ~ 27070, 27360

Femur ~ *continued*
  cyst, excision ~ 27065-27067, 27355-27358
  diaphysectomy ~ 27360
  drainage ~ 27303
  excision ~ 27070, 27360
    epiphyseal bar ~ 20150
  fracture ~ 27244
    closed treatment ~ 27501-27503
    distal ~ 27508, 27510, 27514
    distal, medial or lateral condyle ~ 27509
    epiphysis ~ 27516-27519
    intertrochanteric ~ 27244
    intertrochanteric
      closed treatment ~ 27238
      treatment with implant ~ 27244
      with implant ~ 27245
      with manipulation ~ 27240
    neck
      closed treatment ~ 27230-27232
      open treatment ~ 27236
      percutaneous fixation ~ 27235
    open treatment ~ 27245, 27269,
      27506-27507, 27511-27513
    percutaneous fixation ~ 27509
    pertrochanteric ~ 27244
    pertrochanteric
      closed treatment ~ 27238
      treatment with implant ~ 27244
      with implant ~ 27245
      with manipulation ~ 27240
    proximal end, head
      closed treatment ~ 27267-27268
      open treatment ~ 27269
    shaft ~ 27500, 27502, 27506-27507
    subtrochanteric ~ 27244
    subtrochanteric
      closed treatment ~ 27238
      treatment with implant ~ 27244
      with implant ~ 27245
      with manipulation ~ 27240
    supracondylar ~ 27501-27503, 27509,
      27511-27513
    transcondylar ~ 27501-27503, 27509,
      27511-27513
    trochanteric
      closed treatment ~ 27246
      open treatment ~ 27248
    without manipulation ~ 27501
    with manipulation ~ 27503
  halo ~ 20663
  lesion excision ~ 27062
  osteoplasty
    lengthening ~ 27466-27468
    shortening ~ 27465, 27468
  osteotomywithout fixation ~ 27448
  prophylactic treatment ~ 27187, 27495
  realignment ~ 27454
  reconstruction ~ 27468
    at knee ~ 27442-27443, 27446
    lengthening ~ 27466-27468
    shortening ~ 27465, 27468

Femur ~ *continued*
  repair ~ 27470-27472
    epiphysis ~ 27181, 27475, 27742
    arrest ~ 27185
    muscle transfer ~ 27110
    osteotomy ~ 27140, 27151-27156,
      27161-27165, 27450-27454
    with graft ~ 27170
  saucerization ~ 27070, 27360
  tumor excision ~ 27065-27067, 27355-27358,
    27365
  X-ray ~ 73550
Fenestration, pericardium ~ 33015
Fenestration procedure
  semicircular canal ~ 69820
    revision ~ 69840
  tracheostomy ~ 31610
Fern test ~ 87210
Ferric chloride, urine ~ 81005
Ferrihemoglobin ~ 83045-83050
Ferritin, blood or urine ~ 82728
Ferroxidase ~ (ceruloplasmin) 82390
Fertility control ~ see contraception
Fertility test
  semen analysis ~ 89300-89321
  sperm analysis
    cervical mucus penetration test ~ 89330
    hamster penetration ~ 89329
Fertilization, assisted
  oocyte ~ 89250, 89251
    microtechnique ~ 89280-89281
    with co-culture ~ 89251
Fertilization in vitro ~ 58321-58322
Fetal biophysical profile ~ 76818-76819
Fetal contraction stress test ~ 59020
Fetal hemoglobin ~ 85461
Fetal lung maturity assessment; lecithin
  sphingomyelin ratio ~ 83661
Fetal monitoring ~ 59050-59051, 99500
Fetal non-stress test ~ 59025
  ultrasound ~ 76818
Fetal procedure
  amnioinfusion ~ 59070
  cord occlusion ~ 59072
  fluid drainage ~ 59074
  shunt placement ~ 59076
  unlisted ~ 59897
Fetal testing
  amniotic fluid lung maturity ~ 83661,
    83663-83664
  heart ~ 76825-76826
  Doppler
    complete ~ 76827
    follow-up or repeat study ~ 76828
  hemoglobin ~ 83030-83033, 85460
  ultrasound ~ 76801-76828
    heart ~ 76825
    middle cerebral artery ~ 76821
    umbilical artery ~ 76820
Fetuin ~ 82105-82106
Fever, Australian Q ~ 86000, 86638
Fever, Japanese river ~ 86000

1417

Fibrillation, atrial ~ 33254-33256,
 33265-33266
 documentation ~ 1060F-1061F
Fibrillation, heart ~ see heart, fibrillation
Fibrin
 degradation products ~ 85362-85380
 deposit removal ~ 32150
 stabilizing factor ~ 85290-85291
Fibrinase ~ 85400
Fibrinogen ~ 85384-85385
Fibrinolysin ~ 85400
Fibrinolysins ~ 85390
Fibrinolysis
 alpha-2 antiplasmin ~ 85410
 assay ~ 85396
  activity ~ 85397
  ADAMTS-13 ~ 85397
 plasmin ~ 85400
 plasminogen ~ 85420-85421
 plasminogen activator ~ 85415
 pleural cavity, instillation of agent ~ 32561,
  32562
Fibroadenoma, excision ~ 19120-19126
 ablation
  cryosurgical ~ 19105
Fibroblastoma, arachnoidal ~ 61512, 61519
Fibrocutaneous tags ~ 11200-11201
Fibromatosis, Dupuytren's ~ 26040-26045
Fibromatosis, penile ~ see Peyronie disease
Fibromyoma ~ 58140, 58545-58546, 58561
Fibronectin, fetal ~ 82731
Fibrosis, penile ~ see Peyronie disease
Fibrosis, retroperitoneal ~ 50715
Fibrous cavernitides ~ see Peyronie disease
Fibrous dysplasia ~ 21029, 21181-21184
Fibula ~ see ankle; knee; tibia
 bone graft with microvascular anastomosis ~
  20955
 craterization ~ 27360, 27641
 cyst excision ~ 27635-27638
 diaphysectomy ~ 27360, 27641
 excision ~ 27360, 27641
  epiphyseal bar ~ 20150
 fracture
  malleolus ~ 27786-27814
  shaft ~ 27780-27784
 incision ~ 27607
 osteoplasty lengthening ~ 27715
 repair
  epiphysis ~ 27477-27485, 27730-27742
  nonunion or malunion ~ 27726
  osteotomy ~ 27707-27712
 saucerization ~ 27360, 27641
 tumor excision ~ 27635-27638, 27646
 X-ray ~ 73590
Figure of eight cast ~ 29049
Filariasis ~ 86280
Filtering operation ~ see incision, sclera,
 fistulization
Filtration implant, glaucoma ~ 66180, 66185
Fimbrioplasty ~ 58760
 laparoscopic ~ 58672

Fine needle aspiration ~ 10021-10022
 evaluation ~ 88172-88173
Finger ~ see phalanx, finger
 abscess
  bone, incision and drainage ~ 26034
  incision and drainage ~ 26010-26011
 amputation ~ 26951-26952
  with exploration or removal ~ 26910
 arthrocentesis ~ 20600
 arthrodesis
  interphalangeal joint ~ 26860-26863
  metacarpophalangeal joint ~ 26850-26852
 bone, incision and drainage ~ 26034
 cast ~ 29086
 collection of blood ~ 36415-36416
 decompression ~ 26035
 excision
  constricting ring ~ 26596
  tendon ~ 26180, 26390, 26415
 insertion, tendon graft ~ 26392
 magnetic resonance imaging (MRI) ~ 73221
 reconstruction
  extra digit ~ 26587
  toe to hand transfer ~ 26551-26556
 removal
  implantation ~ 26320
  tube ~ 26392, 26416
 repair
  blood vessel ~ 35207
  claw finger ~ 26499
  extra digit ~ 26587
  macrodactylia ~ 26590
  tendon
   extensor ~ 26415-26434, 26445-26449,
    26460
   flexor ~ 26356-26358, 26440-26442,
    26455
  volar plate ~ 26548
  web finger ~ 26560-26562
 replantation ~ 20816-20822
 reposition ~ 26555
 sesamoidectomy ~ 26185
 splint ~ 29130-29131
 strapping ~ 29280
 tendon sheath
  excision ~ 26145
  incision ~ 26055
  incision and drainage ~ 26020
 tenotomy ~ 26060, 26460
  flexor ~ 26455
 tumor excision ~ 26111-26118
 unlisted services and procedures ~ 26989
 X-ray ~ 73140
Finger flap, tissue transfer ~ 14350
Finger joint ~ see intercarpal joint
Finney operation ~ 43810, 43850-43855
FISH ~ 88365
Fissurectomy, anal ~ 46200
Fissure in ano ~ 46200, 46949-46942
Fistula
 anal, repair ~ 46288, 46706
 autogenous graft ~ 36825

Fistula ~ *continued*
bronchi, repair ~ 32815
carotid-cavernous, repair ~ 61710
chest wall, repair ~ 32906
conjunctiva
without tube ~ 68745
with tube or stent ~ 68750
enterovesical
closure ~ 44660-44661
kidney ~ 50520-50526
lacrimal gland closure ~ 68770
dacryocystorhinostomy ~ 68720
nose repair ~ 30580-30600
oval window ~ 69666
postauricular ~ 69700
rectovaginal
abdominal approach ~ 57305
transperineal approach ~ 57308
with concomitant colostomy ~ 57307
round window ~ 69667
sclera
iridencleisis or iridotasis ~ 66165
sclerectomy with punch or scissors with
iridectomy ~ 66160
thermocauterization with iridectomy ~ 66155
trabeculectomy ab externo in absence
previous surgery ~ 66170
trabeculectomy ab externo with scarring ~
66172
trephination with iridectomy ~ 66150
suture
kidney ~ 50520-50526
ureter ~ 50920-50930
trachea ~ 31755
tracheoesophageal
repair ~ 43305, 43312, 43314
speech prothesis ~ 31611
ureter ~ 50920-50930
urethra ~ 53400-53405
urethrovaginal ~ 57310
with bulbocavernosus transplant ~ 57311
vesicouterine closure ~ 51920-51925
vesicovaginal
closure ~ 51900
transvesical and vaginal approach ~ 57330
vaginal approach ~ 57320
X-ray ~ 76080
Fistulectomy, anal ~ 46060, 46270-46285
Fistulization
conjunction to nasal cavity ~ 68745
esophagus ~ 43350-43352
intestines ~ 44300-44346
lacrimal sac to nasal cavity ~ 68720
penis ~ 54435
pharynx ~ 42955
repair salivary cyst, sublingual ~ 42325-42326
tracheopharyngeal ~ 31755
Fistulization, interatrial ~ 33735-33737
Fistulotomy, anal ~ 46270, 46280
Fitting
cervical cap ~ 57170
contact lens ~ 92071-92072, 92310-92313

Fitting ~ *continued*
diaphragm ~ 57170
low vision aid ~ 92354-92355
ocular prosthesis ~ 92330
spectacles ~ 92340-92342
spectacle prosthesis ~ 92352-92353
Fitzgerald factor ~ 85293
Fixation, interdental without fracture ~ 21497
Fixation, external ~ see external fixation
Fixation, kidney ~ see nephropexy
Fixation, rectum ~ see proctopexy
Fixation, tongue ~ see tongue, fixation
Fixation (device) ~ see application; bone,
fixation; spinal instrumentation
application, external ~ 20690-20692,
20696-20697
pelvic, insertion ~ 22848
removal
external ~ 20694
internal ~ 20670-20680
sacrospinous ligament, vaginal prolapse ~
57282
shoulder ~ 23700
skeletal, humeral epycondyle, percutaneous ~
24566
spinal
insertion ~ 22841-22847
prosthetic ~ 22851
reinsertion ~ 22849
Fixation test, complement ~ 86171
Flank ~ see back/flank
Flap ~ see skin graft and flap
free, breast reconstruction ~ 19364
grafts ~ 15570-15738, 15842
latissimus dorsi breast reconstruction ~ 19361
omentum ~ 49905
omentum, free, with microvascular
anastomosis ~ 49906
transverse rectus abdominis myocutaneous
breast reconstruction ~ 19367-19369
Flatfoot correction ~ 28735
Flea typhus ~ 86000
Fletcher factor ~ 85292
Flow cytometry ~ 88182-88189
diagnostic/pre-treatment ~ 3170F
Flow-volume loop, pulmonary ~ 94375
Fluid
amniotic ~ see amniotic fluid
body ~ 89060
cerebrospinal ~ 86325
collection, incision and drainage, skin ~ 10140
Fluorescein
angiography, ocular ~ 92287
intravenous injection
vascular flow check, graft ~ 15860
Fluorescein angiography ~ 92235
Fluorescent in situ hybridization ~ 88365
Fluoride
blood ~ 82735
urine ~ 82735

1419

Fluoroscopy
bile duct
  calculus removal ~ 74327
  guide catheter ~ 74328, 74330
chest ~ 31628
  bronchoscopy ~ 31622-31640
  complete (four views) ~ 71034
  partial (two views) ~ 71023
drain abscess ~ 75989
GI tract
  guide intubation ~ 74340
hourly ~ 76000-76001
introduction GI tube ~ 74340
larynx ~ 70370
nasogastric ~ 43752
needle biopsy ~ 77002
orogastric ~ 43752
pancreatic duct, guide catheter ~ 74329-74330
pharynx ~ 70370
renal guide catheter ~ 74475
spine/paraspinous, guide catheter/needle ~ 77003
unlisted services and procedures ~ 76496
ureter guide catheter ~ 74480
venous access device ~ 36598, 77001
Flurazepam, blood or urine ~ 82742
Flush aortogram ~ 36251-36254
FNA ~ see fine needle aspiration
Foam stability test ~ 83662
Fold, vocal ~ see vocal cords
Foley operation pyeloplasty ~ 50400-50405, 50544
Foley Y-pyeloplasty ~ 50400-50405
Folic acid ~ 82747
blood ~ 82746
Follicle stimulating hormone (FSH) ~ 80418, 80426, 83001
Folliculin ~ 82679
Follitropin ~ 80418, 80426, 83001
Follow-up inpatient consultations ~ 99251-99255
Follow-up services
post-op ~ 99024
Fontan procedure ~ 33600-33617
Food allergy test ~ 95076, 95079
Foot ~ see metatarsal ~ 28456
amputation ~ 28800-28805
bursa incision and drainage ~ 28001
capsulotomy ~ 28260-28264
cast ~ 29450
fasciectomy ~ 28060
  radical ~ 28060-28062
fasciotomy ~ 28008
  endoscopic ~ 29893
incision ~ 28002-28005
joint ~ see tarsometatarsal joint ~ 28570-28576, 28585
  magnetic resonance imaging (MRI) ~ 73721-73723
lesion excision ~ 28080, 28090
magnetic resonance imaging (MRI) ~ 73718-73720

Foot ~ continued
nerve
  excision ~ 28055
  incision ~ 28035
neuroma excision ~ 28080
reconstruction cleft foot ~ 28360
removal foreign body ~ 28190-28193
repair
  muscle ~ 28250
  tendon ~ 28200-28230, 28234-28238
replantation ~ 20838
sesamoid excision ~ 28315
strapping ~ 29540
suture tendon ~ 28200-28210
tendon sheath excision ~ 28086-28088
tenotomy ~ 28230, 28234
tumor excision ~ 28039-28047
unlisted services and procedures ~ 28899
X-ray ~ 73620-73630
Foot abscess ~ 28005
Forearm ~ see arm, lower ~ 20805
Forehead
reconstruction ~ 21179-21180, 21182-21184
  midface ~ 21159-21160
reduction ~ 21137-21139
Forehead and orbital rim
reconstruction ~ 21172-21180
Foreign body removal
anal ~ 46608
arm
  lower ~ 25248
  upper ~ 24200, 24201
auditory canal, external ~ 69200
  with anesthesia ~ 69205
bronchi ~ 31635
colon ~ 44025, 44390, 45332, 45379
conjunctival, embedded ~ 65210
cornea ~ 65220, 65222
duodenum ~ 44010
external eye ~ 65205
eyelid ~ 67938
finger ~ 26075, 26080
foot ~ 28190, 28193
gum ~ 41805
hand ~ 26070
hip ~ 27033, 27086, 27087
intraocular ~ 65235
knee joint ~ 27310, 27331, 27372
lacrimal duct/gland ~ 68530
larynx ~ 31511, 31530, 31531, 31577
leg, upper ~ 27372
lung ~ 32151
mandible ~ 41806
maxillary sinus ~ 31299
mediastinum ~ 39000, 39010
mouth ~ 40804, 40805
nose ~ 30300
  with anesthesia ~ 30310
  lateral rhinotomy ~ 30320
orbit ~ 61334, 67413, 67430
pancreatic duct ~ 43269
pelvis ~ 27086, 27087

Foreign body removal ~ *continued*
penis ~ 54115
pericardium ~ 33020
  endoscopic ~ 32658
pharynx ~ 42809
pleura ~ 32150, 32151
  endoscopic ~ 32653
rectum ~ 45307, 45915
scrotum ~ 55120
shoulder ~ 23040, 23044
  complicated ~ 23332
  deep ~ 23331
  subcutaneous 23330
skin with debridement ~ 11010-11012
subcutaneous ~ 10120, 10121
  with debridement ~ 11010-11012
ureter ~ 50961, 50980
urethra ~ 52310, 52315
uterus ~ 58562
vagina ~ 57415
Forensic exam ~ 88040
cytopathology ~ 88125
phosphatase, acid ~ 84061
Foreskin of penis ~ 54450
Formycin diphosphate ~ 85362-85380
Fournier's gangrene ~ 11004-11006
Fowler-Stephens orchiopexy ~ 54640, 54650, 54692
Fowler-Stephens procedure ~ 54650
Fox operation ~ 67921-67924
Fraction, factor IX (nine) ~ 85250
Fracture
acetabulum
  closed treatment ~ 27220-27222
    with manipulation ~ 27222
    without manipulation ~ 27220
  open treatment ~ 27226-27228
alveola
  closed treatment ~ 21421
  open treatment ~ 21422-21423
alveolar ridge
  closed treatment ~ 21440
  open treatment ~ 21445
ankle
  bimalleolar ~ 27808-27814
  closed treatment ~ 27816-27818
  lateral ~ 27786-27814, 27792
  medial ~ 27760-27766, 27808-27814
  posterior ~ 27767-27769, 27808-27814
  trimalleolar ~ 27816-27823
ankle bone
  medial ~ 27760-27762
Bennett's thumb fracture
  with dislocation ~ 26645, 26650
  open treatment ~ 26665
bronchi endoscopy ~ 31630
calcaneus
  closed treatment ~ 28400-28405
    with manipulation ~ 28405-28406
    without manipulation ~ 28400
  open treatment ~ 28415-28420
  percutaneous fixation ~ 28436

Fracture ~ *continued*
carpal
  closed treatment
    with manipulation ~ 25624, 25635
    without manipulation ~ 25622, 25630
  open treatment ~ 25628, 25645
carpal scaphoid, closed treatment ~ 25622
cheekbone
  with manipulation ~ 21355
  open treatment ~ 21360-21366
clavicle
  closed treatment
    with manipulation ~ 23505
    without manipulation ~ 23500
  open treatment ~ 23515
  closed treatment ~ 27520
coccyx
  closed treatment ~ 27200
  open treatment ~ 27202
Colles ~ see Colles fracture
Colles-reversed ~ see Smith fracture
elbow
  Monteggia
    closed treatment ~ 24620
    open treatment ~ 24635
  open treatment ~ 24586-24587
femur ~ 27244
  closed treatment ~ 27230, 27238-27240, 27246, 27500-27503, 27508, 27510, 27516-27517
    with manipulation ~ 27232
  distal ~ 27508, 27510, 27514
  epiphysis ~ 27516-27519
  intertrochanteric ~ 27244
    closed treatment ~ 27238
    intramedullary implant ~ 27245
    open treatment ~ 27244
      with implant ~ 27245
    with manipulation ~ 27240
  neck
    closed treatment ~ 27230
      with manipulation ~ 27232
    open treatment ~ 27236
    percutaneous fixation ~ 27235
  open treatment ~ 27245, 27248, 27506-27507, 27511-27514, 27519
  percutaneous fixation ~ 27235, 27509
  pertrochanteric
    closed treatment ~ 27238
      with manipulation ~ 27240
    intramedullary implant shaft ~ 27245, 27500, 27502, 27506-27507
    open treatment ~ 27245, 27245
  subtrochanteric
    closed treatment ~ 27238
      with manipulation ~ 27240
    intramedullary implant ~ 27245
    open treatment ~ 27245
  supracondylar ~ 27501-27503, 27509, 27511-27513
  transcondylar ~ 27501-27503, 27509, 27511-27513

1421

Fracture ~ *continued*
trochanteric
  closed treatment ~ 27246
  open treatment ~ 27248
  with manipulation ~ 27232, 27502-27503, 27510
  without manipulation ~ 27230, 27238, 27246, 27500-27501, 27508, 27516-27517, 27520
fibula
  closed treatment ~ 27780-27781, 27786-27788, 27808-27810
  malleolus ~ 27786-27814
  open treatment ~ 27784, 27792, 27814
  shaft ~ 27780-27786, 27808
  with manipulation ~ 27788, 27810
  without manipulation ~ 27780-27781
frontal sinus, open treatment ~ 21343-21344
great toe
  closed treatment ~ 28490
  without manipulation ~ 28490
heel
  closed treatment
    with manipulation ~ 28405-28406
    without manipulation ~ 28400
  open treatment ~ 28415-28420
humerus
  closed treatment ~ 24500-24505
    with manipulation ~ 23605
    without manipulation ~ 23600
  condyle
    closed treatment ~ 24576-24577
    open treatment ~ 24579
    percutaneous ~ 24582
  epicondyle
    closed treatment ~ 24560-24565
    open treatment ~ 24575
    skeletal fixation, percutaneous ~ 24566
  greater tuberosity fracture
    closed treatment with manipulation ~ 23625
    closed treatment without manipulation ~ 23620
    open treatment ~ 23630
  open treatment ~ 23615-23616
  shaft ~ 24500-24505, 24516
    open treatment ~ 24515
  supracondylar
    closed treatment ~ 24530-24535
    open treatment ~ 24545-24546
    percutaneous fixation ~ 24538
  transcondylar
    closed treatment ~ 24530-24535
    open treatment ~ 24545-24546
    percutaneous fixation ~ 24538
  with dislocation
    closed treatment ~ 23665
    open treatment ~ 23670
  with shoulder dislocation
    closed treatment ~ 23675
    open treatment ~ 23680

Fracture ~ *continued*
hyoid bone
  closed treatment
    manipulation ~ 21494
    without manipulation ~ 21493
  open treatment ~ 21495
ilium
  open treatment ~ 27215, 27218
  percutaneous fixation ~ 27216
knee ~ 27520
  arthroscopic treatment ~ 29850-29851
  open treatment ~ 27524
larynx
  closed treatment
    with manipulation ~ 31586
    without manipulation ~ 31585
  open treatment ~ 31584
malar area
  open treatment ~ 21360-21366
  with bone graft ~ 21366
  with manipulation ~ 21355
mandible
  closed treatment
    interdental fixation ~ 21453
    with manipulation ~ 21451
    without manipulation ~ 21450
  open treatment ~ 21454-21470
    external fixation ~ 21454
    with interdental fixation ~ 21462
    without interdental fixation ~ 21461
  percutaneous treatment ~ 21452
maxilla
  closed treatment ~ 21421
  open treatment ~ 21422-21423
metacarpal
  closed treatment ~ 26600-26605
    with fixation ~ 26607
    with manipulation ~ 26605-26607
    without manipulation ~ 26600
  open treatment ~ 26615
  percutaneous fixation ~ 26608
metatarsal
  closed treatment ~ 28470-28475
    with manipulation ~ 28475-28476
    without manipulation ~ 28450, 28470
  open treatment ~ 28485
  percutaneous fixation ~ 28476
Monteggia ~ see fracture, ulna ~ 24620-24635
nasal bone
  closed treatment ~ 21310-21320
    with manipulation ~ 21315-21320
    without manipulation ~ 21310
  open treatment ~ 21325-21335
nasal septum
  closed treatment ~ 21337
  open treatment ~ 21336
nasal turbinate therapeutic ~ 30930
nasoethmoid
  open treatment ~ 21338-21339
  percutaneous treatment ~ 21340
  with fixation ~ 21340

Fracture ~ *continued*
nasomaxillary
  closed treatment ~ 21345
  open treatment ~ 21346-21348
  with bone grafting ~ 21348
  with fixation ~ 21345-21347
navicular
  closed treatment ~ 25622
  open treatment ~ 25628
  with manipulation ~ 25624
odontoid
  open treatment
    with graft ~ 22319
    without graft ~ 22318
orbit
  closed treatment
    with manipulation ~ 21401
    without manipulation ~ 21400
  open treatment ~ 21406-21408
  blowout fracture ~ 21385-21395
orbital floor
  blow out ~ 21385-21395
palate
  closed treatment ~ 21421
  open treatment ~ 21422-21423
patella
  closed treatment, without manipulation ~ 27520
  open treatment ~ 27524
pelvic ring
  closed treatment ~ 27193-27194
    without manipulation ~ 27193-27194
  open treatment
    anterior ~ 27217
    posterior ~ 27218
  percutaneous fixation ~ 27216
phalanges
  articular
    closed treatment ~ 26740
    open treatment ~ 26746
    with manipulation ~ 26742
  closed treatment ~ 26742, 28510
    articular ~ 26740
    distal ~ 26750
    with manipulation ~ 26755
  distal ~ 26755-26756
    closed treatment ~ 26750
    open treatment ~ 26765
    percutaneous fixation ~ 26756
  finger/thumb
    closed treatment ~ 26720-26725
    with manipulation ~ 26725-26727
    shaft ~ 26720, 26727
  great toe ~ 28490
    closed treatment ~ 28495
    with manipulation ~ 28495-28496
    open treatment ~ 28505
    percutaneous fixation ~ 28496
  open treatment ~ 26735, 26746
    distal ~ 26765

Fracture ~ *continued*
shaft
  closed treatment ~ 26725
  open treatment ~ 26735
  percutaneous fixation ~ 26727
toe
  closed treatment ~ 28515
    with manipulation ~ 28515
    without manipulation ~ 28510
  open treatment ~ 28525
  with manipulation ~ 26742, 26755
  without manipulation ~ 26740, 26750
radius
  closed treatment ~ 25560-25565
  Colles ~ 25600-25605
  distal ~ 25600-25606
    open treatment ~ 25607-25609
    Smith ~ 25600-25605
  head/neck
    closed treatment ~ 24650-24655
    open treatment ~ 24665-24666
  open treatment ~ 25515, 25607-25609
  percutaneous fixation ~ 25606
  shaft ~ 25500, 25525-25526
    closed treatment ~ 25500-25505, 25520
    open treatment ~ 25515, 25525-25526, 25574
  with manipulation ~ 25565, 25605
  without manipulation ~ 25560, 25600
  with ulna ~ 25560-25565
    open treatment ~ 25575
rib
  closed treatment ~ 21800
  external fixation ~ 21810
  open treatment ~ 21805
scaphoid
  closed treatment ~ 25622
  open treatment ~ 25628
  with dislocation
    closed treatment ~ 25680
    open treatment ~ 25685
  with manipulation ~ 25624
scapula
  closed treatment
    with manipulation ~ 23575
    without manipulation ~ 23570
  open treatment ~ 23585
sesamoid
  closed treatment ~ 28530
  foot ~ 28530-28531
  open treatment ~ 28531
skin debridement ~ 11010-11012
skull ~ 62000-62010
sternum
  closed treatment ~ 21820
  open treatment ~ 21825
talus
  closed treatment ~ 28430-28435
  open treatment ~ 28445
  with manipulation ~ 28435-28436
  without manipulation ~ 28430

Fracture ~ continued
tarsal
open treatment ~ 28465
percutaneous fixation ~ 28456
with manipulation ~ 28455-28456
thumb
open treatment ~ 26665
with dislocation ~ 26645-26650
tibia ~ 27759
arthroscopic treatment ~ 29855-29856
closed treatment ~ 27530-27532, 27538,
27750-27752, 27760-27762,
27808-27810, 27824-27825
distal ~ 27824-27828
intercondylar ~ 27538-27540
malleolus ~ 27760-27766, 27808-27814
open treatment ~ 27535-27536, 27540,
27758, 27766, 27814, 27826-27828
percutaneous fixation ~ 27756
plateau ~ 27530-27536, 29855-29856
shaft ~ 27750-27759
with manipulation ~ 27752, 27760-27762,
27810
without manipulation ~ 27530, 27750,
27760-27762, 27808, 27825
trachea, endoscopy ~ 31630
ulna
closed treatment ~ 25560-25565
olecranon
closed treatment ~ 24670-24675
open treatment ~ 24685
open treatment ~ 25574-25575
shaft
closed treatment ~ 25530-25535
open treatment ~ 25545, 25574
styloid process
closed treatment ~ 25650
open treatment ~ 25652
percutaneous fixation ~ 25651
with dislocation ~ 24620, 24635
closed treatment ~ 24620
Monteggia ~ 24620-24635
open treatment ~ 24635
with manipulation ~ 25535, 25565
with radius ~ 25560-25565
open treatment ~ 25575
without manipulation ~ 25530, 25560
vertebra
additional segment, open treatment ~ 22328
cervical, open treatment ~ 22326
closed treatment
with manipulation, casting and/or bracing
~ 22315
without manipulation ~ 22310
lumbar, open treatment ~ 22325
posterior, open treatment ~ 22325-22327
thoracic, open treatment ~ 22327
with shoulder dislocation
closed treatment ~ 23675
open treatment ~ 23680
vertebral process, closed treatment ~ 22305

Fracture ~ continued
wrist, with dislocation
closed treatment ~ 25680
open treatment ~ 25685
zygomatic arch
open treatment ~ 21356-21366
with manipulation ~ 21355
Fragile-X chromosome analysis ~ 88248
Fragility
red blood cell
mechanical ~ 85547
osmotic ~ 85555-85557
Frames, stereotactic ~ 20660
Francisella ~ 86000
antibody ~ 86668
Fredet-Ramstedt procedure ~ 43520
Free E3 ~ 82677
Free skin graft ~ 15050-15157, 15200-15261,
15271-15278, 15757
Free T4 (four) ~ 84439
Frei disease ~ 86729
Frenectomy ~ 40819, 41115
Frenectomy, lingual ~ 41115
Frenotomy ~ 40806, 41010
Frenulectomy ~ 40819
Frenuloplasty ~ 41520
Frenum lip, incision ~ 40806
Frenumectomy ~ 40819
Frickman operation ~ see proctopexy
Frontal craniotomy ~ 61556
Frontal sinus ~ see sinus, frontal
Frontal sinusotomy ~ 31070-31075
Frost suture ~ 67875
Frozen blood preparation ~ 86930-86932
Fructose ~ 84375
semen ~ 82757
Fructose intolerance breath test ~ 91065
Fruit sugar ~ 84375
FSF ~ 85290-85291
FSH ~ 80418, 80426, 83001
FT-4 ~ 84439
Fulguration ~ see destruction
bladder ~ 51020
cystourethroscopy with ~ 52214
lesion ~ 52224
tumor ~ 52234-52240
ureter ~ 50957-50959, 50976-50978
ureterocele
ectopic ~ 52301
orthotopic ~ 52300
Fulguration, endocavitary ~ 17000-17286
Full thickness graft ~ 15200-15261
Function, study, nasal ~ 92512
Function test, lung ~ see pulmonology,
diagnostic
Function test, vestibular ~ see vestibular
function tests
Fundoplasty
esophagogastric ~ 43325
laparoscopic ~ 43279-43282, 43327
via thoracotomy ~ 43328
esophagomyotomy, laparoscopic ~ 43279

Fundoplication ~ **43325**
Fungus
  antibody ~ 86671
  culture
    blood ~ 87103
    hair ~ 87101
    identification ~ 87106
    nail ~ 87101
    other ~ 87102
    skin ~ 87101
    tissue exam ~ 87220
Funnel chest ~ 21740-21743
Furuncle
  incision and drainage ~ 10060-10061
  vulva ~ 56405
Fusion ~ see arthrodesis
  pleural cavity ~ 32560
  thumb in opposition ~ 26820
Fusion, epiphyseal-diaphyseal ~ see epiphyseal arrest
Fusion, joint ~ see arthrodesis
Fusion, joint, interphalangeal, finger ~ 26860-26863

G

Gago procedure ~ 33463-33465
Gait training ~ 97116
Galactogram ~ 77053-77054
  injection ~ 19030
Galactokinase, blood ~ 82759
Galactose
  blood ~ 82760
  urine ~ 82760
Galactose-1-phosphate
  uridyl transferase ~ 82775-82776
Gallbladder ~ see also bile duct
  anastomosis with intestines ~ 47720-47741
  excision ~ 47562-47564, 47600-47620
  exploration ~ 47480
  incision ~ 47490
  incision and drainage ~ 47480
  removal, calculi (stone) ~ 47480
  repair
    with gastroenterostomy ~ 47741
    with intestines ~ 47720-47740
  unlisted services and procedures ~ 47999
  X-ray with contrast ~ 74290-74291
Galvanocautery ~ 17000-17286
Galvanoionization ~ 97033
Gamete intrafallopian transfer ~ see GIFT
Gamete transfer, in vitro fertilization ~ 58976
Gamma camera imaging ~ see nuclear medicine
Gamma glutamyl transferase ~ 82977
Gamma seminoprotein ~ 84152-84153
Gammacorten ~ 80420
Gammaglobulin, blood ~ 82784-82787
Gamulin Rh ~ 90384-90386

Ganglia, trigeminal ~ 61450, 61790
Ganglion cyst ~ 61450, 61790
  aspiration/injection ~ 20612
  drainage ~ 20612
  injection, anesthetic ~ 64505, 64510
  wrist excision ~ 25111-25112
Ganglion, Gasser's ~ 61450, 61790
Ganglion cervicothoracicum ~ 64510
Ganglion pterygopalatinum ~ 64505
Gardner operation ~ 63700-63702
Gardnerella vaginalis detection ~ 87510-87512
Gasserian ganglion
  sensory root
    decompression ~ 61450
    section ~ 61450
  stereotactic ~ 61790
Gasser ganglion ~ 61450, 61790
Gastrectomy
  longitudinal ~ 43775
  partial ~ 43631-43635, 43845
    with gastrojejunostomy ~ 43632
  sleeve ~ 43775
  total ~ 43621-43622
    with esophagoenterostomy ~ 43620
    with gastroduodenostomy ~ 43631
Gastric acid ~ 82930
Gastric analysis test
  secretory study ~ 43755-43757, 89135
Gastric electrodes
  implantation
    laparoscopic, neurostimulator ~ 43647
    open. neurostimulator ~ 43881
  removal
    laparoscopic, neurostimulator ~ 43648
    open, neurostimulator ~ 43882
  replacement
    laparoscopic, neurostimulator ~ 43647
    open, neurostimulator ~ 43881
  revision
    laparoscopic, neurostimulator ~ 43648
    open, neurostimulator ~ 43882
Gastric intubation
  diagnostic ~ 43754-43757
  therapeutic ~ 43753
Gastric lavage, therapeutic ~ 43753
Gastric tests, manometry ~ 91020
Gastric ulcer disease ~ 43610
Gastrin ~ 82938-82941
Gastrocnemius recession, leg, lower ~ 27687
Gastroduodenostomy ~ 43810, 43850-43855
Gastroenterology
  breath hydrogen test ~ 91065
  diagnostic services ~ 91010-91299
  esophagus tests
    acid perfusion ~ 91030
    acid reflux ~ 91032-91033
    balloon distension provocation study ~ 91040
    motility study ~ 91010
  gastroesophageal reflux test ~ 91034-91038
  gastric tests, manometry ~ 91020
  intestine bleeding tube ~ 43460

1425

Gastroenterology ~ *continued*
  manometry ~ 91020
  rectum sensation, tone, compliance ~ 91120
  rectum/anus manometry ~ 91122
  unlisted services and procedures ~ 91299
Gastroenterostomy
  for obesity ~ 43644-43645, 43842-43848
Gastroesophageal reflux test ~ 91034-91038
Gastrointestinal exam
  nuclear medicine
    blood loss study ~ 78278
    protein loss study ~ 78282
    shunt testing ~ 78291
    unlisted services and procedures ~ 78299
Gastrointestinal tract
  imaging intraluminal ~ 91110-91111
  reconstruction ~ 43360-43361
  upper dilation ~ 43249
  X-ray ~ 74240-74245
    with contrast ~ 74246-74249
    guide dilator ~ 74360
    guide intubation ~ 74340
Gastrointestinal, upper
  biopsy, endoscopy ~ 43239
  dilation
    endoscopy ~ 43245
    esophagus ~ 43248
  endoscopy
    catheterization ~ 43241
    destruction lesion ~ 43258
    dilation ~ 43245
    drainage pseudocyst ~ 43240
    exploration ~ 43235
    hemorrhage ~ 43255
    inject varices ~ 43243
    injection ~ 43236
    needle biopsy ~ 43242, 43238
    removal
      foreign body ~ 43247
      lesion ~ 43251
      polyp ~ 43251
      tumor ~ 43251
    stent placement ~ 43256
    thermal radiation ~ 43257
    tube placement ~ 43246
    ultrasound ~ 43237-43238, 43242, 43259, 76975
  exploration endoscopy ~ 43235
  hemorrhage endoscopic control ~ 43255
  injection
    submucosal ~ 43236
    varices ~ 43243
  lesion destruction ~ 43258
  ligation of vein ~ 43244
  needle biopsy, endoscopy ~ 43238, 43242
  removal
    foreign body ~ 43247
    lesion ~ 43250
    polyp ~ 43250-43251
    tumor ~ 43250
  tube placement, endoscopy ~ 43246
  ultrasound endoscopy ~ 43237-43238, 43242, 43259, 76975

Gastrojejunostomy ~ 43860-43865
  conversion from gastostomy tube ~ 49446
  contrast injection ~ 49465
  removal of obstructive material ~ 49460
  replacement of tube ~ 49452
  with duodenal exclusion ~ 48547
  with partial gastrectomy ~ 43632
  with vagotomy ~ 43825
  without vagotomy ~ 43820
Gastroplasty
  Collis ~ 43283, 43338
  evision for obesity ~ 43644-43645, 43842-43848
  wedge gastroplasty ~ 43283, 43338
  with esophagogastric fundoplasty ~ 43842-43843
Gastrorrhaphy ~ 43840
Gastroschises ~ 49605
Gastrostomy
  closure ~ 43870
  laparoscopic, temporary ~ 43653
  temporary ~ 43830
    laparoscopic ~ 43653
    neonatal ~ 43831
  with pancreatic drain ~ 48001
  with pyloroplasty ~ 43640
  with vagotomy ~ 43640
Gastrostomy tube
  change of ~ 43760
  contrast injection ~ 49465
  conversion to gastro-jejunostomy tube ~ 49446
  directed placement, endoscopic ~ 43246
  insertion ~ 49440
  obstructive material removal ~ 49460
  placement, percutaneous
    endoscopic ~ 43246
    nonendoscopic ~ 49440
  replacement ~ 49450
  repositioning ~ 43761
Gastrotomy ~ 43500-43501, 43510
GDH ~ 82965
Gel diffusion ~ 86331
Gel diffusion test ~ 86329-86331
Gene Analysis
  ASPA ~ 81200
  BCKDHB ~ 81205
  BCR/ABL1 ~ 81206-81208
  BLM ~ 81209
  BRAF ~ 81210
  BRCA1 ~ 81214-81215
  BRCA2 ~ 81216-81217
  BRCA1, BRCA1 ~ 81211-81213
  CFTR ~ 81220-81224
  chimerixm analysis ~ 81267-81268
  comparative analysis using short tandem
    repeat makers ~ 81265-81266
  CYP2C19 ~ 81225
  CYP2D6 ~ 81226
  CYP2C9 ~ 81227
  cytogenic constitutional microarray analysis ~ 81228-81229
  F2 ~ 81240

Gene Analysis ~ *continued*
F5 ~ 81241
FANCC ~ 81242
FLT3 ~ 81245
FMR1 ~ 81243-81244
G6PC ~ 81250
GBA ~ 81251
HBA1/HBA2 ~ 81257
HEXA ~ 81255
HFE ~ 81256
HLA class I and II typing
  high resolution ~ 81378
  low resolution ~ 81370-81371
HLA class I typing
  high resolution ~ 81379-81381
  low resolution ~ 81372-81374
HLA class II typing
  high resolution ~ 81382-81383
  low resolution ~ 81375-81377
IGH@ ~ 81261-81263
IGK@ ~ 81264
IKBKAP ~ 81260
JAK2 ~ 81270
KRAS ~ 81275
long QT gene analysis ~ 81280-81282
MCOLN1 ~ 81290
MECP2 ~ 81302-81304
MTHFR ~ 81291
MLH1 ~ 81292-81294
MSH2 ~ 81295-81297
MSH6 ~ 81298-81300
NPM1 ~ 81310
PML/RARalpa ~ 81315-81316
PMS2 ~ 81317-81319
SERPINA1 ~ 81332
SMPD1 ~ 81330
SNRPN/UBE3A ~ 81331
TRB@ ~ 81340-81341
TRG@ ~ 81342
UGT1A1 ~ 81350
VKORC1 ~ 81355
Gene product ~ see protein
Genioplasty ~ 21120-21123
augmentation ~ 21120, 21123
osteotomy ~ 21121-21123
Genitourinary sphincter, artificial ~
53444-53449
Genotype analysis
by nucleic acid
infectious agent
  HIV-1 protease/reverse transcriptase ~ 87901
  hepatitis C virus ~ 87902
Gentamicin ~ 80170
assay ~ 80170
Gentamycin level ~ 80170
Gentiobiase ~ 82963
GERD ~ 91034-91038
German measles ~ 86762, 90706
Gestational trophoblastic tumor ~ 59100, 59870
GGT ~ 82977

GI tract ~ see gastrointestinal tract
Giardia
antigen detection
  immunofluorescence ~ 87269
  enzyme immunoassay ~ 87329
Giardia lamblia
antibody ~ 86674
Gibbons stent ~ 52332
GIF ~ 84307
GIFT (gamete intrafallopian transfer) ~ 58976
Gillies approach
fracture, zygomatic arch ~ 21356
Gill operation ~ 63012
Gingiva ~ see gums
Gingiva, abscess ~ see abscess
fracture ~ see 41800 ~ gums
  zygomatic arch ~ 41800
Gingivectomy ~ 41820
Gingivoplasty ~ 41872
Girdlestone laminectomy ~ see laminectomy
Girdlestone procedure ~ 27120
G1A protein (bone) ~ 83937
Gland ~ see specific gland
Glasses ~ see spectacle services
Glaucoma
cryotherapy ~ 66720
cyclophotocoagulation ~ 66710, 66711
diathermy ~ 66700
fistulization of sclera ~ 66150
provocative test ~ 92140
Glaucoma drainage implant ~ 66180, 66185
GLC ~ 82486
Glenn procedure ~ 33766-33767
bidirectional ~ 33622
Glenohumeral joint
arthrotomy ~ 23040
  with biopsy ~ 23100
  with synovectomy ~ 23105
exploration ~ 23107
removalforeign or loose body ~ 23107
Glenoid Fossa reconstruction ~ 21255
GLN ~ 82975
Globulin
antihuman ~ 86880-86886
corticosteroid-binding ~ 84449
immune ~ 90281-90399
Rh immune ~ 90384-90386
sex hormone binding ~ 84270
thyroxine-binding ~ 84442
Glomerular procoagulant activity ~ see thromboplastin
Glomus caroticum ~ 60600, 60605
Glossectomies ~ see excision, tongue
Glossopexy ~ 41500
Glossorrhaphy ~ see suture, tongue
Glucagon ~ 82943
tolerance panel ~ 80422-80424
tolerance test ~ 82946
Glucose ~ 80422-80424, 80430-80435, 95250
blood test ~ 82947-82950, 82962
body fluid ~ 82945

1427

Glucose ~ *continued*
interstitial fluid continuous monitoring ~ 95250
tolerance test ~ 82951-82952
with tolbutamide ~ 82953
Glucose-6-phosphate dehydrogenase ~ 82955-82960
Glucose phosphate isomerase ~ 84087
Glucosidase ~ 82963
Glucuronide androstanediol ~ 82154
Glue
cornea wound ~ 65286
sclera wound ~ 65286
Glukagon ~ see glucagon
Glutamate dehydrogenase, blood ~ 82965
Glutamate pyruvate transaminase ~ 84460
Glutamic
alanine transaminase ~ 84460
aspartic transaminase ~ 84450
dehydrogenase ~ 82965
Glutamine ~ 82975
Glutamyltransferase, gamma ~ 82977
Glutathione ~ 82978
Glutathione reductase ~ 82979
Glutethimide ~ 82980
Glycanhydrolase, N-acetylmuramide ~ 85549
Glycated hemoglobins ~ 83036
Glycated protein ~ 82985
Glycerol, phosphatidyl ~ 84081
Glycerol, phosphoglycerides ~ 84081
Glycerophosphatase ~ 84075-84080
Glycinate, theophylline sodium ~ 80198
Glycocholic acid ~ 82240
Glycohemoglobin ~ 83036
Glycol, ethylene ~ 82693
Glycosaminoglycan ~ 83864-83866
GMP (guanosine monophosphate), cyclic ~ 83008
Goeckerman treatment ~ 96910-96913
Gol-Vernet operation
pyelotomy, exploration 50120
Gold assay ~ 80172
Goldwaite procedure ~ 27422
Golfer's elbow ~ 24357-24359
Gonadectomy, female ~ 58262-58263, 58291-58292, 58552, 58554, 58661, 58940-58943
Gonadectomy, male ~ 54520, 54522, 54530-54535, 54690
Gonadotropin
chorionic ~ 84702-84704
FSH ~ 83001
ICSH ~ 83002
LH ~ 83002
panel ~ 80426
Gonioscopy ~ 92020
Goniotomy ~ 65820
Gonococcus ~ 87590-87592, 87850
Goodenough Harris drawing test ~ 96100
GOTT ~ 84450
GPUT ~ 82775-82776

Graft ~ see bone graft; bypass graft
anal ~ 46753
aorta ~ 33840-33851, 33860-33877
artery
coronary ~ 33503-33505
bone ~ 38240-38242
harvesting ~ 20900-20902
microvascular anastomosis ~ 20955-20962
osteocutaneous flap with microvascular anastomosis ~ 20969-20973
vascular pedicle ~ 25430
bone and skin ~ 20969-20973
cartilage
ear to face ~ 21235
harvesting ~ 20910-20912
rib to face ~ 21230
conjunctiva ~ 65782
harvesting ~ 68371
cornea, with lesion excision ~ 65426
cornea transplant
allograft preparation ~ 65757
endothelial ~ 65756
in aphakia ~ 65750
lamellar ~ 65710
penetrating ~ 65730
in pseudophakia ~ 65755
dura, spinal cord ~ 63710
endovascular ~ 34900
eye
amniotic membrane ~ 65780
conjunctiva ~ 65782
stem cell ~ 65781
facial nerve paralysis ~ 15840-15845
fascia, cheek ~ 15840
fascia lata, harvesting ~ 20920-20922
gum mucosa ~ 41870
heart ~ 33935, 33945
heart lung ~ 33935
kidney ~ see kidney, transplantation
liver ~ 47135-47136
lung ~ 32851-32854, 33935
muscle, cheek ~ 15841-15845
nail bed reconstruction ~ 11762
nerve ~ 64885-64907
oral mucosa ~ 40818
organ ~ see transplantation
pancreas ~ 48160, 48550, 48554-48556
skin
biological—see Allograft, skin substitute
blood flow check, graft ~ 15860
tendon
finger ~ 26392
hand ~ 26392
harvesting ~ 20924
tissue harvesting ~ 20926
vein cross-over ~ 34520
Grain alcohol ~ see alcohol, ethyl
Granulation tissue cauterization, chemical ~ 17250
Great toe
flap ~ 20973
fracture ~ 28490, 28496, 28505

Great vessels
 graft insertion ~ 33330, 33332, 33335
 shunt
  aorta to pulmonary artery
   ascending ~ 33755
   descending ~ 33762
  central ~ 33764
  subclavian to pulmonary artery ~ 33750
  vena cava to pulmonary artery ~
   33766-33767
 unlisted services and procedures ~ 33999
Great vessels transposition ~ 33770-33781
Greater tuberosity fracture
 with shoulder dislocation
  closed treatment ~ 23665
  open treatment ~ 23670
Greater vestibular gland ~ see Bartholin's
 gland
Green operation ~ (scapulopexy) 23400
Gridley stain ~ 88312
Grippe, Balkan ~ 86000, 86638
Gritti operation ~ 27590-27592
Groin repair, hernia ~ 49550-49557
Group health education ~ 99078
Grouping, blood ~ see blood typing
Growth factors, insulin-like ~ 84305
Growth hormone ~ 83003
 human ~ 80418, 80428-80430, 86277
Growth hormone release inhibiting factor ~
 84307
GTT (hydatidiform mole) ~ 82951, 82952
Guaiac test, blood in feces ~ 82270
Guanosine monophosphate (GMP) ~ 83008
Guanosine monophosphate, cyclic ~ 83008
Guanylic acids ~ 83008
Guard stain ~ 88313
Gullett ~ see esophagus
Gums
 abscess, incision and drainage ~ 41800
 alveolus, excision ~ 41830
 cyst, incision and drainage ~ 41800
 excision
  gingiva ~ 41820
  operculum ~ 41821
 graft, mucosa ~ 41870
 hematoma, incision and drainage ~ 41800
 lesion
  destruction ~ 41850
  excision ~ 41822-41828
 mucosa, excision ~ 41828
 reconstruction
  alveolus ~ 41874
  gingiva ~ 41872
 removal, foreign body ~ 41805
 tumor, excision ~ 41825-41827
 unlisted services and procedures ~ 41899
Gunning-Lieben test ~ 82009-82010
Guthrie test ~ 84030

H

H flu ~ see Hemophilus influenza
HAAb (antibody, hepatitis) ~ 86708, 86709
HAA (hepatitis associated antigen) ~
 87340-87380, 87515-87527
Haemoglobin F ~ see fetal hemoglobin
Haemorrhage ~ see hemorrhage
Haemorrhage rectum ~ see hemorrhage,
 rectum
Hageman factor ~ 85280
Hair
 electrolysis ~ 17380
 KOH examination ~ 87220
 microscopic evaluation ~ 96902
 removal ~ see removal, hair
 transplant
  punch graft ~ 15775-15776
  strip graft ~ 15220-15221
HAI test ~ see hemagglutination inhibition test
Hallux ~ see great toe
Halo
 body cast ~ 29000
 cranial ~ 20661
  for thin skull osteology ~ 20664
 femur ~ 20663
 maxillofacial ~ 21100
 pelvic ~ 20662
 removal ~ 20665
Haloperidol assay ~ 80173
Halsted mastectomy ~ see mastectomy, radical
Halsted hernia repair ~ 49495
Ham test ~ 85475
Hammertoe repair ~ 28285-28286
Hamster penetration test ~ 89329
Hand ~ see also carpometacarpal joint;
 intercarpal joint
 amputation
  at metacarpal ~ 25927
   revision ~ 25924, 25929-25931
  at wrist ~ 25920
   revision ~ 25922
 arthrodesis
  carpometacarpal joint ~ 26843-26844
  intercarpal joint ~ 25820-25825
 bone, incision and drainage ~ 26034
 cast ~ 29085
 decompression ~ 26035-26037
 fracture metacarpal ~ 26600
 insertion tendon graft ~ 26392
 magnetic resonance imaging (MRI) ~
  73218-73223
 reconstruction tendon pulley ~ 26500-26502
 removal
  implantation ~ 26320
   tube/rod ~ 26390-26392, 26416

Hand ~ *continued*
repair
blood vessel ~ 35207
cleft hand ~ 26580
muscle ~ 26591-26593
tendon
extensor ~ 26410-26416, 26426-26428,
26433-26437
flexor ~ 26350-26358, 26440
profundus ~ 26370-26373
replantation ~ 20808
strapping ~ 29280
tendon excision ~ 26390
extensor ~ 26415
tenotomy ~ 26450, 26460
tumor excision ~ 26111-26118
unlisted services and procedures ~ 26989
X-ray ~ 73120-73130
Handling
device ~ 99002
radioelement ~ 77790
specimen ~ 99000-99001
Hand abscess ~ see abscess, hand
Hand phalange ~ see finger, bone
Hanganutziu Deicher antibodies ~ see
antibody, heterophile
Haptoglobin ~ 83010-83012
Hard palate ~ see palate
Harelip operation ~ see cleft lip, repair
Harii procedure ~ 25430
Harrington rod
insertion ~ 22840
removal ~ 22850
Hartmann procedure
open ~ 44143
laparoscopic ~ 44206
Harvesting
bone graft ~ 20900-20902
bone marrow ~ 38230
cartilage graft ~ 20910-20912
conjunctival graft ~ 68371
eggs, in vitro fertilization ~ 58970
endoscopic, vein for bypass graft ~ 33508
fascia lata graft ~ 20920-20922
intestines ~ 44132-44133
kidney ~ 50300-50320, 50547
liver ~ 47133, 47140-47142
lower extremity vein for vascular
reconstruction ~ 35572
stem cell ~ 38205-38206
tendon graft ~ 20924
tissue grafts ~ 20926
upper extremity
artery for coronary artery bypass graft ~
35600
vein for bypass graft ~ 35500
Hauser procedure ~ 27420
Hayem's elementary corpuscle ~ see blood,
platelet
Haygroves procedure ~ 27120, 27122
HBcAb ~ 86704, 86705
HBeAb ~ 86707

HBeAg ~ 87350
HBsAb ~ 86706
HBsAg (hepatitis B surface antigen) ~ 87340
HCG ~ 84702, 84703
HCO3 ~ see bicarbonate
Hct (hematocrit) ~ 85014
HCV antibodies ~ see antibody, hepatitis C
HDL (high density lipoprotein) ~ 83718
Head
angiography ~ 70496, 70544-70546
CT scan ~ 70450-70470, 70496
excision ~ 21015-21070
fracture and/or dislocation ~ 21310-21497
incision ~ 21010, 61316, 62148
introduction or removal ~ 21076-21116
lipectomy, suction assisted ~ 15876
magnetic resonance angiography (MRA) ~
70544-70546
nerve graft ~ 64885-64886
other procedures ~ 21299, 21499
repair/revision and/or reconstruction ~
21120-21296
ultrasound exam ~ 76506, 76536
unlisted services and procedures ~ 21499
X-ray ~ 70350
Head rings, stereotactic ~ see stereotactic
frame
Headbrace
application ~ 21100
application/removal ~ 20661
Heaf TB test ~ 86580
Health and behavior assessment ~
96150-96155
Health risk assessment instrument ~ 99420
Hearing aid
bone conduction
implantation ~ 69710
removal ~ 69711
repair ~ 69711
replacement ~ 69710
check ~ 92592-92593
services
electroacoustic test ~ 92594-92595
examination ~ 92590-92591
Hearing evaluation ~ 92510
Hearing tests ~ see audiologic function tests;
hearing evaluation
Hearing therapy ~ 92507-92510, 92601-92604
Heart
ablation
arrhythmogenic focus ~ 33250-33251, 33261
atrial tissue ~ 33254-33259
endoscopic ~ 33265-33266
anomoly repair ~ 33615, 33617
artificial heart ~ 0051T-0053T
atria ~ see atria
balloon device ~ 33973-33974
biopsy ~ 93505
ultrasound imaging guidance ~ 76932
blood vessel repair ~ 33320-33322

Heart ~ *continued*
  cardiac event recorder ~ 33282, 33284
  cardiac output measurements ~ 93451,
    93561-93562
  cardiac rehabilitation ~ 93797-93798
  cardioassist ~ 92970-92971
  cardiopulmonary bypass
    with aortic aneurysm repair ~ 33877
    with ascending aorta graft ~ 33860,
      33863-33864
    with atrial septectomy/septostomy ~ 33736
    with chamber fistula repair ~ 33500
    with descending thoracic aorta graft ~ 33875
    with lung transplant ~ 32852, 32854
    with operative ablation ~ 33251, 33256,
      33259, 33261
    with pericardiectomy ~ 33031
    with pulmonary artery repair ~ 33910,
      33916, 33922, 33926
    with replacement of ventricular assist ~
      33983
    with sinus of valsalva repair ~ 33702, 33720
    with transcatheter aortic valve replacement
      (TAVR/TAVI) ~ 33367-33369
    with transverse arch graft ~ 33870
    with tumor excision ~ 33120
    with wound repair ~ 33305
  cardioversion ~ 92960-92961
  catheterization ~ see Cardiac catheterization
  cor triatriatum repair ~ 33732
  CT scan ~ 75571-75573
    angiography ~ 75574
  cyst, pericardial, resection ~ 33050
  diagnostic imaging
    acoustic cardiography ~ 0223T-0225T
    blood pool ~ 78472-78473, 78481, 78483,
      78496
    SPECT ~ 78494
    CT scan ~ 75571-75573
      angiography ~ 75574
    myocardial imaging
      infarct avid ~ 78466, 78468-78469
      perfusion ~ 78451-78454
      perfusion study ~ 78491-78492
      PETMetabolic evaluation ~ 78459
    shunt detection ~ 78428
    unlisted cardiovascular diagnostic nuclear
      medicine procedure ~ 78499
  electrophysiologic procedure ~ 93600-93660
  electrode
    insertion ~ 33202-33203, 33210-33211,
      33216-33217, 33224-33225
    removal ~ 33238
      single/dual chamber ~ 33243-33244
    exploration ~ 33310-33315
    foreign body removal ~ 33310
  great vessels ~ see great vessels
  heart-lung bypass ~ see cardiopulmonary
    bypass
  heart-lung transplantation ~ see
    transplantation, heart-lung

Heart ~ *continued*
  hemodynamic monitoring
    non-invasive ~ 93880-93883, 93922-93931,
      93965-93990, 93998
    with pharmacologic agent ~ 93463
    with physiologic exercise study ~ 93464
  implantation
    artificial heart, intracorporeal ~ 0051T
    total replacement heart system,
      intracorporeal ~ 0051T
    ventricular assist device ~ 33975-33976,
      33979
  infundibular stenosis ~ 33476-33478
  intracardiac ischemia monitoring system
    evaluation ~ 0305T-0306T
    insertion ~ 0302T-0304T
    removal ~ 0307T
    removal and replacement ~ 0302T-0304T
  intraoperative pacing and mapping ~ 93631
  ligation, fistula ~ 37607
  magnetic resonance imaging (MRI) ~
    75557-75565
  mitral valve ~ see mitral valve
  muscle ~ see myocardial
  myocardial infarction
    revascularization ~ 92941, 92943-92944
    tissue plasminogen activator (tPA) ~ 4077F
  myocardium
    imaging ~ 78466-78469
    perfusion study ~ 78451-78454
    revascularization ~ 33140-33141
  open chest massage ~ 32160
  output ~ see cardiac output
  pacemaker ~ see also Pacemaker, heart
    conversion ~ 33214
    insertion ~ 33206-33208
    pulse generator ~ 33212-33213, 33221
    removal ~ 33233-33237
    replacement
      catheter ~ 33210
      electrode ~ 33210-33211
      insertion ~ 33206-33208
      pulse generator ~ 33227-33229
  pacing
    arrhythmia induction ~ 93618
    atria ~ 93610
    transcutaneous, temporary ~ 92953
    ventricular ~ 33224-33226, 93612
  pacing cardioverter-defibrillator ~ see
    Cardioverter-defibrillator
  pericardium
    drainage ~ 33025
    pericardiectomy ~ 33030, 33031
    pericardiocentesis ~ 33010-33011
  reconstruction
    atrial septum ~ 33735-33737
    vena cava ~ 34502
  removal
    balloon device ~ 33974
    electrode ~ 33238
    ventricular assist device ~ 33977-33978
      extracorporeal ~ 33990-33993

1431

Heart ~ *continued*
  intracorporeal ~ 33980
  removal single/dual chamber
    electrodes ~ 33243-33244
    pulse generator ~ 33241
    repair ~ 33218-33220
  repair
    anomaly ~ 33615-33617
    aortic sinus ~ 33702-33722
    artificial heart, intracorporeal ~ 0052T,
      0053T
    atrial septum ~ 33641, 33647
    atrioventricular canal ~ 33660-33665
      complete ~ 33670
      prosthetic valve ~ 33670
    atrioventricular valve ~ 33660-33665
    cor triatriatum ~ 33732
    electrode ~ 33218
    fenestration ~ 93580
    infundibular ~ 33476-33478
    mitral valve ~ 33420-33430
    myocardium ~ 33542
    outflow tract ~ 33476-33478
    postinfarction ~ 33542-33545
    prosthetic valve dysfunction ~ 33496
    septal defect ~ 33608-33610, 33660,
      33813-33814, 93581
    sinus of valsalva ~ 33702-33722
    sinus venosus ~ 33645
    tetralogy of Fallot ~ 33692-33697, 33924
    total replacement heart system
      intracorporeal ~ 0052T, 0053T
    tricuspid valve ~ 33463-33468
    ventricle ~ 33611-33612
      obstruction ~ 33619
    ventricular septum ~ 33545, 33647,
      33681-33688, 33692-33697, 93581
    ventricular tunnel ~ 33722
    wound ~ 33300-33305
  replacement
    artificial heart, intracorporeal ~ 0052T,
      0053T
    electrode ~ 33210-33211, 33217
    mitral valve ~ 33430
    total replacement heart system,
      intracorporeal ~ 0052T, 0053T
    tricuspid valve ~ 33465
    ventricular assist device ~ 33981-33983
  repositioning
    electrode ~ 33215, 33217, 33226
    tricuspid valve ~ 33468
  resuscitation ~ 92950
  septal defect ~ see septal defect
  sinus of valsalvus repair ~ 33702-33722
  sinus venosus repair ~ 33645
  tetralogy of fallot repair ~ 33692-33697,
    33924
  thrombectomy ~ see thrombectomy
  transplantation ~ 33935, 33945
    allograft preparation ~ 33933, 33944
  tumor excision ~ 33120-33130
  unlisted services and procedures ~ 33999

Heart ~ *continued*
  valve closure ~ 33600, 33602
  vena cava reconstruction ~ 34502
  ventricle
    commissurotomy, right ventricle ~
      33476-33478
    obstruction removal ~ 33619
    pacing ~ 33224-33226, 93612
    repair ~ 33548, 33611-33612
    tunnel repair ~ 33722
    ventriculomyectomy ~ 33416
    wound repair ~ 33300-33305
**Heart sounds, acoustic recording, with
  computer analysis ~ 93799**
Heart vessels
  angioplasty, percutaneous ~ 92982-92984
  insertion graft ~ 33330-33335
  thrombolysis ~ 92975-92977
  valvuloplasty, percutaneous ~ 92986-92990
Heat unstable haemoglobin ~ see hemoglobin,
  thermolabile
Heavy lipoproteins ~ see lipoprotein
Heavy metal ~ 83015-83018
Heel ~ 36415-36416
  X-ray ~ 73650
Heel bone ~ see calcaneus
Heel fracture ~ see calcaneus, fracture
Heel spur excision ~ 28119
Heine-Medin disease ~ see polio
Heine operation ~ see cyclodialysis
Heinz bodies ~ 85441-85445
Helicobacter pylori
  antibody ~ 86677
  antigen detection enzyme immunoassay ~
    87338-87339
Helicobacter pylori ~ *continued*
  blood test ~ 83009
  breath test ~ 78267-78268, 83013-83014
  stool ~ 87338
  urease activity ~ 83009, 83013-83014
Heller procedure ~ 32665, 43330-43331
Helminth antibody ~ 86682
Hemagglutination inhibition test ~ 86280
Hemangioma ~ 17106-17108
Hemapheresis ~ 36511-36516
Hematochezia ~ 82270, 82274
Hematologic test ~ see blood tests
Hematology and coagulation ~ 85002-85999
Hematoma
  ankle ~ 27603
  arm, lower ~ 25028
  arm, upper, incision and drainage ~ 23930
  brain
    drainage ~ 61154-61156
    evacuation ~ 61312-61315
    incision and drainage ~ 61312-61315
    drain ~ 61108
  ear, external
    complicated ~ 69005
    simple ~ 69000

Hematoma ~ continued
elbow, incision and drainage ~ 23930
epididymis, incision and drainage ~ 54700
gums, incision and drainage ~ 41800
hip ~ 26990
incision and drainage
  neck ~ 21501-21502
  skin ~ 10140
  thorax ~ 21501-21502
knee ~ 27301
leg, lower ~ 27603
leg, upper ~ 27301
mouth ~ 41005-41009, 41015-41018
  incision and drainage ~ 40800-40801
nasal septum, incision and drainage ~ 30020
nose, incision and drainage ~ 30000-30020
pelvis ~ 26990
scrotum, incision and drainage ~ 54700
shoulder, drainage ~ 23030
skin
  incision and drainage ~ 10140
  puncture aspiration ~ 10160
subdural ~ 61108
subungual, evacuation ~ 11740
testis, incision and drainage ~ 54700
tongue ~ 41000-41006, 41015
vagina, incision and drainage ~ 57022-57023
wrist ~ 25028
Hematopoietic stem cell transplantation ~ see
  stem cell, transplantation
Hematopoietin ~ see erythropoietin
Hematuria ~ see blood, urine
Hemic and lymphatic systems, surgical
  procedures ~ 38100-38999
Hemiepiphyseal arrest, elbow ~ 24470
Hemifacial microsomia, reconstruction,
  mandibular condyle ~ 21247
Hemilaminectomy ~ 63020-63044
Hemilaryngectomy ~ 31370-31382
Hemipelvectomies ~ see amputation,
  interpelviabdominal
Hemiphalangectomy, toe ~ 28160
Hemispherectomy
partial ~ 61543
total ~ 61542
Hemocytoblast ~ see stem cell
Hemodialysis ~ 90935-90937
blood flow study ~ 90940
duplex scan of access ~ 93990
Kt/V level ~ 3082F-3084F
plan of care documented ~ 0505F
via catheter ~ 4054F
via functioning arteriovenous
  fistula 4052F
  graft 4053F
Hemodynamic monitoring, non-invasive left
  ventricular ~ 93799
Hemofiltration ~ 90945-90947

Hemoglobin
A1c (HbA1c) level ~ 3044F-3045F
analysis, O2 affinity ~ 82820
carboxyhemoglobin ~ 82375-82376, 88740
chromatography ~ 83021
concentration ~ 85046
electrophoresis ~ 83020
fetal ~ 83030-83033, 85460-85461
fractionation and quantitation ~ 83020
glycosated (A1C) ~ 83036-83037
methemoglobin ~ 83045-83050
  transcutaneous ~ 88741
non-automated ~ 83026
plasma ~ 83051
sulfhemoglobin ~ 83055-83060
thermolabile ~ 83065-83068
transcutaneous ~ 88738, 88740
urine ~ 83069
Hemoglobin, glycosylated ~ see
  glycohemoglobin
Hemoglobin F (fetal)
chemical ~ 83030
qualitative ~ 83033
Hemogram
added indices ~ 85025-85027
automated ~ 85025-85027
manual ~ 85014-85018, 85032
Hemolysins ~ 85475
with agglutinins ~ 86940-86941
Hemolytic complement ~ see complement,
  hemolytic
Hemolytic complement, total ~ see
  complement, hemolytic, total
Hemoperfusion ~ 90997
Hemophil ~ see clotting factor
Hemophilus influenza
antibody ~ 86684
vaccines ~ 90644-90648, 90748
Hemorrhage
abdomen ~ 49002
anal, endoscopic control ~ 46614
chest cavity, endoscopic control ~ 32654
colon, endoscopic control ~ 44391, 45382
colon-sigmoid, endoscopic control ~ 45334
esophagus, endoscopic control ~ 43227
gastrointestinal, upper, endoscopic control ~
  43255
intestines, small, endoscopic control ~ 44366,
  44378
liver, control ~ 47350
lung ~ 32110
nasal
  cauterization ~ 30901-30906
  endoscopic control ~ 31238
nasopharynx ~ 42970-42972
oropharynx ~ 42960-42962
rectum, endoscopic control ~ 45317
throat ~ 42960-42962
uterus, postpartum ~ 59160
vagina ~ 57180

1433

Hemorrhoidectomy
complex ~ 46260
 with fissurectomy ~ 46261-46262
external complete ~ 46250
ligature ~ 46221
simple ~ 46255
 with fissurectomy ~ 46257-46258
Hemorrhoidopexy ~ 46947
Hemorrhoids
destruction ~ 46930
excision ~ 46250-46262, 46320
incision, external ~ 46083
injection, sclerosing solution ~ 46500
ligation ~ 46945-46946
stapling ~ 46947
suture ~ 46945-46946
Hemosiderin ~ 83070-83071
Hemothorax, thoracostomy ~ 32551
Heparin ~ see clotting inhibitors ~ 85520
neutralization ~ 85525
protamine tolerance test ~ 85530
Heparin cofactor I ~ see antithrombin III
Hepatectomy
extensive ~ 47122
left lobe ~ 47125
partial
 donor ~ 47140-47142
 lobe ~ 47120
right lobe ~ 47130
total
 donor ~ 47133
Hepaticodochotomy ~ see hepaticostomy
Hepaticoenterostomy ~ 47802
Hepaticostomy ~ 47400
Hepaticotomy ~ 47400
Hepatic abscess ~ see abscess, liver
Hepatic arteries ~ see artery, hepatic
Hepatic artery aneurysm ~ see artery, hepatic, aneurysm
Hepatic duct
anastomosis, with intestines ~ 47765, 47802
exploration ~ 47400
incision and drainage ~ 47400
removalcalculi (stone) ~ 47400
repair, with intestines ~ 47765, 47802
unlisted services and procedures ~ 47999
Hepatic haemorrhage ~ see hemorrhage, liver
Hepatic portal vein ~ see vein, hepatic portal
Hepatic portoenterostomies ~ see hepaticoenterostomy
Hepatic transplantation ~ see liver, transplantation
Hepatitis A and hepatitis B ~ 90636
Hepatitis antibody
A ~ 86708-86709
B core ~ 86704-86705
B surface ~ 86706
Be ~ 86707
C ~ 86803-86804
delta agent ~ 86692
IgG ~ 86704, 86708
IgM ~ 86704-86705, 86708-86709

Hepatitis antigen
B ~ 87515-87517
B surface ~ 87340-87341
Be ~ 87350
C ~ 87520-87522
delta agent ~ 87380
G ~ 87525-87527
Hepatitis A vaccine
adolescent/pediatric
 2 dose schedule ~ 90633
 3 dose schedule ~ 90634
adult dosage ~ 90632
Hepatitis B and Hib ~ 90748
Hepatitis B vaccine dosage
adolescent ~ 90743
adult ~ 90746
immunosuppressed ~ 90740, 90747
pediatric/adolescent ~ 90744
Hepatitis B virus e antibody ~ see antibody, hepatitis
Hepatitis B virus surface ab ~ see antibody, hepatitis B, surface
Hepatorrhaphy ~ see liver, repair
Hepatotomy
abscess ~ 47010-47011
 percutaneous ~ 47011
cyst ~ 47010-47011
 percutaneous ~ 47011
Hernia repair
abdominal ~ 49590
 incisional ~ 49560
 recurrent ~ 49565
diaphragmatic ~ 39503, 39540--39541
epigastric ~ 49570
 incarcerated ~ 49572
 laparoscopic ~ 49652-49653
femoral ~ 49550
 incarcerated ~ 49553
 recurrent ~ 49555
 recurrent incarcerated ~ 49557
incisional
 incarcerated ~ 49561
 laparoscopic ~ 49654-49657
 thoracoabdominal 43336-43337
inguinal ~ 49491, 49495-49500, 49505
 incarcerated ~ 49492, 49496, 49501, 49507, 49521
 laparoscopic ~ 49650-49651
 recurrent ~ 49520
 sliding ~ 49525
 strangulated ~ 49492
lumbar ~ 49540
lung ~ 32800
orchiopexy ~ 54640
paraesophageal hiatal
 via
  laparotomy ~ 43332-43333
  thoracoabdominal incision ~ 43336-43337
  thoractopy ~ 43334-43335
recurrent incisional
 incarcerated ~ 49566
 reducible ~ 49565

Hernia repair ~ *continued*
  umbilicus
    incarcerated ~ 49582, 49587
    laparoscopic ~ 49652-49653
    reducible ~ 49580, 49585
    with spermatic cord ~ 55540
    spigelian ~ 49590
    ventral, laparoscopic ~ 49652-49653
Hernia, cerebral ~ see encephalocele
Hernia, rectovaginal ~ see rectocele
Hernia, umbilical ~ see omphalocele
Heroin, alkaloid screening ~ 82101
Heroin screen ~ 82486
Herpes simplex
  antibody ~ 86696
  antigen detection
    immunofluorescence ~ 87273-87274
    nucleic acid ~ 87528-87530
    identification smear and stain ~ 87207
Herpes smear and stain ~ 87207
Herpes virus-4 (gamma), human ~ see
  Epstein-Barr virus
Herpes virus-6 (six) detection ~ 87531-87533
Herpetic vesicle destruction ~ 54050-54065
Heteroantibodies ~ see antibody, heterophile
Heterologous transplant ~ see xenograft
Heterologous transplantation ~ see heterograft
Heterophile antibody ~ 86308-86310
Heterotropia ~ see strabismus
Hex b ~ see b-hexosaminidase
Hexadecadrol ~ see dexamethasone
Hexosephosphate isomerase ~ see
  phosphohexose isomerase
Heyman procedure ~ 27179, 28264
Hgb (hemoglobin) ~ 85018
HGH (human growth hormone) ~ 80418,
  80428, 80430, 83003, 86277
Hg factor ~ see glucagon
HHV-4 ~ see Epstein-Barr virus
HIAA (hydroxyindolacetic acid, urine) 83497
Hibb operation ~ 22841
Hib vaccine
  4 dose schedule
    HbOC ~ 90645
    PRP-T ~ 90648
  PRP-D
    booster ~ 90646
  PRP-OMP
    3 dose schedule ~ 90647
Hickmann catheterization ~ see cannulization;
  catheterization, venous, central line;
  venipuncture
Hidradenitis (see also sweat gland)
  excision ~ 11450-11471
  suppurative, incision and drainage ~
    10060-10061
Highly selective vagotomy ~ see vagotomy,
  highly selective
Highmore antrum ~ see sinuses, maxillary
High altitude simulation test ~ 94452-94453
High density lipoprotein ~ 83718
High molecular weight kininogen ~ 85293

Hill procedure
  laparoscopic ~ 43280
Hinton positive ~ 86592, 86593
Hip joint
  arthroplasty ~ 27132
    revision ~ 27134-27138
  arthrotomy ~ 27052
  biopsy ~ 27052
  capsulotomy, with release, flexor muscles ~
    27036
    dislocation ~ 27250-27252
    congenital ~ 27256-27259
    open treatment ~ 27253-27254
    without trauma ~ 27265-27266
  manipulation ~ 27275
  reconstruction, revision ~ 27134-27138
  synovium
    excision ~ 27054
    arthroscopic ~ 29863
  total replacement ~ 27132
Hip ~ see also femur; pelvis
  abscess, incision and drainage ~ 26990
  arthrocentesis ~ 20610
  arthrodesis ~ 27284-27286
  arthrography ~ 73525
  arthroplasty ~ 27130-27132
  arthroscopy ~ 29860-29863, 29914
  arthrotomy ~ 27030-27033
  biopsy ~ 27040-27041
  bone, drainage ~ 26992
  bursa, incision and drainage ~ 26991
  capsulectomy with release, flexor muscles ~
    27036
  cast ~ 29305-29325
  craterization ~ 27070
  cyst, excision ~ 27065-27067
  denervation ~ 27035
  echography, infant ~ 76885-76886
  endoprosthesis ~ see prosthesis, hip
  excision ~ 27070
  exploration ~ 27033
  fasciotomy ~ 27025
  fusion ~ 27284-27286
  hematoma, incision and drainage ~ 26990
  injectio, radiologic ~ 27093-27096
  reconstruction, total replacement ~ 27130
  removal
    cast ~ 29710
    foreign body ~ 27033, 27086-27087
      arthroscopic ~ 29861
    loose body
      arthroscopic ~ 29861
  prosthesis ~ 27090-27091
  repair
    muscle transfer ~ 27100-27105, 27111
    osteotomy ~ 27146-27156
    tendon ~ 27097
  saucerization ~ 27070
  stem prosthesis ~ see arthroplasty, hip
  strapping ~ 29520

CPT PLUS! 2013

Hip ~ *continued*
tenotomy
  abductor tendon ~ 27006
  adductor tendon ~ 27000-27003
  iliopsoas ~ 27005
total replacement ~ 27130-27132
tumor
  excision ~ 27043-27045, 27049, 27059,
    27065-27067
  radical ~ 27075-27076
ultrasound, infant ~ 76885-76886
X-ray ~ 73500-73520, 73540
  with contrast ~ 73525
  intraoperative ~ 73530
Hip stem prostheses ~ see arthroplasty, hip
Hippocampus excision ~ 61566
Histamine ~ 83088
Histamine release test ~ 86343
Histochemistry ~ 88319
Histocompatibility testing ~ see tissue typing
Histoplasma
  antibody ~ 86698
  antigen ~ 87385
**Histoplasma capsulatum, antigen detection,
  enzyme immunoassay** ~ 87385
Histoplasmin test ~ see histoplasmosis, skin
  test
Histoplasmoses ~ see histoplasmosis
Histoplasmosis skin test ~ 86510
History and physical ~ 57410
HIV
  antibody ~ 86701-86703
  confirmation test ~ 86689
HIV-1
  antigen detection
  enzyme immunoassay ~ 87390
HIV-2
  antigen detection
  enzyme immunoassay ~ 87391
HK3 kallikrein ~ see prostate specific antigen
HLA
  crossmatch ~ 86825, 86826
  molecular pathology ~ 81370-81383
  typing ~ 86812-868122
HMRK ~ see Fitzgerald factor
HMW kininogen ~ see Fitzgerald factor
Hoffman apparatus ~ 20690
Hofmeister operation (gastrectomy, total) ~
  43632
Holographic imaging ~ 76375
Holten test ~ 82575
Home health services ~ 99500-99600
  activities of daily living ~ 99509
  anticoagulant management ~ 99363-99364
  apnea care ~ 94774-94777
  catheter care ~ 99507
  enema administration ~ 99511
  established patient ~ 99347-99350
  hemodialysis ~ 99512
  home infusion procedures ~ 99601-99602
  individual or family counseling ~ 99510

Home health services ~ *continued*
  intramuscular injections ~ 99506
  mechanical ventilation ~ 99504
  newborn care ~ 99502
  new patient ~ 99341-99345
  postnatal assessment ~ 99501
  prenatal monitoring ~ 99500
  respiratory therapy ~ 99503
  sleep studies ~ 95805-95811
  stoma care ~ 99505
  unlisted services and procedures ~ 99600
  ventilation assist ~ 94005
Home visits ~ 99341-99350
Homocystine ~ 83090
  urine ~ 82615
Homogenization, tissue ~ 87176
Homograft, skin ~ 15350
Homologous grafts ~ see graft
Homologous transplantation ~ see homograft
Homovanillic acid, urine ~ 83150
Hormone adrenocorticotrophic (ACTH) ~
  80400-80406, 80412, 80418, 82024
  corticotropic-releasing ~ 80412
  growth ~ see human growth hormone
  human growth ~ 80418, 80428, 80430, 86277,
    83003
  interstitial cell-stimulating ~ see luteinizing
    hormone (LH)
  luteinizing hormone (LH) ~ 80418, 80426,
    83002
  parathyroid ~ 83970
  pituitary lactogenic (prolactin) ~ 80418,
    80440, 84146
  placental lactogen ~ 83632
  somatotropin release-inhibiting (somatostatin)
    ~ 84307
  thyroid-stimulating (TSH) ~ 80418,
    80438-80440, 80443
Hormone-binding globulin, sex ~ see globulin,
  sex hormone binding
Hormones, adrenal cortex ~ see corticosteroids
Hormones, antidiuretic ~ see antidiuretic
  hormone
Hormone assay
  ACTH ~ 82024
  aldosterone, blood or urine ~ 82088
  androstenedione, blood or urine ~ 82157
  androsterone, blood or urine ~ 82160
  angiotensin II ~ 82163
  corticosterone ~ 82528
  cortisol, total ~ 82533
  dehydroepiandrosterone ~ 82626
  dihydroelestosterone ~ 82651
  dihydrotestosterone ~ 82651
  epiandrosterone ~ 82666
  estradiol ~ 82670
  estriol ~ 82677
  estrogen ~ 82671-82672
  estrone ~ 82679
  follicle stimulating hormone (FSH) ~ 83001
  growth hormone, human ~ 83003

1436

CPT codes and descriptions only ©2012 American Medical Association. All rights reserved.

Hormone assay ~ *continued*
hydroxyprogesterone ~ 83498-83499
luteinizing hormone ~ 83002
somatotropin ~ 83003
testosterone ~ 84403
vasopressin ~ 84588
Hormone pellet implantation ~ 11980
Hospital discharge services ~ 99238-99239
Hospital services
inpatient services ~ 99238-99239
discharge services ~ 99238-99239,
1110F-1111F
initial care, new or established patient ~
99221-99223
initial hospital care ~ 99221-99223
newborn ~ 99460-99462, 99477
prolonged services ~ 99356-99357
subsequent hospital care ~ 99231-99233
observation
discharge services ~ 99234-99236
initial care ~ 99218-99220
new or established patient ~ 99218-99220
subsequent ~ 99224-99226
same day admission, discharges services ~
99234-99236
subsequent newborn care ~ 99462
subsequent observation care ~ 99224-99226
Hot pack treatment ~ 97010
House calls ~ 99341-99350
Howard test ~ 52005
HPL ~ (lactogen, human placental) 83632
HTLV I antibody
confirmatory test ~ 86689
detection ~ 86687
HTLV II antibody ~ 86688
HTLV III ~ see HIV
HTLV III antibodies ~ see antibody, HIV
HTLV IV ~ see HIV-2
Hubbard tank therapy ~ 97036
Hue test ~ 92283
Huggin operation ~ 54520
Huhner test ~ 89300, 89320
Human chorionic gonadotropin ~ see
chorionic gonadotropin
Human chorionic somatomammotropin ~ see
lactogen, human placental
Human epididymus protein ~ 86305
Human growth hormone(HGH) ~ 80418,
80428-80430
Human herpes virus 4 ~ see Epstein-Barr
virus
Human immunodeficiency virus ~ see HIV
Human immunodeficiency virus 1 ~ see
HIV-1
Human immunodeficiency virus 2 ~ see
HIV-2
Human papillomavirus detection ~
87620-87622
Human placental lactogen ~ 83632
Human T cell leukemia virus I ~ see HTLV I
Human T cell leukemia virus II ~ see HTLV
II

Human T cell leukemia virus I antibodies ~
see antibody, HTLV IHuman T cell
leukemia virus II antibodies ~ see antibody,
HTLV II
**Humeral epicondylitides, lateral (tennis
elbow)** ~ 24357-24359
Humeral fracture ~ see fracture, humerus
Humerus ~ see arm, upper; shoulder
abscess
incision and drainage ~ 23935
craterization ~ 23184, 24140
cyst
excision ~ 23150, 24110
with allograft ~ 23156, 24116
with autograft ~ 23155, 24115
diaphysectomy ~ 23184, 24140
excision ~ 23174, 23184, 23195, 24134,
24140, 24150
fracture
closed treatment ~ 24500-24505
with manipulation ~ 23605
without manipulation ~ 23600
condyle
closed treatment ~ 24576-24577
open treatment ~ 24579
percutaneous fixation ~ 24582
epicondyle
closed treatment ~ 24560-24565
open treatment ~ 24575
skeletal fixation, percutaneous ~ 24566
greater tuberosity fracture
closed treatment with manipulation ~
23625
closed treatment without manipulation ~
23620
open treatment ~ 23630
open treatment ~ 23615-23616
shaft ~ 24500-24505, 24516
open treatment ~ 24515
supracondylar
closed treatment ~ 24530-24535
open treatment ~ 24545-24546
percutaneous fixation ~ 24538
transcondylar
closed treatment ~ 24530-24535
open treatment ~ 24545-24546
percutaneous fixation ~ 24538
with dislocation ~ 23665-23670
osteomyelitis ~ 24134
pinning, wiring ~ 23491, 24498
prophylactic treatment ~ 23491, 24498
radical resection ~ 23220
repair ~ 24430
with graft ~ 24435
nonunion, malunion ~ 24430-24435
osteoplasty ~ 24420
osteotomy ~ 24400-24410
resection head ~ 23195
saucerization ~ 23184, 24140
sequestrectomy ~ 23174, 24134

1437

Humerus ~ *continued*
tumor
  excision ~ 23150, 23220, 24110
    with allograft ~ 23156, 24116
    with autograft ~ 23155, 24115
    radial head or neck ~ 24152
  X-ray ~ 73060
Hummelshein operation ~ see strabismus, repair
Humor shunt, aqueous ~ 66180, 66185
HVA (homovanillic acid) ~ 83150
Hyaluron binding assay ~ 89398
Hybrid approach
  stage 1 ~ 33620-33621
  stage 2 ~ 33622
Hybridization probes, DNA ~ see nucleic acid probe
Hydatid disease ~ see echinococcosis
Hydatidiform mole
  evacuation and curettage ~ 59870
  excision ~ 59100
Hydration ~ 96360-96361
  rehydration oral solution ~ 4056F
  status ~ 2030F-2031F
Hydrocarbons, chlorinated ~ 82441
Hydrocele
  aspiration ~ 55000
  excision
    bilateral, tunica vaginalis ~ 55041
    unilateral
      spermatic cord ~ 55500
      tunica vaginalis ~ 55040
  repair ~ 55060
Hydrochloric acid, gastric ~ see acid, gastric
Hydrochloride, vancomycin ~ see vancomycin
Hydrocodon ~ see dihydrocodeinone
Hydrogen ion concentration ~ see pH
Hydrolase, acetylcholine ~ see acetylcholinesterase
Hydrolase, triacylglycerol ~ see lipase
Hydrolases, phosphoric monoester ~ see phosphatase
Hydrotherapy (Hubbard tank) ~ 97036, 97113
Hydrotubation ~ 58350
Hydroxyacetanilide ~ see acetaminophen
Hydroxycorticosteroid ~ 83491
Hydroxyindolacetic acid ~ 83497
  urine ~ 83497
Hydroxypregnenolone ~ 80406, 84143
Hydroxyprogesterone ~ 80402-80406, 83498-83499
Hydroxyproline ~ 83500-83505
Hydroxytyramine ~ see dopamine
Hygroma, cystic, axillary/cervical, excision ~ 38550-38555
Hymen
  excision ~ 56700
  incision ~ 56442
Hymenal ring, revision ~ 56700
Hymenectomy ~ 56700
Hymenotomy ~ 56442

Hyoid
  bone, fracture
    closed treatment
      with manipulation ~ 21494
      without manipulation ~ 21493
    open treatment ~ 21495
  muscle, incision and suspension ~ 21685
Hyperbaric oxygen pressurization ~ 99183
Hypercycloidal X-ray ~ 76101-76102
Hyperdactylies ~ see supernumerary digit
Hyperglycemic glycogenolytic factor ~ see glucagon
Hypertelorism of orbit ~ see orbital hypertelorism
Hyperthermia therapy ~ see thermotherapy
Hyperthermia treatment ~ 77600-77620
Hypnotherapy ~ 90880
Hypodermis ~ see subcutaneous tissue
Hypogastric plexus
  destruction ~ 64681
  injection
    anesthetic ~ 64517
    neurolytic ~ 64681
Hypoglossal-facial anastomosis ~ see anastomosis, nerve, facial to hypoglossal
Hypoglossal nerve
  anastomosis, to facial nerve ~ 64868
Hypopharynges ~ see hypopharynx
Hypopharynx, biopsy ~ 42802
Hypophysectomy ~ 61546-61548, 62165
Hypophysis ~ see pituitary gland
Hypopyrexia ~ see hypothermia
Hypospadias repair ~ 54300, 54352
  complications ~ 54340-54348
  first stage ~ 54304
    proximal penile or penoscrotal ~ 54332
  one stage
    meatal advancement ~ 54322
    perineal ~ 54336
  urethroplasty
    local skin flaps ~ 54324
    local skin flaps and mobilization of urethra ~ 54326
    local skin flaps, skin graft patch and/or island flap ~ 54328
  urethroplasty for second stage ~ 54308-54316
    free skin graft ~ 54316
  urethroplasty for third stage ~ 54318
Hypoxia
  breathing response ~ 94450
  high altitude simulation test ~ 94452-94453
Hysterectomy
  abdominal
    radical ~ 58210
    resection of ovarian malignancy ~ 58951, 58953-58956
    supracervical ~ 58180
    total ~ 58150, 58200, 58956
      with colpo-urethrocystopexy ~ 58152
      with partial vaginectomy ~ 58200
      with omentectomy ~ 58956

1438

Hysterectomy ~ *continued*
  cesarean
    after cesarean delivery ~ 59525
    with closure of vesicouterine fistula ~ 51925
  laparoscopic ~ 58541-58544
    radical ~ 58548
    total ~ 58570-58573
  removal lesion ~ 59100
  supracervical
    laparoscopic ~ 58541-58544
  vaginal ~ 58260-58270, 58290-58294,
    58550-58554
    with colpectomy ~ 58275-58280
    with colpo-urethrocystopexy ~ 58267, 58293
    laparoscopic ~ 58550, 58570-58573
    radical ~ 58285
    removal tubes/ovaries ~ 58262-58263,
      58291-58292, 58552, 58554
    repair of enterocele ~ 58263, 58292, 58294
Hysterolysis ~ 58559
Hysteroplasty ~ 58540
Hysterorrhaphy ~ 58520, 59350
Hysterosalpingography ~ 74740
  catheterization ~ 58345
  injection procedure ~ 58340
Hysterosalpingostomy ~ see implantation,
  tubouterine
Hysteroscopy
  ablation, endometrial ~ 58563
  diagnostic ~ 58555
  lysis adhesions ~ 58559
  placement fallopian tube implants ~ 58565
  removal
    impacted foreign body ~ 58562
    leiomyomata ~ 58561
  resection of intrauterine septum ~ 58560
  surgical with biopsy ~ 58558
  unlisted services and procedures ~ 58579
Hysterosonography ~ 76831
Hysterotomy ~ 59100
  induced abortion
    with amniotic injections ~ 59852
    with vaginal suppositories ~ 59857
Hysterotrachelectomy ~ 57530

I

I, angiotensin ~ see angiotensin I
1 antibodies, HTLV ~ see antibody, HTLV-1
I, coagulation factor ~ see fibrinogenI, heparin
  cofactor ~ see antithrombin
IIIICCE ~ see extraction, lens, intracapsular
Ichthyosis, sex linked ~ see syphilis test
ICSH ~ see luteinizing hormone (LH)
Identification
  oocyte, from follicular fluid ~ 89254
  sperm
    from aspiration ~ 89257
    from tissue ~ 89264

IDH (isocitric dehydrogenase, blood) ~ 83570
Ig ~ see immune globulins
IgE ~ 86003-86005
IgG ~ 86001
II, coagulation factor ~ see prothrombin
II, cranial nerve ~ see optic nerve
Ileal conduit visualization ~ 50690
Ileoscopy via stoma ~ 44383
Ileostomy ~ 44310, 45136
  continent (Kock procedure) ~ 44316
  revision ~ 44312-44314
Iliac arteries ~ see artery, iliac
Iliac crest (free osteocutaneous flap with
  microvascular anastomosis) ~ 20970
Iliohypogastric nerve, injection anesthetic ~
  64425
Ilioinguinal nerve, injection anesthetic ~
  64425
Ilium
  craterization ~ 27070
  cyst excision ~ 27065-27067
  excision ~ 27070
  fracture, open treatment ~ 27215, 27218
  saucerization ~ 27070
  tumor excision ~ 27065-27067
Ilizarov procedure, Monticelli type ~ (see also
  application, bone fixation device) 20692
Imaging ~ see vascular studies
Imaging, gamma camera ~ see nuclear
  medicine
Imaging, magnetic resonance ~ see magnetic
  resonance imaging (MRI)
Imaging, ultrasonic ~ see echography
Imbrication, diaphragm ~ 39545
Imidobenzyle ~ 80174
Imipramine assay ~ 80174
Immune complex assay ~ 86332
Immune globulins ~ 90281-90399
  antitoxin
    botulinum ~ 90287
    diphtheria ~ 90296
  botulism ~ 90288
  cytomegalovirus ~ 90291
  hepatitis B ~ 90371
  human ~ 90281-90284
  rabies ~ 90375-90376
  respiratory syncytial virus ~ 90378
  Rho (D) ~ 90384-90386
  tetanus ~ 90389
  unlisted immune globulin ~ 90399
  vaccinia ~ 90393
  varicella-zoster ~ 90396
Immune globulin administration ~
  90780-90784
Immune globulin E ~ 86003-86005
Immunization administration
  one vaccine/toxoid ~ 90471, 90473
    with counseling ~ 90460
  each additional vaccine/toxoid ~ 90472, 90474
    with counseling ~ 90461

Immunizations
active
  acellular pertussis ~ 90700, 90721-90723
  BCG ~ 90585, 90586
  cholera ~ 90725
  diphtheria ~ 90700-90702, 90719-90723
  diphtheria, tetanus, pertussis (DTP) ~ 90720
  diphtheria, tetanus, acellular influenza B and
    poliovirus inactivated ~ 90698
  hemophilus influenza B ~ 90645-90648,
    90720-90721, 90748
  hepatitis A ~ 90632-90636
  hepatitis B ~ 90740-90748
  influenza ~ 90655-90660
  influenza B ~ 90645-90648
  Japanese encephalitis ~ 90735
  measles ~ 90705
  measles, mumps, rubella (MMR) ~ 90707
  measles, mumps, rubella, varicella ~ 90710
  measles, rubella ~ 90708
  meingococcal ~ 90733, 90734
  mumps ~ 90704
  plague ~ 90727
  pneumococcal ~ 90732
  poliomyelitis ~ 90713
  poliovirus ~ 90712
  rabies ~ 90675, 90676
  rotavirus vaccine ~ 90680
  rubella ~ 90706
  tetanus ~ 90700-90703, 90715,
    90720-90723
  typhoid ~ 90690-90693
  varicella (chicken pox) ~ 90716
  yellow fever ~ 90717
passive
  hyperimmune serum globulin ~ 90287-90399
  immune serum globulin ~ 90281, 90283
unlisted services and procedures ~ 90749
Immunoassay
analyte ~ 83519-83520
infectious agent ~ 86317-86318, 87449-87451
nonantibody ~ 83516-83519
tumor antigen ~ 86294, 86316
  CA 125 ~ 86304
  CA 15-3 ~ 86300
  CA 19-9 ~ 86301
Immunoblotting, Western ~ see Western Blot
Immunochemical, lysozyme (muramidase) ~
  see lysozyme
Immunocytochemistry ~ 88342
Immunodeficiency virus, human ~ see HIV
Immunodeficiency virus type 1 , human ~ see
  HIV 1
Immunodeficiency virus type 2 , human ~ see
  HIV 2
Immunodiffusion ~ 86329-86331
Immunoelectrophoresis ~ 86320-86327,
  86334-86335
Immunofixation electrophoresis ~
  86334-86335
Immunofluorescent study ~ 88346-88347
Immunogen ~ see antigen

Immunoglobulin ~ 82787
platelet associated ~ 86023
thyroid stimulating ~ 84445
Immunoglobulin E ~ 86003-86005
Immunoglobulin receptor assay ~ 86243
Immunologic skin test ~ see skin, tests
Immunology ~ 86000-86849
Immunotherapies, allergen ~ see allergen
  immunotherapy
Impedance testing ~ (see also audiologic
  function tests) 92567
Imperfectly descended testis ~ 54550, 54560
Implantation
aortic valve
  open thoracic approach ~ 0318T
  transcatheter ~ 33361-33365, 33367-33369
artificial heart, intracorporeal ~ 0051T
artificial sphincter ~ 46762
baroreflex activation device ~ 0266T-0268T
biologic, soft tissue reinforcement ~ 15777
bone, for external speech processor/cochlear
  stimulator ~ 69714-69718
brain, chemotherapy ~ 61517
cardiac event recorder ~ 33282
drug delivery device ~ 11981, 11983, 61517
electrode(s)
  array ~ 0282T-0283T
  brain ~ 61850-61875
  gastric ~ 43647-43648
  nerve ~ 65443-65-4581
  spinal cord ~ 63650-63655
eye
  anterior segment ~ 65920
  aqueous shunt to extraocular placement or
    replacement of pegs ~ 65125
  corneal ring segments ~ 0099T
  posterior segment
    extraocular ~ 67120
    intraocular ~ 67121
  reservoir ~ 66180
  vitreous, drug delivery system ~ 67027
fallopian tube ~ 58565
hearing aid hormone pellet(s)
  bone conduction ~ 69710
hip prosthesis ~ see arthroplasty, hip
hormone pellet ~ 11980
joint ~ see arthroplasty
left atrial appendage ~ 0281T
mesh ~ 49568
  hernia repair ~ 43333, 43335, 43337, 49568,
    49652-49657
  vaginal repair ~ 57267
nerve
  into bone ~ 64787
  into muscle ~ 64787
neurostimulators
  gastric ~ 95980-95982
  pulse generator ~ 61885
  receiver ~ 61886
ovum ~ 58976
pulmonary valve prosthesis ~ 0262T

Implantation ~ *continued*
pulse generator
brain ~ 61885-61886
spinal cord electrode array ~ 63685
receiver
brain ~ 61885-61886
spinal cord ~ 63685
removal ~ 20670-20680
elbow/radius ~ 24164
reservoir vascular access device
declotting ~ 36593
retinal electrode array ~ 0100T
total replacement heart system
intracorporeal ~ 0051T
tubouterine ~ 58752
ventricular assist device ~ 33975-33979
percutaneousl ~ 33990-33991
Implant removal ~ see specific anatomical site
Impression, maxillofacial
auricular prosthesis ~ 21086
definitive obturator prosthesis ~ 21080
facial prosthesis ~ 21088
interim obturator ~ 21079
mandibular resection prosthesis ~ 21081
nasal prosthesis ~ 21087
oral surgical splint ~ 21085
orbital prosthesis ~ 21077
palatal augmentation prosthesis ~ 21082
palatal lift prosthesis ~ 21083
speech aid prosthesis ~ 21084
surgical obturator ~ 21076
In situ hybridization ~ see nucleic acid probe,
cytogenetic studies, morphometric analysis
IM injection ~ see injection, intramuscular
In vitro fertilization ~ 58321-58322
In vivo NMR spectroscopy ~ see magnetic
resonance spectroscopy
Incision ~ see also incision and drainage
abdomen ~ 49000
exploration ~ 58960
abscess, soft tissue ~ 20005
accessory nerve ~ 63191
anal
fistula ~ 46270, 46280
septum ~ 46070
sphincter ~ 46080
ankle ~ 27607
tendon ~ 27605-27606
anus ~ see anus, incision
aortic valve for stenosis ~ 33415
artery, nose ~ 30915-30920
atrial septum ~ 33735-33737
bile duct sphincter ~ 43262, 47460
bladder
catheterization ~ 51045
with destruction ~ 51020-51030
with radiotracer ~ 51020
bladder diverticulum ~ 52305
brachial artery exposure ~ 34834

Incision ~ *continued*
brain
amygdalohippocampectomy ~ 61566
subpial ~ 61567
breast capsules ~ 19370
burn scab ~ 16035-16036
cataract, secondary
laser surgery ~ 66821
stab incision technique ~ 66820
chest, biopsy ~ 32096-32098
colon
exploration ~ 44025
stoma
creation ~ 44320-44322
revision ~ 44340-44346
cornea, for astigmatism ~ 65772
corpus callosum ~ 61541
cricothyroid membrane ~ 31605
dentate ligament ~ 63180-63182
duodenum ~ 44010
ear, inner labyrinth
transcanal ~ 69801
elbow ~ 24000
esophagus ~ 43020, 43045
muscle ~ 43030
exploration
heart ~ 33310-33315
kidney ~ 50010
eye
adhesions ~ 65880
anterior segment ~ 65860-65865
anterior synechiae ~ 65870
corneovitreal ~ 65880
posterior ~ 65875
anterior chamber ~ 65820
trabeculae ~ 65850
eyelid
canthus ~ 67715
sutures ~ 67710
femoral artery
exposure ~ 34812-34813
fibula ~ 27607
finger
decompression ~ 26035
tendon ~ 26060, 26455-26460
tendon sheath ~ 26055
foot ~ 28005
capsule ~ 28260-28264
fasciotomy ~ 28008
for infection ~ 28002-28003
tendon ~ 28230, 28234
frontal lobe ~ 61490
gallbladder ~ 47490
hand decompression ~ 26035-26037
tendon ~ 26450, 26460
heartexploration ~ 33310-33315
hemorrhoids, external ~ 46083
hepatic ducts ~ see hepaticostomy

1441

Incision ~ *continued*
hip
  denervation ~ 27035
  exploration ~ 27033
  fasciotomy ~ 27025
  joint capsule
    for flexor release ~ 27036
  tendon
    abductor ~ 27006
    adductor ~ 27000-27003
    iliopsoas ~ 27005
hymen ~ see hymen, incision
hymenotomy ~ 56442
hyoid muscle ~ 21685
iliac artery exposure ~ 34820, 34833
intercarpal joint dislocation ~ 25670
interphalangeal joint capsule ~ 26525
intestines, small ~ 44010
  biopsy ~ 44020
  creation
    pouch ~ 44316
    stoma ~ 44300-44310, 44314
  decompression ~ 44021
  exploration ~ 44020
  incision ~ 44020
  removal foreign body ~ 44020
  revision stoma ~ 44312
iris ~ 66500-66505
kidney ~ 50010, 50045
knee
  capsule ~ 27435
  exploration ~ 27310
  fasciotomy ~ 27305
  removal of foreign body ~ 27310
lacrimal punctum ~ 68440
lacrimal sac ~ see dacryocystotomy
larynx ~ 31300-31320
leg, lower fasciotomy ~ 27600-27602
leg, upper fasciotomy ~ 27305
  tenotomy ~ 27306-27307, 27390-27392
lip, frenum ~ 40806
liver ~ see hepatotomy
lung
  biopsy ~ 32096-32097
  decortication
    partial ~ 32225
    total ~ 32220
lymphatic channels ~ 38308
mastoid ~ see mastoidotomy
medullary tract ~ 61470
mesencephalic tract ~ 61480
metacarpophalangeal joint capsule ~ 26520
mitral valve ~ 33420-33422
muscle ~ see myotomy
nerve ~ 64575-64580, 64585, 64595,
  64702-64772
  foot ~ 28035
  root ~ 63185-63190
  sacral ~ 64581
  vagus ~ 43640-43641
nose ~ see rhinotomy

Incision ~ *continued*
orbit ~ see orbitotomy
palm fasciotomy ~ 26040-26045
pancreas sphincter ~ 43262
penis
  prepuce ~ 54000-54001
  newborn ~ 54000
pericardium
  with clot removal ~ 33020
  with foreign body removal ~ 33020
  with tube ~ 33015
pharynx stoma ~ 42955
pleura biopsy ~ 32098
pleural cavity
  empyema ~ 32035-32036
  pneumothorax ~ 32551
prostate
  exposure
    bilateral pelvic lymphadenectomy ~ 55865
    insertion radioactive substance ~ 55860
    lymph node biopsy ~ 55862
    transurethral ~ 52450
pterygomaxillary fossa ~ 31040
pulmonary valve ~ 33470-33474
pyloric sphincter ~ 43520
retina, encircling material ~ 67115
sclera
  fistulization
    iridencleisis or iridotasis ~ 66165
    sclerectomy with punch or scissors with
      iridectomy ~ 66160
    thermocauterization with iridectomy ~
      66155
    trabeculectomy ab externo in absence
      previous surgery ~ 66170
    trephination with iridectomy ~ 66150
semicircular canal
  fenestration ~ 69820
  revision ~ 69840
seminal vesicle ~ 55600-55605
  complicated ~ 55605
shoulder
  bone ~ 23035
  capsular contracture release ~ 23020
  removal, calcareous deposits ~ 23000
  tenomyotomy ~ 23405-23406
shoulder joint ~ 23040-23044
sinus
  frontal ~ 31070-31087
  maxillary ~ 31020-31032
    endoscopic ~ 31256-31267
  multiple ~ 31090
  sphenoid
    sinusotomy ~ 31050-31051
skin ~ 10040-10180
skull ~ 61316, 62148
  suture ~ 61550-61552
spinal cord ~ 63200
  tract ~ 63170, 63194-63199

Incision ~ *continued*
stomach
creation, stoma ~ 43830-43832
exploration ~ 43500
pyloric sphincter ~ 43520
synovectomy ~ 26140
temporomandibular joint ~ 21010
tendon, arm, upper ~ 24310
thigh, fasciotomy ~ 27025
thorax
empyema ~ 32035-32036
pneumothorax ~ 32551
thyroid gland ~ see thyrotomy
tibia ~ 27607
toe
capsule ~ 28270-28272
fasciotomy ~ 28008
tendon ~ 28232-28234
tenotomy ~ 28010-28011
tongue, frenum ~ 41010
trachea
emergency ~ 31603-31605
planned ~ 31600-31601
with flaps ~ 31610
tympanic membrane ~ 69420
with anesthesia ~ 69421
ureter ~ 50600
ureterocele ~ 51535
urethra ~ 53000-53010
meatus ~ 53020-53025
uterus, remove lesion ~ 59100
vagina, exploration ~ 57000
vas deferens ~ 55200
for X-ray ~ 55300
vestibule of the mouth ~ see mouth, vestibule
vitreous strands
laser surgery ~ 67031
pars plana approach ~ 67030
wrist ~ 25100-25105
capsule ~ 25085
decompression ~ 25020-25025
tendon sheath ~ 25000-25001
Incisional hernia repair ~ see hernia, repair,
incisional
Incision and drainage ~ see also drainage;
incision
abdomen
fluid ~ 49082-49083
pancreatitis ~ 48000
abscess
abdomen ~ 49020, 49040
open ~ 49040
percutaneous ~ 49021
anal ~ 46045-46050
ankle ~ 27603
appendix ~ 44900
open ~ 44900
percutaneous ~ 44901
arm, lower ~ 25028
arm, upper ~ 23930-23931
auditory canal, external ~ 69020

Incision and drainage ~ *continued*
abscess ~ *continued*
Bartholin's gland ~ 56420
bladder ~ 51080
brain ~ 61320-61321
breast ~ 19020
ear, external
complicated ~ 69005
simple ~ 69000
elbow ~ 23930
epididymis ~ 54700
eyelid ~ 67700
finger ~ 26010-26011
gums ~ 41800
hip ~ 26990
kidney ~ 50020
open ~ 50020
percutaneous ~ 50021
knee ~ 27301
leg, lower ~ 27603
leg, upper ~ 27301
liver ~ 47010
open ~ 47010
percutaneous ~ 47011
lung ~ 32200
percutaneous ~ 32201
lymph node ~ 38300-38305
mouth ~ 40800-40801, 41005-41009,
41015-41018
nasal septum ~ 30020
neck ~ 21501-21502
nose ~ 30000-30020
ovary ~ 58820-58822
abdominal approach ~ 58822
palate ~ 42000
paraurethral gland ~ 53060
parotid gland ~ 42300-42305
pelvis ~ 26990, 45000
perineum ~ 56405
peritoneum ~ 49020
percutaneous ~ 49021
prostrate ~ 55720-55725
rectum ~ 45005-45020, 46040, 46050-46060
retroperitoneal ~ 49060
open ~ 49060
salivary gland ~ 42300-42320
scrotum ~ 54700, 55100
Skene's gland ~ 53060
skin ~ 10060-10061
subdiaphragmatic, percutaneous ~
49040-49041
sublingual gland ~ 42310-42320
submaxillary gland ~ 42310-42320
subphrenic, percutaneous ~ 49040-49041
testis ~ 54700
thorax ~ 21501-21502
throat ~ 42700-42725
tongue ~ 41000-41006, 41015
tonsil ~ 42700
urethra ~ 53040
uvula ~ 42000
vagina ~ 57010

1443

Incision and drainage ~ *continued*
abscess ~ *continued*
  vulva ~ 56405
  wrist ~ 25028
  ankle ~ 27610
  bile duct ~ 47420-47425
  bladder ~ 51040
  bulla, skin, puncture aspiration ~ 10160
  bursa
    ankle ~ 27604
    arm, lower ~ 25031
    elbow ~ 23931
    foot ~ 28001
    hip ~ 26991
    knee ~ 27301
    leg, lower ~ 27604
    leg, upper ~ 27301
    palm ~ 26025-26030
    pelvis ~ 26991
    wrist ~ 25031
  carbuncle
    skin ~ 10060-10061
  carpals ~ 25035, 26034
  comedones
    skin ~ 10040
  cyst
    conjunctiva ~ 68020
    gums ~ 41800
    liver
      open ~ 47010
      percutaneous ~ 47011
    lung ~ 32200
      percutaneous ~ 32201
    mouth ~ 40800-40801, 41005-41009,
      41015-41018
    ovarian ~ 58800-58805
    skin ~ 10040-10061
      pilonidal ~ 10080-10081
      puncture aspiration ~ 10160
      spinal cord ~ 63172-63173
    thyroid gland ~ 60000
    tongue ~ 41000-41006, 41015, 60000
  elbow
    abscess ~ 23935
    arthrotomy ~ 24000
  femur ~ 27303
  fluid collection
    skin ~ 10140
  foreign body, skin ~ 10120-10121
  furuncle ~ 10060-10061
  gallbladder ~ 47480
  hematoma
    ankle ~ 27603
    arm, lower ~ 25028
    arm, upper ~ 23930
    brain ~ 61312-61315
    ear, external
      complicated ~ 69005
      simple ~ 69000
    elbow ~ 23930
    epididymis ~ 54700

Incision and drainage ~ *continued*
  gums ~ 41800
  hip ~ 26990
  knee ~ 27301
  leg, lower ~ 27603
  leg, upper ~ 27301
  mouth ~ 40800-40801, 41005-41009,
    41015-41018
  nasal septum ~ 30020
  neck ~ 21501-21502
  nose ~ 30000-30020
  pelvis ~ 26990
  scrotum ~ 54700
  skin ~ 10140
    puncture aspiration ~ 10160
  skull ~ 61312-61315
  testis ~ 54700
  thorax ~ 21501-21502
  tongue ~ 41000-41006, 41015
  vagina ~ 57022-57023
  wrist ~ 25028
hepatic duct ~ 47400
hip bone ~ 26992, 27030
humerus abscess ~ 23935
interphalangeal joint
  toe ~ 28024
intertarsal joint ~ 28020
kidney ~ 50040, 50125
knee ~ 27303, 27310
lacrimal gland ~ 68400
lacrimal sac ~ 68420
liver
  abscess or cyst ~ 47010-47011
    percutaneous ~ 47011
mediastinum ~ 39000-39010
metatarsophalangeal joint ~ 28022
milia, multiple ~ 10040
onychia ~ 10060-10061
orbit ~ 67405, 67440
paronychia ~ 10060-10061
pelvic bone ~ 26992
penis ~ 54015
pericardium ~ 33025
phalanges, finger ~ 26034
pilonidal cyst ~ 10080-10081
pustules, skin ~ 10040
radius ~ 25035
seroma, skin ~ 10140
shoulder
  abscess ~ 23030
  arthrotomy
    acromioclavicular joint ~ 23044
    sternoclavicular joint ~ 23044
    bursa ~ 23031
    hematoma ~ 23030
shoulder joint, arthrotomy, glenohumeral joint
  ~ 23040
tarsometatarsal joint ~ 28020
tendon sheath
  finger ~ 26020
  palm ~ 26020

Incision and drainage ~ *continued*
thorax
deep ~ 21510
toe ~ 28024
ulna ~ 25035
ureter ~ 50600
vagina ~ 57020
wound infection, skin ~ 10180
wrist ~ 25028, 25040
Inclusion bodies
fluid ~ 88106
smear ~ 87207-87210
Incomplete abortion ~ see abortion, incomplete
Indicator dilution studies ~ 93561-93562
Induced abortion ~ see abortion
Induced hyperthermia ~ see thermotherapy
Induced hypothermia ~ see hypothermia
Induratio penis plastica ~ see Peyronie disease
Infant, newborn, intensive care ~ see intensive care, neonatal
Infantile paralysis ~ see polio
Infection
actinomyces ~ see actinomycosis
bone ~ see osteomyelitis
diagnosis, group A strep test ~ 3210F
filarioidea ~ see filariasis
immunoassay ~ 86317-86318
postoperative wound ~ see postoperative wound infection
rapid test ~ 86403-86406
treatment, antibiotic prescribed ~ 4045F
wound ~ see wound, infection
Infectious agent
antigen detection
direct fluorescence ~ 87265-87272, 87276, 87278, 87280, 87285-87290
bordetella ~ 87265
chlamydia trachomatis ~ 87270
cryptosporidium ~ 87272
cytomegalovirus ~ 87271
enterovirus ~ 87267
giardia ~ 87269
influenza A ~ 87276
legionella pneumophila ~ 87278
respiratory syncytial virus ~ 87280
treponema pallidum ~ 87285
varicella-zoster ~ 87290
enzyme immunoassay
adenovirus ~ 87301
aspergillus ~ 87305
chlamydia trachomatis ~ 87320
clostridium difficile ~ 87324
cryptococcus neoformans ~ 87327
cryptosporidium ~ 87328
cytomegalovirus ~ 87332
entamoeba histolytica dispar group ~ 87336
entamoeba histolytica group ~ 87337
escherichia coli 0157 ~ 87335
giardia ~ 87329
helicobacter pylori ~ 87338-87339

Infectious agent ~ *continued*
hepatitis B surface antigen (HBsAg) ~ 87340
hepatitis B surface antigen (HBsAg) neutralization ~ 87341
hepatitis Be antigen (HBeAg) ~ 87350
hepatitis, delta agent ~ 87380
histoplasma capsulatum ~ 87385
HIV-1 ~ 87390
HIV-2 ~ 87391
influenza A ~ 87400
influenza B ~ 87400
multiple step method ~ 87301-87449, 87451
not otherwise specified ~ 87449, 87451
respiratory syncytial virus ~ 87420
rotavirus ~ 87425
shiga-like toxin ~ 87427
single step method ~ 87450
streptococcus, group A ~ 87430
immunofluorescence ~ 87260, 87273-87275, 87277, 87279, 87281-87283, 87299-87300
adenovirus ~ 87260
herpes simplex ~ 87273-.87274
influenza B ~ 87275
legionella micdadei ~ 87277
not otherwise specified ~ 87299
parainfluenza virus ~ 87279
pneumocystis carinii ~ 87281
polyvalent ~ 87300
rubeola ~ 87283
concentration ~ 87015
detection
by immunoassay
adenovirus ~ 87809
chlamydia trachomatis ~ 87810
clostridium difficile ~ 87803
influenza ~ 87804
neisseria gonorrheae ~ 87850
not otherwise specified ~ 87899
respiratory syncytial virus ~ 87807
streptococcus, group A ~ 87880
streptococcus, group B ~ 87802
trichomonas vaginalis ~ 87808
with direct optical observation ~ 87802-87899
by nucleic acid
bartonella henselae ~ 87470-87472
bartonella quintana ~ 87470-87472
borrelia burgdorferi ~ 87475-87477
candida species ~ 87480-87482
chlamydia pneumoniae ~ 87485-87487
chlamydia trachomatis ~ 87490-87492
clostridium difficile ~ 87493
cytomegalovirus ~ 87495-87497
enterovirus ~ 87498
gardnerella vaginalis ~ 87510-87512
hepatitis B virus ~ 87515-87517
hepatitis B ~ 87520-87522
hepatitis G ~ 87525-87527
herpes simplex virus ~ 87528-87530

Infectious agent ~ *continued*
  herpes virus-6 (six) ~ 87531-87533
  HIV-1 ~ 87534-87536
  HIV-2 ~ 87537-87539
  influenza ~ 87501-87503
  legionella pneumophila ~ 87540-87542
  multiple organisms ~ 87800-87801
  mycobacteria avium-intracellulare ~
    87560-87562
  mycobacteria species ~ 87550-87552
  mycobacteria tuberculosis ~ 87555-87557
  mycoplasma pneumoniae ~ 87580-87582
  neisseria gonorrheae ~ 87590-87592
  not otherwise specified ~ 87797-87799
  papillomavirus, human ~ 87620-87622
  staphylococcus aureus ~ 87640-87641
  streptococcus, group A ~ 87650-87652
  streptococcus, group B ~ 87653
  trichomonas vaginalis ~ 87660
  vancomycin resistance ~ 87500
  enzymatic activity ~ 87905
  genotype analysis by nucleic acid
    hepatitis C virus ~ 87902
    HIV-1 protease/reverse transcriptase ~ 87901
  phenotype analysis
    by nucleic acid
    HIV-1 drug resistance ~ 87903-87904
  phenotype prediction
    by genetic database
    HIV-1 drug resistance ~ 0023T
Infectious mononucleosis virus ~ see
  Epstein-Barr virus
Inflammatory process
  localization
  nuclear medicine ~ 78805-78807
Inflation
  ear, middle
  eustachian tube
    with catheterization ~ 69400
    without catheterization ~ 69401
  eustachian tube
    myringotomy ~ 69420
    anesthesia ~ 69424
Influenza A
  antigen detection
    direct fluorescence ~ 87276
    enzyme immunoassay ~ 87400
Influenza B
  antigen detection
    enzyme immunoassay ~ 87400
    immunofluorescence ~ 87275
Influenza vaccine ~ see vaccines
Influenza virus
  antibody ~ 86710
  by immunoassay
    with direct optical observation ~ 87804
  by nucleic acid ~ 87501-87503
Infraorbital nerve
  avulsion ~ 64734
  incision ~ 64734
  transection ~ 64734
Infrared light treatment ~ 97026

Infratentorial craniectomy ~ 61520-61521
Infusion
  amnion, transabdominal ~ 59072
  cerebral, intravenous, for thrombolysis ~
    37195
  intraosseous ~ 36680
  radioelement ~ 77750
  transcatheter therapy ~ 37202, 37211-37214
Infusion pump
  electronic analysis, spinal cord ~ 62367-62368
  insertion, intra-arterial ~ 36260
  intra-arterial
    removal ~ 36262
    revision ~ 36261
  intravenous
    insertion ~ 36563
    repair ~ 36576
    replacement ~ 36583
  maintenance ~ 95990-95991, 96520-96530
  spinal cord ~ 62361-62362
  ventricular catheter ~ 61215
Infusion therapy ~ 62350-62351, 62360-62362
  arterial catheterization ~ 36640
  chemotherapy ~ 96410-96414, 96422-96425
  home infusion procedures ~ 99601-99602
  intravenous ~ 90780-90781
  pain ~ 62360-62362, 62367-62368
  subcutaneous ~ 96369-96371
  transcatheter therapy ~ 75896
Ingestion challenge test ~ 95076, 95079
Inguinal hernia repair ~ see hernia, repair,
  inguinal
INH ~ see drug assay
Inhalation pentamidine ~ 94642
Inhalation provocation tests ~ see bronchial
  challenge test
Inhalation treatment ~ (see also pulmonology,
  therapeutic) 94640, 94644-94645, 94664,
  99503
Inhibin A ~ 86336
Inhibition test, hemagglutination ~ see
  hemagglutination inhibition test
Inhibition, fertilization ~ see contraception
Inhibitor, alpha 1-protease ~ see alpha-1
  antitrypsin
Inhibitor, alpha 2-plasmin ~ see alpha-2
  antiplasmin
Inhibitory concentration, minimum ~ see
  minimum inhibitory concentration
Initial inpatient consultations ~ see
  consultation, initial inpatient
Injection ~ see allergen immunotherapy;
  infusion
  abdomen
    air ~ 49400
    contrast material ~ 49400
  angiography, pulmonary ~ 75746
  ankle, radial ~ 27648
  antibiotic ~ see antibiotic administration
  antigen (allergen) ~ 95115-95125
  aorta (aortography), radiologic ~ 93567

Injection ~ *continued*
aponeurosis ~ 20550
bladder, radiologic ~ 51600-51610
brain canal ~ 61070
bronchography, segmental ~ 31899
bursa ~ 20600-20610
cardiac catheterization ~ 93563-93568
carpal tunnel, therapeutic ~ 20526
chemotherapy ~ 96400-96450, 96542
cistern, medication or other ~ 61055
contrast, via catheter ~ 49424
corpora cavernosa ~ 54235
cyst
  bone ~ 20615
  kidney ~ 50390
  pelvis ~ 50390
  thyroid ~ 60300
diagnostic, additional sequential, each push ~
  96376
elbow, arthrography, radiologic ~ 24220
epidural ~ see epidural, injection
esophageal varices, endoscopy ~ 43243
esophagus
  sclerosing agent ~ 43204
  submucosal ~ 43201
extremity, pseudoaneurysm ~ 36002
eye
  air ~ 66020
  medication ~ 66030
eyelid, subconjunctional ~ 68200
foot, nerve ~ 64455
ganglion, anesthetic ~ 64505, 64510
ganglion cyst ~ 20612
gastric varices, endoscopy ~ 43243
heart vessels
  cardiac catheterization ~ 93563-93568
  radiologic ~ 93563
hemorrhoids, sclerosing solution ~ 46500
hip, radiologic ~ 27093-27095
insect venom ~ 95130-95134
intervertebral disk
  chemonucleolysis agent ~ 62292
  radiological ~ 62290-62291
intraamniotic ~ 59852
intra-arterial ~ 96373, 96379
  thrombolytic ~ 37184-37186
intradermal, for tattooing ~ 11920-11922
intralesional, skin ~ 11900-11901
intramuscular ~ 96372
  therapeutic ~ 96372, 99506
intravenous ~ 96379
  nuclear diagnostic localization ~ 78808
  thrombolytic ~ 37187-37188
  unlisted ~ 96379
  vascular flow check, graft ~ 15860
intravenous push ~ 96374-96376
joint ~ 20600-20610
kidney
  drugs ~ 50391
  radiologic ~ 50394
knee, radiologic ~ 27370

Injection ~ *continued*
lacrimal gland, radiologic ~ 68850
left heart, radiologic ~ 93565
lesion, skin ~ 11900-11901
ligament ~ 20550
liver ~ 47015
  radiologic ~ 47500-47505
mammary ductogram/galactogram ~ 19030
muscle endplate
  cervical spine ~ 64613
  extremity ~ 64614
  facial ~ 64612
  trunk ~ 64614
nerve
  anesthetic ~ 01991-01992, 64400-64530
  neurolytic agent ~ 64600-64640,
    64680-64681
orbit
  retrobulbar
    alcohol ~ 67505
    medication ~ 67500
  tenon's capsule ~ 67515
pancreatography ~ 48400
paraveretebral facet joint/nerve ~ 64490-64495
penis
  for erection ~ 54235
  Peyronie disease ~ 54200
    with surgical exposure of plague ~ 54205
  radiology ~ 54230
  vasoactive drugs ~ 54231
peritoneal cavity air ~ see pneumoperitoneum
prophylactic, additional sequential, each push
  ~ 96376
radiologic, breast ~ 19030
rectum, sclerosing solution ~ 45520
right heart ~ see cardiac catheterization,
  injection
  radiologic ~ 93566
sacroiliac joint, for arthrography ~ 27096
salivary duct ~ 42660
salivary gland, radiologic ~ 42550
sclerosing agent
  esophagus ~ 43204
  intravenous ~ 36470-36471
sentinel node identification ~ 38792
shoulder, arthrography, radiologic ~ 23350
shunt, peritoneal, venous ~ 49427
sinus tract ~ 20500
  diagnostic ~ 20501
spider veins, telangiectasia ~ 36468-36469
spinal artery ~ 62294
spinal cord
  anesthetic ~ 62310-62319
  blood ~ 62273
  neurolytic agent ~ 62280-62282
  other ~ 62310-62311
  radiological ~ 62284
  steroids, urethral stricture ~ 52283
subcutaneous ~ 96372
  diagnostic ~ 90782
silicone ~ 11950-11954

1447

Injection ~ *continued*
  therapeutic ~ 96372, 90782
  temporomandibular joint, arthrography ~ 21116
  tendon origin, insertion ~ 20551
  tendon sheath ~ 20550
  therapeutic
    extremity pseudoaneurysm ~ 36002
    lung ~ 32960
    thyroid ~ 60300
    turbinate ~ 30200
  thoracic cavity ~ see pleurodesis, chemical
  trachea ~ 31612
    puncture ~ 31612
  transtracheal, bronchography ~ 31899
  trigger point(s)
    one or two muscles ~ 20552
    two or more muscles ~ 20553
  turbinate ~ 30200
  unlisted services and procedures ~ 90799
  ureter
    drugs ~ 50391
    radiologic ~ 50684
  venography ~ 36005
  ventricle
    dye ~ 61120
    medication or other ~ 61026
  vitreous ~ 67028
    fluid substitute ~ 67025
  vocal cords, therapeutic ~ 31513, 31570-31571
  wrist
    carpal tunnel, therapeutic ~ 20526
    radiologic ~ 25246
Inkblot test ~ 96101-96103
Inner ear ~ see ear, inner
Innominate arteries ~ see artery, brachiocephalic
Innominate tumor excision ~ 27077
Inorganic sulfates ~ see sulfate
Insemination, artificial ~ 58321-58322, 89268
Insertion ~ see also implantation; intubation; transplantation
  baffle, ear, middle ~ 69410
  balloon, intra-aortic ~ 33967, 33973
  breast implants ~ 19340-19342
  cannula
    arteriovenous ~ 36810-36815
    ECMO ~ 36822
    extra corporeal circulation for regional chemotherapy of extremity ~ 36823
    thoracic duct ~ 38794
    vein to vein ~ 36800
  catheter
    abdomen ~ 49324, 49419-49421, 49435
    abdominal artery ~ 36245-36248
    aorta ~ 36200
    bile duct ~ 47525-47530, 75982
      percutaneous ~ 47510
    bladder ~ 51045, 51701-51703
    brachiocephalic artery ~ 36215-36218
    brain ~ 61210, 61770

Insertion ~ *continued*
  breast, for interstitial radioelement application ~ 19296-19298
  bronchi ~ 31717
  bronchus, for intracavitary radioelement application ~ 31643
  cardiac ~ see catheterization, cardiac
    flow directed ~ 93503
  ear, middle ~ 69405
  eustachian tube ~ 69405
  gastrointestinal, upper ~ 43241
  intraperitoneal ~ 49418-49419
  jejunum ~ 44015
  kidney ~ 50392
  lower extremity artery ~ 36245-36248
  nasotracheal ~ 31720
  pelvic artery ~ 36245-36248
  pleural cavity ~ 32550
  portal vein ~ 36481
  prostate ~ 55875
  pulmonary artery ~ 36013-36015
  right heart ~ 36013, 93451
  skull ~ 61107
  spinal cord ~ 62350-62351
  suprapubic ~ 51102, 51045
  thoracic artery ~ 36215-36218
  tracheobronchial ~ 31725
  ureter via kidney ~ 50393
  urethra ~ 51701-51703
  vena cava ~ 36010
  venous ~ 36011-36012, 36400-36410, 36420-36425, 36500-36510, 36555-36558, 36568-36569
  cecostomy tube ~ 49442
  cervical dilation ~ 59200
  cochlear device ~ 69930
  colonic tube ~ 49442
  distraction device
    posterior spinous process, lumbar ~ 0171T-0172T
  drug delivery implant ~ 11981, 11983
  duodenostomy tube ~ 49441
  electrode
    brain ~ 61531-61533, 61760, 61850-61875
    heart ~ 33202-33203, 33210-33211, 33216-33217, 33224-33225, 93620-93622
    nerve ~ 64553-64581
    retina ~ 0100T
    sphenoidal ~ 95830
    spinal cord ~ 63650-63655
    stomach
      laparoscopic, neurostimulator ~ 43647
      open, neurostimulator ~ 43881
  endotracheal tube ~ 31500
  gastrostomy tube
    laparoscopic ~ 43653
    percutaneous ~ 43246, 49440
  graft
    aorta ~ 33330-33335
    heart vessel ~ 33330-33335

Insertion ~ *continued*
  guide, kidney pelvis ~ 50395
  guide wire
    endoscopy ~ 43248
    esophagoscopy ~ 43248
    with dilation ~ 43226
  Heyman capsule, uterus
    for brachytherapy ~ 58346
  iliac artery occlusion device ~ 34808
  implant, bone
    for external speech processor/cochlear
      stimulator ~ 69714-69718
  infusion pump
    intra-arterial ~ 36260
    intravenous ~ 36563
    spinal cord ~ 62361-62362
  intracatheter/needle
    aorta ~ 36160
    arteriovenous shunt ~ 36147-36148
    intra-arterial ~ 36100-36140
    intravenous ~ 36000
    kidney ~ 50392
  intraocular lens ~ 66983
    manual or mechanical technique ~ 66982, 66984
    not associated with concurrent cataract removal ~ 66985
  intrauterine device (IUD) ~ 58300
  jejunostomy tube
    endoscopy ~ 44372
    percutaneous ~ 49441
  keel, laryngoplasty ~ 31580
  laminaria ~ 59200
  mesh, pelvic floor ~ 57267
  nasobiliary tube, endoscopy ~ 43267
  nasopancreatic tube, endoscopy ~ 43267
  needle
    bone ~ 36680
    intraosseous ~ 36680
    prostate ~ 55875-55876
  needle wire, trachea ~ 31730
  neurostimulator
    pulse generator ~ 64590
    receiver ~ 64590
  nose, septal prosthesis ~ 30220
  obturator, larynx ~ 31527
  ocular implant
    with/without conjunctival graft ~ 65150
    with foreign material ~ 65155
    muscles attached ~ 65140
    muscles, not attached ~ 65135
    in scleral shell ~ 65130
  orbital transplant ~ 67550
  oviduct
    chromotubation ~ 58350
    hydrotubation ~ 58350
  ovoid, vagina, for brachytherapy ~ 57155
  pacemaker, heart ~ 33206-33208
    pulse generator only ~ 33212-33213, 33221

Insertion ~ *continued*
  pacing cardio-defibrillator
    leads ~ 33216-33220, 33224-33225, 33243-33244
    pulse generator only ~ 33230-33231, 33240
  packing, vagina ~ 57180
  penile prosthesis, inflatable ~ see penile prosthesis, insertion, inflatable
  pessary, vagina ~ 57160
  pin, skeletal traction ~ 20650
  probe, brain ~ 61770
  prostaglandin ~ 59200
  prostate, radioactive substance ~ 55860
  prosthesis
    knee ~ 27438, 27445
    nasal septal ~ 30220
    palate ~ 42281
    pelvic floor ~ 57267
    penis
      inflatable ~ 54401-54405
      noninflatable ~ 54400
    speech ~ 31611
    testis ~ 54660
    urethral sphincter ~ 53444-53445
  pulse generator
    brain ~ 61885-61886
    heart ~ 33212-33213
    spinal cord ~ 63685
  radioactive material
    bladder ~ 51020
    cystourethroscopy ~ 52250
  receiver
    brain ~ 61885-61886
    spinal cord ~ 63685
  reservoir
    brain ~ 61210-61215
    spinal cord ~ 62360
    subcutaneous ~ 49419
  sensor, fetal oximetry
    cervix ~ 0021T
    vagina ~ 0021T
  shunt ~ 36835
    abdomen
      vein ~ 49425
      venous ~ 49426
    intrahepatic portosystemic ~ 37182
  spinal instrument ~ 22849
    spinous process ~ 22841
  spinal instrumentation
    anterior ~ 22845-22847
    internal spinal fixation ~ 22841
    pelvic fixation ~ 22848
    posterior nonsegmental
      Harrington rod technique ~ 22840
    posterior segmental ~ 22842-22844
    prosthetic device ~ 22851
  stent
    bile duct ~ 43268, 47801
      percutaneous ~ 47511
    bladder ~ 51045
    conjunctiva ~ 68750

Insertion ~ *continued*
coronary ~ 92980-92981
esophagus ~ 43219
gastrointestinal, upper ~ 43256
ileum ~ 44383
indwelling ~ 50605
lacrimal duct ~ 68815
pancreatic duct ~ 43268
small intestines ~ 44370, 44379
ureter via kidney ~ 50393
ureteral ~ 50947, 52332
urethral ~ 52282
tamponade, esophagus ~ 43460
tandem uterus for brachytherapy ~ 57155
tendon graft
finger ~ 26392
hand ~ 26392
testicular prosthesis ~ see prosthesis, testicular, insertion
tissue expanders, skin ~ 11960-11971
tube
bile duct ~ 43268
esophagus ~ 43510
gastrointestinal, upper ~ 43241
ileum ~ 44383
kidney ~ 50398
pancreatic duct ~ 43268
small intestines ~ 44379
trachea ~ 31730
ureter ~ 50688
ureteral guide wire ~ 52334
vascular pedicle, carpal bone ~ 25430
venous access device
central ~ 36560-36566
peripheral ~ 36570-36571
ventilating tube ~ 69433
ventricular assist device ~ 33975
wire, skeletal traction ~ 20650
Inspiratory positive pressure breathing ~ see intermittent positive pressure breathing (IPPB)
Instillation
agent for fibrinolysis ~ 32561-32562
agent for pleurodesis ~ 32560
bladder ~ see bladder, instillation
drugs
bladder ~ 51720
kidney ~ 50391
ureter ~ 50391
Instrumentation ~ see application; bone, fixation; spinal instrumentation
spinal
insertion ~ 22840-22848, 22851
reinsertion ~ 22849
removal ~ 22850, 22852-22855
Insufflation, eustachian tube ~ see eustachian tube, inflation
Insulin ~ 80422, 80432-80435
antibody ~ 86337
blood ~ 83525
free ~ 83527

Insulin C-peptide measurement ~ see C-peptide
Insulin like growth factors ~ see somatomedin
Insurance
basic life and/or disability evaluation services ~ 99450
examination ~ 99450-99456
Integumentary system
biopsy ~ 11100-11101
breast
excision ~ 19100-19272
incision ~ 19000-19030
metallic localization clip placement ~ 19295
preoperative placement of needle localization ~ 19290-19291
reconstruction ~ 19316-19396
repair ~ 19316-19396
unlisted services and procedures ~ 19499
burns ~ 15002-15005, 15100-15121, 16000-16036
debridement ~ 11000-11006, 11010-11047
destruction ~ see also dermatology
actinotherapy ~ 96900
benign or premalignant lesion ~ 17000-17250
chemical exfoliation ~ 17360
cryotherapy ~ 17340
electrolysis epilation ~ 17380
malignant lesion ~ 17260-17286
by photodynamic therapy ~ 96567
Mohs micrographic surgery ~ 17311-17315
photodynamic therapy ~ 96567-96571
unlisted services and procedures ~ 17999
drainage ~ 10040-10180
excision
benign lesion ~ 11400-11471
debridement ~ 11000-11006, 11010-11047
malignant lesion ~ 11600-11646
incision ~ 10040-10180
introduction ~ 11900-11980
drug delivery implant ~ 11981, 11983
nails ~ 11720-11765
paring ~ 11055-11057
photography ~ 96904
pressure ulcers ~ 15920-15999
removal, drug delivery implant ~ 11982-11983
repair
adjacent tissue transfer/rearrangement ~ 14000-14350
complex ~ 13100-13160
flaps, other ~ 15740-15776
free skin grafts ~ 15050-15136, 15200-15261, 15271-15278
intermediate ~ 12031-12057
other procedures ~ 15780-15879
simple ~ 12001-12021
skin and/or deep tissue ~ 15570-15738
shaving of epidermal or dermal lesion ~ 11300-11313

Integumentary system ~ *continued*
skin replacement surgery and skin substitute grafts
autograft/tissue cultured autograft ~ 15040-15157
skin substitute graft ~ 15271-15278
surgical preparation ~ 15002-15005
skin tags, removal ~ 11200-11201
Intelligence test ~ 96100
Intensive care
low birthweight infant, subsequent care ~ 99478-99480
neonatal, initial ~ 99477
Intercarpal joint
arthrodesis ~ 25820-25825
dislocation, closed treatment ~ 25660
repair ~ 25447
Intercostal nerve
destruction ~ 64620
injection
anesthetic ~ 64420-64421
neurolytic ~ 64620
Interdental fixation
device application ~ 21110
without fracture ~ 21497
mandibular fracture
closed treatment ~ 21453
open treatment ~ 21462
Interdental papilla ~ see gums
Interdental wire fixation
closed treatment craniofacial separation ~ 21431
Interferometry eye, biometry ~ 92136
Intermediate care facility (ICF) visits ~ 99304-99318
Intermittent positive pressure breathing (IPPB) ~ see continuous positive airway pressure (CPAP); continuous negative pressure breathing (CNPB)
Internal breast prostheses ~ see breast, implants
Internal ear ~ see ear, inner
Internal rigid fixation, reconstruction, mandibular rami ~ 21196
Internet E/M service ~ 98969, 99444
Interphalangeal joint
arthrodesis ~ 26860-26863
arthroplasty ~ 26535-26536
arthrotomy ~ 26080, 28054
biopsy, synovium ~ 26110
capsule
excision ~ 26525
incision ~ 26525
dislocation
closed treatment ~ 26770
with manipulation ~ 26340
open treatment ~ 26785
percutaneous fixation ~ 26776
exploration ~ 26080

Interphalangeal joint ~ *continued*
fracture
closed treatment ~ 26740
with manipulation ~ 26742
open treatment ~ 26746
fusion ~ 26860-26863
great toe
arthrodesis ~ 28755
with tendon transfer ~ 28760
fusion ~ 28755
with tendon transfer ~ 28760
removal of foreign body ~ 26080
repair
collateral ligament ~ 26545
volar plate ~ 26548
synovectomy ~ 26140
toe ~ 28272
arthrotomy ~ 28024
dislocation ~ 28660-28665, 28675
percutaneous fixation ~ 28666
excision ~ 28160
exploration ~ 28024
removal
foreign body ~ 28024
loose body ~ 28024
synovial biopsy ~ 28054
Intersex state
clitoroplasty ~ 56805
vaginoplasty ~ 57335
Intersex surgery
female to male ~ 55980
male to female ~ 55970
Interstitial cell stimulating hormone ~ see luteinizing hormone (LH)
Interstitial cystitides, chronic ~ see cystitis, interstitial
Interstitial cystitis ~ see cystitis, interstitial
Interstitial fluid pressure monitoring ~ 20950
Interstitial cell stimulating hormone ~ see luteinizing hormone (LH)
Intertarsal joint
arthrotomy ~ 28020, 28050
exploration ~ 28020
removal
foreign body ~ 28020
loose body ~ 28020
synovial
biopsy ~ 28050
excision ~ 28070
Interthoracoscapular amputation ~ see amputation, interthoracoscapular
Intertrochanteric femur fracture ~ see femur, fracture, intertrochanteric
Intervertebral chemonucleolysis ~ see chemonucleolysis
Intervertebral disc
annuloplasty ~ 22526-22527
arthroplasty ~ 0092T, 0163T, 22856, 22857
aspiration ~ 62267

Intervertebral disc ~ *continued*
diskography
  cervical ~ 72285
  lumbar ~ 72295
  thoracic ~ 72285
excision
  decompression ~ 63075-63078
  herniated ~ 63020-63044, 63055-63066
injection
  chemonucleolysis agent ~ 62292
  X-ray ~ 62290-62291
  removal ~ 0095T, 0164T, 22864, 22865
  revision ~ 0098T, 0165T, 22861, 22862
Intestinal anastomosis ~ see anastomosis,
  intestines
Intestinal invagination ~ see intussusception
Intestinal peptide, vasoactive ~ see vasoactive
  intestinal peptide
Intestine(s)
allotransplantation ~ 44135-44136
  removal ~ 44137
anastomosis ~ 44625-44626
biopsy ~ 44100
bleeding tube ~ 43460
closure
  enterostomy, large or small ~ 44625-44626
  stoma ~ 44620-44625
excision, donor ~ 44132-44133
exclusion ~ 44700
laparoscopic resection, with anastomosis ~
  44202-44208
lesion excision ~ 44110, 44111
lysis of adhesions, laparoscopic ~ 44200
nuclear medicine imaging ~ 78290
reconstruction
  bladder ~ 50820
  colonic reservoir ~ 45119
repair
  diverticula ~ 44605
  obstruction ~ 44615
  ulcer ~ 44605
  wound ~ 44605
suture
  diverticula ~ 44605
  stoma ~ 44620-44625
  ulcer ~ 44605
  wound ~ 44605
transplantation
  allograft preparation ~ 44715-44721
  donor enterectomy ~ 44132-44133
  removal of allograft ~ 44137
unlisted services and procedures ~ 44238,
  44799
Intestines, large ~ see anus; cecum; colon;
  rectum
Intestines, small
anastomosis ~ 43845, 44130
biopsy ~ 44020
  endoscopy ~ 44361
catheterization jejunum ~ 44015
decompression ~ 44021

Intestines, small ~ *continued*
destruction lesion ~ 44369
  tumor ~ 44369
endoscopy ~ 44364
  biopsy ~ 44361, 44377
  control of bleeding ~ 44366, 44378
  via stoma ~ 44382
  destruction
    lesion ~ 44369
    tumor ~ 44369
  diagnostic ~ 44376
  exploration ~ 44360
  hemorrhage ~ 44366
  insertion
    stent ~ 44370, 44379
    tube ~ 44379
  pelvic pouch ~ 44385-44386
  removal
    foreign body ~ 44363
    lesion ~ 44365
    polyp ~ 44364-44365
    tumor ~ 44364-44365
  via stoma ~ 44380
  tube placement ~ 44372
  tube revision ~ 44373
enterostomy ~ 44300
excision ~ 44120-44128
  partial with anastomosis ~ 44140
exclusion ~ 44700
exploration ~ 44020
gastrostomy tube ~ 44373
hemorrhage ~ 44378
hemorrhage control ~ 44366
ileostomy ~ 44310-44314, 45136
  continent ~ 44316
incision ~ 44020
  creation
    pouch ~ 44316
    stoma ~ 44300-44310, 44314
  decompression ~ 44021
  exploration ~ 44020
  revision
    stoma ~ 44312
    stoma closure ~ 44620-44626
insertion
  catheter ~ 44015
  jejunostomy tube ~ 44372
jejunostomy ~ 44310
  laparoscopic ~ 44201
lysis adhesions ~ 44005
removal foreign body ~ 44020, 44363
repair
  diverticula ~ 44602-44603
  enterocele
    abdominal approach ~ 57270
    vaginal approach ~ 57268
  fistula ~ 44640-44661
  hernia ~ 44050
  malrotation ~ 44055
  obstruction ~ 44050
  ulcer ~ 44602-44603

Intestine, small ~ *continued*
  volvulus ~ 44050
  wound ~ 44602-44603
  revision jejunostomy tube ~ 44373
  suture
    diverticula ~ 44602-44603
    fistula ~ 44640-44661
    plication ~ 44680
    ulcer ~ 44602-44603
    wound ~ 44602-44603
  X-ray ~ 74245, 74249-74251
  guide intubation ~ 74355
Intestinovesical fistula ~ see fistula,
  enterovesical
Intimectomy ~ see endarterectomy
Intra arterial injections ~ see injection,
  intra-arterial
Intra-abdominal voiding pressure studies ~
  51797
Intra-osseous infusion ~ see infusion,
  intraosseous
Intracapsular extraction of lens ~ see
  extraction, lens, intracapsular
Intracardiac echocardiography ~ 93662
Intracranial arterial perfusion, thrombolysis
  ~ 61624
  biopsy ~ 61140
  extracranial ~ 61623
  microdissection ~ 69990
  neoplasm
    acoustic neuroma ~ see brain, tumor,
      excision
    craniopharyngioma ~ see craniopharyngioma
    meningioma ~ see meningioma
Intrafallopian transfer, gamete ~ see GIFT
Intraluminal angioplasty ~ see angioplasty
Intramuscular injection ~ see injection,
  intramuscular
Intraocular lens
  exchange ~ 66986
  insertion ~ 66983
    not associated with concurrent cataract
      removal ~ 66985
    manual or mechanical technique ~ 66982,
      66984
Intratracheal intubation ~ see insertion,
  endotracheal tube
Intrauterine contraceptive device ~ see
  intrauterine device (IUD)
Intrauterine device (IUD)
  insertion ~ 58300
  removal ~ 58301
Intravascular stent ~ see transcatheter,
  placement, intravascular stents
  X-ray ~ 75960
Intravascular ultrasound
  intraoperative ~ 37250-37251
Intravenous infusion
  diagnosis ~ 96365-96368
  hydration ~ 96360-96361
    status documented ~ 2030F-2031F

Intravenous injection ~ see injection,
  intravenous
Intravenous pyelogram ~ see urography,
  intravenous
Intravenous therapy ~ (see also injection,
  chemotherapy) 90780-90781
  pain management ~ 90783-90784
Intravesical instillation ~ see bladder,
  instillation
Intravitreal injection pharmacologic agent ~
  67028
Intrinsic factor ~ 83528
  antibody ~ 86340
Introduction
  breast
    metallic localization clip placement ~ 19295
    preoperative placement, needle ~
      19290-19291
  drug delivery implant ~ 11981, 11983
  gastrointestinal tube ~ 44500
    with fluoroscopic guidance ~ 74340
  tissue expanders, skin ~ 11960-11971
Intubation ~ *see also* insertion
  duodenal, with aspiration ~ 43756-43757
  endotracheal tube ~ 31500
  eustachian tube ~ see catheterization,
    eustachian tube
  gastric, with aspiration ~ 43753-43755
Intubation tube ~ see endotracheal tube
Intussusception
  barium enema ~ 74283
  reduction
    laparotomy ~ 44050
Invagination, intestinal ~ see intussusception
Inversion, nipple ~ see nipples, inverted
Iodide test ~ see nuclear medicine, thyroid,
  uptake
Iodine test ~ see starch granules, feces
Ionization, medical ~ see iontophoresis
Iontophoreses ~ see iontophoresis
Iontophoresis ~ 97033
  sweat collection ~ 89230
IP ~ see allergen immunotherapy
Ipecac administration ~ 99175
IPPB ~ see intermittent positive pressure
  breathing; pulmonology, therapeutic
Iridectomy
  with corneoscleral or corneal section ~ 66600
  by laser surgery ~ 66761
  peripheral for glaucoma ~ 66625
  with sclerectomy with punch or scissors ~ 66160
  with thermocauterization ~ 66155
  with transfixion as for iris bombe ~ 66605
  with trephination ~ 66150
Iridencleisis ~ 66165
Iridodialysis ~ 66680
Iridoplasty ~ 66762
Iridotasis ~ 66165

Iridotomy
excision
with corneoscleral or corneal section ~ 66600
with cyclectomy ~ 66605
optical ~ 66635
peripheral ~ 66625
incision
stab ~ 66500
with transfixion as for iris bombe ~ 66505
by laser surgery ~ 66761
optical ~ 66635
peripheral ~ 66625
sector ~ 66630
by stab incision ~ 66500
Iris
cyst, destruction ~ 66770
excision
iridectomy
with corneoscleral or corneal section ~ 66600
with cyclectomy ~ 66605
optical ~ 66635
peripheral ~ 66625
sector ~ 66630
incision
iridotomy
stab ~ 66500
with transfixion as for iris bombe ~ 66505
lesion, destruction ~ 66770
repair
with ciliary body ~ 66680
suture ~ 66682
revision
laser surgery ~ 66761
photocoagulation ~ 66762
suture, with ciliary body ~ 66682
Iron ~ 83540
absorption ~ 78162
chelatable total body iron ~ 78172
turnover rate ~ 78160
utilization ~ 78170
Iron binding capacity ~ 83550
Iron hematoxylin stain ~ 88312
Iron stain ~ 85536, 88313
Irradiation blood products ~ 86945
Irrigation
bladder ~ 51700
catheter, brain ~ 62194, 62225
corpora cavernosa, priapism ~ 54220
Irrigation ~ *continued*
penis, priapism ~ 54220
peritoneal ~ see peritoneal lavage
shunt, spinal cord ~ 63744
sinus
maxillary ~ 31000
sphenoid ~ 31002
vagina ~ 57150
Irving sterilization (ligation, fallopian tube, oviduct) ~ 58600-58611, 58670

Ischemic stroke
onset ~ 1065F-1066F
tissue plasminogen activator (tPA)
documentation that administration was considered ~ 4077F
Ischial
bursa excision ~ 27060
tumor excision ~ 27075, 27078
Ischiectomy ~ 15941
Islands of Langerhans ~ see Islet cell
Island pedicle flaps ~ 15740
Islet cell
antibody ~ 86341
Isocitrate dehydrogenase ~ see isocitric dehydrogenase
Isocitric dehydrogenase blood ~ 83570
Isolation sperm ~ 89260-89261
Isomerase, glucose 6 (six) phosphate ~ see phosphohexose isomerase
Isopropanol ~ see isopropyl alcohol
Isopropyl alcohol ~ 84600
Isthmusectomy, thyroid gland ~ 60210-60225
IUD ~ see intrauterine device (IUD)
IV infusion therapy ~ see allergen immunotherapy; chemotherapy; infusion; injection, chemotherapy
IV ~ see injection, chemotherapy; intravenous therapy
IVF ~ see artificial insemination; in vitro fertilization
Ivy bleeding time ~ 85002
IV injection ~ see injection, intravenous
IV, coagulation factor ~ see calcium
IX complex, factor ~ see Christmas factor

J

Jaboulay operation ~ 43810, 43850, 43855
Jannetta procedure ~ 61458
Japanese, river fever ~ see scrub typhus
Jatene type procedure ~ 33770-33781
Jaw joint ~ see facial bones; mandible; maxilla
jaws
muscle reduction ~ 21295-21296
X-ray for orthodontics ~ 70355
Jejunostomy
catheterization ~ 44015
contrast ~ 49465
insertion
catheter ~ 44015
percutaneous ~ 49441
laparoscopic ~ 44186-44187
non-tube ~ 44187, 44310
obstructive material removal ~ 49460
replacement ~ 49451
with pancreatic drain ~ 48001

Jejunum
creation, stoma
laparoscopic ~ 44201
transfer
with microvascular anastomosis free ~
43496
Johannsen procedure ~ 53400
Johanson operation ~ see reconstruction,
urethra
Joint ~ see specific joint
arthrocentesis ~ 20600-20610
aspiration ~ 20600-20610
dislocation ~ see dislocation
drainage ~ 20600-20610
finger ~ see intercarpal joint
fixation (surgical) ~ see arthrodesis
injection ~ 20600-20610
nuclear medicine imaging ~ 78300, 78315
radiology stress views ~ 77071
shoulder ~ see glenohumeral joint
survey ~ 77077
wrist ~ see radiocarpal joint
Joint syndrome, temporomandibular ~ see
temporomandibular joint (TMJ)
Jones and Cantarow test ~ see blood urea
nitrogen; urea nitrogen, clearance
Jones procedure ~ 28760
Joplin procedure ~ 28294
Jugal bone ~ see cheek bone
Jugular vein ~ see vein, jugular

K

K-wire fixation, tongue ~ 41500
Kader operation ~ see incision, stomach,
creation, stoma; incision and drainage
Kala Azar smear ~ 87207
Kallidin I /Kallidin 9 ~ see Bradykinin
Kallikreinogen ~ see Fletcher factor
Kallikrein HK3 ~ see antigen, prostate specific
Kasai procedure ~ 47701
Kedani fever ~ see scrub typhus
Keel, insertion/removal, laryngoplasty ~
31580
Keen operation (laminectomy) ~ 63600
Kelikian procedure ~ 28280
Keller procedure ~ 28292
Kelly urethral plication ~ 57220
Keratectomy, partial, for lesion ~ 65400
Keratomileusis ~ 65760
Keratophakia ~ 65765
Keratoplasty
endothelial ~ 65756
allograft preparation ~ 65757
lamellar ~ 65710
penetrating ~ 65730
in aphakia ~ 65750
in pseudophakia ~ 65755
Keratoprosthesis ~ 65770

Keratotomy, radial ~ 65771

Ketogenic steroids ~ 83582
Ketone body, acetone ~ 82009-82010
Ketosteroids ~ 83586-83593
Kidner procedure ~ 28238
Kidney
abscess
incision and drainage
open ~ 50020
percutaneous ~ 50021
anesthesia ~ 00862
biopsy ~ 50200-50205
endoscopic ~ 50555-50559, 52354
catheterization, endoscopic ~ 50572
cyst
ablation ~ 50541
aspiration ~ 50390
excision ~ 50280-50290
injection ~ 50390
X-ray ~ 74470
destruction
calculus ~ 50590
endoscopic ~ 50557, 50576, 52354
dilation ~ 50395
endoscopy
biopsy ~ 50555, 50574-50576, 52354
catheterization ~ 50553, 50572
destruction ~ 50557, 50576, 52354
dilation
intra-renal stricture ~ 52343, 52346
ureter ~ 50553
excision tumor ~ 52355
exploration ~ 52351
lithotripsy ~ 52353
removal
calculus ~ 50561, 50580, 52352
foreign body ~ 50561, 50580
via incision ~ 50562-50580
via stoma ~ 50551-50561
excision
donor ~ 50300-50320, 50547
partial ~ 50240
recipient ~ 50340
transplantation ~ 50370
with ureters ~ 50220-50236
exploration ~ 50010, 50045, 50120
incision ~ 50010, 50045
incision and drainage ~ 50040, 50125
injection
drugs ~ 50391
radiologic ~ 50394
insertion
catheter ~ 50392-50393
guide ~ 50395
intracatheter ~ 50392
stent ~ 50393
tube ~ 50398
instillation drugs ~ 50391
lithotripsy ~ 50590
manometry pressure ~ 50396

1455

Kidney ~ *continued*	**Knee ~** *continued*

Kidney ~ *continued*
mass ablation ~ 50542
needle biopsy ~ 50200
nuclear medicine
function study ~ 78725
imaging ~ 78700-78710
unlisted services and procedures ~ 78799
removal
calculus ~ 50060-50081, 50130, 50561
foreign body ~ 50561, 50580
repair
blood vessels ~ 50100
fistula ~ 50520-50526
horseshoe kidney ~ 50540
renal pelvis ~ 50400-50405
wound ~ 50500
solitary ~ 50405
suture
fistula ~ 50520-50526
horseshoe kidney ~ 50540
transplantation
anesthesia
donor ~ 00862
recipient ~ 00868
allograft preparation ~ 50323-50329
donor ~ 00862
donor nephrectomy ~ 50300-50320, 50547
implantation of graft ~ 50360
recipient nephrectomy ~ 50340, 50365
reimplantation kidney ~ 50380
removal transplant renal autograft ~ 50370
ultrasound ~ 76770-76776
X-ray with contrast guide catheter ~ 74475
Kidney stone ~ see calculus, removal, kidney
Killian operation ~ see sinusotomy, frontal
Kinase, creatine ~ see CPK
Kineplasty ~ see cineplasty
Kinetic therapy ~ 97530
Kininase A ~ see angiotensin converting
enzyme (ACE)
Kininogen ~ 85293
Kininogen, high molecular weight ~ see
Fitzgerald factor
Kleihauer-Betke test ~ 85460
Kloramfenikol ~ see chloramphenicol
Knee ~ see femur; fibula; patella; tibia
abscess ~ 27301
arthrocentesis ~ 20610
arthrodesis ~ 27580
arthroplasty ~ 27440-27445, 27447
revision ~ 27486-27487
arthroscopy
diagnostic ~ 29870
surgical ~ 29866-29868, 29871-29889
arthrotomy ~ 27310, 27330-27335, 27403
autograft, osteochondral, open ~ 27416
biopsy ~ 27323-27324, 27330-27331
synovium ~ 27330
bone, drainage ~ 27303
bursa ~ 27301
excision ~ 27340

Knee ~ *continued*
cyst, excision ~ 27345-27347
disarticulation ~ 27598
dislocation ~ 27550-27552, 27560-27562
open treatment ~ 27556-27558, 27566
drainage ~ 27310
excision
cartilage ~ 27332-27333
ganglion ~ 27347
lesion ~ 27347
synovial lung ~ 27334-27335
exploration ~ 27310, 27331
fasciotomy ~ 27305, 27496-27499
fracture ~ 27520-27524
arthroscopic treatment ~ 29850-29851
fusion ~ 27580
hematoma ~ 27301
incision, capsule ~ 27435
injection, X-ray ~ 27370
magnetic resonance (MRI) ~ 73721-73723
manipulation ~ 27570
meniscectomy ~ 27332-27333
reconstruction ~ 27437-27438
ligament ~ 27427-27429
with prosthesis ~ 27445
removal
foreign body ~ 27310, 27331, 27372
loose body ~ 27331
prosthesis ~ 27488
repair
ligament ~ 27405-27409
collateral ~ 27405
collateral and cruciate ~ 27409
cruciate ~ 27407-27409
meniscus ~ 27403
tendon ~ 27380-27381
replacement ~ 27447
retinacular release ~ 27425
strapping ~ 29530
suture tendon ~ 27380-27381
transplantation
chondrocytes ~ 27412
meniscus ~ 29868
osteochondral
allograft ~ 27415-29867
autograft ~ 27412-29866
tumor excision ~ 27327-27329, 27337-27339,
27365
unlisted services and procedures ~ 27599
X-ray ~ 73560-73564
arthrography ~ 73580
bilateral ~ 73565
X-ray with contrast arthrography ~ 73580
Knee cap
excision ~ 27350
repair, instability ~ 27420-27424
Knee joint arthroplasty ~ 27446
Knee prosthesis ~ see prosthesis, knee
Knock-knee repair ~ 27455-27457
Kocher operation ~ 23650-23680
Kocher pylorectomy ~ see gastrectomy, partial

Kock pouch ~ 44316
  formation ~ 50825
Kock procedure ~ 44316
KOH ~ see hair; nails; tissue, examination for fungi
Kraske procedure ~ 45116
Krause operation ~ see gasserian ganglion, sensory root, decompression
Kroenlein procedure ~ 67420
Krukenberg procedure ~ 25915
Kuhlmann test ~ 96100
Kyphectomy
  more than two segments ~ 22819
  up to two segments ~ 22818

L

L-alanine ~ see aminolevulinic acid (ALA)
L ascorbic acid ~ see ascorbic acid
L aspartate 2 oxoglutarate aminotransferase ~ see transaminase, glutamic oxaloacetic
L glutamine ~ see glutamine
L-leucylnaphthylamidase ~ see leucine aminopeptidase
L/S ratio, amniotic fluid ~ 83661
Labial adhesions, lysis ~ 56441
Laboratory panel
  ACTH stimulation panel ~ 80400
  acute hepatitis panel ~ 80074
  basic metabolic panel ~ 80048
  comprehensive metabolic panel ~ 80053
  corticotropic releasing hormone (CRH) stimulation panel ~ 80412
  electrolyte panel ~ 80051
  general health panel ~ 80050
  glucagon tolerance panel ~ 80422-80424
  gonadotropin releasing hormone stimulation panel ~ 80426
  growth hormone
    stimulation panel ~ 80428
    suppression panel ~ 80430
  hepatic function panel ~ 80076
  insulin
    tolerance panel ~ 80434-80435
    induced C-peptide suppression panel ~ 80432
  lipid panel ~ 80061
  metyrapone panel ~ 80436
  obstetric panel ~ 80055
  renal function ~ 80069
  thyrotropin releasing hormone (TRH) stimulation panel ~ 80438-80440
Laboratory services ~ 8000-8999
  anatomic pathology ~ 88000-88999
  chemistry ~ 82000-84999
  consultations, clinical pathology ~ 80500-80502
  cytogenetic studies ~ 88230-88299
  cytopathology ~ 88104-88199

Laboratory services ~ *continued*
  drug testing ~ 80100-80103
  evocative/suppression testing ~ 80400-80440
  hematology and coagulation ~ 85002-85999
  immunology ~ 86000-86849
  microbiology ~ 87001-87999
  organ or disease oriented panels ~ 80048-80076
  other pathology and laboratory procedures ~ 89050-89240
  reproductive medicine procedures ~ 89250-89356
  surgical pathology ~ 88300-88399
  therapeutic drug assays ~ 80150-80299
  transcutaneous procedures ~ 88720
  transfusion medicine ~ 86850-86999
  urinalysis ~ 81000-81099
Labyrinth ~ see ear, inner
Labyrinthectomy ~ 69905
  with mastoidectomy ~ 69910
  with skull base surgery ~ 61596
Labyrinthotomy
  transcanal ~ 69801
Laceration repair ~ see specific site **
Lacrimal duct
  canaliculi, repair ~ 68700
  exploration ~ 68810
    with anesthesia ~ 68811
    canaliculi ~ 68840
    stent ~ 68815
  insertion, stent ~ 68815
  removal
    dacryolith ~ 68530
    foreign body ~ 68530
  X-ray with contrast ~ 70170
Lacrimal gland
  biopsy ~ 68510
  close fistula ~ 68770
  excision
    partial ~ 68505
    total ~ 68500
  fistulization ~ 68720
  incision and drainage ~ 68400
  injection, X-ray ~ 68850
  nuclear medicine, tear flow ~ 78660
  removal
    dacryolith ~ 68530
    foreign body ~ 68530
  repair, fistula ~ 68770
  tumor, excision
    without closure ~ 68540
    with osteotomy ~ 68550
Lacrimal punctum
  closure
    by plug ~ 68761
    by thermocauterization, ligation or laser surgery ~ 68760
  dilation ~ 68801
  incision ~ 68440
  repair ~ 68705

Lacrimal sac
 biopsy ~ 68525
 excision ~ 68520
 incision and drainage ~ 68420
Lacrimal system, unlisted services and procedures ~ 68899
Lactase deficiency breath test ~ 91065
Lactate ~ 83605
Lactate dehydrogenase ~ see lactic dehydrogenase
Lactic acid ~ 83605
Lactic acid measurement ~83605
Lactic cytochrome reductase ~ see lactic dehydrogenase
Lactic dehydrogenase ~ 83615-83625
Lactiferous duct
 excision ~ 19112
 exploration ~ 19110
Lactoferrin, fecal ~ 83630
Lactogen, human placental ~ 83632
Lactogenic hormone ~ see prolactin
Lactose, urine ~ 83633-83634
Ladd procedure ~ 44055
Lagophthalmos, repair ~ 67912
Laki Lorand factor ~ see fibrin stabilizing factor
Lamblia intestinalis ~ see giardia lamblia
Lambrinudi operation ~ see arthrodesis, foot joint
Lamellar keratoplasties ~ see keratoplasty, lamellar
Laminaria, insertion ~ 59200
Laminectomy ~ 62351, 63001, 63005-63011, 63015-63044, 63180-63200, 63265-63290, 63300-63655
 with facetectomy ~ 63045-63048
 lumbar ~ 22630, 63012
 surgical ~ 63170-63172
Laminoplasty, cervical ~ 63050-63051
Langerhans islands ~ see islet cell
Language evaluation ~ 92506
Language therapy ~ 92507-92508
LAP ~ 83670
Laparoscopic appendectomy ~ see appendectomy, laparoscopic
Laparoscopic biopsy of ovary ~ see biopsy, ovary, laparoscopic
Laparoscopy
 abdominal ~ 49320-49327, 49329
 adrenalectomy ~ 50545
 adrenal gland, biopsy or excision ~ 60650
 appendectomy ~ 44970
 aspiration ~ 49322
 biopsy ~ 47561, 49321
 lymph nodes ~ 38570
 bladder repair ~ 51990, 51992, 51999
 cecostomy ~ 44188
 cholangiography ~ 47560-47561
 cholecystectomy ~ 47562-47564
 cholecystenterostomy ~ 47570

Laparoscopy ~ *continued*
 colectomy
  laparoscopic ~ 44213
  partial ~ 44204-44208, 44213
  total ~ 44210-44212
 colostomy ~ 44188
 destruction, lesion ~ 58662
 drainage, extraperitoneal lymphocele ~ 49323
 ectopic pregnancy ~ 59150
  with salpingectomy and/or oophorectomy ~ 59151
 electrode implantation, gastric ~ 43647, 43648
 electrode removal, gastric ~ 43648
 electrode replacement, gastric ~ 43647
 electrode revision, gastric ~ 43648
 enterectomy ~ 44202
 enterolysis ~ 44180
 enterostomy, closure ~ 44227
 esophageal lengthening ~ 43283
 esophagogastric fundoplasty ~ 43280, 43327-43328
 esophagomyotomy fundoplasty ~ 43279
 fimbrioplasty ~ 58672
 gastrectomy, longitudinal/sleeve ~ 43775
 gastric restrictive procedures ~ 43644-43645, 43770-43775
 gastrostomy, temporary ~ 43653
 hernia repair
  epigastric
   incarcerated or strangulated ~ 49653
   reducible ~ 49652
  incisional
   incarcerated or strangulated ~ 49655
   reducible ~ 49654
  incisional recurrent
   incarcerated or strangulated ~ 49657
   reducible ~ 49656
  inguinal
   initial ~ 49650
   recurrent ~ 49651
  paraesophageal ~ 43281-43282
  spigelian
   incarcerated or strangulated ~ 49653
   reducible ~ 49652
  umbilical
   incarcerated or strangulated ~ 49653
   reducible ~ 49652
  ventral
   incarcerated or strangulated ~ 49653
   reducible ~ 49652
 hysterectomy ~ 58541-58544
  radical ~ 58548
  total ~ 58570-58573
 ileostomy ~ 44187
 incontinence repair ~ 51990-51992
 in vitro fertilization ~ 58976
  retrieve oocyte ~ 58970
  transfer embryo ~ 58974
  transfer gamete ~ 58976
 jejunostomy ~ 44186-44187
 kidney, ablation ~ 50541-50542

Laparoscopy ~ *continued*
ligation, veins, spermatic ~ 55550
liver ablation, tumor ~ 47370-47371
lymphadenectomy ~ 38571-38572
lymphatic ~ 38570-38589
lysis of adhesions ~ 58660
lysis of intestinal adhesions ~ 44180
nephrectomy ~ 50545-50548
partial ~ 50543
omentopexy ~ 49326
orchiectomy ~ 54690
orchiopexy ~ 54692
oviduct surgery ~ 58670-58671, 58679
pelvis ~ 49320
proctectomy
complete ~ 45395
with creation of colonic reservoir ~ 45397
proctopexy, for prolapse ~ 45400-45402
prostatectomy ~ 55866
pyeloplasty ~ 50544
rectum, resection ~ 45395-45397
unlisted ~ 45499
removal
fallopian tubes ~ 58661
leiomyomata ~ 58545-58546
ovaries ~ 58661
spleen ~ 38120
testis ~ 54690
resection, intestines, with anastomosis ~ 44202-44203
salpingostomy ~ 58673
splenectomy ~ 38120-38129
splenic flexure, mobilization ~ 44213
stomach ~ 43647-43659
gastric bypass ~ 43644-63645
gastric restrictive ~ 43770-43775, 43848, 43886-43888
gastroenterostomy ~ 43644-43645
Roux-en-Y ~ 43644
unlisted services and procedures ~ 38129, 38589, 43289, 43659, 44238-44239, 44979, 47379, 47579, 49329, 49659, 50549, 50949, 54699, 55559, 58578-58579, 58679, 59898
ureterolithotomy ~ 50945
ureteroneocystostomy ~ 50947-50948
urethral suspension ~ 51990
vaginal hysterectomy ~ 58550-58554
vaginal suspension ~ 57425
vagus nerves, transection ~ 43651-43652
with X-ray ~ 47560
Laparotomy
with biopsy ~ 49000
exploration ~ 47015, 49000-49002, 58960
hemorrhage control ~ 49002
second look ~ 58960
staging ~ 58960
for staging ~ 49220
Laparotomy, exploratory ~ see abdomen, exploration
Lapidus procedure ~ 28297
Large bowel ~ see anus; cecum; rectum

Laroyenne operation ~ see vagina, abscess, incision and drainage, 57010
Laryngeal function study ~ 92520
Laryngeal sensory testing ~ 92614-92617
Laryngectomy ~ 31360-31382
partial ~ 31367-31382
subtotal ~ 31367-31368
Laryngocele, removal ~ 31300
Laryngofissure ~ 31300
Laryngography ~ 70373
Laryngopharyngectomy ~ see excision, larynx, with pharynx, 31390, 31395
Laryngopharynx ~ see hypopharynx
Laryngoplasty
burns ~ 31588
cricoid split ~ 31587
laryngeal stenosis ~ 31582
laryngeal web ~ 31580
open reduction of fracture ~ 31584
Laryngoscopy
diagnostic ~ 31505
direct ~ 31515-31571
exploration ~ 31505, 31520-31526, 31575
fiberoptic ~ 31575-31579
with stroboscopy ~ 31579
indirect ~ 31505-31513
newborn ~ 31520
operative ~ 31530-31561
Laryngotomy ~ 31300
diagnostic ~ 31320
total ~ 31360-31368
Larynx
aspiration, endoscopy ~ 31515
biopsy, endoscopy ~ 31510, 31535-31536, 31576
dilation, endoscopic ~ 31528-31529
endoscopy
direct ~ 31515-31571
excision ~ 31545-31546
exploration ~ 31505, 31520-31526, 31575
fiberoptic ~ 31575-31579
with stroboscopy ~ 31579
indirect ~ 31505-31513
operative ~ 31530-31561
excision
lesion ~ 31512, 31578
endoscopic ~ 31545-31546
partial ~ 31367-31382
with pharynx ~ 31390-31395
total ~ 31360-31365
exploration, endoscopic ~ 31505, 31520-31526, 31575
fracture, closed treatment
with manipulation ~ 31586
without manipulation ~ 31585
open treatment ~ 31584
insertion, obturator ~ 31527
nerve, destruction ~ 31595
reconstruction
burns ~ 31588
cricoid split ~ 31587

1459

Larynx ~ *continued*
  other ~ 31588
  stenosis ~ 31582
  web ~ 31580
  removal
    foreign body, endoscopic ~ 31511,
      31530-31531, 31577
    lesion, endoscopic ~ 31512, 31545-31546,
      31578
  repair, reinnervation neuromuscular pedicle ~
    31590
  stroboscopy ~ 31579
  tumor excision ~ 31300
    endoscopic ~ 31540-31541
  unlisted services and procedures ~ 31599
  vocal cord(s), injection ~ 31513, 31570-31571
  X-ray ~ 70370
    with contrast ~ 70373
Laser surgery
  anal ~ , 46614, 46917
  cautery, esophagus ~ 43227
  lacrimal punctum ~ 68760
  lens, posterior ~ 66821
  lesion
    mouth ~ 40820
    nose ~ 30117-30118
    penis ~ 54057
    skin ~ 17000-17111, 17260-17286
  myocardium ~ 33140-33141
  prostate ~ 52647-52649
  spine, diskectomy ~ 62287
  tumors, urethra and bladder ~ 52234
  urethra and bladder ~ 52214
Laser treatment ~ see destruction ~
  17000-17286, 96920-96922
Lateral epicondylitis ~ see tennis elbow
Latex fixation ~ 86403-86406
LATS ~ see thyrotropin releasing hormone
  (TRH)
Latzko operation ~ see repair, vagina, fistula;
  revision
LAV ~ see HIV
LAV-2 (two) ~ see HIV-2 (two)
LAV antibodies ~ see antibody, HIV
Lavage
  colon ~ 44701
  lung
    bronchial ~ 31624
    total ~ 32997
  peritoneal ~ 49084
  stomach ~ 43753
LCM ~ see lymphocytic choriomeningitis
LD ~ lactic dehydrogenase, 83615
LDH ~ 83615-83625
LDL ~ 83721
Lead ~ 83655
Leadbetter procedure ~ 53431
Lecithin-sphingomyelin ratio ~ 83661
Lecithinase C ~ see tissue typing
Lee and White test ~ 85345
Leep procedure ~ 57460
Lefort procedure, vagina ~ 57120

Lefort I procedure
  midface reconstruction ~ 21141-21147, 21155,
    21160
  palatal of maxillary fracture ~ 21421-21423
Lefort II procedure
  midface reconstruction ~ 21150-21151
  nasomaxillary complex fracture ~
    21345-21348
Lefort III procedure
  craniofacial separation ~ 21431-21436
  midface reconstruction ~ 21154-21159
Left atrioventricular valve ~ see mitral valve
Left heart cardiac catheterization ~ see
  cardiac catheterization, left heart
Leg
  cast
    rigid total contact ~ 29445
  lower ~ see also ankle; fibula; knee; tibia
    abscess, incision and drainage ~ 27603
    amputation ~ 27598, 27880-27882
      revision ~ 27884-27886
    angiography ~ 73706
    artery, ligation ~ 37618
    biopsy ~ 27613-27614
    bursa, incision and drainage ~ 27604
    bypass graft ~ 35903
    cast ~ 29405-29435, 29450
    CAT scan ~ 73700-73706
    decompression ~ 27600-27602
    exploration, blood vessel ~ 35860
    fasciotomy ~ 27600-27602, 27892-27894
    hematoma, incision and drainage ~ 27603
    lesion, excision ~ 27630
    magnetic resonance imaging (MRI) ~
      73718-73720
    repair
      blood vessel ~ 35226
        with other graft ~ 35286
        with vein graft ~ 35256
      fascia ~ 27656
      tendon ~ 27658-27692
    splint ~ 29515
    strapping ~ 29580
    suture, tendon ~ 27658-27665
    tumor, excision ~ 27615-27619, 27632,
      27634
    unlisted services and procedures ~ 27899
    Unna boot ~ 29580
    X-ray ~ 73592
  upper ~ see femur
    abscess ~ 27301
    amputation ~ 27590-27592
      at hip ~ 27290-27295
      revision ~ 27594-27596
    angiography ~ 73706, 75635
    artery, ligation ~ 37618
    biopsy ~ 27323-27324
    bursa ~ 27301
    bypass graft ~ 35903
    cast ~ 29345-29355, 29365, 29450
    cast brace ~ 29358

Leg ~ *continued*
CT scan ~ 73700-73706, 75635
exploration, blood vessel ~ 35860
fasciotomy ~ 27305, 27496-27499,
27892-27894
halo application ~ 20663
hematoma ~ 27301
magnetic resonance imaging (MRI) ~
73718-73720
neurectomy ~ 27325-27326
removal
cast ~ 29705
foreign body ~ 27372
repair
blood vessel with other graft ~ 35286
blood vessel with vein graft ~ 35256
muscle ~ 27385-27386, 27400, 27430
tendon ~ 27393-27400
splint ~ 29505
strapping ~ 29580
suture, muscle ~ 27385-27386
tenotomy ~ 27306-27307, 27390-27392
tumor, excision ~ 27327-27329,
27337-27339, 27365
unlisted services and procedures ~ 27599
Unna boot ~ 29580
X-ray ~ 73592
wound exploration, penetrating ~ 20103
Legionella
antibody ~ 86713
antigen ~ 87277-87278, 87540-87542
**Legionella micdadei antigen detection,
immunofluorescence ~** 87277
**Legionella pneumophila antigen detection,
direct fluorescence ~** 87278
Leg length measurement X-ray ~ see
scanogram
Leiomyomata, removal ~ 58140, 58545-58546,
58561
Leishmania, antibody ~ 86717
Lengthening, tendon ~ see tendon, lengthening
Lens
extracapsular ~ 66940
intracapsular ~ 66920
dislocated ~ 66930
intraocular
exchange ~ 66986
reposition ~ 66825
prosthesis, insertion ~ 66983
manual or mechanical technique ~ 66982,
66984
not associated with concurrent cataract
removal ~ 66985
removal, lens material
aspiration technique ~ 66840
extracapsular ~ 66940
intracapsular ~ 66920-66930
pars plana approach ~ 66852
phacofragmentation technique ~ 66850

Lens material
aspiration technique ~ 66840
pars plana approach ~ 66852
phacofragmentation technique ~ 66850
Leptomeningioma ~ see meningioma
Leptospira, antibody ~ 86720
Leriche operation ~ (thoracolumbar
sympathectomy) 64809
Lesion ~ see tumor
anal
destruction ~ 46900-46917, 46924
excision ~ 45108, 46922
ankle, tendon sheath ~ 27630
arm, lower
tendon sheath
excision ~ 25110
auditory canal, external
excision
exostosis ~ 69140
radical with neck dissection ~ 69155
radical without neck dissection ~ 69150
soft tissue ~ 69145
bladder, destruction ~ 51030
brain
excision ~ 61534, 61536, 61600-61608,
61615-61616
radiation treatment ~ 77432
brainstem, excision ~ 61575-61576
breast, excision ~ 19120-19126
carotid body, excision ~ 60600-60605
chemotherapy ~ 96405-96406
destruction ~ 67220-67225
ciliary body, destruction ~ 66770
colon
destruction ~ 44393, 45383
excision ~ 44110-44111
conjunctiva
destruction ~ 68135
excision ~ 68110-68130
over 1cm ~ 68115
with adjacent sclera ~ 68130
expression ~ 68040
cornea
destruction ~ 65450
excision ~ 65400
of pterygium ~ 65420-65426
destruction, ureter ~ 52341-52342,
52344-52345, 52354
ear, middle, excision ~ 69540
epididymis, excision ~ 54830
esophagus
ablation ~ 43228
excision ~ 43100-43101
removal ~ 43216
excision ~ 59100
bladder ~ 52224
urethra ~ 52224, 53265
eye, excision ~ 65900

Lesion ~ *continued*
eyelid
destruction ~ 67850
excision
under anesthesia ~ 67808
without closure ~ 67840
multiple, different lids ~ 67805
multiple, same lid ~ 67801
single ~ 67800
facial, destruction ~ 17000-17004, 17280-17286
femur, excision ~ 27062
finger, tendon sheath ~ 26160
foot, excision ~ 28080, 28090
gums
destruction ~ 41850
excision ~ 41822-41828
hand tendon sheath ~ 26160
intestines, excision ~ 44110
intestines, small
destruction ~ 44369
excision ~ 44111
iris, destruction ~ 66770
larynx, excision ~ 31545-31546
leg, lower, tendon sheath ~ 27630
lymph node, incision and drainage ~ 38300-38305
mesentery, excision ~ 44820
mouth
destruction ~ 40820
excision ~ 40810-40816, 41116
vestibule
destruction ~ 40820
repair ~ 40830
nerve, excision ~ 64774-64792
nose, intranasal
external approach ~ 30118
internal approach ~ 30117
orbit, excision ~ 61333, 67412
palate
destruction ~ 42160
excision ~ 42104-42120
pancreas, excision ~ 48120
pelvis, destruction ~ 58662
penis
destruction
cryosurgery ~ 54056
electrodesiccation ~ 54055
extensive ~ 54065
laser surgery ~ 54057
simple ~ 54050-54060
surgical excision ~ 54060
excision ~ 54060
penile plaque ~ 54110-54112
pharynx
destruction ~ 42808
excision ~ 42808
rectum, excision ~ 45108
removal, larynx ~ 31512, 31578
resection ~ 52354

Lesion ~ *continued*
retina
destruction
extensive ~ 67227-67228
localized ~ 67208-67210
radiation by implantation of source ~ 67218
sclera, excision ~ 66130
skin
abrasion ~ 15786-15787
biopsy ~ 11100-11101
destruction
benign ~ 17000-17250
malignant ~ 17260-17286
by photodynamic therapy ~ 96567
excision
benign ~ 11400-11471
malignant ~ 11600-11646
injection ~ 11900-11901
paring or curettement ~ 11055-11057
shaving ~ 11300-11313
skin tags, removal ~ 11200-11201
skull, excision ~ 61500, 61600-61608, 61615-61616
spermatic cord, excision ~ 55520
spinal cord
destruction ~ 62280-62282
excision ~ 63265-63273
stomach, excision ~ 43611
testis, excision ~ 54512
toe, excision ~ 28092
tongue, excision ~ 41110-41114
uvula
destruction ~ 42145
excision ~ 42104-42107
vagina, destruction ~ 57061-57065
vulva
destruction
extensive ~ 56515
simple ~ 56501
wrist tendon, excision ~ 25110
Lesion of sciatic nerve ~ see sciatic nerve, lesion
Leucine aminopeptidase ~ 83670
Leukemia lymphoma virus I (one), adult T cell ~ see HTLV I (one)
Leukemia lymphoma virus II (two) antibodies, human T cell ~ see antibody, HTLV-II (two)
Leukemia lymphoma virus I (one) antibodies, human T cell ~ see antibody, HTLV I (one)
Leukemia virus II (two), hairy cell associated, human T cell ~ see HTLV II (two)
Leukoagglutinins ~ 86021
Leukocyte ~ see also white blood cell
alkaline phosphatase ~ 85540
antibody ~ 86021
count ~ 85032, 85048, 89055
histamine release test ~ 86343
phagocytosis ~ 86344
transfusion ~ 86950
Leu 2 antigens ~ see CD8
Levarterenol ~ see noradrenalin

Levator muscle rep ~ (blepharoptosis, repair) 67901-67909
Leveen shunt
  insertion ~ 49425
  patency test ~ 78291
  revision ~ 49426
Levulose ~ see fructose
LGV ~ (lymphogranuloma venereum) antibody 86729
LH ~ (luteinizing hormone) 80418, 80426, 83002
LHR ~ (leukocyte histamine release test) 86343
Lid suture ~ (blepharoptosis, repair) 67901-67909
Lidocaine, assay ~ 80176
Lift, face ~ see face lift
Ligament ~ see specific site
  collateral repair, knee with cruciate ligament ~ 27409
  dentate
    incision ~ 63180-63182
    section ~ 63180-63182
  injection ~ 20550
  release
    coracoacromial ~ 23415
    transverse carpal ~ 29848
  repair
    elbow ~ 24343-24346
    knee joint ~ 27405-27409
Ligation
  artery
    abdomen ~ 37617
    carotid ~ 37600-37606
    chest ~ 37616
    coronary ~ 33502
    coronary artery ~ 33502
    ethmoidal ~ 30915
    extremity ~ 37618
    fistula ~ 37607
    maxillary ~ 30920
    neck ~ 37615
    temporal ~ 37609
  esophageal varices ~ 43204, 43400
  fallopian tube, oviduct ~ 58600-58611, 58670
  gastroesophageal ~ 43405
  hemorrhoids ~ 46945-46946
  oviducts ~ 59100
  salivary duct ~ 42665
  shunt
    aorta, pulmonary ~ 33924
    peritoneal, venous ~ 49428
  thoracic duct ~ 38380
    abdominal approach ~ 38382
    thoracic approach ~ 38381
  vas deferens ~ 55450
  vein
    clusters ~ 37785
    esophagus ~ 43205, 43244, 43400
    femoral ~ 37650
    gastric ~ 43244
    iliac ~ 37660

Ligation ~ *continued*
  jugular, internal ~ 37565
  perforate ~ 37760-37761
  saphenous ~ 37700-37735, 37780
  vena cava ~ 37619
Ligature strangulation, skin tags ~ 11200-11201
Light coagulation ~ see photocoagulation
Light scattering measurement ~ see nephelometry
Light therapy, UV ~ see actinotherapy
Limb ~ see extremity
Limited lymphadenectomy for staging ~ see lymphadenectomy, limited, for staging
Limited neck dissection, with thyroidectomy ~ 60252
Limited resection mastectomies ~ see breast, excision, lesion
Lindholm operation ~ see tenoplasty
Lingual bone ~ see hyoid bone
Lingual frenectomy ~ see excision, tongue, frenum
Lingual nerve
  avulsion ~ 64740
  incision ~ 64740
  transection ~ 64740
Lingual tonsil ~ see tonsils, lingual
Linton procedure ~ 37760-37761
Lip
  biopsy ~ 40490
  excision ~ 40500-40530
    frenum ~ 40819
  incision, frenum ~ 40806
  reconstruction ~ 40525-40527
  repair ~ 40650-40654
    cleft lip ~ 40700-40761
    fistula ~ 42260
  unlisted services and procedures ~ 40799
Lip, cleft ~ see cleft lip
Lipase ~ 83690
Lipectomies, aspiration ~ see liposuction
Lipectomy ~ 15830-15839
  suction assisted ~ 15876-15879
Lipids, feces ~ 82705-82710
Lipo-lutin ~ see progesterone
Lipolysis, aspiration ~ see liposuction
Lipophosphodiesterase I (one) ~ see tissue typing
Lipoprotein
  (a) ~ 83695
  blood ~ 83695, 83700-83721
  LDL ~ 83700-83704-, 83721
  phospholipase A2 ~ 83698
Lipoprotein, alpha ~ see lipoprotein
Lipoprotein, pre-beta ~ see lipoprotein, blood
Liposuction ~ 15876-15879
Lisfranc operation ~ see amputation, foot; radical resection; replantation
Listeria monocytogenes, antibody ~ 86723
Lithium, assay ~ 80178
Litholapaxy ~ 52317-52318

1463

Lithotripsy ~ see extracorporeal shock wave
   therapy
   bile duct calculi (stone), endoscopy ~ 43265
   bladder ~ 52353
   kidney ~ 50590, 52353
   pancreatic duct calculi (stone), endoscopy ~
      43265
   ureter ~ 52353
   urethra ~ 52353
   with cystourethroscopy ~ 52353
Lithotrity ~ see litholapaxy
Liver ~ see hepatic duct
   ablation, tumor ~ 47380-47382
      laparoscopic ~ 47370-47371
   abscess
      aspiration ~ 47015
      incision and drainage
         open ~ 47010
         percutaneous ~ 47011
      injection ~ 47015
   aspiration ~ 47015
   biopsy ~ 47100
   cyst
      aspiration ~ 47015
      incision and drainage
         open ~ 47010
         percutaneous ~ 47011
   excision
      extensive ~ 47122
      partial ~ 47120, 47125-47130, 47140-47142
      total ~ 47133
   injection ~ 47015
      radiologic ~ 47505
      X-ray ~ 47500
   lobectomy ~ 47125-47130
      partial ~ 47120
   needle biopsy ~ 47000-47001
   nuclear medicine
      imaging ~ 78201-78216
      vascular flow ~ 78206
   repair
      abscess ~ 47300
      cyst ~ 47300
      wound ~ 47350-47362
   suture, wound ~ 47350-47362
   transplantation ~ 47135-47136
      allograft preparation ~ 47143-47147
   trisegmentectomy ~ 47122
   unlisted services and procedures ~ 47379,
      47399
Living activities, daily ~ see activities of daily
   living
Lobectomy
   brain ~ 61323, 61537-61540
   contralateral subtotal, thyroid gland ~ 60212,
      60225
   liver ~ 47120-47130
   lung ~ 32480-32482
      sleeve ~ 32486
   parotid gland ~ 42410-42415
   segmental ~ 32663

Lobectomy ~ *continued*
   sleeve ~ 32486
   temporal lobe ~ 61537-61538
   thyroid gland partial ~ 60210-60212
   total ~ 60220-60225
   total ~ 32663
Lobotomy, frontal ~ 61490
Localization of nodule, radiographic, breast ~
   77032
Local excision mastectomies ~ see breast,
   excision, lesion
Local excision of lesion or tissue of femur ~
   see excision, lesion, femur
Log hydrogen ion concentration ~ see pH
Lombard test ~ see audiologic function test
Long term care facility visits ~ see nursing
   facility services
Longmire operation ~ (anastomosis, hepatic
   duct to intestines) 47765
Long acting thyroid stimulator ~ see
   thyrotropin releasing hormone (TRH)
Loopogram ~ see urography, antegrade
Loose body
   removal
      ankle ~ 27620
      carpometacarpal joint ~ 26070
      elbow ~ 24101
      interphalangeal joint ~ 28020
         toe ~ 28024
      knee joint ~ 27331
      metatarsophalangeal joint ~ 28022
      tarsometatarsal joint ~ 28020
         toe ~ 28022
      wrist ~ 25101
Lord procedure ~ (anal sphincter dilation)
   45905
Louis Bar syndrome ~ see ataxia telangiectasia
Low birth weight intensive care services ~
   99478-99480
Low density lipoprotein ~ see lipoprotein,
   LDL
Low frequency ultrasound ~ 0183T
Low vision aids ~ see spectacle services
   fitting ~ 92354-92355
   supply ~ 92392
Lower extremities ~ see extremity, lower
Lower GI series ~ see barium enema
LRH ~ (luteinizing releasing hormone) 83727
LSD ~ (lysergic acid diethylamide)
   80100-80103, 80299
LTH ~ see prolactin
Lumbar ~ see spine
   aspiration, disk, percutaneous ~ 62287
Lumbar plexus
   decompression ~ 64714
   injection, anesthetic ~ 64449
   neuroplasty ~ 64714
   release ~ 64714
   repair/suture ~ 64862
Lumbar puncture ~ see spinal tap
Lumbar spine fracture ~ see fracture, vertebra,
   lumbar

Lumbar sympathectomy ~ see sympathectomy, lumbar
Lumbar vertebra ~ see vertebra, lumbar
Lumen dilation ~ 74360
Lumpectomy ~ 19301-19302
Lunate
  arthroplasty, with implant ~ 25444
  dislocation
    closed treatment ~ 25690
    open treatment ~ 25695
Lung
  abscess
    incision and drainage
      open ~ 32200
      percutaneous ~ 32200-32201
  aspiration ~ 32405
  biopsy ~ 32096-32097
  bullae
    excision ~ 32141
      endoscopic ~ 32655
  cyst
    incision and drainage
      open ~ 32200
    removal ~ 32140
  decortication
    endoscopic ~ 32651-32652
    partial ~ 32225
    total ~ 32220
    with parietal pleurectomy ~ 32320
  empyema, excision ~ 32540
  excision ~ 32440-32445
    bronchus resection ~ 32486
    completion ~ 32488
    donor
      heart-lung ~ 33930
      lung ~ 32850
    empyema ~ 32540
    lobe ~ 32480-32482
    segment ~ 32484
    tumor ~ 32503-32504
  foreign body, removal ~ 32151
  hemorrhage ~ 32110
  lavage
    bronchial ~ 31624
    total ~ 32997
  lysis, adhesions ~ 32124
  needle biopsy ~ 32405
  nuclear medicine
    imaging, perfusion ~ 78580, 78597, 78598
    imaging, ventilation ~ 78579, 78582, 78598
    unlisted services and procedures ~ 78599
  pneumocentesis ~ 32405
  pneumolysis ~ 32940
  pneumothorax ~ 32960
  puncture ~ 32405
  removal ~ 32440-32445
    bilobectomy ~ thoracoscopic ~ 32670
    bronchial valve ~ 31648-31649
    bronchoplasty ~ 32501
    completion pneumonectomy ~ 32488
    extrapleural ~ 32445

Lung ~ *continued*
  pneumonectomy 32440-32445
    thoracoscopic ~ 32671
    segmentectomy, thoracoscopic ~ 32669
    single lobe ~ 32480
    single segment ~ 32484
    sleeve lobectomy ~ 32486
    sleeve pneumonectomy ~ 32442
    two lobes ~ 32482
    volume reduction ~ 32491
  repair, hernia ~ 32800
  segmentectomy ~ 32484
  tear, repair ~ 32110
  thoracotomy
    biopsy ~ 32096-32097
    cardiac massage ~ 32160
    for post-op complications ~ 32120
    removal
      bullae ~ 32141
      cyst ~ 32140
      intrapleural foreign body ~ 32150
      intrapulmonary foreign body ~ 32151
      repair ~ 32110
  transplantation ~ 32851-32854, 33935
    allograft preparation ~ 32855-32856, 33933
    donor pneumonectomy
      heart-lung ~ 33930
      lung ~ 32850
  unlisted services and procedures ~ 32999
Lung function tests ~ see pulmonology, diagnostic
Lung volume reduction, emphysematous ~ 32491
Lupus anticoagulant assay ~ 85705
Lupus band test ~ see immunofluorescent study
Luteinizing hormone (LH) ~ 80418, 80426, 83002
Luteinizing releasing factor ~ 83727
Luteotropic hormone ~ see prolactin
Luteotropin ~ see prolactin
Luteotropin, placental ~ see lactogen, human placental
Lyme disease ~ 86617-86618
Lyme disease ab ~ see antibody, Lyme disease
Lyme disease vaccine ~ see vaccination
Lymph duct, injection ~ 38790
Lymph nodes
  abscess, incision and drainage ~ 38300-38305
  biopsy ~ 38500, 38510-38530, 38570
    needle ~ 38505
  dissection ~ 38542
  excision ~ 38500, 38510-38530
    abdominal ~ 38747
    inguinofemoral ~ 38760-38765
    laparoscopic ~ 38571-38572
    limited, for staging
      para-aortic ~ 38562
      pelvic ~ 38562
      retroperitoneal ~ 38564
    pelvic ~ 38770

Lymph nodes ~ *continued*
  radical
    axillary ~ 38740-38745
    cervical ~ 38720-38724
    suprahyoid ~ 38720-38724
    retroperitoneal transabdominal ~ 38780
    thoracic ~ 38746
  exploration ~ 38542
  hygroma, cystic
    axillary/cervical excision ~ 38550-38555
  nuclear medicine, imaging ~ 78195
  removal
    abdominal ~ 38747
    inguinofemoral ~ 38760-38765
    pelvic ~ 38770
    retroperitoneal transabdominal ~ 38780
    thoracic ~ 38746
  sentinel, mapping ~ 38900
Lymph vessels
  abdomen, lymphangiography ~ 75805-75807
  arm, lymphangiography ~ 75801-75803
  leg, lymphangiography ~ 75801-75803
  nuclear medicine, imaging ~ 78195
  pelvis, lymphangiography ~ 75805-75807
Lymphadenectomy
  abdominal ~ 38747
  bilateral inguinofemoral ~ 54130, 56632,
    56637
  bilateral pelvic ~ 51575, 51585, 51595, 54135,
    55845, 55865
    total ~ 38571-38572, 57531, 58210
  diaphragmatic assessment ~ 58960
  gastric ~ 38747
  inguinofemoral ~ 38760-38765
  inguinofemoral, iliac and pelvic ~ 56640
  injection, sentinel node ~ 38792
  limited para-aortic, resection of ovarian
    malignancy ~ 58951, 58954
  limited pelvic ~ 55842, 55862, 58954
  limited, for staging
    para-aortic ~ 38562
    pelvic ~ 38562
    retroperitoneal ~ 38564
  mediastinal ~ 21632
  para-aortic ~ 58958
  pelvic ~ 58958
  peripancreatic ~ 38747
  portal ~ 38747
  radical
    axillary ~ 38740-38745
    cervical ~ 38720-38724
    pelvic ~ 54135, 55845, 58548
    suprahyoid ~ 38700
  regional ~ 50230
  retroperitoneal transabdominal ~ 38780
  thoracic ~ 38746
  unilateral inguinofemoral ~ 56631, 56634
Lymphadenitis, incision and drainage ~
  38300-38305
Lymphadenopathy associated antibodies ~ see
  antibody, HIV
Lymphadenopathy associated virus ~ see HIV

Lymphangiogram, abdominal ~ see
  lymphangiography, abdomen
Lymphangiography
  abdomen ~ 75805-75807
  arm ~ 75801-75803
  injection ~ 38790
  leg ~ 75801-75803
  pelvis ~ 75805-75807
Lymphangioma, cystic ~ see hygroma
Lymphangiotomy ~ 38308
Lymphatic channels, incision ~ 38308
Lymphatic cyst ~ see lymphocele
Lymphatic system, unlisted procedure ~
  38999
Lymphatics ~ see specific procedure
Lymphoblast transformation ~ see
  blastogenesis
Lymphocele
  drainage, laparoscopic ~ 49323
  extraperitoneal, open drainage ~ 49062
Lymphocoele ~ see lymphocele
Lymphocyte
  culture ~ 86821-86822
  toxicity assay ~ 86805-86806
  transformation ~ 86353
Lymphocyte, thymus-dependent ~ see T cells
Lymphocytes, CD4 ~ see CD4
Lymphocytes, CD8 ~ see CD8
Lymphocytic choriomeningitis, antibody ~
  86727
Lymphocytotoxicity ~ 86805-86806
Lymphogranuloma venereum, antibody ~
  86729
Lymphoma virus, Burkitt ~ see Epstein-Barr
  virus
Lynch procedure ~ 31075
Lysergic acid diethylamide ~ 80102-80103,
  80299
Lysergide ~ see lysergic acid diethylamide
Lysis
  adhesions
    epidural ~ 62263-62264
    fallopian tube ~ 58740
    foreskin ~ 54450
    intestinal ~ 44005
    labial ~ 56441
    lung ~ 32124
    nose ~ 30560
    ovary ~ 58740
    oviduct ~ 58740
    penile, post-circumcision ~ 54162
    ureter ~ 50715-50725
    urethra ~ 53500
    uterus ~ 58559
  euglobulin ~ 85360
  labial, adhesions ~ 56441
  nose, intranasal synechia ~ 30560
Lysozyme ~ 85549

M

Macewen operation ~ see hernia, repair, inguinal
Machado test ~ (complement, fixation test) 86171
Maclean-De Wesselow test ~ see blood urea nitrogen; urea nitrogen, clearance
Macrodactylia, repair ~ 26590
Madlener operation ~ (tubal ligation) 58600
Magnesium ~ 83735
Magnet operation ~ see eye, removal of foreign body
Magnetic resonance, unlisted services and procedures ~ 76498
Magnetic resonance angiography (MRA)
  abdomen ~ 74185
  arm ~ 73225
  chest ~ 71555
  head ~ 70544-70546
  leg ~ 73725
  neck ~ 70547-70549
  pelvis ~ 72198
  spine ~ 72159
Magnetic resonance imaging (MRI)
  abdomen ~ 74181-74183
  ankle ~ 73721-73723
  arm ~ 73218-73220, 73223
  bone marrow study ~ 77084
  brain ~ 70551-70555
    intraoperative ~ 70557-70559
  breast ~ 77058-77059
  chest ~ 71550-71552
  elbow ~ 73221
  face ~ 70540-70543
  finger joint ~ 73221
  foot ~ 73718-73719
  foot joints ~ 73721-73723
  guidance
    needle placement ~ 77021
    parenchymal tissue ablation ~ 77022
    visceral tissue ablation ~ 76394
  hand ~ 73218-73220, 73223
  heart ~ 75557-75565
  joint
    lower extremity ~ 73721-73723
    upper extremity ~ 73221-73223
  knee ~ 73721-73723
  leg ~ 73718-73720
  neck ~ 70540-70543
  orbit ~ 70540-70543
  pelvis ~ 72195-72197
  radiology, diagnostic, procedures ~ 76499
  spectroscopy ~ 76390
  spine
    cervical ~ 72141-72142, 72156-72158
    lumbar ~ 72148-72158
    thoracic ~ 72146-72147, 72156-72158

Magnetic resonance imaging (MRI) ~ continued
  temporomandibular joint (TMJ) ~ 70336
  toe ~ 73721-73723
  wrist ~ 73221
Magnetic resonance spectroscopy ~ 76390
Magnetic stimulation, transcranial ~ 90867-90868
Magnetoencephalography (MEG) ~ 95965-95967
Magnuson procedure ~ 23450
Magpi operation ~ (hypospadias, repair) 54322
Major vestibular gland ~ see Bartholin's gland
Malar area
  augmentation ~ 21270
  bone graft ~ 21210
  fracture
    with bone graft ~ 21366
    with manipulation ~ 21355
    open treatment ~ 21360-21366
  reconstruction ~ 21270
Malar bone ~ see cheekbone
Malaria antibody ~ 86750
Malaria smear ~ 87207
Malate dehydrogenase ~ 83775
Maldescent, testis ~ see testis, undescended
Male circumcision ~ see circumcision
Male genital system, surgical procedures ~ 54000-55899
Malformation, arteriovenous ~ see arteriovenous malformation
Malic dehydrogenase ~ (malate dehydrogenase) 83775
Malleolus ~ see ankle; fibula; leg, lower; tibia; tibiofibular joint
  metatarsophalangeal joint ~ 27889
Mallet finger repair ~ 26432
Maltose, tolerance test ~ 82951-82952
Malunion repair
  femur
    with graft ~ 27472
    without graft ~ 27470
  metatarsal ~ 28322
  tarsal joint ~ 28320
Mammalian oviduct ~ see fallopian tube
Mammaplasties ~ see breast, reconstruction
Mammary abscess ~ see abscess, breast
Mammary arteries ~ see artery, mammary
Mammary duct
  X-ray with contrast ~ 77053-77054
Mammary ductogram, injection ~ 19030
Mammary stimulating hormone ~ see prolactin
Mammilliplasty ~ see nipples, reconstruction
Mammogram, breast, localization nodule ~ 77032
Mammography ~ 77055-77057
  screening ~ 77057
  with computer-aided detection ~ 77051-77052
Mammoplasty
  augmentation ~ 19324-19325
  reduction ~ 19318

1467

Mammotomy ~ see mastotomy
Mammotropic hormone, pituitary ~ see prolactin
Mammotropic hormone, placental ~ see lactogen, human placental
Mammotropin ~ see prolactin
Mandated services, on call services ~ 99027
Mandible ~ see facial bones; maxilla; temporomandibular joint (TMJ)
 abscess, excision ~ 21025
 bone graft ~ 21215
 cyst, excision ~ 21040, 21046-21047
 fracture
  closed treatment
   with interdental fixation ~ 21453
   with manipulation ~ 21451
   without manipulation ~ 21450
  open treatment ~ 21454-21470
   external fixation ~ 21454
   with interdental fixation ~ 21462
   without interdental fixation ~ 21461
  percutaneous treatment ~ 21452
 osteotomy ~ 21198-21199
 reconstruction, with implant ~ 21244-21246, 21248-21249
 removal, foreign body ~ 41806
 torus mandibularis, excision ~ 21031
 tumor, excision ~ 21040-21047
 X-ray ~ 70100-70110
Mandibular body
 augmentation
  with bone graft ~ 21127
  with prosthesis ~ 21125
Mandibular condyle, fracture, open treatment ~ 21465
 reconstruction ~ 21247
Mandibular condylectomy ~ see condylectomy
Mandibular fracture ~ see fracture, mandible
Mandibular rami
 reconstruction
  with bone graft ~ 21194
  without bone graft ~ 21193
  with internal rigid fixation ~ 21196
  without internal rigid fixation ~ 21195
Mandibular resection prosthesis ~ 21081
Mandibular staple bone plate, reconstruction, mandible ~ 21244
Manganese ~ 83785
Manipulation
 chest wall ~ 94667-94668
 chiropractic ~ 98940-98943
 dislocation and/or fracture ~ 25535
  acetabulum ~ 27222
  acromioclavicular ~ 23545
  ankle ~ 27810, 27818, 27860
  carpometacarpal ~ 26670-26676
  clavicular ~ 23505
  elbow ~ 24300, 24640
  femoral ~ 27232, 27502, 27510, 27517
   pertrochanteric ~ 27240
  fibula ~ 27781, 27788

Manipulation ~ continued
 finger ~ 26725-26727, 26742, 26755
 greater tuberosity, humeral ~ 23625
 hand ~ 26670-26676
 heel ~ 28405-28406
 hip ~ 27257
 hip socket ~ 27222
 humeral ~ 23605, 24505, 24535, 24577
  epicondyle ~ 24565
 hyoid ~ 21494
 intercarpal ~ 25660
 interphalangeal joint ~ 26340, 26770-26776
 larynx ~ 31586
 lunate ~ 25690
 malar area ~ 21355
 mandibular ~ 21451
 metacarpal ~ 26605-26607
 metacarpophalangeal ~ 26700-26706, 26742
 metacarpophlangeal joint ~ 26340
 metatarsal ~ 28475-28476
 nasal bone ~ 21315-21320
 orbit ~ 21401
 phalangeal shaft ~ 26727
  distal, finger or thumb ~ 26755
  phalanges, finger/thumb ~ 26725
 phalanges
  finger ~ 26742, 26755, 26770-26776
  finger/thumb ~ 26727
  great toe ~ 28495-28496
  toes ~ 28515
 radial ~ 24655, 25565
 radial shaft ~ 25505
 radiocarpal ~ 25660
 radioulnar ~ 25675
 scapular ~ 23575
 shoulder ~ 23650-23655
  with greater tuberosity ~ 23665
 shoulder dislocation sternoclavicular ~ 23525
  with surgical or anatomical neck fracture ~ 23675
 talus ~ 28435-28436
 tarsal ~ 28455-28456
 thumb ~ 26641-26650
 tibial ~ 27532, 27752
 trans-scaphoperilunar ~ 25680
 ulnar ~ 24675, 25535, 25565
 vertebral ~ 22315
 wrist ~ 25259, 25624, 25635, 25660, 25675, 25680, 25690
 foreskin ~ 54450
 globe ~ 92018-92019
 hip ~ 27275
 interphalangeal joint, proximal ~ 26742
 knee ~ 27570
 osteopathic ~ 98925-98929
 shoulder, application of fixation apparatus ~ 23700
 spine, with anesthesia ~ 22505
 tibial, distal ~ 27762

Manometric studies
kidney, pressure ~ 50396
rectum/anus ~ 91122
ureter, pressure ~ 50686
ureterostomy ~ 50686
Manometry, rectum ~ 90911
Mantoux test ~ (TB skin test) 86580
Manual therapy ~ 97140
Maquet procedure ~ 27418
Marcellation operation ~ (vaginal
hysterectomy) 58260-58270, 58550
Marrow, bone ~ see bone marrow
Marshall-Marchetti-Krantz procedure ~
51840-51841, 58152, 58267, 58293
Marsupialization ~ 10040
Bartholin's gland cyst ~ 56440
cyst, sublingual salivary ~ 42409
liver, cyst or abscess ~ 47300
pancreatic cyst ~ 48500
urethral diverticulum ~ 53240
Mass, kidney, ablation ~ 50542
Massage, cardiac ~ 32160
therapy ~ 97124
Masseter muscle/bone, reduction ~
21295-21296
**Mass spectrometry and tandem mass
spectrometry**
analyte
qualitative ~ 83788
quantitative ~ 83789
Mastectomy
gynecomastia ~ 19300
modified radical ~ 19307
partial ~ 19301-19302
radical ~ 19305-19306
simple, complete ~ 19303
subcutaneous ~ 19304
Mastectomy, Halsted ~ see radical mastectomy
Mastoid
excision
complete ~ 69502
radical ~ 69511
modified ~ 69505
petrous apicectomy ~ 69530
simple ~ 69501
obliteration ~ 69670
repair
with apicectomy ~ 69605
by excision ~ 69601-69603
fistula ~ 69700
with tympanoplasty ~ 69604
Mastoid cavity, debridement ~ 69220-69222
Mastoidectomy
cochlear device implantation ~ 69930
complete ~ 69502
revision ~ 69601
ossicular chain reconstruction ~ 69605
radical ~ 69511
modified ~ 69505
revision ~ 69602-69603
simple ~ 69501

Mastoidectomy ~ *continued*
with apicectomy ~ 69605
with labyrinthectomy ~ 69910
with petrous apicectomy ~ 69530
with skull base surgery ~ 61590, 61597
decompression ~ 61595
facial nerve ~ 61595
with tympanoplasty ~ 69604, 69641-69646
Mastoidotomy ~ 69635-69637
with tympanoplasty ~ 69635
ossicular chain reconstruction ~ 69636
and synthetic prosthesis ~ 69636
Mastoids
polytomography ~ 76101-76102
X-ray ~ 70120-70130
Mastopexy ~ 19316
Mastotomy ~ 19020
Maternity care and delivery ~ see abortion;
cesarean delivery; ectopic pregnancy;
obstetrical care
Maxilla ~ see facial bones; mandible
bone graft ~ 21210
CT scan ~ 70486-70488
cyst, excision ~ 21048-21049
excision ~ 21030, 21032-21034
fracture
closed treatment ~ 21345, 21421
open treatment ~ 21346-21348, 21422-21423
with fixation ~ 21345-21347
osteotomy ~ 21206
reconstruction, with implant ~ 21245-21246,
21248-21249
tumor, excision ~ 21048-21049
Maxillary arteries ~ see artery, maxillary
Maxillary sinus ~ see sinus, maxillary
Maxillary torus palatinus, tumor excision ~
21032
Maxillectomy ~ 31225-31230
**Maxillofacial fixation, application, halo type
appliance** ~ 21100
Maxillofacial impressions
auricular prosthesis ~ 21086
definitive obturator prosthesis ~ 21080
facial prosthesis ~ 21088
interim obturator prosthesis ~ 21079
mandibular resection prosthesis ~ 21081
nasal prosthesis ~ 21087
oral surgical splint ~ 21085
orbital prosthesis ~ 21077
palatal augmentation prosthesis ~ 21082
palatal lift prosthesis ~ 21083
speech aid prosthesis ~ 21084
surgical obturator prosthesis ~ 21076
**Maxillofacial procedures, unlisted services
and procedures** ~ 21299
Maxillofacial prosthesis ~ 21076-21089
unlisted services and procedures ~ 21089
Maydl operation ~ (colostomy) 45563, 50810
Mayo hernia repair ~ 49580-49587
Mayo operation ~ (varicose vein removal)
37700-37735, 37780, 37785
Mayo procedure ~ 28292

1469

MBC ~ (minimum bactericidal concentration) 87181-87190
McBride procedure ~ 28292
McBurney operation ~ (see also hernia, repair, inguinal) 49495-49500, 49505
McCannel procedure ~ 66682
McDonald operation ~ (repair, cervix, cerclage, abdominal; revision) 57700
McIndoe procedure ~ (vagina, construction) 57291
McKissock surgery ~ (breast, reduction) 19318
McVay operation ~ (hernia, repair, inguinal) 49495-49500, 49505
Measles, German ~ see rubella
Measles uncomplicated ~ see rubeola
Measles vaccine ~ see vaccines
Meat fibers, feces ~ 89160
Meatoplasty ~ 69310
Meatotomy ~ 53020-53025
  contact laser vaporization with/without transurethral resection of prostate ~ 52648
  with cystourethroscopy ~ 52281
  infant ~ 53025
  non-contact laser coagulation prostate ~ 52647
  transurethral electrosurgical resection, prostate ~ 52601
  ureter ~ 52290
  ureteral, cystourethroscopy ~ 52290-52305
Meckel's diverticulum, excision ~ 44800
  unlisted services and procedures ~ 44899
Median nerve
  decompression ~ 64721
  neuroplasty ~ 64721
  release ~ 64721
  repair/suture, motor ~ 64835
  transposition ~ 64721
Median nerve compression ~ see carpal tunnel syndrome
Mediastinal cyst ~ see cyst, mediastinal
Mediastinoscopy ~ 39400
Mediastinotomy
  cervical approach ~ 39000
  transthoracic approach ~ 39010
Mediastinum ~ see chest; thorax
  cyst, excision ~ 32662, 39200
  endoscopy
    biopsy ~ 39400
    exploration ~ 39400
  exploration ~ 39000-39010
  incision and drainage ~ 39000-39010
  needle biopsy ~ 32405
  removal, foreign body ~ 39000-39010
  tumor, excision ~ 32662, 39220
  unlisted procedures ~ 39499
Mediastinum and diaphragm, surgical procedures ~ 39000-39599
Medical disability evaluation services ~ 99455-99456
Medical genetics ~ 96040
Medical nutrition therapy ~ 97802-97804
Medical testimony ~ 99075

Medication management therapy ~ 99605-99607
Medicine, preventive ~ see preventive medicine
Medicine, pulmonary ~ see pulmonology
Medicine services ~ 90281-99602
Medulla, tractotomy ~ 61470
Medullary tract
  incision ~ 61470
  section ~ 61470
Meibomian cyst ~ see chalazion
Membrane, mucous ~ see mucosa
Membrane, tympanic ~ see ear, drum
Membrane oxygenation, extracorporeal ~ see extracorporeal membrane oxygenation
Meninges, tumor, excision ~ 61512, 61519
Meningioma, excision ~ 61512, 61519
  tumor, excision ~ 61512, 61519
Meningitis, lymphocytic benign ~ see lymphocytic choriomeningitis
Meningocele repair ~ 63700-63702
Meningococcal vaccine ~ see vaccines
Meningococcus ~ see neisseria meningitidis
Meningomyelocele ~ see myelomeningocele
Meniscectomy
  knee joint ~ 27332-27333
  temporomandibular joint ~ 21060
Meniscus
  knee
    excision ~ 27332-27333
    repair ~ 27403
    transplantation ~ 29868
Mental nerve
  avulsion ~ 64736
  incision ~ 64736
  transection ~ 64736
Meprobamate ~ 83805
Mercury ~ 83015, 83825
Merskey test ~ see fibrin degradation products
Mesencephalic tract
  incision ~ 61480
  section ~ 61480
Mesencephalon, tractotomy ~ 61480
Mesenteric arteries ~ see artery, mesenteric
Mesentery
  lesion, excision ~ 44820
  repair ~ 44850
  suture ~ 44850
  unlisted services and procedures ~ 44899
Mesh
  implantation, hernia ~ 49568
  insertion, pelvic floor ~ 57267
  removal, abdominal infected ~ 11008
Metabisulfite test ~ (red blood cell (RBC), sickling) 85660
Metabolite ~ 82520
  thromboxane ~ 84431
Metacarpal
  amputation ~ 26910
  craterization ~ 26230
  cyst, excision ~ 26200-26205
  diaphysectomy ~ 26230

Metacarpal ~ *continued*
  fracture
    closed treatment ~ 26605
      with fixation ~ 26607
    open treatment ~ 26615
    percutaneous fixation ~ 26608
    with manipulation ~ 26605-26607
    without manipulation ~ 26600
  ostectomy ~ 26250
  repair
    lengthening ~ 26568
    nonunion ~ 26546
    osteotomy ~ 26565
  saucerization ~ 26230
  tumor
    excision ~ 26200-26205
    radical resection ~ 26250
Metacarpophalangeal joint
  arthrodesis ~ 26850-26852
  arthroplasty ~ 26530-26531
  arthroscopy
    diagnostic ~ 29900
    surgical ~ 29901-29902
  arthrotomy ~ 26075
  biopsy, synovium ~ 26105
  capsule
    excision ~ 26520
    incision ~ 26520
  capsulodesis ~ 26516-26518
  dislocation
    closed treatment ~ 26700
    open treatment ~ 26715
    percutaneous fixation ~ 26705-26706
    with manipulation ~ 26340
  exploration ~ 26075
  fracture
    closed treatment ~ 26740
    open treatment ~ 26746
    with manipulation ~ 26742
  fusion ~ 26516-26518, 26850-26852
  removal of foreign body ~ 26075
  repair, collateral ligament ~ 26540-26542
  synovectomy ~ 26135
Metadrenaline ~ see metanephrines
Metals, heavy ~ see heavy metal
Metamfetamine ~ see methamphetamine
Metanephrines ~ 83835
Metatarsal ~ see foot
  amputation ~ 28810
  condyle, excision ~ 28288
  craterization ~ 28122
  cyst, excision ~ 28104-28107
  diaphysectomy ~ 28122
  excision ~ 28110-28114, 28122, 28140
  fracture
    closed treatment
      with manipulation ~ 28475-28476
      without manipulation ~ 28470
    open treatment ~ 28485
    percutaneous fixation ~ 28476

Metatarsal ~ *continued*
  free osteocutaneous flap with microvascular
    anastomosis ~ 20972
  repair ~ 28322
    lengthening ~ 28306-28307
    osteotomy ~ 28306-28309
  saucerization ~ 28122
  tumor, excision ~ 28104-28107, 28173
Metatarsectomy ~ 28140
Metatarsophalangeal joint
  arthrotomy ~ 28022, 28052
  cheilectomy ~ 28289
  dislocation ~ 28630-28635, 28645
    percutaneous fixation ~ 28636
  exploration ~ 28022
  great toe
    arthrodesis ~ 28750
    fusion ~ 28750
  removal
    of foreign body ~ 28022
    of loose body ~ 28022
  repair, hallux rigidus ~ 28289
  synovial
    biopsy ~ 28052
    excision ~ 28072
  toe ~ 28270
Methadone ~ 83840
Methaemoglobin ~ see methemoglobin
Methamphetamine, blood or urine ~ 82145
Methanol ~ 84600
Methbipyranone ~ see metyrapone
Methemalbumin ~ 83857
Methemoglobin ~ 83045-83050, 88741
Methenamine silver stain ~ 88312
Methopyrapone ~ see metyrapone
Methoxyhydroxymandelic acid ~ see
  vanillylmandelic acid
Methsuximide ~ 83858
Methylamphetamine ~ see methamphetamine
Methylene bichloride ~ see dichloromethane
Methylfluorprednisolone ~ see dexamethasone
Methylmorphine ~ see codeine
Methyl alcohol ~ (methanol) 84600
Metroplasty ~ see hysteroplasty
Metyrapone ~ 80436
MIC ~ (minimum inhibitory concentration)
  87186
Micro-ophthalmia, orbit reconstruction ~
  21256
Microalbumin, urine ~ 82043-82044
Microbiology ~ 0023T, 87001-87999
Microdissection ~ 88380-88381
Microfluorometries, flow ~ see flow cytometry
Microdissection ~ 88380
Microglobulin, beta 2
  blood ~ 82232
  urine ~ 82232
Micrographic surgery, Mohs technique ~
  17311-17315
Micropigmentation, correction ~ 11920-11922
Microscope, surgical ~ see operating
  microscope

1471

Microscopic evaluation, hair ~ 96902
Microscopies, electron ~ see electron microscopy
Microscopy, ear exam ~ 92504
Microsomal antibody ~ 86376
Microsomia, hemifacial ~ see hemifacial microsomia
Microsurgery, operating microscope ~ 69990
Microvascular anastomosis
  bone graft
    fibula ~ 20955
    other ~ 20962
  fascial flap, free ~ 15758
  muscle flap, free ~ 15756
  osteocutaneous flap with, ~ 20969-20973
  skin flap, free ~ 15757
Microvite A ~ see vitamin A
Microwave therapy ~ (see also physical medicine/therapy/occupational therapy) 97020
Midbrain ~ see brain; brainstem; mesencephalon; skull base surgery
Midcarpal medioccipital joint, arthrotomy ~ 25040
Middle cerebral artery velocimetry ~ 76821
Middle ear ~ see ear, middle
Midface
  reconstruction
    with bone graft ~ 21145-21160, 21188
    without bone graft ~ 21141-21143
    forehead advancement ~ 21159-21160
Migration inhibitory factor (MIF) ~ 86378
Mile operation ~ see colectomy, total, with proctectomy
Milia, multiple, removal ~ 10040
Miller procedure ~ 28737
Miller-Abbott intubation ~ 44500, 74340
Minerva cast ~ 29035
  removal ~ 29710
Minimum inhibitory concentration (MIC) ~ 87186
Minimum lethal concentration ~ 87187
Minnesota multiphasic personality inventory ~ see MMPI
Miscarriage
  incomplete abortion ~ 59812
  missed abortion
    first trimester ~ 59820
    second trimester ~ 59821
  septic abortion ~ 59830
Missed abortion ~ see abortion; miscarriage, missed abortion
Mitchell procedure ~ 28296
Mitogen blastogenesis ~ 86353
Mitral valve
  incision ~ 33420-33422
  repair ~ 33420-33427
    incision ~ 33420-33422
  replacement ~ 33430
Mitrofanoff operation ~ (appendico-vesicostomy) 50845
Miyagawanella ~ see Chlamydia

MMPI ~ (Minnesota multiphasic personality inventory) 96100
MMR shots ~ (measles, mumps and rubella vaccines) 90707
Mobilization
  splenic flexure ~ 44139
  stapes ~ 69650
Modified radical mastectomy ~ see mastectomy, modified radical
Mohs micrographic surgery ~ 17311-17315
Molar pregnancy ~ see hydatidiform mole
Mold, culture ~ 87107
Mole, carneous ~ see abortion
Mole, hydatid ~ see hydatidiform mole
Molecular cytogenetics ~ 88271-88275
  interpretation and report ~ 88291
Molecular diagnostics
  reverse transcription and amplified probe
    enterovirus ~ 87498
    hepatitis C ~ 87521
    HIV-1 ~ 87535
    HIV-2 ~ 87538
  reverse transcription and quantification
    hepatitis C ~ 87522
    HIV-1 ~ 87536
    HIV-2 ~ 87539
Molecular oxygen saturation ~ see oxygen saturation
Molecular pathology
  ~ (see also Gene analysis) 81200-81383, 81400-81408
Molluscum contagiosum
  destruction ~ 17110-17111, 46900, 46910, 46916-46917, 54050-54065
  excision
    anus ~ 46922
    penis ~ 54060
Molteno procedure ~ 66180
Monilia ~ see candida
Monitoring
  blood pressure, 24 hour ~ 93784-93790
  electrocardiogram ~ (see also electrocardiography) 93224-93229
  electroencephalogram ~ 95812-95813, 95950-95953, 95956
    with drug activation ~ 95954
    with physical activation ~ 95954
    with WADA activation ~ 95958
  fetal
    during labor ~ 59050-59051, 99500
    interpretation only ~ 59051
  glucose, interstitial fluid ~ 95250
  interstitial fluid pressure ~ 20950
  pediatric apnea ~ 94774-94777
  seizure ~ 61531, 61760
Monitoring, sleep ~ see polysomnography
Monoethylene glycol ~ see ethylene glycol
Mononuclear cell antigen ~ 86356
Mononucleosis virus, infectious ~ see Epstein-Barr virus

Monophosphate
adenosine ~ (adenosine monophosphate (AMP)) 82030
adenosine cyclic ~ (cyclic AMP) 82030
guanosine ~ (guanosine monophosphate (GMP)) 83008
guanosine cyclic ~ (cyclic GMP) 83008
Monospot test ~ (rapid test for infection) 86308
Monoxide, carbon ~ see carbon monoxide
Monteggia fracture ~ 24620-24635
Monticelli procedure ~ (application, bone fixation device) 20690, 20692
Morbilli ~ see rubeola
Morphine methyl ether ~ see codeine
Morphometric analysis
nerve ~ 88356
skeletal muscle ~ 88355
tumor ~ 88358-88361, 88367-88368
Morton's neuroma, excision ~ 28080
Moschcowitz operation ~ see repair, hernia, femoral; revision
Mosenthal test ~ (urinalysis, routine) 81002
Mother cell ~ see stem cell
Motility study, esophagus ~ 91010
Motion analysis
by video and 3-D kinematics ~ 96000, 96004
computer-based ~ 96000, 96004
Mouth
abscess, incision and drainage ~ 40800-40801, 41005-41009, 41015-41018
biopsy ~ 40808, 41108
cyst, incision and drainage ~ 40800-40801, 41005-41009, 41015-41018
excision, frenum ~ 40819
hematoma, incision and drainage ~ 40800-40801, 41005-41009, 41015-41018
lesion
destruction ~ 40820
excision ~ 40810-40816, 41116
vestibule of
destruction ~ 40820
repair ~ 40830
mucosa, excision ~ 40818
reconstruction ~ 40840-40845
removal, foreign body ~ 40804-40805
repair, laceration ~ 40830-40831
unlisted services, procedures ~ 40899, 41599
vestibule of
excision, destruction ~ 40808-40820
incision ~ 40800-40806
other procedures ~ 40899
removal, foreign body ~ 40804
repair ~ 40830-40845
Move ~ see transfer
finger ~ 26555
toe joint ~ 26556
toe to hand ~ 26551-26554
Moynihan test ~ (gastrointestinal tract, X-ray, with contrast) 74246-74249
MPR ~ (multifetal pregnancy reduction) 59866
MRA ~ see magnetic resonance angiography
MRI ~ see magnetic resonance imaging

MSLT ~ (multiple sleep latency testing) 95805
Mucin, synovial fluid ~ 83872
Mucocele sinusotomy, frontal ~ 31075
Mucopolysaccharides ~ 83864-83866
Mucormycoses ~ see mucormycosis
Mucormycosis, antibody ~ 86732
Mucosa
ectopic gastric imaging ~ 78290
excision of lesion
alveolar, hyperplastic ~ 41828
vestibule of mouth ~ 40810-40818
via esophagoscopy ~ 43228
via small intestinal endoscopy ~ 44369
via upper gi endoscopy ~ 43258
periodontal grafting ~ 41870
urethra, mucosal advancement ~ 53450
vaginal biopsy ~ 57100-57105
Mucosa, buccal ~ see mouth, mucosa
Mucous cyst antibody, hand or finger ~ 26160
Mucous membrane ~ see mouth, mucosa
cutaneous
biopsy ~ 11100-11101
excision
benign lesion ~ 11440-11446
malignant lesion ~ 11640-11646
layer closure, wounds ~ 12051-12057
simple repair, wounds ~ 12011-12018
excision, sphenoid sinus ~ 31288
lid margin
correction of trichiasis ~ 67835
nasal test ~ 95065
ophthalmic test ~ 95060
rectum
proctoplasty for prolapse ~ 45505
MUGA (multiple gated acquisition) ~ 78452, 78454, 78473, 78483
Muller procedure ~ see sleep study
Multifetal pregnancy reduction ~ 59866
Multi-leaf collimator (MLC) device ~ 77338
Multiple sleep latency testing (MSLT) ~ 95805
Multiple valve procedures ~ see valvuloplasty
Mumford operation ~ (partial claviculectomy, arthroscopic) 29824
Mumps
antibody ~ 86735
immunization ~ 90704, 90707, 90710
vaccine ~ 90704
MMR ~ 90707
MMRV ~ 90710
Muramidase ~ 85549
Murine typhus ~ 86000
Muscle ~ see specific muscle
abdomen ~ see abdominal wall
biopsy ~ 20200-20206
debridement ~ 11043, 11046
infected ~ 11004-11006
heart ~ see myocardium
neck ~ see neck muscle
oculomotor ~ see eye muscles

Muscle ~ continued
removal, foreign body ~ 20520-20525
repair
   extraocular ~ 65290
   forearm ~ 25260-25274
   wrist ~ 25260-25274
revision, arm, upper ~ 24330-24331
transfer
   arm, upper ~ 24301, 24320
   elbow ~ 24301
   femur ~ 27110
   hip ~ 27100-27105, 27111
   shoulder ~ 23395-23397, 24301, 24320
Muscle compartment syndrome, detection ~
20950
Muscle denervation ~ see denervation
Muscle division
scalenus anticus ~ 21700-21705
sternocleidomastoid ~ 21720-21725
Muscle flaps ~ 15732-15738
free ~ 15756
Muscle grafts ~ 15841-15845
Muscle testing
dynamometry, eye ~ 92260
extraocular multiple muscles ~ 92265
manual ~ 95831-95834
Musculo-skeletal system ~ see musculoskeletal
system
Musculoplasty ~ see muscle, repair
Musculoskeletal system, surgical procedures ~
20005-29999
Musculotendinous (rotator) cuff, repair ~
23410-23412
Mustard procedure ~ (repair, great arteries;
revision) 33774-33777
Myasthenia gravis, tensilon test ~
95857-95858
Mycobacteria
culture ~ 87116
   identification ~ 87118
detection ~ 87550-87562
sensitivity studies ~ 87190
Mycoplasma
antibody ~ 86738
culture ~ 87109
detection ~ 87580-87582
Mycota ~ see fungus
Myectomy, anorectal ~ see myomectomy,
anorectal
Myelencephalon ~ see medulla
Myelin basic protein, cerebrospinal fluid ~
83873
Myelography
brain ~ 70010
spine
   cervical ~ 72240
   lumbosacral ~ 72265
   thoracic ~ 72255
   total ~ 72270

Myelomeningocele, repair ~ 63704-63706
Myeloperoxidase (MPO) ~ 83876
Myelotomy ~ 63170
Myocardial, perfusion imaging ~ 78451-78454
positron emission tomography (PET) ~ 78459
Myocardial imaging ~ 78466-78469
perfusion study
   positron emission tomography (PET) ~
   78491-78492
   single photon emission computed
   tomography (SPECT) ~ 78451-78452
repair, postinfarction ~ 33542
Myocutaneous flaps ~ 15732-15738, 15756
Myofascial pain dysfunction syndrome ~ see
temporomandibular joint (TMJ)
Myofibroma ~ see leiomyomata
Myoglobin ~ 83874
Myomectomy
anorectal ~ 45108
uterus ~ 58140-58146, 58545-58546
Myoplasty ~ see muscle, repair
Myotomy
esophagus ~ 43030
hyoid ~ 21685
Myringoplasty ~ 69620
Myringostomy ~ see myringostomy
Myringotomy ~ 69420-69421
Myxoid cyst ~ see ganglion

N

N. meningitidis ~ see Neisseria meningitidis
Naffziger operation ~ (decompression, orbit;
section) 61330
Nagel test ~ (color vision examination) 92283
Nail(s)
avulsion ~ 11730-11732
biopsy ~ 11755
debridement ~ 11720-11721
evacuation, hematoma, subungual ~ 11740
excision ~ 11750-11752
   cyst, pilonidal ~ 11770-11772
KOH examination ~ 87220
removal ~ 11730-11732, 11750-11752
trimming ~ 11719
Nail bed, reconstruction ~ 11762
repair ~ 11760
Nail fold, excision wedge ~ 11765
Nail plate separation ~ see onychia
Narcosynthesis, diagnostic and therapeutic ~
90865
Nasal abscess ~ see nose, abscess
Nasal area, bone graft ~ 21210
Nasal bleeding ~ see epistaxis

Nasal bone
  fracture
    closed treatment ~ 21310-21320
    open treatment ~ 21325-21335
    with manipulation ~ 21315-21320
    without manipulation ~ 21310
    X-ray ~ 70160
Nasal deformity, repair ~ 40700-40761
Nasal function study ~ 92512
Nasal polyp ~ see nose, polyp
Nasal prosthesis, impression ~ 21087
Nasal septum
  abscess, incision and drainage ~ 30020
  fracture
    closed treatment ~ 21337
    open treatment ~ 21336
  hematoma, incision and drainage ~ 30020
  repair ~ 30630
  submucous resection ~ 30520
Nasal sinuses ~ see sinus; sinuses
Nasal smear, eosinophils ~ 89190
Nasal turbinate fracture, therapeutic ~ 30930
Nasoethmoid complex
  fracture
    open treatment ~ 21338-21339
    percutaneous treatment ~ 21340
  reconstruction ~ 21182-21184
Nasogastric tube, placement ~ 43752
Nasolacrimal duct
  exploration ~ 68810
    with anesthesia ~ 68811
  insertion
    catheter dilation 68816
    stent ~ 68815
  X-ray, with contrast ~ 70170
Nasomaxillary fracture
  closed treatment ~ 21345
  open treatment ~ 21346-21348
  with bone grafting ~ 21348
Nasopharynges ~ see nasopharynx
Nasopharyngoscopy ~ 92511
Nasopharynx ~ see also pharynx
  biopsy ~ 42804-42806
  hemorrhage ~ 42970-42972
  unlisted services and procedures ~ 42999
Natriuretic peptide ~ 83880
Natural ostium sinus
  maxillary ~ 31000
  sphenoid ~ 31002
Navicular
  arthroplasty, with implant ~ 25443
  fracture
    closed treatment ~ 25622
    open treatment ~ 25628
    with manipulation ~ 25624
  repair ~ 25440
Navigation, computer assisted ~ 0054T-0055T, 20985
  repair ~ 25440

Neck
  angiography ~ 70498, 70547-70549
  artery, ligation ~ 37615
  biopsy ~ 21550
  bypass graft ~ 35901
  CT scan ~ 70490-70492, 70498
  dissection, radical ~ see radical neck
    dissection
  exploration
    blood vessel ~ 35800
    lymph nodes ~ 38542
  incision and drainage
    abscess ~ 21501-21502
    hematoma ~ 21501-21502
  lipectomy, suction assisted ~ 15876
  magnetic resonance angiography (MRA) ~
    70547-70549
  magnetic resonance imaging(MRI) ~
    70540-70543
  nerve, graft ~ 64885-64886
  repair, blood vessel ~ 35201
    with other graft ~ 35261
    with vein graft ~ 35231
  skin, revision ~ 15819
  tumor
    excision ~ 21552-21558
    excision/resection ~ 21557-21558
  ultrasound exam ~ 76536
  unlisted services and procedures, surgery ~
    21899
  wound exploration, penetrating ~ 20100
  X-ray ~ 70360
Neck muscle
  division
    scalenus anticus ~ 21700-21705
    sternocleidomastoid ~ 21720-21725
Necropsy
  coroner's exam ~ 88045
  forensic exam ~ 88040
  gross and micro exam ~ 88020-88029
  gross exam ~ 88000-88016
  organ ~ 88037
  regional ~ 88036
  unlisted services and procedures ~ 88099
Needle biopsy ~ see also biopsy
  abdomen mass ~ 49180
  bone ~ 20220-20225
  bone marrow ~ 38221
  breast ~ 19100
  colon, endoscopy ~ 45392
  colon-sigmoid, endoscopy ~ 45342
  CT scan guidance ~ 77012
  epididymis ~ 54800
  esophagus, endoscopy ~ 43232
  fluoroscopic guidance ~ 77002
  gastrointestinal, upper, endoscopy ~ 43238,
    43242
  kidney ~ 50200
  liver ~ 47000-47001
  lung ~ 32405
  lymph nodes ~ 38505

Needle biopsy ~ *continued*
  mediastinum ~ 32405
  muscle ~ 20206
  pancreas ~ 48102
  pleura ~ 32400
  prostate ~ 55700
    transperineal ~ 55706
  retroperitoneal mass ~ 49180
  salivary gland ~ 42400
  spinal cord ~ 62269
  testis ~ 54500
  thyroid gland ~ 60100
  transbronchial ~ 31629, 31633
Needle localization
  breast
    placement ~ 19290-19291
    with lesion excision ~ 19125-19126
    magnetic resonance guidance ~ 77021
Needle manometer technique ~ 20950
Needle wire
  introduction, trachea ~ 31730
  placement, breast ~ 19290-19291
Neer procedure ~ 23470
Neisseria gonorrheae ~ 87590-87592, 87850
Neisseria meningitidis, antibody ~ 86741
Neobladder, construction ~ 51596
Neonatal critical care ~ see also newborn care
  initial ~ 99468
  subsequent ~ 99469
Neoplasm
  cancer photoradiation therapy ~ see photochemotherapy
  cardiac ~ see heart, tumor
  colon ~ see colon, tumor
  esophageal ~ see tumor, esophagus
  spinal cord ~ see spinal cord, neoplasm
  unspecified nature of brain ~ see brain, tumor
Neoplastic growth ~ see tumor
Nephelometry ~ 83883
Nephrectomy
  donor ~ 50300-50320, 50547
  laparoscopic ~ 50545-50548
  partial ~ 50240
    laparoscopic ~ 50543
  recipient ~ 50340
  with ureters ~ 50220-50236, 50546, 50548
Nephrolith ~ see calculus, removal, kidney
Nephrolithotomy ~ 50060-50075
Nephropexy ~ 50400-50405
Nephroplasty ~ see kidney, repair
Nephropyeloplasty ~ see pyeloplasty
Nephrorrhaphy ~ 50500
Nephroscopy ~ see endoscopy, kidney
Nephrostogram ~ 50394
Nephrostolithotomy, percutaneous ~ 50080-50081
Nephrostomy ~ 50040
  change tube ~ 50398
  endoscopic ~ 50562-50570
  percutaneous ~ 52334
  with drainage ~ 50040
  X-ray with contrast, guide dilation ~ 74485

Nephrostomy tract, establishment ~ 50395
Nephrotomogram ~ see nephrotomography
Nephrotomography ~ 74415
Nephrotomy ~ 50040-50045
  with exploration ~ 50045
Nerve
  see also nerves
  biopsy ~ 64795
  neuroma, excision
    cutaneous ~ 64774
    digital ~ 64776, 64778
    foot, other than digital ~ 64782, 64783
    hand, other than digital ~ 64782, 64783
    peripheral ~ 64784
    sciatic ~ 64786
Nerve conduction
  motor nerve ~ 95905, 95907-95913
  preconfigured electrode array ~ 0197T
Nerve graft
  additional nerve ~ 64901-64902
  arm or leg ~ 64892-64893, 64897-64898
  foot or hand ~ 64890-64891, 64895-64896
  head or neck ~ 64885-64886
  neurovascular pedicle ~ 15750
  pedicle ~ 64905, 64907
Nerve root ~ see also cauda equina; spinal cord
  decompression ~ 22856, 63020-63048, 63055-63103
  incision ~ 63185-63190
  section ~ 63185-63190
Nerve stimulation, transcutaneous ~ see application, neurostimulation
Nerve teasing ~ 88362
Nerves
  anastomosis
    facial to hypoglossal ~ 64868
    facial to phrenic ~ 64870
    facial to spinal accessory ~ 64866
  avulsion ~ 64732-64772
  biopsy ~ 64795
  cervical neurostimulator implant ~ 0282T-0283T
  decompression ~ 64702-64727
    cranial ~ 61458, 61460
    laminotomy/laminectomy ~ 0274T-0275T
  denervation ~ 27035
  destruction ~ 64600-64681
    laryngeal, recurrent ~ 31595
  graft ~ 64885-64907
  implantation, electrode ~ 0282T-0283T, 64553-64581
    to bone ~ 64787
    to muscle ~ 64787
  incision ~ 28035, 43640-43641, 64732-64772
  injection
    anesthetic ~ 01991-01992, 64400-64530
    diagnostic agent ~ 0213T, 64493-64495
    neurolytic agent ~ 64600-64681
    therapeutic agent ~ 0213T, 64490-64495
  insertion, electrode ~ 64553-64581
  lesion, excision ~ 64774-64792
  neurofibroma, excision ~ 64788-64792

Nerves ~ *continued*
neurolemmoma, excision ~ 64788-64792
neurolytic, internal ~ 64727
neuroma
  destruction ~ 64632
  excision ~ 64774-64786
  injection ~ 64455
neuroplasty ~ 64702-64721
removal, electrode ~ 64585
repair
  graft ~ 64885-64911
  microdissection ~ 69990
  suture ~ 64831-64876
spinal accessory
  incision ~ 63191
  section ~ 63191
suture ~ 64831-64876
sympathectomy, excision ~ 64802-64818
thoracic neurostimulator implant ~
  0282T-0283T
transection ~ 64732-64772
transposition ~ 64718-64721
unlisted services and procedures ~ 64999
Nerve V, cranial ~ see trigeminal nerve
Nerve VII, cranial ~ see facial nerve
Nerve X, cranial ~ see vagus nerve
Nerve XI, cranial ~ see accessory nerve
Nerve XII, cranial ~ see hypoglossal nerve
Nervous system, surgical procedures ~
  61000-64999
Nesidioblast ~ see islet cell
Neural conduction ~ see nerve conduction
Neural ganglion ~ see ganglion
Neurectomy
foot ~ 28055
gastrocnemius ~ 27326
hamstring muscle ~ 27325
leg, upper ~ 27325
popliteal ~ 27326
tympanic ~ 69676
Neuroendoscopy, intracranial ~ 62160-62165
Neurofibroma
cutaneous nerve, excision ~ 64788
extensive, excision ~ 64792
peripheral nerve, excision ~ 64790
Neurolemmoma
cutaneous nerve, excision ~ 64788
extensive, excision ~ 64792
peripheral nerve, excision ~ 64790
Neurologic system ~ see nervous system
Neurology procedures
brain cortex magnetic stimulation ~ 0310T,
  90867-90868
brain mapping ~ 0310T, 90867, 96020
brain surface electrode stimulation ~
  95961-95962
central motor function mapping ~ 0310T
cognitive performance ~ 96125

Neurology procedures ~ *continued*
diagnostic
  anal sphincter ~ 51785
  autonomic function tests
    heart rate response ~ 95921, 95943
    parasympathetic ~ 95943
    pseudomotor response ~ 95921-95924
    sympathetic function ~ 95921-95924,
     95943
    valsalva maneuver ~ 95922, 95943
  brain surface electrode stimulation ~
    95961-95962
  central motor transcranial motor stimulation
    ~ 95928-95929
  electrocorticogram, intraoperative ~ 95829
  electroencephalogram (EEG) ~ 95812-95827,
    95955
    brain death ~ 95824
    electrode placement ~ 95830
    intraoperative ~ 95955
    monitoring ~ 95812-95813, 95950-95953,
     95956
    physical or drug activation ~ 95954
    sleep ~ 95800-95801, 95822, 95827
    standard ~ 95819
    WADA activation ~ 95958
  electroencephalography (EEG), digital
    analysis ~ 95957
  electromyography
    fine wire dynamic ~ 96004
    ischemic limb exercise test ~ 95875
    needle ~ 51785, 95860-95872
    surface dynamic ~ 96002-96004
  higher cerebral function
    aphasia test ~ 96105
    cognitive function tests ~ 96116
    developmental tests ~ 96110-96111
    neurobehavioral status ~ 96116
    neuropsychological testing ~ 96118-96120
  magnetoencephalography (MEG) ~
    95965-95967
  motion analysis
    by accelerometer and gyroscope ~ 0199T
    by video and 3-D kinematics ~ 96000,
     96004
    computer-based ~ 96000, 96004
  muscle testing, manual ~ 95831-95834
  nerve conduction
    motor and sensory ~ 95905-95913
  neurofunctional testing ~ 96020
  neuromuscular junction tests ~ 95937
  neurophysiological monitoring, intraoperative
    ~ 95940-95941
  neuropsychological testing ~ 96118-96120
    cognitive performance ~ 96125
    computer assisted ~ 96120
  plantar pressure measurements, dynamic ~
    96001, 96004
  polysomnography ~ 95782-95783,
    95808-95811
  range of motion ~ 95851-95852

1477

Neurology procedures ~ continued
reflex
blink reflex ~ 95933
sleep study ~ 96800-95801, 95803-95811
somatosensory testing ~ 95925-95927,
95938-95939
tensilon test ~ 95857
unlisted services and procedures ~ 95999
urethral sphincter ~ 51785
visual evoked potential, CNS ~ 95930
Neurolysis
nerve ~ 64704-64708
internal ~ 64727
Neuroma
acoustic ~ see brain, tumor, excision
excision
cutaneous nerve ~ 64774
digital nerve ~ 64776-64778
foot ~ 28080
foot nerve ~ 64782-64783
hand nerve ~ 64782-64783
interdigital (Morton's) ~ 28080
peripheral nerve ~ 64784
sciatic nerve ~ 64786
injection, anesthetic or steroid ~ 64455
Neuromuscular junction tests ~ 95937
Neuromuscular pedicle reinnervation larynx
~ 31590
Neuromuscular reeducation ~ 97112
Neurophysiologic testing
autonomic nervous function
heart rate response ~ 95921-95924
pseudomotor response ~ 95921-95924
sympathetic function ~ 95921-95924
intraoperative ~ 95940-95941
Neuroplasty
cranial nerve ~ 64716
digital nerve ~ 64702-64704
peripheral nerve
arm ~ 64708
brachial plexus ~ 64713
cranial ~ 64716
lrh ~ 64708
lumbar plexus ~ 64714
median at carpal tunnel ~ 64721
sciatic ~ 64712
ulnar at elbow ~ 64718
ulnar at wrist ~ 64719
Neuropsychological testing ~ 96117
Neurorrhaphy ~ 64831-64876
peripheral nerve
conduit ~ 64910-64911
with graft ~ 64885-64907
Neurostimulation, application ~ 64550, 64566
Neurostimulators
analysis ~ 95970-95982
application ~ 64550
implantation ~ 64553-64565
electrodes ~ 43647, 43881
insertion
pulse generator ~ 61885-61886, 64590
receiver ~ 61885-61886, 64590

Neurostimulators ~ continued
removal
electrodes ~ 43648, 43882, 61880
pulse generator ~ 61888, 64595
receiver ~ 61888, 64595
replacement ~ 61885
electrodes ~ 43647, 43881
Neurotomy, sympathetic ~ see gasserian
ganglion, sensory root, decompression
Neurovascular pedicle flaps ~ 15750
Neutralization test, virus ~ 86382
New patient
domiciliary or rest home visit ~ 99324-99328
emergency department services ~ 99281-99288
home services ~ 99341-99345
hospital inpatient services ~ 99221-99239
hospital observation services ~ 99217-99220
initial office visit ~ 99201-99205
inpatient consultations ~ 99251-99255
office and/or other outpatient consultations ~
99241-99245
Newborn care ~ 99460-99465, 99502
attendance at delivery ~ 99464
birthing room ~ 99460
blood transfusion ~ 36450
circumcision
clamp or other device ~ 54150
surgical excision ~ 54160
history and examination ~ 99460, 99463
laryngoscopy ~ 31520
normal ~ 99460-99463
prepuce slitting ~ 54000
preventive, office ~ 99461
resuscitation ~ 99465
standby for cesarean delivery ~ 99360
subsequent hospital care ~ 99462
umbilical artery catheterization ~ 36660
Nickel ~ 83885
Nicolas-Durand-Favre disease ~ see
lymphogranuloma venereum
Nicotine ~ 83887
Nidation ~ see implantation
Nipples ~ see breast
inverted ~ 19355
reconstruction ~ 19350
Nissen operation ~ see fundoplasty,
esophagogastric
Nissen procedure
laparoscopic ~ 43280
Nitrate reduction test ~ see urinalysis
Nitric Oxide ~ 95012
Nitroblue tetrazolium dye test ~ 86384
Nitrogen, blood urea ~ see blood urea nitrogen
NMR imaging ~ see magnetic resonance
imaging (MRI)
NMR spectroscopies ~ see magnetic resonance
spectroscopy
No man's land, tendon repair ~ 26356-26358
Noble procedure ~ see repair; suture
Nocardia, antibody ~ 86744
Nocturnal penile rigidity test ~ 54250
Nocturnal penile tumescence test ~ 54250

Node, lymph ~ see lymph nodes
Nodes ~ see lymph nodes
Node dissection, lymph ~ see dissection, lymph
   nodes
Non-office medical services ~ 99056
Non-stress test, fetal ~ 59025
Nonunion repairS
   femur
      with graft ~ 27472
      without graft ~ 27470
   metatarsal ~ 28322
   tarsal joint ~ 28320
Noradrenalin
   blood ~ 82383-82384
   urine ~ 82384
Norchlorimipramine ~ see imipramine
Norepinephrine ~ see catecholamines
   blood ~ 82383-82384
   urine ~ 82384
Nortriptyline, assay ~ 80182
Norwood procedure ~ 33611-33612, 33619,
   33622
Nose
   abscess, incision and drainage ~ 30000-30020
   artery, incision ~ 30915-30920
   biopsy, intranasal ~ 30100
   dermoid cyst, excision
      complex ~ 30125
      simple ~ 30124
   displacement therapy ~ 30210
   endoscopy
      diagnostic ~ 31231-31235
      surgical ~ 31237-31297
   excision, rhinectomy ~ 30150-30160
   fracture
      closed treatment ~ 21345
      open treatment ~ 21325-21336,
         21338-21339, 21346-21347
      percutaneous treatment ~ 21340
      with fixation ~ 21330, 21340, 21345-21347
   hematoma, incision and drainage ~
      30000-30020
   hemorrhage, cauterization ~ 30901-30906
   insertion, septal prosthesis ~ 30220
   intranasal lesion
      external approach ~ 30118
      internal approach ~ 30117
   lysis of adhesions ~ 30560
   polyp, excision
      extensive ~ 30115
      simple ~ 30110
   reconstruction
      cleft lip/cleft palate ~ 30460-30462
      dermatoplasty ~ 30620
      primary ~ 30400-30420
      secondary ~ 30430-30450
      septum ~ 30520
   removal
      foreign body ~ 30300
      anesthesia ~ 30310
      lateral rhinotomy ~ 30320

Nose ~ *continued*
   repair
      adhesions ~ 30560
      cleft lip ~ 40700-40761
      fistula ~ 30580-30600, 42260
      rhinophyma ~ 30120
      septum ~ 30540-30545, 30630
      synechia ~ 30560
      vestibular stenosis ~ 30465
   skin
      excision ~ 30120
      surgical planing ~ 30120
   submucous resection turbinate
      excision ~ 30140
   turbinate
      excision ~ 30130-30140
      fracture ~ 30930
      injection ~ 30200
   turbinate mucosa, cauterization ~ 30801-30802
   unlisted services and procedures ~ 30999
Nose bleed ~ (hemorrhage, nasal) 30901-30906
NTD ~ (nitroblue tetrazolium dye test) 86384
Nuclear antigen, antibody ~ 86235
Nuclear imaging ~ see nuclear medicine
Nuclear magnetic resonance imaging ~ see
   magnetic resonance imaging (MRI)
Nuclear magnetic resonance spectroscopy ~
   see magnetic resonance spectroscopy
Nuclear medicine ~ 78012-79999
   adrenal gland imaging ~ 78075
   bladder, residual study ~ 78730
   blood
      flow imaging ~ 78445
      iron
         absorption ~ 78162
         chelatable ~ 78172
         plasma ~ 78160
         red cells ~ 78140
         utilization ~ 78170
      platelet survival ~ 78190-78191
      red cells ~ 78120-78121
      red cells survival ~ 78130-78135
      unlisted services and procedures ~ 78199
      whole blood volume ~ 78122
   bone
      density study ~ 78350-78351
      imaging ~ 78300-78320
      SPECT ~ 78320
      ultrasound ~ 76977
      ultrasound services and procedures ~ 78399
   bone marrow imaging ~ 78102-78104
   brain
      blood flow ~ 78610
      cerebrospinal flow ~ 78630-78650
      imaging ~ 78600-78609
      vascular flow ~ 78610
   endocrine system, unlisted services and
      procedures ~ 78099
   esophagus
      imaging (motility) ~ 78258
      reflux study ~ 78262
   gastric mucosa imaging ~ 78261

1479

Nuclear medicine ~ *continued*
gastrointestinal
  blood loss study ~ 78278
  protein loss study ~ 78282
  shunt testing ~ 78291
  unlisted services and procedures ~ 78299
genitourinary system, unlisted services and
  procedures ~ 78799
heart
  blood flow ~ 78414
  blood pool imaging ~ 78472-78473,
    78481-78483, 78494-78496
  myocardial imaging ~ 78459, 78466-78469
  myocardial perfusion ~ 78451-78454
  shunt detection ~ 78428
  unlisted services and procedures ~ 78499
inflammatory process ~ 78805-78807
intestines imaging ~ 78290
kidney
  function study ~ 78725
  imaging ~ 78700-78707, 78710
lacrimal gland, tear flow ~ 78660
liver
  imaging ~ 78201-78216
  vascular flow ~ 78206
lung
  imaging perfusion ~ 78580, 78597, 78598
  imaging ventilation ~ 78579, 78582, 78598
  unlisted services and procedures ~ 78599
lymph nodes ~ 78195
lymphatics ~ 78195
  unlisted services and procedures ~ 78199
musculoskeletal system, unlisted services and
  procedures ~ 78399
nervous system, unlisted services and
  procedures ~ 78699
parathyroid gland imaging ~ 78070
pulmonary perfusion ~ 78580, 78597-78598
pulmonary ventilation ~ 78579, 78582, 78598
salivary gland function study ~ 78232
  imaging ~ 78230-78231
spleen
  imaging ~ 78185, 78215-78216
  unlisted services and procedures ~ 78199
stomach
  blood loss study ~ 78278
  emptying study ~ 78264
  protein loss study ~ 78282
  reflux study ~ 78262
  vitamin B-12 absorption ~ 78270-78272
testes imaging ~ 78761
therapeutic
  heart ~ 79440
  interstitial ~ 79300
  intra-arterial ~ 79445
  intra-articular ~ 79440
  intracavitary ~ 79200
  intravenous ~ 79101
  intravenous infusion ~ 79403
  oral ~ 79005
  thyroid ~ 79200-79300
  unlisted services and procedures ~ 79999

Nuclear medicine ~ *continued*
thyroid
  imaging for metastases ~ 78015-78018
  imaging with flow ~ 78013
  metastases uptake ~ 78020
  uptake ~ 78012, 78014
tumor imaging
  positron emission tomography (PET) ~
    78811-78816
    with computed tomography ~ 78814-78816
tumor localization ~ 78800-78804
unlisted services and procedures ~ 78999
urea breath test ~ 78267-78268
ureter, reflux study ~ 78740
vein thrombosis imaging ~ 78455-78458
Nucleases, DNA ~ see DNAse
Nucleic acid probe
amplified probe detection, infectious agent
  bartonella henselae ~ 87471
  bartonella quintana ~ 87471
  borrelia burgdorferi ~ 87476
  candida species ~ 87481
  chlamydia pneumoniae ~ 87486
  chlamydia trachomatis ~ 87491
  cytomegalovirus ~ 87496
  enterovirus ~ 87498, 87500
  gardnerella vaginalis ~ 87511
  hepatitis B virus ~ 87516
  hepatitis C ~ 87521
  hepatitis G ~ 87526
  herpes simplex virus ~ 87529
  herpes virus-6 ~ 87532
  HIV-1 ~ 87535
  HIV-2 ~ 87538
  legionella pneumophila ~ 87541
  multiple organisms ~ 87801
  mycobacteria avium-intracellulare ~ 87561
  mycobacteria species ~ 87551
  mycobacteria tuberculosis ~ 87556
  mycoplasma pneumoniae ~ 87581
  neisseria gonorrheae ~ 87591
  not otherwise specified ~ 87798, 87801
  papillomavirus, human ~ 87621
  staphylococcus aureus ~ 87640-87641
  streptococcus, group A ~ 87651
  streptococcus, group B ~ 87653
direct probe detection, infectious agent
  bartonella henselae ~ 87470
  bartonella quintana ~ 87470
  borrelia burgdorferi ~ 87475
  candida species ~ 87480
  chlamydia pneumoniae ~ 87485
  chlamydia trachomatis ~ 87490
  clostridium difficile ~ 87493
  cytomegalovirus ~ 87495
  gardnerella vaginalis ~ 87510
  hepatitis B virus ~ 87515
  hepatitis C ~ 87520
  hepatitis G ~ 87525
  herpes simplex virus ~ 87528
  herpes virus-6 ~ 87531
  HIV-1 ~ 87534

Nucleic acid probe ~ *continued*
HIV-2 ~ 87537
legionella pneumophila ~ 87540
multiple organisms ~ 87800
mycobacteria avium-intracellulare ~ 87560
mycobacteria species ~ 87550
mycobacteria tuberculosis ~ 87555
mycoplasma pneumoniae ~ 87580
neisseria gonorrheae ~ 87590
not otherwise specified ~ 87797
papillomavirus, human ~ 87620
streptococcus, group A ~ 87650
trichomonas vaginalis ~ 87660
genotype analysis, infectious agent
HIV-1 ~ 87901, 87906
hepatitis C virus ~ 87902
in situ hybridization ~ 88120-88121,
88365-88368
phenotype analysis, infectious agent
HIV-1 drug resistance ~ 87903-87904
quantification, infectious agent
bartonella henselae ~ 87472
bartonella quintana ~ 87472
borrelia burgdorferi ~ 87477
candida species ~ 87482
chlamydia pneumoniae ~ 87487
chlamydia trachomatis ~ 87492
cytomegalovirus ~ 87497
gardnerella vaginalis ~ 87512
hepatitis B virus ~ 87517
hepatitis C ~ 87522
hepatitis G ~ 87527
herpes simplex virus ~ 87530
herpes virus-6 ~ 87533
HIV-1 ~ 87536
HIV-2 ~ 87539
legionella pneumophila ~ 87542
mycobacteria avium-intracellulare ~ 87562
mycobacteria species ~ 87552
mycobacteria tuberculosis ~ 87557
mycoplasma pneumoniae ~ 87582
neisseria gonorrheae ~ 87592
not otherwise specified ~ 87799
papillomavirus, human ~ 87622
streptococcus, group A ~ 87652
Nucleolysis, intervertebral disk ~ see
chemonucleolysis
Nucleotidase ~ 83915
Nursemaid elbow ~ 24640
Nursing facility discharge services ~ see
discharge services, nursing facility
Nursing facility services ~ 99304-99318
annual assessment ~ 99318
care plan oversight services ~ 99379-99380
comprehensive assessments
new or established patient ~ 99301-99303
discharge services ~ 99315-99316,
1110F-1111F
subsequent care ~ 99307-99310
Nuss procedure
with thoracoscopy ~ 21743
without thoracoscopy ~ 21742

Nutrition therapy
group ~ 97804
home infusion ~ 99601-99602
initial assessment ~ 97802
reassessment ~ 97803
Nystagmus tests ~ see vestibular function tests
optokinetic ~ 92534, 92544
positional ~ 92532, 92542
spontaneous ~ 92531, 92540-92541

O

O2 (two) saturation ~ see oxygen saturation
Ober-Yount procedure ~ (fasciotomy, hip)
27025
Obliteration
mastoid ~ 69670
vagina
total ~ 57110-57112
vault ~ 57120
Oblongata, medulla ~ see medulla
Observation ~ (see Evaluation and
Management; Hospital Services)
99217-99220, 99224-99225, 99234-99236
Obstetrical care
abortion
induced
by amniocentesis injection ~ 59850-59852
by dilation and curettage ~ 59840
by dilation and evaluation ~ 59841
missed
first trimester ~ 59820
second trimester ~ 59821
spontaneous ~ 59812
therapeutic ~ 59840-59852
antepartum care ~ 59425-59426
cesarean delivery ~ 59618-59622
only ~ 59514
postpartum care ~ 59515
routine ~ 59510
with hysterectomy ~ 59525
curettage, hydatidiform mole ~ 59870
evacuation, hydatidiform mole ~ 59870
external cephalic version ~ 59412
miscarriage, surgical completion ~
59812-59821
placenta delivery ~ 59414
postpartum care ~ 59430, 59514
septic abortion ~ 59830
total (global) ~ 59400, 59610, 59618
unlisted services and procedures ~
59898-59899
vaginal, after cesarean ~ 59610-59614
vaginal delivery ~ 59409-59410
delivery after cesarean ~ 59610-59614
Obstruction ~ see occlusion
Obstruction clearance, venous access device ~
36595-36596
Obstruction colon ~ see colon, obstruction

Obturator nerve
avulsion ~ 64763-64766
incision ~ 64763-64766
transection ~ 64763-64766
Obturator prosthesis ~ 21076
definitive ~ 21080
insertion, larynx ~ 31527
interim ~ 21079
Occipital nerve, greater
avulsion ~ 64744
incision ~ 64744
injection, anesthetic ~ 64405
transection ~ 64744
Occlusion
extracranial, intracranial ~ 61623
fallopian tube, oviduct ~ 58565, 58615
penis, vein ~ 37790
umbilical cord ~ 59072
Occlusive disease of artery ~ see repair, artery;
revision
Occult blood ~ 82270
penis, by hemoglobin immunoassay ~ 82274
Occupational therapy, evaluation ~
97003-97004
Ocular implant ~ see orbital implant
insertion
in scleral shell ~ 65130
muscles attached ~ 65140
muscles, not attached ~ 65135
modification ~ 65125
reinsertion ~ 65150
with foreign material ~ 65155
removal ~ 65175
Ocular muscle ~ see eye muscles
Ocular orbit ~ see orbit
Ocular photoscreening ~ 99174
Ocular prostheses ~ see prosthesis, ocular
Oculomotor muscle ~ see eye muscles
Oddi sphincter ~ see sphincter of Oddi
Odontoid dislocation
open treatment/reduction ~ 22318
with grafting ~ 22319
Odontoid fracture
open treatment/reduction ~ 22318
with grafting ~ 22319
Odontoid process, excision ~ 22548
Oesophageal neoplasm ~ see tumor, esophagus
Oesophageal varices ~ see esophageal varices
Oesophagus ~ see esophagus
Oestradiol ~ see estradiol
Office and/or other outpatient services
established patient ~ 99211-99215
new patient ~ 99201-99205
normal newborn ~ 99461
office visit
established patient ~ 99211-99215
new patient ~ 99201-99205
outpatient visit
established patient ~ 99211-99215
new patient ~ 99201-99205
prolonged services ~ 99354-99355

Office medical services
after hours ~ 99050
emergency care ~ 99058
extended hours ~ 99051
Office or other outpatient consultations ~
99241-99245
Olecranon ~ see elbow; humerus; radius; ulna
bursa, arthrocentesis ~ 20605
cyst, excision ~ 24125-24126
tumor
cyst ~ 24120
excision ~ 24125-24126
Olecranon process
craterization ~ 24147
diaphysectomy ~ 24147
excision ~ 24147
abscess ~ 24138
fracture ~ see elbow; humerus; radius
closed treatment ~ 24670-24675
open treatment ~ 24685
osteomyelitis ~ 24138, 24147
saucerization ~ 24147
sequestrectomy ~ 24138
Oligoclonal immunoglobulins ~ 83916
Omentectomy ~ 49255, 58950-58958
laparotomy ~ 58960
oophorectomy ~ 58943
resection ovarian malignancy ~ 58950-58952
resection peritoneal malignancy ~
58950-58958
resection tubal malignancy ~ 58950-58958
Omentum
excision ~ 49255, 58950-58958
flap ~ 49904-49905
free, with microvascular anastomosis ~
49906
unlisted services and procedures ~ 49999
Omphalectomy ~ 49250
Omphalocele, repair ~ 49600-49611
Omphalomesenteric duct, excision ~ 44800
Omphalomesenteric duct, persistent ~ see
diverticulum, Meckel's
Oncoprotein
des-gamma-carboxyprothrombin (DCP) ~
83951
HER-2/neu ~ 83950
One stage prothrombin time ~ (see also
prothrombin time) 85610-85611
Online medical evaluation ~ 99444
Onychectomy ~ see excision, nails
Onychia, drainage ~ 10060-10061
Oocyte
assisted fertilization, microtechnique ~
89280-89281
biopsy ~ 89290-89291
culture
extended ~ 89272
less than 4 (four) days ~ 89250
with co-culture ~ 89251
identification, follicular fluid ~ 89254
insemination ~ 89268

Oocyte ~ *continued*
  retrieval, for in vitro fertilization ~ 58970
  storage ~ 89346
  thawing ~ 89356
Oophorectomy ~ 58262-58263, 58291-58292,
    58552, 58554, 58661, 58940-58943
  ectopic pregnancy
    laparoscopic treatment ~ 59120
    surgical treatment ~ 59120
Oophorectomy, partial ~ see excision, ovary,
    partial
Oophorocystectomy ~ see cystectomy, ovarian
Open biopsy, adrenal gland ~ see adrenal
    gland, biopsy
Operating microscope ~ 69990
Operation
  Abbe-Estlander ~ 00102, 40527, 40761
  Bischof ~ 63170
  Blalock-Hanlon ~ 33735-33737
  Blalock-Taussig ~ 33750
  Bristow ~ 23460
  Campbell ~ 27422
  Chevron ~ 28296
  Cotte ~ 58400-58410
  Dunn ~ see arthrodesis, foot joint
  Duvries ~ see tenoplasty
  Estes ~ see ovary, transposition
  Foley y-pyeloplasty ~ 50400-50405
  Fontan ~ see repair, heart, anomaly
  Gill ~ 63012
  Green ~ see scapulopexy
  Halsted ~ 49491
  Heller ~ 32665
  Hibb ~ 22610, 22612, 22614
  Jaboulay gastroduodenostomy ~ 43810
  Keller ~ 28292
  Leriche ~ 00622, 64809
  Mumford ~ 29824
  Nissen ~ 43324
  Norwood ~ 33611-33612, 33619
  Potts-Smith ~ 33762
  Ramstedt ~ see pyloromyotomy
  Raskind ~ 33735-33737
  Raz ~ 51845
  Richardson hysterectomy ~ 53460
  Schlatter total gastrectomy ~ 43620-43622
  Swanson ~ 28309
  Swenson ~ 45120
  Takeuchi ~ 33505
  Thiersch ~ 15050
  Winiwarter ~ 47720-47740
  Winter ~ 54435
Operation microscopes ~ see operating
    microscope
Operculectomy ~ 41821
Operculum ~ see gums
Ophthalmic mucous membrane test ~ (see
    also allergy tests) 95060
Ophthalmology services ~ 92002-92499

Ophthalmology, diagnostic
  color vision exam ~ 92283
  computerized scanning ~ 92132-92134
  computerized screening ~ 99172, 99174
  dark adaptation ~ 92284
  electro-oculography ~ 92270
  electromyography, needle ~ 92265
  electroretinography ~ 92275
  endoscopy ~ 66990
  eye exam
    established patient ~ 92012-92014
    new patient ~ 92002-92004
    with anesthesia ~ 92018-92019
    glaucoma provocative test ~ 92140
  gonioscopy ~ 92020
  ocular photography
    external ~ 92285
    internal ~ 92286-92287
  ophthalmoscopy ~ 92225-92226
    with dynamometry ~ 92260
    with fluorescein angiography ~ 92235
    with fluorescein angioscopy ~ 92230
    with fundus photography ~ 92250
    with indocyanine-green angiography ~ 92240
    remote imaging ~ 92227-92228
  photoscreening ~ 99174
  refractive determination ~ 92015
  sensorimotor exam ~ 92060
  tonometry, serial ~ 92100
  ultrasound ~ 76511-76529
  visual acuity screen ~ 99172-99173
  visual field exam ~ 92081-92083
  visual function screen ~ 99172, 99174
Ophthalmoscopy ~ 92225-92226
Opiates ~ 83925
Opinion, second ~ see confirmatory
    consultations
Optic nerve
  decompression ~ 67570
    with nasal/sinus endoscopy ~ 31294
  head evaluation ~ 2027F
Optokinetic nystagmus test ~ see nystagmus
    tests, optokinetic
Oral lactose tolerance test ~ see glucose,
    tolerance test ~ 82951-82953
Oral mucosa ~ see mouth, mucosa
Oral surgical splint ~ 21085
Orbit ~ see orbital contents; orbital floor;
    periorbital region
  biopsy ~ 61332
    exploration ~ 67450
    fine needle aspiration or orbital contents ~ 67415
    orbitotomy without bone flap ~ 67400
  CT scan ~ 70480-70482
  decompression ~ 61330
    bone removal ~ 67414, 67445
  exploration ~ 61332, 67400, 67450
  lesion, excision ~ 61333
  fracture
    closed treatment
      with manipulation ~ 21401
      without manipulation ~ 21400

1483

Orbit ~ *continued*
open treatment ~ 21406-21408
  blowout fracture ~ 21385-21395
incision and drainage ~ 67405, 67440
injection
  retrobulbar ~ 67500-67505
  tenon's capsule ~ 67515
insertion, implant ~ 67550
lesion, excision ~ 67412, 67420
magnetic resonance imaging (MRI) ~ 70540-70543
removal
  decompression ~ 67445
  exploration ~ 61334
  foreign body ~ 61334, 67413, 67430
  implant ~ 67560
  sella turcica ~ 70482
unlisted services and procedures ~ 67599
X-ray ~ 70190-70200
Orbital contents, aspiration ~ 67415
Orbital floor ~ see orbit; periorbital region
fracture, blow out ~ 21385-21395
Orbital hypertelorism, osteotomy
periorbital ~ 21260-21263
Orbital implant ~ see ocular implant
insertion ~ 67550
removal ~ 67560
Orbital prosthesis ~ 21077
Orbital rims, reconstruction ~ 21182-21184
Orbital rim and forehead, reconstruction ~
21172-21180
Orbital transplant ~ 67560
Orbital walls, reconstruction ~ 21182-21184
Orbitocraniofacial reconstruction, secondary
~ 21275
Orbitotomy
with bone flap
  for exploration ~ 67450
  lateral approach ~ 67420
  with drainage ~ 67440
  with removal foreign body ~ 67430
  with removal of bone for decompression ~ 67445
without bone flap
  for exploration ~ 67400
  with drainage only ~ 67405
  with removal lesion ~ 67412
  with removal foreign body ~ 67413
  with removal of bone for decompression ~ 67414
Orbit area reconstruction, secondary ~ 21275
**Orbit wall decompression with nasal/sinus
endoscopy ~ 31292-31293**
Orchidectomies ~ see excision, testis
Orchidopexy ~ see orchiopexy
Orchidoplasty ~ see repair, testis
Orchiectomy
laparoscopic ~ 54690
partial ~ 54522
radical
  abdominal exploration ~ 54535
  inguinal approach ~ 54530
simple ~ 54520

Orchiopexy
abdominal approach ~ 54650
inguinal approach ~ 54640
intra-abdominal testis ~ 54692
Orchioplasty ~ see repair, testis
Organ or disease oriented panels ~
80048-80076
electrolyte ~ 80051
general health panel ~ 80050
hepatic function panel ~ 80076
hepatitis panel ~ 80074
lipid panel ~ 80061
metabolic
  basic ~ 80048
  comprehensive ~ 80053
obstetric panel ~ 80055
renal function ~ 80069
Organic acids ~ 83918-83921
Organ grafting ~ see transplantation
Organ system, neurologic ~ see nervous
system
Ormond disease ~ see retroperitoneal fibrosis
Orogastric tube placement ~ 43752
Oropharynx, biopsy ~ 42800
Orthodontic cephalogram ~ 70350
Orthomyxoviridae ~ see influenza virus
Orthomyxovirus ~ see influenza virus
Orthopantogram ~ 70355
Orthopedic cast ~ see cast
Orthopedic surgery
computer assisted navigation ~ 0054T-0055T,
  20985
stereotaxis, computer assisted ~ 20985
Orthoptic training ~ 92065
Orthoroentgenogram ~ 77073
Orthosis ~ see orthotics
Orthotics
check-out ~ 97703
fitting and training ~ 97504
Osmolality
blood ~ 83930
urine ~ 83935
Osseous survey ~ 77074-77076
Osseous tissue ~ see bone
Ossicles
excision stapes
  with footplate drill out ~ 69661
  without foreign material ~ 69660-69661
reconstruction ossicular chain
  tympanoplasty with antrotomy or
    mastoidotomy ~ 69636-69637
  tympanoplasty with mastoidectomy ~ 69642,
    69644, 69646
  tympanoplasty without mastoidectomy ~
    69632-69633
release, stapes ~ 69650
replacement, with prosthesis ~ 69633, 69637
Ostectomy
metacarpal ~ 26250
metatarsal ~ 28288
phalanges, finger ~ 26260-26262

Ostectomy ~ *continued*
  pressure ulcer
    ischial ~ 15941, 15945
    sacral ~ 15933, 15935, 15937
    trochanteric ~ 15951, 15953, 15958
    scapula ~ 23190
    sternum ~ 21620
Osteocalcin ~ 83937
Osteocartilaginous exostoses ~ see exostosis
Osteochondroma ~ see exostosis
**Osteocutaneous flap, with microvascular
  anastomosis** ~ 20969-20973
Osteoma sinusotomy, frontal ~ 31075
Osteomyelitis ~ 20005
  elbow, incision and drainage ~ 23935
  excision
    clavicle ~ 23180
    facial ~ 21026
    humerus, proximal ~ 23184
    mandible ~ 21025
    scapula ~ 23182
  femur/knee, incision and drainage ~ 27303
  finger incision ~ 26034
  hand incision ~ 26034
  hip incision, deep ~ 26992
  humerus ~ 24134
    incision and drainage ~ 23935
  incision
    foot ~ 28005
    shoulder ~ 23035
    thorax ~ 21510
  olecranon process ~ 24138, 24147
  pelvis incision, deep ~ 26992
  radius ~ 24136, 24145
  sequestrectomy
    clavicle ~ 23170
    humeral head ~ 23174
    scapula ~ 23172
    skull ~ 61501
Osteopathic manipulation ~ 98925-98929
Osteoplasty
  carpal bone ~ 25394
  facial bones
    augmentation ~ 21208
    reduction ~ 21209
  femoral neck ~ 27179
  femur ~ 27179
    lengthening ~ 27466-27468
    shortening ~ 27465, 27468
  fibula, lengthening ~ 27715
  humerus ~ 24420
  metacarpal ~ 26568
  phalanges, finger ~ 26568
  radius ~ 25390-25393
  tibia, lengthening ~ 27715
  ulna ~ 25390-25393
  vertebra ~ 72291-72292
    lumbar ~ 22521-22522
    thoracic ~ 22520-22522

Osteotomy
  calcaneus ~ 28300
  chin ~ 21121-21123
  clavicle ~ 23480-23485
  femur ~ 27140, 27151
    femoral neck ~ 27161
    for slipped epiphysis ~ 27181
    with fixation ~ 27165
    without fixation ~ 27448-27450
    with open reduction of hip ~ 27156
    with realignment ~ 27454
  fibula ~ 27707-27712
  hip ~ 27146-27151
    femoral, with open reduction ~ 27156
    femur ~ 27151
  humerus ~ 24400-24410
  mandible ~ 21198-21199
    extra-oral ~ 21047
    intra-oral ~ 21046
  maxilla ~ 21206
    extra-oral ~ 21049
    intra-oral ~ 21048
  metacarpal ~ 26565
  metatarsal ~ 28306-28309
  orbit reconstruction ~ 21256
  pelvis ~ 27158
  periorbital
    orbital hypertelorism ~ 21260-21263
    osteotomy with graft ~ 21267-21268
  phalanges
    finger ~ 26567
    toe ~ 28299, 28310-28312
  radius
    and ulna ~ 25365, 25375
    distal third ~ 25350
    middle or proximal third ~ 25355
    multiple ~ 25370
  skull base ~ 61582-61585, 61592
  spine
    anterior ~ 22220-22226
    posterior, posterolateral ~ 22206-22208,
      22210-22214
  talus ~ 28302
  tarsal ~ 28304-28305
  tibia ~ 27455-27457, 27705, 27709-27712
  ulna ~ 25360
    multiple ~ 25370
    and radius ~ 25365, 25375
  vertebra
    additional segment, anterior approach ~
      22226
      posterior/posterolateral approach ~ 22216
    cervical
      anterior approach ~ 22220
      posterior/posterolateral approach ~ 22210
    lumbar
      anterior approach ~ 22224
      posterior/posterolateral approach ~ 22214
    thoracic
      anterior approach ~ 22222
      posterior/posterolateral approach ~ 22212

Osteotomy ~ *continued*
  with graft reconstruction periorbital region ~
    21267-21268
Os calcis fracture ~ see calcaneus, fracture
Otolaryngology, diagnostic exam under
  anesthesia ~ 92502
Otomy ~ see incision
Otoplasty ~ 69300
Otorhinolaryngology services ~ 92502-92597
Ouchterlony immunodiffusion ~ 86331
Outer ear ~ see ear, outer
Outpatient visit ~ see history and physical;
  office and/or other outpatient services
Output, cardiac ~ see cardiac output
Ova, smear ~ 87177
Oval window, repair fistula ~ 69666
Oval window fistula ~ see fistula, oval window
Ovarian cyst ~ see cyst, ovarian; ovary, cyst
Ovarian vein syndrome, ureterolysis ~ 50722
Ovariectomies ~ see oophorectomy
Ovariolysis ~ 58740
Ovary
  abscess, incision and drainage ~ 58820-58822
    abdominal approach ~ 58822
  biopsy ~ 58900
  cyst, incision and drainage ~ 58800-58805
  excision ~ 58662, 58720
    cyst ~ 58925
    partial
      oophorectomy ~ 58661, 58940
      ovarian malignancy ~ 58943
      peritoneal malignancy ~ 58943
      tubal malignancy ~ 58943
      wedge resection ~ 58920
    total ~ 58940-58943
  laparoscopy ~ 58660-58662, 58679
  lysis, adhesions ~ 58660, 58740
  radical resection ~ 58950-58952
  transposition ~ 58825
  tumor, resection ~ 58950-58958
  unlisted services and procedures ~ 58679,
    58999
  wedge resection ~ 58920
Oviduct
  anastomosis ~ 58750
  chromotubation ~ 58350
  ectopic pregnancy ~ 59120-59121
  excision ~ 58700-58720
  fulguration, laparoscopic ~ 58670
  hysterosalpingography ~ 74740
  laparoscopy ~ 58679
  ligation ~ 58600-58611
  lysis, adhesions ~ 58740
  occlusion ~ 58615
    laparoscopic ~ 58671
  repair ~ 58752
    anastomosis ~ 58750
    create stoma ~ 58770
  unlisted services and procedures ~ 58679,
    58999
  X-ray with contrast ~ 74740
Ovocyte ~ see oocyte

Ovulation tests ~ 84830
Ovum implantation ~ see implantation
Ovum transfer surgery ~ see gamete
  intrafallopian transfer (GIT)
Oxalate ~ 83945
Oxidase, ceruloplasmin ~ see ceruloplasmin
Oxidoreductase, alcohol-nad+ ~ see
  antidiuretic hormone
Oximetry (noninvasive) ~ see pulmonology,
  diagnostic
  blood O2 saturation, ear or pulse ~
    94760-94762
Oxoisomerase ~ see phosphohexose isomerase
Oxosteroids ~ see ketosteroids
Oxycodinone ~ 80102-80103, 83925
Oxygenation, extracorporeal membrane ~ see
  extracorporeal membrane oxygenation
Oxygen saturation ~ 82805-82810
Oxyproline ~ see hydroxyproline
Oxytocin stress test, fetal ~ 59020

P

P & P ~ (proconvertin) 85230
P-acetamidophenol ~ see acetaminophen
Pacemaker, heart
  conversion ~ 33214
  data analysis ~ 93288, 93293-93294
  electronic analysis ~ 93288
    antitachycardia system ~ 93724
  evaluation and programming
    dual lead ~ 93280, 93286, 93288
    in person ~ 93279-93281, 93286, 93288
    multiple lead ~ 93281, 93286, 93288
    remote ~ 93293-93294, 93296
    single lead ~ 93279, 93286, 93288
  insertion ~ 33206-33208
    electrode ~ 33202-33203, 33210-33211,
      33216-33217, 33224-33225
    pulse generator only ~ 33212-33213, 33221

  lead placement ~ 33202-33203
  removal
    pulse generator only ~ 33233
    transvenous electrodes ~ 33234-33235
    via thoracotomy ~ 33236-33237
  repair, electrode ~ 33218-33220
  replacement
    catheter ~ 33210
    electrode ~ 33210-33211
    insertion ~ 33206-33208
    pulse generator ~ 33227-33229
  repositioning, electrode ~ 33215, 33226
  revise pocket, chest ~ 33222
  telephonic analysis ~ 93293
  upgrade ~ 33214
Pachymetry, eye ~ 76514
Packing, nasal hemorrhage ~ 30901-30906

Pain management
  epidural/intrathecal ~ 62350-62351,
    62360-62362, 99601-99602
  intravenous therapy ~ 90783-90784
Palatal augmentation prosthesis ~ 21082
Palatal lift prosthesis ~ 21083
Palate
  abscess, incision and drainage ~ 42000
  biopsy ~ 42100
  excision ~ 42120, 42145
  fracture
    closed treatment ~ 21421
    open treatment ~ 21422-21423
  lesion
    destruction ~ 42160
    excision ~ 42104-42120
  prosthesis ~ 42280-42281
  reconstruction, lengthening ~ 42226-42227
  repair
    cleft palate ~ 42200-42225
    laceration ~ 42180-42182
    Vomer flap ~ 42235
  unlisted services and procedures ~ 42299
Palate, cleft ~ see cleft palate
Palatoplasty ~ 42200-42225
Palatoschisis ~ see cleft palate
Palm
  bursa, incision and drainage ~ 26025-26030
  fasciectomy ~ 26121-26125
  fasciotomy ~ 26040-26045
  tendon, excision ~ 26170
  tendon sheath
    excision ~ 26145
    incision and drainage ~ 26020
Palsy, seventh nerve ~ see facial nerve
    paralysis
Pancreas
  anastomosis, with intestines ~ 48520-48540
  anesthesia ~ 00794
  biopsy ~ 48100
    needle biopsy ~ 48102
  cyst
    anastomosis ~ 48520-48540
    repair ~ 48500
  debridement, peripancreatic tissue ~ 48105
  excision
    ampulla of vater ~ 48148
    duct ~ 48148
    partial ~ 48140-48146, 48150, 48154, 48160
    peripancreatic tissue ~ 48105
    total ~ 48155-48160
  lesion, excision ~ 48120
  needle biopsy ~ 48102
  placement, drainage ~ 48000-48001
  pseudocyst
    drainage
      open ~ 48510
      percutaneous ~ 48511
  removal, calculi (stone) ~ 48020
  removal transplanted allograft ~ 48556
  repair, cyst ~ 48500
  suture ~ 48545

Pancreas ~ *continued*
  transplantation ~ 48160, 48550, 48554-48556
    allograft preparation ~ 48550-48552
  unlisted services and procedures ~ 48999
  X-ray with contrast ~ 74300-74305
    injection procedure ~ 48400
Pancreas, endocrine only ~ see islet cell
Pancreatectomy
  donor ~ 48550
  partial ~ 48140-48146, 48150-48154, 48160
  total ~ 48155-48160
  with transplantation ~ 48160
Pancreaticojejunostomy ~ 48548
Pancreatic DNAse ~ see DNAse
Pancreatic duct
  destruction, calculi (stone) ~ 43265
  dilation, endoscopy ~ 43271
  endoscopy ~ 43273
    collection, specimen ~ 43260
    destruction
      calculi (stone) ~ 43265
      tumor ~ 43272
    dilation ~ 43271
    removal (endoscopic)
      calculi (stone) ~ 43264
  endoscopy ~ *continued*
      foreign body ~ 43269
      stent ~ 43269
    sphincter pressure ~ 43263
    sphincterotomy ~ 43262
    tube placement ~ 43267-43268
  incision, sphincter ~ 43262
  removal
    calculi (stone) ~ 43264
    foreign body ~ 43269
    stent ~ 43269
  tube placement
    nasopancreatic ~ 43267
    stent ~ 43268
  tumor, destruction ~ 43272
  X-ray with contrast, guide catheter ~
    74329-74330
Pancreatic elastase 1 (PEL1) ~ 82656
Pancreatic islet cell ab ~ see antibody, islet
  cell
Pancreatitis, incision and drainage ~ 48000
Pancreatography
  injection procedure ~ 48400
  intraoperative ~ 74300-74301
  postoperative ~ 74305
Pancreatojejunostomies ~ see
  pancreaticojejunostomy
Pancreatorrhaphy ~ 48545
Pancreatotomy ~ see incision, pancreas
Pancreozymin-secretin test ~ 82938
Panel ~ see organ or disease oriented panel
Panniculectomy ~ see lipectomy
Paper chromatographies ~ see
  chromatography, paper
Papilla, interdental ~ see gums
Pap smears ~ 88141-88155, 88164-88167,
  88174-88175

1487

Papillectomy ~ 46220
Papilloma
  destruction ~ 54050-54065
    anus ~ 46900-46924
    penis ~ 54050-54065
PAPP D ~ see lactogen, human placental
Para-tyrosine ~ see tyrosine
Paracentesis
  abdomen ~ 49082-49083
  eye
    with aqueous aspiration ~ 65800
    with aqueous release ~ 65800
    with discission of anterior hyaloid membrane
      ~ 65810
    with removal
      blood ~ 65815
      vitreous ~ 65810
    thorax ~ 32554-32555
Paracervical nerve
  injection, anesthetic ~ 64435
Paraesophageal hiatal hernia
  repair via
    laparotomy ~ 43332-43333
    thoracoabdominal incision ~ 43336-43337
    thoracotomy ~ 43334-43335
Paraffin bath therapy ~ 97018
Paraganglioma, medullary ~ see
  pheochromocytoma
Parainfluenza virus antigen detection,
  immunofluorescence ~ 87279
Paralysis, facial nerve ~ see facial nerve
  paralysis
Paralysis, infantile ~ see polio
Paranasal sinuses ~ see sinus; sinuses
Parasites
  blood ~ 87207
  examination ~ 87169
  smear ~ 87177
Parasitic worms ~ see helminth
Parathormone ~ 83970
Parathyrin ~ see parathormone
Parathyroidectomy ~ 60500-60505
Parathyroid autotransplantation ~ 60512
Parathyroid gland
  autotransplant ~ 60512
  excision ~ 60500-60502
  exploration ~ 60500-60505
  nuclear medicine, imaging ~ 78070
Parathyroid hormone ~ 83970
Parathyroid hormone measurement ~ see
  parathormone
Parathyroid transplantation ~ see
  transplantation, parathyroid
Paraurethral gland
  abscess, incision and drainage ~ 53060
Paravertebral nerve
  destruction ~ 64633-64636
  injection
    anesthetic ~ 64470-64484
    neurolytic ~ 64633-64636
Parietal cell vagotomies ~ see vagotomy,
  highly selective

Parietal craniotomy ~ 61556
Paring
  skin lesion, benign hyperkeratotic
    more than four lesions ~ 11057
    single lesion ~ 11055
    two to four lesions ~ 11056
Paronychia, incision and drainage ~
  10060-10061
Parotid duct
  diversion ~ 42507-42510
  reconstruction ~ 42507-42510
Parotid gland
  abscess, incision and drainage ~ 42300-42305
  calculi (stone), excision ~ 42330, 42340
  excision
    partial ~ 42410-42415
    total ~ 42420-42426
  tumor, excision ~ 42410-42426
Parotitides, epidemic ~ see mumps
Pars abdominalis aortae ~ see aorta,
  abdominal
Partial
  colectomy ~ see colectomy, partial
  cystectomy ~ see cystectomy, partial
  esophagectomy ~ see esophagectomy, partial
  gastrectomy ~ see excision, stomach, partial
  glossectomy ~ see excision, tongue, partial
  hepatectomy ~ see excision, liver, partial
  mastectomies ~ see breast, excision, lesion
  nephrectomy ~ see excision, kidney, partial
  pancreatectomy ~ see pancreatectomy, partial
  splenectomy ~ see splenectomy, partial
  thromboplastin time ~ see thromboplastin,
    partial, time
  ureterectomy ~ see ureterectomy, partial
Particle agglutination ~ 86403-86406
Parvovirus antibody ~ 86747
Patch allergy tests ~ 95044
Patella
  dislocation ~ 27560-27566
  excision ~ 27350
    with reconstruction ~ 27424
  fracture ~ 27520-27524
  reconstruction ~ 27437-27438
  repair
    chondromalacia ~ 27418
    instability ~ 27420-27424
Patella, chondromalacia ~ see chondromalacia
  patella
Patellar tendon bearing (PTB) cast ~ 29435
Patellectomy with reconstruction ~ 27424
Paternity testing ~ 86910-86911
Patey's operation ~ see mastectomy, radical
Pathologic dilatation ~ see dilation
Pathology and laboratory services ~
  80000-89999
  clinical consultation ~ 80500-80502
  surgical ~ 88300-88399
    consultation ~ 88321-88325
      intraoperative ~ 88329-88334
    decalcification procedure ~ 88311
    electron microscopy ~ 88348-88349

Pathology and laboratory services ~ *continued*
gross and micro exam
level II ~ 88302
level III ~ 88304
level IV (four) ~ 88305
level V (five) ~ 88307
level VI (six) ~ 88309
gross exam, level I ~ 88300
histochemistry ~ 88313-88319
immunocytochemistry ~ 88313, 88342
immunofluorescent study ~ 88346-88347
nerve teasing ~ 88362
special stain ~ 88312-88314, 88319
tissue hybridization ~ 88365
unlisted procedures ~ 88399, 89240
Patterson's test ~ see blood urea nitrogen
Paul-Bunnell test ~ see antibody; antibody
identification; microsomal antibody
P B antibodies ~ see antibody, heterophile
PBG ~ see porphobilinogen
PCP ~ (phencyclidine) 83992
Pean's operation ~ (amputation, upper leg, at
hip) 27290
Pectoral cavity ~ see chest cavity
Pectus carinatum
reconstructive repair ~ 21740-21742
with thoracoscopy ~ 21743
Pectus excavatum
reconstructive repair ~ 21740-21742
with thoracoscopy ~ 21743
Pediatric critical care ~ 99471-99472
Pediatric intensive care ~ 99478
Pedicle fixation insertion ~ 22842-22844
Pedicle flap
formation ~ 15570-15576
island ~ 15740
neurovascular ~ 15750
transfer ~ 15650
PEEP ~ see pressure breathing, positive
Peet operation ~ see nerves, sympathectomy,
excision
Pelvi-ureteroplasty ~ see pyeloplasty
Pelvic adhesions ~ see adhesions, pelvic
Pelvic exam ~ 57410
Pelvic exenteration ~ 51597
Pelvic fixation insertion ~ 22848
Pelvic lymphadenectomy ~ 58240
Pelvimetry ~ 74710
Pelviolithotomy ~ 50130
Pelvis ~ see also hip
abscess, incision and drainage ~ 26990, 45000
angiography ~ 72191
biopsy ~ 27040-27041
bone, drainage ~ 26992
brace application ~ 20662
bursa, incision and drainage ~ 26991
CT scan ~ 72191-72194, 74176-74178
cyst
aspiration ~ 50390
injection ~ 50390
destruction, lesion ~ 58662

Pelvis ~ *continued*
endoscopy
destruction of lesion ~ 58662
lysis of adhesions ~ 58660
oviduct surgery ~ 58670-58671
exclusion, small intestine ~ 44700
exenteration ~ 45126, 58240
fasciotomy, decompression ~ 27027
with debridement ~ 27057
halo ~ 20662
hematoma, incision and drainage ~ 26990
lysis, adhesions ~ 58660
magnetic resonance angiography ~ 72198
magnetic resonance imaging (MRI) ~
72195-72197
removal, foreign body ~ 27086-27087
repair
osteotomy ~ 27158
tendon ~ 27098
ring
dislocation ~ 27193-27194, 27216-27218
fracture ~ 27216-27218
closed treatment ~ 27193-27194
tumor, excision ~ 27043-27045, 27049, 27059
ultrasound ~ 76856-76857
unlisted services and procedures for hips and
hip joint ~ 27299
X-ray ~ 72170-72190, 73540
manometry ~ 74710
Pemberton osteotomy of pelvis ~ see
osteotomy, pelvis
Penectomy ~ see amputation, penis
Penetration keratoplasties ~ see keratoplasty,
penetrating
Penile induration ~ see Peyronie disease
Penile prosthesis
insertion
inflatable ~ 54401-54405
noninflatable ~ 54400
removal
inflatable ~ 54406, 54410-54417
semi-rigid ~ 54415-54417
repair, inflatable ~ 54408
replacement
inflatable ~ 54410-54411, 54416-54417
semi-rigid ~ 54416-54417
Penile rigidity test ~ 54250
Penile tumescence test ~ 54250
Penis
amputation
partial ~ 54120
radical ~ 54130-54135
total ~ 54125
biopsy ~ 54100-54105
circumcision
with clamp or other device ~ 54150
newborn ~ 54150
repair ~ 54163
surgical excision, newborn ~ 54160

Penis ~ *continued*
excision
  partial ~ 54120
  prepuce ~ 54150-54161, 54163
  total ~ 54125-54135
  frenulum, excision ~ 54164
incision, prepuce ~ 54000-54001
incision and drainage ~ 54015
injection
  for erection ~ 54235
  peyronie disease ~ 54200
    surgical exposure plague ~ 54205
  vasoactive drugs ~ 54231
  X-ray ~ 54230
insertion, prosthesis
  inflatable ~ 54401-54405
  noninflatable ~ 54400
irrigation, priapism ~ 54220
lesion
  destruction
    cryosurgery ~ 54056
    electrodesiccation ~ 54055
    extensive ~ 54065
    laser surgery ~ 54057
    simple ~ 54050-54060
    surgical excision ~ 54060
  excision ~ 54060
    penile plague ~ 54110-54112
nocturnal penile tumescence test ~ 54250
occlusion, vein ~ 37790
plaque, excision ~ 54110-54112
plethysmography ~ 54240
prepuce, stretch ~ 54450
reconstruction
  angulation ~ 54360
  chordee ~ 54300-54304, 54328
  complications ~ 54340-54348
  epispadias ~ 54380-54390
  hypospadias ~ 54328-54352
  injury ~ 54440
removal
  foreign body ~ 54115
  prosthesis
    inflatable ~ 54406, 54410-54417
    semi-rigid ~ 54415-54417
repair
  fistulization ~ 54435
  priapism with shunt ~ 54420-54430
  prosthesis, inflatable ~ 54408
replacement, prosthesis
  inflatable ~ 54410-54411, 54416-54417
  semi-rigid ~ 54416-54417
revascularization ~ 37788
rigidity test ~ 54250
test erection ~ 54250
unlisted services and procedures ~ 55899
venous studies ~ 93980-93981
Penis adhesions
lysis, post-circumcision ~ 54162
Penis prostheses ~ see penile prosthesis
Pentagastrin test ~ see gastric analysis test
Pentamidine ~ see inhalation treatment

Peptidase P ~ see angiotensin converting enzyme (ACE)
Peptidase S ~ see leucine aminopeptidase
Peptide, connecting ~ see C-peptide
Peptide, vasoactive intestinal ~ see vasoactive intestinal peptide
Peptidyl dipeptidase A ~ see angiotensin converting enzyme (ACE)
Percutaneous abdominal paracentesis ~ see abdomen, drainage
Percutaneous atherectomies ~ see artery, atherectomy
Percutaneous biopsy, gallbladder/bile ducts ~ see bile duct, biopsy
Percutaneous discectomies ~ see diskectomy, percutaneous
Percutaneous electric nerve stimulation ~ see application, neurostimulation
Percutaneous fixation ~ 25671
Percutaneous lumbar diskectomy ~ see aspiration, nucleus of disk, lumbar
Percutaneous lysis ~ 62263-62264
Percutaneous nephrostomies ~ see nephrostomy, percutaneous
Percutaneous transluminal angioplasty
artery
  aortic ~ 35472
  brachiocephalic ~ 35475
  coronary ~ 92982-92984
  pulmonary ~ 92997-92998
  renal ~ 35471
  tibioperoneal ~ 35470
  visceral ~ 35471
venous ~ 35476
Percutaneous transluminal coronary angioplasty ~ see percutaneous transluminal angioplasty
Pereyra procedure ~ 51845, 57289, 58267
Performance measures
acute bronchitis, interventions
  antibiotics prescribed ~ 4120F-4124F
acute otitis externa/media with effusion
  hearing test ~ 3230F
  history auricular/periauricular pain ~ 1116F
  interventions
    antimicrobial therapy ~ 4131F-4132F
    effusion antihistamines/decongestants ~ 4133F-4134F
    systemic steroids ~ 4135F-4136F
    topical therapy ~ 4130F
  physical exam, membrane motility ~ 2035F
advance care plan ~ 1157F-1158F
age-related eye disease study (AREDS) ~ 4177F
anginal symptom assessment ~ 1002F
antiplatelet therapy ~ 4011F
asthma
  history
    intermittent ~ 1039F
    persistent ~ 1038F
  pharmacologic therapy ~ 4015F
  symptoms ~ 1005F

Performance measures ~ *continued*
   diastolic blood pressure ~ 3078F-3080F
   dyspnea ~ 3450F-3452F
   ECG ~ 3120F
   epilepsy
      EEG ~ 3650F
      MRI/CT scan 3324F
   erythropoietin ~ 3160F
   esophageal biopsy ~ 3150F
   flow cytometry ~ 3170F
   functional expiratory volume ~ 3040F, 3042F
   group B Streptococcus (GBS) ~ 3294F
   hemoglobin A1c ~ 3044F-3046F
   HIV ~ 3490F-3515F
   Kt/V measurement ~ 3082F-3084F
   LDL cholestorel ~ 3048F-3050F
   left ventricular ejection fraction ~ 3021F, 3022F
   left ventricular function ~ 3020F
   lipid panel ~ 3011F
   macroalbuminuria test ~ 3062F
   melanoma ~ 3321F-3322F
   microalbuminuria test 3060F-3061F
   nephropathy treatment ~ 3066F
   oxygen saturation ~ 3028F, 3035F-3037F
   pulmonary function test ~ 3038F
   retinopathy screening ~ 3072F
   rheumatoid arthritis ~ 3470F-3476F
   screening mammography ~ 3014F
   spirometry ~ 3023F-3027F
   Strep A testing ~ 3210F
   suicide risk ~ 3085F
   systolic blood pressure ~ 3074F, 3075F-3077F
   TB ~ 3455F
   thromboembolism ~ 3550F-3552F
   tumor node and metastases staging (TNM) ~3323F
   upper GI endoscopy ~ 3130F, 3132F, 3140F-3142F
   urine protein ~ 3060F-3062F
  end-stage renal disease
   dialysis plan of care ~ 0505F, 0507F
   intervention, AV fistula ~ 4051F-4055F
   test results, Kt/V measurement ~ 3082F-3084F
  epilepsy
   diagnostic screening
      electroencephalogram (EEG) ~ 3650F
      MRI/CT scan ~ 3324F
   follow-up or other outcomes
      surgical therapy considered ~ 5200F
   history
      etiology reviewed, documented ~ 1205F
      seizure type/frequency documented ~ 1200F
   interventions
      childbearing counseling ~ 4340F
      safety counseling ~ 4330F
   patient safety
      anti-epileptic drug (AED) side effects counseling ~ 6070F

Performance measures ~ *continued*
  follow up
   exam communicated ~ 5010F
   fracture documentation ~ 5015F
   mole examination ~ 5005F
   osteoporosis ~ 5015F
  gastro-esophageal reflux disease (GERD)
   history, alarm symptoms ~ 1070F-1071F
   test results
      upper endoscopy ~ 3130F, 3132F
      biopsy for Barrett's esophagus ~ 3140F-3142F, 3150F, 3200F
      barium swallow ~ 3140F-3142F, 3150F, 3200F
  geriatrics (GER)
   fall screening ~ 1100F-1101F
   history
      advance care plan ~ 1123F, 1124F
      medication reconciliation ~ 1110F-1111F
      urinary incontinence ~ 1090F-1091F
   patient management
      urinary incontinence plan ~ 0509F
  heart failure
   assessment ~ 0001F
   examination ~ 2000F-2002F
   history ~ 1003F-1004F
   intervention
      ACE/ARB ~ 4010F, 4480F-4481F
      beta-blocker ~ 4008F
   test results ~ 3020F-3022F
  hematology
   intervention ~ 4090F, 4095F, 4100F
   test results ~ 3155F, 3160F, 3170F
  hepatitis
   intervention
      antiviral therapy ~ 4150F, 4153F
      counseling ~ 4158F, 4159F
      education, alcohol ~ 4158F
      education, contraception ~ 4159F
      hepatitis A vaccination ~ 4148F, 4155F
      hepatitis B vaccination ~ 4149F, 4157F
      peginterferon & ribavirin therapy ~ 4153F
      RNA testing ~ 4150F-4151F
   test results
      genotype testing ~ 3266F
      hepatitis A immunity ~ 3215F
      hepatitis B immunity ~ 3216F
      RNA testing ~ 3218F, 3220F, 3265F
  hydration ~ 2030F-2031F
  hypertension
   blood pressure measurement ~ 2000F
   intervention plan of care ~ 4050F
   test results, plan of care ~ 3074F-3075F, 3077F-3080F
  major despressive disorder
   diagnostic/screening
      depression ~ 3351F-3354F
      severity classification ~ 3088F-3093F
      suicide risk ~ 3085F, 3092F
   history, diagnostic status ~ 1040F
   intervention
      counseling ~ 4000F

1493

Performance measures ~ *continued*
  fundus ~ 2020F-2021F
  hydration status ~ 2018F, 2030F-2031F
  macular ~ 2019F, 2021F
  major depressive disorder clinical interview
    ~ 2060F
  mental status ~ 2014F, 2044F
  optic nerve ~ 2027F
  osteoarthritis assessment ~ 2004F
  skin ~ 2029F
  vital signs ~ 2010F
  volume overload assessment ~ 2002F
  weight ~ 2001F
 prenatal-postpartum care
  diagnosis/screening
    ABO and Rh typing ~ 3293F
    D Rh typing ~ 3290F-3291F
    HIV status ~ 3292F
  patient management ~ 0500F-0503F
 preventive care & screening
  history
    tobacco use ~ 1000F, 1034F-1036F
  intervention
    pharmacologic therapy ~ 4001F
    influenza immunization ~ 4037F
    tobacco use counseling ~ 4000F, 4004F
  test results
    screening mammography ~ 3014F
    colorectal screening ~ 3017F
 statin therapy ~ 4013F
 stroke and stroke rehabilitation
  history
    anticoagulant therapy ~ 1060F-1061F
    tissue plasminogen ~ 1065F-1066F
  intervention
    anticoagulant therapy ~ 4075F
    antiplatelet therapy ~ 4073F
    rehabilitation services ~ 4079F
    thrombosis prophylaxis ~ 4070F
    tissue plasminogen ~ 4077F
  test results
    carotid imaging ~ 3100F
    lesion screening ~ 3110F-3112F
  patient safety
    dysphagia screening ~ 6010F
    swallowing eligibility ~ 6015F
    NPO order ~ 6020F
 therapeutic, preventive or other interventions
  anesthesia ~ 4255F-4256F
  anti-inflammatory/analgesic ~ 4016F
  antibiotic agent ~ 4045F, 4048F. 4049F.
    4120F. 4124F
  anticoagulant therapy ~ 4075F
  antiplatelet therapy ~ 4073F
  arterio-venous fistula ~ 4051F
  aspirin ~ 4084F
  asthma medication ~ 4015F
  beta blocker ~ 4115F
  bisphosphonate therapy ~ 4100F
  dialysis ~ 4052F-4055F
  electroconvulsive therapy ~ 4066F-4067F

Performance measures ~ *continued*
  erythropoietin therapy ~ 4090F-4095F
  gastroenteritis education ~ 4058F
  gastrointestinal prophylaxis for NSAID use
    ~ 4017F
  heart failure education ~ 4003F
  hepatitis vaccination ~ 4148F-4149F, 4275F
  hypertension care plan ~ 4050F
  influenza immunization ~ 4035F-4037F
  inhaled bronchodilator ~ 4025F
  internal mammary artery graft ~ 4110F
  oxygen therapy, long term ~ 4030F
  pharmacologic therapy ~ 4005F,
    4063F-4065F
  pneumococcal immunization ~ 4040F
  psychotherapy services ~ 4060F, 4062F
  pulmonary rehabilitation ~ 4033F
  rehabilitation services ~ 4089F
  rehydration solution ~ 4056F
  statin therapy ~ 4013F
  therapeutic exercise ~ 4018F
  thrombosis prophylaxis ~ 4070F
  tissue plasminogen administration ~ 4077F
  warfarin therapy ~ 4012F
 tobacco use
  assessment ~ 1000F
  counseling ~ 4000F
  pharmacologic therapy ~ 4001
 vital signs, documented and reviewed ~ 2010F
Performance test ~ see physical
  medicine/therapy/occupational therapy
 performance test, physical therapy ~ 97750
 psychological test ~ 96100
Perfusion
 brain, imaging ~ 0042T
 esophagus acid ~ 91030
 myocardial ~ 78451-78454
  imaging ~ 78466-78469
 positron emission tomography (PET),
  myocardial imaging ~ 78491-78492
 pulmonary ~ 78580, 78597-78598
Perfusion, intracranial arterial thrombolysis ~
  61624
Perfusion pump ~ see infusion pump
Pericardectomies ~ see excision, pericardium
Pericardial cyst ~ see cyst, pericardial
Pericardial sac drainage ~ 32659
Pericardial window for drainage ~ 33025
Pericardial window technic ~ see
  pericardiostomy
Pericardiectomy
 complete ~ 33030-33031
 subtotal ~ 33030-33031
Pericardiocentesis ~ 33010-33011
 ultrasound guidance ~ 76930
Pericardiostomy tube ~ 33015
Pericardiotomy
 removal
  clot ~ 33020
  foreign body ~ 33020

Pericardium
biopsy, endoscopic ~ 32604
cyst, excision/resection ~ 32661, 33050
diagnostic thoracoscopy ~ 32601
excision ~ 32659, 33025, 33030-33031
incision
removal
clot ~ 33020
foreign body ~ 33020
with tube ~ 33015
incision and drainage ~ 33025
puncture aspiration ~ 33010-33011
removal
clot, endoscopic ~ 32658
foreign body, endoscopic ~ 32658
tumor, excision ~ 32661, 33050
Peridural anesthesia ~ see anesthesia, epidural
Peridural injection ~ see epidural, injection
Perineal prostatectomy ~ see prostatectomy,
perineal
Perineoplasty ~ 56810
Perineorrhaphy
repair, rectocele ~ 57250
Perineum
abscess, incision and drainage ~ 56405
colposcopy ~ 99170
debridement, infected ~ 11004, 11006
removal, prosthesis ~ 53442
repair ~ 56810
X-ray with contrast ~ 74775
Perionychia ~ see paronychia
Periorbital region
reconstruction, osteotomy with graft ~
21267-21268
repair, osteotomy ~ 21260-21263
Peripheral artery disease (PAD) rehabilitation
~ 93668
Peripheral nerve repair/suture, major ~
64856, 64859
Periprosthetic capsulectomy breast ~ 19371
Peristaltic pumps ~ see infusion pump
Peritoneal dialysis ~ 90945-90947, 4055F
Kt/V level ~ 3082F-3084F
Peritoneal free air ~ see pneumoperitoneum
Peritoneal lavage ~ 49084
Peritoneoscopy ~ see endoscopy, peritoneum
Peritoneum
abscess
incision and drainage ~ 49020
percutaneous ~ 49021
endoscopy
biopsy ~ 47561
drainage, lymphocele ~ 49323
X-ray ~ 47560
exchange, drainage catheter ~ 49423
injection, contrast, via catheter ~ 49424
ligation, shunt ~ 49428
removal
cannula/catheter ~ 49422
foreign body ~ 49402
shunt ~ 49429

Peritoneum ~ *continued*
tumor, resection ~ 58950-58956
unlisted services and procedures ~ 49999
venous shunt, injection ~ 49427
X-ray ~ 74190
Persistent, omphalomesenteric duct ~ see
diverticulum, Meckel's
Persistent truncus arteriosus ~ see truncus
arteriosus
Personal care ~ see self care
Pessary insertion ~ 57160
Pesticides chlorinated hydrocarbons ~ 82441
PET ~ see positron emission tomography
Petrous temporal excision, Apex ~ 69530
Peyronie disease
with graft ~ 54110-54112
injection ~ 54200
surgical exposure ~ 54205
pH ~ *see also* blood
exhaled breath ~ 83987
other fluid ~ 83986
urine ~ 83986
Phacoemulsification
removal
extracapsular cataract ~ 66982, 66984
secondary membranous cataract ~ 66850
Phagocytosis, white blood cells ~ 86344
Phalangectomy
toe ~ 28150
partial ~ 28160
Phalanges (hand)) ~ see finger, bone
Phalanx, finger
craterization ~ 26235-26236
cyst, excision ~ 26210-26215
diaphysectomy ~ 26235-26236
excision ~ 26235-26236
radical, for tumor ~ 26260-26262
fracture
articular
closed treatment ~ 26740
with manipulation ~ 26742
open treatment ~ 26746
distal ~ 26755-26756
closed treatment ~ 26750
open treatment ~ 26765
percutaneous fixation ~ 26756
open treatment ~ 26735
distal ~ 26765
shaft ~ 26720-26727
open treatment ~ 26735
incision and drainage ~ 26034
ostectomy, radical, for tumor ~ 26260-26262
repair
lengthening ~ 26568
nonunion ~ 26546
osteotomy ~ 26567
saucerization ~ 26235-26236
thumb fracture, shaft ~ 26720-26727
tumor, excision ~ 26210-26215

1495

Phalanx, great toe ~ see also phalanx, toe
fracture ~ 28490
  with manipulation ~ 28495-28496
  open treatment ~ 28505
  without manipulation ~ 28490
  percutaneous fixation ~ 28496
Phalanx, toe
condyle, excision ~ 28126
craterization ~ 28124
cyst, excision ~ 28108
diaphysectomy ~ 28124
excision ~ 28124, 28150-28160
fracture
  with manipulation ~ 28515
  without manipulation ~ 28510
  open treatment ~ 28525
repair, osteotomy ~ 28310-28312
saucerization ~ 28124
tumor, excision ~ 28108, 28175
Pharmaceutic preparations ~ see drug
Pharmacotherapies ~ see chemotherapy
Pharyngeal tonsil ~ see adenoids
Pharyngectomy partial ~ 42890
Pharyngolaryngectomy ~ 31390-31395
Pharyngoplasty ~ 42950
Pharyngorrhaphy ~ see suture, pharynx
Pharyngostomy ~ 42955
Pharyngotomy ~ see incision, pharynx
Pharyngotympanic tube ~ see eustachian tube
Pharynx ~ see also nasopharynx; throat
biopsy ~ 42800-42806
cineradiography ~ 70371, 74230
creation, stoma ~ 42955
excision ~ 42145
  with larynx ~ 31390-31395
  partial ~ 42890
  resection ~ 42892-42894
hemorrhage ~ 42960-42962
lesion
  destruction ~ 42808
  excision ~ 42808
reconstruction ~ 42950
removal, foreign body ~ 42809
repair, with esophagus ~ 42953
unlisted services and procedures ~ 42999
video study ~ 70371, 74230
X-ray ~ 70370, 74210
Phencyclidine ~ 83992
Phenobarbital ~ 82205
assay ~ 80184
Phenothiazine ~ 84022
Phenotype
analysis
  by nucleic acid, infectious agent
    HIV-1 drug resistance ~ 87903-87904
prediction
  by genetic database
    HIV-1 drug resistance ~ 0023T
Phenylalanine ~ 84030
Phenylalanine-tyrosine ratio ~ 84030
Phenylketones ~ 84035
Phenylketonuria ~ see phenylalanine

Phenytoin assay ~ 80185-80186
Pheochromocytoma ~ 80424
Pheresis ~ see apheresis
Phlebectasia ~ see varicose vein
Phlebectomy varicose veins ~ 37765-37766
Phlebographies ~ see venography
Phleborrhaphy ~ see suture, vein
Phlebotomy therapeutic ~ 99195
Phoria ~ see strabismus
Phosphatase
alkaline ~ 84075, 84080
blood ~ 84078
forensic examination ~ 84061
Phosphatase acid ~ 84060
blood ~ 84066
Phosphate, pyridoxal ~ see pyridoxal
phosphate
Phosphatidylcholine cholinephosphohydrolase
~ see tissue typing
Phosphatidylglycerol ~ 84081
Phosphatidyl glycerol ~ see
phosphatidylglycerol
Phosphocreatine phosphotransferase, ADP ~
see CPK
Phosphogluconate-6 dehydrogenase ~ 84085
Phosphoglycerides, glycerol ~ see
phosphatidylglycerol
Phosphohexose isomerase ~ 84087
Phosphohydrolases ~ see phosphatase
Phosphokinase, creatine ~ see CPK
Phospholipase C ~ see tissue typing
Phospholipid antibody ~ 86147
Phosphomonoesterase ~ see phosphatase
Phosphoric monoester hydrolases ~ see
phosphatase
Phosphorus ~ 84100
urine ~ 84105
Phosphotransferase, ADP phosphocreatine ~
see CPK
Photo patch allergy test ~ see allergy tests ~
95052
Photochemotherapies, extracorporeal ~ see
photopheresis
Photochemotherapy ~ see dermatology ~
96910-96913
endoscopic light ~ 96570-96571
Photocoagulation
endolaser panretinal, vitrectomy ~ 67040
focal endolaser, vitrectomy ~ 67040
Photocoagulation ~ continued
iridoplasty ~ 66762
lesion
  cornea ~ 65450
  retina ~ 67210, 67227-67228
retinal detachment
  prophylaxis ~ 67145
  repair ~ 67105
Photodynamic therapy ~ 96567-96571
Photography skin, diagnostic ~ 96904
Photography, ocular ~ see ophthalmoscopy,
diagnostic
Photopheresis extracorporeal ~ 36522

Photophoresis ~ see actinotherapy;
  photochemotherapy
Photoradiation therapies ~ see actinotherapy
Photoscreen ocular ~ 99174
Photosensitivity testing ~ see allergy tests ~
  95056
Phototherapies ~ see actinotherapy
Phototherapy, ultraviolet ~ see actinotherapy
Phrenic nerve
  anastomosis, to facial nerve ~ 64870
  avulsion ~ 64746
  incision ~ 64746
  injection, anesthetic ~ 64410
  transection ~ 64746
**Physical medicine/therapy/occupational
  therapy**
  activities of daily living ~ 97535, 99509
  aquatic therapy, with exercises ~ 97113
  athletic training
    evaluation ~ 97005
    re-evaluation ~ 97006
  check-out, orthotic/prosthetic ~ 97762
  cognitive skills development ~ 97532
  community/work reintegration ~ 97537
  evaluation ~ 97001-97006
  kinetic therapy ~ 97530
  manual therapy ~ 97140
  modalities
    contrast baths ~ 97034
    diathermy treatment ~ 97024
    electric simulation
      unattended ~ 97014
      attended, manual ~ 97032
    hot or cold pack ~ 97010
    hydrotherapy (Hubbard tank) ~ 97036
    infrared light treatment ~ 97026
    iontophoresis ~ 97033
    microwave therapy ~ 97024
    paraffin bath ~ 97018
    traction ~ 97012
    ultrasound ~ 97035
    ultraviolet light ~ 97028
    unlisted services and procedures ~ 97039
    vasopneumatic device ~ 97016
    whirlpool therapy ~ 97022
  orthotics training ~ 97760
  osteopathic manipulation ~ 98925-98929
  procedures
    aquatic therapy ~ 97113
    gait training ~ 97116
    group therapeutic ~ 97150
    massage therapy ~ 97124
    neuromuscular reeducation ~ 97112
    physical performance test ~ 97750
    therapeutic exercises ~ 97110
    traction therapy ~ 97140
    work hardening ~ 97545-97546
  prosthetic training ~ 97761
  sensory integration ~ 97533
  therapeutic activities ~ 97530
  unlisted services and procedures ~ 97139,
    97799

**Physical medicine/therapy/occupational
  therapy** ~ *continued*
  wheelchair management/propulsion ~ 97542
  work reintegration ~ 97537
Physician services
  care plan oversight services ~ 99339-99340,
    99374-99380
    documentation of plan, surrogate decision
      maker ~ 1123F, 1124F
    domiciliary facility ~ 99339-99340
    home health agency care ~ 99374
    home or rest home care ~ 99339-99340
    hospice ~ 99377-99378
    nursing facility ~ 99379-99380
  case management services ~ 99366-99368
  direction, advanced life support ~ 99288
  online ~ 99444
  prolonged
    with direct patient contact ~ 99354-99357
      outpatient/office ~ 99354-99355
    with direct patient services inpatient ~
      99356-99357
    without direct patient contact ~ 99358-99359
  standby ~ 99360
  supervision, care plan oversight services ~
    99339-99340, 99374-99380
    documentation of plan, surrogate decision
      maker ~ 1123F, 1124F
  team conference ~ 99367
  telephone ~ 99441-99443
Piercing of ear lobe ~ 69090
Piles ~ see hemorrhoids
Pilonidal cyst
  excision ~ 11770-11772
  incision and drainage ~ 10080-10081
Pin ~ see also wire
  insertion/removal, skeletal traction ~ 20650
  prophylactic treatment
    femur ~ 27187
    humerus ~ 24498
    shoulder ~ 23490-23491
Pinch graft ~ 15050
Pinna ~ see ear, external
Pinworms examination ~ 87172
Pirogoff procedure ~ 27888
Pituitary epidermoid tumor ~ see
  craniopharyngioma
Pituitary gland
  excision ~ 61546-61548
  tumor, excision ~ 61546-61548, 62165
Pituitary growth hormone ~ see growth
  hormone
Pituitary lactogenic hormone ~ see prolactin
Pituitectomy ~ see excision, pituitary gland
PKU ~ see phenylalanine
Placement
  bronchial stent ~ 31636-31637
  catheter
    bile duct ~ 75982
    breast, for interstitial radioelement
      application ~ 19296-19298

1497

Placement ~ *continued*
  bronchus, for intracavitary radioelement
    application (see also catheterization) ~
    31643
  catheter, cardiac (see also catheterization,
    cardiac) ~ 93503
  colonic stent ~ 44397, 45327, 45345, 45387
  drainage, pancreas ~ 48001
  guidance
    catheter
      abscess ~ 75989
      bile ~ 75982
      specimen ~ 75989
    prosthesis
      thoracic aorta ~ 75958-75959
  interstitial device
    abdomen ~ 49327, 49411-49412
    lungs ~ 32553
    omentum ~ 49411-49412
    pelvis ~ 49411-49412
    pleura ~ 32553
    peritoneum ~ 49411-49412
    prostate ~ 55876
    retroperitoneum ~ 49411-49412
  intravascular stent
    coronary ~ 92980-92981
    intracranial ~ 61635
  jejunostomy tube
    endoscopic ~ 44372
    percutaneous ~ 49441
  metallic localization clip, breast ~ 19295
  nasogastric tube ~ 43752
  needle
    bone ~ 36680
    interstitial radioelement application
      genitalia ~ 55920
      head ~ 41019
      muscle ~ 20555
      neck ~ 41019
      pelvic organs ~ 55920
      soft tissue ~ 20555
      prostate ~ 55875
  needle wire, breast ~ 19290-19291
  orogastric tube ~ 43752
  pressure sensor ~ 34806
  radiation delivery device, intracoronary artery
    ~ 92974
  seton, anal ~ 46020
  tracheal stent ~ 31631
  transcatheter pressure sensor ~ 34806
  ureteral stent ~ 50947
Placenta delivery ~ 59414
Placental lactogen ~ see lactogen, human
  placental
Placental villi ~ see chorionic villus
Plagiocephaly ~ 21175
Plague vaccine ~ 90727
Planing nose, skin ~ 30120
Plantar common digital nerve
  destruction, neurolytic ~ 64632
Plantar digital nerve decompression ~ 64726

Plantar pressure measurements dynamic ~
  96001, 96004
Plasma frozen preparation ~ 86927
Plasma prokallikrein ~ see Fletcher factor
Plasma protein-A, pregnancy-associated
  (PAPP-A) ~ 84163
Plasma test volume determination ~
  78110-78111
Plasma thromboplastin
  antecedent ~ 85270
  component ~ 85250
Plasmin ~ 85400
Plasmin antiactivator ~ see alpha-2
  antiplasmin
Plasminogen ~ 85420-85421
Plasmodium antibody ~ 86750
Plastic repair of mouth ~ see mouth, repair
Plate, bone ~ see bone plate
Platelet ~ see also blood cell count, complete
  blood count
  aggregation ~ 85576
  antibody ~ 86022-86023
  assay ~ 85055
  blood ~ 85025
  count ~ 85032, 85049
  neutralization ~ 85597
Platelet cofactor I ~ see clotting factor
Platelet test survival test ~ 78190-78191
Platysmal flap ~ 15825
PLC ~ see tissue typing
Pleoptic training ~ 92065
Plethysmography ~ see also vascular studies
  extremities ~ 93922-93923
  veins ~ 93965
  penis ~ 54240
  pulmonary ~ 94706
Pleura
  biopsy ~ 32098, 32400, 32609
  decortication ~ 32320
  empyema, excision ~ 32540
  excision ~ 32310-32320
    endoscopic ~ 32656
  foreign body, removal ~ 32150-32151
  needle biopsy ~ 32400
  removal, foreign body ~ 32653
  repair ~ 32215
  thoracotomy ~ 32098, 32100
  unlisted services and procedures ~ 32999
Pleural cavity
  aspiration ~ 32554-32555
  catheterization ~ 32550, 32552
  chemotherapy administration ~ see also
    chemotherapy ~ 96440
  incision
    empyema ~ 32035-32036
    pneumothorax ~ 32551
  instillation of agent for
    fibrinolysis ~ 32561-32562
    pleurodesis ~ 32560
  puncture and drainage ~ 32554-32555
  thoracostomy ~ 32035-32036
Pleural endoscopies ~ see thoracoscopy

Pleural scarification for repeat pneumothorax ~ 32215
Pleural tap ~ see thoracentesis
Pleurectomy
anesthesia ~ 00542
parietal ~ 32310-32320
endoscopic ~ 32656
Pleuritis, purulent ~ see abscess, thorax
Pleurocentesis ~ see thoracentesis
Pleurodesis
chemical ~ 32560
endoscopic ~ 32650
Pleurosclerosis ~ see pleurodesis
Plexectomy, choroid ~ see choroid plexus, excision
Plexus, choroid ~ see choroid plexus
Plexus brachialis ~ see brachial plexus
Plexus cervicalis ~ see cervical plexus
Plexus coeliacus ~ see celiac plexus
Plexus lumbalis ~ see lumbar plexus
PLGN ~ see plasminogen
Plication, sphincter, urinary bladder ~ see bladder, repair, neck
Pneumocentesis lung ~ 32405
Pneumocisternogram ~ see cisternography
Pneumococcal vaccine ~ 90669, 90670, 90732
Pneumocystis carinii antigen detection, immunofluorescence ~ 87281
Pneumogastric nerve ~ see vagus nerve
Pneumogram pediatric ~ 94772
Pneumolysis ~ 32940
Pneumonectomy ~ 32440-325445
completion ~ 32488
donor ~ 32850, 33930
sleeve ~ 32442
thoracoscopic ~ 32671
Pneumonology ~ see pulmonology
Pneumonolysis ~ 32940
intrapleural ~ 32652
open intrapleural ~ 32124
Pneumonostomy ~ 32200-32201
Pneumonotomy ~ see incision, lung
Pneumoperitoneum ~ 49400
Pneumothorax
chemical pleurodesis ~ 32560
pleural scarification for repeat ~ 32215
therapeutic, injection intrapleural air ~ 32960
thoracentesis with tube insertion ~ 32555
Polio
antibody ~ 86658
vaccine ~ 90712-90713
Poliovirus vaccine, inactivated ~ see vaccines
Pollicization digit ~ 26550
Polya gastrectomy ~ see gastrectomy, partial
Polydactylism ~ see supernumerary digit
Polydactylous digit
reconstruction ~ 26587
repair ~ 26587
Polydactyly, toes ~ 28344

Polyp
antrochoanal, removal ~ 31032
esophagus, ablation ~ 43228
nose, excision
endoscopic ~ 31237-31240
extensive ~ 30115
simple ~ 30110
sphenoid sinus, removal ~ 31051
urethra, excision ~ 53260
Polypectomy
nose, endoscopic ~ 31237
uterus ~ 58558
Polypeptide, vasoactive intestinal ~ see vasoactive intestinal peptide
Polysomnography ~ 95808-95811
Polyuria test ~ see water load test
Pomeroy's operation ~ (tubal ligation) 58600
Pooling blood products ~ 86965
Popliteal arteries ~ see artery, popliteal
Popliteal synovial cyst ~ see Baker's cyst
Poradenitistras ~ see lymphogranuloma venereum
PORP (partial ossicular replacement prosthesis) ~ 69633, 69637
Porphobilinogen urine ~ 84106-84110
Porphyrin precursors ~ 82135
Porphyrins
feces ~ 84126-84127
urine ~ 84119-84120
Portal vein ~ see vein, hepatic portal
Porter-Silber test ~ see corticosteroid, blood
Portoenterostomies, hepatic ~ see hepaticoenterostomy
Port film ~ 77417
Portoenterostomy ~ 47701
Posadas-Wernicke disease ~ see coccidioidomycosis
Positional nystagmus test ~ see nystagmus tests, positional
Positive-pressure breathing, inspiratory ~ see intermittent positive pressure breathing (IPPB)
Positive end expiratory pressure ~ see pressure breathing, positive
Positron emission tomography (PET)
brain ~ 78608-78609
heart ~ 78459
myocardial imaging, perfusion study ~ 78491-78492
Post-op visit ~ 99024
Postauricular fistula ~ see fistula, postauricular
Postcaval ureter ~ see retrocaval ureter
Postmortem ~ see autopsy
Postoperative wound infection incision and drainage ~ 10180
Postop vas reconstruction ~ see vasovasorrhaphy
Postpartum care
cesarean delivery ~ 59515
after attempted vaginal delivery ~ 59622
previous ~ 59610, 59614-59618, 59622
vaginal delivery ~ 59430
after previous cesarean delivery ~ 59614

1499

Potassium ~ 84132
　urine ~ 84133
Potential, auditory evoked ~ see auditory
　evoked potentials
Potential, evoked ~ see evoked potential
Potts-Smith procedure ~ 33762
Pouch, Kock ~ see Kock pouch
PPP ~ see fibrin degradation products
PRA ~ see cytotoxic screen
Prealbumin ~ 84134
Prebeta lipoproteins ~ see lipoprotein, blood
Pregl's test ~ (cystourethroscopy,
　catheterization, urethral) 52005
Pregnancy
　abortion
　　induced ~ 59855-59857
　　　by amniocentesis injection ~ 59850-59852
　　　by dilation and curettage ~ 59840
　　　by dilation and evaluation ~ 59841
　　　septic ~ 59830
　　therapeutic
　　　by dilation and curettage ~ 59851
　　　by hysterectomy ~ 59852
　　　by saline ~ 59850
　cesarean delivery ~ 59618-59622
　　with hysterectomy ~ 59525
　　only ~ 59514
　　postpartum care ~ 59514-59515
　　routine care ~ 59510
　　vaginal birth after ~ 59610-59614
　ectopic
　　abdominal ~ 59130
　　cervix ~ 59140
　　interstitial
　　　partial resection uterus ~ 59136
　　　total hysterectomy ~ 59135
　　laparoscopy
　　　with salpingectomy and/or oophorectomy
　　　　~ 59151
　　　without salpingectomy and/or
　　　　oophorectomy ~ 59150
　　tubal ~ 59121
　　　with salpingectomy and/or oophorectomy
　　　　~ 59120
　miscarriage
　　surgical completion
　　　any trimester ~ 59812
　　　first trimester ~ 59820
　　　second trimester ~ 59821
　molar ~ see also hydatidiform mole
　multifetal reduction ~ 59866
　placenta delivery ~ 59414
　test ~ 84702-84703
　　urinalysis ~ 81025
　vaginal delivery ~ 59409-59410
　　antepartum care ~ 59425-59426
　　after cesarean delivery ~ 59610-59614
　　postpartum care ~ 59430
　　total obstetrical care ~ 59400, 59610, 59618
Pregnanediol ~ 84135
Pregnanetriol ~ 84138
Pregnenolone ~ 84140

Prekallikrein ~ see Fletcher factor
Prekallikrein factor ~ 85292
Premature, closure, cranial suture ~ see
　craniosynostosis
Prenatal procedure ~ 59897
　amnioinfusion, transabdominal ~ 59070
　drainage, fluid ~ 59074
　occlusion, umbilical cord ~ 59072
　stunt ~ 59076
Prenatal testing
　amniocentesis ~ 59000
　　with amniotic fluid reduction ~ 59001
　chorionic villus sampling ~ 59015
　cordocentesis ~ 59012
　fetal blood sample ~ 59030
　fetal monitoring ~ 59050
　　interpretation only ~ 59051
　non-stress test, fetal ~ 59025, 99500
　oxytocin stress test ~ 59020
　stress test, oxytocin ~ 59020
　ultrasound ~ 76801-76817
　　fetal biophysical profile ~ 76818-76819
　　fetal heart ~ 76825
Prentiss operation ~ see orchiopexy, inguinal
　approach
Preparation
　for transfer, embryo ~ 89255
　thawing
　　embryo, cryopreserved ~ 89352
　　oocytes, cryopreserved ~ 89356
　　reproductive tissue, cryopreserved ~ 89354
　　sperm, cryopreserved ~ 89353
Presacral sympathectomy ~ see
　sympathectomy, presacral
Prescription
　contact lens (see also contact lens services) ~
　　92310-92317
　ocular prosthesis (see also prosthesis, ocular)
　　~ 92330-92335
Pressure, blood ~ see blood pressure
Pressure, venous ~ see blood pressure, venous
Pressure breathing ~ (see also pulmonology,
　therapeutic)
　negative, continuous (CNP) ~ 94662
　positive, continuous (CPAP) ~ 94660
Pressure measurement of sphincter of Oddi ~
　see sphincter of Oddi, pressure measurement
Pressure ulcer (decubitus) ~ see debridement;
　skin graft and flap
Pressure ulcers excision ~ 15920-15999
Pretreatment
　red blood cell
　　antibody identification ~ 86970-86972
　serum
　　antibody identification ~ 86975-86978
Prevention & control ~ see prophylaxis
Preventive medicine ~ 99381-994397
　administration/interpretation of health risk
　　assessment ~ 99420
　counseling and/or risk factor reduction
　　intervention ~ 99401-99429
　　behavior change ~ 99406-99409

1500

Preventive medicine ~ *continued*
   group counseling ~ 99411-99412
   individual counseling ~ 99401-99404
   established patient ~ 99382-99397
   new patient ~ 99381-99387
   newborn care ~ 99461
   respiratory pattern recording ~ 94772
   self-exam for moles ~ 5005F
   unlisted services and procedures ~ 99429
Priapism
   repair
     fistulization ~ 54435
     with shunt ~ 54420-54430
Primidone assay ~ 80188
PRL ~ see prolactin
Pro-insulin C peptide ~ see C-peptide
Proalbumin ~ see prealbumin
Probes, DNA ~ see nucleic acid probe
Probes, nucleic acid ~ see nucleic acid probe
Procainamide assay ~ 80190-80192
Procalcitonin (PCT) ~ 84145
Procedure, Fontan ~ see repair, heart, anomaly
Procedure, maxillofacial ~ see maxillofacial
   procedures
Process, odontoid ~ see odontoid process
Procidentia
   rectum
     excision ~ 45130-45135
     repair ~ 45900
Procoagulant activity, glomerular ~ see
   thromboplastin
Proconvertin ~ 85230
Proctectasis ~ see dilation, rectum
Proctectomy
   partial ~ 45111, 45113-45116, 45123
   total ~ 45110, 45112, 45119-45120
     with colon ~ 45121
     with colectomy ~ 44157-44158
     with ileostomy ~ 44212
Proctocele ~ see rectocele
Proctopexy ~ 45540-45541
   with sigmoid excision ~ 45550
Proctoplasty ~ 45500-45505
Proctorrhaphy ~ see rectum, suture
Proctoscopies ~ see anoscopy
Proctosigmoidoscopy
   ablation, polyp or lesion ~ 45320
   biopsy ~ 45305
   destruction, tumor ~ 45320
   dilation ~ 45303
   exploration ~ 45300
   hemorrhage control ~ 45317
   placement, stent ~ 45327
   removal
     foreign body ~ 45307
     polyp ~ 45308-45315
     tumor ~ 45315
   volvulus repair ~ 45321
Products, gene ~ see protein
Proetz therapy nose ~ 30210
Profibrinolysin ~ see plasminogen
Progenitor cell ~ see stem cell

Progesterone ~ 84144
Progesterone receptors ~ 84234
Progestin receptors ~ see progesterone
   receptors
Proinsulin ~ 84206
Projective test ~ 96100
Prokallikrein ~ see Fletcher factor
Prokallikrein, plasma ~ see Fletcher factor
Prokinogenase ~ see Fletcher factor
Prolactin ~ 80418, 80440, 84146
Prolapse ~ see procidentia
Prolapse, rectal ~ see procidentia, rectum
Prolastin ~ see alpha-1 antitrypsin
Prolonged services ~ 99354-99357, 99360
   without direct patient contact ~ 99358-99359
Prophylactic treatment
   antibiotic ~ 4045F, 4047F-4049F
   antimicrobial ~ 4046F
   cefazolin or cefuroxime ~ 4041F-4043F
   femoral neck or proximal femur
     nailing, pinning or wiring ~ 27187
   femur
     nailing, pinning or wiring ~ 27495
   humerus
     pinning, wiring ~ 24498
   radius
     nailing, pinning, plating or wiring ~ 25490,
     25492
   shoulder
     clavicle ~ 23490
     humerus ~ 23491
   tibia ~ 27745
   ulna
     nailing, pinning, plating or wiring ~
     25491-25492
   venous thromboembolism (VTE) ~ 4044F
Prophylaxis
   anticoagulant therapy ~ 4075F
   deep vein thrombosis (DVT) ~ 4070F
   retina detachment
     cryotherapy, diathermy ~ 67141
     photocoagulation ~ 67145
Prostaglandin ~ 84150
   insertion ~ 59200
Prostanoids ~ see prostaglandin
Prostate
   ablation, cryosurgery ~ 55873
   abscess, drainage ~ 52700
     incision and drainage ~ 55720-55725
   biopsy ~ 55700-55706
     transperineal ~ 55706
   brachytherapy, needle insertion ~ 55875-55976
   coagulation, laser ~ 52647
   destruction
     cryosurgery ~ 55873
     thermotherapy ~ 53850-53852
       microwave ~ 53850
       radio frequency ~ 53852
   enucleation, laser ~ 52649
   excision
     partial ~ 55801, 55821-55831
     perineal ~ 55801-55815

Prostate ~ *continued*
   radical ~ 55810-55815, 55840-55845
   retropubic ~ 55831-55845
   suprapubic ~ 55821
   transurethral ~ 52402, 52601, 52630
  exploration, exposure ~ 55860
   with nodes ~ 55862-55865
  incision
   exposure ~ 55860-55865
   transurethral ~ 52450
  insertion
   catheter or needle ~ 55875
   radioactive substance ~ 55860
  needle biopsy ~ 55700
   transperineal ~ 55706
  placement
   catheter ~ 55875
   dosimeter ~ 55876
   fiducial marker ~ 55876
   interstitial device ~ 55876
   needle ~ 55875
  thermotherapy, transurethral ~ 53850-53852
  ultrasound ~ 76872-76873
  unlisted services and procedures ~ 55899
   urinary system ~ 53899
  urethra, stent insertion ~ 52282, 53855
  vaporization, laser ~ 52648
Prostate specific antigen ~ 84152-84154
Prostatectomy ~ 52601
  laparoscopic ~ 55866
  perineal
   partial ~ 55801
   radical ~ 55810-55815
  retropubic
   partial ~ 55831
   radical ~ 55840-55845, 55866
  suprapubic, partial ~ 55821
  transurethral ~ 52630
Prostatic abscess ~ see abscess, prostate
Prostatotomy ~ 55720-55725
Prosthesis
  augmentation, mandibular body ~ 21125
  auricular ~ 21086
  breast
   insertion ~ 19340-19342
   removal ~ 19328-19330
   supply ~ 19396
  check-out ~ see also physical
   medicine/therapy/occupational therapy ~
   97703
  cornea ~ 65770
  facial ~ 21088
  hernia, mesh ~ 49568
  hip, removal ~ 27090-27091
  intestines ~ 44700
  knee, insertion ~ 27438, 27445
  lens
   not associated with concurrent cataract
   removal ~ 66985
   insertion ~ 66982-66985
   manual or mechanical technique ~
   66982-66984

Prosthesis ~ *continued*
  mandibular resection ~ 21081
  nasal ~ 21087
  nasal septum, insertion ~ 30220
  obturator ~ 21076
   definitive ~ 21080
   interim ~ 21079
  ocular ~ 21077, 65770, 66982-66985,
   92330-92335, 92358, 92393
   fitting and prescription ~ 92330
   loan ~ 92358
   prescription ~ 92335
   supply ~ 92393
  orbital ~ 21077
   partial or total ~ 69633, 69637
  ossicle reconstruction, chain ~ 69633
  palatal augmentation ~ 21082
  palatal lift ~ 21083
  palate ~ 42280-42281
  penile
   insertion ~ 54400-54405
   removal ~ 54406, 54410-54417
   repair ~ 54408
   replacement ~ 54410-54411, 54416-54417
  perineum, removal ~ 53442
  skull plate
   removal ~ 62142
   replacement ~ 62143
  spectacle ~ *continued*
   fitting ~ 92352-92353
   repair ~ 92371
  speech aid ~ 21084
  spinal, insertion ~ 22851
  synthetic ~ 69633, 69637
  temporomandibular joint, arthroplasty ~ 21243
  testicular, insertion ~ 54660
  training ~ 97520
  urethral sphincter
   insertion ~ 53444-53445
   removal ~ 53446-53447
   repair ~ 53449
   replacement ~ 53448
  wrist, removal ~ 25250-25251
Protease F ~ see plasmin
Protein
  C-reactive ~ 86140-86141
  glycated ~ 82985
  myelin basic ~ 83873
  osteocalcin ~ 83937
  prealbumin ~ 84134
  serum ~ 84155, 84165
  total ~ 84155-84160
  urine ~ 84156
  western blot ~ 84181-84182, 88372
Protein analysis, tissue western blot ~ 88371
Protein C activator ~ 85337
Protein C antigen ~ 85302
Protein C assay ~ 85303
Protein C resistance assay ~ 85307
Protein S
  assay ~ 85306
  total ~ 85305

Prothrombase ~ see thrombokinase
Prothrombin ~ 85210
Prothrombinase ~ see thromboplastin
Prothrombin time ~ 85610-85611
Prothrombokinase ~ 85230
Protime ~ see prothrombin time
Proton treatment delivery
    complex ~ 77525
    intermediate ~ 77523
    simple ~ 77520-77522
Protoporphyrin ~ 84202-84203
Protozoa antibody ~ 86753
Provitamin A ~ see vitamin, A
Provocation test ~ see also allergy tests
    for glaucoma ~ 92140
Prower factor ~ see Stuart-Prower factor
PSA ~ see prostate specific antigen
Pseudocyst, pancreas ~ see pancreas,
    pseudocyst
PSG ~ see polysomnography
Psoriasis treatment ~ (see also dermatology;
    photochemotherapy) 96910-96922
Psychiatric diagnosis
    evaluation of records or reports ~ 90885
    evaluation ~ 90791
    with medical services ~ 90792
    interactive complexity ~ 90785
    major depressive disorder (MDD) ~
        3088F-3093F
    psychological testing ~ 96101-96103, 96125
    computer assisted ~ 96103
    suicide risk assessment ~ 3085F
    unlisted services and procedures ~ 90899
Psychiatric treatment
    biofeedback training ~ 90875-90876
    consultation with family ~ 90887
    drug management ~ 90863
    electroconvulsive therapy ~ 90870, 4066F
        referral documented ~ 4067F
    environmental intervention ~ 90882
    family ~ 90846-90849, 99510
    group ~ 90853
    hypnotherapy ~ 90880
    narcosynthesis analysis ~ 90865
    pharmacotherapy
        antidepressant ~ 4063F-4064F
        antipsychotic ~ 4065F
        drug management ~ 90863
    psychoanalysis ~ 90845
    report preparation ~ 90889
    suicide risk assessment ~ 3085F
    transcranial magnetic stimulation ~
        90867-90869
    unlisted services and procedures ~ 90899
Psychoanalysis ~ 90845
Psychophysiologic feedback ~ see biofeedback
Psychotherapy
    family of patient ~ 90846-90847
    for crisis ~ 90839-90840
    group other than multifamily ~ 90853

Psychotherapy ~ *continued*
    individual patient/family member ~
        90832-90834, 90836-90838
    interactive complexity ~ 90785
    major depressive disorder ~ 4060F-4062F
    multifamily ~ 90849
    referral, documented ~ 4062F
    with pharmacologic management ~ 90863
PTA (clotting factor XI (eleven)) ~ 85270
PTA (percutaneous transluminal angioplasty)
    ~ 35471, 85270. 92997, 92998
PTB (patellar tendon bearing) cast ~ 29435
**PTC (clotting factor IX (nine); Christmas
    factor)** ~ 85250
**PTCA (percutaneous transluminal coronary
    angioplasty)**
    aortic ~ 35472
    brachiocephalic ~ 35475
    coronary ~ 92982-92984
    pulmonary ~ 92997-92998
    renal ~ 35471
    visceral ~ 35471
Pteroylglutamic acid ~ see folic acid
Pterygium
    excision ~ 65420
    with graft ~ 65426
Pterygomaxillary fossa incision ~ 31040
Pterygopalatine ganglion ~ see sphenopalatine
    ganglion
PTH ~ see parathormone
Ptosis ~ see blepharoptosis; procidentia
PTT ~ see thromboplastin, partial, time
Ptyalectasis ~ see dilation, salivary duct
Pubic symphysis ~ 27282
Pubis
    craterization ~ 27070
    cyst, excision ~ 27065-27067
    excision ~ 27070
    saucerization ~ 27070
    tumor, excision ~ 27065-27067
Pudendal nerve
    avulsion ~ 64761
    destruction ~ 64630
    incision ~ 64761
    injection
        anesthetic ~ 64430
        neurolytic ~ 64630
    transection ~ 64761
Puestow procedure ~ 48548
Pulled elbow ~ see nursemaid elbow
Pulmonary artery ~ 33690
    banding ~ 33620
    catheterization ~ see also catheterization,
        pulmonary artery
    embolism ~ 33910-33916
    excision ~ 33910-33916
    percutaneous transluminal angioplasty ~
        92997-92998
    reimplantation ~ 33788
    repair ~ 33620, 33690, 33917-33920
        reimplantation ~ 33788

Pulmonary artery ~ continued
shunt
from aorta ~ 33755-33762, 33924
subclavian ~ 33750
from vena cava ~ 33766-33767
transection ~ 33922
Pulmonary function test ~ see pulmonology, diagnostic
Pulmonary hemorrhage ~ see hemorrhage, lung
Pulmonary medical services ~ 94010-94799
Pulmonary perfusion imaging ~ 78580, 78597, 78598
Pulmonary valve
implantation, prosthesis ~ 0262T
incision ~ 33470-33474
repair ~ 33470-33474
replacement ~ 33475
Pulmonary vein
repair
complete ~ 33730
partial ~ 33724
stenosis ~ 33726
stenosis
repair ~ 33726
Pulmonology
diagnostic
airway closing volume ~ 94727
apnea monitoring, pediatric ~ 94774-94777
bronchodilation ~ 94664
bed testing, neonate ~ 94780-94781
car seat testing, neonate ~ 94780-94781
carbon dioxide response curve ~ 94400
carbon monoxide diffusion capacity ~ 94729
expired gas analysis
CO2 ~ 94770
NO ~ 95012
O2 and CO2 ~ 94681
O2 update, direct ~ 94680
O2 uptake, indirect ~ 94690
quantitative ~ 94250
flow-volume loop ~ 94375
hemoglobin O2 affinity ~ 82820
high altitutde simulation test (HAST) ~ 94452-9444-53
hypoxia response curve ~ 94450
inhalation treatment ~ 94640
maximum breathing capacity ~ 94200
maximal voluntary ventilation ~ 94200
membrane compliance ~ 94750
membrane diffusion capacity ~ 94729
oximetry, ear or pulse ~ 94760-94762
resistance to airflow ~ 94726, 94728
spirometry ~ 94010-94070
evaluation ~ 94010-94070
patient initiated with bronchospasm ~ 94014-94016
sputum mobilization with inhalants ~ 94664
stress test ~ 94621
stress test, pulmonary ~ 94620

Pulmonology ~ continued
therapeutic
expired gas analysis ~ 94250
inhalation, pentamidine ~ 94642
inhalation treatment ~ 94640, 94644-94645, 94664, 99503
intrapulmonary surfactant admin ~ 94610
manipulation of chest wall ~ 94667-94668
pressure ventilation
negative CNPB ~ 94662
positive CPAP ~ 94660
unlisted services and procedures ~ 94799
ventilation assist ~ 94002-94005, 99504
unlisted services and procedures ~ 94799
Pulse generator
electronic analysis ~ 95970-95971
heart, insertion/replacement ~ 33212-33213
Pulse rate increased ~ see tachycardia
Pump ~ see chemotherapy, pump services; infusion pump
Pump, infusion ~ see infusion pump
Pump services oxygenator/heat exchanger ~ 99190-99192
Punch graft ~ 15775-15776
Puncture
artery ~ 36600
chest, drainage ~ 32554-32555
cisternal ~ see cisternal puncture
lumbar ~ see spinal tap
lung ~ 32405
pericardium ~ 33010-33011
pleural cavity, drainage ~ 32554-32555
skull, drain fluid ~ 61000-61020
cistern ~ 61050
inject cistern ~ 61055
inject ventricle ~ 61026
shunt
drain fluid ~ 61070
injection ~ 61070
spinal cord
diagnostic ~ 62270
drain fluid ~ 62272
lumbar ~ 62270
tracheal, aspiration and/or injection ~ 31612
Puncture aspiration
abscess, skin ~ 10160
bulla ~ 10160
cyst
breast ~ 19000-19001
skin ~ 10160
hematoma ~ 10160
Pure-tone audiometry ~ 92552, 92553
Pustules removal ~ 10040
Putti-Platt procedure ~ 23450
PUVA ~ (dermatology; photochemotherapy; ultraviolet light therapy) 96912
Pyelogram ~ see urography, intravenous; urography, retrograde
Pyelography ~ 74400, 74425
injection ~ 50394

Pyelolithotomy ~ 50130
  anatrophic ~ 50075
  coagulum ~ 50130
Pyeloplasty ~ 50400-50405, 50544
  repair, horseshoe kidney ~ 50540
  secondary ~ 50405
Pyeloscopy
  with cystourethroscopy ~ 52351
   biopsy ~ 52354
   destruction ~ 52354
   lithotripsy ~ 52353
   removal, calculus ~ 52352
   tumor excision ~ 52355
Pyelostogram ~ 50394
Pyelostolithotomy percutaneous ~
  50080-50081
Pyelostomy ~ 50125, 50400-50405
  change tube ~ 50398
Pyelotomy
  complicated ~ 50135
  with drainage ~ 50125
  endoscopic ~ 50570
  exploration ~ 50120
  with removal calculus ~ 50130
Pyeloureterogram antegrade ~ 50394
Pyeloureteroplasty ~ see pyeloplasty
Pyloric sphincter
  incision ~ 43520
  reconstruction ~ 43800
Pyloromyotomy ~ 43520
  with gastrectomy ~ 43639
Pyloroplasty ~ 43800
  with gastrectomy ~ 43639
  with vagotomy ~ 43640
Pyothorax ~ see abscess, thorax
Pyridoxal phosphate ~ 84207
Pyrophosphate, adenosine ~ see adenosine
  diphosphate
Pyrophosphorylase, Udp galactose ~
  (galactose-one-phosphate, uridyl transferase)
  82775, 82776
Pyruvate ~ 84210-84220

Q

Q fever ~ 86000, 86638
Q fever ab ~ see antibody, coxiella burnetii
Quadriceps repair ~ 27430
**Quantitative sudomotor axon reflex test
(QSART)** ~ 95923
Quick test ~ prothrombin time 85610, 85611
Quinidine assay ~ 80194
Quinine ~ 84228

R

Rabies vaccine ~ 90675-90676
Rachicentesis ~ see spinal tap
Radial head, subluxation ~ see nursemaid elbow
Radial keratotomy ~ 65771
Radiation ~ see irradiation
Radiation physics
  consultation ~ 77336-77370
  unlisted services and procedures ~ 77399
Radiation therapy ~ 77280-77295
  CT scan guidance ~ 77014
  consultation, radiation physics ~ 77336-77370
  dose plan ~ 77300, 77305-77331
   brachytherapy ~ 77326-77328
   intensity modulation ~ 77301
   teletherapy ~ 77305-77321
  field set-up ~ 77280-77295
  multi-leaf collimator (MLC) device ~ 77338
  planning ~ 77261-77263, 77299
  special ~ 77470
  stereotactic
   body ~ 77373
   cerebral lesions ~ 77371-77372
   guidance ~ 77432
  treatment delivery ~ 77371-77373
   intensity modulation ~ 77418
   proton beam ~ 77520-77525
   single ~ 77402-77406
   stereotactic ~ 77371-77373
   superficial ~ 77401
   three or more areas ~ 77412-77416
   two areas ~ 77407-77411
   weekly ~ 77427
  treatment device ~ 77332-77334
  treatment management
   one or two fractions only ~ 77431
   unlisted services and procedures ~ 77499
   weekly ~ 77427
Radical excision of lymph nodes ~ see
  excision, lymph nodes, radical
Radical mastectomies, modified ~ see
  mastectomy, modified radical
Radical neck dissection
  with auditory canal surgery ~ 69155
  laryngectomy ~ 31365-31368
  pharyngolaryngectomy ~ 31390-31395
  with thyroidectomy ~ 60254
  with tongue excision ~ 41135, 41145,
   41153-41155
Radical resection ~ see also resection, radical
  abdomen ~ 51597
  acetabulum ~ 27076
  ankle ~ 27615, 27616
  arm, lower ~ 25077
  calcaneus ~ 27647
  elbow, capsule, soft tissue,
   bone with contracture release ~ 24149

Radical resection ~ continued
face ~ 21015
fibula ~ 27646
finger ~ 26117
foot ~ 28046, 28047
forearm ~ 25077
hand ~ 26115
hip
  soft tissue ~ 27049
  tumor or infection ~ 27075-27076
humerus ~ 23220
innominate ~ 27077
ischial ~ 27078
knee ~ 27329
leg
  lower ~ 27615
  upper ~ 27329
metacarpal ~ 26250
metatarsal ~ 28173
mouth, with tongue excision ~ 41150, 41155
ovarian tumor
  bilateral
    salpingo-oophorectomy-omentectomy ~
      58950-58954
    with radical dissection for debulking ~
      58952-58954
    with total abdominal hysterectomy ~
      58951, 58953-58954
pelvis, soft tissue ~ 27049
peritoneal tumor
  bilateral
    salpingo-oophorectomy-omentectomy ~
      58952-58954
    with radical dissection for debulking ~
      58952-58954
phalanges
  fingers ~ 26260-26262
  toe ~ 28175
radius ~ 25170
scalp ~ 21015
scapula ~ 23210
shoulder ~ 23077
sternum ~ 21630-21632
talus, tumor ~ 27647
tarsal ~ 28171
tibia ~ 27645
tonsil ~ 42842-42845
tumor
  back/flank ~ 21935, 21936
  femur ~ 27365
  knee ~ 27329, 27365
  leg, upper ~ 27329
  neck ~ 21557, 21558
  thorax ~ 21557, 21558
ulna ~ 25170
wrist ~ 25077
Radical vulvectomy ~ see vulvectomy, radical
Radio-cobalt B12 Schilling test ~ see vitamin,
  B-12, absorption study
Radioactive colloid therapy ~ 79200-79300

Radioactive substance
insertion
  kidney ~ 50578
  prostate ~ 55860
  ureteral endoscopic ~ 50978
  urethral endoscopic ~ 50959
Radiocarpal joint
arthrotomy ~ 25040
dislocation, closed treatment ~ 25660
Radiocinematographies ~ see cineradiography
Radioelement
application ~ 77761-77778
  surface ~ 77789
  with ultrasound ~ 76965
handling ~ 77790
infusion ~ 77750
Radioelement substance
catheter placement
  breast ~ 19296-19298
  bronchus ~ 31643
  muscle or soft tissue ~ 20555
  pelvic organ ~ 55920
  prostate ~ 55875
  soft tissue ~ 20555
needle placement
  head/neck ~ 41019
  muscle ~ 20555
  prostate ~ 55875-55876
  soft tissue ~ 20555
Radiography ~ see radiology, diagnostic; X-ray
Radioimmunosorbent test ~ see
  gammaglobulin, blood
Radioisotope brachytherapy ~ see
  brachytherapy
Radioisotope scan ~ see nuclear medicine
**Radiological marker, preoperative placement,
  excision of breast lesion ~** 19125-19126
Radiology services ~ 70010-79999
diagnostic radiology ~ 70010-76499
diagnostic ultrasound ~ 76506-76999
nuclear medicine ~ 78012-79999
radiation oncology ~ 77261-77799
stress views ~ 77071
Radionuclide CT scan ~ see emission
  computerized tomography
Radionuclide imaging ~ see nuclear medicine
Radionuclide therapy
intra-articular ~ 79440
intravascular ~ 79420
intravenous infusion ~ 79403
leukemia ~ 79100
other ~ 79400
polycythemia vera ~ 79100
thyroid gland ~ 79000-79035
unlisted services and procedures ~ 79999
**Radionuclide tomography, single photon
  emission- computed ~** see SPECT
Radiopharmaceutical localization
inflammatory process ~ 78805
injection ~ 78808

Radiopharmaceutical therapy
heart ~ 79440
interstitial ~ 79300
intra-arterial ~ 79445
intra-articular ~ 79440
intracavitary ~ 79200
intravenous ~ 79101, 79403
leukemia ~ 79100
oral ~ 79005
other ~ 79400
polycythemia vera ~ 79100
thyroid gland ~ 79020-79035
unlisted services and procedures ~ 79999
Radiotherapeutic ~ see radiation therapy
Radiotherapies ~ see irradiation
Radiotherapy, surface ~ see application, radioelement, surface
Radioulnar joint
arthrodesis, with resection of ulna ~ 25830
dislocation
closed treatment ~ 25675
open treatment ~ 25676
Radius ~ see also also arm, lower; elbow; ulna
arthroplasty ~ 24365
with implant ~ 24366, 25441
craterization ~ 24145, 25151
cyst, excision ~ 24125-24126, 25120-25126
diaphysectomy ~ 24145, 25151
dislocation
with fracture
closed treatment ~ 24620
open treatment ~ 24635
partial ~ 24640
subluxate ~ 24640
excision ~ 24130, 24136, 24145, 24152
epiphyseal bar ~ 20150
partial ~ 25145
styloid process ~ 25230
fracture ~ 25605
closed treatment ~ 25500-25505, 25520, 25600-25605
with manipulation ~ 25605
without manipulation ~ 25600
distal ~ 25600-25609
open treatment ~ 25607-25609
head/neck
closed treatment ~ 24650-24655
open treatment ~ 24665-24666
open treatment ~ 25515, 25525-25526, 25574
percutaneous fixation ~ 25606
shaft ~ 25500-25526
open treatment ~ 25574
with ulna ~ 25560-25565
open treatment ~ 25575
implant, removal ~ 24164
incision and drainage ~ 25035
osteomyelitis ~ 24136, 24145
osteoplasty ~ 25390-25393
prophylactic treatment ~ 25490, 25492

Radius ~ *continued*
repair
epiphyseal arrest ~ 25450-25455
epiphyseal separation
closed ~ 25600
closed with manipulation ~ 25605
open treatment ~ 25607-25609
percutaneous fixation ~ 25606
with graft ~ 25405, 25420-25426
malunion or nonunion ~ 25400, 25415
osteotomy ~ 25350-25355, 25370-25375
and ulna ~ 25365
saucerization ~ 24145, 25151
sequestrectomy ~ 24136, 25145
tumor, cyst ~ 24120
excision ~ 24125-24126, 25120-25126, 25170
Ramstedt operation ~ see pyloromyotomy
Ramus anterior, nervus thoracicus ~ see intercostal nerve
Range of motion test
extremities or trunk ~ 95851
eye ~ 92018-92019
hand ~ 95852
Rapid heart rate ~ see tachycardia
Rapid plasma reagin test ~ 86592-86593
Rapid test for infection ~ 86308, 86403-86406
monospot test ~ 86308
Rapoport test ~ 52005
Raskind procedure ~ 33735-33737
Rathke pouch tumor ~ see craniopharyngioma
Rat typhus ~ (Murine typhus) 86000
Rays, roentgen ~ see X-ray
Raz procedure ~ (repair, bladder, neck) 51845
RBC ~ see red blood cell (RBC)
RBC ab ~ see antibody, red blood cell
Reaction lip without reconstruction ~ 40530
Reaction, polymerase chain ~ see polymerase chain reaction (PCR)
Realignment
femur with osteotomy ~ 27454
knee extensor ~ 27422
Receptor ~ see CD4; estrogen, receptor; FC receptor; progesterone receptors
Receptor assay
hormone ~ 84233-84235
non hormone ~ 84238
Recession gastrocnemius leg, lower ~ 27687
Reconstruction ~ see revision
abdominal wall
omental flap ~ 49905
acetabulum ~ 27120-27122
anal
congenital absence ~ 46730-46740
fistula ~ 46742
graft ~ 46753
with implant ~ 46762
sphincter ~ 46750-46751, 46760-46762
ankle ~ 27700-27703
apical-aortic conduit ~ 33404

1507

Reconstruction ~ *continued*
atrial
  endoscopic ~ 33265-33266
  open ~ 33254-33256
auditory canal, external ~ 69310-69320
bile duct, anastomosis ~ 47800
bladder
  from colon ~ 50810
  from intestines ~ 50820, 51960
  and urethra ~ 51800-51820
breast ~ 19357-19369
  augmentation ~ 19324-19325
  with free flap ~ 19364
  with latissimus dorsi flap ~ 19361
  mammoplasty ~ 19318-19325
  nipple ~ 19350-19355
  with other techniques ~ 19366
  revision ~ 19380
  with tissue expander ~ 19357
  transverse rectus abdominis myocutaneous
    flap ~ 19367-19369
bronchi ~ 32501
  graft repair ~ 31770
  stenosis ~ 31775
canthus ~ 67950
cardiac anomoly, complex ~ 33622
carpal ~ 25443
carpal bone ~ 25394, 25430
cheekbone ~ 21270
chest wall, omental flap ~ 49904
  trauma ~ 32820
cleft palate ~ 42200-42225
conduit, apical-aortic ~ 33404
conjunctiva ~ 68320-68335
  with flap
    bridge or partial ~ 68360
    total ~ 68362
cranial bone, extracranial ~ 21181-21184
ear, middle
  tympanoplasty with antrotomy or
    mastoidotomy
    with ossicular chain reconstruction ~
      69636-69637
  tympanoplasty with mastoidectomy ~ 69641
    with intact or reconstructed wall ~
      69643-69644
    with ossicular chain reconstruction ~
      69642
    radical or complete ~ 69644-69645
  tympanoplasty without mastoidectomy ~
    69631
    with ossicular chain reconstruction ~
      69632-69633
elbow ~ 24360
  with implant ~ 24361-24362
  total replacement ~ 24363
esophagus ~ 43300, 43310, 43313
  creation, stoma ~ 43350-43352
  esophagostomy ~ 43350
  fistula ~ 43305, 43312, 43314
  gastrointestinal ~ 43360-43361

Reconstruction ~ *continued*
eye
  graft
    conjunctiva ~ 65782
    stem cell ~ 65781
  transplantation
    amniotic membrane ~ 65780
eyelid
  canthus ~ 67950
  second stage ~ 67975
  total ~ 67973-67975
  total eyelid
    lower, one stage ~ 67973
    upper, one stage ~ 67974
  transfer tarsoconjunctival flap from opposing
    eyelid ~ 67971
facial bones, secondary ~ 21275
fallopian tube ~ see repair
femur
  lengthening ~ 27466-27468
  shortening ~ 27465, 27468
fibula, lengthening ~ 27715
finger, polydactylous ~ 26587
foot, cleft ~ 28360
forehead ~ 21172-21180, 21182-21184
glenoid fossa ~ 21255
gums
  alveolus ~ 41874
  gingiva ~ 41872
hand
  tendon pulley ~ 26390, 26500-26502
  toe to finger transfer ~ 26551-26556
heart
  atrial ~ 33253
    endoscopic ~ 33265-33266
    open ~ 33254-33256
  atrial septum ~ 33735-33737
  pulmonary artery shunt ~ 33924
  vena cava ~ 34502
hip
  replacement ~ 27130-27132
  secondary ~ 27134-27138
hip joint, with prosthesis ~ 27125
interphalangeal joint ~ 26535-26536
  collateral ligament ~ 26545
intestines, small, anastomosis ~ 44130
knee ~ 27437-27438
  femur ~ 27442-27443, 27446
  ligament ~ 27427-27429
  prosthesis ~ 27438, 27445
  replacement ~ 27447
  revision ~ 27486-27487
  tibia ~ 27440-27443, 27446
kneecap, instability ~ 27420-27424
larynx
  burns ~ 31588
  cricoid split ~ 31587
  other ~ 31588
  stenosis ~ 31582
  web ~ 31580
lip ~ 40525-40527, 40761

Reconstruction ~ *continued*
lunate ~ 25444
malar augmentation,
  prosthetic material ~ 21270
  with bone graft ~ 21210
mandible, with implant ~ 21244-21246,
  21248-21249
mandibular condyle ~ 21247
mandibular rami
  with bone graft ~ 21194
  without bone graft ~ 21193
  with internal rigid fixation ~ 21196
  without internal rigid fixation ~ 21195
maxilla, with implant ~ 21245-21246,
  21248-21249
metacarpophalangeal joint ~ 26530-26531
midface
  with bone graft ~ 21145-21160, 21188
  without bone graft ~ 21141-21143
  forehead advancement ~ 21159-21160
mouth ~ 40840-40845
nail bed ~ 11762
nasoethmoid complex ~ 21182-21184
navicular ~ 25443
nose
  cleft lip/cleft palate ~ 30460-30462
  dermatoplasty ~ 30620
  primary ~ 30400-30420
  secondary ~ 30430-30450
  septum ~ 30520
orbit ~ 21256
orbit area, secondary ~ 21275
orbit with bone grafting ~ 21182-21184
orbital rim ~ 21172-21180
orbital rims ~ 21182-21184
orbital walls ~ 21182-21184
orbitocraniofacial, secondary revision ~ 21275
oviduct, fimbrioplasty ~ 58760
palate
  cleft palate ~ 42200-42225
  lengthening ~ 42226-42227
parotid duct, diversion ~ 42507-42510
patella ~ 27437-27438
  instability ~ 27420-27424
penis
  angulation ~ 54360
  chordee ~ 54300-54304
  complications ~ 54340-54348
  epispadias ~ 54380-54390
  hypospadias ~ 54332, 54352
    one stage distal with urethroplasty ~
    54324-54328
    one stage perineal ~ 54336
periorbital region, osteotomy with graft ~
  21267-21268
pharynx ~ 42950
pyloric sphincter ~ 43800
radius ~ 24365, 25390-25393, 25441
  arthroplasty, with implant ~ 24366
shoulder joint, with implant ~ 23470-23472

Reconstruction ~ *continued*
skull ~ 21172-21180
  defect ~ 62140-62141, 62145
sternum ~ 21740-21742
  with thoracoscopy ~ 21743
stomach
  with duodenum ~ 43810, 43850-43855,
    43865
  gastric bypass ~ 43846
  with jejunum ~ 43820-43825, 43860
  for obesity ~ 43846-43848
  Roux-en-Y ~ 43846
superior-lateral orbital rim and forehead ~
  21172-21175
supraorbital rim and forehead ~ 21179-21180
symblepharon ~ 68335
temporomandibular joint, arthroplasty ~
  21240-21243
throat ~ 42950
thumb
  from finger ~ 26550
  opponensplasty ~ 26490-26496
tibia
  lengthening ~ 27715
  tubercle ~ 27418
toe
  angle deformity ~ 28313
  extra toes ~ 28344
  hammertoe ~ 28285-28286
  macrodactyly ~ 28340-28341
  polydactylous ~ 26587
  syndactyly ~ 28345
  webbed toe ~ 28345
tongue, frenum ~ 41520
trachea
  carina ~ 31766
  cervical ~ 31750
  fistula ~ 31755
  intrathoracic ~ 31760
trapezium ~ 25445
tympanic membrane ~ 69620
ulna ~ 25390-25393, 25442
  radioulnar ~ 25337
ureter ~ 50700
  with intestines ~ 50840
urethra ~ 53410-53440, 53445
  complications ~ 54340-54348
  hypospadias
    one stage distal with meatal advancement
    ~ 54322
    one stage distal with urethroplasty ~
    54324-54328
  suture to bladder ~ 51840-51841
  urethroplasty for second stage ~
    54308-54316
  urethroplasty for third stage ~ 54318
uterus ~ 58540
vas deferens ~ see vasovasorrhaphy
vena cava ~ 34502
  with resection ~ 37799
wound repair ~ 13100-13160

Reconstruction ~ *continued*
  wrist ~ 25332
    capsulectomy ~ 25320
    capsulorrhaphy ~ 25320
    realign ~ 25335
    zygomatic arch ~ 21255
Rectal bleeding ~ see hemorrhage, rectum
Rectal prolapse ~ see procidentia, rectum
Rectal sphincter dilation ~ 45910
Rectocele repair ~ 45560
Rectopexy ~ see proctopexy
Rectoplasty ~ see proctoplasty
Rectorrhaphy ~ see rectum, suture
Rectovaginal fistula ~ see fistula, rectovaginal
Rectovaginal hernia ~ see rectocele
Rectum ~ see also anus
  abscess, incision and drainage ~ 45005-45020,
    46040, 46060
  biopsy ~ 45100
  dilation, endoscopy ~ 45303
  endoscopy
    destruction, tumor ~ 45320
    dilation ~ 45303
    exploration ~ 45300
    hemorrhage ~ 45317
    removal
      foreign body ~ 45307
      polyp ~ 45308-45315
      tumor ~ 45308-45315
      volvulus ~ 45321
  excision
    with colon ~ 45121
    partial ~ 45111, 45113-45116, 45123
    total ~ 45110, 45112, 45119-45120
  exploration, endoscopic ~ 45300
  hemorrhage, endoscopic ~ 45317
  injection, sclerosing solution ~ 45520
  lesion, excision ~ 45108
  manometry ~ 91122
  prolapse, excision ~ 45130-45135
  removal
    fecal impaction ~ 45915
    foreign body ~ 45307, 45915
  repair
    fistula ~ 45800-45825
    injury ~ 45562-45563
    prolapse ~ 45505-45541, 45900
    rectocele ~ 45560
    stenosis ~ 45500
    with sigmoid excision ~ 45550
  stricture, excision ~ 45150
  suture
    fistula ~ 45800-45825
    prolapse ~ 45540-45541
  tumor
    destruction ~ 45190, 45320, 46937-46938
    excision ~ 45160-45172
  unlisted services and procedures ~ 44239,
    45999
Reductase, glutathione ~ see glutathione
  reductase

Reductase, lactic cytochrome ~ see lactic
  dehydrogenase
Red blood cell (RBC)
  antibody ~ 86850-86870
    pretreatment ~ 86970-86972
  count ~ 85032-85041
  fragility
    mechanical ~ 85547
    osmotic ~ 85555-85557
  hematocrit ~ 85014
  iron utilization ~ 78170
  morphology ~ 85007
  platelet estimation ~ 85007
  sedimentation rate
    automated ~ 85652
    manual ~ 85651
  sequestration ~ 78140
  sickling ~ 85660
  survival test ~ 78130-78135
  volume determination ~ 78120-78121
Red blood cell ab ~ see antibody, red blood
  cell
Reduction
  forehead ~ 21137-21139
  lung volume ~ 32491
  mammoplasty ~ 19318
  masseter muscle/bone ~ 21295-21296
  osteoplasty, facial bones ~ 21209
  pregnancy, multifetal ~ 59866
  skull, craniomegalic ~ 62115-62117
Reflex test
  blink reflex ~ 95933
Reflux study ~ 78262
Refraction ~ 92015
Rehabilitation
  artery, occlusive disease ~ 93668
  auditory
    post-lingual hearing loss ~ 92633
    pre-lingual hearing loss ~ 92630
    status evaluation ~ 92626-92627
  cardiac ~ 93797-93798
  services considered, documentation ~ 4079F
Rehabilitative ~ see rehabilitation
Rehfuss test ~ see gastroenterology diagnostic,
  stomach
Reichstein's substances ~ see deoxycortisol
Reimplantation
  arteries
    aorta prosthesis ~ 35697
    carotid ~ 35691, 35694-35695
    subclavian ~ 35693-35695
    vertebral ~ 35691-35693
    visceral ~ 35697
  kidney ~ 50380
  ovary ~ 58825
  pulmonary artery ~ 33788
  ureters ~ 51565
  ureter, to bladder ~ 50780-50785
Reinnervation larynx, neuromuscular pedicle
  ~ 31590
Reinsch test ~ 83015

Reinsertion
drug delivery implant ~ 11983
spinal fixation device ~ 22849
Relative density ~ see specific gravity
Release
carpal tunnel ~ 64721
elbow contracture, with radical release of
capsule ~ 24149
flexor muscles, hip ~ 27036
muscle, knee ~ 27422
nerve ~ 64702-64726
neurolytic ~ 64727
retina, encircling material ~ 67115
spinal cord ~ 63200
stapes ~ 69650
tarsal tunnel ~ 28035
tendon ~ 24332, 25295
Release-inhibiting hormone, somatotropin ~
see somatostatin
Removal
adjustable gastric restrictive device ~
43772-43774
allograft, intestinal ~ 44137
artificial intervertebral disc
cervical interspace ~ 0095T, 22864
lumbar interspace ~ 22865, 0164T
balloon, intra-aortic ~ 33974
balloon assist device, intra-aortic ~ 33968,
33971
blood clot, eye ~ 65930
blood component, apheresis ~ 36511-36516
breast
capsules ~ 19371
implants ~ 19328-19330
modified radical ~ 19307
partial ~ 19300-19302
radical ~ 19305-19306
simple, complete ~ 19303
subcutaneous ~ 19304
calcareous deposit, subdeltoid ~ 23000
calculi (stone)
bile duct ~ 43264, 47420-47425
percutaneous ~ 47554, 47630
bladder ~ 51050, 52310-52318, 52352
gallbladder ~ 47480
hepatic duct ~ 47400
kidney ~ 50060-50081, 50130, 50561,
50580, 52352
pancreas ~ 48020
pancreatic duct ~ 43264
salivary gland ~ 42330-42340
ureter ~ 50610-50630, 50961, 50980,
51060-51065, 52320-52330, 52352
urethra ~ 52310-52315, 52352
cardiac event recorder ~ 33284
cast ~ 29700-29715
cataract
dilated fundus evaluation ~ 2021F
with replacement
not associated with concurrent ~ 66983
extracapsular ~ 66982, 66984
intracapsular ~ 66983

Removal ~ *continued*
catheter
central venous ~ 36589
fractured ~ 37197
peritoneum ~ 49422
pleural cavity ~ 32552
spinal cord ~ 62355
cerclage, cervix ~ 59871
cerumen, auditory canal, external ~ 69210
clot pericardium ~ 33020
endoscopic ~ 32658
comedones ~ 10040
contraceptive capsules ~ 11976
cranial tongs ~ 20665
cyst ~ 10040
dacryolith
lacrimal duct ~ 68530
lacrimal gland ~ 68530
defibrillator
heart ~ 33244
pulse generator only ~ 33241
via thoracotomy ~ 33243
drug delivery implant ~ 11982-11983
ear wax, auditory canal, external ~ 69210
electrode
brain ~ 61535, 61880
heart ~ 33238
nerve ~ 64585
spinal cord ~ 63661-63664
stomach ~ 43648, 43882
embolus ~ see embolectomy
external fixation system ~ 20694
eye
bone ~ 67414, 67445
with bone ~ 65112
with implant
muscles attached ~ 65105
muscles, not attached ~ 65103
without implant ~ 65101
with muscle or myocutaneous flap ~ 65114
ocular contents
with implant ~ 65093
without implant ~ 65091
orbital contents only ~ 65110
fallopian tube, laparoscopy ~ 58661
fat, lipectomy ~ 15876-15879
fecal impaction, rectum ~ 45915
fibrin deposit ~ 32150
fixation device ~ 20670-20680
foreign bodies ~ 65205-65265
anal ~ 46608
ankle joint ~ 27610, 27620
arm
lower ~ 25248
upper ~ 24200-24201
auditory canal, external ~ 69200
with anesthesia ~ 69205
bile duct ~ 43269
bladder ~ 52310-52315
brain ~ 61570, 62163
bronchi ~ 31635
colon ~ 44025, 44390, 45379

1511

Removal ~ *continued*
colon-sigmoid ~ 45332
conjunctival embedded ~ 65210
cornea
  with slit lamp ~ 65222
  without slit lamp ~ 65220
duodenum ~ 44010
elbow ~ 24000, 24101, 24200-24201
esophagus ~ 43020, 43045, 43215, 74235
external eye ~ 65205
eyelid ~ 67938
finger ~ 26075-26080
foot ~ 28190-28193
gastrointestinal, upper ~ 43247
gum ~ 41805
hand ~ 26070
hip ~ 27033, 27086-27087
hysteroscopy ~ 58562
interphalangeal joint, toe ~ 28024
intertarsal joint ~ 28020
intestines, small ~ 44020, 44363
intraocular ~ 65235
kidney ~ 50561, 50580
knee joint ~ 27310, 27331, 27372
lacrimal duct ~ 68530
lacrimal gland ~ 68530
larynx ~ 31511, 31530-31531, 31577
leg, upper ~ 27372
lung ~ 32151
mandible ~ 41806
mediastinum ~ 39000-39010
metatarsophalangeal joint ~ 28022
mouth ~ 40804-40805
muscle ~ 20520-20525
nose ~ 30300
  anesthesia ~ 30310
  lateral rhinotomy ~ 30320
orbit ~ 61334, 67413, 67430
  with bone flap ~ 67430
  without bone flap ~ 67413
pancreatic duct ~ 43269
patella ~ see patellectomy
pelvis ~ 27086-27087
penile tissue ~ 54115
penis ~ 54115
pericardium ~ 33020
  endoscopic ~ 32658
peritoneum ~ 49402
pharynx ~ 42809
pleura ~ 32150-32151
  endoscopic ~ 32653
posterior segment
  magnetic extraction ~ 65260
  nonmagnetic extraction ~ 65265
rectum ~ 45307, 45915
scrotum ~ 55120
shoulder ~ 23040-23044
  complicated ~ 23332
  deep ~ 23331
  subcutaneous ~ 23330
skin, with debridement ~ 11010-11012
stomach ~ 43500

Removal ~ *continued*
subcutaneous tissue ~ 10120-10121
  with debridement ~ 11010-11012
tarsometatarsal joint ~ 28020
tendon sheath ~ 20520-20525
toe ~ 28022
ureter ~ 50961, 50980
urethra ~ 52310-52315
uterus ~ 58562
vagina ~ 57415
wrist ~ 25040, 25101, 25248
foreign body, elbow ~ 24101
hair, electrolysis ~ 17380
halo ~ 20665
hearing aid, bone conduction ~ 69711
hematoma, brain ~ 61312-61315
implantation ~ 20670-20680
  ankle ~ 27704
  contraceptive capsules ~ 11976
  elbow ~ 24160
  eye ~ 67120-67121
  finger ~ 26320
  hand ~ 26320
  radius ~ 24164
  wrist ~ 25449
infusion pump
  intra-arterial ~ 36262
  intravenous ~ 36590
  spinal cord ~ 62365
intra-aortic balloon ~ 33974
  assist device ~ 33968, 33971
intrauterine device (IUD) ~ 58301
keel, laryngoplasty ~ 31580
lacrimal gland
  partial ~ 68505
  total ~ 68500
lacrimal sac, excision/(optional) ~ 68520
laryngocele ~ 31300
leiomyomata ~ 58545-58546, 58561
lens ~ 66920-66940
lens material ~ 66840-66852
lesion
  conjunctiva ~ 68040
  larynx ~ 31512, 31578
    endoscopic ~ 31545-31546
loose body
  ankle ~ 27620
  carpometacarpal joint ~ 26070
  elbow ~ 24101
  interphalangeal joint, toe ~ 28024
  intertarsal joint ~ 28020
  knee joint ~ 27331
  metatarsophalangeal joint ~ 28022
  tarsometatarsal joint ~ 28020
  toe ~ 28022
  wrist ~ 25101
lung
  apical tumor ~ 32503-32504
  bronchial valve ~ 31648-31649
  bronchoplasty ~ 32501
  completion pneumonectomy ~ 32488
  cyst ~ 32140

Removal ~ *continued*
  extrapleural ~ 32445
  pneumonectomy ~ 32440-32445
  single lobe ~ 32480
  single segment ~ 32484
  sleeve lobectomy ~ 32486
  sleeve pneumonectomy ~ 32442
  two lobes ~ 32482
  volume reduction ~ 32491
  lymph nodes
    abdominal ~ 38747
    inguinofemoral ~ 38760-38765
    pelvic ~ 38770
    retroperitoneal, transabdominal ~ 38780
    thoracic ~ 38746
  mammary implant ~ 19328-19330
  mastoid, air cells ~ 69670
  mesh, abdominal wall ~ 11008
  milia, multiple ~ 10040
  nails ~ 11730-11732, 11750-11752
  neurostimulators
    pulse generator ~ 64595
    receiver ~ 64595
  ocular implant ~ 65175, 65920
  orbital implant ~ 67560
  ovaries, laparoscopy ~ 58661
  pacemaker, heart ~ 33233-33237
  patella, complete ~ 27424
  plate, skull ~ 62142
  polyp
    anal ~ 46610, 46612
    antrochoanal ~ 31032
    colon ~ 44392, 45385
    colon-sigmoid ~ 45333
    endoscopy ~ 44364-44365, 44394
    esophagus ~ 43217, 43250
    gastrointestinal, upper ~ 43250-43251
    rectum ~ 45315
    sphenoid sinus ~ 31051
  prosthesis
    abdomen ~ 49606
    abdominal wall ~ 11008
    hip ~ 27090-27091
    knee ~ 27488
    penis ~ 54406, 54410-54417
    perineum ~ 53442
    skull ~ 62142
    urethral sphincter ~ 53446-53447
    wrist ~ 25250-25251
  pulse generator
    brain ~ 61888
    spinal cord ~ 63688
  pustules ~ 10040
  receiver, brain ~ 61888
    spinal cord ~ 63688
  reservoir, spinal cord ~ 62365
  seton, anal ~ 46030
  shoulder joint, foreign or loose body ~ 23107
  shunt
    brain ~ 62256-62258
    heart ~ 33924
    peritoneum ~ 49429

Removal ~ *continued*
  spinal cord ~ 63746
  skin tags ~ 11200-11201
  sling
    urethra ~ 53442
    vagina ~ 57287
  spinal instrumentation
    anterior ~ 22855
    posterior nonsegmental
      Harrington rod ~ 22850
    posterior segmental ~ 22852
  stent
    bile duct ~ 43269
    pancreatic duct ~ 43269
  suture
    anal ~ 46754
    anesthesia ~ 15850-15851
  thrombus ~ see thrombectomy
  tissue expanders, skin ~ 11971
  transplant intestines ~ 44137
  transplant kidney ~ 50370
  tube
    ear, middle ~ 69424
    finger ~ 26392, 26416
    hand ~ 26392, 26416
  tumor, temporal bone ~ 69970
  ureter, ligature ~ 50940
  urethral stent
    bladder ~ 52310-52315
    urethra ~ 52310-52315
  vein
    clusters ~ 37785
    perforation ~ 37760-37761
    saphenous ~ 37720-37735, 37780
    varicose ~ 37765-37766
  venous access device ~ 36590
    obstruction ~ 75901-75902
  ventilating tube, ear, middle ~ 69424
  ventricular assist device ~ 33977-33978
    extracorporeal ~ 33990-33993
    intracorporeal ~ 33980
  vitreous, anterior approach ~ 67005-67010
  wire, anal ~ 46754
Renal ~ (see also kidney)
  abscess ~ see abscess, kidney
  arteries ~ see artery, renal
  autotransplantation ~ see autotransplantation, renal
  calculus ~ see calculus, removal, kidney
  cyst ~ see cyst, kidney
  dialyses ~ see hemodialysis
  disease services ~ see dialysis
  transplantation ~ see kidney, transplantation
Renin ~ 80408, 80416, 84244
  peripheral vein ~ 80417
Renin-converting enzyme ~ 82164
Reoperation
  carotid thromboendarterectomy ~ 35390
  coronary artery bypass
    valve procedure ~ 33530
  distal vessel bypass ~ 35700

Repair ~ see also revision
abdomen ~ 49900
  hernia ~ 49491-49525, 49565, 49570, 49582-49590
  omphalocele ~ 49600-49611
  suture ~ 49900
abdominal wall ~ 15830, 15847
anal
  anomaly ~ 46744-46748
  fistula ~ 46288, 46706, 46715-46716
  stricture ~ 46700-46705
aneurysm, aorta ~ 0078T-0081T, 33877-33886, 34800-34805, 34825-34832, 75952-75953
  arteriovenous ~ 36832
  iliac artery ~ 75954
  intracranial artery ~ 61697-61708
ankle
  ligament ~ 27695-27698
  tendon ~ 27612, 27650-27654, 27680-27687
aorta ~ 33320-33322, 33802-33803
  coarctation ~ 33840-33851
  graft ~ 33860-33877
  sinus of valsalva ~ 33702-33720
aortic arch
  with cardiopulmonary bypass ~ 33853
  without cardiopulmonary bypass ~ 33852
aortic valve ~ 33400-33403
  obstruction, outflow tract ~ 33414
  septic hypertrophy ~ 33416
  stenosis ~ 33415
arm
  lower ~ 25260-25263, 25270
    fasciotomy ~ 24495
    secondary ~ 25265, 25272-25274
    tendon ~ 25290
    tendon sheath ~ 25275
  muscle ~ 24341
  tendon ~ 24332, 24341, 25280, 25295, 25310-25316
  upper
    muscle revision ~ 24330-24331
    muscle transfer ~ 24301, 24320
    tendon lengthening ~ 24305
    tendon revision ~ 24320
    tendon transfer ~ 24301
    tenotomy ~ 24310
arteriovenous aneurysm ~ 36832
arteriovenous fistula
  abdomen ~ 35182
    acquired or traumatic ~ 35189
  head ~ 35180
    acquired or traumatic ~ 35188
  lower extremity ~ 35184
    acquired or traumatic ~ 35190
  neck ~ 35180
    acquired or traumatic ~ 35188
  thorax ~ 35182
    acquired or traumatic ~ 35189
  upper extremity ~ 35184
    acquired or traumatic ~ 35190

Repair ~ *continued*
arteriovenous malformation
  intracranial ~ 61680-61692
  intracranial artery ~ 61705-61708
  spinal artery ~ 62294
  spinal cord ~ 63250-63252
artery
  angioplasty ~ 75962-75968
  aorta ~ 35452, 35472
  axillary ~ 35458
  brachiocephalic ~ 35458, 35475
  bypass graft ~ 35501-35571, 35601-35683, 35691-35695, 35700
  bypass in-situ ~ 35582-35587
  bypass venous graft ~ 33510-33516, 35510-35525
  femoral ~ 35456
  iliac ~ 34900
  occlusive disease ~ 35001, 35005-35021, 35045-35081, 35091, 35102, 35111, 35121, 35131, 35141, 35151, 35161
  pulmonary ~ 33690
  renal ~ 35450
  renal or visceral ~ 35471
  subclavian ~ 35458
  thromboendarterectomy ~ 35301-35321, 35341-35390
  viscera ~ 35450, 35471
arytenoid cartilage ~ 31400
bile duct ~ 47701
  with intestines ~ 47760, 47780-47785
  wound ~ 47900
bladder
  exstrophy ~ 51940
  fistula ~ 44660-44661, 45800-45805, 51880-51925
  neck ~ 51845
  resection ~ 52500
  wound ~ 51860-51865
blepharoptosis, frontalis muscle technique with fascial sling ~ 67902
blood vessel
  abdomen ~ 35221
    with other graft ~ 35281
    with vein graft ~ 35251
  chest ~ 35211-35216
    with other graft ~ 35271-35276
    with vein graft ~ 35241-35246
  finger ~ 35207
  graft defect ~ 35870
  hand ~ 35207
  kidney ~ 50100
  lower extremity ~ 35226
    with other graft ~ 35286
    with vein graft ~ 35256
  neck ~ 35201
    with other graft ~ 35261
    with vein graft ~ 35231
  upper extremity ~ 35206
    with other graft ~ 35266
    with vein graft ~ 35236

Repair ~ *continued*
body cast ~ 29720
brain, wound ~ 61571
breast, suspension ~ 19316
bronchi, fistula ~ 32815
brow pyrosis ~ 67900
bunion ~ 28290-28299
bypass graft ~ 35901-35907
   fistula ~ 35870
calcaneus, osteotomy ~ 28300
cannula ~ 36860-36861
carpal ~ 25440
carpal bone ~ 25431
cervix
   cerclage ~ 57700
      abdominal ~ 59320-59325
   suture ~ 57720
chest wall ~ 32905
   closure ~ 32810
   fistula ~ 32906
chin
   augmentation ~ 21120, 21123
   osteotomy ~ 21121-21123
clavicle, osteotomy ~ 23480-23485
cleft hand ~ 26580
cleft lip ~ 40525-40527, 40700-40761
   nasal deformity ~ 40700-40701, 40720-40761
cleft palate ~ see cleft palate, repair
colon
   fistula ~ 44650-44661
   hernia ~ 44050
   malrotation ~ 44055
   obstruction ~ 44050
cornea ~ see cornea, repair
coronary chamber fistula ~ 33500-33501
cyst
   Bartholin's gland ~ 56440
   liver ~ 47300
diaphragm
   for eventration ~ 39545
   hernia ~ 39503-39541
   laceration ~ 39501
ductus arteriosus ~ 33820-33824
ear, middle
   oval window fistula ~ 69666
   round window fistula ~ 69667
elbow
   hemiepiphyseal arrest ~ 24470
   ligament ~ 24343-24346
   muscle ~ 24341
   muscle transfer ~ 24301
   tendon ~ 24340-24342
      each ~ 24341
   tendon lengthening ~ 24305
   tendon transfer ~ 24301
   tennis elbow ~ 24357-24359
encephalocele ~ 62121
enterocele
   hysterectomy ~ 58270, 58294
epididymis ~ 54900-54901

Repair ~ *continued*
epispadias ~ 54380-54390
esophagus ~ 43300, 43310, 43313
   esophagogastrostomy ~ 43320
   esophagojejunostomy ~ 43340-43341
   fistula ~ 43305, 43312, 43314, 43420-43425
   fundoplasty ~ 43325, 43327-43328
   muscles ~ 43330-43331
   pre-existing perforation ~ 43405
   varices ~ 43401
   wound ~ 43410-43415
eye
   ciliary body ~ 66680
      suture ~ 66682
   conjunctiva ~ 65270-65273
      wound ~ 65270-65273
   cornea ~ 65275
      astigmatism ~ 65772-65775
      with glue ~ 65286
      wound ~ 65275-65285
   fistula, lacrimal gland ~ 68770
   iris
      with ciliary body ~ 66680
      suture ~ 66682
   lacrimal duct, canaliculi ~ 68700
   lacrimal punctum ~ 68705
   retina, detachment ~ 67101-67113
   sclera
      with glue ~ 65286
      with graft ~ 66225
      reinforcement ~ 67250-67255
      staphyloma ~ 66220-66225
      wound ~ 65286, 66250
   strabismus, chemodenervation ~ 67345
   symblepharon
      division ~ 68340
      with graft ~ 68335
      without graft ~ 68330
   trabeculae ~ 65855
eye muscles
   strabismus
      adjustable sutures ~ 67335
      one horizontal muscle ~ 67311
      one vertical muscle ~ 67314
      posterior fixation suture technique ~ 67334-67335
      previous surgery, not involving extraocular muscles ~ 67331
      release extensive scar tissue ~ 67343
      superior oblique muscle ~ 67318
      two horizontal muscles ~ 67312
      two or more vertical muscles ~ 67316
      wound, extraocular muscle ~ 65290
eyebrow, ptosis ~ 67900
eyelashes
   epilation
      by forceps ~ 67820
      by other than forceps ~ 67825
      incision of lid margin ~ 67830
      with free mucous membrane graft ~ 67835

Repair ~ *continued*
eyelid ~ 21280-21282
  ectropion ~ 67916-67917
    suture ~ 67914
    thermocauterization ~ 67915
  entropion ~ 67924
    excision tarsal wedge ~ 67923
    suture ~ 67921-67924
    thermocauterization ~ 67922
  excisional ~ 67961-67966
  lagophthalmos ~ 67912
  ptosis, conjunctivo-tarso-Muller's
    muscle-levator resection ~ 67908
  frontalis muscle technique ~ 67901-67902
  levator resection ~ 67903-67904
  reduction of overcorrection ~ 67909
  superior rectus technique ~ 67906
  retraction ~ 67911
  wound, suture ~ 67930-67935
facial bones ~ 21208-21209
facial nerve
  paralysis ~ 15840-15845
  suture, intratemporal, lateral to geniculate
    ganglion ~ 69740
  intratemporal, medial to geniculate
    ganglion ~ 69745
fallopian tube ~ 58752
  anastomosis ~ 58750
  create stoma ~ 58770
fascial defect ~ 50728
femur ~ 27470-27472
  epiphysis ~ 27475-27485, 27742
  arrest ~ 27185
  open treatment ~ 27177-27178
  osteoplasty ~ 27179
  osteotomy ~ 27181
  by pinning ~ 27176
  by traction ~ 27175
  with graft ~ 27170
  muscle transfer ~ 27110
  osteotomy ~ 27140, 27151, 27450-27454
  femoral neck ~ 27161
  with fixation ~ 27165
  with open reduction ~ 27156
fibula
  epiphysis ~ 27477-27485, 27730-27742
  nonunion or malunion ~ 27726
  osteotomy ~ 27707-27712
finger
  claw finger ~ 26499
  macrodactylia ~ 26590
  polydactylous ~ 26587
  syndactyly ~ 26560-26562
  tendon
    extensor ~ 26415-26434, 26445-26449
    flexor ~ 26356-26358, 26440-26442
    joint stabilization ~ 26474
    pip joint ~ 26471
  toe transfer ~ 26551-26556
  trigger ~ 26055
  volar plate ~ 26548
  web finger ~ 26560-26562

Repair ~ *continued*
fistula
  carotid-cavernous ~ 61710
  mastoid ~ 69700
  rectovaginal ~ 57308
foot
  fascia ~ 28250
  muscle ~ 28250
  tendon ~ 28200-28226, 28238
gallbladder
  with gastroenterostomy ~ 47741
  with intestines ~ 47720-47740
great arteries ~ 33770-33781
great vessel ~ 33320-33322
hallux valgus ~ 28290-28299
hamstring ~ 27097
hand
  cleft hand ~ 26580
  muscle ~ 26591-26593
  tendon
    extensor ~ 26410-26416, 26426-26428,
      26433-26437
    flexor ~ 26350-26358, 26440
    profundus ~ 26370-26373
hearing aid, bone conduction ~ 69711
heart
  anomaly ~ 33600-33617
  aortic sinus ~ 33702-33722
  artificial heart, intracorporeal ~ 0052T-0053T
  atrioventricular canal ~ 33660-33665
    complete ~ 33670
  atrioventricular valve ~ 33660-33665
  blood vessel ~ 33320-33322
  cor triatriatum ~ 33732
  infundibular ~ 33476-33478
  mitral valve ~ 33420-33427
  myocardium ~ 33542
  outflow tract ~ 33476-33478
  postinfarction ~ 33542-33545
  prosthetic valve ~ 33670, 33852-33853
  prosthetic valve dysfunction ~ 33496
  pulmonary artery shunt ~ 33924
  pulmonary valve ~ 33470-33474
  septal defect ~ 33545, 33608-33610,
    33681-33688, 33692-33697
    atrial and ventricular ~ 33647
    atrium ~ 33641
  sinus of valsalva ~ 33702-33722
  sinus venosus ~ 33645
  tetralogy of Fallot ~ 33692-33697
  total replacement heart system,
    intracorporeal ~ 0052T-0053T
  tricuspid valve ~ 33465
  ventricle ~ 33611-33612
    obstruction ~ 33619
  ventricular tunnel ~ 33722
  wound ~ 33300-33305
hepatic duct, with intestines ~ 47765, 47802
hernia
  abdomen ~ 49565, 49590
    incisional ~ 49560
  epigastric ~ 49570

Repair ~ *continued*
   incarcerated ~ 49572
   epigelian
      incarcerated or strangulated ~ 49653
      reducible ~ 49652
   femoral ~ 49550
      incarcerated ~ 49553
      recurrent ~ 49555
      recurrent incarcerated ~ 49557
      reducible recurrent ~ 49555
   hiatal ~ 43332-43337
   incisional
      incarcerated or strangulated ~ 49561,
         49655
      recurrent incarcerated ~ 49566, 49657
      recurrent reducible ~ 49656
      reducible ~ 49564
   inguinal ~ 49491-49521
      initial ~ 49650
      recurrent ~ 49651
      sliding ~ 49525
   intestinal ~ 44025-44050
   lumbar ~ 49540
   lung ~ 32800
   orchiopexy ~ 54640
   paraesophageal ~ 43332-43337
   reducible ~ 49565, 49570
      femoral ~ 49550
      incisional ~ 49560
      inguinal ~ 49500, 49505
      recurrent ~ 49520
   sliding ~ 49525
   spigelian ~ 49590
      incarcerated or strangulated ~ 49653
      reducible ~ 49652
   umbilical ~ 49580, 49585
      incarcerated ~ 49582, 49587, 49653
      reducible ~ 49580, 49652
   ventral
      incarcerated or strangulated ~ 49653
      reducible ~ 49652
   with spermatic cord ~ 54640
hip
   muscle transfer ~ 27100-27105, 27111
   osteotomy ~ 27146-27156
   tendon ~ 27097
humerus ~ 24420-24430
   with graft ~ 24435
   osteotomy ~ 24400-24410
ileostomy ~ see ileostomy, repair
interphalangeal joint, volar plate ~ 26548
intestines
   enterocele
      abdominal approach ~ 57270
      vaginal approach ~ 57268
   obstruction ~ 44615
intestines, large
   closure enterostomy ~ 44620-44626
   diverticula ~ 44605
   ulcer ~ 44605
   wound ~ 44605

Repair ~ *continued*
   intestines, small
      closure enterostomy ~ 44620-44626
      diverticula ~ 44602-44603
      fistula ~ 44640-44661
      hernia ~ 44050
      malrotation ~ 44055
      obstruction ~ 44025-44050
      ulcer ~ 44602-44603
      wound ~ 44602-44603
   introitus, vagina ~ 56800
   iris, ciliary body ~ 66680
   jejunum
      free transfer, with microvascular anastomosis
         ~ 43496
   kidney
      fistula ~ 50520-50526
      horseshoe ~ 50540
      renal pelvis ~ 50400-50405
      wound ~ 50500
   knee
      cartilage ~ 27403
      instability ~ 27420
      ligament ~ 27405-27409
         collateral ~ 27405
         collateral and cruciate ~ 27409
         cruciate ~ 27407-27409
      meniscus ~ 27403
      tendon ~ 27380-27381
   larynx
      fracture ~ 31584-31586
      reinnervation, neuromuscular pedicle ~
         31590
   leg
      lower
         fascia ~ 27656
         tendon ~ 27658-27692
      upper
         muscle ~ 27385-27386, 27400, 27430
         tendon ~ 27393-27400
   ligament ~ see ligament, repair
   lip ~ 40650-40654
      cleft lip ~ 40700-40761
      fistula ~ 42260
   liver, abscess ~ 47300
      cyst ~ 47300
      wound ~ 47350-47361
   lung
      hernia ~ 32800
      pneumolysis ~ 32940
      tear ~ 32110
   mastoidectomy
      complete ~ 69601
      modified radical ~ 69602
      radical ~ 69603
      with apicectomy ~ 69605
      with tympanoplasty ~ 69604
   maxilla, osteotomy ~ 21206
   mesentery ~ 44850
   metacarpal
      lengthening ~ 26568
      nonunion ~ 26546

1517

Repair ~ *continued*
  osteotomy ~ 26565
metacarpophalangeal joint
  capsulodesis ~ 26516-26518
  collateral ligament ~ 26540-26542
  fusion ~ 26516-26518
metatarsal ~ 28322
  osteotomy ~ 28306-28309
microsurgery ~ 69990
mitral valve ~ 33420-33427
mouth
  laceration ~ 40830-40831
  vestibule of ~ 40830-40845
musculotendinous cuff ~ 23410-23412
nail bed ~ 11760
nasal deformity, cleft lip ~ 40700-40761
nasal septum ~ 30630
navicular ~ 25440
neck muscles
  scalenus anticus ~ 21700-21705
  sternocleidomastoid ~ 21720-21725
nerve ~ 64876
  graft ~ 64885-64907
  microrepair ~ 69990
  suture ~ 64831-64876
nose
  adhesions ~ 30560
  fistula ~ 30580-30600, 42260
  rhinophyma ~ 30120
  septum ~ 30540-30545, 30630
  synechia ~ 30560
  vestibular stenosis ~ 30465
omphalocele ~ 49600-49611
osteotomy
  femoral neck ~ 27161
  radius, and ulna ~ 25365
  ulna, and radius ~ 25365
  vertebra
    additional segment ~ 22216, 22226
    cervical ~ 22210, 22220
    lumbar ~ 22214, 22224
    thoracic ~ 22212, 22222
oviduct ~ 58752
  create stoma ~ 58770
pacemaker, heart
  electrode ~ 33218-33220
palate
  laceration ~ 42180-42182
  vomer flap ~ 42235
pancreas
  cyst ~ 48500
  pseudocyst ~ 48510-48511
    percutaneous ~ 48511
paravaginal defect ~ 57284-57285, 57423
pectus carinatum ~ 21740-21742
  with thoracoscopy ~ 21743
pectus excavatum ~ 21740-21742
  with thoracoscopy ~ 21743
pelvic floor, prosthetic insertion ~ 57267
pelvis
  osteotomy ~ 27158
  tendon ~ 27098

Repair ~ *continued*
penis
  fistulization ~ 54435
  injury ~ 54440
  priapism ~ 54420-54435
  shunt ~ 54420-54430
perineum ~ 56810
periorbital region, osteotomy ~ 21260-21263
phalanx
  finger
    lengthening ~ 26568
    osteotomy ~ 26567
    nonunion ~ 26546
  toe, osteotomy ~ 28310-28312
pharynx, with esophagus ~ 42953
pleura ~ 32215
prosthesis, penis ~ 54408
pulmonary artery ~ 33917-33920
  reimplantation ~ 33788
pulmonary valve ~ 33470-33474
quadriceps ~ see quadriceps, repair
radius
  epiphyseal ~ 25450-25455
  malunion or nonunion ~ 25400, 25415
  osteotomy ~ 25350-25355, 25370-25375
  with graft ~ 25405, 25420-25426
rectocele ~ see rectocele, repair
rectovaginal fistula ~ 57308
rectum
  fistula ~ 45800-45825
  injury ~ 45562-45563
  prolapse ~ 45505-45541, 45900
  rectocele ~ 45560
  stenosis ~ 45500
  with sigmoid excision ~ 45550
retinal detachment with diathermy ~ see
  diathermy, retinal detachment, repair
rotator cuff ~ see rotator cuff, repair
salivary duct ~ 42500-42505
  fistula ~ 42600
scapula
  fixation ~ 23400
  scapulopexy ~ 23400
sclera ~ see sclera, repair
scrotum ~ 55175-55180
septal defect ~ 33813-33814
shoulder, capsule ~ 23450-23466
  cuff ~ 23410-23412
  ligament release ~ 23415
  muscle transfer ~ 23395-23397
  musculotendinous rotator cuff ~
    23415-23420
  tendon ~ 23410-23412, 23430-23440
  tenomyotomy ~ 23405-23406
simple, integumentary system ~ see
  integumentary system, repair, simple
sinus
  ethmoid, cerebrospinal fluid leak ~ 31290
  sphenoid, cerebrospinal fluid leak ~ 31291
sinus of valsalva ~ 33702-33722

Repair ~ *continued*
  skin, wound
    complex ~ 13100-13160
    intermediate ~ 12031-12057
    simple ~ 12020-12021
  skull
    cerebrospinal fluid leak ~ 62100
    encephalocele ~ 62120
  spica cast ~ 29720
  spinal cord ~ 63700
    cerebrospinal fluid leak ~ 63707-63709
    meningocele ~ 63700-63702
    myelomeningocele ~ 63704-63706
  spinal meningocele ~ see meningocele, repair
  spine, osteotomy ~ 22210-22226
  spleen ~ 38115
  stomach
    esophagogastrostomy ~ 43320
    fistula ~ 43880
    fundoplasty ~ 43325, 43327-43328
    laceration ~ 43501-43502
    stoma ~ 43870
    ulcer ~ 43501
  talus, osteotomy ~ 28302
  tarsal ~ 28320
    osteotomy ~ 28304-28305
  testis
    injury ~ 54670
    suspension ~ 54620-54640
    torsion ~ 54600
  throat
    pharyngoesophageal ~ 42953
    wound ~ 42900
  thumb
    muscle ~ 26508
    tendon ~ 26510
  tibia ~ 27720-27725
    epiphysis ~ 27477-27485, 27730-27742
    osteotomy ~ 27455-27457, 27705,
      27709-27712
    pseudoarthrosis ~ 27727
  toe
    bunion ~ 28290-28299
    muscle ~ 28240
    tendon ~ 28240
    webbing ~ 28280, 28345
  toes
    macrodactylia ~ 26590
    polydactylous ~ 26587
  tongue ~ 41250-41252
    fixation ~ 41500
    laceration ~ 41250-41252
    mechanical ~ 41500
    suture ~ 41510
  trachea, fistula ~ 31755
    stenosis ~ 31780-31781
    stoma ~ 31613-31614
      scar ~ 31830
      with plastic repair ~ 31825
      without plastic repair ~ 31820
    with plastic repair ~ 31825

Repair ~ *continued*
    without plastic repair ~ 31820
  wound
    cervical ~ 31800
    intrathoracic ~ 31805
  tricuspid valve ~ 33463-33465
  truncus arteriosus, Rastelli type ~ 33786
  tunica vaginalis, hydrocele ~ 55060
  tympanic membrane ~ 69450, 69610
  ulna
    epiphyseal ~ 25450-25455
    malunion or nonunion ~ 25400, 25415
    osteotomy ~ 25360, 25370-25375,
      25425-25426
    with graft ~ 25405, 25420
  umbilicus, omphalocele ~ 49600-49611
  ureter
    anastomosis ~ 50740-50825
    continent diversion ~ 50825
    deligation ~ 50940
    fistula ~ 50920-50930
    lysis adhesions ~ 50715-50725
    suture ~ 50900
    urinary undiversion ~ 50830
  ureterocele ~ 51535
  urethra
    artificial sphincter ~ 53449
    diverticulum ~ 53240, 53400-53405
    fistula ~ 45820-45825, 53400-53405, 53520
    stoma ~ 53520
    stricture ~ 53400-53405
    urethrocele ~ 57230
    wound ~ 53502-53515
  urethral sphincter ~ 57220
  urinary incontinence ~ 53431-53440, 57284
  uterus
    fistula ~ 51920-51925
    rupture ~ 58520, 59350
    suspension ~ 58400-58410
  vagina
    anterior ~ see colporrhaphy, anterior
    cystocele ~ 57240, 57260
    enterocele ~ 57265
    fistula ~ 46715-46716, 51900
      rectovaginal ~ 57300-57307
      transvesical and vaginal approach ~ 57330
      urethrovaginal ~ 57310-57311
      vesicovaginal ~ 57320-57330
    hysterectomy ~ 58267, 58293
    incontinence ~ 57284, 57288
    pereyra procedure ~ 57289
    postpartum ~ 59300
    prolapse ~ 57282-57284
    rectocele ~ 57250-57260
    suspension ~ 57280, 57284
      laparoscopic ~ 57425
    wound ~ 57200-57210
  vaginal wall prolapse ~ see colporrhaphy
  vas deferens, suture ~ 55400

1519

Repair ~ *continued*
  vein
    angioplasty ~ 35460, 35476, 75978
    femoral ~ 34501
    graft ~ 34520
    pulmonary ~ 33730
    transposition ~ 34510
  vulva, postpartum ~ 59300
  wound
    complex ~ 13100-13160
    intermediate ~ 12031-12057
    simple ~ 12001-12021
  wound dehiscence
    complex ~ 13160
    simple ~ 12020-12021
  wrist ~ 25260-25263, 25270, 25447
    bone ~ 25440
    carpal bone ~ 25431
    cartilage ~ 25107
    removal, implant ~ 25449
    secondary ~ 25265, 25272-25274
    tendon ~ 25280-25316
    tendon sheath ~ 25275
    total replacement ~ 25446
Repeat surgeries ~ see reoperation
Replacement
  aortic valve ~ 33405-33413
  arthroplasties, hip ~ see arthroplasty, hip
  artificial heart, intracorporeal ~ 0052T-0053T
  cerebrospinal fluid shunt ~ 62160, 62194, 62225-62230
  contact lens ~ see contact lens services
  elbow, total ~ 24363
  electrode
    heart ~ 33210-33211, 33216-33217
    stomach ~ 43647
  eye, drug delivery system ~ 67121
  gastrostomy tube ~ 43760
  hearing aid, bone conduction ~ 69710
  hip ~ 27130-27132
    revision ~ 27134-27138
  implant, bone, for external speech processor/cochlear stimulator ~ 69717-69718
  knee, total ~ 27447
  mitral valve ~ 33430
  nerve ~ 64726
  neurostimulator
    pulse generator/receiver
      intracranial ~ 61885
      peripheral nerve ~ 64590
      spinal ~ 63685
  ossicles, with prosthesis ~ 69633, 69637
  ossicular replacement ~ see TORP (total ossicular replacement prosthesis)
  pacemaker ~ 33206-33208
    catheter ~ 33210
    electrode ~ 33210-33211, 33216-33217
  pacing cardioverter-defibrillator
    leads ~ 33243-33244
  pulse generator only ~ 33241

Replacement ~ *continued*
  penile, prosthesis ~ 54410-54411, 54416-54417
  prosthesis, skull ~ 62143
    urethral sphincter ~ 53448
  pulmonary valve ~ 33475
  pulse generator
    brain ~ 61885
    peripheral nerve ~ 64590
    spinal cord ~ 63685
  receiver
    brain ~ 61885
    peripheral nerve ~ 64590
    spinal cord ~ 63685
  skull plate ~ 62143
  spinal cord, reservoir ~ 62360
  tissue expanders, skin ~ 11970
  total replacement ~ see hip, total replacement
  total replacement heart system
    intracorporeal ~ 0052T-0053T
  tricuspid valve ~ 33465
  ureter, with intestines ~ 50840
  venous access device ~ 36582-36583, 36585
    catheter ~ 36578
  venous catheter, central ~ 36580-36581, 36584
  ventricular assist device ~ 33981-33983
Replantation
  arm, upper ~ 20802
  digit ~ 20816-20822
  foot ~ 20838
  forearm ~ 20805
  hand ~ 20808
  thumb ~ 20824-20827
Report preparation
  extended, medical ~ 99080
  psychiatric ~ 90889
Reposition toe to hand ~ 26551-26556
Repositioning
  central venous catheter ~ 36597
  electrode, heart ~ 33215-33217, 33226
  gastrostomy tube ~ 43761
  heart, defibrillator leads ~ 33215-33216, 33226, 33249
  intraocular lens ~ 66825
  tricuspid valve ~ 33468
Reproductive tissue
  cryopreservation
    embryo(s) ~ 89258
    sperm ~ 89259
    testicular tissue ~ 89335
  thawing of cryopreserved
    embryo(s) ~ 89352
    oocytes, each aliquot ~ 89356
    sperm/semen ~ 89353
    testicular/ovarian tissue ~ 89354
  storage
    oocyte(s) ~ 89346
    sperm/semen ~ 89343
    testicular/ovarian ~ 89344
Reprogramming, shunt, brain ~ 62252
Reptilase test ~ 85635
Repilase time ~ see thrombin time

Resection
aortic valve, stenosis ~ 33415
bladder diverticulum ~ 52305
bladder neck, transurethral ~ 52500
brain lobe ~ see lobectomy, brain
chest wall ~ 19260-19272
diaphragm ~ 39560-39561
endaural ~ see ear, inner, excision
humeral head ~ 23195
intestines, small, laparoscopic ~ 44202-44203
lung ~ 32520-32525
mouth, with tongue excision ~ 41153
myocardium
    aneurysm ~ 33542
    septal defect ~ 33545
nasal septum submucous ~ see nasal septum,
    submucous resection
nose
    septum ~ 30520
ovary, wedge ~ see ovary, wedge resection
palate ~ 42120
phalangeal head, toe ~ 28153
prostate transurethral ~ see prostatectomy,
    transurethral
radical
    arm, upper ~ 24077, 24079
    elbow ~ 24077, 24079
        with contracture release ~ 24149
    foot ~ 28046-28047
    humerus ~ 24150
    radius ~ 24152
    tumor
        ankle ~ 27615-27616
        calcaneus or talus ~ 27647
        clavicle ~ 23200
        femur ~ 27329, 27364-27365
        fibula ~ 27646
        humerus ~ 23220
        knee ~ 27329, 27364-27365
        leg, lower ~ 27615-27616
        leg, upper ~ 27329, 27364-27365
        metatarsal ~ 28173
        scapula ~ 23210
        shoulder 23077-23078
        tarsal ~ 28171
        tibia ~ 27645
        wrist ~ 25077-25078
    ribs ~ 19260-19272, 32900
    synovial membrane ~ see synovectomy
    temporal bone ~ 69535
    tumor
        fallopian tube ~ 58957-58958
        ovary ~ 58957-58958
        peritoneum ~ 58957-58958
    ulna, arthrodesis radioulnar joint ~ 25830
    ureterocele
        ectopic ~ 52301
        orthotopic ~ 52300
    vena cava, with reconstruction ~ 37799
Resonance spectroscopy, magnetic ~ see
    magnetic resonance spectroscopy

Respiration, positive-pressure ~ see pressure
    breathing, positive
**Respiratory pattern recording, preventive,
    infant** ~ 94772
Respiratory system, surgical procedures ~
    30000-32999
Respiratory syncytial virus (RSV)
    antibody ~ 86756
    antigen detection
        by direct fluorescence ~ 87280
        by direct optical observation ~ 87807
        by enzyme immunoassay ~ 87420
    immune globulins ~ 90378
Response, auditory evoked ~ see auditory
    evoked potentials
Rest home visit ~ see domiciliary services
Resuscitation
    cardiac ~ see cardiac massage
    cardio-pulmonary ~ see cardio-pulmonary
        resuscitation (CPR)
    newborn ~ 99465
Reticulocyte count ~ 85044-85045
Retina
    incision, encircling material ~ 67115
    lesion
        extensive, destruction ~ 67227-67228
        localized, destruction ~ 67208-67218
    macular/fundus exam, dilated ~ 2019F-2021F
        findings communicated for diabetes
            management ~ 5010F
    repair
        detachment ~ 67113
            by scleral buckling ~ 67112
            cryotherapy or diathermy ~ 67101
            injection of air ~ 67110
            photocoagulation ~ 67105
            by scleral buckling ~ 67112
            scleral dissection ~ 67107
            with vitrectomy ~ 67108, 67112
        prophylaxis, detachment ~ 67141-67145
    retinopathy
        destruction
            cryotherapy, diathermy ~ 67227
        treatment
            photocoagulation ~ 67228, 67229
Retinacular knee release ~ 27425
Retinopathy
    destruction
        cryotherapy, diathermy ~ 67227
    treatment
        photocoagulation, cryotherapy ~ 67228,
            67229
Retraction, clot ~ see clot retraction
Retrieval transcatheter foreign body ~ 37197
Retrocaval ureter ureterolysis ~ 50725
**Retrograde cholangiopancreatographies,
    endoscopic** ~ see cholangiopancreatography
Retrograde cystourethrogram ~ see
    urethrocystography, retrograde
Retrograde pyelogram ~ see urography,
    retrograde

1521

Retroperitoneal area
abscess, incision and drainage
  open ~ 49060
  percutaneous ~ 49061
biopsy ~ 49010
cyst, destruction/excision ~ 49203-49205,
  58957, 58958
endometriomas, destruction/excision ~
  49203-49205, 58957, 58958
exploration ~ 49010
needle biopsy, mass ~ 49180
tumor, destruction/excision ~ 49203-49205,
  58957, 58958
Retroperitoneal fibrosis ureterolysis ~ 50715
Retropubic prostatectomies ~ see
  prostatectomy, retropubic
Revascularization
distal upper extremity with interval ligation ~
  36838
endovascular
  femoral ~ 37224-37227
  iliac ~ 37220-37223
  peroneal ~ 37228-37235
  popliteal ~ 37224-37227
  tibeal ~ 37228-37235
interval ligation distal upper extremity ~
  36838
penis ~ 37788
transmyocardial ~ 33140-33141
Reversal, vasectomy ~ see vasovasorrhaphy
Reverse T3 ~ see triiodothyronine, reverse
Reverse triiodothyronine ~ see
  triiodothyronine, reverse
Revision ~ see reconstruction
aorta ~ 33404
blepharoplasty ~ 15820-15823
bronchial stent ~ 31638
bronchus ~ 32501
bypass graft, vein patch ~ 35685
cervicoplasty ~ 15819
colostomy ~ see colostomy, revision
cornea
  prosthesis ~ 65770
  reshaping
    epikeratoplasty ~ 65767
    keratomileusis ~ 65760
    keratophakia ~ 65765
defibrillator site, chest ~ 33223
ear, middle ~ 69662
external fixation system ~ 20693
eye, aqueous shunt ~ 66185
gastrostomy tube ~ 44373
hip replacement ~ see replacement, hip,
  revision
hymenal ring ~ 56700
ileostomy ~ see ileostomy, revision
infusion pump
  intra-arterial ~ 36261
  intravenous ~ 36576-36578, 36582-36583
iris
  iridoplasty ~ 66762
  iridotomy ~ 66761

Revision ~ *continued*
jejunostomy tube ~ 44373
lower extremity arterial bypass ~ 35879-35881
pacemaker site, chest ~ 33222
rhytidectomy ~ 15824-15829
semicircular canal, fenestration ~ 69840
shunt, intrahepatic portosystemic ~ 37183
sling ~ 53442
stapedectomy ~ see stapedectomy, revision
stomach, for obesity ~ 43848
tracheostomy, scar ~ 31830
urinary-cutaneous anastomosis ~ 50727-50728
vagina
  prosthetic graft ~ 57295-57296
  sling
    stress incontinence ~ 57287
venous access device ~ 36576-36578,
  36582-36583, 36585
ventricle
  ventriculomyectomy ~ 33416
  ventriculomyotomy ~ 33416
Rheumatoid factor ~ 86430-86431
Rhinectomy
partial ~ 30150
total ~ 30160
Rhinomanometry ~ 92512
Rhinopharynx ~ see nasopharynx
Rhinophyma repair ~ 30120
Rhinoplasty
cleft lip/cleft palate ~ 30460-30462
primary ~ 30400-30420
secondary ~ 30430-30450
Rhinoscopy ~ see endoscopy, nose
Rhinotomy lateral ~ 30118, 30320
Rhizotomy ~ 63185-63190
Rho variant du ~ 86905
Rhytidectomy ~ 15824-15829
Rhytidoplasties ~ see face lift
Rh (D) ~ see blood typing
Rh immune globulin ~ see immune globulins,
  Rho (D)
Rib
cartilage, graft to face ~ 21230
excision ~ 21600-21616, 32900
fracture
  closed treatment ~ 21800
  external fixation ~ 21810
  open treatment ~ 21805
resection ~ 19260-19272, 32900
X-ray ~ 71100-71111
Riboflavin ~ 84252
Richardson operation hysterectomy ~ see
  hysterectomy, abdominal, total
Richardson procedure ~ 53460
Rickettsia antibody ~ 86757
Ridell operation ~ see sinusotomy, frontal
Ridge, alveolar ~ see alveolar ridge
Right atrioventricular valve ~ see tricuspid
  valve
Right heart cardiac catheterization ~ see
  cardiac catheterization, right heart
Ripstein operation ~ see proctopexy

Risk factor reduction intervention ~ see
  performance measures, preventive medicine
Risser jacket ~ 29010-29015
  removal ~ 29710
Rocky mountain spotted fever ~ 86000
Roentgenographic ~ see X-ray
Roentgenography ~ see radiology, diagnostic
Roentgen rays ~ see X-ray
Ropes test ~ 83872
Rorschach test ~ 96100
Ross procedure ~ 33413
Rotation flap ~ see skin, adjacent tissue
  transfer
Rotator cuff repair ~ 23410-23420
Rotavirus
  antibody ~ 86759
  antigen detection, enzyme immunoassay ~
    87425
Rotavirus vaccine ~ 90680
Round window repair fistula ~ 69667
Round window fistula ~ see fistula, round
  window
Roux-en-y procedure ~ 43621, 43633-43634,
  43644, 43846, 47740-47741, 47780-47785,
  48540
Rpr ~ 86592-86593
RSV (respiratory syncytial virus)
  antibody ~ 86756
  antigen detection
    by direct fluorescence ~ 87280
    by direct optical observation ~ 87807
    by enzyme immunoassay ~ 87420
  immune globulins ~ 90378
RT3 ~ see triiodothyronine, reverse
Rubbing alcohol ~ see isopropyl alcohol
Rubella
  antibody ~ 86762
  vaccine ~ 90706
Rubella/mumps ~ see vaccines
Rubella HI test ~ see hemagglutination
  inhibition test
Rubeola
  antibody ~ 86765
  antigen detection, immunofluorescence ~
    87283
Rubeolla ~ see rubeola
Russell viper venom time ~ 85612-85613

S

Sac, endolymphatic ~ see endolymphatic sac
Saccomanno technique ~ 88108
Sacral nerve
  implantation, electrode ~ 64561, 64581
  insertion, electrode ~ 64561, 64581
Sacroiliac joint
  arthrodesis ~ 27280
  arthrotomy ~ 27050

Sacroiliac joint ~ *continued*
  biopsy ~ 27050
  dislocation, open treatment ~ 27218
  fusion ~ 27280
  injection for arthrography ~ 27096
  X-ray ~ 72200-72202
Sacrum
  augmentation
    percutaneous ~ 0200T-0201T
    with CT guidance ~ 72292
    with fluoroscopic guidance ~ 72291
  sacroplasty, percutaneous ~ 0200T-0201T
  tumor, excision ~ 49215
  X-ray ~ 72220
Salabrasion ~ 15810-15811
Salicylate assay ~ 80196
Saline-solution abortion ~ see abortion,
  induced, by saline
Salivary duct
  catheterization ~ 42660
  dilation ~ 42650-42660
  ligation ~ 42665
  repair ~ 42500-42505
  fistula ~ 42600
Salivary gland virus ~ see Cytomegalovirus
Salivary glands
  abscess, incision and drainage ~ 42310-42320
  biopsy ~ 42405
  calculi (stone), excision ~ 42330-42340
  cyst
    creation, fistula ~ 42325-42326
    drainage ~ 42409
    excision ~ 42408
  injection, X-ray ~ 42550
  needle biopsy ~ 42400
  nuclear medicine
    function study ~ 78232
    imaging ~ 78230-78231
  parotid, abscess ~ 42300-42305
  unlisted services and procedures ~ 42699
  X-ray ~ 70380-70390
    with contrast ~ 70390
Salmonella antibody ~ 86768
Salpingectomy ~ 58262-58263, 58291-58292,
  58552, 58554, 58661, 58700
  ectopic pregnancy
    laparoscopic treatment ~ 59151
    surgical treatment ~ 59120
  oophorectomy ~ 58943
Salpingo-oophorectomy ~ 58720
  resection ovarian malignancy ~ 58950-58956
  resection peritoneal malignancy ~
    58950-58956
  resection tubal malignancy ~ 58950-58956
Salpingohysterostomy ~ see implantation,
  tubouterine
Salpingolysis ~ 58740
Salpingoneostomy ~ 58673, 58770
Salpingoplasty ~ see fallopian tube, repair
Salpingostomy ~ 58673, 58770
  laparoscopic ~ 58673

Salter osteotomy of the pelvis ~ see osteotomy, pelvis
Sampling ~ see biopsy; brush biopsy; needle biopsy
Sang-Park procedure ~ 33735-33737
Sao Paulo typhus ~ see Rocky Mountain spotted fever
Saucerization
  calcaneus ~ 28120
  clavicle ~ 23180
  femur ~ 27070, 27360
  fibula ~ 27360, 27641
  hip ~ 27070
  humerus ~ 23184, 24140
  ileum ~ 27070
  metacarpal ~ 26230
  metatarsal ~ 28122
  olecranon process ~ 24147
  phalanges, finger ~ 26235-26236
  toe ~ 28124
  pubis ~ 27070
  radius ~ 24145, 25151
  scapula ~ 23182
  talus ~ 28120
  tarsal ~ 28122
  tibia ~ 27360, 27640
  ulna ~ 24147, 25150
Saundby test ~ see blood, feces
Scabies ~ see tissue, examination for ectoparasites
Scalenotomy ~ see muscle division, scalenus anticus
Scalenus anticus division ~ 21700-21705
Scaling ~ see exfoliation
Scalp tumor resection, radical ~ 21015
Scalp blood sampling ~ 59030
Scan ~ see specific site, nuclear medicine
  abdomen ~ see abdomen, CT scan
  CT ~ see CT scan
  MRI ~ see magnetic resonance imaging
  PET ~ see positron emission tomography
  radionuclide ~ see emission computerized tomography
Scanning, radioisotope ~ see nuclear medicine
Scanogram ~ 77073
Scaphoid fracture
  closed treatment ~ 25622
  open treatment ~ 25628
  with manipulation ~ 25624
Scapula
  craterization ~ 23182
  cyst excision ~ 23140
    with allograft ~ 23146
    with autograft ~ 23145
  diaphysectomy ~ 23182
  excision ~ 23172, 23190
    partial ~ 23182
  fracture
    closed treatment
      with manipulation ~ 23575
      without manipulation ~ 23570
    open treatment ~ 23585

Scapula ~ *continued*
  ostectomy ~ 23190
  repair
    fixation ~ 23400
    scapulopexy ~ 23400
  saucerization ~ 23182
  sequestrectomy ~ 23172
  tumor
    excision ~ 23140, 23210
    with allograft ~ 23146
    with autograft ~ 23145
    radical resection ~ 23210
  X-ray ~ 73010
Scapulopexy ~ 23400
Scarification pleural ~ 32215
Scarification of pleura ~ see pleurodesis
Schanz operation ~ see femur, osteotomy
Schauta operation ~ see hysterectomy, vaginal, radical
Schede procedure ~ 32905-32906
Scheie procedure ~ see iridectomy
Schilling test ~ see vitamin B-12 absorption study ~ 78270
Schlatter operation total gastrectomy ~ see excision, stomach, total
Schlicter test ~ (bactericidal titer, serum) 87197
Schocket procedure ~ (aqueous shunt) 66180
Schonbein test ~ see blood, feces
Schuchard procedure osteotomy, maxilla ~ 21206
Schwannoma, acoustic ~ see brain, tumor, excision
Sciatic nerve
  decompression ~ 64712
  injection, anesthetic ~ 64445-64446
  lesion, excision ~ 64786
  neuroma, excision ~ 64786
  neuroplasty ~ 64712
  release ~ 64712
  repair/suture ~ 64858
Scintigraphy ~ see nuclear medicine
  computed tomographic ~ see emission computerized tomography
Scissoring skin tags ~ 11200-11201
Sclera
  excision, sclerectomy with punch or scissors ~ 66160
  fistulization
    iridencleisis or iridotasis ~ 66165
    sclerectomy with punch or scissors with iridectomy ~ 66160
    thermocauterization with iridectomy ~ 66155
    trabeculectomy ab externo in absence of previous surgery ~ 66170
    trephination with iridectomy ~ 66150
  incision, fistulization
    iridencleisis or iridotasis ~ 66165
    sclerectomy with punch or scissors with iridectomy ~ 66160
    thermocauterization with iridectomy ~ 66155
    trabeculectomy ab externo in absence of previous surgery ~ 66170

ALPHABETICAL INDEX

Sclera ~ *continued*
trephination with iridectomy ~ 66150
lesion, excision ~ 66130
repair
reinforcement
with graft ~ 67255
without graft ~ 67250
staphyloma
with graft ~ 66225
without graft ~ 66220
with glue ~ 65286
wound
operative ~ 66250
tissue glue ~ 65286
Scleral buckling operation ~ see retina, repair, detachment
Scleral ectasia ~ see staphyloma, sclera
Sclerectomy ~ 66160
Sclerotherapy venous ~ 36468-36471
Sclerotomy ~ see incision, sclera
Screening, drug ~ see drug screen
Scribner cannulization ~ 36810
Scrotal varices ~ see varicocele
Scrotoplasty ~ 55175-55180
Scrotum
abscess, incision and drainage ~ 54700, 55100
excision ~ 55150
exploration ~ 55110
hematoma, incision and drainage ~ 54700
removal, foreign body ~ 55120
repair ~ 55175-55180
ultrasound ~ 76870
unlisted services and procedures ~ 55899
Scrub typhus ~ 86000
Second look surgery ~ see reoperation
Second opinion ~ see confirmatory
consultations
Section ~ see also decompression
cesarean ~ see cesarean delivery
cranial nerve ~ 61460
spinal access ~ 63191
dentate ligament ~ 63180-63182
gasserian ganglion, sensory root ~ 61450
medullary tract ~ 61470
mesencephalic tract ~ 61480
nerve root ~ 63185-63190
spinal accessory nerve ~ 63191
spinal cord tract ~ 63194-63199
tentorium cerebelli ~ 61440
vestibular nerve
transcranial approach ~ 69950
translabyrinthine approach ~ 69915
Sedation with or without analgesia ~ 99141-99142
Seddon-Brookes procedure ~ 24320
Sedimentation rate
blood cell
automated ~ 85652
manual ~ 85651
Segmentectomy
breast ~ 19301-19302
lung ~ 32484

Seidlitz powder test ~ see X-ray, with contrast
Selective cellular enhancement technique ~ 88112
Selenium ~ 84255
Self care ~ see physical
medicine/therapy/occupational therapy
training ~ 97535, 99509
Sella turcica
CT scan ~ 70480-70482
X-ray ~ 70240
Semen ~ see sperm
Semen analysis ~ 89300-89322
sperm analysis ~ 89331
antibodies ~ 89325
with sperm isolation ~ 89260-89261
Semenogelase ~ see antigen, prostate specific
Semicircular canal incision
fenestration ~ 69820
revised ~ 69840
Semilunar bone ~ see lunate
ganglion ~ see gasserian ganglion
Seminal vesicle(s)
cyst, excision ~ 55680
excision ~ 55650
incision ~ 55600-55605
mullerian duct, excision ~ 55680
unlisted services and procedures ~ 55899
vesiculography ~ 74440
X-ray with contrast ~ 74440
Seminin ~ see antigen, prostate specific
Semiquantitative ~ 81005
Sengstaaken tamponade esophagus ~ 43460
Senning procedure ~ (repair/revision, great arteries) 33774-33777
Senning type ~ 33774-33777
Sensitivity study
antibiotic
agar ~ 87181
disc ~ 87184
enzyme detection ~ 87185
macrobroth ~ 87188
MIC (minimum inhibitory concentration) ~ 87186
microtiter ~ 87186
MLC (minimum lethal concentration) ~ 87187
mycobacteria ~ 87190
antiviral drugs, HIV-1, tissue culture ~ 87904
Sensor, fetal oximetry
cervix ~ 0021T
vagina ~ 0021T
Sensorimotor exam ~ 92060
Sensory nerve common, repair/suture ~ 64834
Sentinel node injection procedure ~ 38792
Separation, craniofacial
closed treatment ~ 21431
open treatment ~ 21432-21436
Septal defect
repair ~ 33813-33814
ventricular
closure ~ 33675-33688
open ~ 33675-33688

1525

Septectomy
  atrial ~ 33735-33737
    balloon (Rashkind type) ~ 92992
    blade method (Park) ~ 92993
    closed ~ see septostomy, atrial
    submucous nasal ~ see nasal septum,
      submucous resection
Septic abortion ~ see abortion, septic
Septoplasty ~ 30520
Septostomy, atrial ~ 33735-33737
    balloon (Rashkind type) ~ 92992
    blade method (Park) ~ 92993
Septum, nasal ~ see nasal septum
Sequestrectomy
  carpal ~ 25145
  clavicle ~ 23170
  humeral head ~ 23174
  humerus ~ 24134
  olecranon process ~ 24138
  radius ~ 24136, 25145
  scapula ~ 23172
  skull ~ 61501
  ulna ~ 24138, 25145
Serialography aorta ~ 75625
Serodiagnosis, syphilis ~ see serologic test for
    syphilis
Serologic test for syphilis ~ 86592-86593
Seroma incision and drainage, skin ~ 10140
Serotonin ~ 84260
Serum
  albumin ~ see albumin, serum
  antibody identification, pretreatment ~
    86975-86978
  CPK ~ see creatine kinase, total
  serum immune globulin ~ 90281-90283
Sesamoid bone
  excision ~ 28315
  finger, excision ~ 26185
  foot, fracture ~ 28530-28531
  thumb, excision ~ 26185
Sesamoidectomy toe ~ 28315
Sever procedure ~ see contracture, palm,
    release
Severing of blepharorrhaphy ~ see
    tarsorrhaphy, severing
Sex change operation
  female to male ~ 55980
  male to female ~ 55970
Sex chromatin identification ~ 88130-88140
Sex hormone binding globulin ~ 84270
Sex-linked ichthyoses ~ see syphilis test
SGOT ~ 84450
SGPT ~ 84460
Shaving skin lesion ~ 11300-11313
SHBG (sex hormone binding globulin) ~
    84270
Shelf procedure ~ (see also osteotomy, hip)
    27146-27151
**Shiga-like toxin antigen detection, enzyme
    immunoassay** ~ 87427
Shigella antibody ~ 86771

Shirodkar operation ~ (repair, cervix, cerclage,
    abdominal) 57700
Shock wave (extracorporeal) therapy ~
    0019T-0020T
Shock wave, lithotripsy ~ 50590
Shock wave, ultrasonic ~ see ultrasound
Shop typhus of Malaya ~ see Murine typhus
Shoulder ~ see also clavicle; scapula
  abscess, drainage ~ 23030
  amputation ~ 23900-23921
  arthrocentesis ~ 20610
  arthrodesis ~ 23800
    with autogenous graft ~ 23802
  arthrography, injection, radiologic ~ 23350
  arthroscopy
    diagnostic ~ 29805
    surgical ~ 29806-29828
      biceps tenodesis ~ 29828
  arthrotomy, with removal loose or foreign
    body ~ 23107
  biopsy
    deep ~ 23066
    soft tissue ~ 23065
  blade ~ see scapula
  bone
    excision
      acromion ~ 23130
      clavicle ~ 23120-23125
    incision ~ 23035
    tumor, excision ~ 23140-23146
  bursa, drainage ~ 23031
  capsular contracture release ~ 23020
  cast
    figure eight ~ 29049
    removal ~ 29710
    spica ~ 29055
    velpeau ~ 29058
  disarticulation ~ 23920-23921
  dislocation, closed treatment, with
    manipulation ~ 23650-23655
  exploration ~ 23107
  hematoma, drainage ~ 23030
  manipulation, application of fixation apparatus
    ~ 23700
  prophylactic treatment ~ 23490-23491
  radical resection ~ 23077
  removal
    calcareous deposits ~ 23000
    cast ~ 29710
    foreign body
      complicated ~ 23332
      deep ~ 23331
      subcutaneous ~ 23330
    foreign or loose body ~ 23107
  repair
    capsule ~ 23450-23466
    ligament release ~ 23415
    muscle transfer ~ 23395-23397
    rotator cuff ~ 23410-23420
    tendon ~ 23410-23412, 23430-23440
    tenomyotomy ~ 23405-23406

Shoulder ~ *continued*
strapping ~ 29240
surgery, unlisted services and procedures ~ 23929
tumor, excision ~ 23071-23078
unlisted services and procedures ~ 23929
X-ray ~ 73020-73030
X-ray with contrast ~ 73040
Shoulder joint ~ see also clavicle; scapula
arthroplasty, with implant ~ 23470-23472
arthrotomy
  with biopsy ~ 23100-23101
  with synovectomy ~ 23105-23106
dislocation
  with greater tuberosity fracture
    closed treatment ~ 23665
    open treatment ~ 23670
  open treatment ~ 23660
  with surgical or anatomical neck fracture
    closed treatment with manipulation ~ 23675
dislocation ~ *continued*
  open treatment ~ 23680
excision, torn cartilage ~ 23101
exploration ~ 23040-23044
incision and drainage ~ 23040-23044
removal, foreign body ~ 23040-23044
X-ray ~ 73050
Shunt(s)
aqueous
  to extraocular reservoir ~ 66180
    revision ~ 66185
arteriovenous ~ see arteriovenous shunt
brain
  creation ~ 62180-62223
  removal ~ 62256-62258
  replacement ~ 62160, 62194, 62225-62230, 62258
  reprogramming ~ 62252
cerebrospinal fluid ~ see cerebrospinal fluid shunt
creation
  arteriovenous
    direct ~ 36821
    ECMO ~ 36822
    Thomas shunt ~ 36835
    transposition ~ 36818-36820
    with bypass graft ~ 35686
    with graft ~ 36825-36830
  cerebrospinal fluid ~ 62200
  Thomas shunt ~ 36835
  fetal ~ 59076
  great vessel
    aorta to pulmonary artery, ascending ~ 33755
    descending ~ 33762
    central ~ 33764
    subclavian pulmonary artery ~ 33750
    systemic to pulmonary ~ 33924
    vena cava to pulmonary artery ~ 33766-33767

Shunt(s) ~ *continued*
intra-atrial ~ 33735-33737
Levenn
  insertion ~ 49425
  patency test ~ 78291
  revision ~ 49426
nonvascular, X-ray ~ 75809
peritoneal, venous
  injection ~ 49427
  ligation ~ 49428
  removal ~ 49429
peritoneal X-ray ~ 75809
pulmonary artery
  from aorta ~ 33755-33762, 33924
  subclavian ~ 33750
  from vena cava ~ 33766-33767
revision, arteriovenous ~ 36832
spinal cord
  creation ~ 63740-63741
  irrigation ~ 63744
  removal ~ 63746
  replacement ~ 63744
superior mesenteric-caval ~ see anastomosis, caval to mesenteric
ureter to colon ~ 50815
ventriculocisternal with valve ~ (ventriculocisternostomy) 62180, 62200, 62201
Shuntogram ~ 75809
Sialic acid ~ 84275
Sialodochoplasty ~ 42500-42505
Sialogram ~ see sialography
Sialography ~ 70390
Sickling electrophoresis ~ 83020
Siderocytes ~ 85536
Siderophilin ~ see transferrin
Sigmoid ~ see colon-sigmoid
Sigmoid bladder cystectomy ~ 51590
Sigmoidoscopy
ablation
  polyp ~ 45339
  tumor ~ 45339
biopsy ~ 45331
collection, specimen ~ 45331
exploration ~ 45330, 45335
hemorrhage control ~ 45334
injection, submucosal ~ 45335
needle biopsy ~ 45342
placement, stent ~ 45345
removal
  foreign body ~ 45332
  polyp ~ 45333, 45338
  tumor ~ 45333, 45338
repair, volvulus ~ 45337
ultrasound ~ 45341-45342
Signal-averaged electrocardiography ~ see electrocardiogram
Silica ~ 84285
Silicon dioxide ~ see silica
Silicone contouring injections ~ 11950-11954
Silver operation ~ see Keller procedure
Silver procedure ~ 28290

Simple mastectomies ~ see mastectomy
Single photon absorptiometry ~ see
  absorptiometry, single photon
Single photon emission computed tomography
  (SPECT) ~ *see also* emission computed
  tomography
  abscess localization ~ 78807
  bone ~ 78320
  cerebrospinal fluid ~ 78647
  heart ~ 78451-78454
  kidney ~ 78710
  liver ~ 78205
  tumor localization ~ 78803
Sinus
  ethmoidectomy, excision ~ 31254
  pilonidal ~ see cyst, pilonidal
Sinus of valsalva repair ~ 33702-33722
Sinus venosus repair ~ 33645
Sinusectomy, ethmoid ~ see ethmoidectomy
Sinuses
  endoscopy, with dilation ~ 31295-31297
  ethmoid
    excision ~ 31200-31205
      with nasal/sinus endoscopy ~ 31254-31255
      repair of cerebrospinal leak ~ 31290
  frontal
    destruction ~ 31080-31085
    exploration ~ 31070-31075
      with nasal/sinus endoscopy ~ 31276
    fracture, open treatment ~ 21343-21344
    incision ~ 31070-31087
  injection ~ 20500
    diagnostic ~ 20501
  maxillary
    antrostomy ~ 31256-31267
    excision ~ 31225-31230
    exploration ~ 31020-31032
      with nasal/sinus endoscopy ~ 31233
    incision ~ 31020-31032, 31256-31267
    irrigation ~ 31000
    skull base ~ 61581
    surgery ~ 61581
  multiple
    incision ~ 31090
    paranasal, incision ~ 31090
  sphenoid
    biopsy ~ 31050-31051
    exploration ~ 31050-31051
      with nasal/sinus endoscopy ~ 31235
    incision ~ 31050-31051
      with nasal/sinus endoscopy ~ 31287-31288
    irrigation ~ 31002
    repair of cerebrospinal leak ~ 31291
    sinusotomy ~ 31050-31051
    skull base surgery ~ 61580-61581
  unlisted services and procedures ~ 31299
  X-ray ~ 70210-70220
Sinusoidal rotational testing ~ see ear, nose
  and throat
Sinusoscopy
  maxillary sinus ~ 31233
  sphenoid sinus ~ 31235

Sinusotomy ~ see also sinus, multiple
  combined ~ 31090
  frontal sinus
    exploratory ~ 31070-31075
    nonobliterative ~ 31086-31087
    obliterative ~ 31080-31085
  maxillary ~ 31020-31032
  multiple, paranasal ~ 31090
  sphenoid sinus ~ 31050-31051
Sisi test ~ 92564
Sistrunk operation ~ see cyst, thyroid gland,
  excision
Size reduction, breast ~ see breast, reduction
Skeletal fixation humeral epicondyle,
  percutaneous ~ 24566
Skeletal traction, insertion/removal pin/wire ~
  20650
Skene's gland abscess
  destruction ~ 53270
  excision ~ 53270
  incision and drainage ~ 53060
Skilled nursing facilities (SNF) services
  initial care ~ 99304-99306
  discharge services ~ 99315-99316
  other services ~ 99318
  subsequent care ~ 99307-99310
Skin
  abrasion ~ 15786-15787
    chemical peel ~ 15788-15793
    dermabrasion ~ 15780-15783
    salabrasion ~ 15810-15811
  abscess ~ see abscess, skin
  adjacent tissue transfer ~ 14000-14350
  autograft ~ see autograft, skin
  biopsy ~ 11100-11101
  chemical exfoliation ~ 17360
  complete physical examination ~ 2029F
  cyst ~ see cyst, skin
  debridement ~ 11000-11006, 11010-11047
    eczematous ~ 11000-11001
    infected ~ 11000-11006
    subcutaneous tissue ~ 11042, 11045
      infected ~ 11004-11006
    with open fracture and/or dislocation ~
      11010-11012
  decubitus ulcer(s) ~ see pressure ulcer
    (decubitus)
  desquamation ~ see exfoliation
  destruction
    benign lesions
      fifteen or more lesions ~ 17004
      first lesion ~ 17000
      two-fourteen lesions ~ 17003
    flat warts ~ 17110-17111
    lesions ~ 17106-17108
    malignant lesions ~ 17260-17286
      by photodynamic therapy ~ 96567
    premalignant lesions
      by photodynamic therapy ~ 96567
      fifteen or more lesions ~ 17004
      first lesion ~ 17000
      two-fourteen lesions ~ 17003

Skull ~ *continued*
  drain fluid ~ 61070
  injection ~ 61070
  subdural ~ 61000-61001
  ventricular fluid ~ 61020
  reconstruction ~ 21172-21180
  defect ~ 62140-62141, 62145
  reduction, craniomegalic ~ 62115-62117
  removal
    plate ~ 62142
    prosthesis ~ 62142
  repair
    cerebrospinal fluid leak ~ 62100
    encephalocele ~ 62120
  replacement
    plate ~ 62143
    prosthesis ~ 62143
  stereotactic navigational procedure ~
    61781-61783
  tumor, excision ~ 61500
  X-ray ~ 70250-70260
Skull base surgery
  anterior cranial fossa
    bicoronal approach ~ 61586
    craniofacial approach ~ 61580-61583
    extradural ~ 61600-61601
    Lefort 1 osteotomy approach ~ 61586
    orbitocranial approach ~ 61584-61585
    transzygomatic approach ~ 61586
  carotid aneurysm ~ 61613
  carotid artery ~ 61610
    transection/ligation ~ 61609-61612
  craniotomy ~ 62121
  dura, repair of cerebrospinal fluid leak ~
    61618-61619
  middle cranial fossa
    extradural ~ 61605, 61607
    infratemporal approach ~ 61590-61591
    intradural ~ 61606, 61608
    orbitocranial zygomatic approach ~ 61592
  posterior cranial fossa
    extradural ~ 61615
    intradural ~ 61616
    transcondylar approach ~ 61596-61597
    transpetrosal approach ~ 61598
    transtemporal approach ~ 61595
Sleep study ~ 95800-95801, 95806-95807
  actigraphy ~ 95803
  latency testing ~ 95805
  polysomnography ~ 95808-95811
Sliding inlay graft, tibia ~ see ankle; tibia,
  repair
Sling operation
  incontinence ~ 53440
    removal ~ 53442
  stress incontinence ~ 51992, 57287
  vagina ~ 57287-57288
Small bowel ~ see intestines, small
  neoplasm ~ see tumor, intestines, small
Smas flap ~ 15829
Smear cervical ~ see cervical smears
  Papanicolaou ~ see Pap smears

Smear and stain ~ see also cytopathology,
  smears
  cornea ~ 65430
  fluorescent ~ 87206
  gram or giesma ~ 87205
  ova, parasites ~ 87177
  parasites ~ 87207
  wet mount ~ 87210
Smith fracture ~ 25600-25605
Smith-Robinson operation ~ see arthrodesis,
  vertebra
Smithwick operation ~ see excision, nerve,
  sympathetic
SO4 ~ see sulfate
Soave procedure ~ 45120
Sodium ~ 84295, 84302
  urine ~ 84300
Sodium glycinate, theophylline ~ see
  theophylline
Sofield procedure ~ 24410
Soft tissue ~ see tissue, soft
Solar plexus ~ see celiac plexus
Solitary cyst ~ see bone, cyst
Somatomammotropin, chorionic ~ 83632
Somatomedin ~ 84305
Somatosensory testing
  lower limbs ~ 95926
  trunk or head ~ 95927
  upper limbs ~ 95925
Somatostatin ~ 84307
Somatotropin ~ 83003
Somatotropin release inhibiting hormone ~
  see somatostatin
Somatropin ~ see growth hormone, human
Somnographies ~ see polysomnography
Somophyllin T ~ see theophylline
Sonography ~ see echography
Sonohysterography ~ 76831
  saline infusion, injection procedure ~ 58340
Sore, bed ~ see pressure ulcer (decubitus)
Spasm eyelid ~ see blepharospasm
Special services, procedures and reports ~
  99000-99091
  after hours medical services ~ 99050
  analysis, remote physiologic data ~ 99091
  computer data analysis ~ 99090, 0206T
  device handling ~ 99002
  emergency care in office ~ 99058
  emergency care out of office ~ 99060
  extended hours, medical services ~
    99051-99053
  group education ~ 99078
    self-management ~ 98961-98962
  hyperbaric oxygen ~ 99183
  individual education, self management ~
    98960
  medical testimony ~ 99075
  non-office medical services ~ 99056
  on call services ~ 99026-99027
  phlebotomy ~ 99199
  post-op visit ~ 99024

Special services, procedures, reports ~ *continued*
pump services ~ 99190-99192
reports and forms
  medical, extended ~ 99080
  psychiatric ~ 90889
specimen handling ~ 99000-99001
supply of materials ~ 99070
  educational ~ 99071
unlisted services and procedures ~ 99199
unusual travel ~ 99082
Specific gravity body fluid ~ 84315
Specimen concentration ~ 87015
Specimen handling ~ 99000-99001
SPECT
abscess localization ~ 78807
bone ~ 78320
brain imaging ~ 78607
cerebrospinal fluid ~ 78647
heart ~ 78451-78454, 78469, 78494
kidney ~ 78710
liver ~ 78205
parathyroid gland ~ 78071-78072
tumor localization ~ 78803
Spectacle services
fitting
  low vision aid ~ 92354-92355
  spectacle prosthesis ~ 92352-92353
  spectacles ~ 92340-92342
repair ~ 92370-92371
Spectrometry, mass
analyte
  qualitative ~ 83788
  quantitative ~ 83789
Spectrophotometry ~ 84311
atomic absorption ~ see atomic absorption spectroscopy
Spectroscopy
atomic absorption ~ 82190
expired breath analysis ~ 94799
magnetic resonance ~ 76390
Spectrum analyses ~ see spectrophotometry
Speech evaluation ~ 92506
cine ~ 70371
for prosthesis ~ 92597, 92607-92608
video ~ 70371
Speech prosthesis ~ 21084, 92609
creation ~ 31611
evaluation for speech ~ 92597, 92607-92608
insertion ~ 31611
Speech therapy ~ 92507-92508
Sperm
cryopreservation ~ 89259
evaluation ~ 89329-89331
storage ~ 89343
thawing ~ 89353
washing ~ 58323
Sperm analysis
antibodies ~ 89325
cervical mucus penetration test ~ 89330
count ~ 89310, 89320, 89322

Sperm analysis ~ *continued*
forensic ~ 88125
hamster penetration test ~ 89329
hyaluron binding assay ~ 89398
identification, aspiration ~ 89257
  from testis tissue ~ 89264
isolation ~ 89260-89261
motility ~ 89300, 89310, 89320-89322
Sperm evaluation, cervical mucus penetration test ~ see Huhner test
Spermatic cord
hydrocele, excision ~ 55500
laparoscopy ~ 55559
lesion, excision ~ 55520
repair, veins ~ 55530-55540
  abdominal approach ~ 55535
  with hernia repair ~ 55540
varicocele, excision ~ 55530-55540
Spermatic veins
excision ~ 55530-55540
ligation ~ 55550
Spermatocele excision ~ 54840
Spermatocystectomy ~ (spermatocele excision) 54840
Sphenoid sinus ~ see sinuses, sphenoid
Sphenoidotomy excision, with nasal/sinus endoscopy ~ 31287-31288
Sphenopalatine ganglion injection, anesthetic ~ 64505
Sphincter ~ see specific sphincter
anal ~ see anal sphincter
artificial genitourinary ~ see prosthesis, urethral sphincter
pyloric ~ see pyloric sphincter
Sphincter of Oddi pressure measurement, endoscopy ~ 43263
Sphincteroplasty
anal ~ 46750-46751, 46760-46761
  with implant ~ 46762
bile duct ~ 47460
bladder neck ~ see bladder, repair, neck
Sphincterotomy ~ 52277
anal ~ 46080
bile duct ~ 47460
Spica cast
hip ~ 29305-29325
repair ~ 29720
shoulder ~ 29055
Spinal accessory nerve
anastomosis to facial nerve ~ 64866
incision ~ 63191
injection, anesthetic ~ 64412
section ~ 63191
Spinal column ~ see spine
Spinal cord ~ see also cauda equina; nerve root
biopsy ~ 63275-63290
cyst
  aspiration ~ 62268
  incision and drainage ~ 63172-63173
decompression ~ 63001-63103
  with cervical laminoplasty ~ 63050-63051

Spinal cord ~ *continued*
drain fluid ~ 62272
exploration ~ 63001-63044
graft, dura ~ 63710
implantation
 electrode ~ 63650-63655
 pulse generator ~ 63685
 receiver ~ 63685
incision ~ 63200
 dentate ligament ~ 63180-63182
 tract ~ 63170, 63194-63199
injection
 anesthetic ~ 62310-62319
 blood ~ 62273
 CT scan ~ 62284
 neurolytic agent ~ 62280-62282
 other ~ 62310-62311
 X-ray ~ 62284
insertion
 electrode ~ 63650-63655
 pulse generator ~ 63685
 receiver ~ 63685
lesion
 destruction ~ 62280-62282
 excision ~ 63265-63273, 63300-63308
needle biopsy ~ 62269
neoplasm, excision ~ 63275-63290
puncture (tap) ~ *continued*
 diagnostic ~ 62270
 drain fluid ~ 62272
 lumbar ~ 62270
release ~ 63200
reconstruction, dorsal spine elements ~ 63295
removal
 catheter ~ 62355
 electrode ~ 63661-63664
 pulse generator ~ 63688
 pump ~ 62365
 receiver ~ 63688
 reservoir ~ 62365
repair
 cerebrospinal fluid leak ~ 63707-63709
 meningocele ~ 63700-63702
 myelomeningocele ~ 63704-63706
section
 dentate ligament ~ 63180-63182
 tract ~ 63194-63199
shunt
 create ~ 63740-63741
 irrigation ~ 63744
 removal ~ 63746
 replacement ~ 63744
stereotaxis
 aspiration ~ 63615
 biopsy ~ 63615
 creation lesion ~ 63600
 excision lesion ~ 63615
 stimulation ~ 63610
syrinx, aspiration ~ 62268
tumor, excision ~ 63275-63290
Spinal fluid ~ see cerebrospinal fluid
Spinal fracture ~ see fracture, vertebra

Spinal instrumentation
anterior ~ 22845-22847
 removal ~ 22855
internal fixation ~ 22841
pelvic fixation ~ 22848
posterior nonsegmental, Harrington rod
 technique ~ 22840
 removal ~ 22850
posterior segmental ~ 22842-22844
 removal ~ 22852
prosthetic device ~ 22851
reinsertion of spinal fixation device ~ 22849
Spinal manipulation ~ see manipulation, chiropractic
Spinal nerve
avulsion ~ 64772
transection ~ 64772
Spinal tap ~ see cervical puncture; cisternal puncture; subdural tap; ventricular puncture
drainage fluid ~ 62272
lumbar ~ 62270
Spine ~ see also spinal cord; vertebra; vertebral body; vertebral process
allograft
 morselized ~ 20930
 structural ~ 20931
arthroplasty, lumbar ~ 22856-22865
aspiration ~ 62267
autograft
 local ~ 20936
 morselized ~ 20937
 structural ~ 20938
biopsy ~ 20250-20251
chemotherapy administration ~ (see also chemotherapy) 96450
CT scan
 cervical ~ 72125-72127
 lumbar ~ 72131-72133
 thoracic ~ 72128-72130
fixation ~ 22842
fusion
 anterior ~ 22808-22812
 anterior approach ~ 22548-22585, 22812
 exploration ~ 22830
 lateral extracavitary ~ 22532-22534
 posterior approach ~ 22590-22802
insertion, instrumentation ~ 22840-22848, 22851
kyphectomy ~ 22818-22819
magnetic resonance angiography ~ 72159
magnetic resonance imaging
 cervical ~ 72141-72142, 72156-72158
 lumbar ~ 72148-72158
 thoracic ~ 72146-72147, 72156-72158
manipulation, with anesthesia ~ 22505
myelography
 cervical ~ 72240
 lumbosacral ~ 72265
 thoracic ~ 72255
 total ~ 72270
reconstruction, dorsal spine elements ~ 63295
reinsertion, instrumentation ~ 22849

Spine ~ *continued*
removal, instrumentation ~ 22850,
22852-22855
repair, osteotomy
anterior ~ 22220-22226
posterior ~ 22210-22214
cervical laminoplasty ~ 63050-63051
posterolateral ~ 22216
ultrasound ~ 76800
unlisted services and procedures, surgery ~
22899
X-ray ~ 72020, 72090
absorptiometry ~ 77080-77082
cervical ~ 72040-72052
lumbosacral ~ 72100-72120
standing ~ 72069
thoracic ~ 72070-72074
thoracolumbar ~ 72080
total ~ 72010
with contrast
cervical ~ 72240
lumbosacral ~ 72265
thoracic ~ 72255
total ~ 72270
Spirometry ~ (see also pulmonology,
diagnostic) 94010-94070
patient initiated ~ 94014-94016
Splanchnicectomy ~ see nerves,
sympathectomy, excision
Spleen
excision ~ 38100-38102
laparoscopic ~ 38120
injection, radiologic ~ 38200
nuclear medicine, imaging ~ 78185,
78215-78216
repair ~ 38115
Splenectomy
laparoscopic ~ 38120
partial ~ 38101
partial with repair, ruptured spleen ~ 38115
total ~ 38100
en bloc ~ 38102
Splenoplasty ~ see repair, spleen
Splenoportography ~ 75810
injection procedures ~ 38200
Splenorrhaphy ~ 38115
Splint ~ see casting; strapping
arm
long ~ 29105
short ~ 29125-29126
finger ~ 29130-29131
leg
long ~ 29505
short ~ 29515
oral surgical ~ 21085
ureteral ~ see ureteral splinting
Split grafts ~ 15100-15121
Split renal function test ~ see
cystourethroscopy, catheterization, ureteral
Splitting blood products ~ 86985
Spontaneous abortion ~ see abortion

Sprengel's deformity ~ 23400
Spring water cyst ~ see cyst, pericardial
Spur, bone ~ see exostosis
calcaneal ~ see heel spur
Sputum analysis ~ 89220
SRH ~ (somatostatin) 84307
Ssabanejew-Frank operation ~ (incision,
stomach, creation, stoma) 43830-43832
Stabilizing factor, fibrin ~ see fibrin stabilizing
factor
Stable factor ~ 85230
Stallard procedure ~ see
conjunctivorhinostomy
Stamey procedure ~ (repair, bladder, neck)
51845
Standby services physician ~ 99360
Stanford-Binet test ~ see psychiatric diagnosis
Stanftan ~ (Binet test) 96101-96103
Stapedectomy
revision ~ 69662
with footplate drill out ~ 69661
without foreign material ~ 69660
Stapedotomy
revision ~ 69662
with footplate drill out ~ 69661
without foreign material ~ 69660
Stapes
excision
with footplate drill out ~ 69661
without foreign material ~ 69660
mobilization ~ see mobilization, stapes
release ~ 69650
revision ~ 69662
Staphyloma
sclera repair
with graft ~ 66225
without graft ~ 66220
State operation ~ see proctectomy
Statin therapy ~ see performance measures
Statistics/biometry ~ see biometry
Steindler stripping ~ 28250
Stellate ganglion injection, anesthetic ~ 64510
Stem cell
concentration ~ 38215
count ~ 86587
cryopreservation ~ 38207, 88240
donor search ~ 38204
harvesting ~ 38205-38206
limbal, allograft ~ 65781
plasma depletion ~ 38214
platelet depletion ~ 38213
red blood cell depletion ~ 38212
T-cell depletion ~ 38210
thawing ~ 38208-38209, 88241
transplantation ~ 38240-38242
tumor cell depletion ~ 38211
washing ~ 38209
Stem, brain ~ see brainstem
Stenger test ~ (audiologic function test; ear,
nose and throat) 92565, 92577

Stenosis
aortic ~ see aortic stenosis
bronchi ~ 31641
    reconstruction ~ 31775
excision, trachea ~ 31780-31781
laryngoplasty ~ 31582
reconstruction, auditory canal, external ~
    69310
repair, trachea ~ 31780-31781
tracheal ~ see trachea stenosis
urethral ~ see urethral stenosis
Stensen duct ~ see parotid duct
Stent
indwelling insertion, ureter ~ 50605
placement
    bronchoscopy ~ 31631, 31636-31637
    colonoscopy ~ 45387
        via stoma ~ 44397
    endoscopy, gastrointestinal, upper ~ 43256
    enteroscopy ~ 44370
    proctosigmoidoscopy ~ 45327
    sigmoidoscopy ~ 45345
    transcatheter, intravascular ~ 37205-37208,
        37215, 37216
        extracranial ~ 0075T-0076T
    ureteroneocystomy ~ 50947-50948
revision, bronchoscopy ~ 31638
urethra ~ 52282
    prostatic ~ 53855
Stent, intravascular ~ see transcatheter,
    placement, intravascular stents
Stents, tracheal ~ see tracheal stent
Stereotactic frame application/removal ~
    20660
Stereotaxis
aspiration
    brain lesion ~ 61750
        with CT scan and/or MRI ~ 61751
    spinal cord ~ 63615
biopsy
    aspiration, brain lesion ~ 61750
    brain ~ 61750
        with CT scan and/or MRI ~ 61751
    breast ~ 77031
    prostate ~ 55706
    spinal cord ~ 63615
catheter placement, brain
    infusion ~ 0169T
    radiation source ~ 61770
computer assisted
    cranial ~ 61781-61782
    orthopedic surgery ~ 0054T-0055T, 20985
    spinal ~ 61783
creation lesion
    brain
        deep ~ 61720-61735
        percutaneous ~ 61790
    gasserian ganglion ~ 61790
    spinal cord ~ 63600
    trigeminal tract ~ 61791

Stereotaxis ~ *continued*
CT scan
    aspiration ~ 61751
    biopsy ~ 61751
excision lesion
    brain ~ 61750
    spinal cord ~ 63615
focus beam, radiosurgery ~ 77371-77373
    cranial ~ 61796-61799
    spinal ~ 63620-63621
    stereotactic frame application ~ 20660,
        61800
radiation therapy ~ 77421, 77432-77435
stimulation, spinal cord ~ 63610
target volume guidance ~ 77421
Sterile coverings ~ see dressings
Sternal fracture ~ see fracture, sternum
Sternoclavicular joint
arthrotomy ~ 23044
    with biopsy ~ 23101
    with synovectomy ~ 23106
dislocation
    closed treatment
        with manipulation ~ 23525
        without manipulation ~ 23520
    open treatment ~ 23530-23532
        with fascial graft ~ 23532
Sternocleidomastoid division ~ 21720-21725
Sternotomy closure ~ 21750
Sternum
debridement ~ 21627
excision ~ 21620, 21630-21632
fracture
    closed treatment ~ 21820
    open treatment ~ 21825
ostectomy ~ 21620
radical resection ~ 21630-21632
reconstruction ~ 21740-21742, 21750
    with thoracoscopy ~ 21743
X-ray ~ 71120-71130
Steroid-binding protein, sex ~ see globulin,
    sex hormone binding
Steroids
anabolic ~ see androstenedione
injection, urethral stricture ~ 52283
ketogenic, urine ~ 83582
STH (somatotropic hormone) ~ see growth
    hormone
Stimulating antibody, thyroid ~ see
    immunoglobulin, thyroid stimulating
Stimulation
electric ~ see electrical stimulation
lymphocyte ~ see blastogenesis
spinal cord, stereotaxis ~ 63610
transcutaneous electric ~ see application,
    neurostimulation
Stimulator, long-acting thyroid ~ see
    thyrotropin releasing hormone (TRH)
Stimulators, cardiac ~ see heart, pacemaker
Stimulus evoked response ~ 51792
Stoffel operation ~ (rhizotomy) 63185, 63190

Stoma
creation
  bladder ~ 51980
  kidney ~ 50551-50561
  stomach, neonatal ~ 43831
    temporary ~ 43830-43831
  ureter ~ 50860
  ureter, endoscopy via ~ 50951-50961
Stomach
anastomosis
  with duodenum ~ 43810, 43850-43855
  with jejunum ~ 43820-43825, 43860-43865
biopsy ~ 43605
creation
  stoma
    temporary ~ 43830-43831
    laparoscopic ~ 43653
electrogastrography ~ 91132-91133
excision
  partial ~ 43631-43639, 43845
  total ~ 43620-43622
exploration ~ 43500
gastric bypass ~ 43644-43645, 43846
  revision ~ 43848
incision ~ 43830-43832
  exploration ~ 43500
  pyloric sphincter ~ 43520
  removal, foreign body ~ 43500
nuclear medicine
  blood loss study ~ 78278
  emptying study ~ 78264
  imaging ~ 78261
  protein loss study ~ 78282
  reflux study ~ 78262
  vitamin B-12 absorption ~ 78270-78272
reconstruction
  for obesity ~ 43644-43645, 43842-43847
  Roux-en-Y ~ 43644, 43846
removal, foreign body ~ 43500
repair ~ 48547
  fistula ~ 43880
  fundoplasty ~ 43325
    laparoscopic ~ 43279-43282
  laceration ~ 43501-43502
  stoma ~ 43870
  ulcer ~ 43501
suture
  fistula ~ 43880
  for obesity ~ 43842-43843
  stoma ~ 43870
  ulcer ~ 43840
  wound ~ 43840
tumor, excision ~ 43610-43611
ulcer, excision ~ 43610
unlisted services and procedures ~ 43659, 43999
Stomatoplasty ~ see mouth, repair
Stone, kidney ~ see calculus, removal, kidney
Stookey-Scarff procedure ~
  (ventriculocisternostomy) 62200
Stool blood ~ see blood, feces

Storage
embryo ~ 89342
oocyte ~ 89346
reproductive tissue ~ 89344
sperm ~ 89343
Strabismus
chemodenervation ~ 67345
repair
  adjustable sutures ~ 67335
  extraocular muscles ~ 67340
  one horizontal muscle ~ 67311
  one vertical muscle ~ 67314
  posterior fixation suture technique ~
    67334-67335
  previous surgery, not involving extraocular
    muscles ~ 67331
  release extensive scar tissue ~ 67343
  superior oblique muscle ~ 67318
  transposition ~ 67320
  two horizontal muscles ~ 67312
  two or more vertical muscles ~ 67316
Strapping ~ see cast; splint
ankle ~ 29540
back ~ 29799
chest ~ 29200
elbow ~ 29260
finger ~ 29280
foot ~ 29540
hand ~ 29280
hip ~ 29520
knee ~ 29530
shoulder ~ 29240
thorax ~ 29200
toes ~ 29550
unlisted services and procedures ~ 29799
Unna boot ~ 29580
wrist ~ 29260
Strassman procedure ~ 58540
Strayer procedure leg, lower ~ 27687
Streptococcus pneumoniae vaccine ~ see
  vaccines
Streptococcus
group A
  antigen detection
    enzyme immunoassay ~ 87430
    nucleic acid ~ 87650-87652
    direct optical observation ~ 87880
group B
  antigen detection by immunoassay with
    direct optical observation ~ 87802
  prenatal screening ~ 3294F
Streptokinase, antibody ~ 86590
Stress tests
cardiovascular ~ 93015-93024
multiple gated acquisition (MUGA) ~
  78472-78473
myocardial perfusion imaging ~ 78451-78454
pulmonary ~ see pulmonology, diagnostic ~
  94620-94621
Stricture repair, urethra ~ 53400-53405
Stricturoplasty intestines ~ 44615
Stroboscopy larynx ~ 31579

1535

STS ~ (syphilis test) 86592-86593
Stuart-Prower factor ~ 85260
Study, color vision ~ see color vision
  examination
Sturmdorf procedure ~ 57520
Styloid process radial, excision ~ 25230
Styloidectomy radial ~ 25230
Stypven time ~ see Russell viper venom time
Subacromial bursa arthrocentesis ~ 20610
Subclavian arteries ~ see artery, subclavian
Subcutaneous injection ~ see injection,
  subcutaneous
Subcutaneous mastectomies ~ see mastectomy,
  subcutaneous
Subcutaneous tissue excision ~ 15830-15839,
  15847
Subdiaphragmatic abscess ~ see abscess,
  subdiaphragmatic
Subdural electrode
  insertion ~ 61531-61533
  removal ~ 61535
Subdural hematoma ~ see hematoma, subdural
Subdural puncture ~ 61105-61108
Subdural tap ~ 61000-61001
Sublingual gland
  abscess, incision and drainage ~ 42310-42320
  calculi (stone), excision ~ 42330
  cyst
    drainage ~ 42409
    excision ~ 42408
  excision ~ 42450
Subluxation elbow ~ 24640
Submandibular gland
  calculi (stone), excision ~ 42330-42335
  excision ~ 42440
Submaxillary gland abscess, incision and
  drainage ~ 42310-42320
Submucous resection of nasal septum ~ see
  nasal septum, submucous resection
Subperiosteal implant reconstruction
  mandible ~ 21245-21246
  maxilla ~ 21245-21246
Subphrenic abscess ~ see abscess,
  subdiaphragmatic
Substance S, Reichstein's ~ see deoxycortisol
Subtrochanteric fracture ~ see femur, fracture,
  subtrochanteric
Sucrose hemolysis test ~ see red blood cell
  (RBC), fragility, osmotic
Suction lipectomies ~ see liposuction
Sudiferous gland ~ see sweat gland
Sugar water test ~ see red blood cell (RBC),
  fragility, osmotic
Sugars ~ 84375-84379
Sugiura procedure ~ see esophagus, repair,
  varices
Sulfate
  chondroitin ~ see chondroitin sulfate
  DHA ~ see dehydroepiandrosterone sulfate
  urine ~ 84392
Sulfation factor ~ see somatomedin
Sulphates ~ see sulfate

Sumatran mite fever ~ see scrub typhus
Superficial musculoaponeurotic system
  (SMAS) flap rhytidectomy ~ 15829
Supernumerary digit
  reconstruction ~ 26587
  repair ~ 26587
Supply
  chemotherapeutic agent ~ (see also
    chemotherapy) 96545
  contact lenses ~ 92391, 92396
  educational materials ~ 99071
  low vision aids ~ (see also spectacle services)
    92392
  materials ~ 99070
  ocular prosthesis ~ 92393
  prosthesis, breast ~ 19396
  spectacle prosthesis ~ 92395
  spectacles ~ 92390
Suppositories, vaginal ~ see pessary
Suppression ~ 80400-80408
Suppression/testing ~ see evocative/suppression
  test
Suppressor T lymphocyte marker ~ see CD8
Suppurative hidradenitides ~ see hidradenitis,
  suppurative
Suprahyoid lymphadenectomy ~ 38700
Supraorbital nerve
  avulsion ~ 64732
  incision ~ 64732
  transection ~ 64732
Supraorbital rim and forehead reconstruction
  ~ 21179-21180
Suprapubic prostatectomies ~ see
  prostatectomy, suprapubic
Suprarenal
  gland ~ see adrenal gland
  vein ~ see vein, adrenal
Suprascapular nerve injection, anesthetic ~
  64418
Suprasellar cyst ~ see craniopharyngioma
Surface CD4 receptor ~ see CD4
Surface radiotherapy ~ see application,
  radioelement, surface
Surgeries
  breast-conserving ~ see breast, excision, lesion
  conventional ~ see celiotomy
  laser ~ see laser surgery
  Mohs ~ see Mohs micrographic surgery
  repeat ~ see reoperation
Surgery services ~ 10000-69999
  auditory system ~ 69000-69979
  cardiovascular system ~ 33000-37799
  digestive system ~ 40490-49999
  endocrine system ~ 60000-60699
  eye and ocular adnexa ~ 65091-68899
  female genital system ~ 56405-58999
  hemic and lymphatic systems ~ 38100-38999
  integumentary system ~ 10000-19999
  intersex surgery ~ 55970-55980
  male genital system ~ 54000-55899
  maternity care and delivery ~ 59000-59899
  mediastinum and diaphragm ~ 39000-39599

Suture ~ *continued*
  wound
    cervical ~ 31800
    intrathoracic ~ 31805
  ulcer ~ 44604-44605
  ureter ~ 50900
    deligation ~ 50940
    fistula ~ 50920-50930
  urethra
    fistula ~ 45820-45825, 53520
    stoma ~ 53520
    to bladder ~ 51840-51841
    wound ~ 53502-53515
  uterus
    fistula ~ 51920-51925
    rupture ~ 58520, 59350
    suspension ~ 58400-58410
  vagina
    cystocele ~ 57240, 57260
    enterocele ~ 57265
    fistula
      rectovaginal ~ 57300-57307
      transvesical and vaginal approach ~ 57330
      urethrovaginal ~ 57310-57311
      vesicovaginal ~ 51900, 57320-57330
    rectocele ~ 57250-57260
    suspension ~ 57280, 57283
    wound ~ 57200-57210
  vas deferens ~ 55400
  vein, femoral ~ 37650
    iliac ~ 37660
  wound ~ 44604-44605
Swallowing evaluation ~ 92526, 92610-92613, 92616-92617
  cine ~ 74230
  treatment ~ 92526
  video ~ 74230
Swanson procedure ~ 28309
Sweat collection iontophoresis ~ 89230
Sweat glands, excision
  axillary ~ 11450-11451
  inguinal ~ 11462-11463
  perianal ~ 11470-11471
  perineal ~ 11470-11471
  umbilical ~ 11470-11471
Sweat test ~ (chloride, blood) 82435
Swenson procedure ~ 45120
Syme procedure ~ 27888
Sympathectomy
  artery
    digital ~ 64820
    radial ~ 64821
    superficial palmar arch ~ 64823
    ulnar ~ 64822
  cervical ~ 64802
  cervicothoracic ~ 64804
  digital artery, with magnification ~ 64820
  lumbar ~ 64818
  presacral ~ 58410
  thoracic ~ 32664
  thoracolumbar ~ 64809
  with rib excision ~ 21616

Sympathetic nerve
  excision ~ 64802-64818
  injection, anesthetic ~ 64508, 64520-64530
Sympathins ~ see catecholamines
Symphysiotomy horseshoe kidney ~ 50540
Symphysis, pubic ~ see pubic symphysis
Syncytial virus, respiratory ~ see respiratory syncytial virus
Syndactylism, toes ~ see webbed, toe
Syndactyly repair ~ 26560-26562
Syndesmotomy ~ see ligament, release
Syndrome
  andrenogenital ~ see adrenogenital syndrome
  ataxia-telangiectasia ~ see ataxia telangiectasia
  Bloom ~ see Bloom syndrome
  carpal tunnel ~ see carpal tunnel syndrome
  Costen's ~ see temporomandibular joint (TMJ)
  Eerb-Goldflam ~ see myasthenia gravis
  ovarian vein ~ see ovarian vein syndrome
  synechiae, intrauterine ~ see adhesions, intrauterine
  Treacher Collins ~ see Treacher-Collins syndrome
  urethral ~ see urethral syndrome
Syngesterone ~ see progesterone
Synostosis (cranial) ~ see craniosynostosis
Synovectomy
  arthrotomy with, glenohumeral joint ~ 23105
    sternoclavicular joint ~ 23106
  elbow ~ 24102
  excision
    carpometacarpal joint ~ 26130
    finger joint ~ 26135-26140
    hip joint ~ 27054
    interphalangeal joint ~ 26140
    knee joint ~ 27334-27335
    metacarpophalangeal joint ~ 26135
    palm ~ 26145
  wrist ~ 25105, 25118-25119
    radical ~ 25115-25116
Synovial
  bursa ~ see bursa
  cyst ~ see ganglion
  membrane ~ see synovium
  popliteal space ~ see baker's cyst
Synovium
  biopsy
    carpometacarpal joint ~ 26100
    interphalangeal joint ~ 26110
    knee joint ~ 27330
    metacarpophalangeal joint, with synovial biopsy ~ 26105
  excision
    carpometacarpal joint ~ 26130
    finger joint ~ 26135-26140
    hip joint ~ 27054
    interphalangeal joint ~ 26140
    knee joint ~ 27334-27335
Syphilis ab ~ see antibody, Treponema pallidum
Syphilis test ~ 86592-86593
Syrinx spinal cord, aspiration ~ 62268

System
 endocrine ~ see endocrine system
 hemic ~ see hemic system
 lymphatic ~ see lymphatic system
 musculoskeletal ~ see musculoskeletal system
 nervous ~ see nervous system

T

T cell leukemia virus I antibodies, adult ~ 86687, 86689
T cell leukemia virus, I, human ~ 86687, 86689
T cell leukemia virus II antibodies, human ~ 86688
T cell leukemia virus II , human ~ 86688
T lymphotropic virus type III antibodies, human ~ 86689, 86701-86703
T-3 ~ see triiodothyronine
T-4 ~ 84436-84439, 86360
T-7 index ~ 84436
T-8 ~ 86360
T-cells CD4, absolute ~ 86361
 count ~ 86359
 ratio ~ 86360
T- cell T8 antigens ~ 86360
T- phyl ~ 80198
T3 free ~ 84481
T4 molecule ~ 86360
T4 total ~ 84436
Taarnhoj Procedure ~ see section ~ 61450
Tachycardia heart, recording ~ 93609
Tacrolimus drug assay ~ 80197
Tag, skin ~ see skin, tags
Tail bone
 excision ~ 27080
 fracture ~ 27200-27202
Takeuchi Procedure ~ 33505
Talectomy ~ see astragalectomy
Talotarsal joint dislocation ~ 28570-28575, 28585
 percutaneous fixation ~ 28576
Talus
 arthrodesis
 pantalar ~ 28705
 subtalar ~ 28725
 triple ~ 28715
 arthroscopy
 surgical ~ 29891-29892
 subtalar ~ 29904-29907, 29915-29916
 autograft, osteochondral ~ 28446
 craterization ~ 28120
 cyst, excision ~ 28100-28103
 diaphysectomy ~ 28120
 excision ~ 28120, 28130
 fracture
 open treatment ~ 28445
 percutaneous fixation ~ 28436

Talus ~ *continued*
 with manipulation ~ 28435-28436
 without manipulation ~ 28430
 repair
 osteochondritis dissecans ~ 29892
 osteotomy ~ 28302
 saucerization ~ 28120
 tumor, excision ~ 27647, 28100-28103
Tap
 cisternal ~ see cisternal puncture
 lumbar diagnostic ~ see spinal tap
Tarsal fracture
 percutaneous fixation ~ 28456
Tarsal bone ~ see ankle bone
Tarsal joint ~ see foot
 arthrodesis ~ 28730-28735, 28740
 with advancement ~ 28737
 with lengthening ~ 28737
 craterization ~ 28122
 cyst, excision ~ 28104-28107
 diaphysectomy ~ 28122
 dislocation ~ 28540-28545, 28555
 percutaneous fixation ~ 28545-28546
 excision ~ 28116, 28122
 fracture
 open treatment ~ 28465
 with manipulation ~ 28455-28456
 without manipulation ~ 28450
 fusion ~ 28730-28735, 28740
 with advancement ~ 28737
 with lengthening ~ 28737
 repair ~ 28320
 osteotomy ~ 28304-28305
 saucerization ~ 28122
 tumor, excision ~ 28104-28107, 28171
Tarsal strip procedure ~ 67917-67924
Tarsal tunnel release ~ 28035
Tarsal wedge procedure ~ 67916-67923
Tarsometatarsal joint
 arthrodesis ~ 28730-28735, 28740
 arthrotomy ~ 28020, 28050
 dislocation ~ 28600-28605, 28615
 percutaneous fixation ~ 28606
 exploration ~ 28020
 fusion ~ 28730-28735, 28740
 removal
 foreign body ~ 28020
 loose body ~ 28020
 synovial
 biopsy ~ 28050
 excision ~ 28070
Tarsorrhaphy ~ 67875
 median ~ 67880
 severing ~ 67710
 with transposition of tarsal plate ~ 67882
Tattoo
 cornea ~ 65600
 skin ~ 11920-11922
TB test, antigen response ~ 0010T
 skin test ~ 86580-86585
TBG ~ see thyroxine binding globulin
TBS ~ see Bethesda system

TCT ~ see thrombin time
TD shots ~ see tetanus immunization; vaccines
Team conference case management services ~ 99366-99368
Tear duct ~ see lacrimal duct
Tear gland ~ see lacrimal gland
Technique
  pericardial window ~ see pericardiostomy
  projective ~ see projective test
Teeth X-ray ~ 70300-70320
Telangiectasia
  chromosome analysis ~ 88248
  injection ~ 36468
Telangiectasia, cerebello-oculocutaneous ~ see ataxia telangiectasia
Telephone
  evaluation and management services
    non-physician ~ 98966-98968
    physician ~ 99441-99443
  pacemaker analysis ~ 93293
Teletherapy dose plan ~ 77305-77321
Temperature gradient studies ~ 93740
Temporal arteries ~ 37609
Temporal bone
  electromagnetic bone conduction hearing device
    implantation/replacement ~ 69710
    removal/repair ~ 69711
  excision ~ 69535
  resection ~ 69535
  tumor, removal ~ 69970
  unlisted services and procedures ~ 69979
Temporal, petrous
  excision, apex ~ 69530
Temporomandibular joint (TMJ)
  arthrocentesis ~ 20605
  arthrography ~ 70328-70332
    injection ~ 21116
  arthroplasty ~ 21240-21243
  arthroscopy
    diagnostic ~ 29800
    surgical ~ 29804
  arthrotomy ~ 21010
  cartilage, excision ~ 21060
  condylectomy ~ 21050
  coronoidectomy ~ 21070
  dislocation
    closed treatment ~ 21480-21485
    open treatment ~ 21490
  injection, radiologic ~ 21116
  magnetic resonance imaging (MRI) ~ 70336
  manipulation ~ 21073
  meniscectomy ~ 21060
  prostheses ~ see prosthesis, temporomandibular joint
  reconstruction ~ see reconstruction, temporomandibular joint
  X-ray with contrast ~ 70328-70332
Tenago Procedure ~ 53431
Tendinosuture ~ see suture, tendon

Tendon
  Achilles ~ see Achilles tendon
  arm, upper, revision ~ 24320
  excision
    forearm ~ 25109
    finger, excision ~ 26180
    forearm, repair ~ 25260-25274
    graft, harvesting ~ 20924
    insertion, biceps tendon ~ 24342
  lengthening
    ankle ~ 27685-27686
    arm, upper ~ 24305
    elbow ~ 24305
    finger ~ 26476, 26478
    forearm ~ 25280
    hand ~ 26476, 26478
    leg, lower ~ 27685-27686
    leg, upper ~ 27393-27395
    toe ~ 28240
    wrist ~ 25280
  palm, excision ~ 26170
  release
    arm, lower ~ 25295
    arm, upper ~ 24332
    wrist ~ 25295
  shortening
    ankle ~ 27685-27686
    finger ~ 26477, 26479
    hand ~ 26477, 26479
    leg, lower ~ 27685-27686
  transfer
    arm, lower ~ 25310-25312, 25316
    arm, upper ~ 24301
    elbow ~ 24301
    finger ~ 26497-26498
    hand ~ 26480-26489
    leg, lower ~ 27690-27692
    leg, upper ~ 27400
    pelvis ~ 27098
    thumb ~ 26490-26492, 26510
    wrist ~ 25310-25312, 25316
  transplant, leg, upper ~ 27396-27397
  wrist, repair ~ 25260-25274
Tendon origin insertion, injection ~ 20551
Tendon pulley reconstruction of hand ~ see hand, reconstruction, tendon pulley
Tendon sheath
  arm, lower, repair ~ 25275
  finger
    incision ~ 26055
    incision and drainage ~ 26020
    lesion ~ 26160
  foot, excision ~ 28086-28088
  hand lesion ~ 26160
  injection ~ 20550
  palm, incision and drainage ~ 26020
  removal, foreign body ~ 20520-20525
  wrist
    excision, radical ~ 25115-25116
    incision ~ 25000-25001
    repair ~ 25275
Tenectomy, tendon sheath ~ 25110

Tennis elbow repair ~ 24357-24359
Tenodesis
  biceps tendon
    arthroscopic ~ 29828
    at elbow ~ 24340
    shoulder ~ 23430
    finger ~ 26471-26474
    wrist ~ 25300-25301
Tenolysis
  ankle ~ 27680-27681
  arm, lower ~ 25295
  arm, upper ~ 24332
  finger
    extensor ~ 26445-26449
    flexor ~ 26440-26442
  foot ~ 28220-28226
  hand extensor ~ 26445-26449
    flexor ~ 26440-26442
  leg, lower ~ 27680-27681
  wrist ~ 25295
Tenomyotomy, shoulder ~ 23405-23406
Tenon's capsule injection ~ 67515
Tenoplasty anesthesia ~ 01714
Tenorrhaphy ~ see suture, tendon
Tenosuspension ~ see tenodesis
Tenosuture ~ see suture, tendon
Tenotomy
  Achilles tendon ~ 27605-27606
  ankle ~ 27605-27606
  arm, lower ~ 25290
  arm, upper ~ 24310
  finger ~ 26060, 26455-26460
  foot ~ 28230, 28234
  hand ~ 26450, 26460
  hip, iliopsoas tendon ~ 27005
  hip, abductor ~ 27006
  hip, adductor ~ 27000-27003
  leg, upper ~ 27306-27307, 27390-27392
  toe ~ 28010-28011, 28232-28234, 28240
  wrist ~ 25290
TENS ~ see physical medicine/therapy/
    occupational therapy ~ 64550
Tensilon test ~ 95857-95858
Tension, ocular ~ see glaucoma
Tentorium cerebelli section ~ 61440
Terman-Merrill test ~ 96100
Termination, pregnancy ~ see abortion
Test
  antiglobulin ~ 86880
  aphasia ~ 96105
  Bender visual-motor Gestalt ~ 96101-96103
  Binet ~ 96101-96103
  blood ~ see blood tests
  blood coagulation ~ see coagulation
  breath ~ see breath test
  cervical mucus penetration ~ 89330
  clinical chemistry ~ 84999
  complement fixation ~ 86171
  exercise ~ 93015-93018
  fern ~ 87210
  fetal, nonstress ~ 59025

Test ~ *continued*
  function, vestibular ~ see vestibular function
    tests
  gel diffusion ~ 86329-86331
  glucose tolerance ~ 82951-82952
  hearing ~ see audiologic function tests
  hemagglutination inhibition ~ 86280
  ink blot ~ see inkblot test
  intelligence ~ 96101-96102
  lung function ~ see pulmonology, diagnostic
  neutralization ~ 86382
  Papanicolaou ~ 88141-88155, 88164-88167,
    88174-88175
  pregnancy ~ 84702-84703
  quick ~ 85610-85611
  radioimmunosorbent ~ 82784-82787
  Rorschach ~ 96101
  Schilling ~ 78270
  skin ~ see skin, tests
  Stanford-Binet ~ see psychiatric diagnosis
  tuberculin ~ 86580
Test tube fertilization ~ 58321-58322
Tester, color vision ~ 92283
Testes
  cryopreservation ~ 89335
  nuclear medicine
    imaging ~ 78761
  undescended ~ 54550-54560
Testicular vein ~ 55530-55540
Testimony, medical ~ 99075
Testing, histocompatibility ~ see tissue typing
Testing, neurophysiologic intraoperative ~
    95940-95941
Testing, neuropsychological ~ 96117
Testing, range of motion ~ see range of
    motion test
Testis
  abscess, incision and drainage ~ 54700
  biopsy ~ 54500-54505
  excision
    laparoscopic ~ 54690
    partial ~ 54522
    radical ~ 54530-54535
    simple ~ 54520
  hematoma, incision and drainage ~ 54700
  insertion, prosthesis ~ 54660
  lesion, excision ~ 54512
  needle biopsy ~ 54500
  repair
    injury ~ 54670
    suspension ~ 54620-54640
    torsion ~ 54600
  suture
    injury ~ 54670
    suspension ~ 54620-54640
  transplantation, to thigh ~ 54680
  tumor, excision ~ 54530-54535
  undescended, exploration ~ 54550-54560
  unlisted services and procedures ~ 54699,
    55899

Testosterone ~ 84402
  response ~ 80414
    stimulation ~ 80414-80415
    total ~ 84403
Testosterone estradiol binding globulin ~
  84270
Tetanus ~ 86280
  antibody ~ 86774
  immunoglobulin ~ 90389
  vaccine ~ 90703
Tetrachloride, carbon ~ 84600
Tetralogy of Fallot ~ 33692-33697, 33924
Thal-Nissen Procedure ~ 43325
Thawing ~ 86930-86932
  cryopreserved
    embryo ~ 89352
    oocytes ~ 89356
    reproductive tissue ~ 89354
    sperm ~ 89353
  previously frozen cells ~ 38208-38209
Thawing and expansion of frozen cell ~
  88241
THBR ~ 84479
Theleplasty ~ 19350
Theophylline assay ~ 80198
Therapeutic
  abortion ~ 59850-59852
  apheresis ~ 36511-36516
  drug assays ~ 80150-80299
  mobilization ~ see mobilization
  photopheresis ~ 36522
  radiology ~ see radiology, therapeutic
Therapies
  cold ~ see cryotherapy
  exercise ~ 97110-97113
  family ~ 90846-90849, 99510
  language ~ 92507-92508
  milieu ~ 90882
  occupational ~ 97003-97004
  photodynamic ~ 96910-96913
  photoradiation ~ 96900
  physical ~ see physical
    medicine/therapy/occupational therapy
  speech ~ 92507-92508
  tocolytic ~ 59412
  ultraviolet ~ 96900
Therapy
  radiation, brachytherapy ~ 0182T
Thermocauterization
  ectropion, repair ~ 67922
  lesion, cornea ~ 65450
Thermocoagulation ~ 17000-17286
Thermotherapy
  prostate ~ 53850-53852
    microwave ~ 53850
    radiofrequency ~ 53852
Thiamine ~ 84425
Thiersch Operation ~ 15050
Thiersch Procedure ~ 46753
Thigh fasciotomy ~ see femur; leg, upper ~
  27025

Thin layer chromatographies ~ 82489
Thiocyanate ~ 84430
Third disease ~ 86762, 90706
Third opinion ~ see confirmatory consultations
Thompson Procedure ~ 27430
Thompson test ~ see smear and stain, routine
Thoracectomy ~ 32905
Thoracentesis ~ 32554-32555
Thoracic
  anterior ramus ~ see intercostal nerve
  arteries ~ 36215-36218
  cavity ~ see chest cavity
  duct ~ see lymphatics
    cannulation ~ 38794
    ligation ~ 38380
      abdominal approach ~ 38382
      thoracic approach ~ 38381
    suture
      abdominal approach ~ 38382
      cervical approach ~ 38380
      thoracic approach ~ 38381
  empyema ~ 21501-21502
  surgery, video-assisted ~ see thoracoscopy
  vertebra ~ 22101, 22112
  wall ~ see chest wall
Thoracocentesis ~ 32554-32555
Thoracoplasty ~ 32905
  with closure bronchopleural fistula ~ 32906
Thoracoscopy
  diagnostic
    with biopsy ~ 32604, 32606, 32607-32609
    without biopsy ~ 32601
  surgical ~ 32650-32674
    with control traumatic hemorrhage ~ 32654
    with creation pericardial window ~ 32659
    with diagnostic wedge resection ~ 32668
    with esophagomyotomy ~ 32665
    with excision mediastinal cyst, tumor and/or
      mass ~ 32662
    with excision pericardial cyst, tumor and/or
      mass ~ 32661
    with lobectomy ~ 32663
    with mediastinal lymphadenectomy ~ 32674
    with parietal pleurectomy ~ 32656
    with partial pulmonary decortication ~
      32651
    with pleurodesis ~ 32650
    with regional lymphadenectomy ~ 32674
    with removal intrapleural foreign body ~
      32653
    with removal of clot/foreign body ~ 32658
    with resection of thymus ~ 32673
    with resection/plication of bullae ~ 32655
    with sternum reconstruction ~ 21743
    with therapeutic wedge resection ~ 32666,
      32667
    with thoracic sympathectomy ~ 32664
    with total pulmonary decortication ~ 32652
Thoracostomy empyema ~ 32035-32036
  tube, with/without water seal ~ 32551

Thoracotomy
  cardiac massage ~ 32160
  for post-op complications ~ 32120
  hemorrhage ~ 32110
  lymphadenectomy, thoracic ~ 38746
  removal
    bullae ~ 32141
    cyst ~ 32140
    defibrillator ~ 33243
    electrodes ~ 33238
    foreign body
      intrapleural ~ 32150
      intrapulmonary ~ 32151
    pacemaker ~ 33236-33237
  resection
    diagnostic wedge ~ 32507
    therapeutic wedge ~ 32505-32506
  revascularization ~ 33140-33141
  transmyocardial laser
    with biopsy ~ 32096-32097
    with lung repair ~ 32110
    with open intrapleural pneumolysis ~
      32124
    with resection-plication of bullae ~ 32141
Thorax ~ see chest; chest cavity; mediastinum
  angiography ~ 71275
  bioimpedance ~ 93701
  biopsy ~ 21550
  CT scan ~ 71250-71275
  incision, empyema ~ 32035-32036
    pneumothorax ~ 32551
  incision and drainage
    abscess ~ 21501-21502
    deep ~ 21510
    hematoma ~ 21501-21502
  strapping ~ 29200
  tumor
    excision ~ 21552-21558
    excision/resection ~ 21557, 21558
  unlisted services and procedures, surgery ~
    21899
Three glass test ~ 81020
Three-day measles ~ 86762, 90706
Throat ~ see pharynx
  abscess, incision and drainage ~ 42700-42725
  biopsy ~ 42800-42806
  hemorrhage ~ 42960-42962
  reconstruction ~ 42950
  removal, foreign body ~ 42809
  repair
    pharyngoesophageal ~ 42953
    wound ~ 42900
  suture, wound ~ 42900
  unlisted services and procedures ~ 42999
Thrombectomy ~ see also
    thromboendarterectomy
  aortoiliac artery ~ 34151-34201
  arteriovenous fistula, graft ~ 36870
  axillary artery ~ 34101
  axillary vein ~ 34490
  brachial artery ~ 34101

Thrombectomy ~ *continued*
  bypass graft, other than hemodialysis graft or
    fistula ~ 35875-35876
  carotid artery ~ 34001
  celiac artery ~ 34151
  dialysis graft ~ 36831, 36833
  femoral ~ 34201
  femoropopliteal vein ~ 34421-34451
  iliac ~ 34151-34201
  iliac vein ~ 34401-34451
  innominate artery ~ 34001-34101
  mesenteric artery ~ 34151
  percutaneous
    coronary artery ~ 92973
    fluoroscopic guidance ~ 37184-37188
    mechanical arterial ~ 37184-37186
    mechanical venous ~ 37187-37188
  peroneal artery ~ 34203
  popliteal artery ~ 34201-34203
  radial artery ~ 34111
  renal artery ~ 34151
  subclavian artery ~ 34001-34101
  subclavian vein ~ 34471-34490
  tibial artery ~ 34203
  ulnar artery ~ 34111
  vena cava ~ 34401-34451
  vena caval ~ 50230
Thrombin inhibitor I ~ 85300-85301
Thrombin time ~ 85670-85675
Thrombocyte (platelet) ~ see blood, platelet
Thrombocyte AB ~ 86022-86023
Thromboendarterectomy ~ see thrombectomy
  aorta, abdominal ~ 35331
  aortoiliofemoral artery ~ 35363
  axillary artery ~ 35321
  brachial artery ~ 35321
  carotid artery ~ 35301, 35390
  celiac artery ~ 35341
  femoral artery ~ 35302, 35371-35372
  iliac artery ~ 35351, 35361-35363
  iliofemoral artery ~ 35355, 35363
  innominate artery ~ 35311
  mesenteric artery ~ 35341
  peroneal artery ~ 35305-35306
  popliteal artery ~ 35303
  renal artery ~ 35341
  subclavian artery ~ 35301-35311
  superficial femoral artery ~ 35302
  tibial artery ~ 35305-35306
  tibioperoneal trunk artery ~ 35304
  vertebral artery ~ 35301
Thrombokinase ~ 85260
Thrombolysin ~ 85400
Thrombolysis
  catheter exchange, arterial ~ 37211-37214
  cerebral, intravenous infusion ~ 37195
  coronary vessels ~ 92975-92977
  cranial vessels ~ 37195
Thrombolysis biopsy intracranial arterial
  perfusion ~ 61624

1543

Thrombolysis intracranial ~ see ciliary body; cornea; eye, removal, foreign body; iris; lens; retina; sclera; vitreous ~ 65205
Thrombomodulin ~ 85337
Thromboplastin
  inhibition ~ 85705
  inhibition test ~ 85347
  partial time ~ 85730-85732
Thromboplastin antecedent, plasma ~ 85270
Thromboplastinogen ~ 85210-85293
Thromboplastinogen B ~ 85250
Thromboxane, urine ~ 84431
Thumb ~ 26720-26727
  amputation ~ 26910, 26952
  arthrodesis, carpometacarpal joint ~ 26841-26842
  dislocation
    with fracture ~ 26645-26650
      open treatment ~ 26665
    with manipulation ~ 26641
  fracture
    with dislocation ~ 26645-26650
      open treatment ~ 26665
  fusion, in opposition ~ 26820
  reconstruction
    from finger ~ 26550
    opponensplasty ~ 26490-26496
  repair
    muscle ~ 26508
    muscle transfer ~ 26494
    tendon transfer ~ 26510
  replantation ~ 20824-20827
  sesamoidectomy ~ 26185
  unlisted services and procedures ~ 26989
Thymectomy ~ 60520-60521
  sternal split/transthoracic approach ~ 60521-60522
  transcervical approach ~ 60520
Thymotaxin ~ 82232
Thymus gland ~ 60520
  excision ~ 60520-60521
Thyramine ~ 82145
Thyrocalcitonin ~ 80410, 82308
Thyroglobulin ~ 84432
  antibody ~ 86800
Thyroglossal duct cyst, excision ~ 60280-60281
Thyroid gland
  cyst
    aspiration ~ 60300
    excision ~ 60200
    incision and drainage ~ 60000
    injection ~ 60300

Thyroid gland ~ *continued*
  excision
    for malignancy
      limited neck dissection ~ 60252
      radical neck dissection ~ 60254
    partial ~ 60210-60225
    secondary ~ 60260
    total ~ 60240, 60271
      cervical approach ~ 60271
      removal all thyroid tissue ~ 60260
      sternal split/transthoracic approach ~ 60270
      transcervical approach ~ 60520
  metastatic cancer, nuclear imaging ~ 78015-78018
  needle biopsy ~ 60100
  nuclear medicine
    imaging for metastases ~ 78015-78018
    imaging with flow ~ 78013
    metastases uptake ~ 78020
    uptake ~ 78012, 78014
  tumor, excision ~ 60200
Thyroid hormone binding ratio ~ 84479
Thyroid hormone uptake ~ 84479
Thyroid stimulating hormone (TSH) ~ 80418, 80438-80440, 84443
Thyroid stimulating hormone receptor AB ~ 80438-80439
Thyroid stimulating immune globulins ~ 84445
Thyroid stimulator, long acting ~ 80438-80439
Thyroid suppression test ~ 78012, 78014
Thyroidectomy
  partial ~ 60210-60225
  secondary ~ 60260
  total ~ 60240, 60271
    cervical approach ~ 60271
    for malignancy
      limited neck dissection ~ 60252
      radical neck dissection ~ 60254
    removal all thyroid tissue ~ 60260
    sternal split/transthoracic approach ~ 60270
Thyrolingual cyst ~ 60000, 60280-60281
Thyrotomy ~ 31300
Thyrotropin receptor AB ~ 80438-80439
Thyrotropin releasing hormone (TRH) ~ 80438-80439
Thyroxine
  free ~ 84439
  neonatal ~ 84437
  total ~ 84436
  true ~ 84436
Thyroxine binding globulin ~ 84442
Tibia ~ see ankle
  arthroscopy surgical ~ 29891-29892
  craterization ~ 27360, 27640
  cyst, excision ~ 27635-27638
  diaphysectomy ~ 27360, 27640
  excision ~ 27360, 27640
    epiphyseal bar ~ 20150

Tibia ~ *continued*
fracture ~ 27759
fracture
arthroscopic treatment ~ 29855-29856
plafond ~ 29892
closed treatment ~ 27824-27825
distal ~ 27824-27828
intercondylar ~ 27538-27540
malleolus ~ 27760-27766, 27808-27814
open treatment ~ 27535-27536,
27758-27759, 27826-27828
plateau ~ 29855-29856
closed treatment ~ 27530-27536
shaft ~ 27752-27759
with manipulation ~ 27825
without manipulation ~ 27824
incision ~ 27607
osteoplasty, lengthening ~ 27715
prophylactic treatment ~ 27745
reconstruction ~ 27418
at knee ~ 27440-27443, 27446
repair ~ 27720-27725
epiphysis ~ 27477-27485, 27730-27742
osteochondritis dissecans arthroscopy ~
29892
osteotomy ~ 27455-27457, 27705,
27709-27712
pseudoarthrosis ~ 27727
saucerization ~ 27360, 27640
tumor, excision ~ 27635-27638, 27645
X-ray ~ 73590
Tibial
arteries ~ see artery, tibial
nerve
neurostimulation ~ 64566
repair/suture, posterior ~ 64840
Tibiofibular joint
arthrodesis ~ 27871
dislocation ~ 27830-27832
disruption, open treatment ~ 27829
fusion ~ 27871
TIG ~ see immune globulins, tetanus
Time
bleeding ~ 85002
prothrombin ~ 85610-85611
reptilase ~ 85670-85675
Tinnitus assessment ~ 92625
Tissue
culture
chromosome analysis ~ 88230-88239
homogenization ~ 87176
non-neoplastic disorder ~ 88230, 88237
skin grafts ~ 15100-15121, 15342-15343
solid tumor ~ 88239
toxin/antitoxin ~ 87230
virus ~ 87252-87253
dissection, macroscopic ~ 88387-88388
enzyme activity ~ 82657
examination
for ectoparasites ~ 87220
for fungi ~ 87220
macroscopic ~ 88387-88388

Tissue ~ *continued*
expander
breast reconstruction with ~ 19357
insertion, skin ~ 11960
removal, skin ~ 11971
replacement, skin ~ 11970
grafts, harvesting ~ 20926
granulation ~ 17250
homogenization ~ 87176
hybridization in situ ~ 88365-88368
mucosal ~ see mucosa
preparation
drug analysis ~ 80103
macroscopic ~ 88387-88388
skin harvest for culture ~ 15040
soft, abscess ~ 20005
transfer
adjacent
eyelids ~ 67961
skin ~ 14000-14350
facial muscles ~ 15845
finger flap ~ 14350
toe flap ~ 14350
typing
culture ~ 87140-87158
HLA antibodies ~ 86812-86817
HLA crossmatch ~ 86825-86826
lymphocyte culture ~ 86821-86822
Tissue factor ~ see thromboplastin
TLC ~ 82489
screen ~ 84375
TMJ ~ see temporomandibular joint (TMJ)
prostheses ~ 21243
Tobramycin assay ~ 80200
Tocolysis ~ 59412
Tocopherol ~ 84446
Toe ~ see phalanx ~ 28270, 28272
amputation ~ 28810-28825
capsulotomy ~ 28270-28272
fasciotomy ~ 28008
fracture ~ see fracture, phalanges, toe
lesion, excision ~ 28092
reconstruction
angle deformity ~ 28313
extra toes ~ 28344
hammer toe ~ 28285-28286
macrodactyly ~ 28340-28341
syndactyly ~ 28345
webbed toe ~ 28345
repair
bunion ~ 28290-28299
muscle ~ 28240
tendon ~ 28232-28234, 28240
webbed ~ 28280
webbed toe ~ 28345
tenotomy ~ 28010-28011, 28232-28234
unlisted services and procedures ~ 28899
Toe flap tissue transfer ~ 14350

Toes
arthrocentesis ~ 20600
dislocation ~ see specific joint**
magnetic resonance imaging (MRI) ~
73721-73723
reconstruction, extra digit ~ 26587
repair
extra digit ~ 26587
macrodactylia ~ 26590
reposition to hand ~ 26551-26556
strapping ~ 29550
X-ray ~ 73660
Tolbutamide tolerance test ~ 82953
Tolerance test
glucagon ~ 82946
glucose ~ 82951-82952
with tolbutamide ~ 82953
heparin-protamine ~ 85530
insulin ~ 80434-80435
maltose ~ 82951-82952
tolbutamide ~ 82953
Tomodensitometries ~ see CT scan
Tomographic scintigraphy, computed ~ 78607
Tomographic spect myocardial imaging ~
78469
Tomographies, computed X-ray ~ see CT scan
Tomography, computerized axial abdomen ~
74150-74175, 75635
head ~ 70450-70470, 70496
Tomography, emission computed ~ see
positron emission tomography
single photon ~ 78607
Tompkins metroplasty ~ 58540
Tongue
ablation, submucosal tongue base ~ 41530
abscess, incision and drainage ~ 41000-41006,
41015
base suspension ~ 41512
biopsy ~ 41100-41105
cyst, incision and drainage ~ 41000-41006,
41015, 60000
excision
complete ~ 41140-41155
frenum ~ 41115
partial ~ 41120-41135
with mouth resection ~ 41150-41153
with radical neck ~ 41135, 41145,
41153-41155
fixation ~ 41500
hematoma, incision and drainage ~
41000-41006, 41015
incision, frenum ~ 41010
lesion, excision ~ 41110-41114
reconstruction, frenum ~ 41520
repair ~ 41250-41252
laceration ~ 41250-41252
suture ~ 41510
suture ~ 41510
unlisted services and procedures ~ 41599
Tonometry, serial ~ 92100
Tonsil, pharyngeal ~ see adenoids
Tonsillectomy ~ 42820-42826

Tonsils
abscess, incision and drainage ~ 42700
excision ~ 42825-42826
lingual ~ 42870
radical ~ 42842-42845
tag ~ 42860
with adenoids ~ 42820-42821
lingual, destruction ~ 42870
unlisted services and procedures ~ 42999
Topiramate assay ~ 80201
Torek Procedure ~ see orchiopexy
Torkildsen Procedure ~ 62180
TORP (total ossicular replacement prosthesis) ~
69633, 69637
Torsion swing test ~ 92546
Torula ~ see cryptococcus
Torus mandibularis tumor excision ~ 21031
Total
abdominal hysterectomy ~ 58150, 58200,
58956
bilirubin level ~ 82247-82248, 88720
catecholamines ~ 82382
cystectomy ~ 51570, 51580, 51590-51597
dacryoadenectomy ~ 68500
elbow replacement ~ 24363
esophagectomy ~ 43107-43113, 43124
gastrectomy ~ 43620-43622
hemolytic complement ~ 86162
hip arthroplasty ~ 27130-27132
knee arthroplasty ~ 27438, 27445
mastectomies ~ see mastectomy
ostectomy of patella ~ 27424
splenectomy ~ 38100
Touroff Operation ~ 37615
Toxicology screen ~ 80100-80103
Toxin assay ~ 87230
Toxin, botulinum ~ see chemodenervation
Toxoplasma antibody ~ 86777-86778
Trabeculectomies ~ 65855
Trabeculectomy ab externo
in absence of previous surgery ~ 66170
with scarring previous surgery ~ 66172
Trabeculoplasty by laser surgery ~ 65855
Trabeculotomy AB externo eye ~ 65850
Trachea
aspiration ~ 31720
catheter ~ 31720-31725
dilation ~ 31630-31631, 31636-31638
endoscopy, via tracheostomy ~ 31615
excision, stenosis ~ 31780-31781
fistula
with plastic repair ~ 31825
without plastic repair ~ 31820
fracture, endoscopy ~ 31630
incision
emergency ~ 31603-31605
planned ~ 31600-31601
with flaps ~ 31610
introduction, needle wire ~ 31730
puncture, aspiration and/or injection ~ 31612

Trachea ~ *continued*
reconstruction
  carina ~ 31766
  cervical ~ 31750
  fistula ~ 31755
  intrathoracic ~ 31760
repair
  cervical ~ 31750
  fistula ~ 31755
  intrathoracic ~ 31760
  stoma ~ 31613-31614
revision, stoma, scars ~ 31830
scar, revision ~ 31830
stenosis
  excision ~ 31780-31781
  repair ~ 31780-31781
stoma
  repair
    with plastic repair ~ 31825
    without plastic repair ~ 31820
  revision, scars ~ 31830
tumor
  excision
    cervical ~ 31785
    thoracic ~ 31786
unlisted services and procedures, bronchi ~ 31899
wound, suture
  cervical ~ 31800
  intrathoracic ~ 31805
Tracheal stent, placement ~ 31631
tubes ~ 31500
Trachelectomy ~ 57530
radical ~ 57531
Tracheloplasty ~ 15819
Trachelorrhaphy ~ 57720
Tracheo-esophageal fistula ~ see fistula, tracheoesophageal
Tracheobronchoscopy through tracheostomy ~ 31615
Tracheoplasty
cervical ~ 31750
intrathoracic ~ 31760
tracheopharyngeal fistulization ~ 31755
Tracheostoma revision ~ 31613-31614
Tracheostomy
emergency ~ 31603-31605
planned ~ 31600-31601
revision, scar ~ 31830
surgical closure
  with plastic repair ~ 31825
  without plastic repair ~ 31820
tracheobronchoscopy through ~ 31615
with flaps ~ 31610
Tracheotomy tube change ~ 31502
Tracking tests (ocular) ~ 92545
Tract, urinary ~ 74400-74425
Traction therapy ~ 97140
manual ~ 97140
mechanical ~ 97012

Tractotomy
medulla ~ 61470
mesencephalon ~ 61480
Training
activities of daily living ~ 97535, 99509
biofeedback ~ 90901-90911
cognitive skills ~ 97532
community/work reintegration ~ 97537
home management ~ 97535, 99509
orthoptic/pleoptic ~ 92065
orthotics ~ 97504
prosthetics ~ 97520
self care ~ 97535, 99509
sensory integration ~ 97533
walking (physical therapy) ~ 97116
wheelchair management/propulsion ~ 97542
Tram flap
breast reconstruction ~ 19367-19369
Trans-scaphoperilunar fracture/dislocation
closed treatment ~ 25680
open treatment ~ 25685
Transaminase
glutamic oxaloacetic ~ 84450
glutamic pyruvic ~ 84460
Transcatheter
biopsy ~ 37200
closure
  percutaneous
    heart ~ 93580-93581
embolization, percutaneous ~ 37204
  cranial ~ 61624-61626
occlusion, percutaneous ~ 37204
  cranial ~ 61624-61626
placement
  intravascular stents ~ 0075T-0076T, 37205-37208, 37215-37216, 75960, 92980-92981
  sensor, pressure ~ 34806
therapy
  embolization ~ 75894
  infusion ~ 37202, 37211-37214, 75896-75898
  perfusion, cranial ~ 61624-61626
  retrieval ~ 37197
Transcatheter foreign body retrieval ~ 37197
Transcortin ~ 84449
Transcranial Doppler study (TCP) ~ 93886-93893
stimulation, motor ~ 95928-95929
Transcutaneous electric nerve stimulation ~ 64550
Transdermal electrostimulation ~ 64550
Transection
artery, carotid ~ 61610, 61612
blood vessel, kidney ~ 50100
brain, subpial ~ 61567
carotid, with skill base surgery ~ 61609
nerve ~ 64732-64772
  vagus ~ 43640-43641
pulmonary artery ~ 33922
Transesophageal Doppler echocardiography ~ 93312-93318

1547

Transfer
blastocyst ~ 58974-58976
gamete intrafallopian ~ see GIFT
jejunum, with microvascular anastomosis, free ~ 43496
preparation, embryo ~ 89255
cryopreserved ~ 89352
surgical ~ see transposition
tendon ~ see tendon, transfer
toe to hand ~ 26551-26556
Transferase
aspartate amino ~ 84450
glutamic oxaloacetic ~ 84450
Transferrin ~ 84466
Transformation lymphocyte ~ 86353
Transfusion blood ~ 36430
exchange ~ 36450-36455
fetal ~ 36460
push, infant ~ 36440
blood parts, exchange ~ 36511-36516
unlisted services and procedures ~ 86999
white blood cells ~ 86950
Transfusion medicine ~ 86850-86999
Transluminal
angioplasty, arterial ~ 75962-75968
coronary balloon dilatation ~ 92982-92984
Transmyocardial laser revascularization ~ 33140-33141
Transosteal bone plate reconstruction, mandible ~ 21244
Transpeptidase, gamma-glutamyl ~ 82977
Transplant ~ see graft
bone ~ see bone graft
hair ~ see hair, transplant
Transplantation ~ see graft
autologous ~ see autograft
bone marrow ~ 38240-38242
cartilage, knee
allograft ~ 27415, 29867
autograft ~ 27412, 29866
chondrocytes, knee ~ 27412
conjunctiva ~ 65782
cornea
autograft/homograft
allograft preparation ~ 65757
endothelials ~ 65756
lamellar ~ 65710
penetrating ~ 65730-65755
for aphakia ~ 65750
eye
amniotic membrane ~ 65780
conjunctiva ~ 65782
stem cell ~ 65781
hair
punch graft ~ 15775-15776
strip ~ 15220-15221
heart ~ 33945
allograft preparation ~ 33933, 33944
heart-lung ~ 33935

Transplantation ~ *continued*
intestines
allograft preparation ~ 44715-44721
allotransplantation ~ 44135-44136
donor enterectomy ~ 44132-44133
removal of allograft ~ 44137
liver ~ 47135
allograft preparation ~ 47143-47147
heterotopic ~ 47136
lung
allograft preparation ~ 32855-32856, 33933
anesthesia ~ 00580
donor pneumonectomy ~ 32850
double, with cardiopulmonary bypass ~ 32854
double, without cardiopulmonary bypass ~ 32853
single, with cardiopulmonary bypass ~ 32852
single, without cardiopulmonary bypass ~ 32851
meniscus, knee ~ 29868
pancreas ~ 48160, 48550, 48554-48556
allograft preparation ~ 48551-48552
parathyroid ~ 60512
renal
allograft preparation ~ 50323-50329
allotransplantation ~ 50360
with recipient nephrectomy ~ 50365
autotransplantation ~ 50380
donor nephrectomy ~ 50300-50320, 50547
recipient nephrectomy ~ 50340
removal transplanted renal allograft ~ 50370
skin ~ see dermatology
stem cells ~ 38240-38241
cell concentration ~ 38215
cryopreservation ~ 38207
harvesting ~ 38205-38206
plasma depletion ~ 38214
platelet depletion ~ 38213
red blood cell depletion ~ 38212
T-cell depletion ~ 38210
thawing ~ 38208
tumor cell depletion ~ 38211
washing ~ 38209
testis ~ 38208
to thigh ~ 54680
tissue, harvesting ~ 20926
Transpleural thoracoscopy ~ see thoracoscopy
Transposition
arteries
carotid ~ 0037T, 35691, 35694-35695
subclavian ~ 0037T, 35693-35695
vertebral ~ 35691-35693
cranial nerve ~ 64716
eye muscles ~ 67320
great arteries, repair ~ 33770-33781
nerve ~ 64718-64721
ovary ~ 58825
peripheral nerve
major ~ 64856
vein valve ~ 34510

Transthoracic echocardiography ~ 93303-93318, 93350
Transthyretin ~ 84134
Transureteroureterostomy ~ 50770
Transurethral procedure ~ see specific procedure**
prostate
incision ~ 52450
resection ~ 52630
thermotherapy ~ 53850-53852
microwave ~ 53850
radiofrequency ~ 53852
Trapezium arthroplasty with implant ~ 25445
Travel, unusual ~ 99082
Treacher-Collins syndrome midface reconstruction ~ 21150-21151
Treatment, tocolytic ~ 59412
Trendelenburg Operation ~ 37785
Trephine procedure sinusotomy, frontal ~ 31070
Treponema pallidum
antibody, confirmation test ~ 86780
antigen detection, direct fluorescence ~ 87285
TRH ~ see thyrotropin releasing hormone (TRH)
Triacylglycerol ~ 84478
Triacylglycerol hydrolase ~ 83690
Tributyrinase ~ 83690
Trichiasis repair ~ 67825
epilation, by forceps ~ 67820
epilation, by other than forceps ~ 67825
incision of lid margin ~ 67830
with free mucous membrane graft ~ 67835
Trichina ~ 86784, 96902
Trichinella
antibody ~ 86784
trichogram ~ 96902
Trichomonas vaginalis
antigen detection
nucleic acid ~ 87660
by immunoassay with direct optical observation ~ 87808
Trichrome stain ~ 88313
Tricuspid valve
excision ~ 33460
repair ~ 33463-33465
replacement ~ 33465
repositioning ~ 33468
Tridymite ~ 84285
Trigeminal ganglia ~ see Gasserian ganglion
Trigeminal nerve
destruction ~ 64600-64610
injection
anesthetic ~ 64400
neurolytic ~ 64600-64610
Trigeminal tract stereotactic, create lesion ~ 61791
Trigger finger repair ~ 26055
Trigger point injection
one or two muscles ~ 20552
two or more muscles ~ 20553
Triglyceridase ~ 83690

Triglyceride lipase ~ 83690
Triglycerides ~ 84478
Trigonocephaly ~ 21175
Triiodothyronine
free ~ 84481
reverse ~ 84482
total ~ 84480
true ~ 84480
Triolean hydrolase ~ 83690
Trioxopurine ~ 84550, 84560
Tripcellim ~ 84485, 84488-84490
Trisegmentectomy ~ 47122
Trocar biopsy bone marrow ~ 38221
Trochanteric femur fracture ~ 27246, 27248
Trophoblastic tumor GTT ~ 59100, 59870
Troponin ~ 84484
qualitative ~ 84512
quantitative ~ 84484
Truncal vagotomies ~ 43640
Truncus arteriosus repair ~ 33786
Truncus brachiocephalicus ~ see artery, brachiocephalic
Trunk, brachiocephalic ~ see artery, brachiocephalic
Trypanosomiases ~ 86171, 86280
Trypanosomiasis ~ 86171, 86280
Trypsin
duodenum ~ 84485
feces ~ 84488-84490
Trypsin inhibitor, alpha 1-antirypsin ~ see alpha-1 antitrypsin
Trypure ~ 84485, 84488-84490
Tsalicylate intoxication ~ 80196
TSH ~ see thyroid stimulating hormone
TSI ~ see thyroid stimulating immunoglobulin
Tsutsugamushi disease ~ 86000
TT ~ see thrombin time
TT-3 ~ see triiodothyronine, true
TT-4 ~ see thyroxine, true
Tuba auditoria (auditiva) ~ see eustachian tube
Tubal embryo stage transfer ~ see embryo transfer
Tubal ligation ~ 58600
laparoscopic ~ 58670
with cesarean section ~ 58611
Tubal occlusion ~ 58615
with cesarean delivery ~ see occlusion ~ 58615
creat lesion ~ 58565, 58615
Tubal pregnancy ~ 59121
with salpingectomy and/or oophorectomy ~ 59120
Tube change
colonic ~ 49450
duodenostomy ~ 49451
gastro-jejunostomy ~ 49452
gastrostomy ~ 43760, 49446
jejunostomy ~ 49451
tracheotomy ~ 31502

Tube placement
cecostomy tube ~ 44300, 49442
duodenostomy tube ~ 49441
endoscopic
bile duct, pancreatic duct ~ 43268
jejunostomy tube, percutaneous ~ 49441
nasobiliary, nasopancreatic
for drainage ~ 43267
enterostomy tube ~ 44300
gastrostomy tube ~ 43246, 49440
nasogastric tube ~ 43752
orogastric tube ~ 43752
Tube, fallopian ~ see fallopian tube
Tubectomy ~ 58700, 58720
Tubed pedicle flap formation ~ 15570-15576
Tubercle bacilli culture ~ 87116
Tubercleplasty tibia, anterior ~ 27418
Tuberculin test ~ 85480
Tuberculosis
antigen response test ~ 86480
culture ~ 87116
skin test ~ 86580
Tuberculosis vaccine (BCG) ~ 90585-90586
Tubes
endotracheal ~ 31500
gastrostomy ~ 43246, 43760-43761
Tudor "rabbit ear" ~ see urethra, repair
Tuffier vaginal hysterectomy ~ 58260-58270,
58290-58294, 58550-58554
Tumor
abdomen, destruction/excision ~ 49203-49205,
58957, 58958
abdominal wall, excision ~ 22900-22905
acetabulum, excision ~ 27076
ankle ~ 27615-27619, 27632, 27634
arm, lower ~ 25071-25078
arm, upper, excision ~ 24071-24079
back/flank
excision ~ 21930-21936
radical resection ~ 21935, 21936
bile duct
destruction ~ 43272
extrahepatic ~ 47711
intrahepatic ~ 47712
bladder ~ 52234-52240
excision ~ 51530, 52355
bone, ablation ~ 20982
brain ~ 61510
excision ~ 61518, 61520-61521,
61526-61530, 61545, 62164
breast, excision ~ 19120-19126
bronchi, excision ~ 31640
calcaneus ~ 28100-28103
excision ~ 27647
carpal ~ 25130-25136
cheekbone ~ 21030, 21034
chest wall, excision ~ 19260-19272
clavicle excision ~ 23140, 23200
with allograft ~ 23146
with autograft ~ 23145
coccyx ~ 49215

Tumor ~ *continued*
colon, destruction ~ 44393, 45383
cranial bone, reconstruction ~ 21181-21184
destruction
chemosurgery ~ 17311-17315
urethra ~ 53220
ear, middle
extended ~ 69554
transcanal ~ 69550
transmastoid ~ 69552
elbow, excision ~ 24071-24079
esophagus, ablation ~ 43228
excision, femur ~ 27355-27358
face or scalp
excision ~ 21011-21014
radical resection ~ 21015-21016
facial bone ~ 21029-21030, 21034
fallopian tube, resection ~ 58950,
58952-58958
femoral ~ 27355-27358
femur ~ 27065-27067
excision ~ 27365
fibroid ~ 58140, 58545-58546, 58561
fibula ~ 27635-27638
excision ~ 27646
finger, excision ~ 26111-26118
foot ~ 28039-28047
forearm, radical resection ~ 25077
gastrostomy ~ see lesion
gums, excision ~ 41825-41827
hand, excision ~ 26111-26118
heart, excision ~ 33120-33130
hip ~ 27043-27045, 27049, 27059,
27065-27067
excision ~ 27075-27076
humerus excision ~ 23150, 23220, 24110
with allograft ~ 23156, 24116
with autograft ~ 23155, 24115
ileum ~ 27065-27067
immunoassay for antigen ~ 86294, 86316
CA 125 ~ 86304
CA 15-3 ~ 86300
CA 19-9 ~ 86301
innominate, excision ~ 27077
intestines, small, destruction ~ 44369
ischial, excision ~ 27078
kidney, excision ~ 50562, 52355
knee, excision ~ 27327-27329, 27337-27339,
27365
lacrimal gland, excision
frontal approach ~ 68540
with osteotomy ~ 68550
larynx
excision ~ 31300
endoscopic ~ 31540-31541, 31578
incision ~ 31300
leg, lower ~ 27615-27619, 27632, 27634
leg, upper, excision ~ 27327-27329,
27337-27339, 27365
localization, nuclear medicine ~ 78800-78804
mandible ~ 21044-21047

Tumor ~ *continued*
  maxilla ~ 21030, 21034, 21048-21049
  maxillary torus palatinus ~ 21032
  mediastinal, excision ~ 39220
  mediastinum ~ 32662
  meningioma ~ 61512
    excision ~ 61519
  metacarpal ~ 26200-26205, 26250
  metatarsal ~ 28104-28107
    excision ~ 28173
  neck
    excision ~ 21552-21558
    radical resection ~ 21557, 21558
  olecranon, excision ~ 24120
  olecranon process
    with allograft, excision ~ 24126
    with autograft, excision ~ 24125
  ovary, resection ~ 58950-58958
  pancreatic duct, destruction ~ 43272
  parotid gland, excision ~ 42410-42426
  pelvis ~ 27043-27045, 27049, 27059
  pericardial
    endoscopic ~ 32661
    excision ~ 33050
  peritoneum, resection ~ 58950-58958
  phalanges
    finger ~ 26210-26215, 26260-26262
    toe ~ 28108
    excision ~ 28175
  pituitary gland, excision ~ 61546-61548,
    62165
  positron emission tomography (PET) ~
    78811-78816
  pubis ~ 27065-27067
  pulmonary
    ablation ~ 32998
  radiation therapy ~ 77295
  radius ~ 25120-25126, 25170
    excision ~ 24120
    with allograft, excision ~ 24126
    with autograft, excision ~ 24125
  rectum
    destruction ~ 45190, 45320, 46937-46938
    excision ~ 45160-45172
  resection
    face ~ 21015
    scalp ~ 21015
    with cystourethroscopy ~ 52355
  retroperitoneal, destruction/excision ~
    49203-49205, 58957, 58958
  sacrum ~ 49215
  scapula
    excision ~ 23140, 23210
    with allograft ~ 23146
    with autograft ~ 23145
  shoulder, excision ~ 23071-23078
  skull, excision ~ 61500
  soft tissue
    elbow, excision ~ 24071-24079
    finger, excision ~ 26115
    forearm, radical resection ~ 25077

Tumor ~ *continued*
  hand, excision ~ 26115
  wrist
    excision ~ 25071-25078
    radical resection ~ 25077, 25078
  spinal cord, excision ~ 63275-63290
  stomach, excision ~ 43610-43611
  talus ~ 28100-28103
    excision ~ 27647
  tarsal ~ 28104-28107
    excision ~ 28171
  temporal bone, removal ~ 69970
  testis, excision ~ 54530-54535
  thorax
    excision ~ 21552-21558
    radical resection ~ 21557, 21558
  thyroid, excision ~ 60200
  tibia ~ 27365, 27635-27638
    excision ~ 27645
  torus mandibularis ~ 21031
  trachea, excision
    cervical ~ 31785
    thoracic ~ 31786
  ulna ~ 25120-25126, 25170
    excision ~ 24120
    with allograft, excision ~ 24126
    with autograft, excision ~ 24125
  ureter, excision ~ 52355
  urethra ~ 52234-52240, 53220
    excision ~ 52355
  uterus
    excision ~ 58140-58146
    resection ~ 58950-58958
  vagina, excision ~ 57135
  vertebra, additional segment
    excision ~ 22116
    cervical, excision ~ 22100
    lumbar ~ 22102
    thoracic, excision ~ 22101
  wrist ~ 25071-25078, 25135-25136
    radical resection ~ 25077
Tunica vaginalis hydrocele
  aspiration ~ 55000
  excision ~ 55040-55041
  repair ~ 55060
Turbinate
  excision ~ 30130-30140
  fracture, therapeutic ~ 30930
  injection ~ 30200
  submucous resection, nose excision ~ 30140
Turbinate mucosa cauterization ~
    30801-30802
Turcica, sella ~ 70240, 70480-70482
Turnbuckle jacket ~ 29020-29025
  removal ~ 29715
TURP ~ 52630
Tylectomy ~ *see* breast, excision, lesion
Tylenol urine ~ 82003
Tympanic membrane
  create stoma ~ 69433-69436
  incision ~ 69420-69421

Tympanic membrane ~ *continued*
reconstruction ~ 69620
repair ~ 69450, 69610
Tympanic nerve excision ~ 69676
Tympanolysis ~ 69450
Tympanomastoidectomy ~ see tympanoplasty
Tympanometry ~ see audiologic function tests
~ 92550, 92567, 92570
Tympanoplasty ~ 69620
radical or complete ~ 69645
with ossicular chain reconstruction ~ 69646
with antrotomy or mastoidotomy ~ 69635
with ossicular chain reconstruction ~ 69636
and synthetic prosthesis ~ 69637
with mastoidectomy ~ 69641
with intact or reconstructed wall ~ 69643
and ossicular chain reconstruction ~ 69644
with ossicular chain reconstruction ~ 69642
without mastoidectomy ~ 69631
with ossicular chain reconstruction ~ 69632
and synthetic prosthesis ~ 69633
Tympanostomy ~ 69433-69436
Tympanotomy ~ 69420-69421
Typhoid vaccine ~ 90690-90693
AKD ~ 90693
oral ~ 90690
polysaccharide ~ 90691
Typhus
endemic ~ 86000
mite-bone ~ 86000
Sno Paulo ~ 86000
tropical ~ 86000
Typing, blood ~ see blood typing
Typing, HLA ~ 86812-86817
Typing, tissue ~ see tissue typing
Tyrosine ~ 84510
Tzank smear ~ 87207

U

Uchida Procedure ~ 58600
UDP galactose pyrophosphorylase ~
82775-82776
UFR ~ 51736-51741
Ulcer
anal ~ 46200, 46940-46942
decubitus ~ see debridement; skin graft and
flap ~ 15920-15999
pinch graft ~ 15050
pressure ~ 15920-15999
stomach, excision ~ 43610
Ulcerative, cystitis ~ 52260-52265
Ulna ~ see arm, lower; elbow; humerus; radius
arthrodesis, radioulnar joint, with resection ~
25830
arthroplasty, with implant ~ 25442
centralization or wrist ~ 25335
craterization ~ 24147, 25150-25151

Ulna ~ *continued*
cyst, excision ~ 24125-24126, 25120-25126
diaphysectomy ~ 24147, 25150-25151
excision ~ 24147
abscess ~ 24138
complete ~ 25240
epiphyseal bar ~ 20150
partial ~ 25145..2515, 1, 25240
fracture
closed treatment ~ 25530-25535
olecranon ~ 24670-24675
open treatment ~ 24685
open treatment ~ 25545
shaft ~ 25530-25545
open treatment ~ 25574
styloid
closed treatment ~ 25650
open treatment ~ 25652
percutaneous fixation ~ 25651
with dislocation
closed treatment ~ 24620
open treatment ~ 24635
with manipulation ~ 25535
with radius ~ 25560-25565
open treatment ~ 25575
without manipulation ~ 25530
incision and drainage ~ 25035
osteoplasty ~ 25390-25393
prophylactic treatment ~ 25491-25492
reconstruction, radioulnar ~ 25337
repair
epiphyseal arrest ~ 25450-25455
malunion or nonunion ~ 25400, 25415
osteotomy ~ 25360, 25370-25375
and radius ~ 25365
with graft ~ 25405, 25420-25426
saucerization ~ 24147, 25150-25151
sequestrectomy ~ 24138, 25145
tumor
cyst ~ 24120
excision ~ 24125-24126, 25120-25126,
25170
Ulnar arteries ~ see artery, ulnar
Ulnar nerve
decompression ~ 64718
neuroplasty ~ 64718-64719
reconstruction ~ 64718-64719
release ~ 64718-64719
repair/suture, motor ~ 64836
transposition ~ 64718-64719
Ultrasonic ~ see ultrasound
Ultrasonic cardiography ~ see
echocardiography
Ultrasonic procedure ~ 52325
Ultrasonography ~ see echography
Ultrasound ~ see echocardiography; echography
abdomen ~ 76700-76705
artery
intracranial ~ 93886-93893
middle cerebral ~ 76821
umbilical ~ 76820

Ultrasound ~ *continued*
bladder ~ 51798
bone density study ~ 76977
breast ~ 76645
bronchi, endoscopy ~ 31620
chest ~ 76604
colon, endoscopic ~ 45391-45392
colon-sigmoid, endoscopic ~ 45341-45342
drainage, abscess ~ 75989
echoencephalography ~ 76506
esophagus, endoscopy ~ 43231-43232
extremity(s) ~ 76881-76882
eye ~ 76510-76513
  biometry ~ 76516-76519
  foreign body ~ 76529
  pachymetry ~ 76514
fetus ~ 76818-76828
follow-up ~ 76970
for physical therapy ~ 97035
gastrointestinal ~ 76975
gastrointestinal, upper, endoscopic ~
  43237-43238, 43242, 43259
guidance
  amniocentesis ~ 59001, 76946
  amnioinfusion ~ 59070
  arteriovenous fistulae ~ 76936
  chorionic villus sampling ~ 76945
  cryosurgery ~ 55873
  drainage, fetal fluid ~ 59074
  endometrial ablation ~ 58356
  fetal cordocentesis ~ 76941
  fetal transfusion ~ 76941
  heart biopsy ~ 76932
  needle biopsy ~ 43232, 43238, 43242,
    45342, 45392, 76942
  occlusion, umbilical cord ~ 59072
  ova retrieval ~ 76948
  pericardiocentesis ~ 76930
  pseudoaneurysm ~ 76936
  radiation therapy ~ 76950
  radioelement ~ 76965
  shunt placement, fetal ~ 59076
  thoracentesis ~ 76942
  tissue ablation ~ 76490
  vascular access ~ 76937
head ~ 76506, 76536
heart, fetal ~ 76825
hips, infant ~ 76885-76886
hysteronsonography ~ 76831
intraoperative ~ 76998
intravascular, intraoperative ~ 37250-37251
kidney ~ 76770-76776
leg ~ 0183T
neck ~ 76536
non-coronary, intravascular ~ 75945-75946
pelvis ~ 76856-76857
pregnant uterus ~ 76801-76817
prostate ~ 76873
rectal ~ 76872-76873
retroperitoneal ~ 76770-76775
scrotum ~ 76870

Ultrasound ~ *continued*
sonohysterography ~ 76831
spine ~ 76800
stimulation to aid bone healing ~ 20979
umbilical artery ~ 76820
unlisted services and procedures ~ 76999
uterus, tumor ablation ~ 0071T-0072T
vagina ~ 76830
Ultraviolet light therapy dermatology
ultraviolet A ~ 96912
ultraviolet B ~ 96910
for dermatology ~ 96900
for physical medicine ~ 97028
Umbilectomy ~ 49250
Umbilical
artery ultrasound ~ 76820
hernia ~ 49600-49611
vein catheterization ~ 36510
Umbilical cord occlusion ~ 59072
Umbilicus
excision ~ 49250
repair
  hernia ~ 49580-49587
  omphalocele ~ 49600-49611
Undescended testicle ~ 54550-54560
Unfertilized egg ~ 87177
Unguis ~ see nails
Unilateral simple mastectomy ~ see
  mastectomy
Unlisted services and procedures ~ 99499,
  99600
abdomen ~ 22999, 49329, 49999
allergy/immunology ~ 95199
anal ~ 46999
anesthesia ~ 01999
arm ~ 25999
arthroscopy ~ 29999
autopsy ~ 88099
bile duct ~ 47999
brachytherapy ~ 77799
breast ~ 19499
bronchi ~ 31899
cardiac ~ 33999
cardiovascular studies ~ 93799
casting ~ 29799
cervix ~ 58999
chemistry procedure ~ 84999
chemotherapy ~ 96549
chest ~ 32999
coagulation ~ 85999
colon ~ 44799
conjunctiva surgery ~ 68399
craniofacial ~ 21299
CT scan ~ 76497
cytogenetic study ~ 88299
cytopathology ~ 88199
pdermatology ~ 96999
dialysis ~ 90999
diaphragm ~ 39599
ear, external ~ 69399
  inner ~ 69949
  middle ~ 69799

Unlisted services and procedures ~ *continued*
endocrine system ~ 60699
epididymis ~ 55899
esophagus ~ 43289, 43499
evaluation and management services ~ 99499
eye muscle ~ 67399
eye surgery
  anterior segment ~ 66999
  posterior segment ~ 67299
eyelid ~ 67999
fluoroscopy ~ 76496
forearm ~ 25999
gallbladder ~ 47999
gastroenterology test ~ 91299
gum ~ 41899
hand ~ 26989
hemic system ~ 38999
hepatic duct ~ 47999
hip joint ~ 27299
home services ~ 99600
hysteroscopy ~ 58579
immunization ~ 90749
immunology ~ 86849
injection ~ 90799
injection of medication ~ 90799
intestine ~ 44238, 44799
kidney ~ 53899
lacrimal system ~ 68899
laparoscopy ~ 38129, 38589, 43289, 43659,
  44238-44239, 44979, 47379, 47579,
  49329, 49659, 50549, 50949, 54699,
  55559, 58578, 58679, 59898, 60659
larynx ~ 31599
lip ~ 40799
liver ~ 47379, 47399
lungs ~ 32999
lymphatic system ~ 38999
magnetic resonance ~ 76498
maxillofacial ~ 21299
maxillofacial prosthetics ~ 21089
Meckel's diverticulum ~ 44899
mediastinum ~ 39499
mesentery surgery ~ 44899
microbiology ~ 87999
mouth ~ 40899, 41599
musculoskeletal ~ 25999, 26989
musculoskeletal surgery, abdominal wall ~
  22999
  neck ~ 21899
  spine ~ 22899
  thorax ~ 21899
musculoskeletal system ~ 20999
  ankle ~ 27899
  arm, upper ~ 24999
  elbow ~ 24999
  head ~ 21499
  knee ~ 27599
  leg, lower ~ 27899
  leg, upper ~ 27599
necropsy ~ 88099
nervous system surgery ~ 64999

Unlisted services and procedures ~ *continued*
neurology/neuromuscular testing ~ 95999
nose ~ 30999
nuclear medicine ~ 78999
  blood ~ 78199
  bone ~ 78399
  endocrine system ~ 78099
  genitourinary system ~ 78799
  heart ~ 78499
  hematopoietic system ~ 78199
  lymphatic system ~ 78199
  musculoskeletal system ~ 78399
  nervous system ~ 78699
  therapeutic ~ 79999
obstetrical care ~ 59898-59899
omentum ~ 49329, 49999
ophthalmology ~ 92499
orbit ~ 67599
otorhinolaryngology ~ 92700
ovary ~ 58679, 58999
oviduct ~ 58679, 58999
palate ~ 42299
pancreas surgery ~ 48999
pathology ~ 89240
pelvis ~ 27299
penis ~ 55899
peritoneum ~ 49329, 49999
pharynx ~ 42999
physical therapy ~ 97039, 97139, 97799
pleura ~ 32999
pressure ulcer ~ 15999
preventive medicine ~ 99429
prostate ~ 55899
psychiatric ~ 90899
pulmonology ~ 94799
radiation physics ~ 77399
radiation therapy ~ 77499
  planning ~ 77299
radiology, diagnostic ~ 76499
radionuclide therapy ~ 79999
radiopharmaceutical therapy ~ 79999
rectum ~ 44239, 45999
reproductive medicine, lab procedure ~ 89398
salivary gland ~ 42699
scrotum ~ 55899
seminal vesicle ~ 55899
shoulder surgery ~ 23929
sinuses ~ 31299
skin ~ 17999
special services and reports ~ 99199
spine ~ 22899
stomach ~ 43659, 43999
strapping ~ 29799
surgical pathology ~ 88399
temporal bone ~ 69979
testis ~ 54699, 55899
throat ~ 42999
tongue ~ 41599
tonsil/adenoid ~ 42999
trachea ~ 31899
transfusion ~ 86999

Ureteral
  catheterization ~ see catheterization, ureter
  guide wire insertion ~ 52334
  meatotomy ~ 52290
  splinting ~ 50400-50405
  stent insertion ~ 52332
Ureterectomy ~ 50650-50660
  partial ~ 50220, 50546
  total ~ 50548
Ureterocalycostomy ~ 50750
Ureterocele
  excision ~ 51535
  fulguration
    ectopic ~ 52301
    orthotopic ~ 52300
  incision ~ 51535
  repair ~ 51535
  resection, ectopic ~ 52301
    orthotopic ~ 52300
Ureterocolon conduit ~ 50815
Ureteroenterostomy ~ 50800
  revision ~ 50830
Ureterography injection procedure ~ 50684
Ureteroileal conduit ~ 50820
  cystectomy ~ 51590
  removal ~ 50830
Ureterolithotomy ~ 50610-50630
  laparoscopy ~ 50945
  transvesical ~ 51060
Ureterolysis
  for ovarian vein syndrome ~ 50722
  for retrocaval ureter ~ 50725
  for retroperitoneal fibrosis ~ 50715
Ureteroneocystostomy ~ 50780-50785, 50830, 51565
  laparoscopic ~ 50947-50948
Ureteroplasty ~ 50700
Ureteropyelography ~ 50951, 52005
  injection procedure ~ 50684, 50690
Ureteropyelostomy ~ 50740
Ureteroscopy
  dilation
    intra-renal stricture ~ 52346
    ureter ~ 52344-52345
  third stage with cystourethroscopy ~ 52351
    biopsy ~ 52354
    destruction ~ 52354
    lithotripsy ~ 52353
    removal, calculus ~ 52352
    tumor excision ~ 52355
Ureterosigmoidostomy ~ 50810
  revision ~ 50830
Ureterostomy ~ 50860, 50951
  injection procedure ~ 50684
  manometric studies ~ 50686
Ureterostomy tube change ~ 50688
Ureterotomy ~ 50600
  insertion indwelling stent ~ 50605
Ureteroureterostomy ~ 50760-50770, 50830

Urethra
  abscess, incision and drainage ~ 53040
  adhesions, lysis ~ 53500
  artificial sphincter, repair ~ 53449
  biopsy ~ 52204, 53200
  cystourethroscopy ~ 52204-52315
  destruction ~ 52214-52224
  dilation ~ 52260-52265, 53600-53621
    general ~ 53665
    suppository and/or instillation ~ 53660-53661
  diverticulum ~ 53240
  drainage, extravasation ~ 53080-53085
  endoscopy ~ 52000
    biopsy ~ 52204, 52354
    catheterization ~ 52010
    destruction ~ 52354, 52400
    evacuation, clot ~ 52001
    excision, tumor ~ 52355
    exploration ~ 52351
    incision, ejaculatory duct ~ 52402
    injection of implant material ~ 51715
    lithotripsy ~ 52353
    removal, calculus ~ 52352
    resection, ejaculatory duct ~ 52402
    vasectomy ~ 52402
    vasotomy ~ 52402
  excision
    diverticulum ~ 53230-53235
    total
      female ~ 53210
      male ~ 53215
  incision ~ 53000-53010
    meatus ~ 53020-53025
  incision and drainage ~ 53060
  insertion, stent ~ 52282, 53855
  lesion
    destruction ~ 53265
    excision ~ 53260
  paraurethral gland, incision and drainage ~ 53060
  polyp
    destruction ~ 53260
    excision ~ 53260
  pressure profile ~ 51727, 51729
  prolapse
    destruction ~ 53275
    excision ~ 53275
    repair ~ 53275
  proximal, micro-remodeling ~ 53860
  radiotracer ~ 52250
  reconstruction ~ 53410-53440, 53445
    and bladder ~ 51800-51820
    complications ~ 54340-54348
    hypospadias
      one stage ~ 54322-54328
      second stage ~ 54308-54316
      third stage ~ 54318
    meatus ~ 53450-53460

Urethra ~ *continued*
removal
  calculus ~ 52310-52315
  foreign body ~ 52310-52315
  sling ~ 53442
  urethral stent ~ 52310-52315
repair
  diverticulum ~ 53240, 53400-53405
  fistula ~ 45820-45825, 53400-53405, 53520
  sphincter ~ 57220
  stricture ~ 53400-53405
  urethrocele ~ 57230
  wound ~ 53502-53515
Skene's gland, incision and drainage ~ 53060
sphincter ~ 52277
  electromyography ~ 51784-51785
    needle ~ 51785
  insertion, prosthesis ~ 53444
  reconstruction ~ 53445
  removal, prosthesis ~ 53446-53447
  repair, prosthesis ~ 53449
  replacement, prosthesis ~ 53448
stent
  insertion
    premanent ~ 52282
    temporary ~ 53855
suture
  fistula ~ 45820-45825, 53520
  to bladder ~ 51840-51841
  wound ~ 53502-53515
tumor
  destruction ~ 53220
  excision ~ 53220
unlisted services and procedures ~ 53899
urethrocystography ~ 74450-74455
urethrotomy ~ 52270-52276
X-ray with contrast ~ 74450-74455
Urethral
diverticulum
  marsupialization ~ 53240
  meatus, dorsal ~ see epispadias
sphincter
  biofeedback training ~ 90911
  insertion, prosthesis ~ 53444
  removal, prosthesis ~ 53446-53447
  replacement, prosthesis ~ 53448
stenosis, dilation ~ 52281
stent
  insertion ~ 0084T, 52282
  removal
    bladder ~ 52310-52315
    urethra ~ 52310-52315
stricture
  dilation ~ 52281, 53600-53621
  injection, steroids ~ 52283
syndrome, cystourethroscopy ~ 52285
Urethrectomy total
female ~ 53210
male ~ 53215
Urethrocele ~ 53275

Urethrocystography ~ 74450-74455
contrast and/or chain ~ 51605
retrograde ~ 51610
voiding ~ 51600
Urethrocystopexy ~ 51840-51841
Urethromeatoplasty ~ 53450-53460
Urethropexy ~ 51840-51841
Urethroplasty ~ 46744-46746
first stage ~ 53400
one stage, hypospadias ~ 54322-54328
reconstruction
  female urethra ~ 53430
  male anterior urethra ~ 53410
  prostatic/membranous urethra
    first stage ~ 53420
    one stage ~ 53415
    second stage ~ 53425
second stage ~ 53405
hypospadias ~ 54308-54316
third stage, hypospadias ~ 54318
Urethrorrhaphy ~ 53502-53515
Urethroscopy ~ 52000
Urethrostomy ~ 53000-53010
Urethrotomy ~ 53000-53010
direct vision, with cystourethroscopy ~ 52276
internal ~ 52601, 52647-52648
with cystourethroscopy
  female ~ 52270
  male ~ 52275
Uric acid
blood ~ 84550
other source ~ 84560
urine ~ 84560
Uridyltransferase
galactose-1-phosphate ~ 82775-82776
galactosephosphate ~ 82775-82776
Urinalysis ~ 81000-81099
automated ~ 81001, 81003
glass test ~ 81020
microalbumin ~ 82043-82044
microscopic ~ 81015
pregnancy test ~ 81025
qualitative ~ 81005
routine ~ 81002
screen ~ 81007
semiquantitative ~ 81005
unlisted services and procedures ~ 81099
volume measurement ~ 81050
without microscopy ~ 81002
Urinary bladder ~ see bladder
Urinary catheter irrigation ~ 62194, 62225
Urinary sphincter, artificial ~ 53444-53449
Urinary system, surgical procedures ~ 50010-53899
Urinary tract X-ray w contrast ~ 74400-74425
Urine
albumin ~ 82042-82044
blood ~ 83491
colony count ~ 87086
pregnancy test ~ 81025
tests ~ 81001

1557

Urobilinogen
  feces ~ 84577
  urine ~ 84578-84583
Urodynamic tests
  bladder capacity, ultrasound ~ 51798
  cystometrogram ~ 51725-51729
  electromyography studies, needle ~ 51785
  residual urine, ultrasound ~ 51798
  stimulus evoked response ~ 51792
  urethra pressure profile ~ 51727, 51729
  uroflowmetry ~ 51736-51741
  voiding pressure studies
    bladder ~ 51728, 51729
    intra-abdominal ~ 51797
Uroflowmetry ~ 51736-51741
Urography
  antegrade ~ 74425
  infusion ~ 74410-74415
  intravenous ~ 74400-74415
  retrograde ~ 74420
Uroporphyrin ~ 84120
Urothromboplastin ~ see thromboplastin
Uterine
  adhesion ~ 58559
  cervix ~ see cervix
  endoscopies ~ see endoscopy, uterus
  haemorrhage ~ 59160
Uterus
  ablation
    endometrium ~ 58353-58356
    tumor, ultrasound, focused ~ 0071T-0072T
  biopsy
    endometrium ~ 58100-58110
    endoscopic ~ 58558
  catheterization, X-ray ~ 58340
  chromotubation ~ 58350
  curettage ~ 58356
    postpartum ~ 59160
  dilation and curettage ~ 58120
    postpartum ~ 59160
  ectopic pregnancy
    interstitial
      partial resection uterus ~ 59136
      total hysterectomy ~ 59135
  endoscopy
    endometrial ablation ~ 58563
    exploration ~ 58555
    surgery ~ 58558-58565
    treatment ~ 58558-58565
  excision
    laparoscopic ~ 58541-58544, 58550
      with removal of ovaries ~ 58262-58263,
        58291-58293, 58552, 58554
    total ~ 58570-58573
    partial ~ 58180
    radical
      laparoscopic ~ 58548
      open ~ 58210, 58285
    removal of tubes and/or ovaries ~
      58262-58263, 58291-58293, 58552,
      58554

Uterus ~ *continued*
  total ~ 58150-58152, 58200, 58570-58573,
    58953-58956
  vaginal ~ 58260-58270, 58290-58294,
    58550-58554
    with colpectomy ~ 58275-58280
    with colpo-urethrocystopexy ~ 58267
    with repair of enterocele ~ 58270, 58294
  hemorrhage, postpartum ~ 59160
  hydatidiform mole, excision ~ 59100
  hydrotubation ~ 58350
  hysterosalpingography ~ 74740
  incision, removal lesion ~ 59100
  insertion
    Heyman capsule, for brachytherapy ~ 58346
    intrauterine device (IUD) ~ 58300
    tandem, for brachytherapy ~ 57155
  laparoscopy ~ 58570-58578
  lesion, excision ~ 58545-58546, 59100
  reconstruction ~ 58540
  removal, intrauterine device (IUD) ~ 58301
  repair
    fistula ~ 51920-51925
    rupture ~ 58520, 59350
    suspension ~ 58400
      with presacral sympathectomy ~ 58410
  sonohysterography ~ 76831
  suture, rupture ~ 59350
  tumor
    ablation, ultrasound, focused ~ 0071T-0072T
    excision
      abdominal approach ~ 58140, 58146
      vaginal approach ~ 58145
    unlisted services and procedures ~ 58578,
      58999
  X-ray with contrast ~ 74740
UTP hexose 1 phosphate uridylyltransferase
  ~ 82775-82776
UV light therapy ~ 96900
Uvula
  abscess, incision and drainage ~ 42000
  biopsy ~ 42100
  excision ~ 42140-42145
  lesion
    destruction ~ 42145
    excision ~ 42104-42107
  unlisted services and procedures ~ 42299
Uvulectomy ~ 42140

V

**V flap procedure one stage distal
  hypospadias repair** ~ 54322
V, cranial nerve ~ see trigeminal nerve
V-Y operation, bladder, neck ~ 51845
V-Y plasty ~ 14000-14350
Vaccination ~ see allergen immunotherapy;
  immunization; vaccines

Vaccines and toxoids
adenovirus ~ 90476-90477
anthrax ~ 90581
chicken pox ~ 90716
cholera, injectable ~ 90725
diphtheria and tetanus (Td) ~ 90714
diphtheria toxoid ~ 90719
diphtheria, tetanus (DT) ~ 90702
diphtheria, tetanus, acellular pertussis (DTaP)
    ~ 90700
diphtheria, tetanus, acellular pertussis and
    hemophilus influenza B (Hib) (DTaP-Hib)
    ~ 90721
diphtheria, tetanus, acellular pertussis,
    haemophilus influenza type B, and
    inactivated poliovirus (DTaP-Hib-IPV) ~
    90698
diphtheria, tetanus, acellular pertussis, and
    inactivated polivirus (DTaP-IPV) ~ 90696
diphtheria, tetanus, acellular pertussis, hepatitis
    B, and inactivated poliovirus
    (DTaP-HepB-IPV) ~ 90723
diphtheria, tetanus, and acellular pertussis
    (TdaP) ~ 90715
diphtheria, tetanus, whole cell pertussis and
    hemophilus influenza B (HIB) (DTP-Hib)
    ~ 90720
encephalitis, Japanese ~ 90735
    inactivated ~ 90738
hemophilus influenza B ~ 90644-90648
hepatitis A ~ 90632-90634
hepatitis A and hepatitis B ~ 90636
hepatitis B ~ 90739-90747
hepatitis B and hemophilus influenza B
    (HepB-HIB) ~ 90748
human papilloma virus (HPV) ~ 90649, 90650
influenza ~ 90653-90664, 90666-90668, 90672
H1N1 ~ 90633
    pandemic ~ 90664, 90666-90668
measles ~ 90705
measles and rubella ~ 90708
measles, mumps and rubella (MMR) ~ 90707
measles, mumps and rubella and varicella
    (MMRV) ~ 90710
meningococcal ~ 90733-90734
meningococcal conjugate, serogroups C and Y,
    hemophilus influenza B (Hib-MenCY) ~
    90644
mumps ~ 90704
plague ~ 90727
pneumococcal
    7-valent ~ 90669
    13-valent ~ 90670
    polysaccharide 23-valent ~ 90732
poliovirus, inactivated ~ 90713
poliovirus, live, oral ~ 90712
rabies ~ 90675-90676
rotavirus ~ 90680, 90681

Vaccines and toxoids ~ *continued*
rubella ~ 90706
tetanus and diphtheria ~ 90714
tetanus toxoid ~ 90703
tetanus, diphtheria, and acellular pertussis
    (TDaP) ~ 90715
tuberculosis (BCG) ~ 90585-90586
typhoid ~ 90690-90693
unlisted vaccine/toxoid ~ 90749
varicella (chicken pox) ~ 90716
yellow fever ~ 90717
zoster (shingles) ~ 90736
Vagina
abscess, incision and drainage ~ 57010
amines test ~ 82120
biopsy
    colposcopy ~ 57421
    endocervical ~ 57454
    extensive ~ 57105
    simple ~ 57100
closure ~ 57120
colposcopy ~ 57420-57421, 57455-57456,
    57461
construction
    without graft ~ 57291
    with graft ~ 57292
cyst, excision ~ 57135
dilation ~ 57400
endocervical
    biopsy ~ 57454
    exploration ~ 57452
excision
    closure ~ 57120
    complete
        with removal of paravaginal tissue ~
            57111
        with removal of paravaginal tissue with
            lymphadenectomy ~ 57112
        with removal of vaginal wall ~ 57110
    partial
        with removal of paravaginal tissue ~
            57107
        with removal of paravaginal tissue with
            lymphadenectomy ~ 57109
        with removal of vaginal wall ~ 57106
    total ~ 57110
    with hysterectomy ~ 58275-58280
        with repair of enterocele ~ 58280
exploration
    endocervical ~ 57452
    incision ~ 57000
hematoma, incision and drainage ~
    57022-57023
hemorrhage ~ 57180
hysterectomy ~ 58290, 58550-58554
incision and drainage ~ 57020
insertion
    ovoid, for brachytherapy ~ 57155
    packing for bleeding ~ 57180
    pessary ~ 57160
    radiation afterloading appliance ~ 57156
    sensor, fetal oximetry ~ 0021T

1559

Vagina ~ *continued*
irrigation ~ 57150
lesion
  destruction ~ 57061-57065
    extensive ~ 57065
    simple ~ 57061
prolapse, sacrospinous ligament fixation ~ 57282
removal
  foreign body ~ 57415
  prosthetic graft ~ 57295-57296, 57426
  sling, stress incontinence ~ 57287
repair ~ 56800
  cystocele ~ 57240, 57260
    combined anteroposterior ~ 57260-57265
    posterior ~ 57240
  enterocele ~ 57265
  fistula ~ 51900
    rectovaginal ~ 57300-57308
    transvesical and vaginal approach ~ 57330
    urethrovaginal ~ 57310-57311
    vesicovaginal ~ 51900, 57320-57330
  hysterectomy ~ 58267, 58293
  incontinence ~ 57284, 57288
  obstetric ~ 59300
  paravaginal defect ~ 57284-57285, 57423
  Pereyra Procedure ~ 57289
  prolapse ~ 57282-57284, 57423
  prosthesis insertion ~ 57267
  rectocele
    combined anteroposterior ~ 57260-57265
    posterior ~ 57250
  suspension ~ 57280-57283
    laparoscopic ~ 57425
  urethral sphincter ~ 57220
  wound ~ 57200-57210
    colpoperineorrhaphy ~ 57210
    colporrhaphy ~ 57200
revision
  prosthetic graft ~ 57295-57296, 57426
  sling, stress incontinence ~ 57287
septum, excision ~ 57130
suspension ~ 57280-57283
  laparoscopic ~ 57425
suture
  cystocele ~ 57240, 57260
  enterocele ~ 57265
  fistula ~ 51900, 57300-57330
  rectocele ~ 57250-57260
  wound ~ 57200-57210
tumor, excision ~ 57135
ultrasound ~ 76830
unlisted services and procedures ~ 58999
X-ray with contrast ~ 74775
Vaginal delivery ~ 59400, 59610-59614
after previous cesarean delivery ~ 59610-59612
  attempted ~ 59618-59622
  antepartum care ~ 59400
  cesarean delivery after attempted ~ 59618
    delivery only ~ 59620
    postpartum care ~ 59622

Vaginal delivery ~ *continued*
delivery after previous, vaginal delivery only, postpartum care ~ 59614
delivery only ~ 59409
external cephalic version ~ 59412
placenta ~ 59414
postpartum care ~ 59410
routine care ~ 59400
Vaginal hysterectomy ~ 58552-58554
Vaginal smear ~ 88141-88155, 88164-88167, 88174-88175
Vaginal suppositories
induced abortion ~ 59855
  with dilation and curettage ~ 59856
  with hysterectomy ~ 59857
Vaginectomy ~ see colpectomy
Vaginoplasty intersex state ~ 57335
Vaginorrhaphy ~ see colporrhaphy
Vaginoscopy
biopsy ~ 57454
exploration ~ 57452
Vaginotomy ~ see colpotomy
Vagotomy
abdominal ~ 64760
highly selective ~ 43641
parietal cell ~ 43641, 64755
selective ~ 43640
transthoracic ~ 64752
truncal ~ 43640
with gastroduodenostomy revision, reconstruction ~ 43855
with gastrojejunostomy revision, reconstruction ~ 43865
with partial distal gastrectomy ~ 43635
Vagus nerve
avulsion
  abdominal ~ 64760
  selective ~ 64755
  thoracic ~ 64752
incision ~ 43640-43641
  abdominal ~ 64760
  implantation ~ 64568
  selective ~ 64755
  thoracic ~ 64752
injection, anesthetic ~ 64408
removal, neurostimulator ~ 64570
revision or replacement ~ 64569
transection ~ 43640-43641
  abdominal ~ 64760
  selective ~ 43652, 64755
  thoracic ~ 64752
  truncal ~ 43651
Valentine's test ~ 81020
Valproic acid ~ 80164
Valproic acid measurement ~ 80164
Valsalva sinus ~ 33702-33722
Valva atrioventricularis sinistra (valva mitralis) ~ see mitral valve

Valve
aortic ~ 33405-33414
bicuspid ~ see mitral valve
mitral ~ see mitral valve
pulmonary ~ 33470-33475
tricuspid ~ 33460, 33463-33465, 33468
Valve stenoses, aortic ~ 33415, 33417
Valvectomy tricuspid valve ~ 33460
Valvotomy
mitral valve ~ 33420-33422
pulmonary valve ~ 33470-33474
reoperation ~ 33530
Valvuloplasty
aortic valve ~ 33400-33403
femoral vein ~ 34501
mitral valve ~ 33425-33427
percutaneous balloon
aortic valve ~ 92986
mitral valve ~ 92987
pulmonary valve ~ 92990
prosthetic valve ~ 33496
reoperation ~ 33530
tricuspid valve ~ 33463-33465
Van Deen test ~ 82270, 82272
Van Den Bergh test ~ 82247-82248
Vancomycin assay ~ 80202
Vanillylmandelic acid urine ~ 84585
Vanilmandelic acid ~ 84585
Varicella (chicken pox) ~ 90716
Varicella-zoster
antibody ~ 86787
antigen detection, direct fluorescence ~ 87290
Varices esophageal ~ 43205, 43400-43401
Varicocele spermatic cord, excision ~ 55530-55540
Varicose vein
ablation ~ 36475-36479
removal ~ 37765-37785
secondary varicosity ~ 37785
with tissue excision ~ 37735-37761
Vas deferens
anastomosis
to epididymis ~ 54900-54901
excision ~ 55250
incision ~ 55200
for X-ray ~ 55300
ligation ~ 55450
repair, suture ~ 55400
unlisted services and procedures ~ 55899
vasography ~ 74440
X-ray with contrast ~ 74440
Vascular flow check, graft ~ 15860
Vascular injection unlisted services and procedures ~ 36299
Vascular lesion
cranial, excision ~ 61600-61608, 61615-61616
cutaneous, destruction ~ 17106-17108
Vascular malformation
cerebral, repair ~ 61710
finger, excision ~ 26115
hand, excision ~ 26115

Vascular procedure(s)
angioscopy, non-coronary vessels ~ 35400
brachytherapy, intracoronary artery ~ 92974
endoscopy, surgical ~ 37500
harvest, lower extremity vein ~ 35572
intravascular ultrasound
coronary vessels ~ 92978-92979
non-coronary vessels ~ 75945-75946
stent, intracoronary ~ 92980-92981
thrombolysis
coronary vessels ~ 92975-92977
cranial vessels ~ 37195
Vascular rehabilitation ~ 93668
Vascular studies ~ see Doppler scan, Duplex, Plethysmography
angioscopy, non-coronary vessels ~ 35400
aorta ~ 93978-93979
arterial studies (non-invasive)
extracranial ~ 93880-93882
extremities ~ 93922-93924
intracranial ~ 93886-93890
lower extremity ~ 93925-93926
middle cerebral artery, fetal ~ 76821
umbilical artery, fetal ~ 76820
artery studies, upper extremity ~ 93930-93931
bioimpedance cardiovascular analysis ~ 93701
blood pressure monitoring, 24 hour ~ 93784-93790
cardiac catheterization, imaging ~ 93452-93461
hemodialysis access ~ 93990
kidney
multiple study, with pharmacological intervention ~ 78709
single study, with pharmacological intervention ~ 78708
penile vessels ~ 93980-93981
spectroscopy, catheter based ~ 0205T
temperature gradient ~ 93740
unlisted services and procedures ~ 93799
venous studies
extremity ~ 93965-93971
venous pressure ~ 93770
visceral studies ~ 93975-93979
Vascular surgery
arm, upper, anesthesia ~ 01770-01782
elbow, anesthesia ~ 01770-01782
endoscopy ~ 37500
unlisted services and procedures ~ 37799
Vasectomy ~ 55250
contact laser vaporization with/without transurethral resection, of prostate ~ 52648
non-contact laser coagulation of prostate ~ 52647
reversal ~ 55400
transurethral, cystourethroscopic ~ 52402
transurethral electrosurgical resection of prostate ~ 52601, 52648
Vasoactive drugs injection, penis ~ 54231
Vasoactive intestinal peptide ~ 84586
Vasogram ~ 74440
Vasography ~ 74440

1561

Vasointestinal peptide ~ 84586
Vasopneumatic device therapy ~ see physical
medicine/therapy/occupational therapy ~
97016
Vasopressin ~ 84588
Vasotomy ~ 55200, 55300
transurethral, cystourethroscopic ~ 52402
Vasovasorrhaphy ~ 55400
Vasovasostomy ~ 55400
VATS ~ see thoracoscopy
VDRL ~ 86592-86593
Vein
ablation, endovenous ~ 36475-36479
adrenal, venography ~ 75840-75842
anastomosis
caval to mesenteric ~ 37160
intrahepatic portosystemic ~ 37182-37183
portocaval ~ 37140
reniportal ~ 37145
saphenopopliteal ~ 34530
splenorenal ~ 37180-37181
to vein ~ 37140-37160, 37182-37183
angioplasty ~ 75978
transluminal ~ 35460
arm
harvest of vein for bypass graft ~ 35500
venography ~ 75820-75822
axillary, thrombectomy ~ 34490
biopsy, transcatheter ~ 75970
cannulization
to artery ~ 36810-36815
to vein ~ 36800
catheterization
central insertion ~ 36555-36558
organ blood ~ 36500
peripheral insertion ~ 36568-36569
removal ~ 36589
repair ~ 36575
replacement ~ 36578-36581, 36584
umbilical ~ 36510
endoscopic harvest, for bypass graft ~ 33508
external cannula, declotting ~ 36860-36861
extremity, non-invasive studies ~ 93965-93971
femoral, repair ~ 34501
femoropopliteal, thrombectomy ~ 34421-34451
guidance
fluoroscopic ~ 77001
ultrasound ~ 76937
hepatic portal
splenoportography ~ 75810
venography ~ 75885-75887
iliac, thrombectomy ~ 34401-34451
injection, sclerosing agent ~ 36468-36471
interrupt
femoral ~ 37650
iliac ~ 37660
jugular, venography ~ 75860
leg
harvest for vascular reconstruction ~ 35572
venography ~ 75820-75822

Vein ~ *continued*
ligation
clusters ~ 37785
esophagus ~ 43205
jugular ~ 37565
perforation ~ 37760-37761
saphenous ~ 37700-37735, 37780
secondary ~ 37785
liver, venography ~ 75889-75891
neck, venography ~ 75860
nuclear medicine, thrombosis imaging ~
78455-78458
orbit, venography ~ 75880
portal, catheterization ~ 36481
pulmonary, repair ~ 33730
removal
clusters ~ 37785
saphenous ~ 37720-37735, 37780
varicose ~ 37765-37766
renal, venography ~ 75831-75833
repair
aneurysm ~ 36832
angioplasty ~ 75978
graft ~ 34520
sampling, venography ~ 75893
sinus, venography ~ 75870
skull, venography ~ 75870-75872
spermatic
excision ~ 55530-55540
ligation ~ 55550
splenic, splenoportography ~ 75810
stripping, saphenous ~ 37720-37735
subclavian, thrombectomy ~ 34471-34490
thrombectomy, other than hemodialysis graft
or fistula ~ 35875-35876
unlisted services and procedures ~ 37799
valve transposition ~ 34510
vena cava
thrombectomy ~ 34401-34451
venography ~ 75825-75827
Velpeau cast ~ 29058
Vena cava
catheterization ~ 36010
filter
insertion ~ 37191
repositioning ~ 37192
retreival ~ 37193
ligation ~ 37619
reconstruction ~ 34502
resection with reconstruction ~ 37799
Vena caval thrombectomy ~ 50230
Venereal disease research laboratory ~ see
VDRL
Venesection ~ 99195
Venipuncture ~ see catheterization ~ 36821
child/adult
cutdown ~ 36425
percutaneous ~ 36410
infant
cutdown ~ 36420
percutaneous ~ 36400-36406
routine ~ 36415

Venography
  adrenal ~ 75840-75842
  arm ~ 75820-75822
  epidural ~ 75872
  hepatic portal ~ 75885-75887
  injection ~ 36005
  jugular ~ 75860
  leg ~ 75820-75822
  liver ~ 75889-75891
  neck ~ 75860
  nuclear medicine ~ 78445, 78457-78458
  orbit ~ 75880
  renal ~ 75831-75833
  sagittal sinus ~ 75870
  vena cava ~ 75825-75827
  venous sampling ~ 75893
Venorrhaphy ~ see suture, vein
Venotomy ~ 99195
Venous access device
  blood collection ~ 36591-36592
  declotting ~ 36593
  fluoroscopic guidance ~ 77001
  insertion
    central ~ 36560-36566
    peripheral ~ 36570-36571
  irrigation ~ 96523
  obstruction clearance ~ 36595-36596
    guidance ~ 75901-75902
  removal ~ 36590
  repair ~ 36576
  replacement ~ 36582-36583, 36585
    catheter only ~ 36578
Venous blood pressure ~ 93770
Venovenostomy ~ 34530
Ventilating tube
  insertion ~ 69433
  removal ~ 69424
Ventilation assist ~ 94002-94005, 99504
Ventricular puncture ~ 61020-61026,
    61105-61120
Ventriculocisternostomy ~ 62180, 62200-62201
Ventriculography
  anesthesia
    brain ~ 00214
    cardiac ~ 01920
  nuclear imaging ~ 78635
Ventriculomyectomy ~ 33416
Ventriculomyotomy ~ 33416
Vermiform appendix ~ see appendix
Vermilionectomy ~ 40500
Verruca plana ~ 17110-17111
Verruca(e) ~ 17110-17111
Version, cephalic ~ 59412
Vertebra ~ see spinal cord; spine; vertebral
  body ~ 22315
  additional segment, excision ~ 22103, 22116
  arthrodesis
    anterior ~ 22548-22585
    exploration ~ 22830
    lateral extracavitary ~ 22532-22534
    posterior ~ 22590-22802

Vertebra ~ *continued*
  spinal deformity
    anterior approach ~ 22808-22812
    posterior approach ~ 22800-22804
  cervical, excision, for tumor ~ 22100, 22110
    fracture ~ 23675-23680
  fracture/dislocation
    additional segment, open treatment ~ 22328
    cervical, open treatment ~ 22326
    lumbar, open treatment ~ 22325
    thoracic, open treatment ~ 22327
  kyphectomy ~ 22818-22819
  lumbar
    distraction device ~ 0171T-0172T
    excision, for tumor ~ 22102, 22114
  osteoplasty, CT scan ~ 72292
    fluoroscopy ~ 72291
    lumbar ~ 22521-22522
    thoracic ~ 22520-22522
  osteotomy, additional segment, anterior
      approach ~ 22226
    posterior/posterolateral approach ~ 22216
    cervical, anterior approach ~ 22220
    posterior/posterolateral approach ~ 22210
    lumbar,
      anterior approach ~ 22224
    posterior/posterolateral approach ~ 22214
    thoracic, anterior approach ~ 22222
    posterior/posterolateral approach ~ 22212
  thoracic, excision, for tumor ~ 22101, 22112
Vertebrae ~ see vertebra
  arthrodesis, anterior ~ 22548-22585
  lateral extracavitary ~ 22532-22534
  spinal deformity ~ 22818-22819
Vertebral arteries ~ see artery, vertebral
  body
    biopsy ~ 20250-20251
    excision
      decompression ~ 63081-63103
      lesion ~ 63300-63308
      with skull base surgery ~ 61597
    fracture/dislocation
      closed treatment ~ 22305
        without manipulation ~ 22310
    kyphectomy ~ 22818-22819
  column ~ see spine
  corpectomy ~ 63081-63103, 63300-63308
  fracture ~ see fracture, vertebra
  process
    fracture/dislocation
      closed treatment
        with manipulation, casting and/or bracing
          ~ 22315
Vesication ~ see bulla
Vesicle, seminal ~ see seminal vesicle
Vesico-psoas hitch ~ 50785
Vesicostomy cutaneous ~ 51980
Vesicourethropexy ~ 51840-51841
Vesicovaginal fistula ~ 51900, 57320, 57330
Vesiculectomy ~ 55650
Vesiculogram, seminal ~ 55300, 74440
Vesiculography ~ 55300, 74440

Vesiculotomy ~ 55600-55605
  complicated ~ 55605
Vessel, blood ~ see blood vessels
Vessels transposition, great ~ 33770-33781
Vestibular function tests ~ see ear, nose and
  throat
  additional electrodes ~ 92547
  basic ~ 92540
  caloric test ~ 92533
  caloric vestibular tests ~ 92543
  nystagmus
    optokinetic ~ 92534, 92544
    positional ~ 92532, 92542
    spontaneous ~ 92531, 92540-92541
  posturography ~ 92548
  sinusoidal rotational testing ~ 92546
  torsion swing test ~ 92546
  tracking test ~ 92545
Vestibular nerve
  section
    transcranial approach ~ 69950
    translabyrinthine approach ~ 69915
Vestibule of mouth ~ see mouth, vestibule of
Vestibuloplasty ~ 40840-40845
Vidal Procedure ~ 55530-55540
Video
  esophagus ~ 74230
  pharynx ~ 70371, 74230
  speech evaluation ~ 70371
  swallowing evaluation ~ 74230
Video-assisted thoracoscopic surgery ~ see
  thoracoscopy
Videoradiography unlisted services and
  procedures ~ 76120-76125
VII, coagulation factor ~ 85230
VII, cranial nerve ~ see facial nerve
VIII, coagulation factor ~ 85210-85293
Villus, chorionic ~ 59015
Villusectomy ~ see synovectomy
VIP ~ see vasoactive intestinal peptide
Viral antibodies ~ 86280
Viral warts ~ 17110-17111
Virus
  AIDS ~ 87390
  Burkitt lymphoma ~ 86663-86665
  human immunodeficiency ~ 86689,
    86701-86703
  influenza ~ 86710, 87804
  respiratory syncytial ~ see respiratory syncytial
    virus
  salivary gland ~ see cytomegalovirus
Virus identification immunofluorescence ~
  87254
Virus isolation ~ 87250-87255
Visceral larval migrans ~ 86280
Viscosities, blood ~ 85810
Visit, home ~ 99341-99350
Visual acuity screen ~ 99172-99173
Visual field exam ~ 92081-92083
Visual function screen ~ 99172, 1055F
Visual reinforcement audiometry ~ see
  audiologic function tests ~ 92579

Visualization ileal conduit ~ 50690
Vital capacity measurement ~ 94150
Vitamin ~ 84591
  A ~ 84590
  B complex ~ 78270-78272
  B-1 ~ 84425
  B-12 ~ 82607-82608
    absorption study ~ 78270-78272
  B-2 ~ 84252
  B-6 ~ 84207
  B-6 measurement ~ 84207
  BC ~ 82747
  C ~ 82180
  D
    25-hydroxy measurement ~ 82306
    1, 25 dihydroxy ~ 82652
    counseling ~ 4019F
  D-2 ~ 82307
  D-3 ~ 82306
  E ~ 84446
  K ~ 84597
  K dependent bone protein ~ 83937
  K-dependent protein S ~ 85305-85306
Vitelline duct ~ 44800
Vitrectomy
  anterior approach, partial ~ 67005
  for retinal detachment ~ 67112-67113
  pars plana approach ~ 67036-67043
  subtotal ~ 67010
  with endolaser panretinal photocoagulation ~
    67040
  with epiretinal membrane stripping ~
    67041-67043
  with focal endolaser photocoagulation ~ 67039
  with implantation or replacement, drug
    delivery system ~ 67027
Vitreous
  aspiration ~ 67015
  excision
    pars planta approach ~ 67036
    with epiretinal membrane stripping ~
      67041-67043
    with focal endolaser photocoagulation ~
      67039
  implantation, drug delivery system ~ 67027
  incision, strands ~ 67030-67031
  injection
    fluid substitute ~ 67025
    pharmacologic agent ~ 67028
  removal
    anterior approach ~ 67005
    subtotal ~ 67010
  replacement, drug delivery system ~ 67027
  strands
    discission ~ 67030
    severing ~ 67031
    subtotal ~ 67010
VLDL ~ 83695-83721
VMA ~ 84585

Vocal cords
    injection, endoscopy ~ 31513
        therapeutic ~ 31570-31571
Voice box ~ see larynx
Voice button ~ 31611
Voiding pressure studies
    abdominal ~ 51797
    bladder ~ 51728, 51729
    rectum ~ 51797
Volatiles ~ 84600
Volkman contracture ~ 25315-25316
Volume reduction, lung ~ 32491
Von Kraske proctectomy ~ 45111,
    45113-45116, 45123
VP ~ see voiding pressure studies
Vulva
    abscess, incision and drainage ~ 56405
    colposcopy ~ 56820
        biopsy ~ 56821
    excision
        complete ~ 56625, 56633-56640
        partial ~ 56620, 56630-56632
        radical ~ 56630-56631, 56633-56640
            complete ~ 56633-56640
            partial ~ 56630-56632
        simple
            complete ~ 56625
            partial ~ 56620
    lesion, destruction ~ 56501-56515
    perineum
        biopsy ~ 56605-56606
        incision and drainage ~ 56405
    repair, obstetric ~ 59300
Vulvectomy
    complete ~ 56625, 56633-56640
    partial ~ 56620, 56630-56632
    radical ~ 56630-56631, 56633-56640
        complete
            with bilateral inguinofemoral
                lymphadenectomy ~ 56637
            with inguinofemoral, iliac, and pelvic
                lymphadenectomy ~ 56640
            with unilateral inguinofemoral
                lymphadenectomy ~ 56634
        partial
            with bilateral inguinofemoral
                lymphadenectomy ~ 56632
            with unilateral inguinofemoral
                lymphadenectomy ~ 56631
    simple, complete ~ 56625
        partial ~ 56620
VZIG ~ 90396

W

W-plasty ~ see skin, adjacent tissue transfer
WADA activation test ~ 95958
WAIS-R ~ 96100
Waldius Procedure ~ 27445
Wall, abdominal ~ see abdominal wall
Walsh modified radical prostatectomy ~
    52601
Warts, flat, destruction ~ 17110-17111
Washing sperm ~ 58323
Wasserman test ~ 86592-86593
Wassmund Procedure osteotomy, maxilla ~
    21206
Water wart ~ 17110-17111, 54050-54065
Waterston Procedure ~ 33755
Watson-Jones Procedure ~ 27695-27698
Wave, ultrasonic shock ~ see ultrasound
WBC ~ see white blood cell
Webbed toe, repair ~ 28280
Wedge excision osteotomy ~ 21122
Wedge resection ovary ~ 58920
Well-baby care ~ 99381, 99391, 99461
Wellness behavior ~ see evaluation and
    management, health behavior
Wernicke-posadas disease ~ 86490
West Nile virus ~ **86788-86789**
Westergren test ~ 85651-85652
Western blot
    HIV ~ 86689
    protein ~ 84181-84182
    tissue analysis ~ 88371-88372
Wheelchair management/propulsion ~ 97542
    training ~ 97542
Wheeler knife procedure ~ 66820-66821
Wheeler Procedure ~ 15820-15823
    discission secondary membranous cataract ~
        66820
Whipple Procedure ~ 48150
Whirlpool therapy ~ 97022
White blood cell
    alkaline phosphatase ~ 85540
    antibody ~ 86021
    count ~ 85032, 85048, 89055
    differential ~ 85004-85007, 85009
    histamine release test ~ 86343
    phagocytosis ~ 86344
    transfusion ~ 86950
Whitemead Operation ~ 46260
Whitman astragalectomy ~ 28120, 28130
Whitman Procedure ~ 27120
Wick catheter technique ~ 20950
Widal serum test ~ 86000
Window
    oval ~ 69666
    round ~ 69667
Window technic, pericardial ~ 33015
Windpipe ~ see trachea
Winiwarter Operation ~ 47720-47740

1565

Winter Procedure ~ 54435
Wintrobe test ~ 85651-85652
Wire ~ see pin
  insertion/removal, skeletal traction ~ 20650
  interdental, without fracture ~ 21497
Wiring prophylactic treatment, humerus ~ 24498
Wirsung duct ~ see pancreatic duct
Witzel Operation ~ see incision, stomach, creation, stoma; incision and drainage ~ 43500, 43520, 43830-43832
Womb ~ see uterus
Wood alcohol ~ 84600
Work hardening ~ see physical medicine/therapy/occupational therapy ~ 97545-97546
Work related evaluation services ~ 99455-99456
Worm ~ 86682
Wound
  debridement
    non-selective ~ 97602
    selective ~ 97597-97598
  dehiscence, repair ~ 12020-12021, 13160
  exploration
    penetrating
      abdomen/flank/back ~ 20102
      chest ~ 20101
      extremity ~ 20103
      neck ~ 20100
    penetrating trauma ~ 20100-20103
  infection, incision and drainage, postoperative ~ 10180
  negative pressure therapy ~ 97605-97606
  repair
    complex ~ 13100-13160
    intermediate ~ 12031-12057
    simple ~ 12001-12021
    urethra ~ 53502-53515
  suture
    bladder ~ 51860-51865
    kidney ~ 50500
    trachea
      cervical ~ 31800
      intrathoracic ~ 31805
    urethra ~ 53502-53515
  vagina repair ~ 57200-57210
Wrist ~ **see arm, lower; carpal bone**
  abscess ~ 25028
  arthrocentesis ~ 20605
  arthrodesis ~ 25800
    with graft ~ 25810
    with sliding graft ~ 25805
  arthrography ~ 73115
  arthroplasty ~ 25332, 25443, 25447
    revision ~ 25449
    total replacement ~ 25446
    with implant ~ 25441-25442, 25444-25445
  arthroscopy, diagnostic ~ 29840
    surgical ~ 29843-29848

Wrist ~ *continued*
  arthrotomy ~ 25040, 25100-25105
    for repair ~ 25107
  biopsy ~ 25065-25066, 25100-25101
  bursa
    excision ~ 25115-25116
    incision and drainage ~ 25031
  capsule, incision ~ 25085
  cast ~ 29085
  cyst ~ 25130-25136
  decompression ~ 25020-25025
  disarticulation ~ 25920
    reamputation ~ 25924
    revision ~ 25922
  dislocation
    closed treatment ~ 25660
    intercarpal ~ 25660
      open treatment ~ 25670
    open treatment ~ 25670, 25676
    percutaneous fixation ~ 25671
    radiocarpal ~ 25660
      open treatment ~ 25670
    radioulnar
      closed treatment ~ 25675
      percutaneous fixation ~ 25671
    with fracture
      closed treatment ~ 25680
      open treatment ~ 25685
    with manipulation ~ 25259, 25660, 25675
  excision
    carpal ~ 25210-25215
    cartilage ~ 25107
  exploration ~ 25040, 25101
  fasciotomy ~ 25020-25025
  fracture ~ 25645
    closed treatment ~ 25622, 25630
    open treatment ~ 25628
    with dislocation ~ 25680-25685
    with manipulation ~ 25259, 25624, 25635
  ganglion cyst, excision ~ 25111-25112
  hematoma ~ 25028
  incision ~ 25040, 25100-25105
    tendon sheath ~ 25000-25001
  injection
    carpal tunnel, therapeutic ~ 20526
    X-ray ~ 25246
  joint ~ 25040, 25660
  lesion, tendon sheath, excision ~ 25110
  magnetic resonance imaging (MRI) ~ 73221
  reconstruction
    capsulectomy ~ 25320
    capsulorrhaphy ~ 25320
    carpal bone ~ 25394, 25430
    realign ~ 25335
  removal
    foreign body ~ 25040, 25101, 25248
    implant ~ 25449
    loose body ~ 25101
    prosthesis ~ 25250-25251

X

X-ray ~ continued
standing, spine ~ 72069
sternum ~ 71120-71130
teeth ~ 70300-70320
tibia ~ 73590
toe ~ 73660
total body, foreign body ~ 76010
unlisted services and procedures ~
76120-76125
upper GI series ~ 3142F, 3200F
with contrast
ankle ~ 73615
aorta ~ 0080T-0081T, 75600-75630,
75952-75953
artery
abdominal ~ 75726
additional vessels ~ 75774
adrenal ~ 75731-75733
arm ~ 75710-75716
arteriovenous shunt ~ 75791
brachial ~ 75658
head and neck ~ 36221-36226
iliac ~ 75953
leg ~ 75710-75716
mammary ~ 75756
pelvic ~ 75736
pulmonary ~ 75741-75746
renal ~ 36251-36254
spine ~ 75705
transcatheter therapy ~ 75894-75898
bile duct ~ 74300-74320
calculus removal ~ 74327
catheterization ~ 75982-75984
drainage ~ 75980-75982
guide catheter ~ 74328, 74330
bladder ~ 74430, 74450-74455
brain ~ 70010-70015
bronchi ~ 76499
colon, barium enema ~ 74270-74280
corpora cavernosa ~ 74445
elbow ~ 73085
epididymis ~ 74440
gallbladder ~ 74290-74291
gastrointestinal tract ~ 74246-74249
hip ~ 73525
iliofemoral artery ~ 75630
intervertebral disk
cervical ~ 72285
lumbar ~ 72295
thoracic ~ 72285
joint, stress views ~ 77071
kidney
cyst ~ 74470
guide catheter ~ 74475
knee ~ 73560-73564, 73580
lacrimal duct ~ 70170
larynx ~ 70373

X-ray ~ continued
lymph vessel
abdomen ~ 75805-75807
arm ~ 75801-75803
leg ~ 75801-75803
nasolacrimal duct ~ 70170
guide dilation ~ 74485
oviduct ~ 74740
pancreas ~ 74300-74305
pancreatic duct, guide catheter ~
74329-74330
perineum ~ 74775
peritoneum ~ 74190
salivary gland ~ 70390
seminal vesicles ~ 74440
shoulder ~ 73040
spine
cervical ~ 72240
lumbosacral ~ 72265
thoracic ~ 72255
total ~ 72270
temporomandibular joint (TMJ) ~
70328-70332
ureter
guide catheter ~ 74480
guide dilation ~ 74485
urethra ~ 74450-74455
urinary tract ~ 74400-74425
uterus ~ 74740
vas deferens ~ 74440
vein
adrenal ~ 75840-75842
arm ~ 75820-75822
hepatic portal ~ 75810, 75885-75887
jugular ~ 75860
leg ~ 75820-75822
liver ~ 75889-75891
neck ~ 75860
orbit ~ 75880
renal ~ 75831-75833
sampling ~ 75893
sinus ~ 75870
skull ~ 75870-75872
splenic ~ 75810
vena cava ~ 75825-75827
wrist ~ 73115
wrist ~ 73100-73110
X-ray tomography, computed ~ see CT scan
XA, coagulation factor ~ 85260
Xenoantibodies ~ 86308-86310
XI, coagulation factor ~ 85270
XI, cranial nerve ~ see accessory nerve
XII, coagulation factor ~ 85280
XII, cranial nerve ~ see hypoglossal nerve
XIII, coagulation factor ~ 85290-85291
Xylose absorption test
blood ~ 84620
urine ~ 84620

Y

Yeast culture ~ 87106
Yellow fever vaccine ~ 90717
Yersinia antibody ~ 86793

Z

Ziegler Procedure discission secondary
   membranous cataract ~ 66820
Zinc ~ 84630
Zinc manganese leucine aminopeptidase ~
   83670
Zygoma ~ see cheekbone
Zygomatic arch fracture
  open treatment ~ 21356-21366
  with manipulation ~ 21355

Options for the use of these codes include the use of one of the other hospital daily services codes from the evaluation and management series 99231-99233 and perhaps using a code that has a higher value than the routine hospital visit.

REFERRAL

A referral is the transfer of the total care or specific portion of care of a patient from one physician to another. A referral is not a request for consultation. If a patient is referred to the physician for total care or a portion of their care, use evaluation and management visit codes, and other CPT codes if appropriate, to report the services provided. If a patient is sent to the physician for a consultation, use evaluation and management consultation codes to report the services provided.

SEPARATE OR MULTIPLE PROCEDURES

It is appropriate to designate multiple procedures that are rendered on the same date by separate entries. For example: if a proctosigmoidoscopy was performed in addition to a hospital visit, the proctosigmoidoscopy would be considered a SEPARATE procedure and listed in addition to the hospital visit on the health insurance claim form. Another example would be individual medical psychotherapy rendered in addition to a brief subsequent hospital service. In this instance, both services would be coded.

SUPPLIES AND MATERIALS SUPPLIED BY THE PHYSICIAN

The CPT coding system includes specific codes for identifying certain supplies and materials provided by the physician. These supply codes are used to report supplies and materials that are not included in the definition of the basic service.

CPT CODES FOR SUPPLIES AND MATERIALS

92310-92371   Supply of spectacles, contact lenses, low vision aids and ocular prosthesis.

95144-95170   Provision of antigens for allergen immunotherapy.

99070   Supplies and materials (except spectacles) provided by the physician.

99071   Educational supplies, such as books, tapes, and pamphlets, provided by the physician for the patient's education at cost to physician.

PURCHASED DIAGNOSTIC SERVICES

It is common for physicians to bill patients and health insurance companies for diagnostic services that were procured or ordered on behalf of the patient but not